D1212990

THE AMERICAN PSYCHIATRIC PRESS

TEXTBOOK OF NEUROPSYCHIATRY

Second Edition

Edited by

Stuart C. Yudofsky, M.D.
Robert E. Hales, M.D.

Editorial Board

THE AMERICAN PSYCHIATRIC PRESS

TEXTBOOK OF NEUROPSYCHIATRY

Second Edition

Edited by

Stuart C. Yudofsky, M.D.
D. C. and Irene Ellwood Professor and Chairman,
Department of Psychiatry and Behavioral Sciences, Baylor College of Medicine;
Psychiatrist-in-Chief, The Methodist Hospital,
Houston, Texas

Robert E. Hales, M.D.
Clinical Professor of Psychiatry, University of California, San Francisco;
Chairman, Department of Psychiatry, California Pacific Medical Center,
San Francisco, California

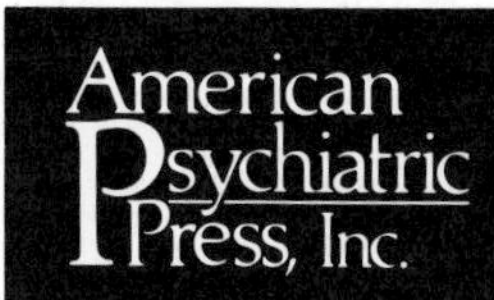

Washington, DC   London, England

Note: The Editors and contributors have worked to ensure that all information in this book concerning drug dosages, schedules, and routes of administration is accurate as of the time of publication and consistent with standards set by the U.S. Food and Drug Administration and the general medical community. As medical research and practice advance, however, therapeutic standards may change. For this reason and because human and mechanical errors sometimes occur, we recommend that readers follow the advice of a physician who is directly involved in their care or the care of a member of their family.

Cover design by Paine Blvett Paine, Inc.
Composition by Harper Graphics
Manufactured by Quebecor America Book Group/Semline, Inc.

Manufactured in the United States of America on acid-free paper.

Second Edition

95 94 93 92 4 3 2 1

American Psychiatric Press, Inc.
1400 K Street, N.W., Washington, DC 20005

Library of Congress Cataloging-in-Publication Data

The American Psychiatric Press textbook of neuropsychiatry / edited by
Stuart C. Yudofsky, Robert E. Hales. — 2nd ed.
p. cm.
Includes bibliographical references and index.
ISBN 0-88048-387-3
1. Neuropsychiatry. I. Yudofsky, Stuart C. II. Hales, Robert E.
III. American Psychiatric Press. IV. Title: Textbook of
neuropsychiatry.
[DNLM: 1. Nervous System Diseases. 2. Neuropsychology.
3. Organic Mental disorders. WM 220 A512]
RC341.A44 1992
616.8—dc20
DNLM/DLC
for Library of Congress 91–41381
CIP

British Library Cataloguing in Publication Data

A CIP record is available from the British Library.

Contents

Section V: Neuropsychiatric Treatments

Contributors

D. Frank Benson, M.D.

The Augustus S. Rose Professor of Neurology, Department of Neurology, University of California, Los Angeles, School of Medicine, Los Angeles, California

William Borden, Ph.D.

Assistant Professor, Department of Psychiatry and School of Social Service Administration, The University of Chicago; Research Associate, Illinois State Psychiatric Institute, Chicago, Illinois

George T. Brandt, M.D.

Instructor, Department of Psychiatry, Uniformed Services University of Health Sciences, Bethesda, Maryland; Assistant Chief, Psychiatry Consultation Liaison Service, Walter Reed Army Medical Center, Washington, DC

William G. Brose, M.D.

Assistant Professor, Department of Anesthesia, Director, Pain Management Service, Stanford University School of Medicine, Stanford, California

Edwin H. Cook, Jr., M.D.

Assistant Professor of Psychiatry and Pediatrics, Director, Laboratory of Developmental Neurochemistry, Child and Adolescent Psychiatry, The University of Chicago, Chicago, Illinois

Jeffrey L. Cummings, M.D.

Associate Professor of Neurology, Psychiatry, and Biobehavioral Sciences, University of California, Los Angeles, School of Medicine; Chief, Behavioral Neuroscience Section, Psychiatry Service, West Los Angeles Veterans Affairs Medical Center, Los Angeles, California

John Cutting, M.D.

Consultant Psychiatrist and Teacher, University of London, London, United Kingdom

David G. Daniel, M.D.
Associate Clinical Professor of Psychiatry, George Washington University; Guest Researcher, Clinical Brain Disorders Branch, Division of Intramural Research Programs, National Institute of Mental Health, Washington, DC; Director, Clinical Neuroscience Service, HCA-Dominion Hospital, Falls Church, Virginia

Steven L. Dubovsky, M.D.
Professor of Psychiatry and Medicine, Vice-Chairman, Department of Psychiatry, University of Colorado School of Medicine, Denver, Colorado

Barry S. Fogel, M.D.
Associate Professor of Psychiatry and Human Behavior, Associate Director, Center for Gerontology and Health Care Research, Brown University, Providence, Rhode Island

David V. Forrest, M.D.
Associate Professor of Clinical Psychiatry, Consultation-Liaison Psychiatrist in Neurology, Faculty, Columbia Psychoanalytic Center, Columbia University College of Physicians and Surgeons, New York, New York

Richard J. Frances, M.D.
Professor of Clinical Psychiatry, Vice-Chairman, Department of Psychiatry, New Jersey Medical School, Newark, New Jersey

John E. Franklin, Jr., M.D.
Assistant Professor of Clinical Psychiatry, Department of Psychiatry, New Jersey Medical School, Newark, New Jersey

Robert P. Friedland, M.D.
Associate Professor of Neurology, Psychiatry, and Radiology, Case Western Reserve University School of Medicine; Clinical Director, Alzheimer Center, University Hospitals of Cleveland, Cleveland, Ohio

Felicia B. Gershberg, Sc.B.
Graduate student, University of California, Berkeley, Berkeley, California

Kenneth L. Goetz, M.D.
Assistant Professor of Psychiatry, Medical College of Pennsylvania, Allegheny Campus; Associate Director, Inpatient Psychiatry, Allegheny General Hospital, Pittsburgh, Pennsylvania

Morris B. Goldman, M.D.
Assistant Professor of Psychiatry, Pritzker School of Medicine; Associate Director for Research, The University of Chicago Research Program at Illinois State Psychiatric Institute, Chicago, Illinois

Lawrence S. Gross, M.D.
Associate Professor of Clinical Psychiatry and the Behavioral Sciences, University of Southern California School of Medicine; Director, Adult Psychiatric Outpatient Clinic, Los Angeles County and University of Southern California Medical Center, Los Angeles, California

Robert E. Hales, M.D.

Clinical Professor of Psychiatry, University of California, San Francisco; Chairman, Department of Psychiatry, California Pacific Medical Center, San Francisco, California

Diane B. Howieson, Ph.D.

Assistant Professor of Neurology and Medical Psychology, Oregon Health Sciences University; Head, Neuropsychology Section, Portland Department of Veterans Affairs Medical Center, Portland, Oregon

Charles A. Kaufmann, M.D.

Associate Professor of Clinical Psychiatry, Columbia University, College of Physicians and Surgeons; Head, Laboratory of Molecular Neurobiology, Scientific Director, Schizophrenia Research Unit, New York State Psychiatric Institute, New York, New York

David J. Kupfer, M.D.

Professor and Chairman, Department of Psychiatry, University of Pittsburgh School of Medicine, Western Psychiatric Institute and Clinic, Pittsburgh, Pennsylvania

Bennett L. Leventhal, M.D.

Professor of Psychiatry and Pediatrics, Director of Child and Adolescent Psychiatry, Interim Chairman, Department of Psychiatry, The University of Chicago, Chicago, Illinois

Muriel D. Lezak, Ph.D.

Associate Professor of Neurology, Psychiatry, and Neurosurgery, Head, Neuropsychology Section, Department of Neurology, Oregon Health Sciences University, Portland, Oregon

Mark R. Lovell, Ph.D.

Assistant Professor of Psychiatry (Psychology), Medical College of Pennsylvania, Allegheny Campus; Chief of Neuropsychological Services, Allegheny General Hospital, Allegheny Neuropsychiatric Institute, Pittsburgh, Pennsylvania

Robert W. McCarley, M.D.

Professor of Psychiatry, Director, Neuroscience Laboratory, Department of Psychiatry, Harvard Medical School, Brockton Veterans Affairs Medical Center, Brockton, Massachusetts

Dolores Malaspina, M.D.

Assistant Professor of Clinical Psychiatry, Columbia University, College of Physicians and Surgeons; Unit Chief, Schizophrenia Research Unit, New York State Psychiatric Institute, New York, New York

John C. Markowitz, M.D.

Assistant Professor of Psychiatry, Cornell University Medical College, New York, New York

Frederick E. Miller, M.D., Ph.D.
Assistant Professor, Department of Psychiatry and Behavioral Sciences, Northwestern University, Chicago, Illinois

Robert M. Nagy, M.D.
Assistant Professor of Clinical Psychiatry and the Behavioral Sciences, University of Southern California School of Medicine; Ward Chief, Psychiatric Hospital, Los Angeles County and University of Southern California Medical Center, Los Angeles, California

Henry A. Nasrallah, M.D.
Professor of Psychiatry and Neurology, Chairman, Department of Psychiatry, The Ohio State University College of Medicine, Columbus, Ohio

Vernon M. Neppe, M.D., Ph.D.
Associate Professor of Psychiatry and Behavioral Sciences, Director, Division of Neuropsychiatry, University of Washington School of Medicine, Seattle, Washington

Thomas C. Neylan, M.D.
Medical Director, Inpatient Psychiatry, California Pacific Medical Center, San Francisco California

Fred Ovsiew, M.D.
Assistant Professor of Clinical Psychiatry, Chief, Clinical Neuropsychiatry, Department of Psychiatry, The University of Chicago, Chicago, Illinois

Samuel W. Perry, M.D.
Professor of Psychiatry, Cornell University Medical College, Associate Director; Consultation-Liaison Division, The New York Hospital, New York, New York

Trevor R. P. Price, M.D.
Professor of Psychiatry and Medicine, Chairman, Department of Psychiatry, Medical College of Pennsylvania, Allegheny Campus, Pittsburgh, Pennsylvania

H. Matthew Quitkin, A.B.
Stanley Scholar, Columbia University, College of Physicians and Surgeons; Research Associate, New York State Psychiatric Institute, New York, New York

Stephen G. Rayport, M.D., Ph.D.
Assistant Professor of Psychiatry, Neurobiology and Behavior, Anatomy and Cell Biology, Columbia University; Director, Laboratory of Neurophysiology, New York State Psychiatric Institute, New York, New York

Charles F. Reynolds III, M.D.
Professor of Psychiatry and Neurology, Director, Sleep and Chronobiology Center, Western Psychiatric Institute and Clinic, University of Pittsburgh School of Medicine, Pittsburgh, Pennsylvania

Robert G. Robinson, M.D.

Professor and Head, Department of Psychiatry, University of Iowa College of Medicine, Iowa City, Iowa

Arthur P. Shimamura, Ph.D.

Associate Professor, Department of Psychology, University of California, Berkeley, Berkeley, California

Jonathan M. Silver, M.D.

Assistant Professor of Clinical Psychiatry, College of Physicians and Surgeons, Columbia University; Director of Neuropsychiatry, Columbia-Presbyterian Medical Center, New York, New York

Robert I. Simon, M.D.

Clinical Professor of Psychiatry, Director, Program in Psychiatry and Law, Georgetown University School of Medicine, Washington, DC

David Spiegel, M.D.

Professor, Department of Psychiatry and Behavioral Sciences, Director, Psychosocial Treatment Laboratory, Stanford University School of Medicine, Stanford, California

Sergio E. Starkstein, M.D., Ph.D.

Chief, Department of Behavioral Neurology, Director, Institute of Neurological Research Raúl Carrea, Buenos Aires, Argentina

Christopher Starratt, Ph.D.

Assistant Professor of Psychiatry (Psychology), Medical College of Pennsylvania, Allegheny Campus; Director of Neuropsychology, Allegheny Neuropsychiatric Institute, Pittsburgh, Pennsylvania

Andrea B. Stone, M.D.

Assistant Professor of Psychiatry, University of Massachusetts Medical School, Director, Premenstrual Syndrome Clinic, Ambulatory Psychiatry, University of Massachusetts Medical Center, Worcester, Massachusetts

Milton E. Strauss, Ph.D.

Professor, Departments of Psychology, Neurology, and Psychiatry, Director, Clinical Psychology Program, Case Western Reserve University, Cleveland, Ohio

Richard L. Strub, M.D.

Clinical Professor of Neurology, Tulane University; Chairman, Department of Neurology, Ochsner Clinic, New Orleans, Louisiana

Daniel Tranel, Ph.D.

Associate Professor of Neurology, Chief, Benton Neuropsychology Laboratory, Division of Behavioral Neurology and Cognitive Neuroscience, Department of Neurology, University of Iowa, Iowa City, Iowa

Gary J. Tucker, M.D.
Professor and Chairman, Department of Psychiatry and Behavioral Sciences, University of Washington School of Medicine, Seattle, Washington

Daniel R. Weinberger, M.D.
Chief, Clinical Brain Disorders Branch, Division of Intramural Research Programs, National Institute of Mental Health, National Institute of Mental Health, Neurosciences Center at Saint Elizabeths, Washington, DC

Peter J. Whitehouse, M.D., Ph.D.
Associate Professor of Neurology, Director, Alzheimer's Center, University Hospitals of Cleveland; Chief, Division of Geriatric and Behavioral Neurology, Case Western Reserve University, Cleveland, Ohio

Michael G. Wise, M.D.
Clinical Professor of Psychiatry, Tulane School of Medicine; Chairman, Department of Psychiatry, Ochsner Clinic, New Orleans, Louisiana

Stuart C. Yudofsky, M.D.
D. C. and Irene Ellwood Professor and Chairman, Department of Psychiatry and Behavioral Sciences, Baylor College of Medicine; Psychiatrist-in-Chief, The Methodist Hospital, Houston, Texas

Jeffrey R. Zigun, M.D.
Senior Staff Fellow, Clinical Brain Disorders Branch, Division of Intramural Research Programs, National Institute of Mental Health, Neurosciences Center at Saint Elizabeths, Washington, DC

Preface

FROM PUBLISHING *The American Psychiatric Press Textbook of Psychiatry* in 1988, we learned the value of having a distinguished, scholarly, and active editorial board. For the second edition of the *Textbook of Neuropsychiatry*, we have such a group whose names are listed on page ii. All chapters were reviewed not only by the two of us, but also by one or more members of the editorial board. The dedicated board members worked diligently to ensure that each chapter is accurate, relevant, and substantive. Many suggestions for changes were advanced, almost all of which resulted in modifications and improvements. Most chapters underwent several revisions before final acceptance. Consequently, we believe that this peer review process greatly assisted us in ensuring the highest quality product for our readers.

Many changes have been made in the second edition of *The American Psychiatric Press Textbook of Neuropsychiatry*. The text has been expanded from 25 chapters to 33, an increase of 32%. In addition, the number of contributors has increased from 42 to 56, a 33% increase. This edition of the *Textbook of Neuropsychiatry* is also vastly revised with many new chapter authors (only 15 of the original contributors in the first edition are contributors in the second).

Those of you who purchased the first edition will note a reorganization of the chapters. Whereas the first edition had four sections, Evaluation and Basic Principles, Organic Mental Disorders, Neuropsychiatric Disorders, and Treatment Issues in Neuropsychiatry, this edition has five sections with different foci. The first section, Basic Principles of Neuroscience, is a lucid review and is followed by the sections Neuropsychiatric Assessment and Neuropsychiatric Symptomatologies. In the fourth section, Neuropsychiatric Disorders, we include a new chapter on the neuropsychiatry of schizophrenia. The final section, Neuropsychiatric Treatments, retains chapters by outstanding contributors to the previous edition, including Steven Dubovsky, David Forrest, and Mark Lovell. They discuss respectively, psychopharmacological treatment, psychotherapy, and cognitive rehabilitation and behavior therapy from the specific perspective of neuropsychiatry. We also added a chapter for family caregivers, and were fortunate to have Robert Simon, the editor of the American Psychiatric Press Review of Clinical Psychiatry in the Law series, as the author of the ethical and legal issues chapter.

For every section of the second edition, we were fortunate to be able to attract some of the outstanding scientists and neuropsychiatrists in the field. The authors spent many hours in organizing the latest information in their respective areas. We begin the book with a review of the cellular and molecular biology of the neuron by Stephen Rayport, followed by Robert McCarley's chapter on human electrophysiology and Daniel Tranel's seminal chapter on functional neuroanatomy. The section on neuropsychiatric assessment features a highly practical chapter on bedside neuropsychiatry by Fred Ovsiew and a pivotal chapter on the neuropsychological evaluation by Diane Howieson and Muriel Lezak, who is the author of the standard textbook in the field. We then included two chapters on other diagnostic techniques: electroencephalography by Thomas Neylan and colleagues and neuroimaging by the distinguished National Institute of Mental Health scientist Daniel Weinberger and colleagues David Daniel and Jeffrey Zigun. Columbia University's Charles Kaufmann prepared a comprehensive and up-to-date chapter on genetics and epidemiology of neuropsychiatric disorders. The neuropsychiatric symptomatologies section comprises outstanding chapters from contributors in the United States and Great Britain. It includes chapters written not only by psychiatrists but also by outstanding neurologists: Richard Strub, Frank Benson, and Barry Fogel (also a psychiatrist). As in the previous edition, this central section features chapters on the major neuropsychiatric disorders, written, we believe, by the leaders in their respective areas.

Our goal in this edition has been to prepare not only a comprehensive text, but also a volume that is clinically relevant and practical to use. We hope that this textbook will be used by psychiatrists, neurologists, neuropsychologists, residents, and trainees in other specialties who work in a variety of clinical settings. Although much of the material may be relevant to those who work in general hospital settings, clinicians and other health professionals practicing in other settings—such as outpatient offices or clinics, community mental health centers, alcohol and drug treatment programs, and state hospitals—should find the information helpful in the care of their patients.

We learned from readers' comments about the first edition that very few people read the textbook from cover to cover. Most read only one or several chapters during any particular period. Consequently we strived to ensure that each chapter would be complete in itself. As a result, there is some overlap among chapters, but we have judged that this was necessary from an information-retrieval standpoint, to prevent readers from having to "jump" from section to section and to allow different authors to provide varying perspectives. For example, although you will find some overlap between Michael Wise's chapter on delirium and John Cutting's chapter on stupor and coma, each presents quite differing perspectives, with Dr. Cutting presenting a classical British point of view and Dr. Wise advancing an American one. Similarly, Jeffrey Cummings's authoritative chapter on the neuropsychiatric aspects of Alzheimer's disease and other dementing illnesses focuses on the clinician's role in making an appropriate diagnosis and treatment recommendations, whereas Arthur Shimamura's and Felicia Gershberg's chapter on the neuropsychiatric aspects of memory and amnesia emphasizes the symptom-related features and research findings.

We are pleased that two of the authors of other outstanding textbooks of neuropsychiatry have contributed chapters to our book. Gary Tucker, who co-authored with Jonathan Pincus *Behavioral Neurology,* wrote the chapter with Vernon Neppe on the neuropsychiatric aspects of seizure disorders. Additionally, Jeffrey Cummings, who authored *Clinical Neuropsychiatry,* wrote the chapter on Alzheimer's disease and other dementing illnesses. Their extraordinary books remain standard references in the field today and have paved the way for this multiauthored text. It should also be emphasized that since the publication of the first edition of *The American Psychiatric Press Textbook of Neuropsychiatry,* the *Journal of Neuropsychiatry and Clinical Neurosciences* began publication. The *Journal* (which we co-edit) is now completing its third year of publication, and many of the articles submitted to us were authored by contributors to this edition of the *Textbook of Neuropsychiatry.* We believe that the *Journal of Neuropsychiatry and Clinical Neurosciences* is a fine complement to this textbook in that the basic information and clinical approaches presented here will be refined and expanded by current research discovery that will appear regularly in the *Journal.*

This book would not have been possible without the help and support of many people. First we thank the many chapter authors who labored diligently to produce contributions that we consider unique, scholarly, and enjoyable to read. Chapter authors displayed remarkable good humor in responding to the many suggestions they received from us and the members of the editorial board. Their good sportsmanship and responsiveness during the sometime laborious and tense process of editing and revising are much appreciated.

We also wish to acknowledge one of our longtime mentors, Evelyn Stone, who unfortunately died during our work on this book. Evelyn, along with her devoted colleague, Shervert Frazier, was one of our earliest and strongest supporters on the American Psychiatric Press Editorial Board, and we would not have been able to produce the first edition, let alone the second, without their wise counsel and advice. Evelyn will be sorely missed by both of us and many, many others in our field.

Consistent with previous projects and experiences, Ron McMillen and his excellent staff at the American Psychiatric Press were enormously helpful and responsive to us. The project editor, Ed Winkleman, displayed remarkable calm and understanding at our many requests and suggestions. Claire Reinburg, Editorial Director for the Books Division, provided much encouragement to us in getting the second edition completed in a timely fashion, as did Karen Loper, the Press's gifted Director of Sales and Marketing, who always does a marvelous job in promoting not only our books but all the excellent publications from the Press. Because production headquarters for this book shifted from Washington to Chicago, Kay Miller deserves special praise and thanks for her persistence with the almost infinite details, ensuring that we had good communication with chapter authors and that all chapters were submitted in a timely fashion and according to the manuscript guidelines.

We thank our wives, Beth Yudofsky, M.D., and Dianne Hales, for their support, encouragement, and assistance concerning many aspects of this book. They also permitted us the additional time (countless hours on the weekends and evenings) for planning, writing, and editing.

Finally, and most importantly, we would like to thank the many people who purchased the first edition, making the second edition possible. We are also grateful for the many letters and cards from psychiatrists, neurologists, neuropsychologists, and other mental health professionals who gave us suggestions and who communicated to us that they found the textbook useful in their clinical practices and teaching duties. We hope that our efforts and those of our chapter authors, editorial board, and the staff of the American Psychiatric Press will be translated into another useful book for professionals who wish to learn more about how to understand, diagnose, and care for patients with neuropsychiatric disorders.

Stuart C. Yudofsky, M.D.
Houston, Texas

Robert E. Hales, M.D.
San Francisco, California

Introduction

ALTHOUGH THERE IS CONSIDERABLE disagreement about just what neuropsychiatry comprises, fundamental to any definition is the indelible inseparability of brain and thought, of mind and body, and of mental and physical. Neuropsychiatry spans these interrelationships to enlarge our understanding of cognitive, emotional, and behavioral function and dysfunction.

❑ WHAT IS NEUROPSYCHIATRY?

It is a fascinating paradox that modern neuropsychiatry, which derives from 19th century social dissension, anatomical dissection, and nosological differentiation, should, as manifested by its very name, be essentially a collaborative and integrative enterprise. Neuropsychiatry bridges the conventional boundaries imposed between mind and matter, between intention and function, and between the guildlike clinical considerations of the professional disciplines of neurology and psychiatry. Most importantly, however, neuropsychiatry vaults the limiting and misleading demarcations of traditional conceptual models of illness. For example, although Parkinson's disease is classified as a movement disorder under the professional aegis of neurology, selected scientific studies show that more than one-third of patients with this disorder have depression (Mayeux 1981), and that dementia and other prominent behavioral and cognitive impairments occur, depending on the study, in from 10% to more than 50% of afflicted patients (Brown and Marsden 1984; Mayeux 1981). Similarly, schizophrenia, conventionally considered a psychiatric illness, is associated with elevated dopamine, subtype 2 (D_2), receptors in caudate nuclei (Wong et al. 1986), and with pathology in frontal, midbrain, diencephalic, and other regions of the brain (Andreasen et al. 1986; Weinberger et al. 1983). Scientific efforts using animal models have succeeded in determining the nucleotide sequence of the genes that code for D_2 receptors that have been implicated in both Parkinson's disease and schizophrenia (Bunzow et al. 1988). The future consequences of such scientific advances may be to compel a clinical reconceptualization of both Parkinson's disease and schizophrenia as neuropsychiatric disorders. This would help to cast light and focus on disabling symptomatologies that often remain dimly recognized and untreated in the shadowy margins of psychiatry and neurology when the disorders or the specialties are too narrowly defined.

This Introduction to the second edition of *The American Psychiatric Press Textbook of Neuropsychiatry* is adapted from an editorial in *The Journal of Neuropsychiatry and Clinical Neurosciences* (Yudofsky SC, Hales RE: The reemergence of neuropsychiatry: definition and direction. Journal of Neuropsychiatry and Clinical Neurosciences 1:1–6, 1989).

Conditions and Symptomatologies Subsumed

Although there is no universally accepted definition of neuropsychiatry, it is our hope that the second edition of *The American Psychiatric Press Textbook of Neuropsychiatry*, through its considerations and emphases, will define and strengthen this concept. A prominent focus of neuropsychiatry is the assessment and treatment of patients with psychiatric illnesses or symptoms associated with brain lesions or dysfunction. These include neuropsychiatric aspects of the following: traumatic brain injury; cerebral vascular disease; seizure disorders; central nervous system (CNS) degenerative diseases, including Alzheimer's disease and other dementias; brain tumors; infectious and inflammatory diseases of the CNS; alcohol and other substance-induced organic mental disorders; and developmental disorders involving the brain. Neuropsychiatry also encompasses those symptoms that lie in the "gray zone" between the specialties of neurology and psychiatry: impairment of attention, alertness, perception, memory, language, and intelligence. Fundamental to neuropsychiatry is the effort to link psychopathology with measurable brain deficits. Where psychiatric symptoms are likely to stem from brain disorders, but where the state of technology has not developed sufficiently to establish brain-syndrome linkages, neuropsychiatry must assume the leadership in pursuing such associations.

There are several syndromes that currently are conceptualized as neuropsychiatric disorders, and for many of these conditions, recent discoveries in even the basic neurosciences are also effecting far-reaching reconceptualizations. For example, new molecular biologic techniques have characterized the amino acid sequence associated with the synthesis of the amyloid protein that is found in neurofibrillary tangles in the brains of certain (although not all) patients with Alzheimer's disease (Kang et al. 1987). The gene responsible for the synthesis of this amyloid protein has been localized on chromosome 21 (St. George-Hyslop et al. 1987). In that the presence of amyloid and other brain pathology similar to that found in Alzheimer's patients is nearly always present in brains of older individuals with trisomy 21 disorder (Down's syndrome), this genetic localization could have implications for the diagnosis, treatment, and perhaps even the prevention of both illnesses. Thus modern molecular genetics may redefine two neuropsychiatric disorders—one conceptualized as a developmental disorder of young people (i.e., Down's syndrome) and the second conceptualized as a dementing illness of old age (i.e., Alzheimer's disease)—that heretofore were loosely linked by symptomatologies (dysfunction of memory, cognition, social judgment, and so on) and neuropathology (amyloid protein and neurofibrillary tangles).

Many human conditions that currently are not considered to be in the province of medicine, will, by virtue of neuroscience discovery, eventually become regarded as neuropsychiatric disorders. This reconceptualization will be of historic and monumental significance to the individuals who suffer from these conditions and to society. Examples range from impulsive murderers and other types of criminal offenders to people who suffer from chemical dependencies. Presently, people with alcoholism are cared for by professionals and programs largely outside traditional medical specialties and hospital structures. Nonetheless, recent evidence is associating alcoholism with the D_2 receptor gene (Blum et al. 1990; Cloninger 1991; Comings et al. 1991). If such a link is ultimately established, the door will open wider to more fundamental involvement by psychiatrists and other medical specialists in the diagnosis and treatment of people who are alcohol dependent.

The Clinical and Philosophical Approach

Neuropsychiatry is an historic clinical discipline—arising in the mid-19th century and falling from prominence early in the 20th century—that is currently reemerging as a subspecialty of psychiatry and neurology. Not dissimilar to the clinical approaches of most other medical specialties or subspecialties, the following is considered by us to be the essence of neuropsychiatric intervention: 1) prevention (e.g., prenatal counseling and treatment of alcoholic expectant mothers to obviate alcohol-induced encephalopathy in infants); 2) early detection of neuropsychiatric symptoms (e.g., recognizing major depression in a poststroke patient with aphasia); 3) focused assessment and operationalization of neuropsychiatric dysfunction (e.g., utilization of the Overt Aggression Scale [Yudofsky et al. 1986] to describe, quantify, and monitor the dyscontrol of rage and violent behavior secondary to traumatic brain injury); 4) specific localization, where possible, in brain tissue, chemistry, physiology, and so on, of "causative" deficits (e.g., detecting an epileptogenic focus in the temporal lobe of a patient who experiences depersonalization and fugue states) and early and specific treatment, where possible, of such deficits; and 5) the use of multiple therapeutic modalities to enable the patients to adapt to those neuropsychiatric deficits that are not reversible.

One philosophical perspective of neuropsychiatry advanced in the second edition of *The American Psychiatric Association Textbook of Neuropsychiatry* is that neuropsychiatric treatment is inherently complex and must, therefore, be comprehensive and collaborative. Thus clinical neuropsychiatry should be an organized, integrated, and multidisciplinary approach that must include not only many professional disciplines, the patient, and the patient's family, but also those enlightened organizations that act as advocates for those who are ravaged by neuropsychiatric disorders.

❑ WHY THE RENAISSANCE OF NEUROPSYCHIATRY?

Neuropsychiatric Disorders Are Common and Disabling

Among the many reasons for the revival of neuropsychiatry is that the disorders subsumed under this rubric are so common and disabling. Although documentation of the prevalence of neuropsychiatric disorders and the comparison of their prevalence to those of other medical illnesses are beyond the scope of this introduction, compelling statistics and confirmatory data are included in the introductions to most of the chapters in this edition of the *Textbook of Neuropsychiatry*. In addition, the neuropsychiatric aspects of most of these disorders, including traumatic brain injury, alcohol-induced organic mental disorders, cerebral vascular disease, and seizure disorders, have been shown by many investigators to be among their most prominent, disabling dimensions (Cummings 1985; Oddy et al. 1985; Robinson et al. 1987; West et al. 1984). With the aging of the population, many of these conditions will become even more prevalent.

A Neuropsychiatric Paradigm Reduces Stigma

A second reason for revitalizing the neuropsychiatric paradigm is to reduce the stigma associated with psychiatric symptoms like delusions, hallucinations, manic and depressive mood changes, confusion, impaired memory, disinhibited behavior, and so on. Appropriate focus on the underlying brain lesions and the biochemical or pathophysiological processes that produce psychiatric symptoms bolsters reconceptualization of symptom complexes as neuropsychiatric disorders. A neuropsychiatric conceptualization not only enlarges and refines the understanding and treatment of such disorders, but also avoids limiting and damaging misconceptions that stem from too-narrow, discipline-based perspectives. A notorious example is schizophrenia—an illness with a predominantly psychiatric conceptualization—wherein the concept of the schizophrenogenic mother erroneously emerged and became widely accepted as a prominent cause of the disorder. This conceptualization incorrectly ascribes causality and, therefore, painful culpability to families who were already under great stress from a tragic and relentless disease. Fortunately, scientific evidence indicating genetic transmission of schizophrenia and the effectiveness of psychopharmacological treatment eventually resulted in the abandonment of the "schizophrenogenic causality" by our field—but not before psychiatry had alienated many patients and family members. A neuropsychiatric reconceptualization of schizophrenia would place greater emphasis on the underlying genetics and disorders of brain tissue, chemistry, and physiology, thereby rendering iatrogenic stigmatization far less likely.

Let us recall that prior to 1914, when Lewy (see Roth and Kroll 1986) traced the neuropathology of paralysis agitans (Parkinson's disease) to the basal ganglia of the brain, this illness was generally considered to be a mental disease, often associated with disparaging religious overtones. For example, even the great neurologist Charcot considered the disease to develop from "violent moral emotions" caused by political unrest prevalent in France in 1877. Even though today's better understanding of Parkinson's disease has documented prominent "mental" symptoms—dementia, depression, and psychosis—our acceptance of the neuropathological basis of the disorder discourages stigma and renders such damaging conceptualizations as a "parkinsonogenic parent" untenable.

Although many psychiatrists (including us) have profound concerns that an increased focus on biology could cause the conceptual pendulum to swing to a reductionist extreme wherein psychosocial aspects of neuropsychiatric disorders are dangerously deemphasized, we nonetheless believe that neurobiological emphasis has, on balance, more advantages than disadvantages for our profession and the patients whom we serve. As Sir Martin Roth and Jerome Kroll so persuasively argue in their brilliant treatise *The Reality of Mental Illness* (Roth and Kroll 1986), critics of psychiatry (i.e., those who contend the profession "invents" mental illness to advance our own interests and material status) separate the mind from the body to bolster their contention that mental illness does not exist. Not only does the neuropsychiatric paradigm parry such attacks (i.e., stigmatization of the patient and the psychiatrist) from "outside" the profession, but, more importantly, it reduces "the attacks from within" (i.e., shame and embarrassment of the patient and family).

Although the psychobiological conceptualization of mental illness was clearly formulated and promulgated by Adolf Meyer over 65 years ago (see Winters 1951) and although a biopsychosocial model was brilliantly advanced for all of medicine over 15 years ago by George Engel (1977), the stigmatization of the mentally ill today remains pervasive. Those who work in the general hospital setting experience daily the reluctance of many individuals with highly disabling psychiatric disorders (e.g., major depression secondary to stroke or dependence on narcotic analgesics) to be transferred from general medical units to excellent, dedicated psychiatric services because "I'm not crazy." It is not uncommon for a patient with symptoms originally thought to be derivative of such chronic, disabling disorders as multiple sclerosis or even a brain tumor to express disappointment when told the underlying disorder is a treatable psychiatric condition such as depression. Political candidates in the United States vehemently deny ever having received psychiatric treatment and refrain from publicly stating, "So what if I, as have millions of other Americans, received treatment for a psychiatric disorder? Does this make me any less qualified to serve?" The unqualified protestations of politicians are obvious indications of their own and their advisers' perceptions of the voting public's negative views of mental illness and its treatment. Could it be that we have been far more successful in communicating and convincing ourselves of the integrity and applicability of our models of mental illness than we have our patients, their families, and society—all of whom still feel that shame is associated with our labels and paradigms? Is it not possible that, where appropriate and accurate, new models and paradigms, based on neuropsychiatric perspectives, would be not only more precise but also more palatable to those who suffer such illnesses?

The Revolution in Neuroscience Research

Lewis Judd, M.D., while Director of the National Institute of Mental Health in 1988, stated at the American Psychiatric Association Annual Meeting that 95% of what we know about the brain as it relates to behavior has been discovered in the past 5 years. This statement highlights the recent, unprecedented advances in the brain sciences. In many important respects, progress in medicine is linked to technological advancement. Before the refinement of the lens and the development of the microscope, a cohesive and broadly accepted conceptualization of infectious illness was not likely to occur. Likewise, without the technological capacity to measure brain waves through the electroencephalogram, a modern conceptualization of seizure disorders—with the many ensuing social and therapeutic benefits—would not be possible. An explosive proliferation of technological advances is under way, the rate and implications of which are heretofore unparalleled. Applied to neuropsychiatric assessment, these advances have resulted in such useful innovations as computed tomography (CT), magnetic resonance imaging (MRI), positron-emission tomography (PET), single photon emission tomography (SPECT), regional cerebral blood flow (rCBF), and a large array of neuroimmunological techniques. The net result of future applications of technological advances will be the inexorable transformation and redefinition of illnesses that had previously been conceptualized as *mental* or *functional* into the neuropsychiatric paradigm. Coincident with this transformation and redefinition, it is critical that the sensitivity, humanity, and ethical bases so inherent to psychosocial models continue to remain prominent. The challenges presented by acquired immunodeficiency syndrome (AIDS) clearly demonstrate how technological, psychological, and interpersonal perspectives are inseparable in understanding and intervening in this devastating disorder. For the second edition of the *Textbook of Neuropsychiatry*, we have chosen topics and chapter authors who incorporate both the recent discoveries and technological advances related to neuroscience research as well as psychosocial and ethical considerations into their chapters.

The renaissance in neuropsychiatry, for the reasons expressed above, will not only enhance the efficacy and integrity of the fields of psychiatry and neurology, but also will have even broader implications. For the silver lining of the scourge of neuropsychiatric illness is that these devastating diseases provide both the impetus and substrate whereby we can explore ourselves. Through understanding Alzheimer's disease, we will eventually gain vital insights into the minute particles of matter and complex spatial and electrical arrangements that regulate unimpaired memory and learning. Through our neurobiological investigation of bipolar illness, we will gain vital insights into the chemistry and physics of healthy feelings, temperament, and mood. It is thus one of life's bitter paradoxes that, through the painful and disabling lesions treated by psychiatrists and neurologists, we are discovering ourselves. In the course of such discovery, we will ultimately not only approach relief from illness, but we may also free ourselves from the limitations—ranging from anxiety to aging—that have been accepted for millennia as the human condition.

Stuart C. Yudofsky, M.D.
Houston, Texas

Robert E. Hales, M.D.
San Francisco, California

❑ REFERENCES

Andreasen N, Nasrallah HA, Dunn V, et al: Structural abnormalities in the frontal system in schizophrenia. Arch Gen Psychiatry 43:136–144, 1986

Blum K, Noble EP, Sheridan PJ, et al: Allelic associations of human dopamine D_2 receptor gene in alcoholism. JAMA 263:2055–2059, 1990

Brown GR, Marsden CD: How common is dementia in Parkinson's disease? Lancet 2:1262–1265, 1984

Bunzow JR, Van Tol HHM, Grandy DK, et al: Cloning and expression of a rat D_2 dopamine receptor cDNA. Nature 336:783–787, 1988

Cloninger CR: D_2 dopamine receptor gene is associated but not linked with alcoholism. JAMA 226:1835–1836, 1991

Comings DE, Comings BG, Muhleman D, et al: The dopamine D_2 receptor locus as a modifying gene in neuropsychiatric disorders. JAMA 226:1793–1800, 1991

Cummings JL: Epilepsy: ictal and interictal behavioral alterations, in Clinical Neuropsychiatry. Edited by Cummings JL. Orlando, FL, Grune & Stratton, 1985, pp 95–116

Engel GL: The need for a new medical model: a challenge for biomedicine. Science 196:129–136, 1977

Kang J, Lemaire H-G, Unterbeck A, et al: The precursor of Alzheimer's disease amyloid A4 protein resembles a cell-surface receptor. Nature 325:733–736, 1987

Mayeux R: Depression and dementia in Parkinson's disease, in Neurology 2: Movement Disorders. Edited by Marsden CD, Fahn S. London, Butterworth, 1981, pp 75–91

Oddy M, Coughlan T, Tyerman A, et al: Social adjustment after closed head injury: a further follow-up seven years after injury. J Neurol Neurosurg Psychiatry 48: 564–568, 1985

Robinson RG, Bolduc P, Price TR: A two-year longitudinal study of poststroke mood disorders: diagnosis and outcome at one and two years. Stroke 18:837–843, 1987

Roth M, Kroll J: The Reality of Mental Illness. Cambridge, England, Cambridge University Press, 1986

St. George-Hyslop PH, Tanzi RE, Polinksy RJ, et al: The genetic defect causing familial Alzheimer's disease maps on chromosome 21. Science 235:885–889, 1987

Weinberger DR, Wagner RL, Wyatt RJ: Neuropathological studies of schizophrenia: a selective review. Schizophr Bull 9:193–212, 1983

West LJ, Maxwell DS, Nobel EP, et al: Alcoholism. Ann Intern Med 100:405–416, 1984

Winters EE (ed): The Collected Papers of Adolf Meyer, Vol 3: Medical Teaching. Baltimore, MD, Johns Hopkins Press, 1951

Wong DF, Wagner HN Jr, Tune LE, et al: Positron emission tomography reveals elevated D_2 dopamine receptors in drug-naive schizophrenics. Science 234:1558–1563, 1986

Yudofsky SC, Silver JM, Jackson M, et al: The Overt Aggression Scale: an operationalized rating scale for verbal and physical aggression. Am J Psychiatry 143:35–39, 1986

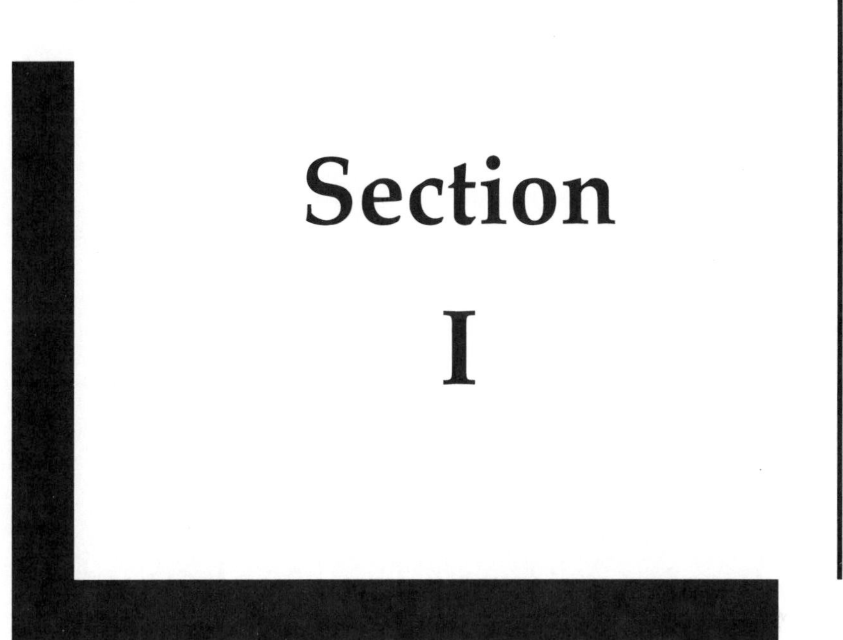

Section I

Basic Principles of Neuroscience

Chapter

1

Cellular and Molecular Biology of the Neuron

Stephen G. Rayport, M.D., Ph.D.

WE NOW HAVE AN increasingly comprehensive understanding of neurons as cells. Major strides are being made toward elucidating neuronal functioning in molecular terms. These advances in neural science have tremendous importance for neuropsychiatry (Barondes 1990; Pardes 1986). They provide a language to describe how neuropsychiatric diseases arise and evolve. Already, knowledge of neurons and their synapses provides the basis for understanding psychopharmacology (Cooper et al. 1986). In time, knowledge of how neurons function is certain to provide insights into higher mental functioning.

Indeed, it was the realization of the critical dependence of the neuron on glucose for its energy (Reivich et al. 1979) that led to the use of positron-emission tomography (PET) for studying the encoding of mental events in the brain. PET scans can identify the selective activation of brain regions involved in language comprehension, speech, or the making of simple verbal associations (Petersen et al. 1988). In patients with schizophrenia, aberrant patterns of frontal lobe activation can be detected (Weinberger 1987), and this goes along with other advances in brain imaging that have clearly shown neuropathology in schizophrenia (Roberts 1990; Suddath et al. 1990). A further understanding of the pathogenesis of schizophrenia awaits an increased understanding of the aberrant development of neurons and the role of experience. In other neuropsychiatric disorders, insight into defects in cellular regulation may prove to be of paramount importance.

Knowing about neurons will prove essential to integrating molecular genetic advances that are likely to underlie the major neuropsychiatric disorders (see Chapter 8). By way of linkage studies, over the last few years researchers have determined where the genes involved in Huntington's chorea, Alzheimer's disease, and neurofibromatosis are likely to be found. For neurofibromatosis type 1, the gene has been identified and cloned (Ponder 1990), and it appears to be involved in the regulation of cell proliferation (Buchberg et al. 1990; Wigler 1990), although exactly how and what consequences this has are the subject of intense research. Localization

Supported by National Institute of Mental Health Grant MH-00705.

and identification of genes for other neuropsychiatric disorders will surely follow in the near future.

To understand how abnormal genes affect higher mental functioning, we need to know how they affect the development and function of neurons. Nonfatal genetic mutations of the sort underlying neuropsychiatric disease probably act by coding for subtly altered molecules made in brain cells. If such aberrant molecules act during development, they could lead to generation of misshapen neurons, the migration of neurons to incorrect locations, or the formation of inappropriate synaptic connections. On the other hand, if their role is in adulthood, genetically aberrant proteins could underlie defects in cellular regulation, synaptic transmission, or intracellular signalling, for example.

Neuropsychiatric disorders may also arise from aberrant experience that permanently alters neuronal connectivity. This is most likely to occur during development when normal environmental input is essential for the fine-tuning of neuronal connections. Studies of the developing visual system have shown that the abnormal visual experience of young animals, during the critical period, results in the permanent pathological connectivity of the animal's visual system (Hubel et al. 1977). This holds true for humans as well. Similar, but more muted, changes occur in the mature nervous system during learning. Work on the simpler nervous systems of organisms, such as the marine snail *Aplysia* (Kandel 1989), has shown that alterations in the strength of synaptic connections encode memory. Here too, pathological experience may permanently alter patterns of neuronal connectivity. Similar experience-dependent changes are likely to occur in the human brain. At present, we can only surmise how these contribute to neuropsychiatric disorders. Evidently, it will be crucial to understand how groups of neurons interconnect to form systems for the control of behavior and how these may be affected by pathological experience.

To make the jump from neurons to higher mental functioning, we may take a lead from developments in information theory, semiotics, and neural network simulations (Edelman 1989; Minsky 1986; Olds 1990). Information theory and semiotics help to clarify the relationship between brain and mind. Neural network research has proved particularly exciting by showing in specific terms how computer-based assemblies of digital elements, with a simple rule for the modification of the strength of their interconnections (back propagation), might produce brainlike behavior (Sejnowksi et al. 1988). Already, neural network approaches have offered a way of understanding complexities in higher mental functioning that have eluded previous conceptualizations, such as the distinction between the thought disorders of schizophrenia and mania (Hoffman 1987) and insight into thought-processing abnormalities in schizophrenia (Servan-Schreiber et al. 1990). As we extend our insights into the cellular workings of the human brain, we will better know what therapeutic interventions best counter aberrant neuronal connections produced by pathological experiences during development or offset genetic defects.

In this chapter, I focus on the properties of neurons: how they develop, connect, and communicate with one another. From the rapid pace of developments, we can be confident that molecular genetic interventions or therapies based on knowledge of how to effectively normalize patterns of neuronal connectivity will lead to better ways of treating and eventually of preventing neuropsychiatric disease. In short, the science of neurons is energizing the renaissance of neuropsychiatry. In the decade to come it should transform the field.

❑ CELLULAR FUNCTION OF NEURONS

Individual neurons in the brain receive signals from thousands of neurons and in turn convey information to thousands of other neurons. Although activity in sensory neurons in the peripheral nervous system may represent particular bits of information, in the central nervous system (CNS), the activity of networks of neurons represents integrated sensory and associational information. CNS neurons may be seen as part of ephemeral, ever changing networks, shifting their participation from network to network as information is drawn from one task and used in another, often simultaneously following a parallel-distributed processing model. The sophistication of these networks depends in part on the neurons that make them up.

Cellular Makeup of the Brain

There are two principal types of brain cells: neurons and glia (Kandel and Schwartz 1985). Neurons process information; glia guide neurons during development and provide key support functions later on. There are three classes of glial cells: astrocytes, oligodendrocytes, and microglia. Astrocytes have three functions: providing the scaffolding of the brain, forming the blood-brain barrier, and guiding neuronal migration during development. Oligodendrocytes produce the myelin sheath that speeds the conduction of information along axons. Microglia act as the macrophages of the brain, remaining quiescent until activated by brain injury.

Neurons are the most differentiated and among the largest cells in the body, with processes stretching as long as a meter. There are also a great number of them in our brains, and the number of interconnections is astronomical. Compare the nervous system of the invertebrate *Aplysia*, with its 10^4–10^5 neurons, to the human brain, with its 10^{12}–10^{13} neurons. If each neuron forms an average of 10^3 connections, the human CNS likely has as many as 10^{15}–10^{16} synapses, or almost a billion times as many as the brain of the *Aplysia*. Surprisingly perhaps, neurons are much the same in snails as they are in man. Although neurons acquire a somewhat increased sophistication as one ascends the phylogenetic scale, the conservation of basic features reinforces the notion that our mental capacities arise primarily from the large number of neurons in our brains and the complexity of their interconnections.

Neuronal Shape

Neurons share a common organization dictated by their function, which is to process and convey information. They come in various sizes and shapes, but all have four well-defined regions: dendrites, cell body, axon, and axon terminals (Figure 1–1). Dendrites receive signals from other neurons. From the dendrites, the signals spread passively, or with an active boost, to the cell body. The cell body serves as an integrating site for signals coming from all the dendrites. In addition, as in other cells, the cell body in a neuron contains the genetic information (in the nucleus) that codes for the fabrication of all the necessary elements of cellular functioning, as well as sites for their manufacture, processing, and transport. The axon conveys information from the cell body to other neurons, often over long distances. At the axon terminals, the neuron makes contact with other neurons or effector cells, in turn eliciting signals in their dendrites. For central neurons, the flow of information is initiated by synaptic input onto dendrites.

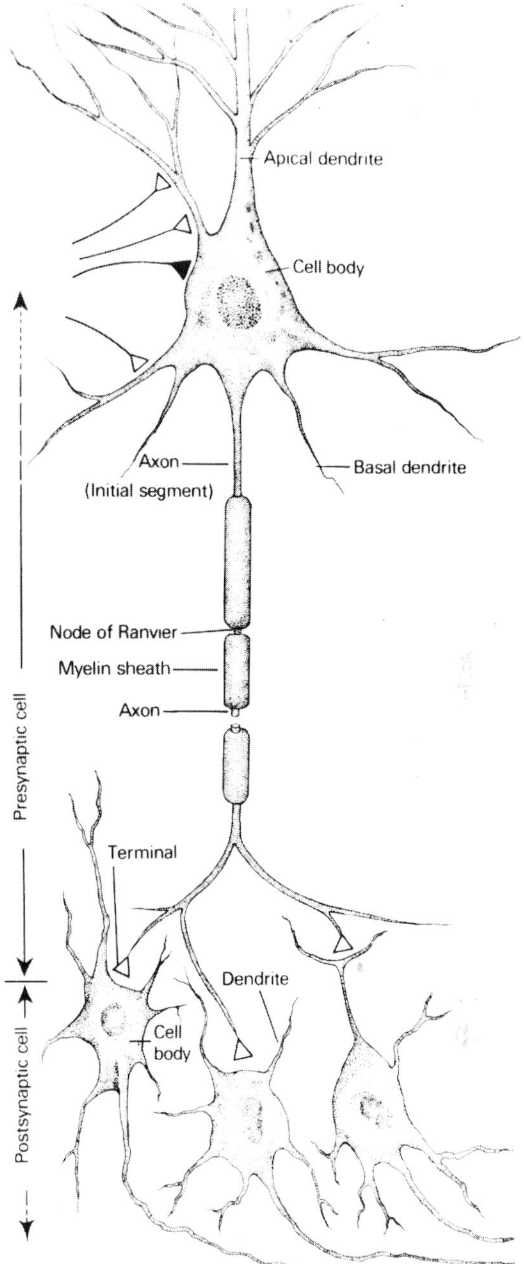

Figure 1–1. Basic shape of the neuron. Neurons have four well-defined cellular regions: dendrites, cell body, axon, and axon terminals. Electrical signals from other neurons impinge on the dendrites. An integration of signals from all dendrites occurs in the cell body and initial segment of the axon. When signals exceed the threshold of the initial segment, an action potential is initiated that travels down the axon to reach the terminal zone. Axon terminals synapse with postsynaptic cells, starting the cycle of information flow anew. (Reprinted from Kandel ER, Schwartz JH: Principles of Neural Science, 2nd Edition. New York, Elsevier, 1985, p 15. Used with permission.)

Signalling Mechanisms Within the Neuron

The neuron carries information electrically. Information enters the cell through synapses on its dendrites. Because the plasma membrane is an excellent insulator, electrical signals spread passively over some distance, often reaching the cell body in this way. Longer dendrites may also contain an amplification mechanism to boost distal inputs to the cell body; this amplification occurs through regenerative mechanisms in the membrane similar to those that give rise to the action potential (discussed below). In the cell body, signals from several dendrites combine. This grand postsynaptic potential (PSP) depolarizes the initial segment of the axon (the part of the axon closest to the cell body), which has the lowest threshold for activation. When threshold is reached, the striking all-or-none electrical explosion of the action potential is initiated. The action potential, or spike, propagates as an electrical wave down the axon at high speed, ultimately spreading into the axon terminals. At specialized sites in the terminals called active zones, electrical activity triggers the release of chemical neurotransmitters, which activate closely apposed postsynaptic receptors on the dendrites of other neurons (or muscle end plates in the case of motor neurons).

The ability of neurons to generate an action potential derives from the presence of ionic gradients across the membrane, in particular of sodium (Na^+) and chloride (Cl^-), which are high outside, and potassium (K^+), which is high inside. These gradients are generated by the continuous action of membrane pumps. Also in the membrane are specialized proteins called membrane channels which regulate the flow of ions, such as Na^+, K^+, Cl^-, and calcium (Ca^{2+}) across the membrane. At rest, the membrane is selectively permeable to K^+ and Cl^-, which causes the cell to be negative inside by about –50 to –75 mV. When the cell is active, this permeability is reversed in favor of Na^+, causing the cell membrane to be depolarized to about +50 mV.

The permeability of Na^+ channel proteins depends on membrane voltage and time. Because inflow of Na^+ depolarizes the membrane, this confers a regenerative property; once a threshold potential is reached, increased Na^+ influx leads to depolarization, which further opens Na^+ channels, further enhancing Na^+ influx, and so on (Figure 1–2). The result is that at threshold, the membrane potential rapidly switches to +50 mV. The membrane potential only stays so depolarized for about a millisecond because the Na^+ channels then show a time-dependent inactivation. Additionally, voltage-dependent K^+ channels, which are also activated by depolarization (but more slowly), increase the K^+ permeability and repolarize the membrane. Therefore, the membrane potential peaks at a depolarized level determined by the Na^+ gradient and then rapidly returns to the resting potential, determined once again by the K^+ gradient. Once the neuron is repolarized, the Na^+ inactivation wears off (the time this takes accounts for the refractory period of the neuron, a brief period when the threshold for firing an action potential is elevated), and the cell can fire again.

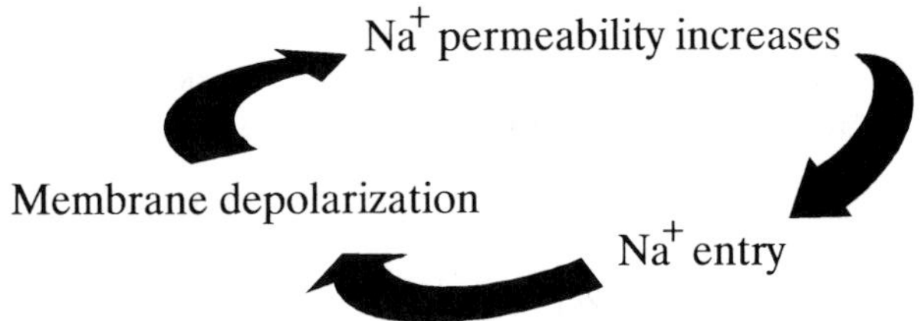

Figure 1–2. The initiation of the action potential. Neurons use fast electrical signals called action potentials. These arise through a regenerative mechanism; once the membrane exceeds threshold, the illustrated loop is engaged and the neuronal membrane rapidly depolarizes. Na^+ = sodium ion.

The regenerative property of the action potential serves not only to amplify threshold potentials (its principal function in dendrites), but also confers long-distance signalling capabilities (Figure 1–3). When the membrane potential peaks under the control of the increase in Na^+ permeability, adjacent regions of the axon become sufficiently depolarized so that they are in turn brought to threshold and generate an action potential. As successive axonal segments are depolarized, the action potential conducts at great speed down the axon, like a wave. This is further enhanced by myelination, which increases the rate of conduction severalfold by limiting the amount of current flow required for action potential conduction. Because of its all-or-none characteristics and ability to conduct over long distances, the action potential provides a high-quality digital signalling mechanism in the neuron.

Although the information that a neuron integrates depends on its synaptic input, how the neuron processes that information depends on its intrinsic properties (Llinás 1988). Many CNS neurons have the ability to generate their own patterns of

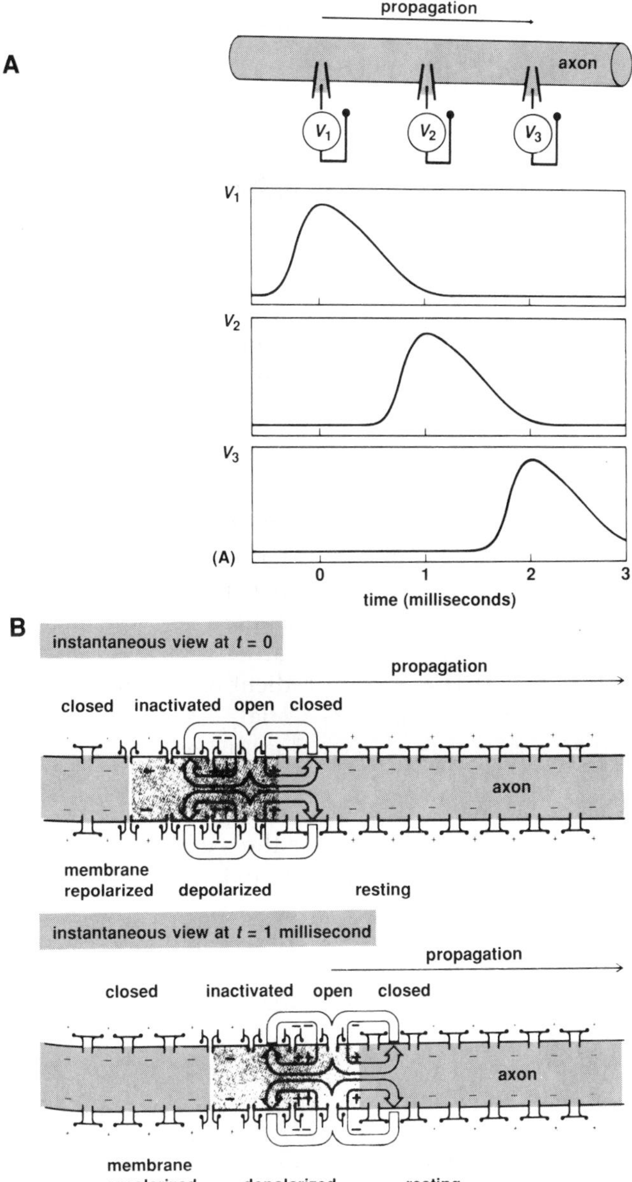

Figure 1–3. Action potential conduction. The regenerative property of ion channels in neuronal membranes mediates the rapid spread of the action potential down the axon. *Panel A:* Electrodes (V_1, V_2, and V_3) placed along the axon show the action potential traveling unchanged down the axon at high speed. *Panel B:* The action potential conducts as a wave. As each segment of the axon is depolarized, the spike it fires in turn depolarizes the subsequent segment. Therefore, as the action potential travels to the right, channels go from closed to open to inactivated to closed. In this way activation of the initial segment of the axon initiates an action potential that conducts all the way to the axon terminals. (Reprinted from Alberts B, Bray D, Lewis J, et al: Molecular Biology of the Cell, 2nd Edition. New York, Garland, 1989, p 1071. Used with permission.)

activity even in the absence of synaptic input, firing either at a regular rate (pacemaker firing) or in clusters of spikes (burst firing). This endogenous activity is driven by specialized ion channels, with their own voltage and time dependence, which periodically bring the initial segment of the axon to threshold (Figure 1–4; *panel A*) and can be visualized by imaging techniques that reveal fluctuating Ca^{2+} levels (Figure 1–4; *panel B*) (Tank et al. 1988). These channels giving rise to autorhythmicity may be modulated by the membrane potential of the cell or second messenger systems. Further, CNS neurons may profoundly change how they respond to a given synaptic input as a function of slight changes in resting potential (Figure 1–4; *panel C*) (Llinás and Jahnsen 1982). For instance, a thalamic neuron fires as a pacemaker when stimulated from slightly depolarized levels, whereas it fires in bursts of action potentials when stimulated from somewhat hyperpolarized levels. Changes in second messenger levels may also profoundly affect the activity or response properties of neurons. This confers a much greater repertoire to the functioning of individual neurons. So, in addition to evoking a response in a postsynaptic neuron, synaptic activity can shape intrinsic firing patterns, causing a cell to shift from one mode of activity to another, or alter the cell's response to other synaptic inputs.

Signalling Between Neurons

Neurons communicate with one another via chemical neurotransmitters at specialized sites of close membrane apposition called synapses. The prototypic synapse connects presynaptic axon terminals with postsynaptic dendrites. This arrangement (Shepherd and Koch 1990) is typical for projection neurons: cells conveying information from one region of the brain to another or, in the case of spinal motor neurons, from the ventral horn to skeletal muscles. By contrast, local circuit neurons, or interneurons, interact only with their neighbors. Like projection neurons, they too make axodendritic connections. In addition, they form several other kinds of synaptic contacts that greatly increase their functional sophistication (Figure 1–5). Dendrites may synapse with dendrites (dendrodendritic connections), or cell bodies on cell bodies (somasomatic), forming local neural circuits that convey information without action potential firing. Axons may synapse onto the axon terminals of other axons (axoaxonal connections) and thereby modulate

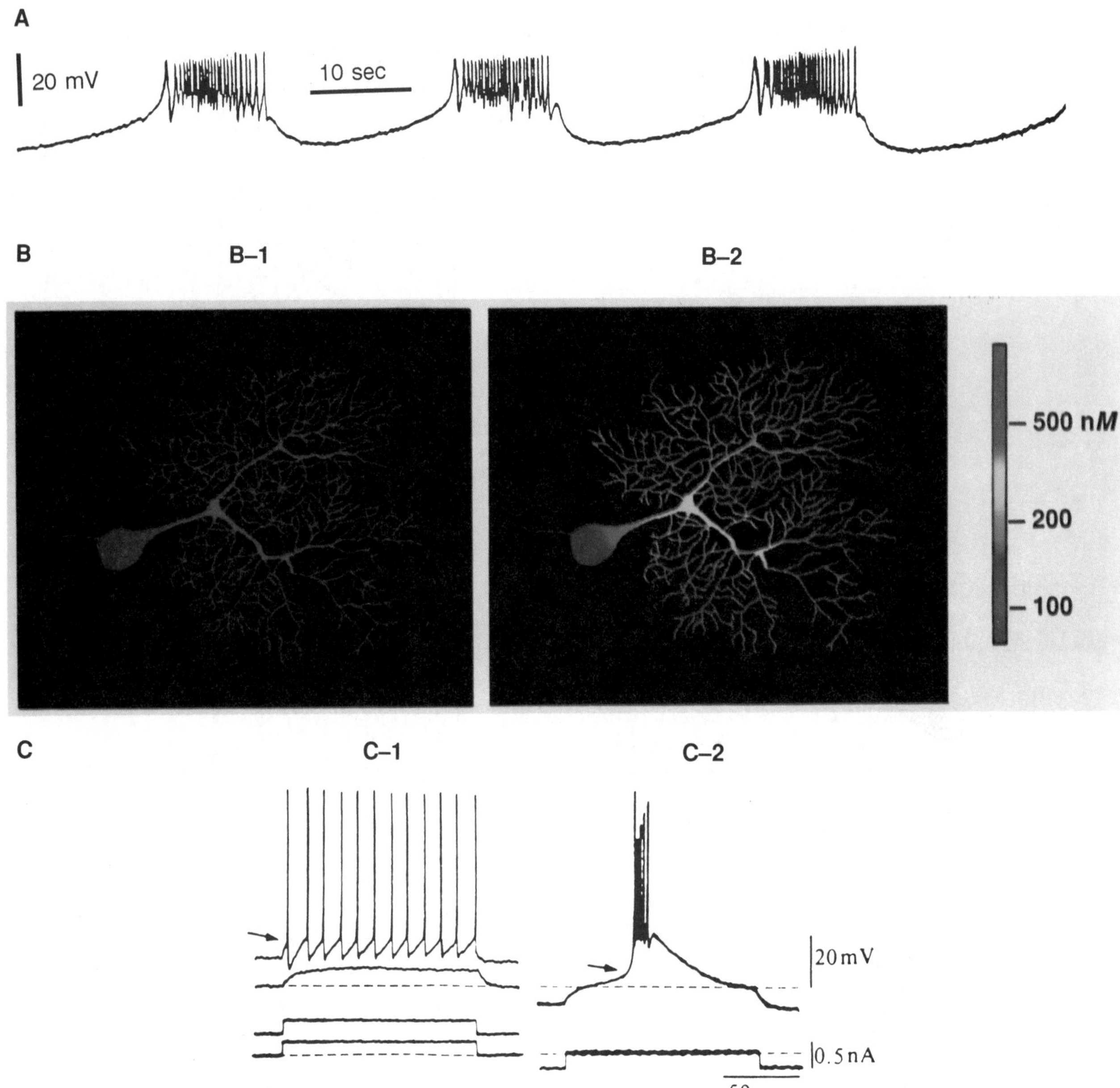

Figure 1–4. Intrinsic electrical properties of mammalian neurons. *Panel A:* Central nervous system neurons frequently show oscillations of membrane potential that trigger rhythmic firing. Here a cerebellar Purkinje cell fires in bursts of about 25 spikes every 20 seconds (the top halves of the action potentials have been cropped). *Panel B:* Purkinje cell bursting and oscillation in dendritic calcium (Ca^{2+}) levels. Ca^{2+}-sensitive dyes can be used to visualize changes in Ca^{2+} levels under fluorescence microscopy. For the cell whose activity is shown in *panel A*, snapshots of Ca^{2+} levels are shown on a flame scale. During quiescent intervals between bursts, dendritic Ca^{2+} levels are low (*B–1*). When burst firing, dendritic Ca^{2+} levels are high (*B–2*). These dendritic Ca^{2+} conductances trigger burst firing. (Reprinted from Tank DW, Sugimori M, Connor JA, et al: Spatially resolved calcium dynamics of mammalian Purkinje cells in cerebellar slice. Science 242:773–777, 1988. Used with permission.) *Panel C:* Thalamic neurons respond differently to a depolarizing step depending on their resting potential. In *C–1,* the lower traces of each pair show that when depolarized from the resting potential (*dashed line*), only a passive response is seen (i.e., there is no action potential firing). However, when the cell is tonically depolarized, the same step initiates regular pacemaker firing (upper traces in each pair). In *C–2,* if the cell is tonically hyperpolarized, the same step initiates burst firing. Each mode of firing has its own threshold indicated by the arrows. (Reprinted from Llinás R, Jahnsen H: Electrophysiology of mammalian thalamic neurones in vitro. Nature 297:406–408, 1982. Used with permission.)

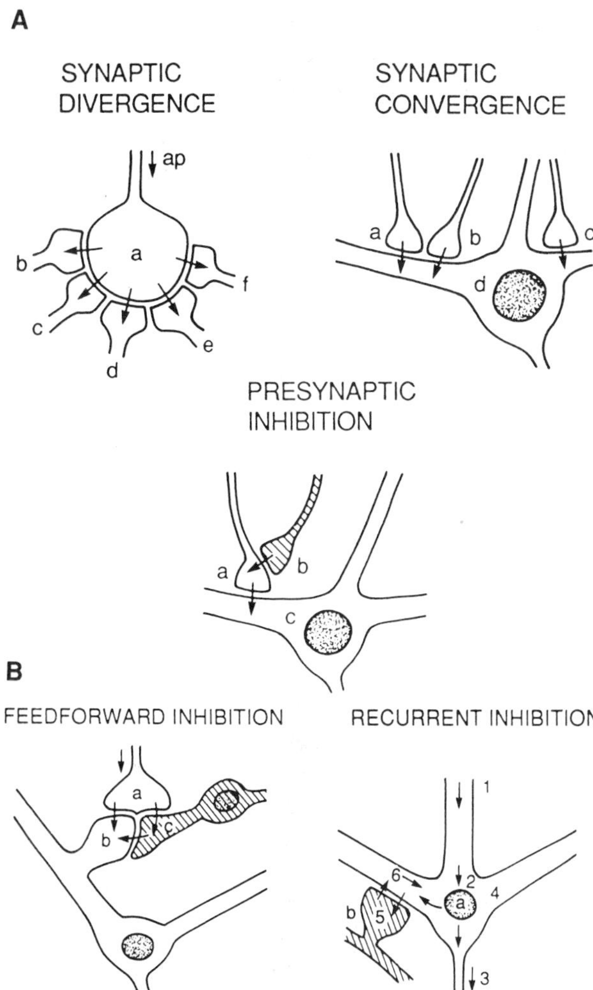

Figure 1–5. Local neuronal signalling in microcircuits. *Panel A:* Different connection patterns dictate how information flows between neurons. In synaptic divergence, an action potential (ap) in one neuron (a) may disseminate information to several postsynaptic cells (b, c, d, e, and f) simultaneously. Alternatively, in the case of synaptic convergence, a single neuron (d) may receive input from an array of presynaptic neurons (a, b, and c). In presynaptic inhibition, one neuron (a) can modulate information flowing between two other neurons (from a to c) by influencing release from the presynaptic neuron's terminals; this can be inhibitory (as shown) or facilitatory (as shown in Figures 1–8 and 1–9). *Panel B:* Neurons may modulate their own actions. In feedforward inhibition, the presynaptic cell (a) may directly activate a postsynaptic cell (b) and at the same time modulate its effects by also activating an inhibitory cell (c), which in turn inhibits cell b. In recurrent inhibition (information flow is shown numerically), a presynaptic cell (a) activates an inhibitory cell (b) that synapses back onto it, limiting the duration of its activity. (Reprinted from Shepherd GM, Koch C: Introduction to synaptic circuits, in The Synaptic Organization of the Brain, 3rd Edition. Edited by Shepherd GM. New York, Oxford, 1990, pp 9, 12. Used with permission.)

transmitter release from the postsynaptic presynaptic terminal. Additionally, some neurons may function both like interneurons and projection neurons.

A minority of local connections (mostly dendrodendritic and somasomatic) are mediated by electrical synapses. Here, multisubunit channels called gap junctions link the cytoplasm of adjacent cells (Bennett et al. 1991), allowing both small molecules and ions carrying electrical signals to flow from one cell to the other. Because they have no ability for amplification, electrical synapses typically join similar sized cells (as do gap junctions connecting cardiac muscle fibers), and unlike the prototypic chemical synapse they usually connect identical regions of the adjoining cells, either dendrite to dendrite or cell body to cell body. The ability to pass small molecules, including some second messengers, gives rise to chemical coupling which is probably principally important during development for setting up morphogenic gradients (Fraser et al. 1987). In the mature CNS, electrical synapses appear to function primarily to synchronize the electrical activity of groups of neurons or where particularly high-frequency transmission of signals is required (Bennett 1977).

Most CNS synaptic connections are chemically mediated (Figure 1–6). Although chemical synapses are somewhat slower than electrical ones, they allow for a significant amplification of signals, may be inhibitory as well as excitatory, are susceptible to a wide range of modulation, and can through the release of transmitters activating second messenger cascades in turn modulate the activity of other cells. One can think of chemical synapses as highly specialized microglands—ones that release their contents just in the synaptic zone. Like glands they hold neurotransmitter molecules (their secretory substance) in numerous, small membrane-bound granules or synaptic vesicles, each containing several thousand molecules. When the presynaptic action potential invades the terminal region or varicosity, it activates voltage-dependent Ca^{2+} channels. The resulting rise in the intracellular Ca^{2+} concentration increases the probability of vesicles fusing with the membrane. The result is that at several active zones, when Ca^{2+} levels rise, there is a near synchronous fusion of synaptic vesicles with the plasma membrane and release of transmitter into the synaptic cleft. Transmitter then has to diffuse only a short distance before it binds to postsynaptic receptors.

Transmitter action is typically limited in dura-

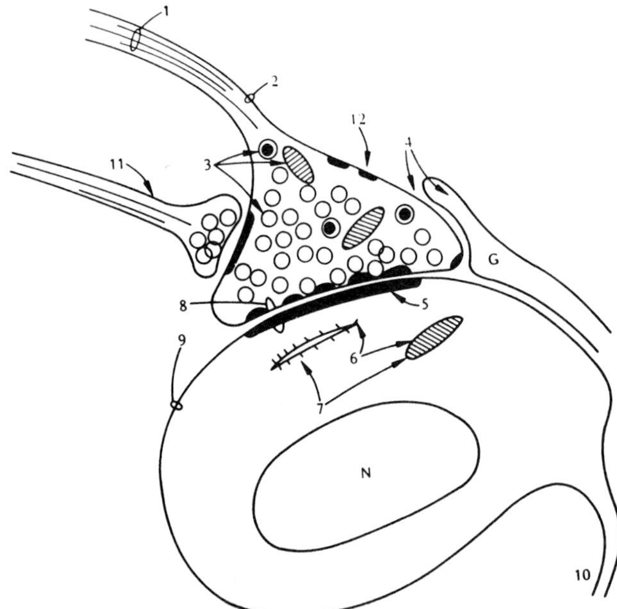

Figure 1–6. Chemical synaptic transmission. The essentials of the chemical synapse are revealed in 12 steps: 1) molecular components of the synapse get to the terminal by axonal transport; 2) an action potential invades the terminal, leading to a local influx of calcium (Ca^{2+}), which triggers release of synaptic vesicles into the cleft; 3) synaptic organelles and enzymes synthesize and package neurotransmitter; 4) extracellular enzymes and glia (G) and neurons limit transmitter action by degradation and reuptake of transmitter; 5) released transmitter impinges on postsynaptic receptors to initiate postsynaptic signals; 6) organelles in the postsynaptic neuron respond to transmitter binding by release of Ca^{2+}, for example; 7) second messengers initiated by receptor binding may influence DNA transcription (in the nucleus [N]) leading to longer-term responses and structural changes; 8) patterns of activity may lead to transient or enduring changes in the efficacy of the synapse; 9) electrical activity in the postsynaptic membrane continues the cycle of information flow; 10) this may lead to generation of action potentials in the postsynaptic cell and signalling to other cells; 11) the functioning of the presynaptic terminal may be influenced by presynaptic modulatory inputs; and 12) the presynaptic terminal may be regulated by its own transmitter through autoreceptors (receptors to the cell's own transmitter). (Reprinted from Cooper JR, Bloom FE, Roth RH: The Biochemical Basis of Neuropharmacology, 5th Edition. New York, Oxford University Press, 1986, p 44. Used with permission.)

tion by one of several mechanisms that rapidly remove the released transmitter from the postsynaptic region (Cooper et al. 1986). Transmitter may be broken down as is the case for acetylcholine, which is hydrolyzed by the enzyme acetylcholinesterase (acetylcholinesterase is bound to the postsynaptic membrane adjacent to the postsynaptic receptors). The monoamine and amino acid neurotransmitters are also metabolized, but, in addition, they are removed from the synaptic cleft by rapid reuptake mechanisms. Highly specific membrane pumps carry the transmitter back into the presynaptic terminal, the postsynaptic cell, or adjacent glial cells where it is repackaged in synaptic vesicles or metabolized or both. Both tricyclic antidepressants and psychostimulants increase synaptic levels of monoamines by inhibiting uptake. Neuropeptide transmitters may act for longer times because they are neither taken up nor rapidly broken down. Instead, they diffuse away from synaptic sites where they are subsequently cleaved by extracellular proteases into inactive peptides.

Rapid Postsynaptic Response Mechanisms

Postsynaptic receptors activated by the binding of neurotransmitter fall into two classes. In the case of ligand-gated channel receptors, the channel is an intrinsic part of the receptor protein complex. Receptor activation directly increases the ionic permeability of the postsynaptic membrane through a change in the shape (allosteric) of the receptor complex. This results in either depolarization giving rise to an excitatory postsynaptic potential (EPSP) or hyperpolarization generating an inhibitory postsynaptic potential (IPSP). The neuromuscular junction is the prototypic excitatory synapse; simultaneous binding of two acetylcholine molecules opens a receptor channel permeable to both Na^+ and K^+. This results in a strong depolarization of the postsynaptic membrane mediated by Na^+ influx and moderated by K^+ efflux. Ligand-gated channels are found at synapses such as the neuromuscular junction where rapid and reliable activation of the postsynaptic cell is required. For motor neurons, the coupling between pre- and postsynaptic cells is strong enough that one motor neuron spike reliably causes the muscle cell to contract.

In the CNS, glutamate receptors mediate most fast excitatory transmission; γ-aminobutyric acid (GABA) and glycine are the most common inhibitory transmitters. GABA and glycine receptors are members of a superfamily of receptors modelled on the nicotinic acetylcholine receptor (Schofield et al. 1990); glutamate receptors form a separate family (Keinänen et al. 1990). Unlike motor neurons, central neurons function in groups so that generally no individual cell has so strong a synaptic connection with another cell that it alone brings it to threshold; rather, groups of neurons—active in concert—converge on a postsynaptic neuron to generate several PSPs. These may summate within regions of the postsynaptic neuron (spatial summation) if they occur close enough together in time (temporal summation) to cause the postsynaptic neuron to fire. As a rule, fast ligand-gated channels mediate the flow of detailed information, such as patterns of sensory input, associations between sensory modalities, or motor output.

Longer-Term Postsynaptic Response Mechanisms

Longer-term modulatory effects are generally mediated by non-channel-linked receptors. This class of receptors is akin to cell-surface hormone receptors where agonist binding regulates cell function via second messenger cascades. Although non-channel-linked receptors may be catalytic or G protein linked, only the latter are known in the CNS. G protein linked receptors are so named because they couple to intracellular guanosine triphosphate (GTP)-binding regulatory proteins (or G proteins for short). G proteins are formed from a complex of three membrane-bound proteins; when the receptor is activated, the α subunit (G_α) binds GTP and dissociates from a complex of the β and γ subunits ($G_{\beta\gamma}$). Both G_α and $G_{\beta\gamma}$ may go on to trigger subsequent events. Activated G proteins have a lifetime of seconds to minutes; G_α autoinactivates by hydrolyzing its bound GTP, after which it reaggregates with $G_{\beta\gamma}$, returning to the resting state. Continued transmitter binding to the receptor may reinitiate the cycle.

G proteins are the first link in signalling cascades that achieve their effects either through activation of protein kinases, enzymes that phosphorylate cellular proteins (Huganir and Greengard 1987), or via changes in the level of intracellular Ca^{2+}, which in turn can trigger protein phosphorylation (Kennedy 1989a). Phosphorylation of cellular proteins may either activate or inactivate them or change their shape profoundly. Proteins affected may include membrane channels, structural elements, and transcriptional regulators for the expression of genes. In this way modulatory actions mediated by second messengers may affect most cellular processes. The potential for amplification, combined with divergence and convergence of signals, provides the requisite mechanisms for enduring changes in neuronal function, in particular the changes essential in learning and memory and during development.

G proteins are links in four major second messenger cascades (Figure 1–7) (Neer and Clapham 1988); although in some cases a cascade may function in isolation, most often they interact, conferring a complexity of action (Role and Schwartz 1989), our knowledge of which is still incomplete.

1. G proteins may link directly to nearby membrane channels to regulate their permeability. In dorsal root ganglion cells, for example, both norepinephrine and GABA act via a G protein to inhibit incoming sensory information by reducing the presynaptic Ca^{2+} influx required to trigger transmitter release (Holz et al. 1986).
2. They may either up- or down-regulate adenylate or guanylate cyclase to change cyclic adenosine monophosphate (cAMP) or cyclic guanosine monophosphate (cGMP) levels, which can directly modulate membrane channels. However, cAMP more commonly binds to the regulatory subunit of cAMP-dependent protein kinase (A-kinase), releasing the catalytic subunit, which phosphorylates membrane channels or other intracellular proteins (Alberts et al. 1989).
3. G proteins may activate the inositol phospholipid system (Berridge and Irvine 1989). In this case, two second messengers are generated. Binding of transmitter by the receptor activates phospholipase C (PLC) via a G protein that hydrolyzes the membrane phospholipid phosphatidylinositol-bis-phosphate (PIP_2) to produce inositol triphosphate (IP_3) and diacylglycerol (DAG). IP_3 stimulates the release of Ca^{2+} from intracellular stores. Ca^{2+} may in turn activate Ca^{2+}-dependent enzymes, including kinases. Additionally, Ca^{2+} triggers translocation of C-kinase from the cytoplasm to the cell membrane. Once translocated, membrane-bound DAG (also produced by PLC) activates C-kinase, which, among many actions, phosphorylates membrane channels.
4. G proteins may couple to phospholipase A_2 forming arachidonic acid (AA) by hydrolysis of membrane phospholipids (Axelrod et al. 1988; Piomelli and Greengard 1990; Piomelli et al. 1987). AA may act either as a second messenger or as a precursor that may be hydrolyzed by lipoxygenase, epoxygenase, or cyclooxygenase enzymes. The cyclooxygenase pathway is principally important outside the brain in producing prostaglandins.

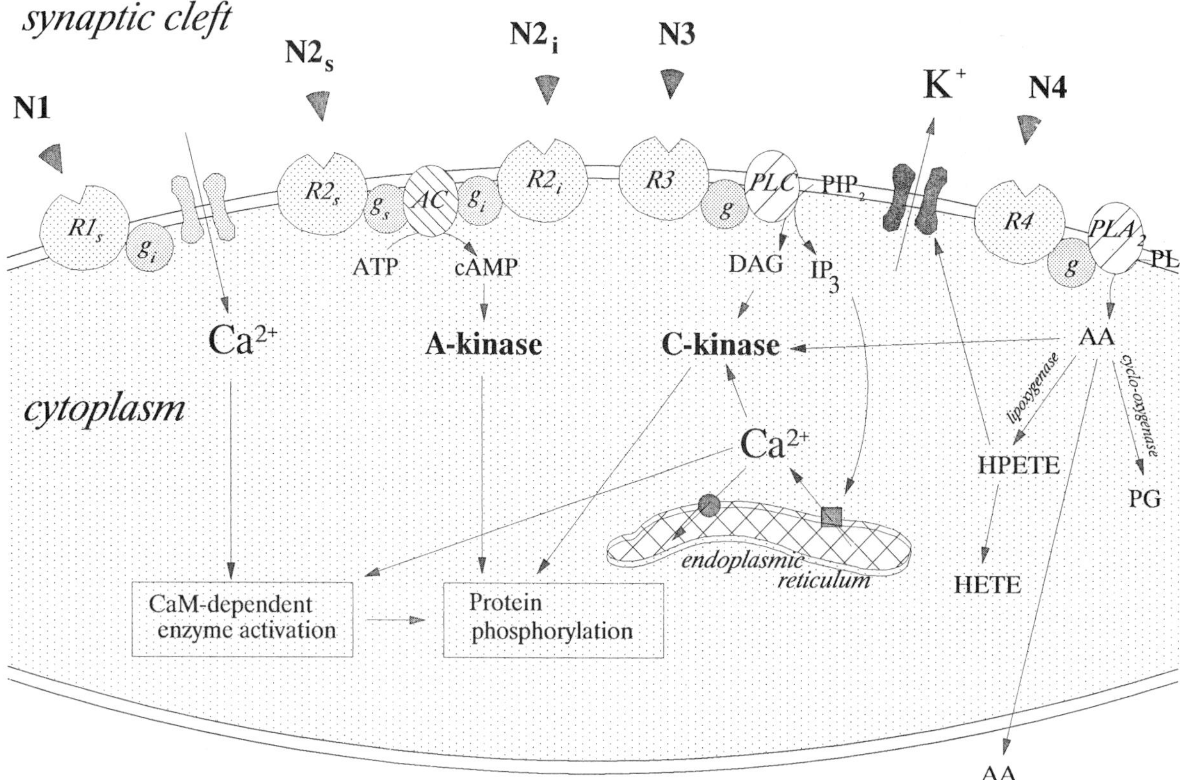

Figure 1–7. Second messenger cascades in neuronal signalling. Neurotransmitters (N1, N2, N3, and N4) activate specific receptors (R1, R2, R3, and R4). These receptors are coupled by G proteins to four postsynaptic signalling systems:

1. N1 inhibits membrane channels through its G protein (g_i) link; among those that may be inhibited are those regulating calcium (Ca^{2+}) entry, which serves as a second messenger with many effects mediated by calmodulin (CaM)-dependent enzyme activation.
2. Adenylate cyclase (AC) can be either stimulated ($N2_s$) or inhibited ($N2_i$) through separate G protein links (g_s and g_i); these actions can lead to an increase in synthesis of cyclic adenosine monophosphate (cAMP), which in turn controls the activity of A-kinase. A-kinase, like other kinases, controls cellular functions through protein phosphorylation.
3. N3 activates phospholipase C (PLC), which hydrolyzes phosphatidylinositol-bis-phosphate (PIP_2) producing two second messengers, diacylglycerol (DAG) and inositol trisphosphate (IP_3). IP_3 triggers the release of Ca^{2+} from the endoplasmic reticulum. Ca^{2+} in turn triggers the translocation of C-kinase to the cell membrane where it is activated by DAG. Because it becomes membrane bound with activation, C-kinase may be especially important in the modulation of membrane channels. Ca^{2+} released from intracellular stores may act similarly to Ca^{2+} that enters from outside the cell; however, because cells maintain Ca^{2+} at low levels, increases in Ca^{2+} levels are generally restricted.
4. N4 works through phospholipase A_2 (PLA_2) to trigger the production of arachidonic acid (AA) by hydrolysis of membrane phospholipids (PL). Unlike other second messengers, AA and its metabolites (hydroxyeicosatetraenoic [HETE] acids) and (hydroperoxyeicosatetraenoic [HPETE] acids) are membrane permeable so they can leave the postsynaptic cell to influence nearby cells; this may be important in long-term potentiation.

K^+ = potassium ion; ATP = adenosine phosphate; PG = prostaglandins. (Adapted from Piomelli et al. 1987; Ross and Gilman 1985.)

Binding of cAMP to membrane channels or their phosphorylation often underlies long-lasting modulatory PSPs. In contrast to the channel-linked receptors where activation leads to the rapid opening of channels, second messenger modulation often leads to the closure of membrane channels generating decreased conductance PSPs. In contrast to increases in conductance, which tend to short-circuit other synaptic input, decreased conductance PSPs have the opposite effect. Synaptic inputs exerting rapid control over the activity of the postsynaptic cell are almost invariably mediated by increases in permeability, whereas modulatory inputs are more often of the decreased conductance type, which can indirectly augment the strength of other inputs.

Second messenger modulation may have more subtle and wider ranging effects. Often no PSP is generated at all; rather, second messengers change the response properties of other receptors. In the retina, for example, dopamine appears to exert a modulatory role underlying dark adaptation (Dowling 1987). Dopamine is contained in a small population of interplexiform cells. These cells, partly under central influence, modulate the efficacy of information flow from receptor cells to horizontal cells, cells that regulate receptive field size and thus light sensitivity. In addition, the electrical coupling between horizontal cells, mediated by gap junctions, is reduced. Dopamine achieves both effects through dopamine, subtype 1 (D_1), receptors coupled to adenylate cyclase. Together these effects can increase retinal sensitivity severalfold, however, at the expense of acuity. In the CNS, several modulatory actions have been ascribed to dopaminergic projections.

Synaptic Modulation in Learning and Memory

Second messengers profoundly increase the range of responses a neuron may show to synaptic input. They activate kinases, which by phosphorylating other proteins act to both amplify and prolong signals. Receptor activation may induce kinase activity that lasts beyond agonist binding, enduring until the kinase is inactivated and phosphatases reverse phosphorylation. Because second messengers trigger numerous cellular functions, activation of a single receptor may trigger a coordinated cellular response involving several systems. This may include activity-dependent modulation of genomic transcription leading to enduring changes in cellular function. Learning and memory require both short- and long-term changes in neurons, and, as has been shown in studies in *Aplysia,* this occurs at synapses.

***Simple learning in* Aplysia.** Animals like the marine mollusk *Aplysia californica* have proved fundamental to studies of cellular mechanisms of learning and memory because changes in such animals' behavior can be traced to specific alterations in signalling between neurons (Kandel 1989). *Aplysia* has several essential features that have been key to this work. Its nervous system is composed of about 10^4–10^5 neurons arranged in ganglia. These are few enough to be tractable, but enough that the animal is capable of a significant range of behavior; indeed, *Aplysia* shows habituation, dishabituation, and sensitization, as well as associative learning. Furthermore, its neurons are giants—up to a millimeter in diameter (more than ten times the size of mammalian neurons)–making single neurons accessible to both physiological and biochemical study. As is more often the case in invertebrates, cells are identified (i.e., they can be recognized as individuals in all members of the species). This makes examination of individual neurons and neural circuits from animal to animal possible.

Behavioral studies have shown that *Aplysia* exhibits a simple defensive behavior called the gill withdrawal reflex, which can be modified by experience. When the siphon, a part of the body wall covering the gill, is stimulated by water turbulence the gill contracts. Repeated mild stimulation of the siphon leads to habituation of the reflex. If on the other hand the animal is aroused by a shock to the tail, the reflex shows sensitization, and subsequently the gill is withdrawn more briskly in response to the same siphon stimulation. If the same shock is administered to *Aplysia* when the reflex is habituated, the responsiveness also increases, showing dishabituation. Habituation and sensitization show both short and long memory. A single training trial may alter the reflex for at most a period of hours, but if training is repeated several times, habituation and sensitization may last for weeks. The animal is also capable of associative learning. If siphon stimulation is immediately followed by tail shock, it will show an increased gill withdrawal to siphon stimulation. In effect, it learns that siphon stimulation signals tail shock.

The essential features of the neural circuit for gill withdrawal reflex are encompassed in a 3-cell circuit (Figure 1–8). Siphon stimulation activates sensory neurons that make direct connections to gill motor neurons. This mediating pathway is under the influence of modulatory interneurons activated by sensory input from the tail (as well as other parts of the body), which synapse onto the presynaptic terminals of the sensory neurons. Thus the terminals of the sensory neurons are both pre- and postsynaptic depending on whether the mediating or modulatory pathway is considered. Gill withdrawal is triggered when siphon stimulation elicits action potentials in the peripheral branches of sensory neurons. These spikes conduct to the abdominal ganglion where sensory cells make synaptic connections with motor neurons. The essential neuronal

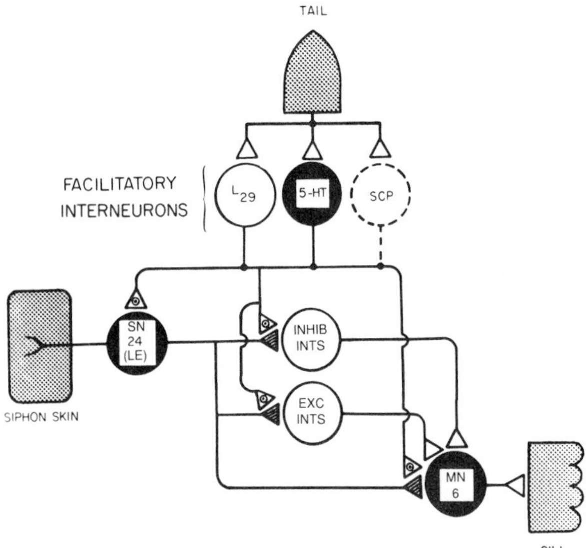

Figure 1–8. *Aplysia* gill withdrawal neural circuit. The marine snail *Aplysia* exhibits a simple defensive behavior, the gill withdrawal reflex, which shows habituation, sensitization, and associative learning. The reflex is mediated by a small number of neurons falling into three classes; the essential cells are shown by *dark circles*. These are sensory, motor, and modulatory interneurons. Sensory neurons (SN; of which there are a total of 24 in the LE cluster) pick up stimuli from the siphon skin. They activate gill motor neurons (MN; of which there are 6), to cause gill contraction. Facilitatory interneurons control the strength of the contraction; sensitizing stimuli to the tail activate neuron L29, and other neurons that use 5-hydroxytryptamine (5-HT; serotonin) or small cardioactive peptide (SCP) as transmitters, to presynaptically increase transmitter release from the sensory neuron terminals (*shaded*), producing heterosynaptic facilitation. Other inhibitory (INHIB INTS) and excitatory interneurons (EXC INTS) may shape the response or mediate a heterosynaptic component of habituation or sensitization. The site of plasticity underlying learning in the reflex is in the presynaptic terminals of the sensory cells (*shaded*). (Reprinted from Kandel ER: Genes, nerve cells, and the remembrance of things past. Journal of Neuropsychiatry and Clinical Neurosciences 1:103–125, 1989. Used with permission.)

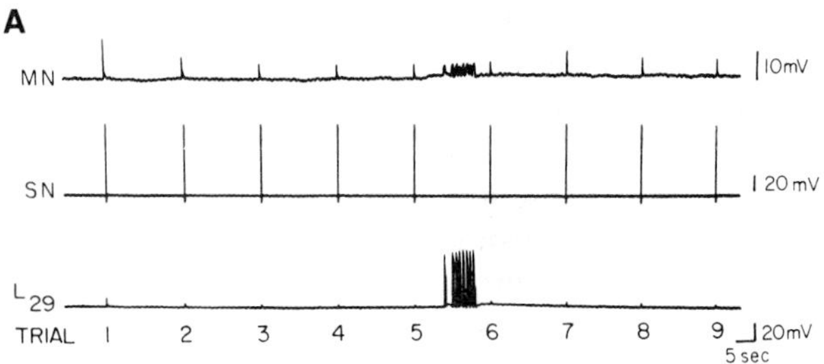

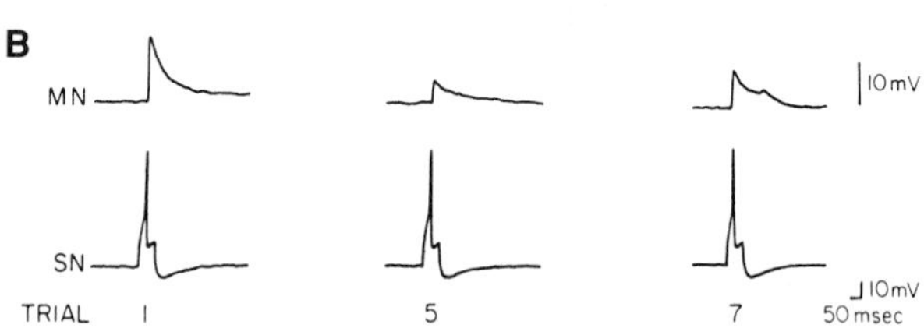

Figure 1–9. Cell culture of minimal 3-cell circuit for gill withdrawal. Single representative sensory, motor, and facilitator neurons can reestablish their normal relationships in vitro. In such an isolated 3-cell circuit, the cellular correlates of habituation and dishabituation may be seen. The continuous record is shown in *panel A;* selected stimulations are shown on a faster time scale in *panel B.* At 10-second intervals, a spike is evoked in the sensory neuron (SN) with a brief depolarizing step. An excitatory postsynaptic potential (EPSP) is recorded in the motor neuron (MN); the SN also makes a minor connection with the facilitator neuron, L29. With repeated SN spikes, the MN EPSP decreases in amplitude; this underlies habituation of the reflex. Then, between stimuli 5 and 6 a series of spikes are evoked in L29, mimicking the effects of sensitizing stimulation (L29 activity has no apparent effect on the SN, but does excite the MN). The result is an increase in the MN EPSP, which takes several seconds to build up, reaching a peak with stimulus 7. This heterosynaptic (or presynaptic) facilitation underlies dishabituation and sensitization and contributes to activity-dependent enhancement of presynaptic facilitation, the cellular mechanism underlying classical conditioning. (Reprinted from Hawkins RD, Schacher S: Identified facilitator neurons L29 and L28 are excited by cutaneous stimuli used in dishabituation, sensitization, and classical conditioning of *Aplysia.* J Neurosci 9:4236–4245, 1989. Used with permission.)

elements in the circuit can be grown in dissociated cell culture (Figure 1–9) (Hawkins and Schacher 1989; Rayport and Schacher 1986). At the sensory axonal terminals, Ca^{2+} influx triggers the release of neurotransmitter, producing an EPSP in the motor neuron. If the sensory-motor connection is strong enough, the motor neuron fires and its action potential conducts to gill muscle producing contraction and withdrawal. More often, however, several nearly synchronous spikes in one or more sensory neurons are required to bring the postsynaptic motor neuron to threshold. The increases in Ca^{2+} resulting from repeated activation of sensory neurons cause inactivation of presynaptic Ca^{2+} channels, resulting in a reduction of Ca^{2+} influx and a decrease in transmitter release. This process, whereby repeated activation of a synapse leads to a reduction in efficacy, is called homosynaptic depression—it is the cellular basis of habituation.

Sensitizing stimuli to the head activate facilitator interneurons. These cells release serotonin and peptide cotransmitters at synapses on to the sensory neuron terminals. Firing of the facilitator cells does not in itself cause gill withdrawal. However, when the siphon is subsequently stimulated, the efficacy of the sensory transmission is increased. This process in which activity in a third neuron increases the strength of the connection between another pair of neurons is termed heterosynaptic facilitation—it underlies sensitization and results from increased transmitter release by the sensory neuron. The facilitatory transmitters mediate facilitation via activation of adenylate cyclase through a G protein link (Figure 1–10; *panel A*). cAMP binds to the regulatory subunit of A-kinase, releasing the catalytic subunit, which phosphorylates a class of voltage dependent K^+ channels, sensitive to serotonin, known as S-K^+ channels. Because the falling phase of the action potential is mediated by an influx of K^+, closing S-K^+ potassium channels results in an action potential of increased duration, one that evokes a greater influx of Ca^{2+} and thus more transmitter release. This mechanism only works when Ca^{2+} channels are active (as in sensitization).

A

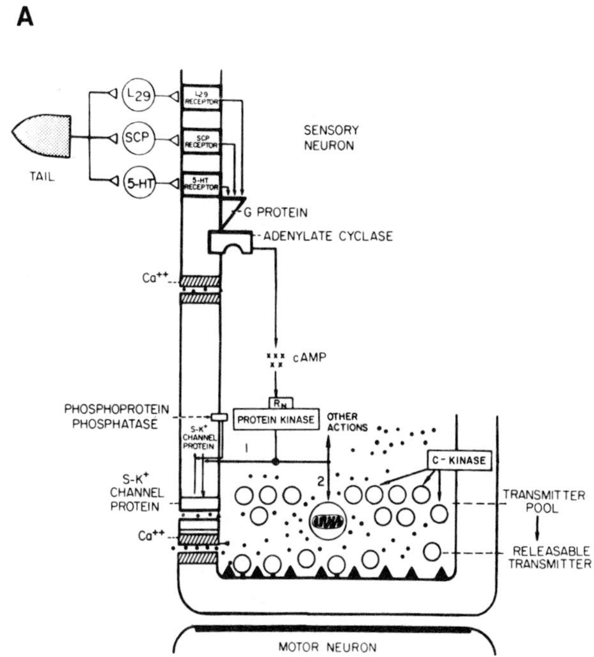

B

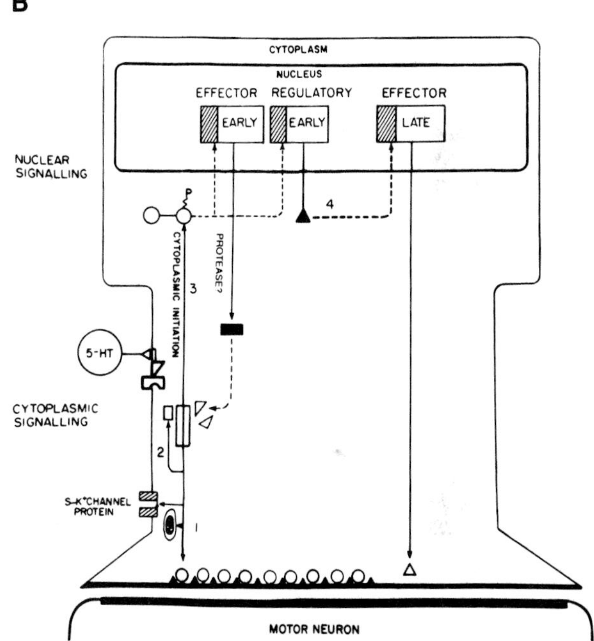

Figure 1–10. Molecular events underlying heterosynaptic facilitation. *Panel A:* Short-term facilitation. Sensitizing stimuli to the tail of *Aplysia* activate facilitatory interneurons that act through a G protein link to activate adenylate cyclase and increase presynaptic levels of cyclic adenosine monophosphate (cAMP). cAMP binds to the regulatory subunit (R_N) of protein kinase (A-kinase here) to release the catalytic subunit which phosphorylates S-K^+ channels and inactivates them. With a decrease in counterbalancing potassium ion (K^+) currents, calcium (Ca^{2+}) influx into the presynaptic terminal increases with the spike, leading to greater transmitter release. Facilitatory input also causes a translocation of C-kinase to the membrane, which appears to increase the pool of sensory neuron transmitter readily available for release; this seems particularly important for dishabituation when transmitter release is depressed. These short-term modulations all involve the covalent modification of existing proteins in the presynaptic terminals. L_{29} = facilitator neuron; SCP = small cardioactive peptide; 5-HT = 5-hydroxytryptamine (serotonin). *Panel B:* Long-term facilitation. Short-term changes underlying facilitation shown in *panel A* (1) can also trigger longer-term memory. For example, kinases can be self-phosphorylating or autocatalytic, leading to changes in activity lasting hours (2). Enduring memory depends on initiating de novo protein transcription, which is initiated by the phosphorylation (P) of immediate early genes (3). One such protein appears to be a protease that breaks down the regulatory subunits of A-kinase, leading to its prolonged activation. Later activated effector genes (4) most likely code for structural proteins allowing for remodeling of synapses, which is known to occur with long-term sensitization or habituation. (Reprinted from Kandel ER: Genes, nerve cells, and the remembrance of things past. Journal of Neuropsychiatry and Clinical Neuroscience 1:103–125, 1989. Used with permission.)

When the sensory-motor synapse is depressed, and Ca^{2+} channels largely inactivated, another mechanism becomes primary. Serotonin activates C-kinase, which is thought to increase the pool of readily releasable sensory neurotransmitter, enhancing the action of a reduced Ca^{2+} influx and thus boosting transmitter release. Associative learning appears to result from a synergistic action of spike-triggered Ca^{2+} influx and serotonin-activated second messenger systems, leading to enhanced C-kinase activity (Braha et al. 1990). In sensitization, dishabituation, and activity-dependent enhancement of presynaptic facilitation (the cellular mechanism of associative learning), the penultimate effect is mediated by a phosphorylation of existing proteins. A covalent modification of existing proteins thus appears to be the molecular basis for short-term memory in *Aplysia.*

In contrast, long-term memory appears to require changes in transcription. Intriguingly, the mechanisms for short-term sensitization (which has been best studied) also contribute to long-term memory, in a continuum. In long-term, as in short-term, sensitization, the memory is encoded by a strengthening of sensory-motor synapses (Figure 1–10; *panel B*), there is increased transmitter release, S-K^+ channels are closed leading to increased Ca^{2+} influx, serotonin and cAMP are the first and second messengers, and a characteristic set of proteins are phosphorylated (Sweatt and Kandel 1989). For long-term memory there is an absolute requirement for gene transcription and the synthesis of new proteins, which leads to structural changes at sensory-motor synapses. Blocking transcription triggered by cAMP-responsive elements blocks mechanisms underlying long- but not short-term sensitization (Dash et al. 1990). Ultimately the changes triggered by repeated tail stimulation, activation of facilitatory interneurons, serotonin application, or cAMP injection lead to structural changes involving the growth of new processes and increased numbers and size of active zones. This is specific to sensory neuron branches contacting postsynaptic motor neurons (Glanzman et al. 1990). These structural changes are likely to be orchestrated by interactions among several second messenger systems, through regulation of transcription.

Hippocampal long-term potentiation. In examining learning and memory in the mammalian nervous system, the hippocampus has been a particular focus because of its essential role in memory—bilateral hippocampectomy almost completely blocks the establishment of long-term memories. Brief high-frequency activation of hippocampal synapses permanently increases their strength through a phenomenon called long-term potentiation (LTP) (Kennedy 1989b; Malenka et al. 1989). LTP has thus proved particularly intriguing as a model of cellular plasticity that is likely to mediate memory function in the mammalian CNS. Strikingly, many of the mechanisms that mediate long-term sensitization in *Aplysia* contribute to enhancement of hippocampal synaptic connections, but in different ways.

Although all three major synaptic links in the hippocampus show LTP, the CA_3-to-CA_1 synapse is better understood (Figure 1–11). Here, the crucial initiating step in the induction of LTP is Ca^{2+} entry localized to the postsynaptic zone. Glutamate released from presynaptic CA_3 cells acts on two classes of postsynaptic receptors on CA_1 cells, the *N*-methyl-D-aspartate (NMDA) and α-amino-3-hydroxy-5-methyl-4-isoxazole propionic acid (AMPA) receptors (also known as kainate or quisqualate receptors). Cloning experiments have revealed that AMPA receptors subsume four different receptor types (Keinänen et al. 1990), each of which can exist in either flip or flop forms (Sommer et al. 1990). Both forms mediate postsynaptic depolarization, but AMPA receptor activation causes depolarization via Na^+ influx, whereas NMDA receptors do so via both Na^+ and Ca^{2+} entry. NMDA receptors differ crucially from AMPA receptors in requiring an initial depolarization before they will respond to neurotransmitter. Both NMDA and AMPA receptors are localized to postsynaptic dendritic spines, but because of the NMDA receptor's depolarization requirement, only AMPA receptors are activated by low-frequency firing of the presynaptic cell, so that little Ca^{2+} enters. In contrast, stronger or higher-frequency activation activates more AMPA receptors, causes a larger postsynaptic depolarization, and is then able to also activate NMDA receptors. NMDA receptors then mediate a localized increase in intracellular Ca^{2+} in the postsynaptic dendritic spine. Ca^{2+} acting as a second messenger initiates a selective enhancement in synaptic efficacy. Because they operate only during strong stimulation, NMDA receptors are crucial for the triggering, but not the expression, of LTP. Their requirement for the conjunction of transmitter and postsynaptic depolariza-

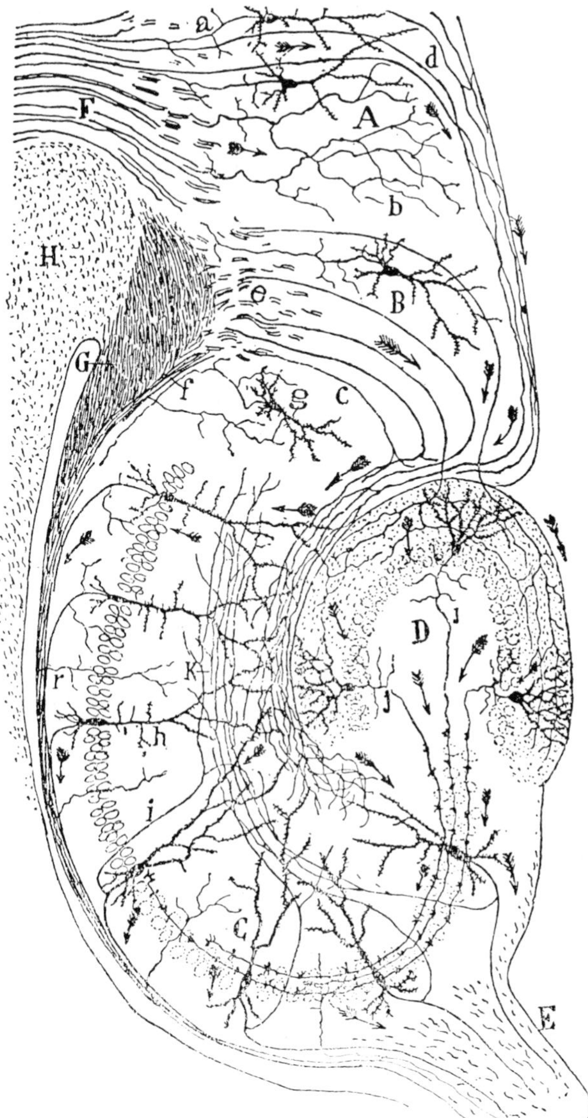

Figure 1–11. The hippocampus in cross-section. Inputs to the hippocampus arise from entorhinal cortex (A and B) and project to granule cells in the dentate gyrus (D; 1st synapse). Granule cells give rise to the mossy fibers that synapse with CA_3 pyramidal cells (C; 2nd synapse). CA_3 cells in turn project to CA_1 cells (h) via the Schaffer collaterals (k; 3rd synapse). Both CA_3 and CA_1 cells are output neurons, sending their axons into the fimbria (E). These three synaptic links exhibit an enduring increase in synaptic efficacy after high-frequency stimulation, called long-term potentiation (LTP). The glutamatergic CA_3-to-CA_1 link has been best studied; LTP is initiated by *N*-methyl-D-aspartate (NMDA) receptor activation and Ca^{2+} influx into the postsynaptic dendrite. (Reprinted from Ramón y Cajal S: Histologie du Système Nerveux de l'Homme & des Vertébrés, Vol II. Madrid, Consejo Superior de Investigaciones Cientificas, reprinted 1972, p 753. Used with permission.)

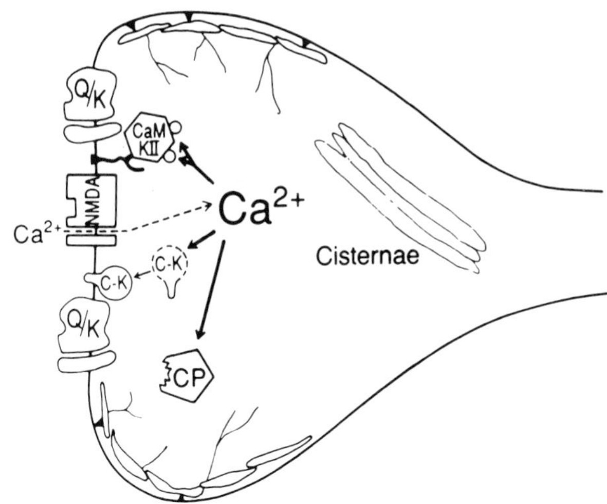

Figure 1–12. Initiation of long-term potentiation (LTP). CA_1 cells have two classes of glutamate receptors, those responding to quisqualate or kainate (Q/K)—also known as α-amino-3-hydroxy-5-methyl-4-isoxazole propionic acid (AMPA) receptors—and those selectively activated by *N*-methyl-D-aspartate (NMDA) when the membrane is depolarized. AMPA receptors mediate a sodium (Na^+)-dependent excitatory postsynaptic potential; with lower-frequency synaptic activity no calcium (Ca^{2+}) enters. However, the conjunction of depolarization and glutamate activates NMDA receptors, which mediate Ca^{2+} entry. Postsynaptic Ca^{2+} may trigger LTP through several mechanisms. It may activate calmodulin-dependent protein kinase II (CaM-KII), C-kinase (C-K), or calpain (CP). C-kinase may also trigger arachidonic acid production (not shown), which may increase presynaptic transmitter release and appears to be essential for the maintenance of LTP. (Reprinted from Kennedy MB: Regulation of neuronal function by calcium. Trends Neurosci 11:417–420, 1989a. Used with permission.)

tion appears to confer both the specificity and associativity of LTP.

Increased postsynaptic Ca^{2+} activates a cascade of intracellular messengers, which could mediate LTP (Figure 1–12). These include Ca^{2+}/calmodulin-dependent protein kinase II (CaM-KII), C-kinase and Ca^{2+}-dependent proteases. The relative importance of each remains open to question. For example, CaM-KII is localized to the postsynaptic membrane where it could phosphorylate postsynaptic AMPA receptors, increasing their response to transmitter. Because CaM-KII can be autoactivating once activated by Ca^{2+}, it might serve to maintain an increased receptor response over a course of minutes to hours. LTP also requires C-kinase activation; C-kinase may mediate transcriptional changes necessary for more permanent synaptic strengthening.

Ca^{2+}-dependent proteases may also be important; they may induce structural changes in the postsynaptic spine to increase the effectiveness of synapses on just that spine.

Whereas LTP is triggered postsynaptically, at the CA_3-to-CA_1 synapse, the expression of LTP appears to be mediated presynaptically through an increased release of glutamate (Bekkers and Stevens 1990; Malinow and Tsien 1990). Indeed, tetanization sufficient to elicit LTP is associated with an increased glutamate release that can be measured for several hours (Bliss et al. 1986); this would most likely occur if each presynaptic action potential elicited more transmitter release. Another line of evidence reveals that although both induction and expression of LTP can be blocked by protein kinase inhibitors, injection of a kinase inhibitor into just the postsynaptic cell blocks the induction of LTP, but not its continued expression (Malinow et al. 1989). These results suggest that immediately after the tetanus, postsynaptic mechanisms triggered by a rise in intracellular Ca^{2+} and involving protein kinase activity boost synaptic strength. Later on, presynaptic kinase activity appears to be crucial, acting to increase transmitter release.

A membrane-permeable second messenger that could diffuse across the synapse and act on the presynaptic terminal seems to be required if postsynaptic signals are to trigger presynaptic changes (Lynch et al. 1989). Among the several second messengers considered in this chapter, only arachidonic acid (AA) is membrane permeable. Furthermore, AA levels rise after stimulation that induces LTP (Lynch et al. 1989). Specificity of action would be explained, if simultaneous presynaptic activity (this would be a second associative site) was required for its action. Indeed, AA application alone is ineffectual. However, delivery of a weak tetanus (one not sufficient to generate LTP itself) in combination with AA results in a slowly developing potentiation occurring over a course of 15–30 minutes (Williams et al. 1989). Potentiation occurs despite blockade of AA metabolism, indicating that the effect is mediated by AA itself and not its metabolites. Furthermore, potentiation cannot be blocked by NMDA antagonists (which block LTP), showing that AA production is a subsequent step in the pathway after NMDA receptor activation. As in LTP, AA application leads to an activity-dependent increase in glutamate release. Either maximal stimulation or AA-induced potentiation precludes further potentiation by the other intervention, supporting further the key role of AA as a membrane-permeable second messenger. How AA mediates increased release is not known, but its activity dependence seems to assure that only simultaneously tetanized presynaptic terminals will show increased glutamate release and thus LTP.

❑ NEURONAL DEVELOPMENT

How neurons are able to modify their connections with experience probably reflects a small fraction of the mechanisms harnessed during CNS development. If synapse modification in the adult resembles or uses developmental mechanisms, other forms of plasticity may exist in the adult that are vestiges of development. Neuropsychiatric disorders might result from aberrant activation of such mechanisms. For example, the gene for Huntington's chorea might code for developmentally programmed cell death; activated aberrantly, it might trigger death of a specific cell population. Alternatively, because there is evidence for an excitotoxic mechanism via glutamate receptors, other developmental mechanisms may be important (Wexler et al. 1991). Numerous developmental disorders result from aberrant growth of neurons forming deficient or aberrant connections. Schizophrenia has been suggested to be rooted in a failure of mesocortical dopaminergic neurons to connect with frontal cortex (Weinberger 1987). Consequently, an insight into developmental mechanisms is likely to be fundamental to elucidating the causes of neuropsychiatric diseases.

Birth and Migration of Neurons

Neurons are largely defined by the place and timing of their birth. Cells destined to become CNS neurons arise from stem cells in the neural tube on a very exact schedule. Within a region, those neurons sharing the same birthday generally follow the same pattern of differentiation, remaining members of a distinct class of cells. Stem cells disappear once they have generated their sets of cells, so there is no further neuronal proliferation in the mature CNS. The adjustment of cell numbers to the requirements of different functions occurs through selective cell death.

Having completed their final cell divisions, neurons migrate to their definitive locations, guided by physical and chemical signals (Figure 1–13). In the

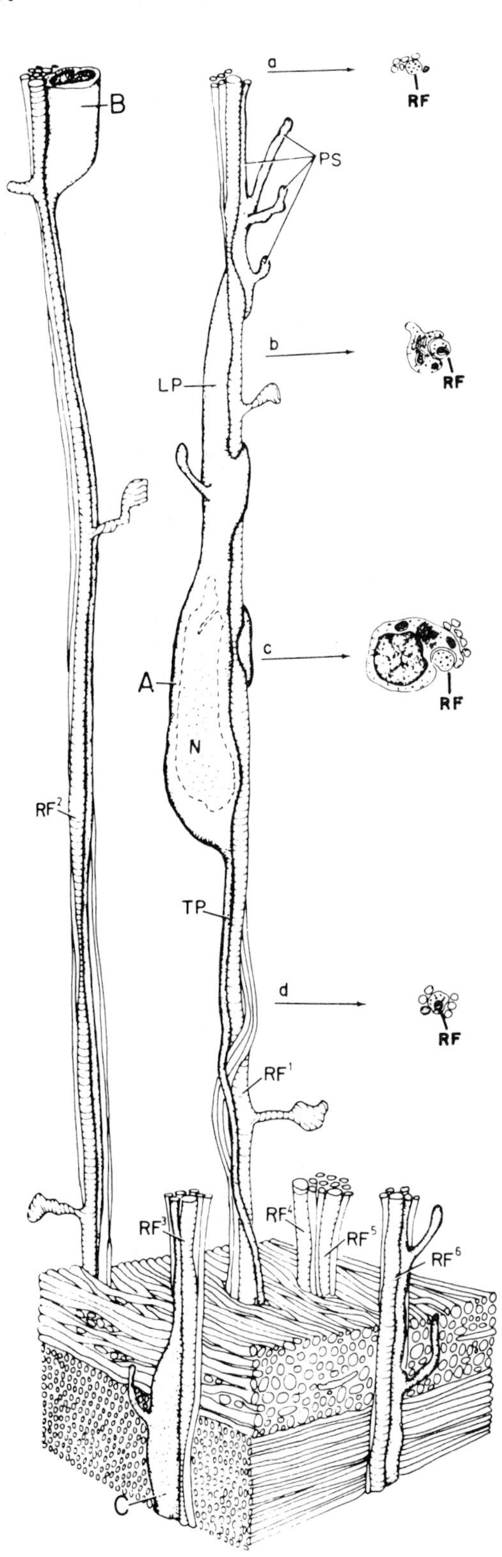

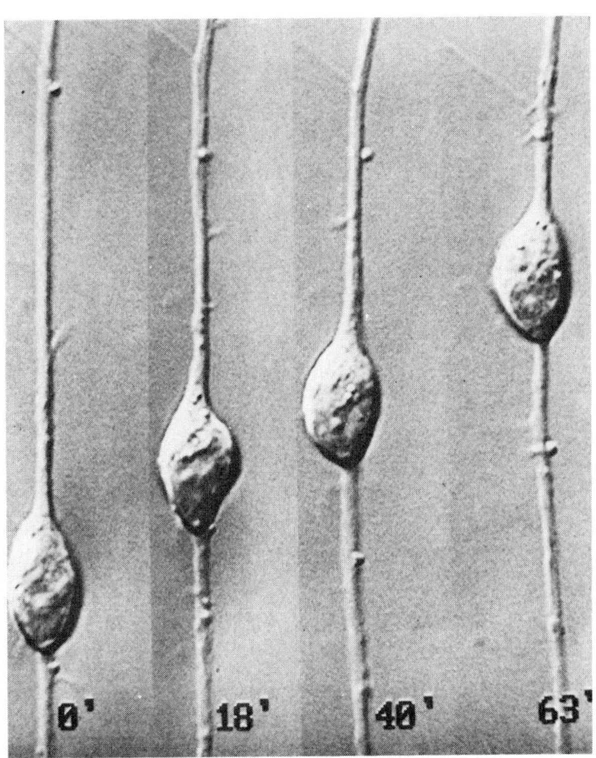

Figure 1–13. Neuronal migration during development. *Panel A:* Three-dimensional reconstruction of migrating neurons in the developing cerebral cortex. Neurons (A, B, and C) arise deep to the cortex (*bottom of schematic*) in the subventricular zone and migrate superficially along radial glial fibers (RF^{1-6}). The migratory neuron (A) is characterized by a leading process (LP) with filopodia (PS), a trailing process (TP), and a nucleus (N) pushed back toward the trailing end of the cell body. Cross-sections of the migratory profile (a, b, c, and d) shown at different levels reveal the close association between neuron and glial cell characteristic of migration. (Reprinted from Rakic P: Mode of cell migration to the superficial layers of fetal monkey neocortex. J Comp Neurol 145:61–84, 1972. Used with permission.) *Panel B:* Developing neurons and glia recombined in culture show migration profiles. Successive frames (at about 20-minute intervals) of a migrating hippocampal neuron are shown. The neuron moves in a stop-and-go fashion along the radial glial fiber. A leading process (extending above the cell) has numerous highly active filopodial extensions. As in the reconstruction (*panel A*), both a TP and posteriorly displaced N are also evident. Neurons will migrate on glia from different brain regions (glia in this figure are from the developing cerebellum), suggesting that there is a general molecular recognition system used throughout the brain in guiding neuronal migration. (Reprinted from Hatten ME: Riding the glial monorail: a common mechanism for glial-guided neuronal migration in different regions of the developing mammalian brain. Trends Neurosci 13:179–184, 1990. Used with permission.)

cortex, for example, a temporary scaffolding of radial glial cells forms (Rakic 1972), which may be fundamental to the later columnar organization of the cortex. When cells complete their final division, they attach to these guides, and move from proliferative zones in the subventricular zone to the superficial surface of the cortex. The radial glial guides define radial units linking a given region of the subventricular proliferative zone to a corresponding cortical column (Rakic 1988). Migration requires cell-adhesion molecules (Jessell 1988; Takeichi 1991). For example, astrotactin, produced by migrating neurons, mediates their attachment to radial glial guides (Hatten 1990). After arriving at their definitive locations, neurons elaborate processes and complete their maturation. Some neurons, such as cerebellar granule cells, migrate a second time, so that rather than growing out their processes from their definitive location, they lay down a process—the parallel fiber—behind them as they migrate.

Neurons seem to know their identity shortly after their final cell division and consequently make connections based on their birthday and birthplace rather than their definitive location. For example, in the neurological mutant mouse reeler (Caviness 1982), named for its unsteady gait, there is a failure in migration of cortical neurons so that cells that should have migrated to the most superficial layers remain in the deepest ones. Despite this extensive reorganization, individual neurons develop into the same cell types they would have if they had migrated successfully. Moreover, they largely make the correct connections. As a result, the cortex of reeler appears inverted. Although the animal's behavior is not entirely normal (it has an unsteady gait), what is remarkable is that cells in this inverted cortex can function at all. This ability of neurons to recognize their targets reflects neuronal specificity and is likely mediated by cell surface molecules that allow developing neurons to recognize one another.

Process Outgrowth

Having migrated to their definitive locations, neurons start to elaborate processes. A specialized structure called the growth cone forms at the end of extending processes. The growth cone controls the insertion of new membrane elements into the cell membrane, it releases proteolytic enzymes to open a pathway through the extracellular matrix, and it extends very fine processes (filopodia) to guide the growing process to its proper target (Purves and Lichtman 1985). Growth cones may extend as much as a millimeter a day. As the growth cone advances, a cytoskeleton of microtubules and neurofilaments is laid down in the elongation process. In addition to maintaining the structure of the growing process, cytoskeletal elements also transport membrane and structural proteins from synthetic sites in the cell body to the newly generated process and transport trophic substances back to the cell body.

Growing processes depend on several cues acting in concert to reach their targets. At different stages, different cues become important. Initially, growth cones depend on intrinsic adhesiveness of neighboring cells. Later on, they are guided by their targets or intermediate stepping-stone cells. Targets may release signalling factors, thereby establishing chemoaffinity gradients, or direct cell-to-cell contact may provide the signal. The definitive target ultimately validates correctly connecting cells by provision of trophic substances that support the survival of the innervating neurons. Cells that fail to make the appropriate connections die for lack of such substances.

The formation of specific connections has been extensively studied in grasshopper limb sensory neurons. These cells are born in the periphery and subsequently send axons into the developing CNS (Goodman et al. 1984). The first neurons to send out processes form the pioneer fibers. Later-developing neurons are guided by adhesive interactions with pioneer fibers. Particular cells in the epithelia, stepping-stone cells, serve as intermediate targets. The growth cones of pioneer fibers identify stepping-stone cells through the extension of chemosensitive filopodia. These filopodia transiently make gap junctional contact with the stepping-stone cells probably exchanging small molecules that act as intracellular signals. If these filopodia are disrupted pharmacologically, growth continues but in an undirected fashion (Bentley and Toroian-Raymond 1986). The pioneer fibers proceed from stepping-stone to stepping-stone until they reach their ultimate targets. The stepping-stone cells themselves develop into neurons, which interestingly send their own processes into the CNS following the pioneer fibers they guided.

Recent work has shown that similar developmental mechanisms operate in the formation of the mammalian CNS. In developing spinal cord, commissural neurons in the dorsolateral spinal cord orient chemotactically to the floor plate in the ventral cord; on reaching the floor plate, the processes use it as a stepping-stone, changing direction and growing into the contralateral spinothalamic tract (Tessier-Lavigne et al. 1988). Similarly, in the developing brain stem, after corticospinal pioneer fibers have extended into the spinal cord, secondary processes arise that innervate the pons; during just this developmental stage, the pons releases a trophic factor that stimulates the outgrowth of pontine collaterals (Heffner et al. 1990).

Neurotrophic Factors

Several neurotrophic factors have now been characterized. These proteins stimulate the outgrowth of neuronal processes, attract growth cones, and support the survival of cells that take them up. Nerve growth factor (NGF) was the first discovered. Brain-derived neurotrophic factor (BDNF) followed; its amino acid sequence shows a significant homology with that of NGF. Together they begin to define a superfamily of neurotrophic factors (Barde 1989). This prompted a further search, which resulted in the discovery of a third member of the family, neurotrophin-3 (Hohn et al. 1990; Maisonpierre et al. 1990), with its own distinctive profile of neurotrophic activity. Other unrelated neurotrophic factors whose action is not necessarily restricted to the nervous system include insulin-like growth factors, fibroblast growth factor, ciliary neurotrophic factor, purpurin, and activin (Schubert et al. 1990).

NGF is the best studied of the neurotrophic factors (Barde 1989). It is released peripherally by the targets of sensory and sympathetic neurons and is necessary for their survival. Indeed, the injection of anti-NGF antibodies into neonatal mice results in a chemical sympathectomy. Among sympathetic targets, NGF is found in extremely high concentration in mouse and snake salivary glands; these have provided quantities sufficient for extensive study. Processes of developing neurons will grow into areas where NGF concentration is high. NGF receptors bind NGF, leading to its endocytic uptake. It is then transported back to the cell body (by retrograde fast axonal transport), where it supports neuronal survival.

Muscle cells also release a factor, similar to NGF in function but as yet uncharacterized, which regulates the survival of their innervating sensory neurons. Early in development, dorsal root ganglia at all levels have similar numbers of neurons. Later on, those ganglia innervating the limbs are considerably larger (having many more cells) than those connected to the trunk. The role of the neurotrophic factors is revealed by provision of exogenous NGF or transplantation of a supernumerary limb bud. Both interventions lead to the survival of neurons in connected sympathetic or dorsal root ganglia that grow to be abnormally large. Although their functions in the CNS are not as well understood, NGF and NGF receptors are selectively distributed. Furthermore, NGF is now known to promote the survival of cholinergic neurons in the basal nucleus of Meynert, the same neurons that are lost with Alzheimer's disease (Thoenen et al. 1987). Similarly, BDNF was recently shown to support the survival of substantia nigra dopaminergic neurons whose loss underlies Parkinson's disease (Hyman et al. 1991).

Neurotrophic and Neurotoxic Actions of Neurotransmitters

Neurotransmitters themselves may have trophic or toxic roles in the shaping of neurons and their interconnections (Lipton and Kater 1989). The progress of growth cones is regulated by local intracellular levels of Ca^{2+}. Ca^{2+} acts within a narrow window. When levels are low, growth cones are quiescent; they move when levels rise. Past a certain level, Ca^{2+} arrests growth and leads to retraction or destruction of neuronal processes (Kater et al. 1989; Silver et al. 1989). Glutamate can regulate the growth of neuronal processes through the control of Ca^{2+} influx. This can be countered by inhibitory neurotransmitters, as well as by provision of increased amounts of trophic factors (Mattson and Kater 1989; Mattson et al. 1989). Dopamine acting at D_1 receptors can inhibit growth cone motility by activating adenylate cyclase and raising intracellular cAMP concentrations (Lankford et al. 1988).

Higher levels of glutamate produce excitotoxicity, perhaps reflecting the pathological functioning of these developmental signalling systems (Kater et al. 1989). Alternatively, excitotoxicity might have a normal function in regulating cell numbers and connectivity. Excitotoxicity appears to be mediated acutely by the entry of Na^+ (through AMPA channels), which leads to neuronal swelling (resulting in brain edema) and, in a delayed mode (through NMDA receptor channels), by sustained Ca^{2+} entry, which kills neurons probably by activation of intracellular proteases. In addition to mediating Na^+ influx and swelling, AMPA receptors may be coupled to the IP_3-DAG pathway, leading also to increases in intracellular Ca^{2+} and C-kinase activation. The NMDA receptor, which is most strongly implicated in excitotoxicity (Choi 1988; Choi and Rothman 1990), is coupled to a high conductance channel for Na^+ and Ca^{2+}, which is blocked by magnesium ions (Mg^{2+}) at resting membrane potentials. Activation of the NMDA receptor requires membrane depolarization (which dislodges the Mg^{2+}) in conjunction with glutamate binding. Competitive antagonists that block NMDA receptors include 2-amino-5-phosphonovalerate (APV). Noncompetitive antagonists block the open channel; these include phencyclidine (PCP), dextrorphan, and MK-801.

Excitotoxicity is likely to underlie neuronal loss in strokes, status epilepticus, hypoglycemia, and head trauma (Choi and Rothman 1990). These brain insults are linked in that all lead to neuronal depolarization, which results in excessive electrical activity, evoking excessive increases in glutamate release. In each case, elevated extracellular glutamate levels can be detected in experimental models. The cytopathology can be mimicked by intracerebral injections of excitatory amino acids. The same neurons spared in the disease states are also less affected in the experimental models, probably because they have fewer excitatory amino acid receptors or have better intracellular Ca^{2+} buffering abilities. Injured neurons show increased intracellular Ca^{2+} levels, and excitatory amino acid antagonists, especially those blocking NMDA receptors or channels, prevent or dramatically reduce neuronal loss in these conditions.

Suggestive evidence supporting a role for excitatory amino acid toxicity in neurodegenerative disorders is less complete (Choi 1988). One rare neurological disease, uniformly fatal in childhood, appears to be due to a deficiency in sulfite oxidase, resulting in elevations of the excitatory amino acid l-sulfo-cysteine (Olney et al. 1975). A recessive form of olivopontocerebellar degeneration, fatal in adult life, is associated with glutamate dehydrogenase deficiency. Two geographically localized neurodegenerative disorders have been tied to the ingestion of excitotoxins. Guam amyotrophic lateral sclerosis-parkinsonism-dementia results from ingestion of the excitatory amino acid β-n-methyl-amino-l-alanine (BMAA) found in the cycad plant (Spencer et al. 1987). Lathyrism, found in regions of Africa fraught with famine, is causally related to ingestion of the chick pea excitotoxin, β-n-oxalyl-amino-l-alanine (BOAA) (Spencer et al. 1986).

Similarities in other neuropsychiatric disorders to idiopathic neurodegenerative disorders suggest a role for excitotoxic mechanisms. Intriguingly, a growing body of findings implicate excitotoxic mechanisms in the pathology of Huntington's disease. The neuropathology of Huntington's disease is mimicked by excitatory amino acid injections; in particular, certain classes of striatal neurons are spared in both cases (Choi 1988; Wexler et al. 1991). Furthermore, measures of striatal NMDA receptors in patients dying of Huntington's disease revealed a selective loss of cells bearing these receptors, supporting the role of NMDA-mediated excitotoxicity in the pathogenesis of the disorder (Young et al. 1988). It is noteworthy that the unique properties of NMDA channels are both central to long-term potentiation and important in neurodegenerative diseases and in aspects of development.

Synapse Formation

When the growth cone approaches the target cell, a complex series of interactions commence. The growth cone functions like a protosynapse in that it releases neurotransmitter when its parent cell is electrically active. Uninnervated postsynaptic cells have transmitter receptors distributed over much of their surface (that later concentrate with innervation). Within minutes of initial contact, a rudimentary form of synaptic transmission starts. Over subsequent days, connections become stronger and stabilize as the growth cone matures into a presynaptic terminal, gathering the cellular elements that are necessary for focused release of neurotransmitter at active zones. In parallel, the postsynaptic cell concentrates receptors opposite the innervating process, removing them from other regions, and over the course of days, postsynaptic specializations develop.

Maturation of the postsynaptic cell requires de novo protein synthesis, much as do learning dependent long-term changes. Immediate early response genes (Morgan and Curran 1989) are among the first genes activated with postsynaptic depolarization by elevations in Ca^{2+}, cAMP, cGMP, IP_3, or DAG. The prototype of this family of proto-oncogenes is c-fos. The transcription of these proto-oncogenes leads to the synthesis of proteins (e.g., fos) that modulate or induce transcription of other genes that directly or indirectly induce structural changes in the cell. For example, NGF synthesis may be controlled by c-fos transcription; lesion of the sciatic nerve leads to a rapid increase in fos levels, which by binding to the transcription initiation site for NGF causes NGF production (Hengerer et al. 1990). Long-term sensitization in *Aplysia* (Barzilai et al. 1989) and hippocampal long-term potentiation (Cole et al. 1989; Wisden et al. 1990) are associated with the specific activation of other immediate early response genes.

The provision of NGF or other neurotrophic factors by postsynaptic cells ensures the survival of successfully innervating presynaptic neurons. More subtle regulation of presynaptic cells occurs as well. In the developing sympathetic nervous system, young neurons are exclusively noradrenergic before synapse formation. Depending on the target tissue, they may become cholinergic, retaining only traces of the noradrenergic phenotype (Landis 1990). This target-dependent effect is mediated by the release of a soluble cholinergic differentiation factor (CDF) by the postsynaptic cells. Once synaptic contact is established, cholinergic activation of the postsynaptic cell by presynaptic spikes suppresses CDF release. Thus synapse formation may trigger far-reaching changes both pre- and postsynaptically, extending as far as the choice of neurotransmitter by a presynaptic neuron.

As in associative learning, simultaneous electrical activity of pre- and postsynaptic elements leads to the strengthening of connections, whereas discordant activity results in the elimination of synapses. As a general pattern, both an excessive number of neurons and synaptic connections arise in the developing nervous system; then, through a combination of activity-dependent competition, trophic factor requirements, and possibly excitotoxic mechanisms, cells and synapses are pruned until the highly defined pattern of innervation of the adult is formed (Purves 1988). This complexity of mechanisms may have arisen because, given even the whole human genome, there is not enough information to code for every connection in the brain. In fact, only about 10% of human genes are brain specific. Therefore, interacting programs, feedback mechanisms, and environmental input are required to provide ways of refining a genetically initiated general pattern of connectivity.

A further rationale for this seemingly wasteful pattern may be drawn from evolution. Throughout phylogeny, changes in neuron number and connectivity would have had to match alterations in limb shape or function. Simultaneous changes in both genes for limb size and neuron number would be quite improbable. Instead, during development the nervous system has the potential to adjust to considerable changes in body shape and, even in the example of a transplanted supernumerary limb, the potential to innervate an extra limb altogether. During later stages of development, these mechanisms also allow for the fine tuning of synaptic connections by environmental input, and they continue to be important throughout the life span in the maintenance of appropriate synaptic connections (Purves 1988).

Sensory Input and Synaptic Plasticity

Sensory experience is essential to the normal maturation of specific neural connections. In the visual system, where this has been most extensively studied, overlapping visual input from the two eyes must be combined in an orderly way to maximize acuity and stereopsis. In animals with binocular vision (e.g., humans, cats, and monkeys), visual stimuli striking the retina activate neurons in the ipsilateral visual cortex. This means that neurons in the left hemiretinas of right and left eyes both convey signals to the left cortex, and similarly neurons in the right hemiretinas do so to the right cortex (Figure 1–14; *panel A*). Thus visual information emanating from the same external source ends up in the contralateral hemisphere regardless of the fact that it is temporarily separated into right and left eye specific pathways.

How is this converging visual information recombined? In visual cortex, inputs from the two eyes project alternately to stripes dominated by one eye or the other forming ocular dominance columns (Hubel and Wiesel 1977). The pattern of stripes resembles those of a zebra (Figure 1–14; *panel B*). Output neurons in the ocular dominance columns project to prestriate visual areas where the visual information derived from inputs to both eyes is recombined and stereopsis clues extracted. How separate signals from each eye are handled in parallel, recombined, and separated again is representative of a more general pattern in the processing of visual information (Livingstone and Hubel 1988).

During development, the ocular dominance columns arise in a crude way independent of visual input (Hubel et al. 1977). Initially, axons carrying information from both eyes extend over all of visual cortex, after which during a critical period they begin to segregate out. During this period, the pattern of sharp stripes, evenly divided between the

A

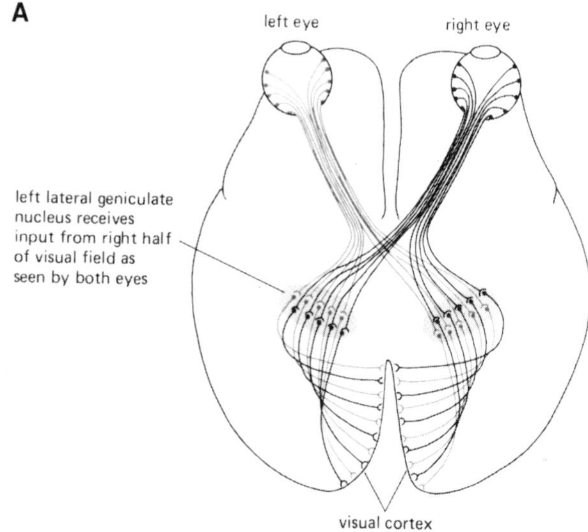

C

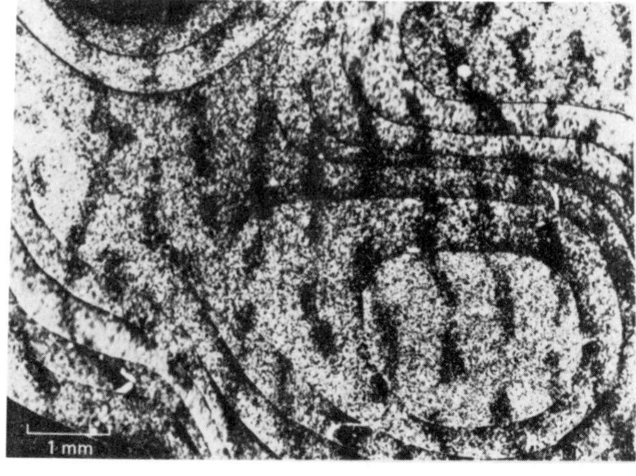

B

1 mm

Figure 1–14. Ocular dominance columns in visual cortex. *Panel A:* Human visual pathway. Optic fibers from each eye split at the chiasm with half going to each side of the brain. Fibers conveying visual information from the right or left sides of each retina project to the lateral geniculate nucleus on the same side of the brain and subsequently to ipsilateral cortex. In this way, left visual field information goes to the right cortex and vice versa. This arrangement raises the question of how the optic radiations from each eye combine in cortex to produce a single image and stereopsis. (Reprinted from Alberts B, Bray D, Lewis J, et al: Molecular Biology of the Cell, 2nd Edition. New York, Garland, 1989, p 1129. Used with permission.) *Panel B:* Visual inputs form ocular dominance columns. In a normal monkey, one eye was injected with a radioactive tracer which is transported transynaptically along the visual pathways. Cortical areas receiving input from the injected eye show up as white. An alternating pattern of stripes is revealed, equally divided between the two eyes. *Panel C:* Monocular deprivation alters ocular dominance column development. Although alternating stripes of ocular dominance arise in the absence of visual input, the sharpening of the pattern depends on experience and activity-dependent competition. Blocking vision in one eye places it at a disadvantage in such a process so that it ends up controlling a minority of cortex. In this plate, the nondeprived eye was injected with the transynaptic tracer showing that it has come to control most of cortex. Normal visual experience is prerequisite to the correct wiring of the cortex. (*Panels B* and *C* reprinted from Hubel DH, Wiesel TN: Ferrier lecture: functional architecture of macaque monkey visual cortex. Proc R Soc Lond [Biol] 198:1–59, 1977. Used with permission.)

two eyes, depends on normal visual experience. If vision in one eye is impaired or there is strabismus, input from the normal or dominant eye comes to control most of visual cortex and the other eye becomes functionally blind (Figure 1–14; *panel C*). In the cortex, the ocular dominance columns of the normal or dominant eye expand at the expense of those of the impaired eye. The segregation of the optic fibers into columns is activity dependent (Constantine-Paton et al. 1990; Miller et al. 1989). It depends on discordant inputs from the two eyes; segregation fails if either visual input to cortex is blocked (with the Na^{+} channel blocker tetrodotoxin) or it is artificially synchronized in both eyes (by simultaneous electrical stimulation).

Different patterns of electrical activity in each optic radiation, as occurs normally, mediate segregation. Segregation also requires activity of postsynaptic cortical cells; infusion of the inhibitory drug muscimol (a GABA-A agonist) causes a reversal of dominance so that, paradoxically, the weak rather than the strong eye gains the larger columns (Reiter and Stryker 1988). Apparently, appropriate segregation of cortical inputs requires both normal presynaptic activity and postsynaptic responses. A similar activity dependence is also found in retinal axons impinging on lateral geniculate cells, the thalamic relay cells projecting to visual cortex (Shatz and Stryker 1988). Indeed, activity-dependent segregation of visual inputs into ocular dominance columns appears to be an inherent property of topographic projections in sensory systems. In frogs, which do not have binocular vision (nor ocular dominance columns), if an extra eye is transplanted into a tadpole, the optic fibers from the third eye will compete with the other eye innervating that side of the brain to produce ocular dominance columns (Constantine-Paton and Law 1978).

Pairing of presynaptic activity with postsynaptic depolarization appears to be required for activity-dependent segregation of sensory inputs, perhaps just as it is necessary for the induction of LTP (Constantine-Paton et al. 1990). As in LTP, this pairing dependence is mediated by the NMDA receptor, which requires both agonist and depolarization (to remove the Mg^{2+} block of the channel) for activation. Infusion of the specific NMDA antagonist APV into developing visual cortex prevents both normal segregation of visual inputs and the effects of unbalanced activity from the two eyes during the critical period (Kleinschmidt et al. 1987). During the critical period, APV significantly blocks visual cortical activity; later on, however, its effectiveness decreases considerably, paralleling the increasing resistance to ocular dominance shifts in more mature animals (Fox et al. 1989). NMDA infusion, on the other hand, increases the sharpness of segregation (Cline and Constantine-Paton 1990). In older animals (once the critical period is past), infusion of NMDA can restore the immature level of plasticity characteristic of the critical period (Udin and Scherer 1990).

❑ PERSPECTIVES

The cellular and molecular language of neurons has powerful explanatory power: the action of psychotropic drugs is understood in this context (Barondes 1990; Cooper et al. 1986). The early antipsychotic reserpine acts in the presynaptic terminal to reduce stores of catecholamine neurotransmitters (which in excess may underlie psychotic symptoms). Current antipsychotics block synaptic transmission in the mesolimbic dopamine system (reducing the effects of catecholamines), possibly specifically at the newly discovered D_3 receptor (Sokoloff et al. 1990). Tricyclic antidepressants block catecholamine reuptake, whereas monoamine oxidase inhibitors block their breakdown, both leading to increased synaptic levels. Anxiolytics modulate the GABA receptor. Lithium modulates the inositol phospholipid system, thereby reducing its activity when it is overactive (Baraban et al. 1989; Berridge et al. 1989). Agents selectively acting in second messenger pathways may prove to be the next generation of psychotropics.

A shared molecular language is emerging for activity-dependent segregation of visual inputs, LTP, excitotoxicity, and the shaping of growing neurites (Brown et al. 1990; Choi and Rothman 1990; Constantine-Paton et al. 1990; Hawkins and Kandel 1984; Lipton and Kater 1989). The key player is the NMDA receptor, which requires both agonist and depolarization for activation. This appears to be the essential requirement for pairing specificity, a mode of synaptic plasticity initially postulated by Hebb (1949), whereby simultaneous activation of pre- and postsynaptic elements strengthens connections. Correlation of presynaptic activity with postsynaptic inhibition may selectively weaken connections (Reiter and Stryker 1988). The Ca^{2+} influx mediated by the NMDA receptor may trigger changes in the effectiveness of synapses, in time leading to structural changes. At higher levels, Ca^{2+} may arrest the growth of neurites, cause their retraction, or selectively lesion the susceptible cell.

Neuropsychiatric disorders, as well, will increasingly come to be understood in the language of neurons. Among the examples mentioned above, striatal degeneration in Huntington's chorea may be a result of NMDA receptor mediated excitotoxicity (Wexler et al. 1991). Striatal cells expressing NMDA receptors appear to be preferentially lost in the brains of patients with Huntington's chorea, and glutamate infusions in animals produce a pattern of neuronal dropout reminiscent of the disease. In Parkinson's disease, a selective loss of dopaminergic neurons in the substantia nigra may be the delayed result of a viral process, lesioning by dopaminergic neurotoxins exemplified by 1-methyl-4-phenyl-1,2,3,4-tetrahydropyridine (MPTP), or a deficiency in the neurotrophic factor BDNF, which may be essential for survival of dopaminergic neurons. In Alzheimer's disease, the loss of cholinergic neurons may result from a NGF deficiency in regions that they innervate or perhaps aberrant handling of NGF once it is taken up by the basal forebrain neurons. Once molecular explanations can be integrated into detailed functional knowledge of neurons and the neuronal systems of which they are part, a unified picture of brain functioning and pathology may emerge.

❑ REFERENCES

Alberts B, Bray D, Lewis J, et al: Molecular Biology of the Cell, 2nd Edition. New York, Garland, 1989

Axelrod J, Burch RM, Jelsema CL: Receptor-mediated activation of phospholipase A_2 via GTP-binding proteins: arachidonic acid and its metabolites as second messengers. Trends Neurosci 11:117–123, 1988

Baraban JM, Worley PF, Snyder SH: Second messenger systems and psychoactive drug action: focus on the phosphoinositide system and lithium. Am J Psychiatry 146:1251–1260, 1989

Barde Y-A: Trophic factors and neuronal survival. Neuron 2:1524–1534, 1989

Barondes SH: The biological approach to psychiatry: history and prospects. J Neurosci 10:1707–1710, 1990

Barzilai A, Kennedy TE, Sweatt JD, et al: 5-HT modulates protein synthesis and the expression of specific proteins during long-term facilitation in *Aplysia* sensory neurons. Neuron 2:1577–1586, 1989

Bekkers JM, Stevens CF: Presynaptic mechanism for long-term potentiation in the hippocampus. Nature 346:724–729, 1990

Bennett MVL: Electrical transmission: a functional analysis and comparison to chemical transmission, in Handbook of Physiology, Vol I: The Nervous System. Edited by Kandel ER. Bethesda, MD, American Physiological Society, 1977, pp 357–416

Bennett MVL, Barrio LC, Bargiello TA, et al: Gap junctions: new tools, new answers, new questions. Neuron 6:305–320, 1991

Bentley D, Toroian-Raymond A: Disoriented pathfinding by pioneer neurone growth cones deprived of filopodia by cytochalasin treatment. Nature 323:712–715, 1986

Berridge MJ, Irvine RF: Inositol phosphates and cell signalling. Nature 341:197–205, 1989

Berridge MJ, Downes CP, Hanley MR: Neural and developmental actions of lithium: a unifying hypothesis. Cell 59:411–419, 1989

Bliss TVP, Douglas RM, Errington ML, et al: Correlation between long-term potentiation and release of endogenous amino acids from dentate gyrus of anaesthetized rats. J Physiol (Lond) 377:391–408, 1986

Braha O, Dale N, Hochner B, et al: Second messengers involved in the two processes of presynaptic facilitation that contribute to sensitization and dishabituation in *Aplysia* sensory neurons. Proc Natl Acad Sci U S A 87:2040–2044, 1990

Brown TH, Kairiss EW, Keenan CL: Hebbian synapses: biophysical mechanisms and algorithms. Annu Rev Neurosci 13:475–511, 1990

Buchberg AM, Cleveland LS, Jenkins NA, et al: Sequence homology shared by neurofibromatosis type-1 gene and IRA-1 and IRA-2 negative regulators of the RAS cyclic AMP pathway. Nature 347:291–294, 1990

Caviness VS: Neocortical histogenesis in normal and reeler mice: a developmental study based on [^{3}H]thymidine autoradiography. Dev Brain Res 4:293–302, 1982

Choi DW: Glutamate neurotoxicity and diseases of the nervous system. Neuron 1:623–634, 1988

Choi DW, Rothman SM: The role of glutamate neurotoxicity in hypoxic-ischemic neuronal death. Annu Rev Neurosci 13:171–182, 1990

Cline HT, Constantine-Paton M: The differential influence of protein kinase inhibitors on retinal arbor morphology and eye-specific stripes in the frog retinotectal system. Neuron 4:899–908, 1990

Cole AJ, Saffen DW, Baraban JM, et al: Rapid increase of an immediate early gene messenger RNA in hippocampal neurons by synaptic NMDA receptor activation. Nature 340:474–476, 1989

Constantine-Paton M, Law MI: Eye-specific termination bands in tecta of three-eyed frogs. Science 202:639–641, 1978

Constantine-Paton M, Cline HT, Debski E: Patterned activity, synaptic convergence, and the NMDA receptor in developing visual pathways. Annu Rev Neurosci 13:129–154, 1990

Cooper JR, Bloom FE, Roth RH: The Biochemical Basis of Neuropharmacology, 5th Edition. New York, Oxford University Press, 1986

Dash PK, Hochner B, Kandel ER: Injection of the cAMP-responsive element into the nucleus of *Aplysia* sensory neurons blocks long-term facilitation. Nature 345:718–721, 1990

Dowling JE: The Retina: An Approachable Part of the Brain. Cambridge, MA, Harvard University Press, 1987

Edelman GM: The Remembered Present: A Biological Theory of Consciousness. New York, Basic Books, 1989

Fox K, Sato H, Daw N: The location and function of NMDA receptors in cat and kitten visual cortex. J Neurosci 9:2443–2454, 1989

Fraser SE, Green CR, Bode HR, et al: Selective disruption of gap junctional communication interferes with a patterning process in *Hydra*. Science 237:49–55, 1987

Glanzman DL, Kandel ER, Schacher S: Target-dependent structural changes accompanying long-term synaptic facilitation in *Aplysia* neurons. Science 249:799–802, 1990

Goodman CS, Bastiani MJ, Doe CQ, et al: Cell recognition during development. Science 225:1271–1279, 1984

Hatten ME: Riding the glial monorail: a common mechanism for glial-guided neuronal migration in different regions of the developing mammalian brain. Trends Neurosci 13:179–84, 1990

Hawkins RD, Kandel ER: Is there a cell-biological alphabet

for simple forms of learning? Psychol Rev 91:375–391, 1984

Hawkins RD, Schacher S: Identified facilitator neurons L_{29} and L_{28} are excited by cutaneous stimuli used in dishabituation, sensitization, and classical conditioning of *Aplysia.* J Neurosci 9:4236–4245, 1989

Hebb DO: The Organization of Behavior: A Neuropsychological Theory. New York, Wiley, 1949

Heffner CD, Lumsden AGS, O'Leary DDM: Target control of collateral extension and directional axon growth in the mammalian brain. Science 247:217–220, 1990

Hengerer B, Lindholm D, Heumann R, et al: Lesion-induced increase in nerve growth factor mRNA is mediated by c-fos. Proc Natl Acad Sci U S A 87:3899–3903, 1990

Hoffman RE: Computer simulations of neural information processing and the schizophrenia-mania dichotomy. Arch Gen Psychiatry 44:178–188, 1987

Hohn A, Leibrock J, Bailey K, et al: Identification and characterization of a novel member of the nerve growth factor/brain-derived neurotrophic factor family. Nature 344:339–341, 1990

Holz GG, Rane SG, Dunlap K: GTP-binding proteins mediate transmitter inhibition of voltage-dependent calcium channels. Nature 319:670–672, 1986

Hubel DH, Wiesel TN: Ferrier lecture: functional architecture of macaque monkey visual cortex. Proc R Soc Lond [Biol] 198:1–59, 1977

Hubel DH, Wiesel TN, LeVay S: Plasticity of ocular dominance columns in monkey striate cortex. Philos Trans R Soc Lond [Biol] 278:377–409, 1977

Huganir RL, Greengard P: Regulation of receptor function by protein phosphorylation. Trends Pharmacol Sci 8: 472–477, 1987

Hyman C, Hofer M, Barde Y-A, et al: BDNF is a neurotrophic factor for dopaminergic neurons of the substantia nigra. Nature 350:230–232, 1991

Jessell TM: Adhesion molecules and the hierarchy of neural development. Neuron 1:3–13, 1988

Kandel ER: Genes, nerve cells, and the remembrance of things past. J Neuropsychiatry Clin Neurosci 1:103–125, 1989

Kandel ER, Schwartz JH: Principles of Neural Science, 2nd Edition. New York, Elsevier, 1985

Kater SB, Mattson MP, Guthrie PB: Calcium-induced neuronal degeneration: a normal growth cone regulating signal gone awry? Ann N Y Acad Sci 568:252–261, 1989

Keinänen K, Wisden W, Sommer B, et al: A family of AMPA-selective glutamate receptors. Science 249:556–560, 1990

Kennedy MB: Regulation of neuronal function by calcium. Trends Neurosci 11:417–420, 1989a

Kennedy MB: Regulation of synaptic transmission in the central nervous system: long-term potentiation. Cell 59:777–787, 1989b

Kleinschmidt A, Bear MF, Singer W: Blockade of NMDA receptors disrupts experience-dependent plasticity of kitten striate cortex. Science 238:355–358, 1987

Landis SC: Target regulation of neurotransmitter phenotype. Trends Neurosci 13:344–350, 1990

Lankford KL, DeMello FG, Klein WL: D1-type dopamine receptors inhibit growth cone motility in cultured retina neurons: evidence that neurotransmitters act as morphogenic growth regulators in the developing central nervous system. Proc Natl Acad Sci U S A 85:4567–4571, 1988

Lipton SA, Kater SB: Neurotransmitter regulation of neuronal outgrowth, plasticity and survival. Trends Neurosci 12:265–270, 1989

Livingstone M, Hubel D: Segregation of form, color, movement, and depth: anatomy, physiology, and perception. Science 240:740–749, 1988

Llinás R: The intrinsic electrophysiological properties of mammalian neurons: insights into central nervous system function. Science 242:1654–1664, 1988

Llinás R, Jahnsen H: Electrophysiology of mammalian thalamic neurones in vitro. Nature 297:406–408, 1982

Lynch MA, Errington ML, Bliss TVP: Nordihydroguaiaretic acid blocks the synaptic component of long-term potentiation and the associated increases in release of glutamate and arachidonate: an in vivo study in the dentate gyrus of the rat. Neuroscience 30:693–701, 1989

Maisonpierre PC, Belluscio L, Squinto S, et al: Neurotrophin-3: a neurotrophic factor related to NGF and BDNF. Science 247:1446–1451, 1990

Malenka RC, Kauer JA, Perkel DJ, et al: The impact of postsynaptic calcium on synaptic transmission: its role in long-term potentiation. Trends Neurosci 12:444–450, 1989

Malinow R, Tsien RW: Presynaptic enhancement shown by whole-cell recordings of long-term potentiation in hippocampal slices. Nature 346:177–180, 1990

Malinow R, Schulman H, Tsien RW: Inhibition of postsynaptic PKC or CaMKII blocks induction but not expression of LTP. Science 245:862–866, 1989

Mattson MP, Kater SB: Excitatory and inhibitory neurotransmitters in the generation and degeneration of hippocampal neuroarchitecture. Brain Res 478:337–348, 1989

Mattson MP, Murrain M, Guthrie PB, et al: Fibroblast growth factor and glutamate: opposing roles in the generation and degeneration of hippocampal neuroarchitecture. J Neurosci 9:3728–3740, 1989

Miller KD, Keller JB, Stryker MP: Ocular dominance column development: analysis and simulation. Science 245:605–615, 1989

Minsky M: The Society of Mind. New York, Simon & Schuster, 1986

Morgan JI, Curran T: Stimulus-transcription coupling in neurons: role of cellular immediate-early genes. Trends Neurosci 12:459–462, 1989

Neer EJ, Clapham DE: Roles of G protein subunits in transmembrane signalling. Nature 333:129–134, 1988

Olds DD: Brain-centered psychology: a semiotic approach. Psychoanalysis and Contemporary Thought 13:331–363, 1990

Olney JW, Misra CH, deGubareff T: Cysteine-S-sulfate: brain damaging metabolite in sulfite oxidase deficiency. J Neuropathol Exp Neurol 34:167–177, 1975

Pardes H: Neuroscience and psychiatry: marriage or coexistence. Am J Psychiatry 143:1205–1212, 1986

Petersen SE, Fox PT, Posner MI, et al: Positron emission tomographic studies of the cortical anatomy of single-word processing. Nature 331:585–589, 1988

Piomelli D, Greengard P: Lipoxygenase metabolites of arachidonic acid in neuronal transmembrane signalling. Trends Pharmacol Sci 11:367–373, 1990

Piomelli D, Volterra A, Dale N, et al: Lipoxygenase metabolites of arachidonic acid as second messengers for presynaptic inhibition of *Aplysia* sensory cells. Nature 328:38–43, 1987

Ponder B: Neurofibromatosis gene cloned. Nature 346: 703–704, 1990

Purves D: Body and Brain: A Trophic Theory of Neural Connections. Cambridge, MA, Harvard University Press, 1988

Purves D, Lichtman JW: Principles of Neural Development. Sunderland, MA, Sinauer, 1985

Rakic P: Mode of cell migration to the superficial layers of fetal monkey neocortex. J Comp Neurol 145:61–84, 1972

Rakic P: Specification of cerebral cortical areas. Science 241:170–176, 1988

Ramón y Cajal S: Histologie du Système Nerveux de l'Homme & des Vertébrés, Vol II. Madrid, Consejo Superior de Investigaciones Cientificas, reprinted 1972

Rayport SG, Schacher S: Synaptic plasticity in vitro: cell culture of identified *Aplysia* neurons mediating short-term habituation and sensitization. J Neurosci 6:759–763, 1986

Reiter HO, Stryker MP: Neural plasticity without postsynaptic action potentials: less-active inputs become dominant when kitten visual cortical cells are pharmacologically inhibited. Proc Natl Acad Sci U S A 85: 3623–3627, 1988

Reivich M, Kuhl D, Wolf A, et al: The (^{18}F)fluorodeoxyglucose method for the measurement of local cerebral glucose utilization in man. Circ Res 44:127–137, 1979

Roberts GW: Schizophrenia: the cellular biology of a functional psychosis. Trends Neurosci 13:207–211, 1990

Role LW, Schwartz JH: Cross-talk between signal transduction pathways. Trends Neurosci 12 (11): centerfold, 1989

Ross EM, Gilman AG: Pharmacodynamics: mechanisms of drug action and the relationship between drug concentration and effect, in The Pharmacological Basis of Therapeutics, 7th Edition. Edited by Gilman AG, Goodman LS, Rall TW, et al. New York, Macmillan, 1985, pp 35–48

Schofield PR, Shivers BD, Seeburg PH: The role of receptor subtype diversity in the CNS. Trends Neurosci 13:8–11, 1990

Schubert D, Kimura H, LaCorbiere M, et al: Activin is a nerve cell survival molecule. Nature 344:868–870, 1990

Sejnowski TJ, Koch C, Churchland PS: Computational neuroscience. Science 241:1299–1306, 1988

Servan-Schreiber D, Printz H, Cohen JD: A network model of catecholamine effects: gain, signal-to-noise ratio, and behavior. Science 249:892–895, 1990

Shatz CJ, Stryker MP: Prenatal tetrodotoxin infusion blocks segregation of retinogeniculate afferents. Science 242:87–89, 1988

Shepherd GM, Koch C: Introduction to synaptic circuits, in The Synaptic Organization of the Brain, 3rd Edition. Edited by Shepherd GM. New York, Oxford, 1990, pp 3–31

Silver RA, Lamb AG, Bolsover SR: Elevated cytosolic calcium in the growth cone inhibits neurite elongation in neuroblastoma cells: correlation of behavioral states with cytosolic calcium concentration. J Neurosci 9: 4007–4020, 1989

Sokoloff P, Giros B, Martres M-P, et al: Molecular cloning and characterization of a novel dopamine receptor (D3) as a target for neuroleptics. Nature 347:146–151, 1990

Sommer B, Keinänen K, Verdoorn, et al: Flip and flop: a cell-specific functional switch in glutamate-operated channels of the CNS. Science 249:1580–1585, 1990

Spencer PS, Ludolph A, Dwivedi MP, et al: Lathyrism: evidence for role of the neuroexcitatory amino acid BOAA. Lancet 2:1066–1067, 1986

Spencer PS, Nunn PB, Hugon J, et al: Guam amyotrophic lateral sclerosis-parkinsonism-dementia linked to a plant excitant neurotoxin. Science 237:517–522, 1987

Suddath RL, Christison GW, Fuller-Torrey E, et al: Anatomical abnormalities in the brains of monozygotic twins discordant for schizophrenia. N Engl J Med 322: 789–794, 1990

Sweatt JD, Kandel ER: Persistent and transcriptionally-dependent increase in protein phosphorylation in long-term facilitation of *Aplysia* sensory neurons. Nature 339:51–54, 1989

Takeichi M: Cadherin cell adhesion receptors as a mophogenetic regulator. Science 251:1451–1455, 1991

Tank DW, Sugimori M, Connor JA, et al: Spatially resolved calcium dynamics of mammalian Purkinje cells in cerebellar slice. Science 242:773–777, 1988

Tessier-Lavigne M, Placzek M, Lumsden AGS, et al: Chemotropic guidance of developing axons in the mammalian central nervous system. Nature 336:775–778, 1988

Thoenen H, Bandtlow C, Heumann R: The physiological function of nerve growth factor in the central nervous system: comparison with the periphery. Rev Physiol Biochem Pharmacol 109:145–178, 1987

Udin SB, Scherer WJ: Restoration of the plasticity of binocular maps by NMDA after the critical period in Xenopus. Science 249:669–672, 1990

Weinberger DR: Implications of normal brain development for the pathogenesis of schizophrenia. Arch Gen Psychiatry 44:660–669, 1987

Wexler NS, Rose EA, Housman DE: Molecular approaches to hereditary diseases of the nervous system: Huntington's Disease as a paradigm. Annu Rev Neurosci 14:503–529, 1991

Wigler M: GAPs in understanding Ras. Nature 346:696–697, 1990

Williams JH, Errington ML, Lynch MA, et al: Arachidonic acid induces a long-term activity-dependent enhancement of synaptic transmission in the hippocampus. Nature 341:739–742, 1989

Wisden W, Errington ML, Williams S, et al: Differential expression of immediate early genes in the hippocampus and spinal cord. Neuron 4:603–614, 1990

Young AB, Greenamyre JT, Hollingsworth Z, et al: NMDA receptor losses in putamen from patients with Huntington's Disease. Science 241:981–983, 1988

Chapter

2

Human Electrophysiology: Basic Cellular Mechanisms and Control of Wakefulness and Sleep

Robert W. McCarley, M.D.

THE FIRST PART OF THIS CHAPTER is designed as a brief review and update on fundamental mechanisms important for understanding neuronal activity and communication at the level of single cells. A more detailed account, with a different emphasis, appears in Chapter 1. There follows a brief note on evoked potential (EP) and electroencephalogram (EEG) analysis. These sections were primarily written for the reader with some knowledge of cellular neurophysiology (even in the far distant past) who wishes a brief review of fundamental concepts and an update on recent advances. Many examples of physiologically important mechanisms in Part I have been chosen with respect to their relevance to Part II of this chapter. Part II is a survey of current concepts in the regulation of sleep and wakefulness, an area of recent advances in understanding funda-

This work was supported by grants from the Department of Veterans Affairs, Medical Research Service, and the National Institute of Mental Health (R37 MH39-683 and R01 MH40-799).

mental mechanisms relevant to behavior and to pathology. The two parts may be read independently of each other.

PART I: BASICS OF NEUROPHYSIOLOGY

❑ INTRODUCTION

The *neuron* is a cell specialized for the use of electrical signalling for information transmission; it may be viewed as an evolutionary outgrowth of the need for more rapid transmission and more precise selection of target elements than was possible with humoral transmission (the release of chemical agents into blood or extracellular fluid). The reader is cautioned that the description in this section is a simplified account and one that is primarily based on mammalian systems; more complete accounts can be found in textbooks such as those by Kandel and Schwartz (1985) and Smith (1989).

All neurons have a *cell body* (or *soma)* and are distinguished from other body cells by the presence of dendrites and axons. The *dendrites* may be thought of as an extension of the "input zone" on the cell body, and their shape often appears tailored to their inputs, with the pyramidal cell dendritic structure being typical of many neurons in regularly layered structures of the brain such as the cerebral cortex, where there are distinct input zones. The more spherical dendritic tree found in brain stem reticular neurons tends to occur in structures without a distinct ordering of different input zones. Figure 2–1 illustrates these two examples of neuronal shape. The axon is a long extension of the neuron that forms the "output element" for transmitting the electrical activation of the soma to a target neuron; it may have numerous branches, called collaterals. Electrical signals traveling down the axon form a propagating wave of depolarization termed the *action potential;* this originates in the soma when the electrical potential on the membrane is sufficiently reduced (membrane depolarization). Thus understanding the mechanisms controlling soma membrane polarization is essential for understanding electrical signalling in the brain.

❑ CONTROL OF NEURONAL MEMBRANE POLARIZATION

The cell *membrane* is a bilayer (double layer) of lipids that separates the interior of the cell from its environment. The cell membrane itself acts as a nonconducting capacitor with the cell interior electrically negative with respect to the outside. Most mammalian neurons, when not being stimulated, have a "resting" membrane polarization of about –70 millivolts (mV). By convention the membrane polarization level is always given in terms of the difference between the interior voltage and the exterior voltage, with the exterior voltage taken to be zero.

Not all of the cell membrane is a nonconductive lipid bilayer; incorporated in the membrane are specialized large protein molecules that form membrane-spanning channels that permit the passage of ions such as potassium ions (K^+). These *ion channels* are usually selective in allowing the flow of only certain ions. The "resting potential" of the neuron arises because of the differences in distribution of electrically charged ions on the inside and outside of the neuronal membrane.

Most of the inside negativity of the resting membrane potential is due to K^+. This negative membrane polarization can be thought of as occurring in the following way: K^+ concentration is greater on the inside of the cell than on the outside, and thus K^+ tends to flow down its concentration gradient, from the inside to the outside (Figure 2–2). That is, excess internal K^+ concentration leads to flow of the K^+ through a particular set of potassium channels to the outside of the membrane. Negatively charged proteins and amino acids (referred to here collectively as anions) on the inside of the cell are too large to pass through the ion channels, and thus there is a concentration of negative charges on the inside of the neuron and of positive charges on the outside of the neuron. The migration of K^+ from inside to outside continues until the buildup of electrical charge resulting from separation of K^+ and the anions (positive electrical charges on the outside and negative charges on the inside) is strong enough to balance exactly the driving force from the K^+ concentration difference. The membrane potential at which balance is achieved is called the K^+ equilibrium potential and is close to the membrane resting potential.

Sodium ions (Na^+) also contribute to the resting membrane potential, although much less than K+ because of the lesser permeability of the membrane to Na^+, even though these ions are much more heavily concentrated on the outside than on the inside. The low interior concentration of Na^+ is maintained by an active (energy-consuming) pump that transports Na^+ to the outside and exchanges three Na^+

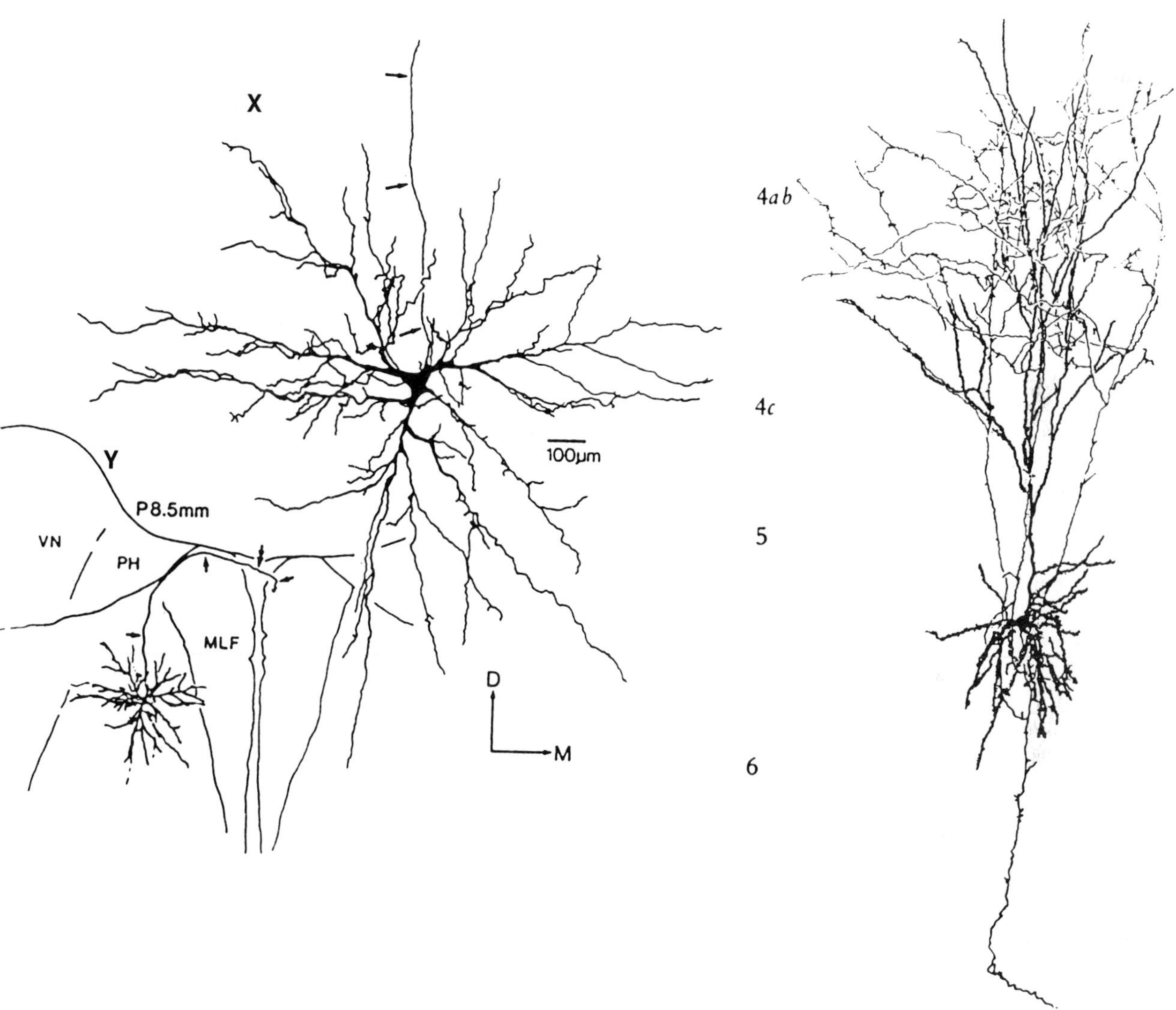

Figure 2–1. *Panel A:* Depiction of a giant neuron of the cat bulbar reticular formation, a region without regular spatial orientation of neurons and their dendrites. Note the extension of dendrites in all directions in the enlarged view of the neuron X; Y shows the axon (arrows) turning to enter the medial longitudinal fasciculus, a fiber bundle comprised of similar spinal cord-projecting neurons. The giant neurons of the brain stem reticular formation are among the largest in the nervous system and likely mediate quick reflex responses. *Panel B:* A pyramidal cell of the rhesus monkey primary visual cortex. The neocortex has many such regularly arranged, radially oriented neurons, with a characteristic apical dendrite orientation in layer 4 and the pyramidal cell body in layer 6. The axon of this neuron is shown leaving the cortex in its path to the lateral geniculate nucleus. It is a corticothalamic projection neuron and part of a feedback loop, because geniculocortical neurons send axons to the cortex that synapse on the dendrites of the illustrated neuron. (*Panel A* is a camera lucida drawing by A. Mitani in the author's laboratory; *Panel B* is adapted from Nauta and Feirtag 1986.)

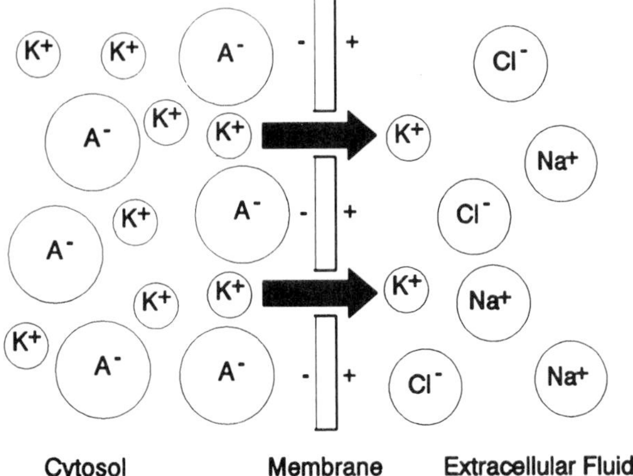

Figure 2–2. Schematic of generation of the resting membrane potential. The concentration gradient causes potassium ions (K^+) to move out of the cell (*arrows*) until this force is balanced by a counteracting electrical potential difference, positive charges on the outside and negative charges on the inside of the membrane. Most of the potential is attributable to K^+; contributions from other ions have been omitted for simplicity. A^- = anions (negatively charged ions; amino acids and proteins); Na^+ = sodium ions; Cl^- = chloride ions.

ions for two K^+ ions. In most neurons, chloride ions do not play a role in resting membrane potential generation because they are in electrical and concentration equilibrium. Calcium ions (Ca^{2+}) are important in many signalling processes but do not play a large role in the resting membrane potential because the permeability of the membrane is low to these ions at the resting potential level.

❑ ACTION POTENTIAL GENERATION

The *action potential* consists of a membrane depolarization followed by a repolarization (Figure 2–3). During the depolarization the inside of the membrane loses its negative charge with respect to the outside and actually becomes slightly positive, about +10 to +30 mV relative to the outside of the neuronal membrane. This depolarization is followed by a repolarization, a return of the membrane potential to its resting level.

As noted above, the most important channel for the resting membrane potential is the potassium channel. This is called a *passive ion channel* because it is not voltage sensitive. The channels important

A

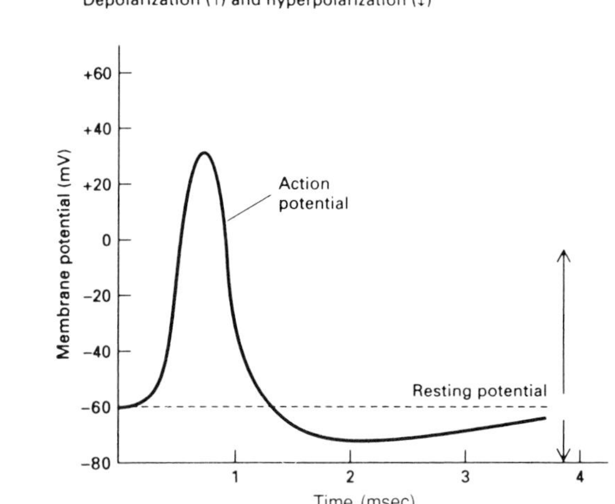

B

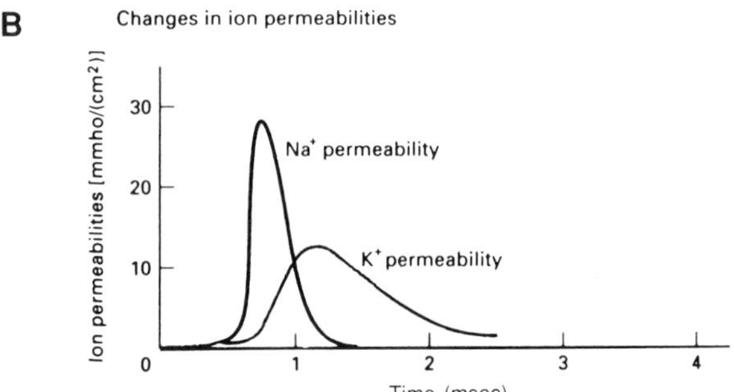

C

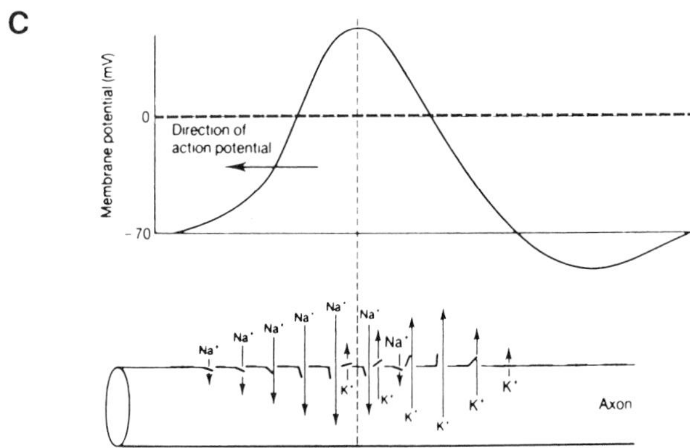

Figure 2–3. *Panel A:* The time course of action potential voltage. *Panel B:* The time course of depolarizing inward sodium current (Na^+) and the repolarizing outward potassium current (K^+); currents are expressed in terms of the permeability (conductance) of the membrane for the two ions. Note the after-hyperpolarization following the action potential (*panel A*) is due to the persistence of the outward K^+ current. (Adapted from Hodgkin and Huxley 1952; Darnell et al. 1990). *Panel C:* Action potential travelling down an axon, flow is right to left. The depolarizing leading edge consists of inrushing sodium currents and the repolarizing trailing edge consists of outward, repolarizing potassium currents. (Adapted from Smith 1989.)

for the action potential are *voltage-sensitive channels*, that is, their conductivity to ions varies with membrane potential voltage.

The sodium channel and Na^+ are of primary importance in the depolarization. The generation of the action potential proceeds in the following way. There is an initial small depolarization of the membrane potential that may be due to excitatory input from other neurons. As the membrane depolarizes the voltage sensitive sodium channels begin to open, and Na^+ flows from the region of high concentration outside the neuron through the channels into the neuron. The inrush of positive charges tends to depolarize the neuron. As long as the initial depolarization is not too great and does not exceed a certain threshold, the membrane potential is restored to its resting level by an efflux of K^+ through the channels described above. However, with stronger initial depolarization, the voltage-sensitive sodium channels allow more Na^+ to enter the neuron, and sufficient Na^+ enters so that the efflux of K^+ cannot keep up with the rate of Na^+ entry.

The more Na^+ that enters the cell, the more the membrane is depolarized, the more Na^+ is admitted by the voltage-sensitive Na^+ channels, and so on. Thus there is a positive feedback resulting in an avalanche of Na^+ entry. This leads to the membrane potential's becoming positive at the peak of the action potential. Schematically,

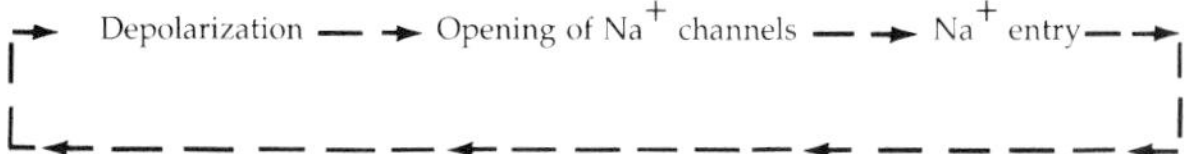

The membrane repolarization part of the action potential is due to two main factors:

1. As the membrane potential depolarizes *voltage-sensitive potassium channels* slowly open. (This is a different potassium channel than the passive channel responsible for the membrane potential.) This delayed-opening potassium channel allows K^+ to flow out of the neuron's interior to the outside, reducing the number of positive charges on the inside and thus tending to repolarize the membrane. (At the height of the action potential the cell interior is positive, and the driving forces on K^+ flow are both this positive voltage and the internal concentration level.) These open potassium channels close as the membrane potential repolarizes.
2. The *voltage-dependent sodium channels* close as a result of the depolarization, a process known as inactivation.

❑ NEUROTRANSMITTER RELEASE BY DEPOLARIZATION OF THE NERVE TERMINAL

Most neurons use electrical conduction (propagation of the action potential down the axon) as the first step in influencing target neurons. The second step is release of packets of neurotransmitters at the nerve terminal. The packets of neurotransmitter molecules are stored in the *presynaptic* terminal in structures called vesicles. When the membranes of the vesicles fuse with the exterior cell membrane, the contents of the vesicle (the neurotransmitters) are released and diffuse across the *synapse*, the small gap between nerve terminal and the target neuron. The release of neurotransmitters at the presynaptic terminal occurs because the action potential depolarizes the terminal and this depolarization opens *voltage-sensitive calcium channels*. Ca^{2+} entry into the terminal triggers the fusion of vesicles with the membrane of the terminal and neurotransmitter release into the synaptic gap between the presynaptic and postsynaptic neuron. The resulting alterations of membrane potential in the postsynaptic neuron are called *postsynaptic potentials (PSPs)*.

❑ ACTION OF NEUROTRANSMITTERS AT RECEPTORS

Neurotransmitters act on specialized membrane structures in the postsynaptic neuron called *receptors*. Receptor is a generalized term for the membrane sites that bind the neurotransmitter molecules. (In general cell biology, receptor is used even more generally to include all structures, including those on the interior of the cell, that preferentially bind a variety of molecules, including circulating hormones and even viruses.) Molecular biological techniques have led to structural identification of membrane receptor components and to physical models of how receptors act. In general, receptors are composed of proteins that coil in and out of the neuronal membrane and have specialized exterior portions for binding neurotransmitters. Receptors may be classified by their mode of action on the target neuron. The classification of signal elements (or messengers) in Table 2–1 illustrates some of the different modes of action. The fundamental notion is that the *first messengers*, the neurotransmitters, may cause the production of second or third mes-

TABLE 2–1. CLASSIFICATION OF SIGNAL ELEMENTS (MESSENGERS)

Messenger type	*Example*	*Site*	*Mode of action*
First messengers	Neurotransmitters	Synapse	Gates ion channels
Second messengers	cAMP	Cytosol	Affects cell metabolism
Third messengers	c-fos	Nucleus	Regulates DNA transcription

Note. cAMP = cyclic adenosine monophosphate.

sengers, which have additional actions on the target neuron, usually acting to prolong responses.

First Messengers: Neurotransmitters

Neurotransmitter-receptor binding may **directly** affect ion channels. The term for a substance that binds at a receptor is a *ligand*, and ion channels of this class are called *ligand-gated ion channels.* An example is the nicotinic receptor, in which binding of acetylcholine (the ligand) leads to a direct change in receptor conformation that allows passage of certain positively charged ions (cations), typically Na^+ and K^+. The molecular structure of this receptor is shown in Figure 2–4. As might be suspected from the direct coupling, this class of receptor is characterized by rapid opening of the ion channel and hence a quick responsiveness.[1]

Depolarizing PSPs are called *excitatory PSPs (EPSPs)* because the neuron is brought closer to the threshold for discharge of an action potential. EPSPs result from a net increased internal positivity, which may arise either from an influx of positive ions or a decrease in an ongoing efflux of positive ions. *Inhibitory PSPs (IPSPs)* hyperpolarize the membrane, make the interior more negative, and thus move the membrane potential farther from action potential discharge threshold. IPSPs may result from an influx of negative ions or from an increased efflux of positive ions.

Second Messengers: cAMP and Intracellular Intermediaries

Neurotransmitter-receptor binding may **indirectly** affect ion channels and also cellular metabolism. In this class of receptor the binding of the neurotransmitter to the receptor induces a cascade of effects that culminates in effects on the ion channel and/or may induce changes in the cell metabolism. This action may occur via second messengers acting in the cytosol and/or through *a guanine nucleotide-binding protein (G protein)* in the cell membrane. Perhaps the best known example is the β_2-adrenergic receptor (Figure 2–5). At this receptor, binding of the neurotransmitter norepinephrine activates a G protein in the neuronal membrane; this G protein in turn regulates the activity of the catalytic subunit of the enzyme adenylate cyclase, which in turn catalyzes the synthesis of *cyclic adenosine monophosphate (cAMP).* (See the sketch of dynamics of G protein activation in Figure 2–5.)

The cAMP is the *second messenger,* acting in the cytosol of the neuron. The cAMP activates a cAMP-dependent protein kinase. The consequences of this activation depend on the substrate for the particular protein kinase that is activated. One consequence may be the phosphorylation of proteins constituting or closely associated with the ion channel, with consequent alterations in permeability (Figure 2–5). Other effects of the second messengers may include regulation of proteins involved in transmitter synthesis and release. Schematically,

Neurotransmitter-receptor binding
→ G protein activation
→ adenylate cyclase activation
→ second messenger production (such as cAMP)
→ protein kinase activation
→ phosphorylation of ion channel and/or metabolic effects

This particular schematic is for the G protein involved in *stimulation* of the second messenger system, G_s. Other effects may include *inhibition* through activation of another class of G proteins, G_i.

An example of β receptor effect is the reduction of the slow-onset hyperpolarization that follows an action potential in hippocampal pyramidal neurons

---

[1]Part of the powerful excitatory effect of brain stem pontogeniculooccipital (PGO) wave input on thalamic neurons in the lateral geniculate nucleus during rapid-eye-movement (REM) sleep (see Part II of this chapter) is thought to be mediated by nicotinic receptors (McCormick 1989), which cause a depolarization because of the influx of positive ions brought about by the ligand-gated opening of the ion channel.

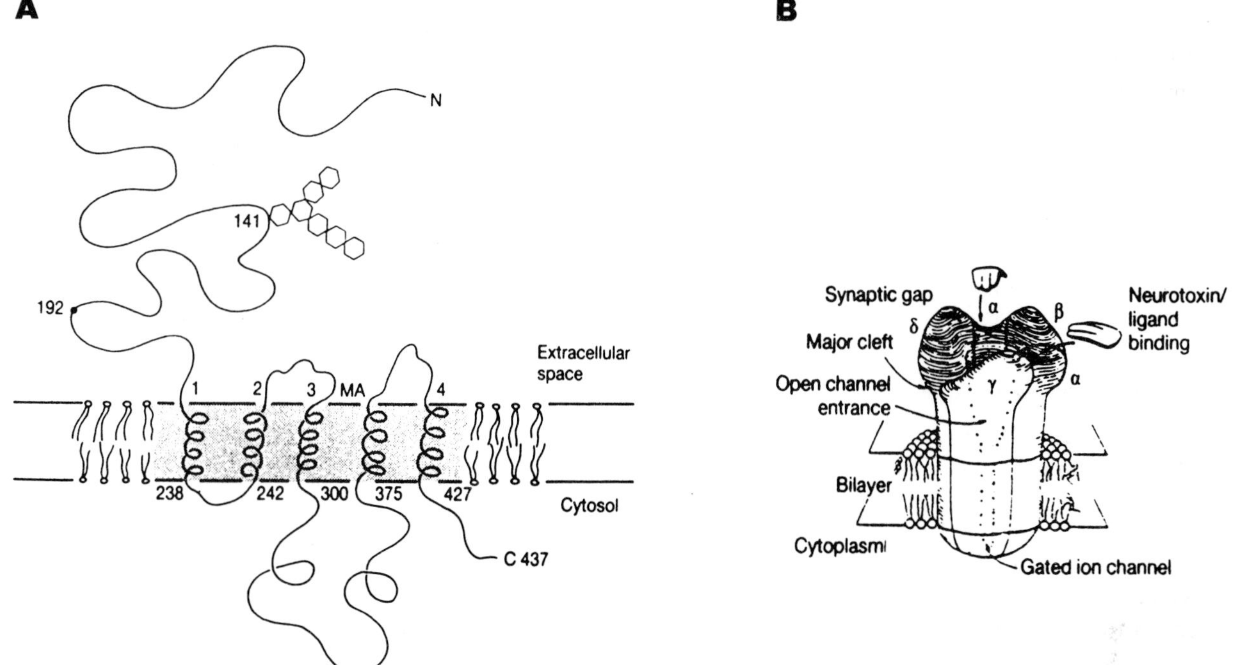

Figure 2–4. Nicotinic acetylcholine receptor. *Panel A:* Schematic of the human subunit of this receptor and its coils in and out of the cell membrane. The binding site for acetylcholine is near amino acid residue number 192. *Panel B:* Schematic of the entirety of this ligand-gated receptor. There are 5 subunits. Note the proximity to the gated ion channel of the unit containing the binding site for acetylcholine and other ligands. (Adapted from Smith 1989.)

and causes a "shutting down" or *accommodation* of repetitive discharges. This reduction of the after-hyperpolarization is mediated by the chain of events schematized above, with activation of the protein kinase A, which, in turn, modifies and reduces ion flow in the potassium channel responsible for the after-hyperpolarization (Nicoll 1988).

The *muscarinic acetylcholine receptor* also indirectly affects the ion channel—an action that is in contrast with the direct effects mediated by the nicotinic acetylcholine receptor. At least five subtypes of the muscarinic receptor are known. The M1 subtype is defined by its high affinity for the antagonist pirenzepine; at the M1 receptor acetylcholine binding leads to membrane G_i protein activation and inhibition of adenylate cyclase and cAMP production. Other receptor subtypes have a lower affinity for pirenzepine. The M2 receptor also works through a G protein coupled system but with a different mode of action on the ion channel than either the M1 or β_2-adrenergic receptor: the entire complex of acetylcholine/M2 receptor/G protein/guanosine triphosphate (GTP) interacts with a potassium ion channel to decrease the outward flow of K^+ and hence to depolarize the cell (Yatani et al. 1987).

Brain stem muscarinic receptors are important in the production of rapid-eye-movement (REM) sleep. A non-M1 muscarinic receptor increases the excitability of *pontine reticular formation (PRF)* neurons by shutting off the outward flow of K^+ (Greene and McCarley 1990).

Calcium as a second messenger: excitatory amino acid receptors, long-term potentiation, synaptic plasticity, and learning. The importance of intracellular calcium as a second messenger should be emphasized, and there are many examples of the important role of calcium in general cellular physiology. They include triggering secretion (insulin and digestive enzymes), contraction (muscle), and conversion of glycogen to glucose. Because of the importance of the phenomenon for psychiatry, the role of calcium in initiating *long-term potentiation (LTP)* is emphasized here (see also Cotman et al.

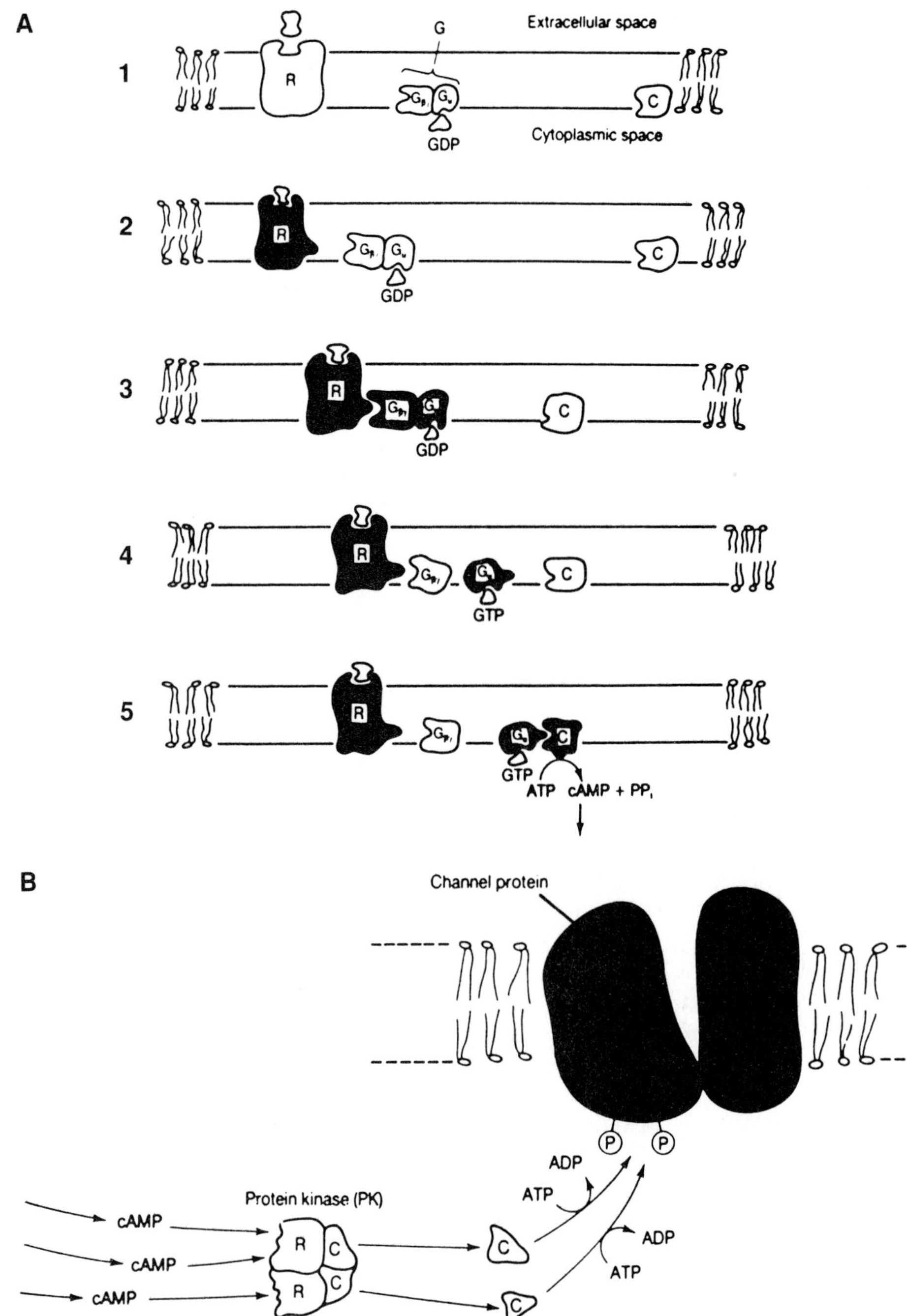

Figure 2–5. β–Adrenergic receptor: G protein and cyclic adenosine monophosphate (cAMP) coupling. *Panel A:* Dynamics of collision-coupling of β-adrenergic receptor with G proteins. 1) and 2) The binding of norepinephrine to the receptor (R) activates it by altering its conformation (solid portions of the sketch represent component activation). 3) When the activated receptor comes into contact with G protein β and γ subunits it couples to them and causes a conformational change. 4) This conformational change frees the Gα subunit and causes the Gα subunit to release its guanosine diphosphate (GDP) in exchange for guanosine triphosphate (GTP). 5) The Gα subunit now sticks to and activates the membrane bound adenylate cyclase (C), which in turn catalyzes the dephosphorylation of adenosine triphosphate (ATP) to cAMP, one of the most important second messengers. *Panel B:* Schematic of cAMP second messenger effects on ion channels. cAMP in the cytosol acts on the regulatory subunit (R) of a protein kinase (PK); this enables the catalytic subunits (C) to phosphorylate a channel protein and thereby change conformation and affect ion permeability. ADP = adenosine diphosphate. (Adapted from Smith 1989.)

1989; Mayer and Miller 1990). (This is an area of intense current work, and some important questions about the mechanisms of LTP remain unresolved.)

Briefly, LTP can be viewed as an elementary form of "associative learning." Coupling of weak input with a strong input to hippocampal neurons leads to a "long-term potentiation" of the weak input, a potentiation that lasts days or even weeks. The role of increased intracellular calcium is thought to be critical.

Before discussing LTP further, it is useful to say a few words about the receptor that mediates it. This is one of the receptors for the amino acid glutamate (or aspartate); the glutamate/aspartate receptor types are collectively known as *excitatory amino acid (EAA)* receptors, because of their excitatory action.

The *N*-methyl-D-aspartate *(NMDA)* EAA receptor (Figure 2–6) is especially important in LTP because the ion channel associated with it is permeable to Ca^{2+}. Other types of EAA receptors are kainate receptors and α-amino-3-hydroxy-5-methyl-4-isoxazole propionic acid (AMPA) receptors (AMPA receptors are also called quisqualate receptors); kainate and AMPA receptors are collectively termed *non-NMDA receptors* and do not admit Ca^{2+} ions.

Opening of the NMDA ion channel allows Ca^{2+} to flow down the concentration gradient and enter the neuron; there is, however, a voltage dependency of the permeability of the NMDA channel to Ca^{2+}, due to a voltage-dependent blockade of the channel by magnesium. At membrane potentials near resting voltages, the blockade is nearly complete. However as the membrane becomes more depolarized the blockade lessens. This voltage dependence makes the necessity of pairing inputs with weak effects with stronger inputs to produce LTP understandable: the strong inputs depolarize the neuron via kainate and AMPA (non-NMDA) channels and this depolarization allows increased Ca^{2+} entry because of decreased magnesium blockade of the NMDA ion channel. Both the NMDA and non-NMDA receptors are ligand-gated, but the Ca^{2+} admitted by the NMDA receptor plays the role of a second messenger and is likely critical for the production of the long-term alterations underlying LTP. The secondary responses mediated by a rise in intracellular Ca^{2+} include changes in other second messengers, such as the stimulation of phospholipases to produce diacylglycerol, inositol triphosphate, and arachidonic acid—factors that may be important in the initiation and maintenance of LTP.

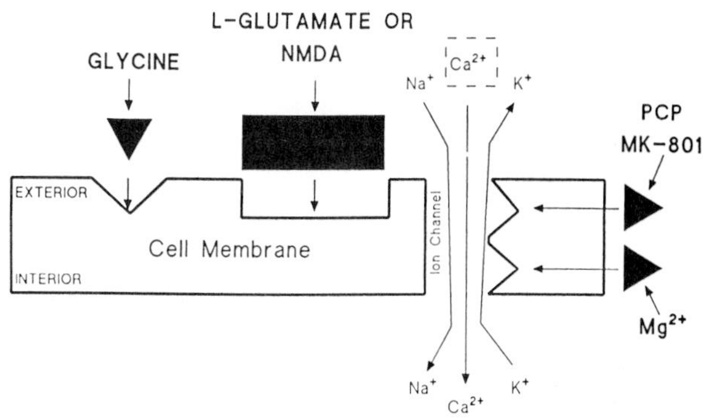

Figure 2–6. Schematic of the *N*-methyl-D-aspartate (NMDA) receptor-ion channel complex. The agonist for the receptor site is NMDA or L-glutamate. The attachment of the agonist to the receptor site (rectangle) leads to opening of the ion channel in the neuronal membrane. A key feature of the NMDA receptor ion channel, in contrast to other excitatory amino acid receptor channels, is that it allows the passage of calcium ions (Ca^{2+}, highlighted) from outside to inside the neuron (in addition to allowing the entry of sodium ions [Na^+ and the exit of potassium ions [K^+]. As described in the text, Ca^{2+} is important both in excitotoxicity and in long-term alterations of neuronal properties such as long-term potentiation. Both phencyclidine (PCP, "angel dust") and MK-801 are noncompetitive blockers of the ion channel. NMDA neurotransmission has a distinctive nonlinear property in that the effect of opening the NMDA channel is dependent on the degree of membrane polarization. At membrane polarization voltages typical of the cell at rest, about –70 mV, the magnesium ion (Mg^{2+}) blocks the channel nearly completely; however this blockage is voltage-dependent, becoming progressively less with membrane depolarization. This progressive decrease in Mg^{2+} blockage produces a positive feedback for NMDA neurotransmission. With opening of the ion channel, the membrane potential is depolarized by the inrush of Na^+ and Ca^{2+}. This depolarization reduces the Mg^{2+} channel blockage, with consequent admission of more Na^+ and Ca^{2+}, more membrane depolarization, less Mg^{2+} blockade, more depolarization, and so on. The glycine site is included in the schematic because this glycine receptor modulates the effect of NMDA.

Still another important EAA receptor type is the "metabotropic" EAA receptor; these receptors are not coupled to an ion channel, but rather act to cause a G protein stimulated release of Ca^{2+} from intracellular stores, an action mediated by inositol triphosphate. This receptor has recently been cloned and found to be structurally distinctive, with no sequence similarity to other G protein coupled receptors; it has extensive expression in hippocampus and cerebellum (Masu et al. 1991).

Calcium and growth and development of neurons. Not only does intracellular Ca^{2+} appear to play an important role in adult synaptic plasticity, it is also important in neurotransmitter-mediated regulation of neuronal growth and development (Lipton and Kater 1989). Intracellular calcium concentrations have an inverted U functional relationship to neuronal growth; at lower levels increasing Ca^{2+} increases growth whereas at higher levels Ca^{2+} increases lead to destruction of neuronal processes. In the visual system (optic tectum) of amphibians, specificity of input from each eye is maintained by glutamate acting at NMDA receptors.

Calcium and excitotoxicity. An important area of current interest is the toxic effects of excessive EAA receptor stimulation, a phenomenon called *excitotoxicity,* which is likely responsible for much of the cellular damage that occurs following decreased oxygenation and/or decreased glucose supply to brain, such as occurs during stroke. The basic concept is that these conditions favor membrane depolarization and hence increased Ca^{2+} entry, with the increased intracellular Ca^{2+} being toxic to the neurons. Increased Ca^{2+} entry occurs both as a result of decreased magnesium blockade of NMDA receptors and/or through voltage-sensitive Ca^{2+} channels. Excitotoxicity may also be important in degenerative diseases, where there may be abnormal sensitivity to NMDA or some form of dysregulation of EAA channels. Such a mechanism has been proposed for Huntington's chorea (see Cotman et al. 1989). More recently a dysregulation of EAA channels has been hypothesized for schizophrenia (McCarley et al. 1991), with the important additional consideration that EAA receptor dysregulation may also interfere with normal neural development (see discussion above and in Chapter 1).

Third Messengers: c-fos and jun

Immediate early genes. An important recent development has been the realization that neurotransmitters may activate mechanisms regulating the transcription of DNA, the genetic material. The induction of the *immediate early genes (IEGs)* such as "c-fos" and "jun" is one example of this mechanism. The term *fos* was first used to describe the oncogene encoded by the Finkel-Biskis-Jenkins murine osteogenic sarcoma virus. The normal cellular sequences from which the viral oncogene (v-fos) was derived are referred to as the *fos proto-oncogene* or *c-fos.* In normal cells the level of the protein product of the c-fos gene, Fos, is highly regulated; many stimuli, some associated with cellular differentiation and some linked with neuronal excitation, lead to a transient induction of c-fos messenger RNA (mRNA). The name for the IEG jun was derived in similar fashion from the oncogene carried by the avian sarcoma virus ASV17; *ju-nana* is the Japanese word for 17. (For an extensive recent discussion of stimulus-transcription coupling, see Morgan and Curran 1989, 1991.) Schematically,

Neurotransmitter-receptor binding
- → change in second messenger levels
- → induction of transcription of the genes c-fos and jun
- → c-fos and jun mRNAs present in cytoplasm for about 1–2 hours
- → translation of Fos and Jun proteins
- → possible alterations in posttranslational modification (e.g., phosphorylation) of Fos by stimuli
- → translocation to nucleus and formation of a Fos-Jun dimer (Fos has half life of about 2 hours)
- → Fos-Jun dimer complex binds to DNA regulatory element (AP-1 site)
- → increase in transcription of DNA
- → increase in production of a particular protein

This area is one of intense current work and hence of great flux in defining both which neurotransmitters and stimuli lead to the IEG production and which proteins are regulated by this transcriptional control, a much more difficult question. Neurotransmitters-receptors reported to modulate c-fos expression include EAAs (especially NMDA, but also kainate), dopamine, opioids, cholecystokinin, progesterone, interleukin-1 (IL-1), and nicotine. Stimuli and conditions known to activate c-fos include heat shock, dehydration, electrical stimulation, seizures (especially in hippocampus), manipulation of internal calcium concentration, treadmill locomotion, and stimulation with light (see Morgan and Curran 1991). Although this list is long, it should not be assumed that all cellular activation leads to c-fos production and that c-fos production is nonspecific.

There appears to be a relatively specific production of c-fos in the hypothalamic suprachiasmatic nucleus (SCN). The SCN contains the basic mechanisms of the circadian clock, which regulates the circadian oscillations of many body systems including temperature and sleep. This clock may be reset to an earlier time (this kind of resetting is called phase advancing) in response to a light stimulus occurring just before the expected onset of light in the environment. Several groups of investigators have found that light stimuli applied at this time—but not at other circadian times that do not induce the same phase reset—have the capability of inducing c-fos. Although it has been hypothesized that the transcriptional regulation of DNA is important in resetting the circadian clock, this has not yet been proven.

The induction of IEGs may be very important for psychiatry because this process may mediate long-term alterations important for behavior. Obviously the key step to understanding the functional significance of IEG stimulation of transcription is knowing which protein is being transcribed; unfortunately this is also the most difficult step.

cAMP-inducible genes. Stimulation of the second messenger cAMP by neurotransmitters may, as discussed above, control DNA transcription *indirectly* through induction of c-fos and other IEGs. There are also genes that are *directly* regulated by cAMP, including those for the neurotransmitter peptides somatostatin and vasointestinal peptide (VIP) (Montminy et al. 1990). This regulation is thought to be accomplished via cAMP-induced release of the active C subunit of protein kinase A; the C subunit moves to the nucleus where it phosphorylates a cAMP responsive element binding protein (CREB). The consequent conformational change in CREB allows it to interact with a target protein and stimulate gene production.

❑ EVOKED POTENTIALS AND THE EEG

The previous sections have detailed basics of cellular electrophysiology and cellular communication. Obviously recording of individual neurons can only be done in humans under very special circumstances, and much of our knowledge of human systems electrophysiology comes through recordings of EPs and the EEG. These techniques use large electrodes and do not record the activity of individual neurons but rather the summated activity of many neural elements. We here briefly outline the essential concepts relevant to EP and EEG generation, taking the EP first. EPs may be thought of as summations of the voltage alterations generated by populations of neural elements in response to a stimulus, typically an external sensory stimulus.

Most of the components of the EP arise from PSPs and not action potentials, which generally are too brief and too asynchronous to summate and produce an EP. (Some of the very short latency [< 10 milliseconds] brain stem auditory EP components are derived from synchronous volleys of action potentials and are an important exception to this rule.)

Figure 2–7 illustrates a depolarizing PSP in the soma; this PSP is generated by the influx of positive ions. The influx of positive ions defines the soma as a current "sink" in this case because, by convention, current is composed of positive ion flow. In contrast, the apical dendrites act as a "source" of current flow. This current flow pattern defines a dipole, literally a "two pole" with the positive pole in the dendrites and the negative in the soma. In the case of a hyperpolarizing PSP in the soma, the dipole polarity would be reversed, with source (positive pole) in the soma and sink in the dendrites; it will be recalled that membrane hyperpolarization arises as the consequence of an net efflux of positive ions. In cerebral structures with a regular laminar structure such as the cortex and hippocampus, such a simple dipole model repeated over many constituent neurons provides a reasonable first approxima-

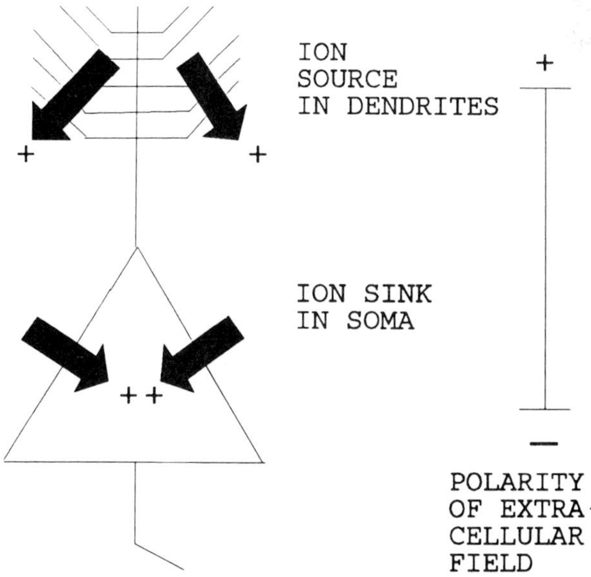

Figure 2–7. Dipole generated by soma depolarization in a pyramidal neuron. (See text for discussion.)

tion to how EPs are generated. Many investigators are currently exploring the use of modelling "equivalent dipoles" as a representation of the average amplitude and polarity within a cerebral region, such as the sensory receiving areas of the cortex.

Practical constraints to localizing the source of EPs include the use of scalp recordings and the consequent "smearing" of current flow as the boundaries between zones of different conductivities are traversed. For example, the brain and its extracellular fluid is a much better conductor than the scalp. Recent studies by Cohen, Cuffin, and associates Cohen et al. (1990) have applied an experimental approach to the question of the accuracy of source localization possible with electrical signals. Using patients who had deep electrodes implanted to locate the seizure source before surgery, these investigators passed a low-level signal through two deep electrodes (a true dipole source!) and then examined how closely the signal source within the brain could be localized from scalp electrode recordings. Brain localization was found to be surprisingly good, being correct on the average to within about 1 cm. Another rather surprising finding of this study was the failure of the magnetoencephalogram (MEG) to localize the source with any significantly greater accuracy than the EEG.[2]

Finally, it is important to emphasize that the biological EP signals recorded from the scalp are of quite low level, often a few microvolts; thus signal averaging is typically used for EP recording to extract the signal from the ongoing EEG and from noise sources, such as muscle activity.

The EEG can be understood as the record of spontaneous voltage fluctuations, as "endogenously generated EPs," although the brain source of the recorded fluctuations is often difficult to pinpoint, with the important exceptions of large amplitude changes due to pathological synchronization of neural elements, such as spikes from seizure discharge. The EEG serves a very useful purpose in pinpointing changes in alertness and sleep stages by changes in its frequency content, a topic discussed in Part II of this chapter.

[2]The MEG is a recording of the magnetic field generated by neural activity and is analogous to the electrical field recorded by the EEG. There currently is considerable debate over whether the MEG will show greater localizing power than the EEG for EPs. The MEG is particularly useful in detecting generating dipoles that are tangentially oriented to the brain surface, but is not sensitive to radially oriented dipoles. The EEG is equally sensitive to tangential and radial dipoles.

The *alpha rhythm* has a frequency range of 8–13 Hz, occurs during wakefulness, appears on eye closure, disappears with eye opening, and is best recorded over the occipital scalp region. Depth recordings in animals indicate alpha rhythm frequencies may also be present in visual thalamus (lateral geniculate body, pulvinar) and the cortical component appears to be generated in relatively small cortical areas that act as epicenters. Unfortunately, there are as yet almost no cellular studies bearing on the genesis of this rhythm, although interaction of corticocortical and thalamocortical neurons has been postulated (Steriade et al. 1990).

PART II: CONTROL OF SLEEP AND WAKEFULNESS

❑ SLEEP ARCHITECTURE

Sleep is divided into two phases. *Rapid-eye-movement (REM) sleep* is usually associated with vivid dreaming, and a high level of brain activity is consistently present. The other phase of sleep, called *non-REM (NREM) sleep* or *slow-wave sleep (SWS)* is associated with reduced neuronal activity. Thought content during this state in humans is, unlike dreams, usually nonvisual and consists of ruminative thoughts.

As shown in Figure 2–8, as one goes to sleep the low-voltage fast EEG of waking gradually gives way to a slowing of frequency. Moreover, as sleep moves toward the deepest stages, there is an abundance of *delta waves*: EEG waves with a frequency of 0.5–4 Hz and of high amplitude. The first REM period usually occurs about 70 minutes after the onset of sleep. REM sleep in humans is defined by the presence of low-voltage fast EEG activity, suppression of muscle tone (usually measured in the chin muscles), and the presence, of course, of rapid eye movements. The first REM sleep episode in humans is short. After this episode, the sleep cycle repeats itself with the appearance of NREM sleep, and then about 90 minutes after the start of the first REM period another REM sleep episode occurs. This rhythmic cycling persists throughout the night. The REM sleep cycle lasts 90 minutes in humans and each REM sleep episode after the first is approximately 30 minutes long.[3] Over the course of the

[3]This time course is schematized in Figure 2–16.

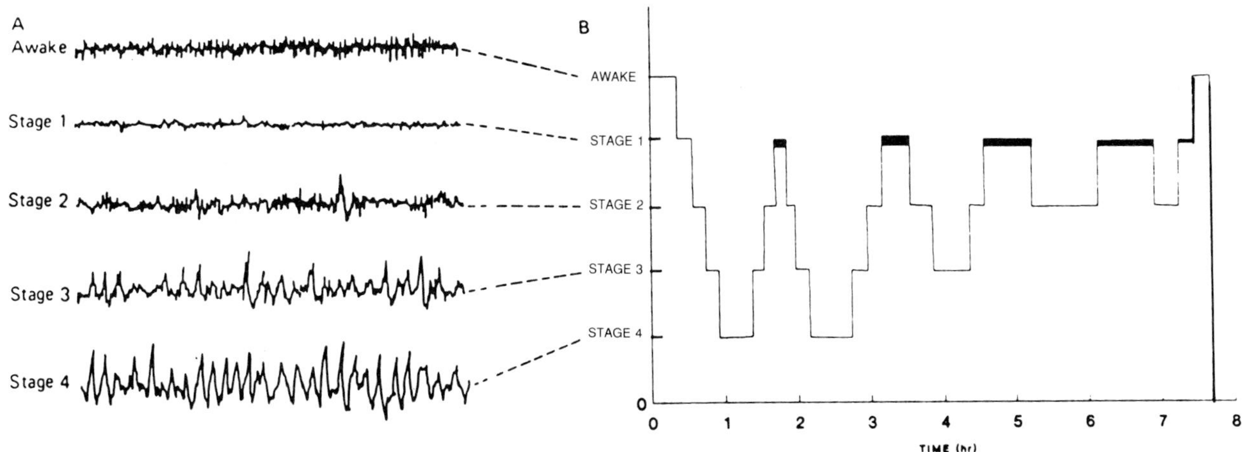

Figure 2–8. Examples of electroencephalogram (EEG) patterns associated with the stages of sleep and the time course of sleep stages. During wakefulness there is a low-voltage fast EEG pattern, often with alpha waves. Stage 1 descending has a low-voltage fast EEG. As sleep deepens the EEG wave frequency slows. During stage 3 delta waves (0.5–4 Hz) appear, and in stage 4 they are present more than 50% of the time. Stage 1 ascending represents rapid-eye-movement (REM) sleep (*black bar*). Often stages 2, 3, and 4 are lumped together as "non-REM sleep." Note that during REM sleep the EEG pattern returns to a low-voltage fast pattern. The percentage of time spent in REM sleep increases with successive sleep cycles whereas the percentage of stages 3 and 4 decreases. (EEG is recorded from the vertex, and each trace is about 30 seconds duration. Adapted from Kandel and Schwarz 1985.)

night, delta wave activity tends to diminish and NREM sleep has waves of higher frequencies and lower amplitude.

❑ SLEEP ONTOGENY AND PHYLOGENY

Periods of immobility and "rest" are present in many lower animals, including insects and lizards. Because of the absence of a cortical brain structure like that of humans, it is difficult to say whether the absence of slow waves in these animals means they are not having the equivalent of human SWS or whether this is present but expressed in a different form not detectable with EEG recordings. REM sleep is present in all mammals, except for monotremes (egg-laying mammals) such as the echidna (spiny anteater). Birds have very brief bouts of REM sleep. REM sleep cycles vary in duration according to the size of the animal, with elephants having the longest cycle and smaller animals having shorter cycles. For example, the cat has a sleep cycle of approximately 22 minutes, whereas the rat cycle is about 12 minutes.

In utero, mammals spend a large percentage of time in REM sleep, ranging from 50% to 80% of a 24-hour day. At birth, animals born with immature nervous systems have a much higher percentage of REM sleep than do the adults of the same species. For example, sleep in the human newborn occupies two-thirds of a 24-hour day, with REM sleep occupying one-half of the total sleep time or about one-third of the entire 24-hour period. The percentage of REM sleep declines rapidly in early childhood so that by approximately age 10 the adult percentage of REM sleep is reached, 20% of total sleep time. Obviously, the predominance of REM sleep in the young suggests an important function in promoting nervous system growth and development (see discussion below on Functions of Sleep).

Delta sleep is minimally present in the newborn but increases over the first years of life, reaching a maximum at about age 10 and declining thereafter. Feinberg et al. (1990) noted that the time course of the level of delta activity over the first three decades can be fit by a gamma distribution. Furthermore, the same developmental time course is found for synaptic density and positron-emission tomography (PET) measurements of metabolic rate in human frontal cortex. Feinberg and colleagues speculated that the reduction in these three variables may reflect a pruning of redundant cortical synapses, and that this is a key factor in cognitive maturation, allowing greater specialization and sustained problem solving.

❑ SLEEP ONSET AND SLEEPINESS

Sleep onset and sleepiness are determined by circadian time of day[4] and by prior wakefulness.

Circadian factors in sleepiness. In adult humans, the period of maximal sleepiness occurs at the time of the circadian low point of the temperature rhythm (Figure 2–9). It is no accident that accidents are most frequent at the time near circadian temperature minima because this is the time of maximal sleepiness. The risk for truck accidents, per vehicle mile, is greatest at this time, and the nuclear reactor incidents at both Chernobyl and Three Mile Island also occurred in the early morning hours. There is a secondary peak of sleepiness that occurs about 3 P.M. (Figure 2–9), corresponding to a favored time for naps. The main functional consequence of deprivation of sleep seems to be the presence of "microsleeps," that is, very brief episodes of sleep during which sensory input from the outside is diminished and cognitive function is markedly altered. Human newborns do not have a strong circadian modulation of sleep, and some species, such as the cat, do not have much circadian modulation even as adults.

Prior wakefulness. The second factor determining sleepiness is the extent of prior wakefulness. Mathematical models of sleep propensity have been developed by Kronauer et al. (1982), who emphasized circadian control, and by Borbély et al. (1982), who emphasized the extent of prior wakefulness. The model by Borbély and associates postulates that the intensity and amplitude of delta wave activity (as measured by power spectral analysis) indexes the level of sleep factor(s) and SWS drive. In this model, the time course of delta activity over the night, a declining exponential, reflects the dissipation of the sleep factor(s). These researchers have not specified the nature of the underlying sleep factor(s).

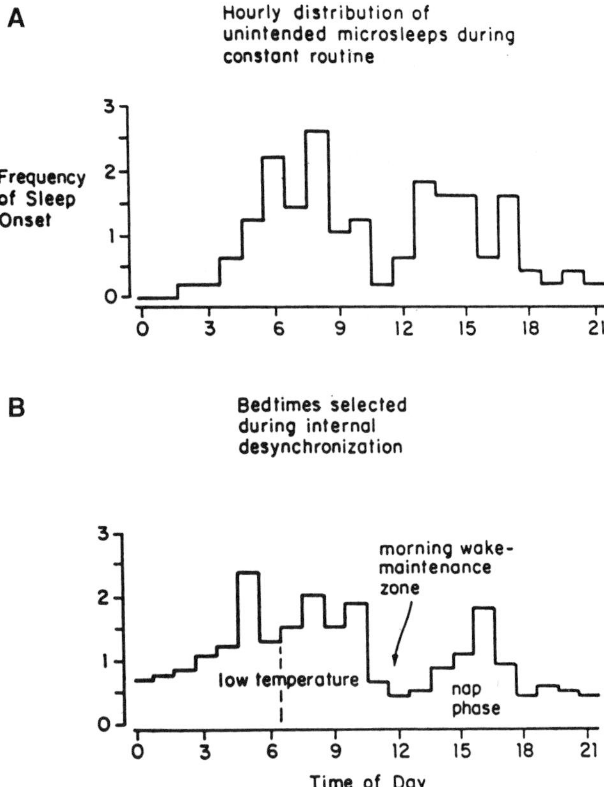

Figure 2–9. Circadian control of sleepiness and sleep onset. *Panel A:* Sleepiness at various clock times for subjects on a constant routine. Sleepiness was measured by Carskadon (see Strogatz 1986) as frequency of unintended microsleeps in subjects instructed to stay awake, with a frequency of 1 indicating the average across all measurements. Note the major peak about 6 A.M., at the presumptive time of temperature minimum, and a secondary peak about 3 P.M., a favored time for a nap. *Panel B:* Sleep propensity measured as the number of self-selected bedtimes (sleep onsets) in subjects in whom temperature was continuously monitored. Note that, as in *panel A*, the maximum number of sleep onsets occur near temperature minimum, and a secondary peak occurs at a circadian phase corresponding to about 3 P.M. These subjects were maintained without circadian cues and showed decoupling of the activity and the temperature rhythms (internal desynchronization) that are otherwise synchronized by external circadian cues, such as dawn and dusk. The sleep onsets were converted to approximate times of day by assuming a temperature minimum at 6:30 A.M. (Adapted from Strogatz 1986.)

[4]Circadian means "about a day" (from the Latin "circa" [about] and "dies" [day]), and the human circadian rhythm can be thought of as a sine wave function with a minimum that occurs between 4:00 and 7:00 A.M. in persons with a normal daytime activity schedule.

❑ THE FACTORS AND EEG PHENOMENA OF SWS

SWS Factors

Several humoral factors have been proposed to account for NREM sleep—alternatively termed slow-wave sleep in this chapter and in the literature, although, properly speaking, stage 2 sleep has few slow waves. The present status of these factors is one of uncertaintly as to whether they participate in the natural regulation of sleep, although they are certainly active as pharmacological agents that decrease wakefulness and increase SWS.

Pappenheimer, Karnovsky, and Krueger (see Krueger 1990) demonstrated that *muramyl peptides* were concentrated in the cerebrospinal fluid and urine of sleep-deprived animals. These muramyl peptides have the capability of reliably inducing SWS when injected into the lateral ventricles or into the basal part of the forebrain. The compounds also induce hyperthermia. They are derived from bacterial cell walls, and it has been theorized they may act like "vitamins" for the production of sleep. Another sleep factor is IL-1, which is a cytokine produced in response to infections (and also by injections of components of bacterial cell walls such as muramyl peptides). It increases SWS and also produces hyperthermia. Hyperthermia itself may increase SWS, but blocking the hyperthermic effects of IL-1 does not block the SWS-inducing effects (Krueger 1990). The argument that IL-1 and muramyl peptides are important in the hypersomnia associated with infections is thus strong, although determination that they are natural sleep factors awaits further research. Hayaishi (1988) found that injections of prostaglandin D_2 into the third ventricle reliably produced SWS and proposed that it is a natural sleep regulatory factor. However, Krueger (1990) was unable to confirm these data. Delta sleep inducing peptide (DSIP) has been proposed as a sleep factor by Monnier and associates, although the literature does not suggest a robust effect. (For a review of this work and of other proposed sleep factors, see Borbély and Tobler 1989.)

EEG Synchronization and Desynchronization: Neural Substrates

The high-voltage slow-wave activity in cortex during NREM sleep–called *EEG synchronization*—contrasts sharply with the low-voltage fast pattern—called *desynchronized* or *activated*—characteristic of both waking and REM sleep and consisting of frequencies in the beta range (approximately 16–32 Hz). One of the major advances of the past few years has been the establishment of the importance of a cholinergic-activating system in EEG desynchronization. This is likely the major component of the *ascending reticular activating system (ARAS;* see below), a concept that arose before methods were available for labelling of neurons using specific neurotransmitters. We now know that a group of the neurons in the brain stem cholinergic nuclei at the pons-midbrain junction have high discharge rates in waking and REM sleep and low discharge rates in SWS. Figure 2–10 indicates the location of the cholinergic laterodorsal tegmental and pedunculopontine tegmental (LDT/PPT) nuclei. There is also extensive anatomical evidence that these cholinergic neurons project to thalamic nuclei important in EEG desynchronization and synchronization. Both in vitro and in vitro neurophysiological studies have indicated that the target neurons in the thalamus re-

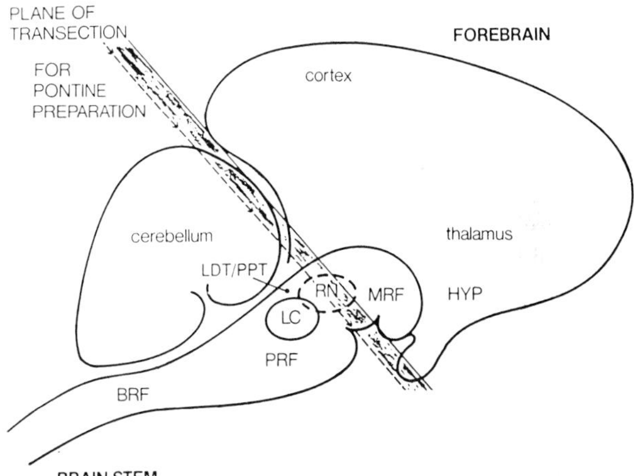

Figure 2–10. Schematic of a sagittal section of a mammalian brain (cat) showing the plane of transection that preserves rapid eye movement (REM) sleep signs caudal to the transection but abolishes them rostral to the transection. BRF = bulbar reticular formation; PRF = pontine reticular formation; MRF = midbrain reticular formation; LDT/PPT = laterodorsal and pedunculopontine tegmental nucleus—the principal site of cholinergic (acetylcholine-containing) neurons important for REM sleep and electroencephalogram (EEG) desynchronization; LC = locus coeruleus—where most norepinephrine-containing neurons are located; RN = dorsal raphe nucleus—the site of many serotonin-containing neurons; HYP = hypothalamus. (Adapted from McCarley 1989.)

spond to cholinergic agonists in a way consistent with EEG activation.

It is likely that cholinergic systems are not the exclusive substrate of EEG desynchronization; brain stem reticular neuronal projections to thalamus (likely using EAAs) and noradrenergic projections from locus coeruleus (for waking, because these neurons are silent in REM sleep) may also play important roles. In addition to brain stem cholinergic systems, cholinergic input to thalamus from the basal forebrain cholinergic nucleus basalis of Meynert (nBM) is also important for EEG desynchronization.

SWS at the Cellular Level in the Thalamus: The "Burst Mode" of Relay Cell Discharge and Failure of Information Transmission

Extracellular recordings by McCarley and Benoit demonstrated that dorsal lateral geniculate neurons discharged in stereotyped bursts during NREM sleep but not during waking or REM sleep. Subsequent investigations in vivo by Steriade and associates and in vitro by McCormick and associates indicated the bursting occurs on a background of membrane hyperpolarization. (For literature references and a more detailed description, see Steriade and McCarley 1990.) This hyperpolarization removes the inactivation of particular Ca^{2+} channels and enables the production of a "calcium spike" (i.e., an inrush of depolarizing calcium ions) when a small depolarization occurs. This depolarizing calcium spike is called a *low-threshold spike (LTS)* to distinguish it from other calcium currents with different triggering thresholds. The LTS depolarizes the neuron sufficiently to reach the threshold for fast sodium action potentials, and a burst of these action potentials rides on the LTS. Figure 2–11 illustrates the role of cholinergic input from LDT/PPT in abolishing the burst mode: the relay neuron is depolarized by a muscarinically mediated potassium current reduction, while the hyperpolarizing γ-aminobutyric acid (GABA)ergic influence of interneurons is lessened by muscarinically mediated hyperpolarization of the interneuron. The net result of relay neuron depolarization is to inactivate the LTS and permit faithful following of high-frequency input.

Spindles. Spindles occur during stage 2 of human sleep and in the light SWS phase of animals; they are composed of waves of approximately 10–12 Hz frequency whose amplitudes wax and wane over the spindle duration of 1–2 seconds. Wave frequency varies with species and is higher in primates. Spindles are relatively well understood at the cellular level. Studies by Steriade and associates (see Steriade and McCarley 1990) indicated that spindle waves arise as the result of interactions of spindle pacemaker GABAergic thalamic nucleus reticularis (RE) neurons and thalamocortical neurons. As schematized in Figure 2–11, spindle waves are blocked by cholinergic brain stem-thalamus projections, which act to hyperpolarize the RE neurons, most likely through a muscarinically mediated potassium conductance increase. The forebrain nucleus basalis also provides cholinergic and hyperpolarizing GABAergic input to RE that assists brain stem input in disrupting the spindles.

Delta EEG activity. The cellular basis of delta waves is not as well known as that of spindles, although recent data indicate the importance of membrane potential oscillations that occur in thalamocortical neurons that are at a hyperpolarized membrane potential level. It is known with some certainty that the delta waves are suppressed by cholinergic activity in brain stem systems and by activity of cholinergic neurons in the forebrain nucleus basalis (Steriade and McCarley 1990). Thus delta waves occur during inactivity of cholinergic and reticular systems and likely represent oscillations occurring in the absence of activating inputs.

❑ REM SLEEP PHYSIOLOGY AND RELEVANT BRAIN ANATOMY

The brain physiology and neurotransmitters important for generation of REM sleep are better understood than those for SWS, although many important questions about REM sleep mechanisms and especially about function remain unanswered.

Transection studies show that the brain stem contains the neural machinery of the REM sleep rhythm. As illustrated in Figure 2–10, a transection made just above the junction of the pons and midbrain produces a state in which periodic occurrence of REM sleep can be found in recordings made in the isolated brain stem, whereas recordings in the isolated forebrain show no sign of REM sleep. These lesion studies by Jouvet (reviewed in Steriade and McCarley 1990) in France established the importance of the brain stem in REM sleep.

Brain stem reticular formation neurons are important as effectors in the production of the physiological events of REM sleep. As in humans, the cardinal signs of REM sleep in lower animals are muscle atonia, EEG desynchronization (low-voltage fast pattern), and rapid eye movements. *PGO waves* (defined below) are also an important component of REM sleep found in recordings from deep brain structures in many animals. (They are visible in the cat recordings in Figure 2–12.) There is suggestive evidence that PGO waves are present in humans, but the depth recordings necessary to establish their existence have not been done. However, their features have been extensively described in animals. PGO waves are spiky EEG waves that arise in the *p*ons and are transmitted to the thalamic lateral *g*eniculate nucleus (a visual system nucleus) and to the visual *o*ccipital cortex, hence the name PGO waves. PGO waves represent an important mode of brain stem activation of the forebrain during REM sleep and are also present in nonvisual thalamic nuclei.

Most of the physiological events of REM sleep have effector neurons located in the brain stem reticular formation, with important neurons especially concentrated in the pontine reticular formation (PRF). Thus PRF neuronal recordings are of special interest for information on mechanisms of production of these events. Intracellular recordings of PRF neurons show that these neurons have relatively hyperpolarized membrane potentials and generate almost no action potentials during NREM sleep. As illustrated in Figure 2–12, PRF neurons begin to depolarize even before the occurrence of the first EEG sign of the approach of REM sleep, the PGO waves that occur 30–60 seconds before the onset of the rest of the EEG signs of REM sleep. As PRF neuronal depolarization proceeds and the threshold for action potential production is reached, these neurons begin to discharge (generate action potentials). Their discharge rate increases as REM sleep is approached and the high level of discharge is maintained throughout REM sleep, due to the maintenance of a membrane depolarization.

Throughout the entire REM sleep episode, almost the entire population of PRF neurons remains depolarized. The resultant increased action potential activity leads to the production of those REM sleep physiological signs that have their physiological bases in PRF neurons. Figure 2–13 provides a schematic overview of REM sleep as arising from increases in activity of the various populations of reticular formation neurons that are important as effectors of REM sleep phenomena. PRF neurons are important for the rapid eye movements (the generator for saccades is in PRF); the PGO waves (a different group of neurons) and a group of dorsolateral PRF neurons control the muscle atonia of REM sleep (these neurons become active just before the onset of muscle atonia). Neurons in *midbrain reticular formation (MRF*; see Figure 2–10) are especially important for EEG desynchronization, for the low-voltage fast EEG pattern. As noted above, these MRF neurons were originally described as making up the ARAS, the set of neurons responsible for EEG desynchronization. Subsequent work has enlarged this original ARAS concept to include cholinergic neurons.

Cholinergic mechanisms are important for REM sleep. Work during the last few years has led to an appreciation of the importance of the neurotransmitter acetylcholine for REM sleep and to the nature of the anatomy and physiology of the cholinergic influences on REM sleep. The essential data supporting this conclusion are outlined below. (For detailed references to the literature, see Steriade and McCarley 1990.)

1. Injection of compounds that are acetylcholine agonists into the PRF produces a REM-like state that very closely mimics natural REM sleep. The latency to onset and duration are dose dependent. Muscarinic receptors appear to be especially critical, with nicotinic receptors of lesser importance.
2. There are naturally occurring cholinergic projections to reticular formation neurons. These arise in the two nuclei at the pons-midbrain junction (Figure 2–14): the LDT nucleus and the PPT nucleus.
3. In vitro recordings in the PRF slice preparation showed that a majority (80%) of reticular formation neurons are excited by cholinergic agonists, with muscarinic effects being especially pronounced. These studies also showed that the increased excitability and membrane depolarization produced by cholinergic agonists is a direct effect, because it persists when synaptic input has been abolished by addition of tetrodotoxin.
4. Experiments lesioning the LDT/PPT nuclei confirm their importance in producing REM sleep phenomena. Destruction of the cell bodies of

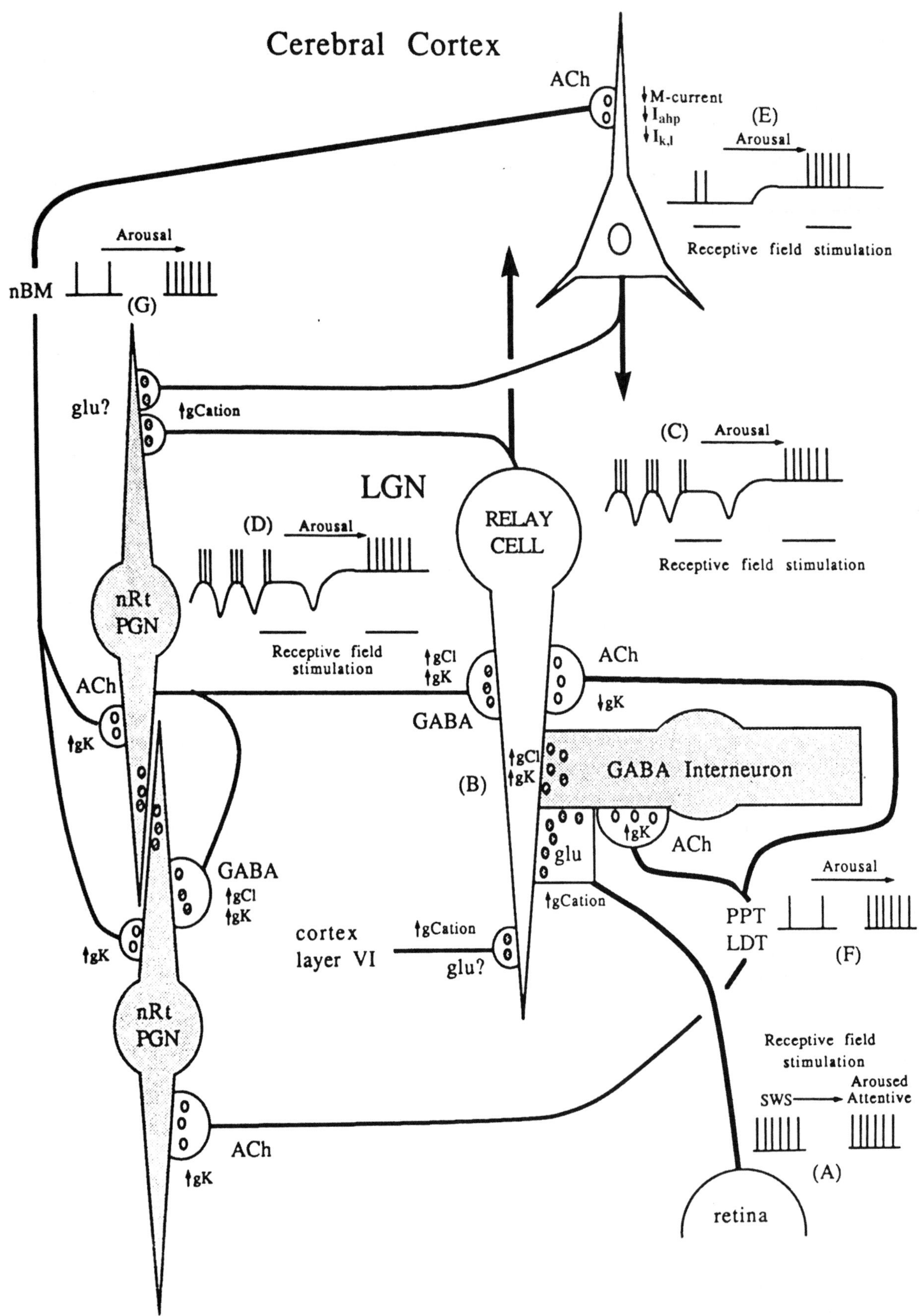

Cerebral Cortex
ACh
M-current
I_{ahp}
$I_{k,l}$
(E)
Arousal
Receptive field stimulation
Arousal
nBM
(G)
glu?
gCation
(C)
Arousal
LGN
RELAY CELL
Receptive field stimulation
(D)
Arousal
nRt PGN
Receptive field stimulation
gCl
gK
ACh
ACh
gK
GABA
gK
GABA Interneuron
gCl
gK
(B)
glu
ACh
gK
GABA
gCl
gK
Arousal
gCation
PPT LDT
cortex layer VI
gCation
glu?
(F)
gK
nRt PGN
Receptive field stimulation
SWS
Aroused Attentive
ACh
gK
(A)
retina

LDT/PPT neurons by local injections of EAAs leads to a marked reduction of REM sleep.

5. A group of LDT/PPT neurons discharges selectively in REM sleep, and the onset of activity begins before the onset of REM sleep. This LDT/PPT discharge pattern and the presence of excitatory projections to the PRF suggest that these cholinergic neurons may be important in producing the depolarization of reticular effector neurons for REM sleep events. The group of LDT/PPT and reticular formation neurons that become active in REM sleep are often referred to as *REM-on neurons.*
6. Cholinergic neurons are important in production of the low-voltage fast EEG pattern (representing "cortical activation") in both REM sleep and in waking. A different group of cholinergic neurons in LDT/PPT is active during this low-voltage fast pattern in both REM and waking. As described, this cholinergic system is especially important in generating the low-voltage fast EEG pattern, often called the "activated EEG." Also playing a role in forebrain activation are projections from MRF neurons and aminergic neurons, especially those in locus coeruleus. Together these neuronal groups form the ARAS. Evidence that multiple systems are involved in EEG desynchronization comes from the inability of lesions of any single one of these systems to disrupt EEG desynchronization on a permanent basis.

Finally, it is worth noting the many *peptides* that are co-localized with the neurotransmitter acetylcholine in LDT/PPT neurons; this co-localization likely also means they have synaptic co-release with acetylcholine. The peptide substance P is found in about 40% of LDT/PPT neurons and, overall, more than 15 different co-localized peptides have been described. The role of these peptides in modulating acetylcholine activity relevant to wakefulness and sleep remains to be elucidated, but it should be emphasized that the co-localized peptide VIP has been reported by several different investigators to enhance REM sleep percentages when it is injected intraventricularly.

REM-off neurons may suppress REM sleep phenomena. *REM-on neurons* are those neurons that become active in REM sleep, compared with SWS and waking, and presumably have a protagonist role in production of REM sleep phenomena. Neurons with an opposite discharge time course that become inactive in REM sleep are called *REM-off*

Figure 2–11. (*facing page*) The effect of ascending cholinergic systems on information processing in the visual system during wakefulness and sleep. Schematic diagram of the interconnections of the retina, lateral geniculate nucleus (LGN), the thalamic reticular-perigeniculate nucleus (nRt/PGN), and the cerebral cortex. Stimulation of a retinal ganglion cell's receptive field results in a train of action potentials being generated and sent to the LGN, even during slow-wave sleep (SWS) (A). Each action potential causes an EPSP mediated by glutamate (glu) in both the LGN relay neuron (B), which projects to cortex and other visual system areas, and the GABAergic interneuron. Activation of the GABAergic interneuron rapidly inhibits the relay cell and increases conductance such that the retinal EPSP is shunted (B).
Burst firing in SWS: As illustrated in (C) and (D) burst firing, sometimes rhythmic, is present in both nRt and the relay cell; this results from both intrinsic properties of the neurons (low-threshold calcium spike; see text) and the connectivity between relay cell and nRt/PGN, as well as the interconnections within the nRt/PGN. Stimulation of the cells receptive field during burst generation will generate only a weak output from the LGN neuron and may temporarily disrupt ongoing burst rhythms (C; left response, horizontal bar). The activity from the retina is further reduced in cortical neurons due to relatively uninhibited M-current (a hyperpolarizing current) and the slow after-hyperpolarization current (I_{ahp}), which underlie spike frequency adaptation (E; left response).
Effects of cholinergic activation: On arousal from SWS and in rapid eye movement (REM) sleep, the cholinergic neurons of the pedunculopontine tegmental (PPT) and laterodorsal tegmental (LDT) nuclei, as well as those of the cholinergic nucleus basalis of Meynert (nBM), increase their rate of spontaneous activity (F and G). Increased activity of these cholinergic neurons disrupts burst generation in the thalamus by depolarizing the relay neurons—through a muscarinically mediated decrease in a resting potassium conductance (gK) (C)—and also activates the cerebral cortical pyramidal neurons through a decrease in M-current, I_{ahp}, and a resting outward potassium conductance, $I_{k,l}$. Thus during wakefulness and REM sleep both the LGN relay neurons as well as the GABAergic neurons of the nRt/PGN are depolarized toward single spike-firing threshold (the low-threshold calcium spike responsible for bursts is inactivated), while the effectiveness of intrageniculate GABAergic inhibitory interneurons is decreased by an acetylcholine (ACh)-mediated increase in gK. In wakefulness stimulation of the receptive field is faithfully reproduced on the output of the LGN relay neuron (C; second horizontal bar). Due to the actions of ACh in the cerebral cortex, the input responsiveness of cortical pyramidal neurons is also increased (E; second horizontal bar). EPSP = excitatory postsynaptic potential; GABA = γ-aminobutyric acid. (Adapted from McCormick 1990.)

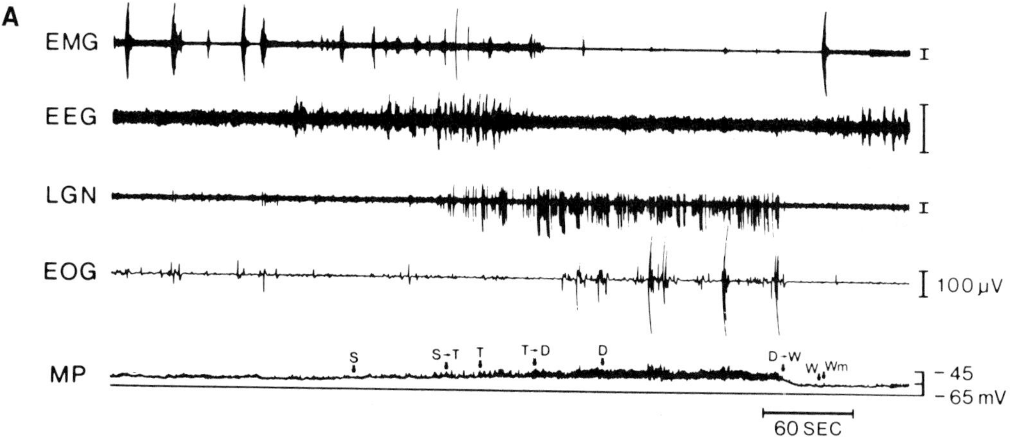

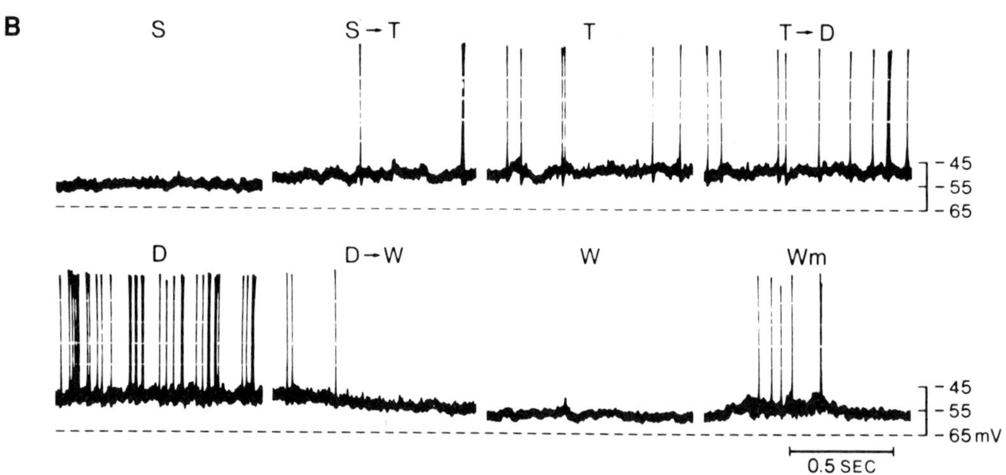

Figure 2–12. Changes in action potential frequency and membrane potential alteration of an intracellularly recorded medial pontine reticular formation neuron in cat over a sleep-wake cycle. *Panel A* shows the inkwriter record defining state and the record of membrane potential (MP) with action potentials filtered out. *Panel B* shows cathode ray oscilloscope photographs taken at the indicated points in the inkwriter record. The record in *panel A* begins in waking (W): note there is eye movement activity in the EOG record, a low-voltage fast EEG, and activity in the EMG record, indicating somatic movement. In W the membrane potential was about –60 mV and remained at approximately the same level with the onset of slow-wave sleep (see S label in MP record, note EEG slow-wave activity). Postsynaptic potential (PSP) activity in slow-wave sleep (S) was low. Even before the onset of the first PGO wave in the LGN record (*panel A*), the MP record showed a gradual onset of MP depolarization. By the time of the first LGN-PGO wave indicated by the S→T label, the PSP activity increased and there was one action potential. With the advent of more PGO waves (segment T, transition period) and the onset of REM sleep (indicated by the letter D for desynchronized sleep, another name for REM sleep), there was further MP depolarization and an accompanying increase in action potentials and PSPs (*panel B* segments labeled T and T→D). The increase in PSPs is visible as the thickening of the inkwriter MP trace in *panel A*. With the onset of full REM sleep (record segment labeled D) and during runs of the phasic activity of PGO waves and REMs, there were storms of depolarizing PSP activity and corresponding action potentials. The MP remained tonically depolarized at about –50 mV throughout REM sleep, with further phasic depolarizations. With the end of REM sleep and the onset of W (segment labeled D→W) there was a membrane repolarization to about the same tonic level seen in the initial W episode. At the point labeled Wm, there was a somatic movement that was accompanied by increased PSPs, a transient (phasic) membrane depolarization, and a burst of action potentials, before the MP returned to its baseline W polarization level. EMG = nuchal electromyogram; EEG = sensorimotor cortex electroencephalogram; LGN = EEG record from lateral geniculate nucleus; EOG = electrooculogram; PGO waves = pontogeniculooccipital waves; REM sleep = rapid-eye-movement sleep; T = transition period from slow-wave sleep to REM sleep. (Data from K. Ito and R. W. McCarley; adapted from Steriade and McCarley 1990.)

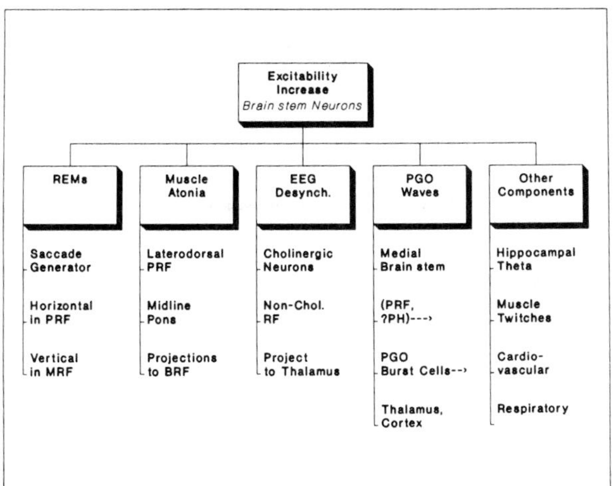

Figure 2–13. Schematic of REM sleep control. Increasing the excitability (activity) of brain stem neuronal pools subserving each of the major components of the state causes the occurrence of this component. For example, the neuronal pool important for the rapid eye movements is suggested to be the brain stem saccade generating system whose main machinery is in paramedian PRF. Although vertical saccades are fewer in REM sleep, their presence suggests similar involvement of the MRF. Information under the other system components sketches the major features of the anatomy and projections of neuronal pools important for muscle atonia, EEG desynchronization, and PGO waves; the last part of the diagram lists other components of REM sleep. BRF = bulbar reticular formation; EEG = electroencephalogram; MRF = midbrain reticular formation (midbrain reticular formation is primary region for EEG desynchronization); PGO waves = pontogeniculooccipital waves; PH = prepositus hypoglossi nucleus; PRF = pontine reticular formation; REM = rapid eye movement.

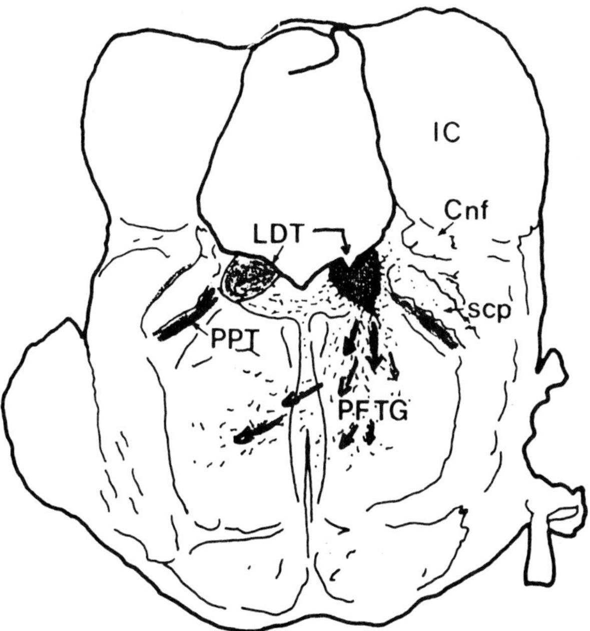

Figure 2–14. Frontal section of the brain stem at the pons-midbrain junction showing the location of the acetylcholine-containing neurons most important for rapid-eye-movement (REM) sleep in laterodorsal tegmental nucleus/pedunculopontine tegmental nucleus (LDT/PPT), and a schematic of projections of LDT to pontine reticular formation (PRF). PFTG = one component of PRF; IC = inferior colliculus; Cnf = cuneiform nucleus; scp = superior cerebellar peduncle. (Adapted from Mitani et al. 1988.)

neurons. REM-off neurons are most active in waking, have discharge activity that declines in SWS, and are virtually silent in REM until they resume discharge toward the later portion of the REM sleep episode. This inverse pattern of activity to REM-on neurons and to REM sleep phenomena such as PGO waves has led to the hypothesis that these neurons may be REM suppressive and interact with REM-on neurons in control of the REM sleep cycle (Figure 2–15). This concept is supported by production of REM sleep from cooling (inactivating) the nuclei where REM-off neurons are found and by some in vivo pharmacological studies (reviewed in Steriade and McCarley 1990). An important recent advance has been the documentation of the inhibitory influence on cholinergic LDT neurons likely important in REM sleep in the in vitro preparation by Luebke et al. (in press); this influence is direct, as indicated by its persistence in the presence of a blocker of synaptic transmission (tetrodotoxin).

The following classes of neurons are REM-off (see Figure 2–10 for anatomy):

- *Norepinephrine-containing neurons* are principally located in the locus coeruleus, called the "blue spot" because of its appearance in unstained brain.
- *Serotonin-containing neurons* are located in the *raphe system* of the brain stem, the midline collection of neurons that extends from the bulb to the midbrain, with higher concentrations of serotonin-containing neurons in the more rostral neurons.
- *Histamine-containing neurons* are located in the posterior hypothalamus.

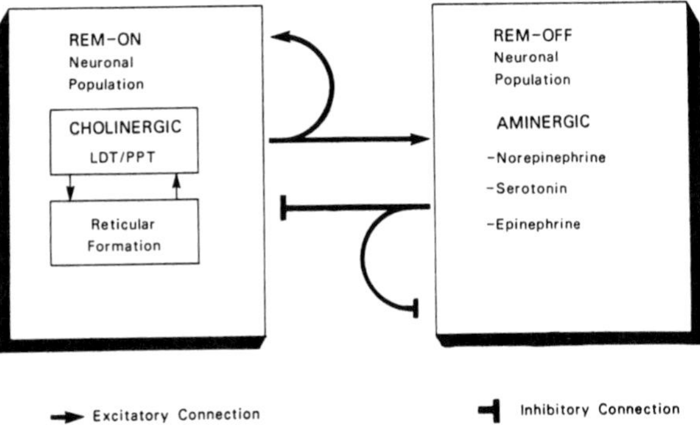

Figure 2–15. Reciprocal interaction model of rapid-eye-movement (REM) sleep control. Cholinergic neurons activate reticular formation neurons in a positive feedback interaction to produce the onset of REM sleep. REM sleep is terminated by the inhibitory activity of REM-off aminergic neurons *(right box)*, which become active at the end of a REM sleep period due to their recruitment by REM-on activity. REM-off neuronal activity decreases in slow-wave sleep and becomes minimal at the onset of REM sleep due to self-inhibitory feedback. This decreased REM-off activity disinhibits REM-on neurons and allows the onset of a REM sleep episode. The cycle then repeats itself. LDT/PPT = laterodorsal tegmental nucleus/pedunculopontine tegmental nucleus.

The histamine system has been conceptualized as one of the wakefulness-promoting systems, in agreement with drowsiness as a common side effect of antihistamines. Transection studies indicate, however, that the histaminergic neurons are not essential for the REM sleep oscillation.

A mathematical and structural model of the occurrence of REM sleep based on interaction of REM-off and REM-on neurons. A recent version of the reciprocal interaction model, originally proposed by Hobson and McCarley (see review by Steriade and McCarley 1990), rather accurately predicts the timing and percentage of REM sleep over a night of human sleep and its variation with the circadian temperature rhythm. The results of McCarley and Massaquoi's recent limit cycle mathematical formulation (McCarley and Massaquoi 1986) are sufficiently faithful to the actual human sleep data to furnish a good schematic, and Figure 2–16 provides a description of the model dynamics. A more extensive presentation appears in Steriade and McCarley (1990).

❑ THE FORM OF DREAMS AND THE BIOLOGY OF REM SLEEP

REM sleep is strongly associated with dreaming, with about 80% of awakenings during the REM state producing a dream report. In experiments involving awakenings at random intervals throughout the night, 80% of all such randomly elicited dream reports have been found to occur in REM sleep. Those dreams that do occur in NREM sleep have been found to be less vivid and intense than REM sleep dreams, suggesting they may represent a pre-REM state in which brain stem neuronal activity is approximating that of REM sleep but the EEG has not yet changed.

Dreams have long been of interest both in popular culture and in psychiatry. Sigmund Freud (1900; relationship to biology discussed in McCarley and Hobson 1977), writing before the presence of the biological state of REM sleep was known, suggested that dreams represented a symbolic disguise of an unacceptable unconscious wish, such as a sexual or aggressive wishes. The purpose of the disguise was to prevent the disruption of sleep that would occur with consciousness of the undisguised wish. Today the activation of the neural systems responsible for REM sleep would seem to be a more accurate and simple explanation for the instigation of the dream state that is linked to the cyclic appearance of REM sleep. There remains the question, however, of why dreams have their own distinctive characteristics and are different from waking consciousness.

The *activation-synthesis hypothesis* proposed by Hobson and McCarley (1977) suggested that many of the characteristic formal features of dreams are isomorphic with (i.e., "parallel to") distinctive features of the physiology of REM sleep. The term *formal features* means universal aspects of dreams, distinct from the dream content particular to an individual (McCarley and Hoffman 1981). As an example of a formal feature of a dream consider the presence of motor activity in dreams. At the physiological level it is known that motor systems, both at the motor cortex and at the brain stem level, are activated during REM sleep episodes. Paralleling motor system activation at the physiological level is the finding that movement in dreams is extremely common, with almost one-third of all verbs used in dream descriptions indicating movement and 80% of dreams having some occurrence of leg movement

A

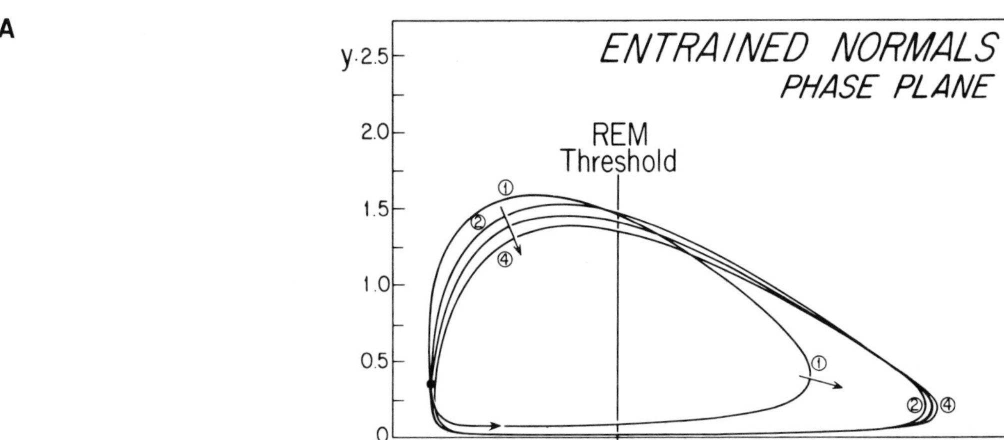

B

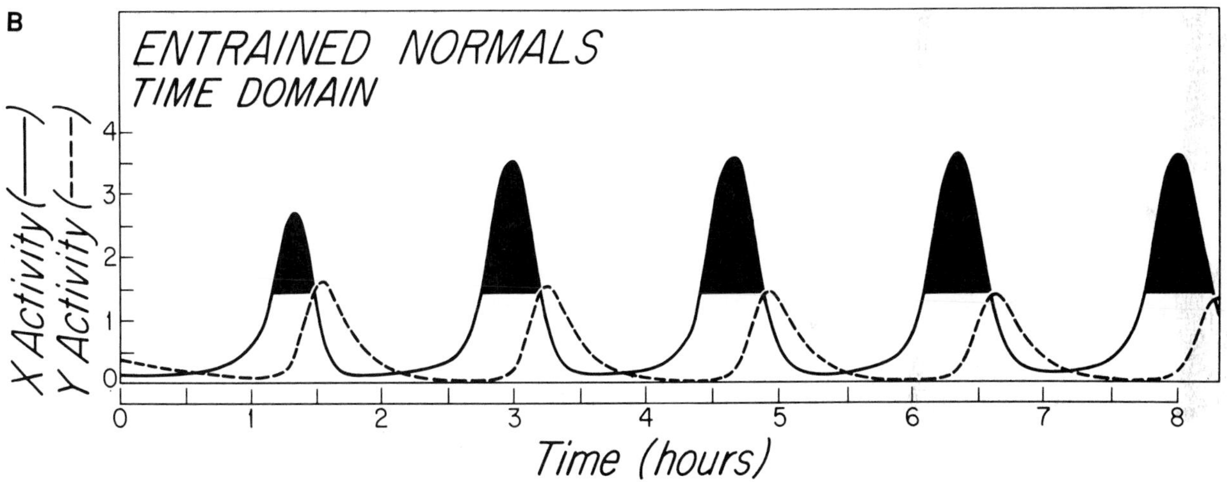

Figure 2–16. Model simulation of a night's course of rapid-eye-movement (REM) sleep in "normal" humans illustrating the variation in REM sleep over the night in subjects entrained to the circadian rhythm. (The limit cycle mathematical model whose results are illustrated is derived from the structural model in Figure 2–15, and the REM sleep variation over the night tracks very closely that actually observed in human sleep.) *Panel B:* A time domain representation following sleep onset (time 0). X Activity = REM-on (REM-promoting activity); Y Activity = REM-off (REM-suppressive neuronal activity). The solid portions of the X graph show those portions of the night with REM sleep; REM occurs at a certain threshold of X activity. The height of these REM activity peaks indicates the intensity of the REM sleep episode. Note the short-duration, lesser intensity first REM episode; subsequent variations of REM are less. The dynamics of REM-off and REM-on interaction are described in the legend to Figure 2–15. *Panel A:* A phase plane representation of the same X (REM-on) and Y (REM-off) activity. In this time graph, is represented by successive points on the X, Y positions. The dot indicates the starting point and the arrow the initial part of this first REM sleep cycle (labeled 1); note this initial portion of the curve is interior to the trajectories of subsequent REM cycles, labeled 2, 3, and 4, in the order of their occurrence (for simplicity sleep cycle 5 has not been graphed in the phase plane). The basic idea of this model is that the duration and intensity of the first REM episode varies according to whether the "limit cycle" is approached from the interior or exterior. This, in turn, depends on the rapidity of release of the REM-on population from REM-off suppression; variations occur with disease (weakening of aminergic influence may be present in depression) or with the circadian phase. The smaller variations in sleep cycles 2 through 4 are due to circadian modulation of other limit cycle parameters. (Adapted from McCarley and Massaquoi 1986.)

(a movement that was easily and reliably scored in dream reports).

Similarly there is activation of sensory systems during REM sleep. The visual system is intensely activated in REM and all dreams have visual experiences; indeed, these are one of the defining features of a dream. An important source of visual system activation during REM sleep is from the PGO waves. The activation synthesis theory suggests that this intense activation of visual and other sensory systems are the substrate for dream sensory experiences. Supporting this theory is the rather frequent occurrence—about 9% of all REM sleep dreams—of dreams with intense "vestibular sensations" (i.e., dreams of flying, floating, falling, soaring, or tumbling), easily relatable to the vestibular system functions of sensing position of the body in space and changes of position. The presence of dreams with vestibular sensations was highly atypical of the daytime sensory experience of the subjects whose dream reports were examined and is thus incompatible with any dream theory linked to a simple "recall" of previous experiences. Rather, the dream experience may reflect the intense REM sleep vestibular system activation, followed by its elaboration and synthesis into dream content. The final product, the dream, thus represents the synthesis of both the brain stem-induced motor and sensory activation with the particular memories and personality characteristics of the dreamer.

Lesion-induced release of REM sleep motor activity supports the presence of neural commands for patterned motor activity in REM sleep and a direct correspondence of the motor system commands and the subjective content of the dream. Activation of motor systems in REM can be observed in cats with a lesion of the muscle atonia zone of the PRF and a consequent *REM sleep without atonia,* a state in which motor activity is released but all of the other signs of REM sleep are present. The failure of muscle atonia is also observed in a human disorder called *REM sleep behavior disorder.* In individuals with this disorder, the muscle activity observed has been found always to parallel the dreamed activity. This close linkage between the physiology and psychology of REM sleep and dreams supports the activation-synthesis hypothesis.

When the activation-synthesis hypothesis was first proposed, it aroused considerable controversy, perhaps because it seemed to threaten psychological interpretation of dreams. Although this theory clearly places instigation of the dream state as a concomitant of a basic biological rhythm, in my opinion there appears to be more than ample room for the addition of personal characteristics in the process of synthesis of brain stem-instigated activation. For example, interpretations of the Rorschach cards are rich sources of information on personality, although the images on the cards themselves were certainly not generated by psychologically meaningful mechanisms.

Finally, it should be noted that as more is learned about forebrain processing during REM sleep, a more complete and complex theory will emerge. Crick and Mitchison (1983) have proposed that REM sleep is a state in which unwanted processing modes are eliminated; chief among these are cortical "parasitic oscillations," a kind of neural analog to obsessive thoughts. In this theory, the PGO wave activity acts to reset and redirect the unwanted neural loops. However, a full test of this theory will have to be postponed until our ability to monitor complex neural processing has greatly increased.

In a more empirical vein, recent neuroimaging studies in both human and cat have indicated activation of the limbic system, suggesting a biological basis of activation of memories and emotions in REM sleep and, perhaps, a mechanism of their linkage. Winson (1990) built on his own work in hippocampal systems to suggest a basis of dreams and a function of REM sleep. Extracellular recordings of CA_1 neurons indicated that CA_1 neurons that had been active during the day in encoding "place fields" (spatial position), fired at a significantly higher rate in REM sleep than CA_1 neurons that had not mapped place fields during the day. Winson suggested that a general function of REM sleep is "off-line" processing of information acquired during the day by comparison with other information acquired throughout the individual's lifetime. In humans dreams may come by their unusual character as a result of the complex associations that are culled from memory.

❑ FUNCTION(S) OF NREM AND REM SLEEP

There are many theories but relatively few solid data on the function of sleep. Here I summarize some of the most plausible functional theories for each sleep phase; some of these theories have been previously discussed.

NREM Sleep

Rest theory. Neuronal recordings and brain metabolic studies indicate the presence of rest on the neural level as well as the behavioral level during NREM sleep.

Behavioral immobilization or "out of harm's way." This theory suggests that sleep evolved as a way of arresting behavior at a time when it might not be advantageous, such as night activity in animals with poor night vision and vulnerability to predators.

REM Sleep

The following theories are not mutually exclusive. Indeed it seems a cogent argument that a complex behavioral state such as REM sleep may have multiple functions, and, as for wakefulness, it may not be meaningful to speak of "the" function of REM sleep.

Promotion of growth and development of the nervous system. The abundance of this metabolically and neurally active state in the young argues for this hypothesis. The recent discovery of NMDA receptors in the PRF offers a potential mechanism (see discussion in Part I) for regulation of neuronal growth and development in this region with high activation during REM sleep (Stevens et al. 1990). The French scientist Jouvet (1979) suggested that the stereotyped motor command patterns of REM sleep are useful in promoting epigenetic development of these circuits.

A "circuit exercise-maintenance function" in the adult. It has been postulated that maintenance of neural circuits requires use and that with increasing diversity of behaviors possible in more advanced animals REM sleep serves as a failsafe mode for ensuring activation and consequent maintenance of sensorimotor circuits. Crick and Mitchison (1983) suggested that the REM sleep activity involved removal of unwanted, "parasitic" modes of neural circuit processing.

Memory processing. Memories may be consolidated and processed during sleep. Hippocampal neurons that encode spatial location and that are activated during wakefulness are preferentially activated in subsequent REM periods compared with the non-wake-activated neurons; the inference is that "memories" are being related to other brain information (Winson 1990).

❑ PROSPECTS FOR THE FUTURE

As is detailed in Chapter 18 of this book, investigation of the sleep alterations associated with psychiatric disorders has proven to be one of the richer fields of clinical research. The vistas for future clinical applications appear even more promising as we come to know the basic neurobiology of both the REM and the NREM phases of sleep. It will become increasingly important for clinical researchers to know about these neurobiological advances to be able to pose the most relevant questions in their studies of disordered human sleep. The ultimate prospect is for a clinical science of psychiatry that is firmly rooted in basic neurobiology.

❑ REFERENCES

Borbély AA: A two process model of sleep regulation. Human Neurobiology 1:195–204, 1982

Borbély AA, Tobler I: Endogenous sleep-promoting substances and sleep regulation. Physiol Rev 69:605–670, 1989

Cohen D, Cuffin BN, Yunokuchi MS, et al: MEG versus EEG localization test using implanted sources in the human brain. Ann Neurol 28:811–817, 1990

Cotman CW, Bridges RJ, Taube JS, et al: The role of the NMDA receptor in central nervous system plasticity and pathology. Journal of NIH Research 1:65–74, 1989

Crick F, Mitchison G: The function of dream sleep. Nature 304:111–114, 1983

Darnell J, Lodish H, Baltimore D: Molecular Cell Biology, 2nd Edition. New York, Scientific American Books, 1990

Feinberg I, Thode HC, Chugani HT, et al: Gamma function describes maturational curves for delta wave amplitude, cortical metabolic rate and synaptic density. J Theor Biol 142:149–161, 1990

Freud S: The interpretation of dreams (1900), in Complete Psychological Works, Standard Edition, Vols 4 and 5. Translated and edited by Strachey J. London, Hogarth, 1966

Greene RW, McCarley RW: Cholinergic neurotransmission in the brainstem: implications for behavioral state control, in Brain Cholinergic Systems. Edited by Steriade M, Biesold D. New York, Oxford University Press, 1990, pp 224–235

Hayaishi O: Sleep-wake regulation by prostaglandins D_2 and E_2. J Biol Chem 263:14593–14596, 1988

Hobson JA, McCarley RW: The brain as a dream state generator: an activation-synthesis hypothesis of the dream process. Am J Psychiatry 134:1335–1348, 1977

Hodgkin AL, Huxley AF: A quantitative description of membrane current and its application to conduction and excitation in nerve. J Physiol 117:500–544, 1952

Jouvet M: What does a cat dream about? Trends Neurosci 2:15–16, 1979

Kandel E, Schwarz JH (eds): Principles of Neural Science. New York, Elsevier, 1985

Kronauer RE, Czeisler CA, Pilato SF, et al: Mathematical model of the human circadian system with two interacting oscillators. Am J Physiol 242 (Regulatory Integrative Comp Physiol 11):R3–R17, 1982

Krueger JM: Somnogenic activity of immune response modifiers. Trends Pharmacol Sci 11:122–126, 1990

Lipton SA, Kater SB: Neurotransmitter regulation of neuronal outgrowth, plasticity and survival. Trends Neurosci 12:265–270, 1989

Leubke JI, Greene RW, Semba K, et al: Serotonin hyperpolarizes cholinergic low threshold burst neurons in the rat laterodorsal tegmental nucleus in vitro. Proc Nat Acad Sci U S A (in press)

McCarley RW: The biology of dreaming sleep, in Principles and Practice of Sleep Medicine. Edited by Kryger MH, Roth T, Dement WC. New York, Saunders, 1989 pp 173–183

McCarley RW, Hobson JA: The neurobiological origins of psychoanalytic dream theory. Am J Psychiatry 134: 1211–1221, 1977

McCarley RW, Hoffman EA: REM sleep dreams and the activation-synthesis hypothesis. Am J Psychiatry 138: 904–912, 1981

McCarley RW, Massaquoi SG: A limit cycle mathematical model of the REM sleep oscillator system. Am J Physiol 251:R1011–R1029, 1986

McCarley RW, Faux SF, Shenton ME, et al: Event-related potentials in schizophrenia: their biological and clinical correlates and a new model of schizophrenic pathophysiology. Schiz Res 4:209–231, 1991

McCormick DA: Cholinergic and noradrenergic modulation of thalamocortical processing. Trends Neurosci 12: 215–221, 1989

McCormick DA: Cellular mechanisms of cholinergic control of neocortical and thalamic neuronal excitability, in Brain Cholinergic Systems. Edited by Steriade M, Biesold D. New York, Oxford University Press, 1990, pp 236–264

Masu M, Tanabe Y, Tsuchida K, et al: Sequence and expression of a metabotropic glutamate receptor. Nature 349:760–765, 1991

Mayer ML, Miller RJ: Excitatory amino acid receptors, second messengers and regulation of intracellular Ca^{2+} in mammalian neurons. Trends Pharmacol Sci 11:254–260, 1990

Montminy MR, Gonzalez GA, Yamamoto KK: Regulation of cAMP-inducible genes by CREB. Trends Neurosci 13:184–188, 1990

Morgan JI, Curran T: Stimulus-transcription coupling in neurons: role of cellular immediate-early genes. Trends Neurosci 12:459–462, 1989

Morgan TJ, Curran T: Stimulus-transcription coupling in the nervous system: involvement of the inducible proto-oncogenes fos and jun, in Annual Review of Neuroscience. Edited by Cowan WM, Shooter EM, Stevens CF, et al. Palo Alto, CA, Annual Reviews, 1991, pp 421–451

Mitani A, Ito K, Hallanger AH, et al: Cholinergic projections from the laterodorsal and pedunculopontine tegmental nuclei to the pontine gigantocellular tegmental field in the cat. Brain Res 451:397–402, 1988

Nauta WJH, Feirtag M: Fundamental Neuroanatomy. New York, WH Freeman, 1986

Nicoll RA: The coupling of neurotransmitter receptors to ion channels in the brain. Science 241:545–551, 1988

Smith CUM: Elements of Molecular Neurobiology. New York, Wiley, 1989

Stevens DS, Greene RW, McCarley RW: Pontine reticular formation neurons: excitatory amino acid receptor-mediated responses. European Sleep Research Society Abstracts 10:332, 1990

Steriade M, McCarley RW: Brainstem Control of Wakefulness and Sleep. New York, Plenum Press, 1990

Steriade M, Gloor P, Llinás RR, et al: Basic mechanisms of cerebral rhythmic activities. Electroencephalogr Clin Neurophysiol 76:481–508, 1990

Strogatz SH: The Mathematical Structure of the Human Sleep-Wake Cycle. New York, Springer-Verlag, 1986

Winson J: The meaning of dreams. Sci Am 263(November):86–96, 1990

Yatani A, Codina J, Brown AM, et al: Direct activation of mammalian atrial muscarinic potassium channels by GTP regulatory protein Gk. Science 235:207–211, 1987

❑ ANNOTATED REFERENCES

Darnell J, Lodish H, Baltimore D: Molecular Cell Biology, 2nd Edition. New York, Scientific American Books, 1990

Introductory text on molecular biology.

Kandel E, Schwarz JH (eds): Principles of Neural Science. New York, Elsevier, 1985

One of the most widely used neuroscience texts; especially useful for cellular neurophysiology.

Kryger MH, Roth T, Dement WC (eds): Principles and Practice of Sleep Medicine. New York, Saunders, 1989

Edited book, excellent text for sleep pathology. Covers descriptive aspects of sleep and other topics also.

Morgan TJ, Curran T: Stimulus-transcription coupling in the nervous system: involvement of the inducible proto-oncogenes fos and jun, in Annual Review of Neuroscience. Edited by Cowan WM, Shooter EM, Stevens CF, et al. Palo Alto, CA, Annual Reviews, 1991, pp 421-451

Recent summary of work on immediate early genes.

Nauta WJH, Feirtag M: Fundamental Neuroanatomy. New York, WH Freeman, 1986

Excellent introduction to the principles of neuroanatomy.

Regan D: Human Brain Electrophysiology. New York, Elsevier, 1989

Standard text on evoked potentials; emphasizes short-latency potentials.

Smith CUM: Elements of Molecular Neurobiology. New York, Wiley, 1989

Excellent text for the molecular neurobiological aspects of receptors and signaling.

Steriade M, McCarley RW: Brainstem Control of Wakefulness and Sleep. New York, Plenum Press, 1990

A comprehensive review, with an emphasis on neurophysiology and mechanisms; covers most of the topics in the second part of this review at an advanced level and has an extensive bibliography.

Chapter

3

Functional Neuroanatomy: Neuropsychological Correlates of Cortical and Subcortical Damage

Daniel Tranel, Ph.D.

DYSFUNCTION OF NEUROANATOMICAL systems in the human brain can lead to a wide variety of cognitive and behavioral manifestations, including changes in intellect, memory, language, perception, judgment and decision making, and personality. Recent advances in neuroanatomical analysis (H. Damasio et al. 1990) and neuropsychological measurement (e.g., see Chapter 5 this volume) have revealed a number of orderly relationships between neural and psychological systems. The precision of knowledge regarding such relationships has reached a level that was only hinted at in the work of two or three decades past. It is now possible to describe, with accuracy and detail, the salient neuropsychological correlates of damage to a number of neuroanatomical regions. This chapter focuses on a variety of such correlates and is keyed to regions that 1) are frequently involved in neurological disease, 2) have relatively clear demarcation from other neural sectors, and 3) have well-studied and specific neuropsychological correlates.

It is important to note at the outset that the discussion makes a number of assumptions that may place certain restrictions on the range of appli-

This work was supported by National Institute of Neurological Disorders and Stroke Grant P01-NS19632. The author thanks Dr. Antonio Damasio for his unwavering encouragement and support, and Dr. Hanna Damasio for her kind assistance with the figures.

cation of the principles and conclusions reviewed. It is assumed, unless otherwise indicated, that the human brain under consideration is endowed with conventional hemispheric dominance, that is, with speech and linguistic functions lateralized to the left hemisphere (e.g., Levy 1990). Furthermore, the discussion assumes normal acquisition and development of cognitive capacities; thus the principles may not apply to persons with developmental learning disabilities, inadequate educational opportunity, and the like.

Finally, the findings presented here are derived for the most part from research that has used the lesion method as the primary paradigm of scientific inquiry. This method (H. Damasio and Damasio 1989, 1990; see also Anderson et al. 1990b) is centered on cognitive experimentation in adult humans with focal brain lesions. In general, such lesions are caused by cerebrovascular disease, surgical ablation of nonmalignant cerebral tumors, some viral infections of the central nervous system, traumatic brain injury, and degenerative disease. Dating back to the innovative formulations of Geschwind (1965), there has been a resurgence of interest in the lesion method, and it now enjoys widespread acceptance and utilization. Much of this renewed popularity can be traced to the advent of modern neuroimaging techniques in the mid-1970s, beginning with computed tomography (CT) and continuing with the emergence of magnetic resonance imaging (MRI) in the early 1980s. These procedures have greatly increased the precision and reliability of neuroimaging definition and, together with increased sophistication of neuropsychological experimentation (e.g., Benton 1988), have allowed more powerful analysis of brain-behavior relationships and more detailed and elaborate theoretical specification (cf. A. R. Damasio 1989). Such advances have enhanced the viability of the lesion method as a technique for scientific inquiry and, in particular, have helped overcome the limitations of small subject groups and single case studies.

❑ THE TEMPORAL LOBES

This discussion focuses on several major subdivisions within the temporal lobe: 1) the posterior portion of the superior temporal gyrus (area 22), which, on the left side, forms the heart of what is traditionally known as *Wernicke's area*; 2) the lateral aspect inferior to the superior temporal gyrus, which comprises the human inferior temporal (IT) region (for the purposes of this discussion, this region is extended posteriorly to include the occipitotemporal junction and anteriorly to include the temporal pole); and 3) the mesial aspect, especially the hippocampal system formed by the entorhinal cortex, amygdala, and hippocampus proper. Figure 3–1 illustrates the neuroanatomical arrangement of these structures, highlighting the lateral/inferior region (which is divided into posterior and anterior components) and the mesial sector. Neuropsychological manifestations of the lateral/inferior and mesial subdivisions are summarized in Table 3–1 and are discussed in detail immediately below. The correlates of area 22 are considered later, together with other language-related regions.

Lateral/Inferior Temporal Region

Posterior component. As depicted in Figure 3–1, the posterior portion of the IT region comprises the posterior parts of the middle, inferior, and fourth temporal gyri, an area that corresponds primarily to cytoarchitectonic field 37. This discussion considers this region together with the posteriorly adjacent occipitotemporal junction, formed by the lower part of cytoarchitectonic fields 18 and 19 and the subjacent white matter. Lesions to posterior IT, especially bilateral ones, can produce unimodal, visually based disorders of recognition. When the lesions extend posteriorly into the inferior portion of the visual association cortices formed by areas 18 and 19, patients lose their ability to recognize visual stimuli at the level of unique identity. Because basic visual perception is unaltered, the presentation conforms to the classic notion of associative agnosia, that is, a normal percept stripped of its meaning (Teuber 1968). The disturbance can affect any number of visual stimuli that normally require recognition at a unique level (e.g., faces, buildings, and automobiles), but the best studied and most common form is agnosia for faces, known as prosopagnosia.

Prosopagnosia is hallmarked by an inability to recognize the identity of previously known faces and an inability to learn new ones. The defect is severe, as patients lose the ability to recognize faces of family members, close friends, and even their own face in a mirror, but it is confined to the visual channel, and exposure to the voice that belongs to

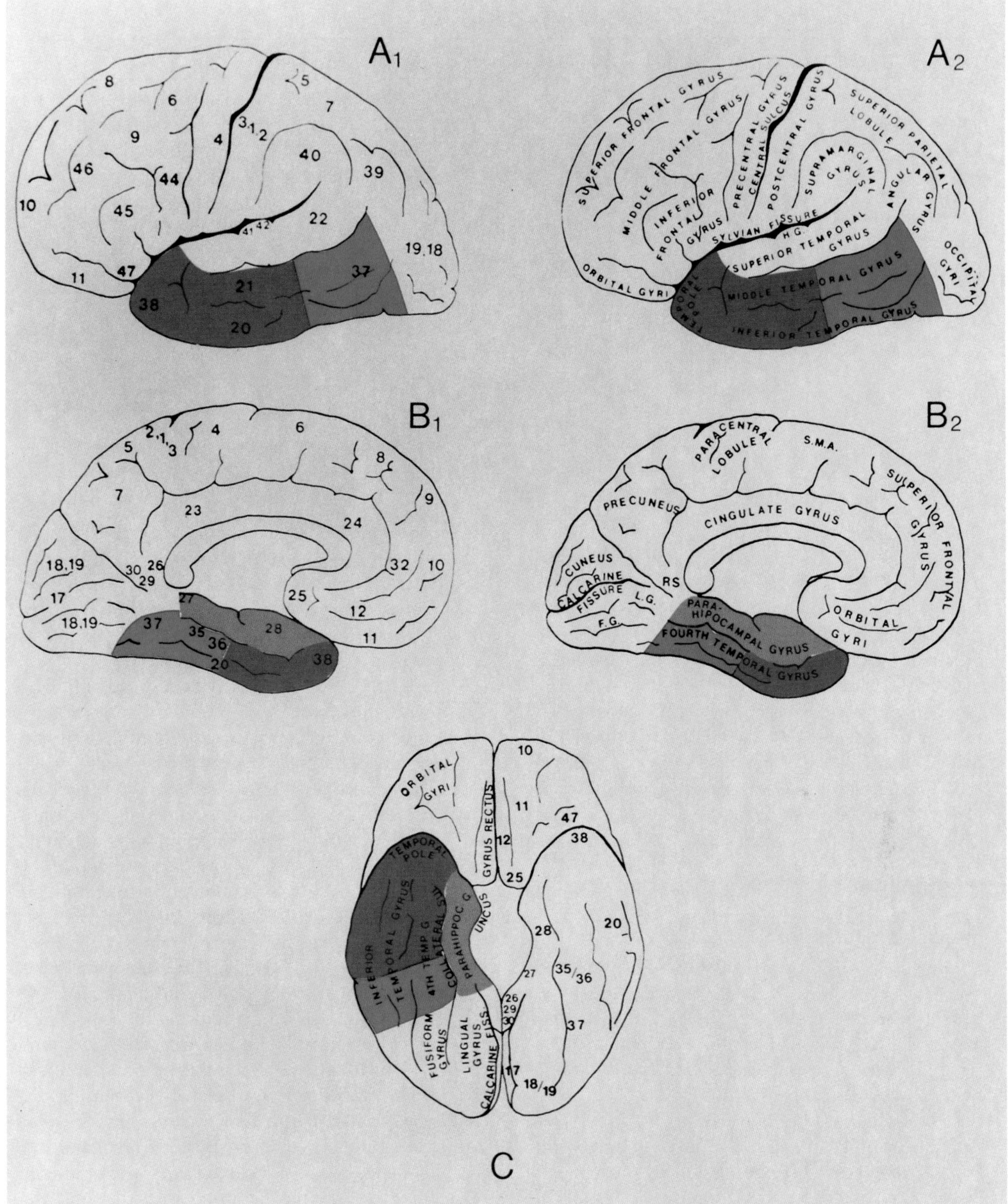

Figure 3–1. Three major subdivisions of the temporal lobe: posterior inferotemporal region (shown in green); anterior inferotemporal region (shown in red); mesial region (shown in yellow). Numbers corresponding to Brodmann's cytoarchitectonic areas are depicted on A_1, B_1, and the right side (left hemisphere) of *C*, and standard gyri names are shown on corresponding A_2, B_2, and the left side (right hemisphere) of *C*. Lateral (A_1 and A_2), mesial (B_1 and B_2), and inferior (*C*) views are represented.

TABLE 3–1. NEUROPSYCHOLOGICAL MANIFESTATIONS OF TEMPORAL LOBE LESIONS

	Hemispheric side of lesion		
Region	*Left*	*Right*	*Bilateral*
Lateral/inferior			
Posterior	"Deep" prosopagnosia; mild defects in category-level object recognition	Transient prosopagnosia; mild defects in category-level object recognition	Severe, permanent prosopagnosia; associative visual agnosia; severe defects in category-level object recognition
Anterior	Anomia; restricted naming impairments; defective proper naming	Anomia for facial expressions	Anomia; retrograde amnesia
Mesial	Anterograde amnesia for verbal material	Anterograde amnesia for nonverbal material	Severe anterograde amnesia for verbal and nonverbal material

the unrecognized face will elicit prompt and accurate recognition. For most persons with prosopagnosia, the ability to recognize facial expressions and to judge gender and estimate age from face information is well preserved (Bruyer et al. 1983; Davidoff and Landis 1990; Tranel et al. 1988). Also, many prosopagnosic individuals remain capable of recognizing identity based on visual but nonfacial information, such as characteristics of gait or posture (Damasio et al. 1982b, 1990b). Some persons with prosopagnosia have impaired perception of texture (Newcombe 1979), and defects in color perception are common (Damasio et al. 1980; Meadows 1974a).

Full-blown "associative" prosopagnosia is nearly always associated with bilateral lesions to posterior IT and the inferior sector of fields 18 and 19 (Benton 1990; Damasio et al. 1982b, 1990b; Meadows 1974b). An MRI of a patient with this type of prosopagnosia is presented in Figure 3–2. Prosopagnosia following unilateral right-sided lesions nearly always has a substantial perceptual component, thus constituting a more "apperceptive" form of the condition (see section on Apperceptive Visual Agnosia below). Unilateral occipitotemporal lesions usually do not cause severe and lasting prosopagnosia, although such lesions may cause significant disturbances in face recognition. On the left, such lesions can produce a partial recognition defect that has been termed *deep prosopagnosia* (Damasio et al. 1988), in which target faces are misidentified as someone who is very similar to the correct person in terms of gender, age, or activity (e.g., recognizing Betty Grable as Marilyn Monroe, or recognizing Magic Johnson as Michael Jordan). Right-sided occipitotemporal lesions may cause slow and erratic face recognition, but not pervasive prosopagnosia (Damasio et al. 1990b).

In addition to disturbances of recognition of unique visual stimuli, lesions to IT can also produce impairments in the visual recognition of stimuli as members of a specific category. For example, when confronted with the picture of a fox or lion, patients may indicate that it is an "animal," but the specific type will elude them. Shown a robin, a patient might respond "bird." This impairment goes beyond the identity recognition defect of prosopagnosia and extends to the level of basic objects, that is, the patients can only recognize the superordinate category to which the entity belongs, but not the subordinate, basic object level (as defined by Rosch et al. 1976). Evidence available thus far indicates that the defect is most pronounced with bilateral IT lesions and less severe (albeit still present) with unilateral left- or right-sided lesions. An especially intriguing discovery is that the impairment does not affect all types of entities equally, but instead is related in a general sense to the conceptual-lexical category to which entities belong. For example, several laboratories have reported patients who have far greater recognition impairment for natural entities such as animals and fruits or vegetables, and much less impairment for manmade entities such as tools and utensils (Damasio 1990; Damasio et al. 1990e; Farah

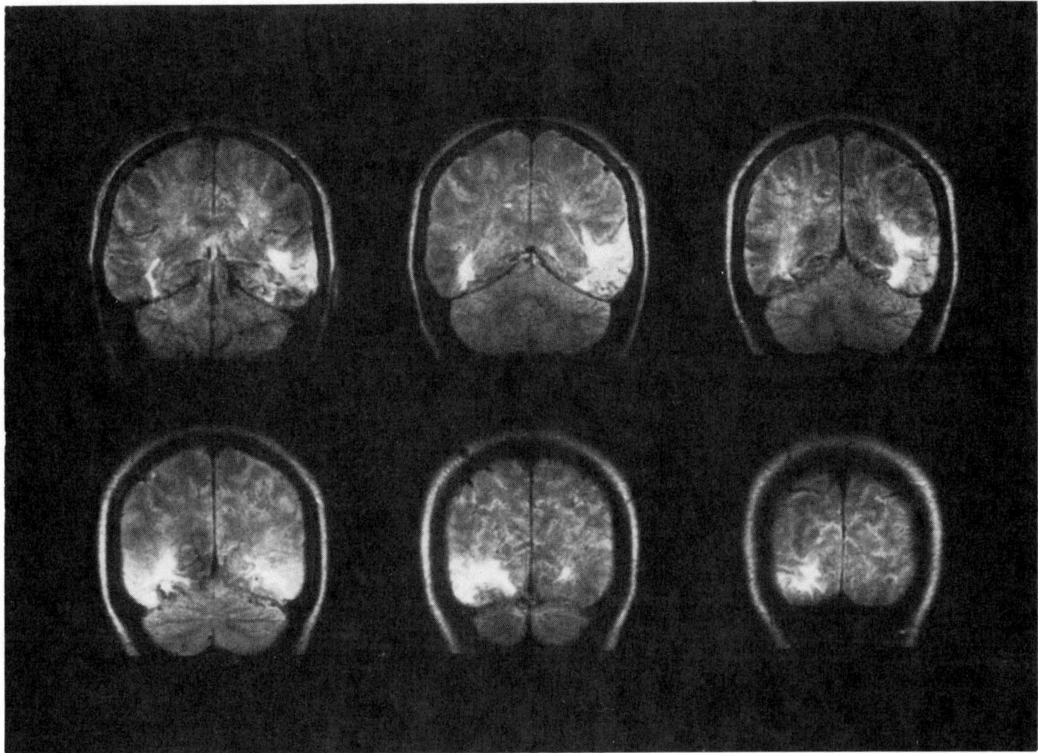

Figure 3–2. T2-weighted magnetic resonance image (MRI) of a 67-year-old, right-handed woman, which shows bilateral occipitotemporal lesions (showing as white, or "bright" signal). In these coronal cuts, the left hemisphere is on the right, and the most anterior cut is in the upper left-hand corner of the figure. The woman developed severe, permanent prosopagnosia after sustaining these lesions.

et al. 1989; Warrington and McCarthy 1987; Warrington and Shallice 1984; Young et al. 1989).

Anterior component. The anterior component of the lateral/inferior temporal lobe (Figure 3–1) is formed by the anterior portion of the middle, inferior, and fourth temporal gyri (comprised by cytoarchitectonic fields 21 and 20), together with the temporal pole (area 38). For many decades, the prevailing wisdom has been that lesions to the left anterolateral temporal lobe, provided they did not encroach into mesial structures or too far posteriorly, would not cause memory defects or deficits in speech or language (e.g., Penfield and Roberts 1959). Although an occasional report appeared indicating that some of these patients may develop anomia (e.g., Heilman et al. 1972; Stafiniak et al. 1990), the consensus has been that even naming impairments were rare following anterior left temporal lesions (Hermann and Wyler 1988). Recent observations, however, have cast an entirely new light on the situation, and it is now abundantly clear that left anterolateral temporal lesions do cause naming deficits, although such defects may be restricted to certain conceptual-lexical categories (Damasio 1990; Damasio et al. 1990e; Tranel 1991a). Defects in other aspects of language operation are not present; in particular, repetition is unaffected, and grammatical structure is entirely normal.

Confrontation naming defects, and even category-specific anomia, have been described in a variety of patients (Hart et al. 1985; McCarthy and Warrington 1988; Miceli et al. 1991; Semenza and Zettin 1988), but the neural correlates of such defects have remained elusive. Recent evidence, however, has firmly established the left anterolateral temporal region as a cortical area subserving access to the reference lexicon (Damasio et al. 1990e; Graff-

Radford et al. 1990a). Depending on the precise location of damage within this region, naming defects may be confined in relatively specific fashion to certain conceptual-lexical categories; patients may have highly defective naming of natural entities (animals and fruits or vegetables), whereas naming of manmade entities (tools and utensils) may be relatively or entirely spared. Additional fractionations have been reported. For example, patients may lose the ability to produce proper names, while preserving the capacity to produce common names (Semenza and Zettin 1989). Based on available evidence, the neural correlate for the selective disruption of proper naming appears to be the most anterior sector of the left temporal lobe, that is, area 38 in the temporal pole (Damasio et al. 1990e). Figure 3–3 shows a depiction of a left anterior/inferior temporal lobe lesion in a patient with a severe naming impairment.

Neuropsychological correlates of damage to the right anterolateral temporal region are less well understood. In one recent case with this type of lesion (Rapcsak et al. 1989), the patient had a selective defect in naming facial expressions such as happiness, sadness, surprise, and fear. The patient did not have difficulty naming other entities, such as objects and actions, and there was no defect in proper naming (famous faces and buildings). In additon, the patient did not have an impairment in recognition, even with regard to the emotional facial expressions that were not correctly named. For example, the patient could match facial expressions to emotional prosody and to emotional scenes at a normal level.

Other recent observations have indicated that the right anterolateral temporal region may play a crucial role in retrograde episodic memory (i.e., in the retrieval of entities and events that are highly specific and unique to an individual's autobiography). Several patients have been studied, for example, in whom there is marked retrograde amnesia in connection with lesions largely circumscribed to right mesial and nonmesial temporal lobe structures (A. R. Damasio, D. Tranel, and H. Damasio, unpublished observations, October 1990; P. J. Eslinger, N. Butters, and A. R. Damasio, personal communica-

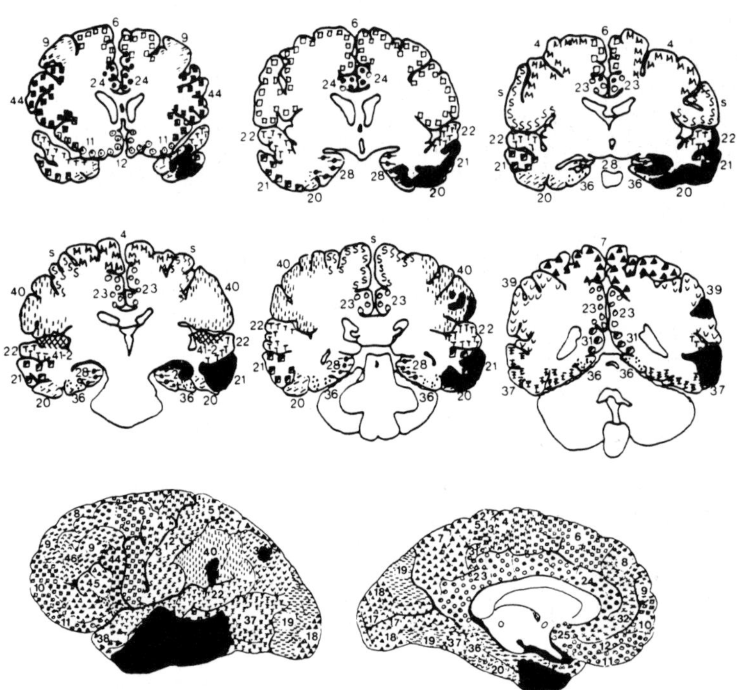

Figure 3–3. Depiction of the lesion of a 22-year-old, right-handed man. The area of damage in the left anterior/inferior temporal lobe is marked in black on the coronal sections (left hemisphere on the right), and on the lateral and mesial views of the left hemisphere. The man had severe anomia, associated with this lesion.

tion, February 10, 1991). The role of mesial temporal structures in retrograde memory has also been explored in nonhuman primates (Horel 1978; Murray et al. 1988; Zola-Morgan and Squire 1986; Zola-Morgan et al. 1988).

Mesial Temporal Region

The mesial sector of the temporal lobe is formed by the parahippocampal gyrus (cytoarchitectonic areas 28 and 27), and by the adjoining hippocampal system including the amygdala, entorhinal cortex, and hippocampus proper (Figure 3–1). Since the landmark report by Scoville and Milner (1957) on patient H. M., who became severely amnesic after bilateral mesial temporal lobe resection for control of intractable seizures, the mesial aspect of the temporal lobes has been linked unequivocally to memory function. More than three decades of research on H. M. (for summary, see Corkin 1984; also see Gabrieli et al. 1988; Sagar et al. 1990), and studies in similar patients, have demonstrated that the hippocampus in particular is critical for the acquisition of new information (i.e., for anterograde memory). Patient R. B. (Zola-Morgan et al. 1986), who had pathologically confirmed bilateral lesions limited to the CA_1 sector of the hippocampus, is another important example of the marked anterograde amnesia that can occur following circumscribed bilateral hippocampal lesions. Another source of evidence comes from patient Boswell (Damasio et al. 1985a), who has bilateral damage to the entire mesial sector of the temporal lobes (hippocampus, amygdala, and entorhinal cortex), and also nonmesial damage (in areas 38, 20, 21, and 37). Boswell's lesions are depicted in Figure 3–4. In the anterograde compartment, Boswell's memory profile is quite similar to the patterns reported for H. M. and R. B.; however, on the retrograde side, unlike H. M. and R. B., Boswell also has a severe impairment (Damasio et al. 1985a, 1987, 1989c; Haist et al. 1990).

With respect to the nature of the amnesia associated with hippocampal damage, several relation-

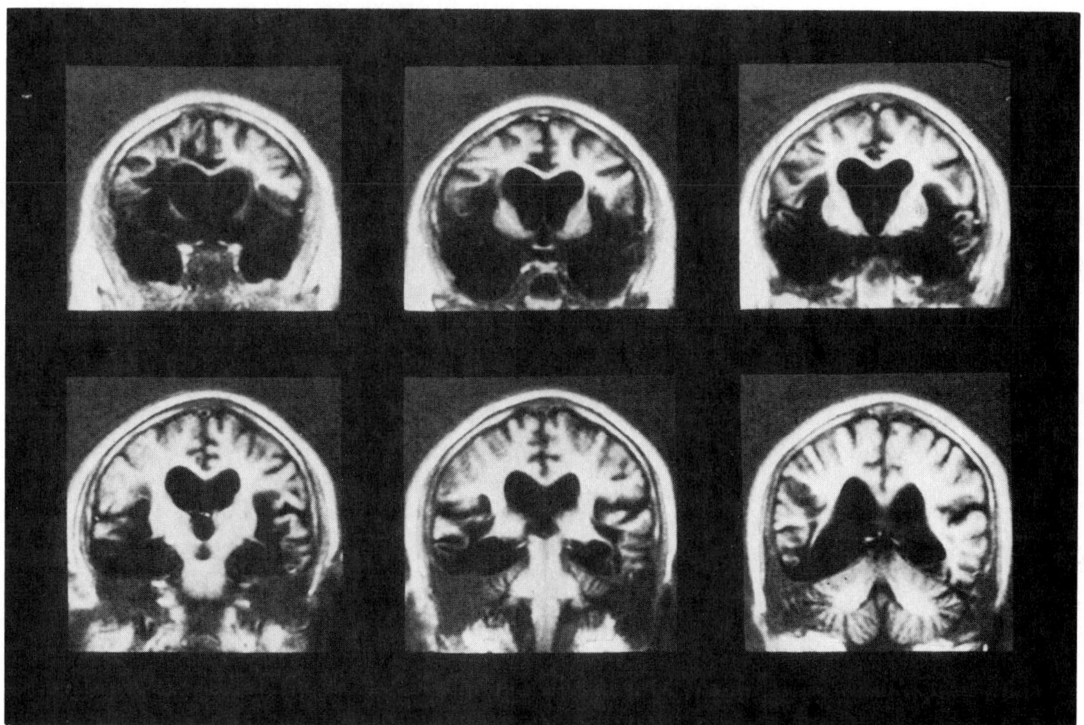

Figure 3–4. T1-weighted magnetic resonance image (MRI) of patient Boswell, who developed severe global amnesia after suffering herpes simplex encephalitis. In these coronal sections, the left hemisphere is on the right, and the most anterior cut is in the upper left-hand corner of the figure. The lesions, which show as black areas, include the anterior temporal regions (amygdala, hippocampus, parahippocampal gyrus, and temporal pole [area 38]), and the anterior portion of the inferior, middle, and superior temporal gyri (areas 20, 21, and anterior 22).

ships have been firmly established. First, there is a consistent relationship between the side of the lesion and the type of learning impairment. Specifically, damage to the left-hippocampal system produces an amnesic syndrome that affects verbal material (e.g., spoken words and written material), but spares nonverbal material; conversely, damage to the right-hippocampal system affects nonverbal material (e.g., complex visual and auditory patterns), but spares verbal material (Frisk and Milner 1990; Milner 1968, 1972; Smith and Milner 1989; Tranel 1991a). A second point is that the hippocampal system does not appear to play a role in the learning of perceptuomotor skills or what is known as *nondeclarative memory*. Patient H. M., for example, can learn skills such as mirror drawing and mirror reading (Corkin 1965, 1968), even though he has no recall of the situation in which the learning of those skills took place. Similar findings have been reported for patient Boswell (Damasio et al. 1989c); in fact, not only can Boswell acquire perceptuomotor skills such as rotor pursuit and mirror tracing at a normal level, but he retains those skills for many years after the initial learning, despite the fact that he cannot recall any shred of knowledge regarding the circumstances of the learning situations.

Another source of evidence comes from patients with Alzheimer's disease. In the early and middle stages of the disease, patients with Alzheimer's disease develop a marked impairment of anterograde memory that (as in patients H. M. and Boswell) spares the learning of nondeclarative information such as new perceptuomotor skills (Eslinger and Damasio 1986; Mickel et al. 1986). The neural hallmark in patients with Alzheimer's disease is damage to the hippocampal system (Hyman et al. 1984; Van Hoesen and Damasio 1987; Van Hoesen et al. 1986).

A final comment pertains to the role of the hippocampus in the retrieval of old information (retrograde memory). Milner (1972) argued that the hippocampus was not needed at all for the retrieval of remote memories. Findings for H. M. and R. B., neither of whom had defects in the retrograde compartment, support this contention. Patient Boswell is also consistent with this notion, inasmuch as the severe defects he shows in the retrograde compartment have been ascribed to his extensive nonmesial, anterior temporal lobe damage (Damasio et al. 1985a, 1989c). However, a recent patient studied by Victor and Agamanolis (1990) was noted to have both anterograde and retrograde defects, in connection with a lesion that was reportedly confined to the mesial temporal lobes. Nonetheless, the weight of the evidence points to the conclusion that the hippocampal system is not the principal repository for old memories.

The role of the amygdala in memory has been a source of controversy. Studies in nonhuman primates have yielded conflicting results, with some laboratories reporting that the amygdala is critical for normal learning (Mishkin 1978; Murray 1990; Murray and Mishkin 1984, 1985, 1986), whereas others maintain that the amygdala does not play a crucial role (Zola-Morgan et al. 1989). Results in the few human cases available are also equivocal. In one recent case, there was a memory defect in connection with pathology circumscribed to both amygdala (Tranel and Hyman 1990). Others, however, have not observed memory defects in patients with bilateral amygdala damage (e.g., Lee et al. 1988).

❑ THE OCCIPITAL LOBES

The neuroanatomical arrangement of structures in and near the occipital lobes is depicted in Figure 3–5. On the lateral aspect of the hemispheres, the occipital lobes comprise the visual association cortices in areas 18 and 19. These areas continue in the mesial aspect. The mesial sector also includes the primary visual cortices (area 17), formed by the cortex immediately above and below the calcarine fissure. For purposes of establishing neuropsychological correlates of the occipital lobes, the region can be subdivided in the vertical plane at the level of the calcarine fissure so that dorsal (superior) and ventral (inferior) components can be designated (Figure 3–5). Each of these sectors is dealt with in turn below. Neuropsychological manifestations of occipital lobe lesions are summarized in Table 3–2.

Dorsal Component

The dorsal component of the occipital lobes comprises the primary visual cortex superior to the calcarine fissure (area 17) and the superior portion of the visual association cortices (areas 18 and 19). For the purposes of this discussion, this region is considered in combination with the anteriorly adjacent parietal areas, including the posterior part of the superior parietal lobule (area 7) and the posterior part of the angular gyrus (area 39) (Figure 3–5). When situated in the primary visual cortex of area

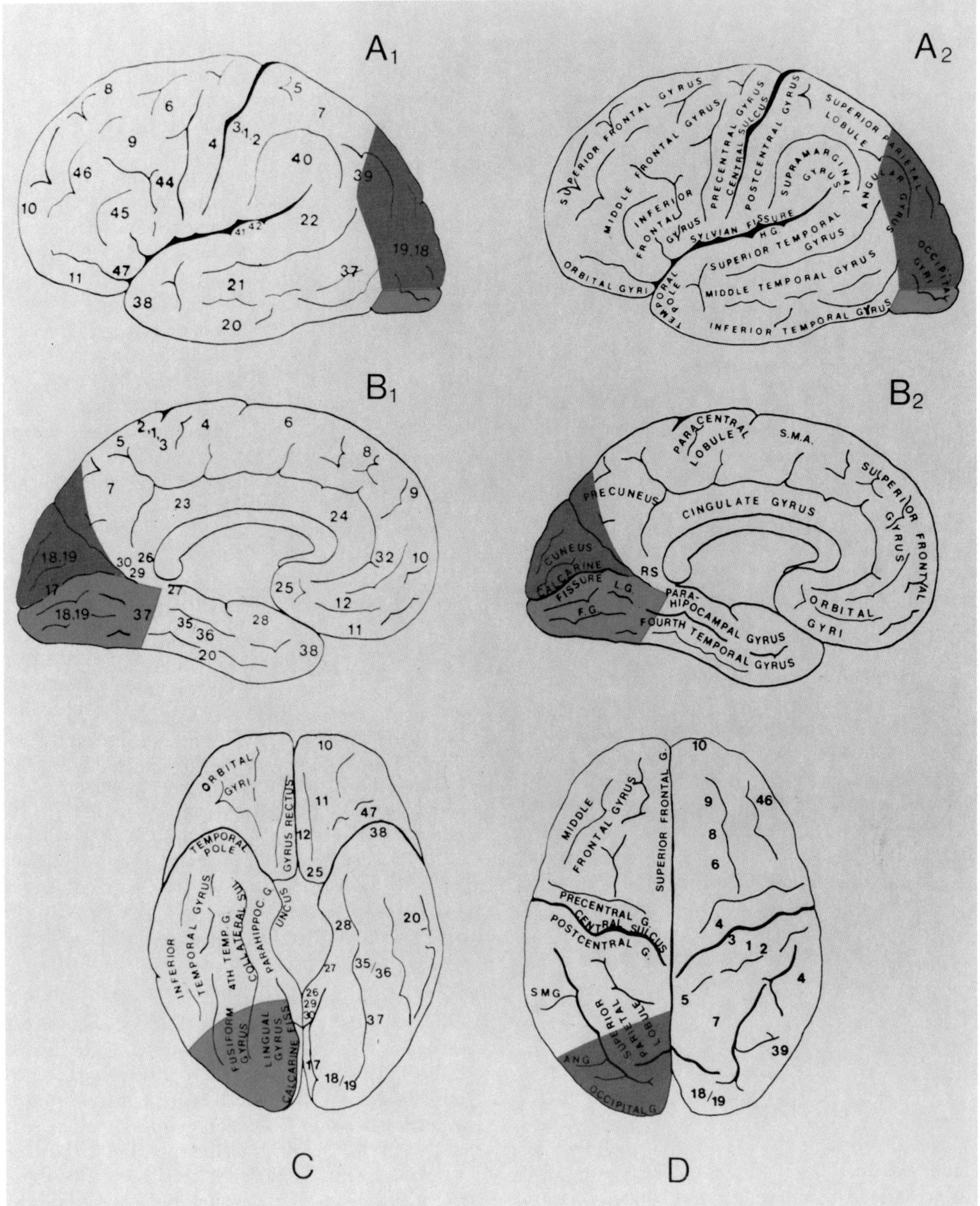

Figure 3–5. Two major subdivisions of the occipital lobe: dorsal (superior) component (shown in red); ventral (inferior) component (shown in green). Numbers corresponding to Brodmann's cytoarchitectonic areas are depicted on A_1, B_1, and the right side (left hemisphere) of C and D, and standard gyri names are shown on corresponding A_2, B_2, and the left side (right hemisphere) of C and D. Lateral (A_1 and A_2), mesial (B_1 and B_2), inferior (C), and superior (D) views are represented.

TABLE 3–2. NEUROPSYCHOLOGICAL MANIFESTATIONS OF OCCIPITAL LOBE LESIONS

	Hemispheric side of lesion		
Region	*Left*	*Right*	*Bilateral*
Dorsal	Partial or mild Balint's syndrome	Partial or mild Balint's syndrome	Balint's syndrome (visual disorientation, ocular apraxia, optic ataxia); defective motion perception; astereopsis
Ventral	Right hemiachromatopsia; "pure" alexia	Left hemiachromatopsia; apperceptive visual agnosia (especially when dorsal sector of right occipital cortices is also damaged); defective facial imagery	Full-field achromatopsia; associative visual agnosia; prosopagnosia

17 and/or its connections, lesions to the dorsal sector of the occipital region lead to a loss of form vision (i.e., blindness) in the inferior visual field contralateral to the lesion, and bilateral lesions of this type will produce an inferior altitudinal hemianopia.

A more intriguing presentation, however, occurs when the lesions spare the primary visual cortex and involve the association cortices of areas 18 and 19. When such lesions encroach into the adjacent parietal region comprised by areas 39 and 7, patients commonly develop a constellation of defects known as *Balint's syndrome.* A CT of a patient with this type of presentation is shown in Figure 3–6. Balint's syndrome is based on the presence of three components: visual disorientation (also known as *simultanagnosia*), ocular apraxia (also known as *psychic gaze paralysis*), and optic ataxia. The key constituent in the syndrome, however, is visual disorientation, and there is considerable variability in the emphasis that is placed on the other components (Damasio 1985; Newcombe and Ratcliff 1989).

Visual disorientation. Visual disorientation (simultanagnosia) can be conceptualized as an inability to attend to more than a very limited sector of the visual field at any given moment. Patients report that they can see clearly in only a small part of the field, the rest being "out of focus" and in a sort of "fog." The sector of clear vision, moreover, is unstable and may shift without warning in any direction, so that patients experience a literal "jumping about" of their visual perception. Such patients are incapable of constructing a spatially coherent visual field, and they cannot follow trajectories of stimuli or place stimuli in their proper locations in space. Because perception of motion is often impaired, such patients may fail to notice objects that have moved about in their visual field or fail to recognize the meaning of movements they have otherwise perceived correctly. For example, patients may fail to recognize a familiar gait or stride or to understand pantomime (Damasio et al. 1989b, 1990a). Isolated disturbances of motion detection, however, are quite rare; one of the few such cases was described by Zihl et al. (1983). Patients with visual disorientation can perceive color and shape normally, so long as objects are appreciated within a clear sector of the visual field.

Ocular apraxia. Ocular apraxia (psychic gaze paralysis) is a deficit of visual scanning. It consists of an inability to direct gaze voluntarily toward a stimulus located in peripheral vision, so as to bring it into central vision. Thus patients fail to direct saccades toward stimuli that have appeared in the panorama of their visual fields, or they produce saccades that are inaccurate and miss the target. Ocular apraxia is not necessary for the development of visual disorientation (Girotti et al. 1982; Newcombe and Ratcliff 1989; Rizzo and Hurtig 1987), although it always occurs together with either visual disorientation or optic ataxia (Damasio 1985).

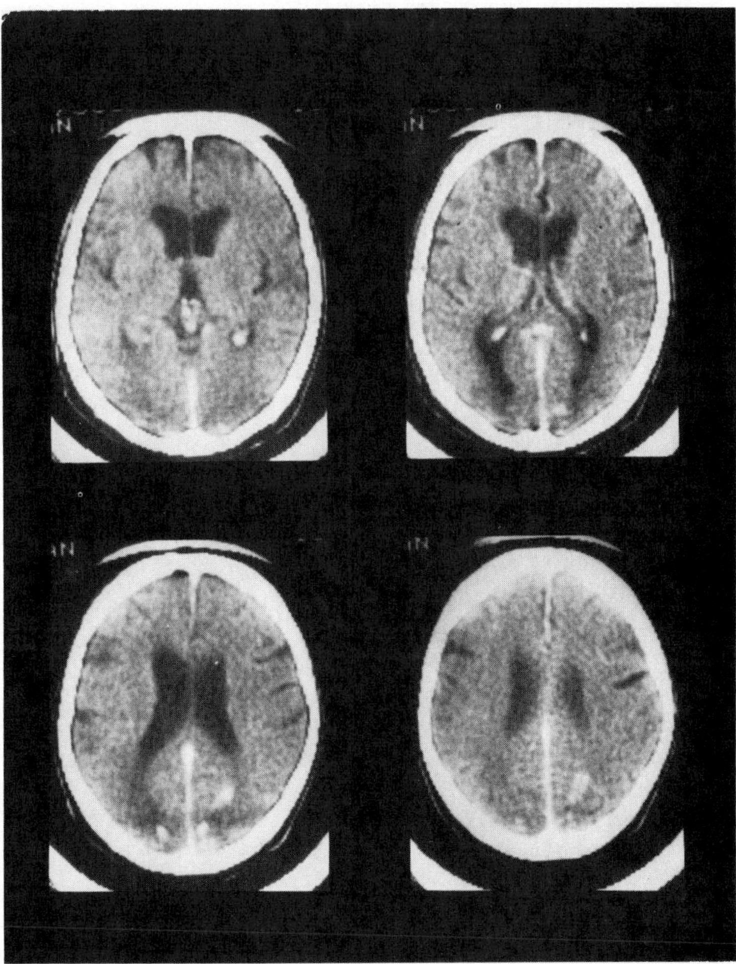

Figure 3–6. Contrast-enhanced computed tomography (CT) scan of a 74-year-old, right-handed man, showing bilateral lesions (areas of increased density) in the superior occipital region, corresponding to the supracalcarine visual association cortices. The man developed a complex visual disturbance (Balint's syndrome) in connection with these lesions.

Optic ataxia. Optic ataxia is a disturbance of visually guided reaching behavior. Patients are not able to point accurately at a target under visual guidance (e.g., they cannot point precisely to the examiner's fingertip or to items such as a cup or coin). Interestingly, pointing to targets on their own body does not pose a problem, as this can be accomplished on the basis of somatosensory information. Also, the patients have no difficulty pointing to sound sources (Damasio and Benton 1979). Optic ataxia can occur in isolation, particularly when lesions are at the border of the occipital and parietal regions, or in the parietal region exclusively.

As alluded to above, the full Balint's syndrome is generally associated with bilateral occipitoparietal lesions, although unilateral lesions can also produce the syndrome, especially when they are on the right. When lesions are confined to the superior occipital cortices without extension into the parietal region, visual disorientation is likely to occur without associated ocular apraxia or optic ataxia. The defects in motion perception that are frequent in patients with Balint's syndrome are probably related to damage in the lower-parietal/lateral-occipital region (i.e., in the region formed by area 39). Many patients with Balint's syndrome have an impairment of stereopsis, that is, the process of recovery of depth from visual information dependent on binocular visual interaction, although complete astereopsis is seen only in the setting of bilateral lesions (Rizzo 1989; Rizzo and Hurtig 1987).

Ventral Component

The ventral component of the occipital lobes comprises the primary visual cortex immediately below the calcarine fissure (area 17) and the inferior portion of the visual association cortices (areas 18 and 19). The latter component corresponds to the lingual and fusiform gyri (see Figure 3–5; C). For the discussion presented below, this region is considered together with the posterior part of area 37 (i.e., the occipitotemporal junction). Damage to primary visual cortex and/or its connections in the inferior bank of the calcarine fissure produces a form vision defect (blindness) in the contralateral superior visual field. Damage to nearby structures may spare vision for form, either partly or entirely, while producing a number of other higher-order visual impairments. Several examples are elaborated below, including acquired achromatopsia, apperceptive visual agnosia, and acquired alexia.

Acquired achromatopsia. Acquired (or "central") achromatopsia is a disorder of color perception involving all or part of the visual field, with preservation of form vision, caused by damage to the inferior visual association cortex and/or its subjacent white matter (Damasio 1985; Damasio et al. 1980; Meadows 1974a). Patients lose color vision in a quadrant, a hemifield, or the entire visual field. The loss may be partial, whereby patients complain that colors appear "washed out" or "dirty," or entire, whereby all forms are seen in shades of black and white. However, perception of form, per se, is unaltered, and the depth and motion perception are also normal. It is important to note that the disorder is acquired, that is, it is not a hereditary (retinal) disorder of color vision, such as the red-green color blindness that is common among males; thus the designation *central achromatopsia.* Also, the inability to name colors is not part of the disorder; such patients have, instead, *color anomia.* Nor is achromatopsia a disturbance of color association (a disorder known as *color agnosia*); achromatopsic patients can answer prompts such as "the color of grass is _____ [green]," or "the color of blood is ______ [red]."

The "purest" form of the disorder is a left hemiachromatopsia associated with a unilateral right occipitotemporal lesion, unaccompanied by other neuropsychological defects. A comparable lesion on the left will produce right hemiachromatopsia but most of those patients will typically also have alexia (see below). A CT of the latter type of patient is shown in Figure 3–7. As the case in Figure 3–7 illustrates, an upper quadrant form vision defect is generally encountered in the colorless hemifield. This is because the occipitotemporal lesion generally disrupts optic radiations or encroaches into primary visual cortex on the inferior bank of the calcarine fissure. Bilateral occipitotemporal lesions may cause full-field achromatopsia, and such patients frequently also manifest associative visual agnosia (especially prosopagnosia).

A recent study reported by Damasio et al. (1989a) pinpointed even further the neural correlates of achromatopsia. Specifically, achromatopsia was associated with lesions to the middle third of the lingual gyrus and with infracalcarine lesions that damaged the white matter immediately behind the posterior tip of the lateral ventricle. Lesions confined to the fusiform gyrus or to the white matter beneath the ventricle did not produce achromatopsia. These findings are consistent with recent data from positron-emission tomography (PET) studies in control subjects (Corbetta et al. 1990; Lueck et al. 1989), which have suggested a similar "color center." Additionally, the results support the extensive body of work in nonhuman primates, which has indicated that separate cellular channels within area 17 are differently dedicated to the processing of color, form, and motion (Hubel and Livingstone 1987; Livingstone and Hubel 1984, 1987, 1988) and that some visual association cortices have an important specialization for color processing (Van Essen and Maunsell 1983; Zeki 1973).

Apperceptive visual agnosia. Apperceptive agnosia was originally attributed to the disturbed integration of otherwise normally perceived components of a stimulus (Lissauer 1890), and in general the concept has persisted as a useful designation for recognition defects in which there is a substantial perceptual component (e.g., Bauer and Rubens 1985). In associative agnosia, perception is entirely or mostly normal. Both conditions involve defective recognition of familiar stimuli. Distinguishing apperceptive and associative agnosia as involving primarily perceptual and mnestic factors, respec-

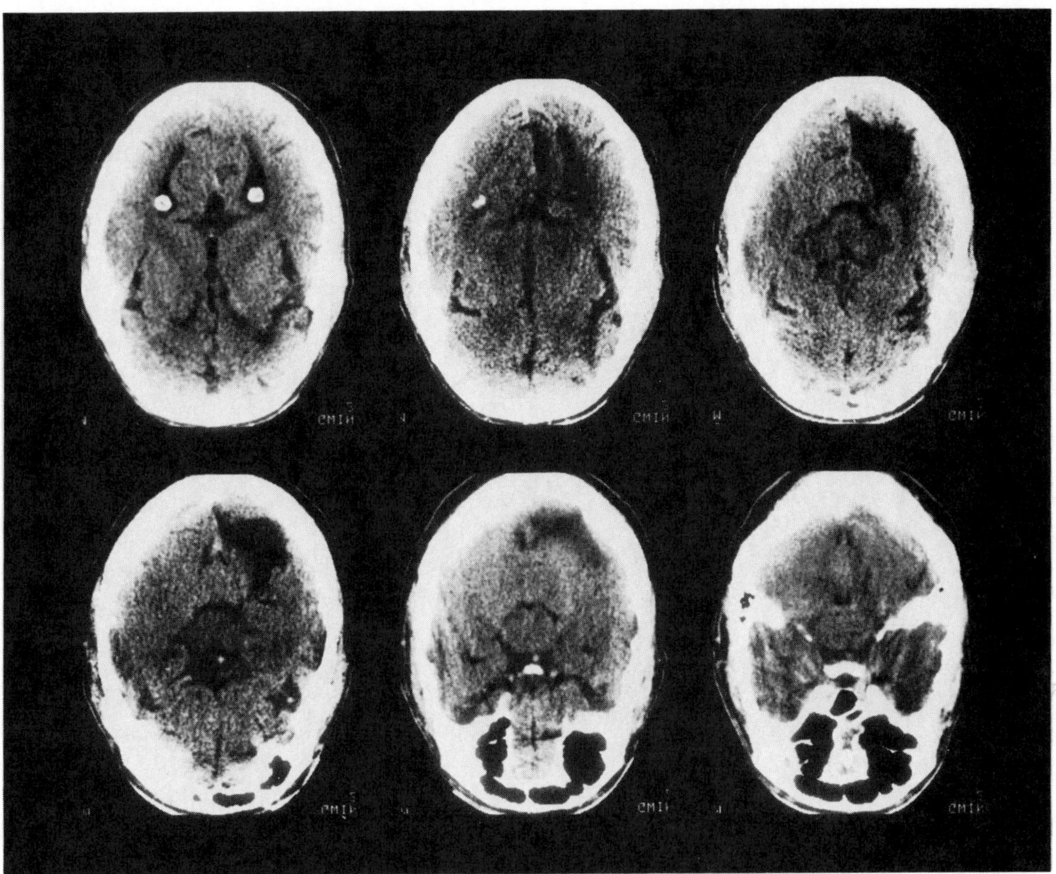

Figure 3–7. Computed tomography (CT) scan of a 67-year-old, right-handed man, showing a lesion (area of decreased density) in the left infracalcarine visual association cortices. The man had a right superior quadrantanopia. In the lower right field, form vision was normal, but he was unable to see color (achromatopsia). He also had acquired (or "pure") alexia.

tively, is of practical value, provided it is understood that perception and recognition are not discrete processes but rather operate on a physiological continuum.

A common form of apperceptive agnosia occurs in the visual modality, in connection with right-sided lesions involving both the inferior and superior sectors of the posterior visual association cortices. Figure 3–8 depicts the lesion of a man with apperceptive prosopagnosia. Several authors have described cases of prosopagnosia following this type of lesion (Damasio et al. 1989b, 1990b; De Renzi 1986; Landis et al. 1986; Michel et al. 1986; Sergent and Villemure 1989). Patients with apperceptive visual agnosia have difficulty perceiving all parts of a visual array simultaneously and in generating the image of a whole entity, given a part. When shown a part of a house, or a car, the patient will be unable to imagine the whole object to which the part must belong and thus fail to recognize the stimulus. A related defect is the inability to assemble parts of a model into a meaningful ensemble (e.g., the patient may be unable to assemble various face parts to form a spatially correct whole). This type of defect has been described in connection with faces (Damasio et al. 1990b) and other objects (Davidoff and Donnelly, in press). Many such patients also report an inability to image faces (Farah 1989). Unlike patients with associative prosopagnosia, patients with apperceptive agnosia will fail many standard neuropsychological tests of visual perception, such as matching differently lit photographs of faces

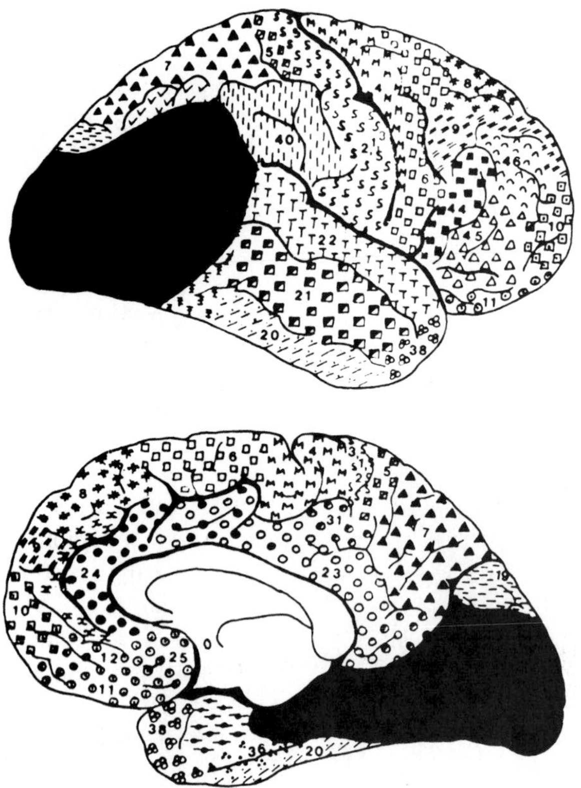

Figure 3–8. Depiction of the lesion of a 68-year-old, right-handed man who suffered an infarction that destroyed right posterior parietal and occipital cortices. Note that the lesion (marked in black) includes visual association cortices both above and below the calcarine fissure. The man had apperceptive prosopagnosia.

and mentally assembling puzzle pieces to form a whole object.

Acquired alexia. Lesions that disconnect both visual association cortices from the dominant, language-related temporoparietal cortices can produce a complete or partial impairment in reading, a condition known as *acquired* (or "pure") *alexia.* Acquired alexia can be caused by a single lesion in the region behind, beneath, and under the occipital horn of the left lateral ventricle, by damaging pathways en route from the callosum and pathways en route from the left visual association cortex (Damasio and Damasio 1983). Another setting is the combination of a lesion in the corpus callosum, which disconnects right-to-left visual information transfer, and a lesion in the left occipital lobe, which disconnects left visual association cortex from left language cortex (e.g., Geschwind 1965; Greenblatt 1983). Such lesions are likely to produce a right hemianopia, and this sign is a frequent, although not invariable (e.g., Greenblatt 1973), accompaniment of pure alexia.

The "purity" of the condition stems from the fact that patients with these lesions do not develop disturbances in writing or other aspects of speech and language operation, which separates this type of alexia from the types of reading defects that are common in aphasic patients (Benson 1979; Benson et al. 1971). In this sense, pure alexia can be construed as a disturbance of visual pattern recognition. Pure alexia is also known as *alexia without agraphia,* or *pure word blindness.*

Patients with pure alexia are unable to read most words and sentences, and in severe cases even reading of single letters is impaired. The problem is not one of visual acuity; the fact that the patient can see the sentences, words, and letters he or she cannot read can be readily demonstrated by having the patient copy those stimuli, a task that will be executed normally. Thus most patients with pure alexia have normal visual acuity, although a quadrantanopia or hemianopia may be present (as mentioned above), and most have normal recognition of nonverbal visual stimuli such as objects and faces.

❑ THE PARIETAL LOBES

On the lateral aspect of the cerebral hemisphere, the parietal lobes comprise a large expanse of cortex that is bounded by the central (Rolandic) sulcus anteriorly, the fissure of Sylvius inferiorly, and the occipital cortices posteriorly (Figure 3–9). It is important to maintain a clear distinction between the right and left hemispheres, as many correlates of the parietal region are highly lateralized. In the discussion below, no strict demarcation is implemented with regard to neighboring regions because many of the neuropsychological manifestations to be considered here are connected to regions that are both in and near the parietal cortices. Principal neuropsychological manifestations of lesions in these regions are summarized in Table 3–3.

Temporoparietal Junction

In the left hemisphere, an area of cortex formed by the posterior part of the superior temporal gyrus

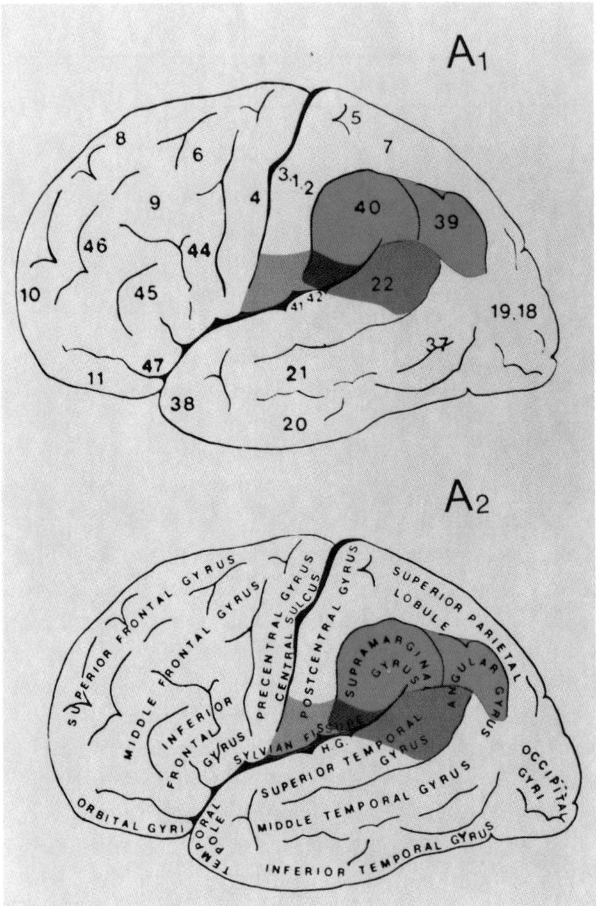

Figure 3–9. Subdivisions of the parietal lobe and nearby regions. The temporoparietal junction, formed by the posterior part of the superior temporal gyrus (area 22), is shown in red. The inferior parietal lobule (shown in green) is formed by the angular (area 39) and supramarginal (area 40) gyri. The parietal operculum is formed by the inferior aspect of the postcentral gyrus (shown in yellow) and a bit of the anteroinferior aspect of the supramarginal gyrus (shown in overlapping yellow and green). Numbers corresponding to Brodmann's cytoarchitectonic areas are depicted on A_1, and standard gyri names are shown on the corresponding A_2. The figures depict a lateral view.

(posterior area 22) constitutes the core of a region known as *Wernicke's area* (Figure 3–9). The posterior part of the inferior parietal lobule (including parts of the angular [area 39] and supramarginal [area 40] gyri) is usually included as part of "greater Wernicke's area." As the name indicates, this region is firmly linked to a constellation of speech and language functions, whose disruption constitutes the syndrome known as *Wernicke's aphasia* (e.g., Benson 1989). The syndrome is hallmarked by fluent, paraphasic speech production; impaired repetition; and defective aural comprehension. Patients can produce speech without hesitation, and the phrase length and melodic contour of utterances are normal; however, there are frequent errors in the choice of individual words used to express an idea (paraphasias). Phonemic (e.g., *sephalot* for elephant) and verbal (e.g., *superintendent* for president) paraphasias are both common. Repetition is impaired, always for sentences and often for digits as well, and may be limited to single words or even less. The comprehension defect can be quite severe as well and frequently involves both aural and written forms of language. The typical lesion associated with Wernicke's aphasia is depicted in Figure 3–10.

In the right hemisphere, lesions in the region of the temporoparietal junction do not cause disturbances of propositional speech and language, but instead may impair the processing of music and other spectral auditory information. A recent patient of this type was reported by Damasio et al. (1990c). After a lesion to the right temporoparietal region, the patient developed a severe defect in the recognition of music. The case was of particular interest because the patient was a trained musician and singer, and the loss of the ability to identify specific singing voices and musical arrangements was especially striking.

Another intriguing neuropsychological correlate of this region is the ability to recognize familiar voices. Van Lancker and colleagues (Van Lancker and Kreiman 1988; Van Lancker et al. 1988) have reported that lesions to the right parietal cortices disrupt this function, even though auditory acuity is fundamentally unaltered, a condition the authors have termed *phonagnosia*. More inferior lesions, confined to the temporal cortices, tend to disrupt perception of auditory spectral information (Robin et al. 1990), but may not disrupt voice recognition (Van Lancker et al. 1989).

Bilateral lesions to the posterior part of the superior temporal gyrus lead to the syndrome of auditory agnosia, in which the patient is unable to recognize both speech and nonspeech sounds (e.g., Vignolo 1982). Almost always caused by stroke, the condition involves the sudden and complete inability to identify the meaning of verbal and nonverbal auditory signals (e.g., spoken words, familiar environmental sounds such as a telephone ringing or a

TABLE 3–3. NEUROPSYCHOLOGICAL MANIFESTATIONS OF PARIETAL LOBE LESIONS

	Hemispheric side of lesion		
Region	*Left*	*Right*	*Bilateral*
Temporoparietal junction (including posterior part of superior temporal gyrus)	Wernicke's aphasia	Amusia; defective music recognition; "phonagnosia"	Auditory agnosia
Inferior parietal lobule	Conduction aphasia; tactile agnosia	Neglect; anosognosia; anosodiaphoria; tactile agnosia	?

Note. ? = Neuropsychological correlates of such a lesion pattern are not well established.

knock on the door). Full-blown auditory agnosia is rare, and in virtually all cases there is a good deal of perceptual impairment together with a recognition defect (cf. Anderson et al. 1990a). The term *agnosia* must be applied with caution and qualification.

Inferior Parietal Lobule

The inferior parietal lobule comprises the supramarginal (area 40) and angular gyri (area 39) (Figure 3–9). On the left side, lesions to the supramarginal gyrus and the neighboring parietal operculum (the area of cortex formed by the most inferior portion of the postcentral gyrus), and/or the underlying white matter, cause a speech and language disturbance known as *conduction aphasia* (e.g., Benson et al. 1973). A CT of such a patient is illustrated in Figure 3–11. The core feature of this aphasia is a marked defect in verbatim repetition, which is disproportionately severe when compared with other speech and language defects. Speech production is fluent but is dominated by phonemic paraphasic errors, and comprehension may be only mildly compromised. Naming is defective and dominated by phonemic errors (i.e., substitution of incorrect phonemes into target naming responses). Reading aloud is impaired, but reading comprehension may be normal. Another distinctive feature of conduction aphasia is that patients cannot write to dictation but are able to write with minimal error when writing spontaneously or to copy.

Conduction aphasia has also been reported with lesions that damage the primary auditory cortex (areas 41 and 42) and extend into the insular cortex and underlying white matter (Damasio and Damasio 1980). Another interesting example is a case described by Hyman and Tranel (1989), in which conduction aphasia occurred together with a complete right hemianesthesia. The lesion in this patient was in the white matter subjacent to the inferior parietal and posterior temporal cortices, with extension into the posterior part of the insula.

On the right side, the most consistent and striking neuropsychological correlates of lesions to the inferior parietal lobule are *neglect* and *anosognosia*. Neglect, associated especially with temporoparietal lesions that include the angular (area 39) and supramarginal (area 40) gyri (e.g., Heilman et al. 1983), refers to a condition whereby the patient fails to attend to stimuli in the contralateral hemispace. In the visual modality, for example, the patient will not attend to the left hemifield and will fail to report stimuli from that side even when it can be demonstrated that there is no impairment of form vision (hemianopia). In principle, neglect can occur in relationship to any sensory modality, but in practice the visual and auditory varieties are most common. Some investigators (e.g., Heilman et al. 1985; Weintraub and Mesulam 1989) have attributed neglect to an impairment of the attentional mechanisms necessary for normal perception. Figure 3–12 shows an MRI of a patient with a large right-hemisphere lesion that includes the inferior parietal lobule, who had severe neglect, anosognosia, and visuospatial impairments.

Neglect can involve intrapersonal as well as extrapersonal space. For example, patients may fail to use, or even deny the existence of, the contralateral arm and leg, even when there is no motor impairment. Representations conjured up in recall can also be affected (e.g., when asked to imagine or draw an

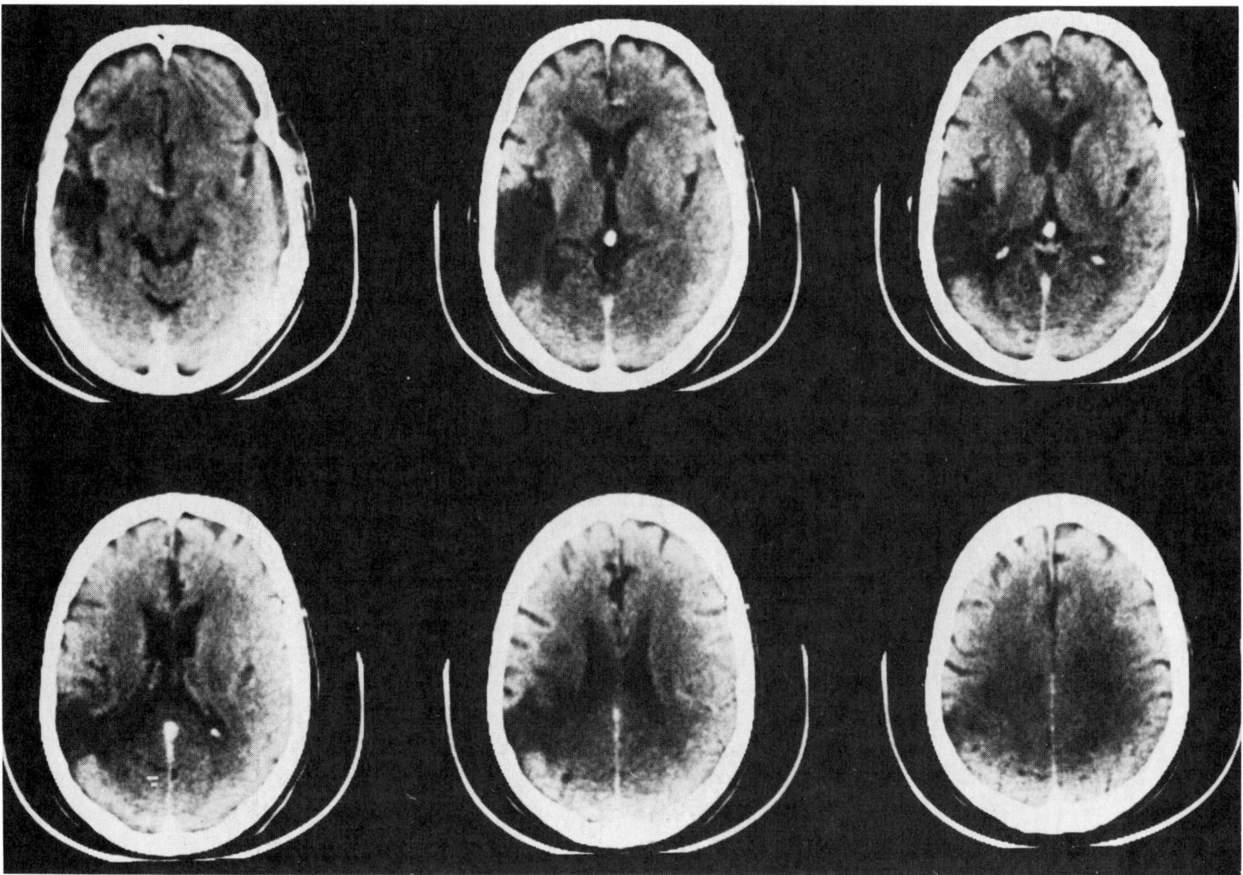

Figure 3–10. Computed tomography (CT) scan of a 56-year-old, right-handed man who developed Wernicke's aphasia following a left middle cerebral artery infarction. The lesion (area of low density) is centered squarely in Wernicke's area, including the posterior superior temporal gyrus (*top row*) and part of the inferior parietal lobule (*bottom row*).

object, the patient will omit the left half, as though it did not exist). Asked to describe well-known scenes from memory, patients may report only the elements from the right side of the representation. The omissions, however, are specific to the patient's perspective, and it can be demonstrated that the patient does have the capacity to access the full array of information. Bisiach and Luzzatti (1978), for example, asked patients to describe a well-known scene from a particular perspective; they then rotated the perspective by 180° and asked the patients again to describe the scene. In the first description, patients reported information only from the right side of the scene. In the second condition, the patients again reported information only from the right side of the scene, but because the perspective had been rotated, this was precisely the same information that had been neglected in the first description.

Anosognosia is another frequent correlate of damage to the right inferior parietal lobule. The term was originally applied to patients who denied that a paretic limb was in fact paretic or that it even belonged to them (Babinski 1914). Denial of sensory loss (e.g., a visual field defect) and cognitive disturbance have also been included under the concept of anosognosia (e.g., Anderson and Tranel 1989). Although popular, the concept *denial of illness* is not equivalent to *anosognosia*, as the latter term denotes a true recognition defect in which the patient is unaware, in terms of internal experience, of acquired motor, sensory, or cognitive deficits. By

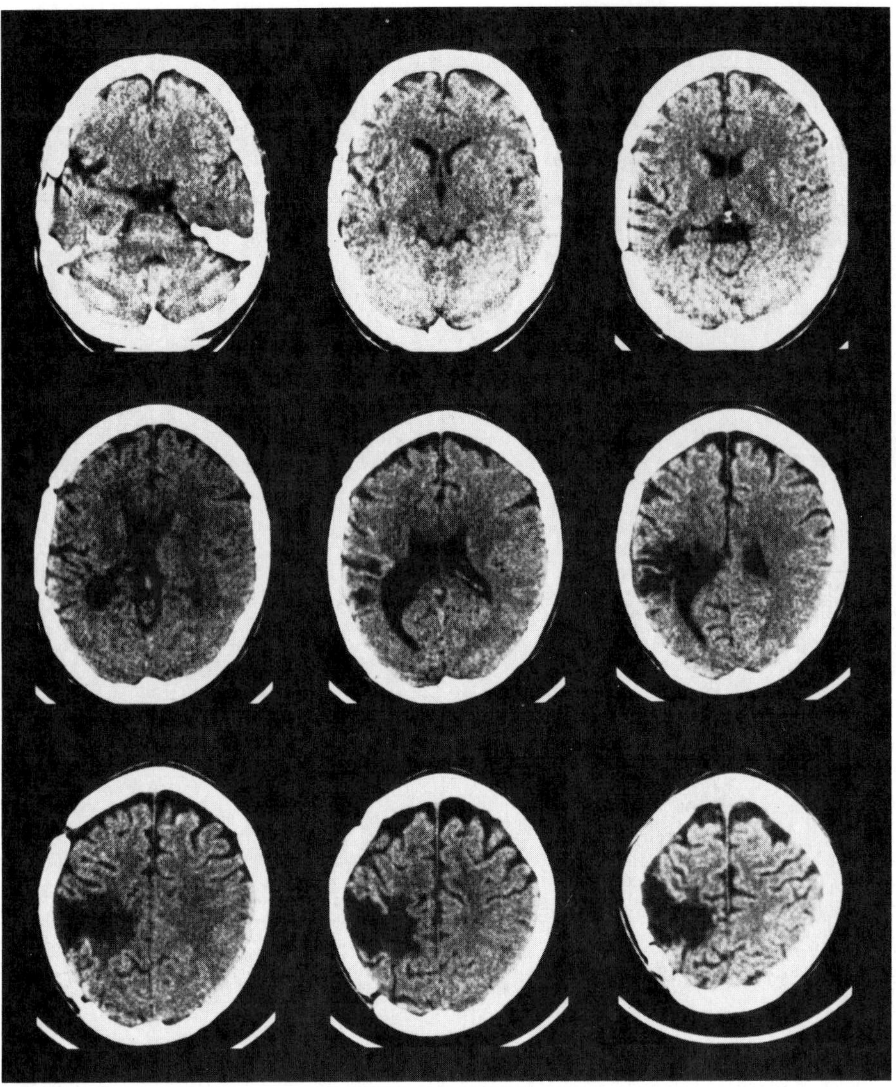

Figure 3–11. Computed tomography (CT) scan of a 35-year-old, right-handed woman, showing a lesion (area of low density) in the left supramarginal gyrus (area 40). Note that the lesion spares the primary auditory cortex and the main part of Wernicke's area (posterior area 22). The woman had conduction aphasia.

contrast, denial of illness may refer to the adaptive psychological condition that allows patients under severe stress to adapt to the calamitous consequences of disease. In any event, anosognosia can be operationally defined as a significant discrepancy between the patient's report of his or her disabilities and the objective evidence regarding his or her level of functioning.

A related term is *anosodiaphoria,* which refers to the condition in which patients appear unconcerned with or minimize the significance of neurological deficits. It is common for patients to manifest anosognosia early in the course of illness, and then for this to gradually evolve into anosodiaphoria. In both conditions, common neuropsychological correlates are defects in visuospatial and visuoconstructional abilities and left hemispatial neglect (Benton 1985; Benton and Tranel, in press).

One other intriguing condition, which has been described in connection with lesions to the inferior

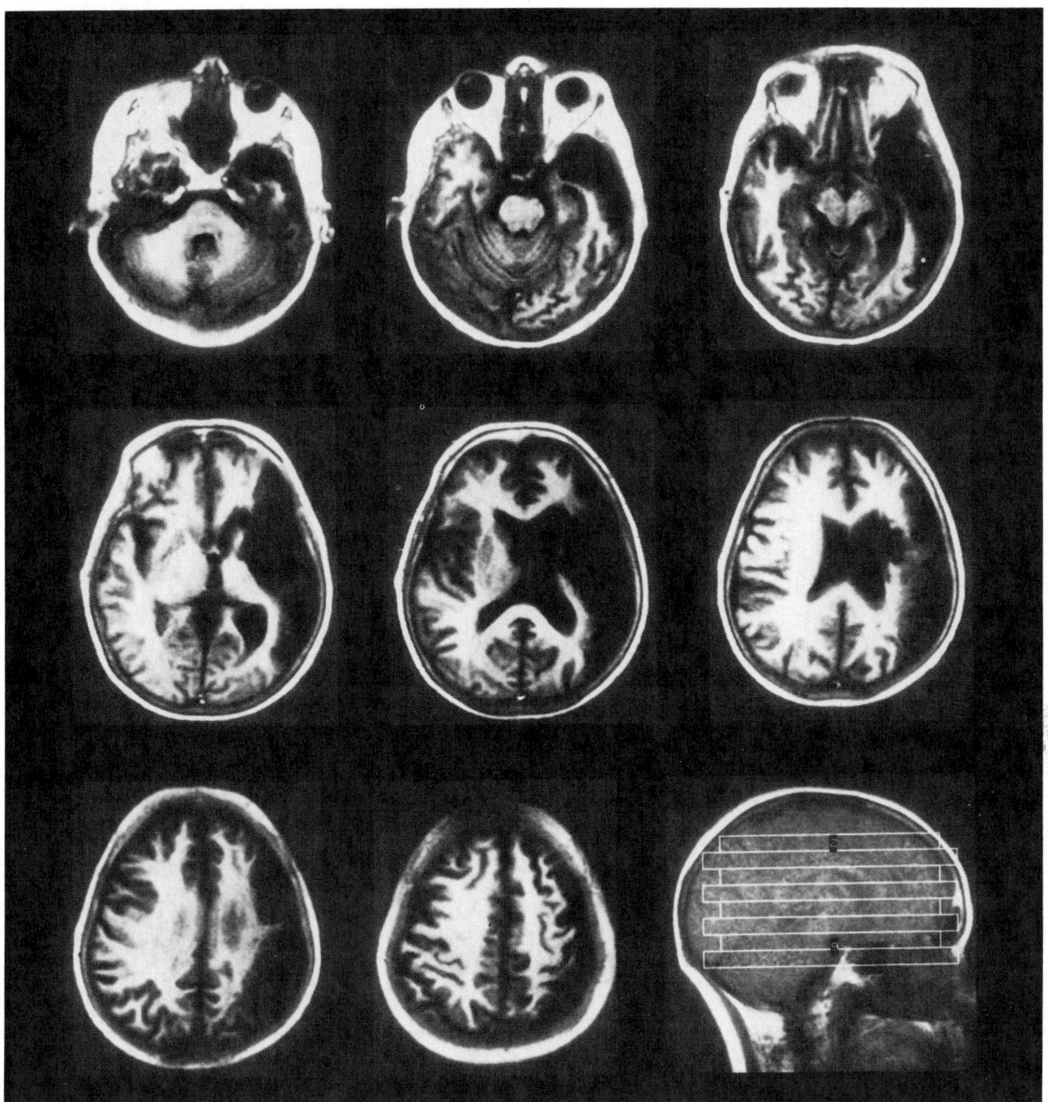

Figure 3–12. T1-weighted magnetic resonance image (MRI) of a 34-year-old, right-handed woman, showing a large right middle cerebral artery infarction. The lesion (showing as a black region) includes a significant portion of the inferior parietal lobule (areas 39 and 40). The woman had severe left-sided neglect, anosognosia, and visuospatial deficits.

parietal lobule and nearby posterior/superior temporal cortices on either the right or left side, is *tactile agnosia* (Caselli 1991). Patients lose the ability to recognize objects presented via the tactile modality, even when basic aspects of somatosensory function are normal or near normal. It is important to note that the condition is different from prosopagnosia in that it involves a disruption of recognition at the basic object level, rather than at the level of unique identity (Tranel 1991b). Thus patients with tactile agnosia cannot recognize stimuli such as keys, pencils, and eating utensils when those items are presented in the somatosensory modality. The condition is far less disabling than a disorder such as prosopagnosia, and many patients with tactile agnosia will not even complain of a defect; in fact, the impairment may only be demonstrable in careful laboratory testing conditions.

❑ THE FRONTAL LOBES

The frontal lobes can be divided into several distinct anatomical regions (Figure 3–13). Each of these areas has a number of relatively specific neuropsychological manifestations; these are summarized in Table 3–4.

Frontal Operculum

The frontal operculum is formed by areas 44, 45, and 47 (Figure 3–13). On the left side, the heart of this region (areas 44 and 45) is known as *Broca's area*. The region is dedicated to a set of speech and language functions whose disruption produces a distinctive pattern of aphasia termed *Broca's aphasia*. Patients with Broca's aphasia have nonfluent speech, characterized by short utterances, long response latencies, flat melodic contour, and agrammatism. Paraphasias are common, usually involving omission of phonemes or addition of incorrect phonemes (phonemic paraphasia), and in severe cases, speech may be virtually unintelligible. A defect in repetition is invariably present, and most patients with Broca's aphasia have defective naming and impaired writing. By contrast, language comprehension is relatively preserved. Individuals with Broca's aphasia are usually able to comprehend simple conversations, and they can comprehend and execute two- and even three-step commands. Reading comprehension may also be relatively preserved. A CT of a typical person with Broca's aphasia is illustrated in Figure 3–14.

When lesions are confined to Broca's area, speech and language recovery can be fairly extensive (Mohr et al. 1978). Lesions that involve other frontal fields in the dorsolateral sector (in addition to Broca's area), or that cut deeper into frontal white matter, lead to a poorer pattern of recovery (Mohr et al. 1978). When lesions involve the lower motor or premotor cortices, or the subjacent white matter, aphemia rather than aphasia results (Schiff et al. 1983), that is, patients may develop articulatory defects and hesitant speech, but a true linguistic impairment is not present. Lesions in structures anterior, superior, and deep to Broca's area, but sparing most or all of areas 44 and 45, will commonly produce transcortical motor aphasia (Rubens 1976), which resembles Broca's aphasia except that a repetition defect is absent.

In the right hemisphere, lesions to the frontal operculum have been linked to defects in paralinguistic communication, but propositional speech and language are not affected (Ross 1981). Specifically, patients may lose the ability to implement normal patterns of prosody and gesturing; their communication is characterized by flat, monotone speech, loss of spontaneous gesturing, and impaired ability to repeat affective contours (e.g., to implement emotional tones in speech, such as happiness or sadness).

TABLE 3–4. NEUROPSYCHOLOGICAL MANIFESTATIONS OF FRONTAL LOBE LESIONS

	Hemispheric side of lesion	
Region	*Left*	*Right*
Frontal operculum	Broca's aphasia	"Expressive" aprosodia
Superior mesial region	Akinetic mutism[a]	Akinetic mutism[a]
Inferior mesial region		
Basal forebrain	Anterograde and retrograde amnesia with confabulation; worse for verbal stimuli	Anterograde and retrograde amnesia with confabulation; worse for nonverbal stimuli
Orbital	Defective social conduct; "acquired" sociopathy[a]	Defective social conduct; "acquired" sociopathy[a]
Lateral prefrontal region	Impaired verbal intellect; defective recency and frequency judgments for verbal material; defective verbal fluency; impaired "executive functions"	Impaired nonverbal intellect; defective recency and frequency judgments for nonverbal material; defective design fluency; impaired "executive functions"

[a]Condition is similar for left-sided and right-sided lesions; bilateral lesions produce a more severe version of the same condition.

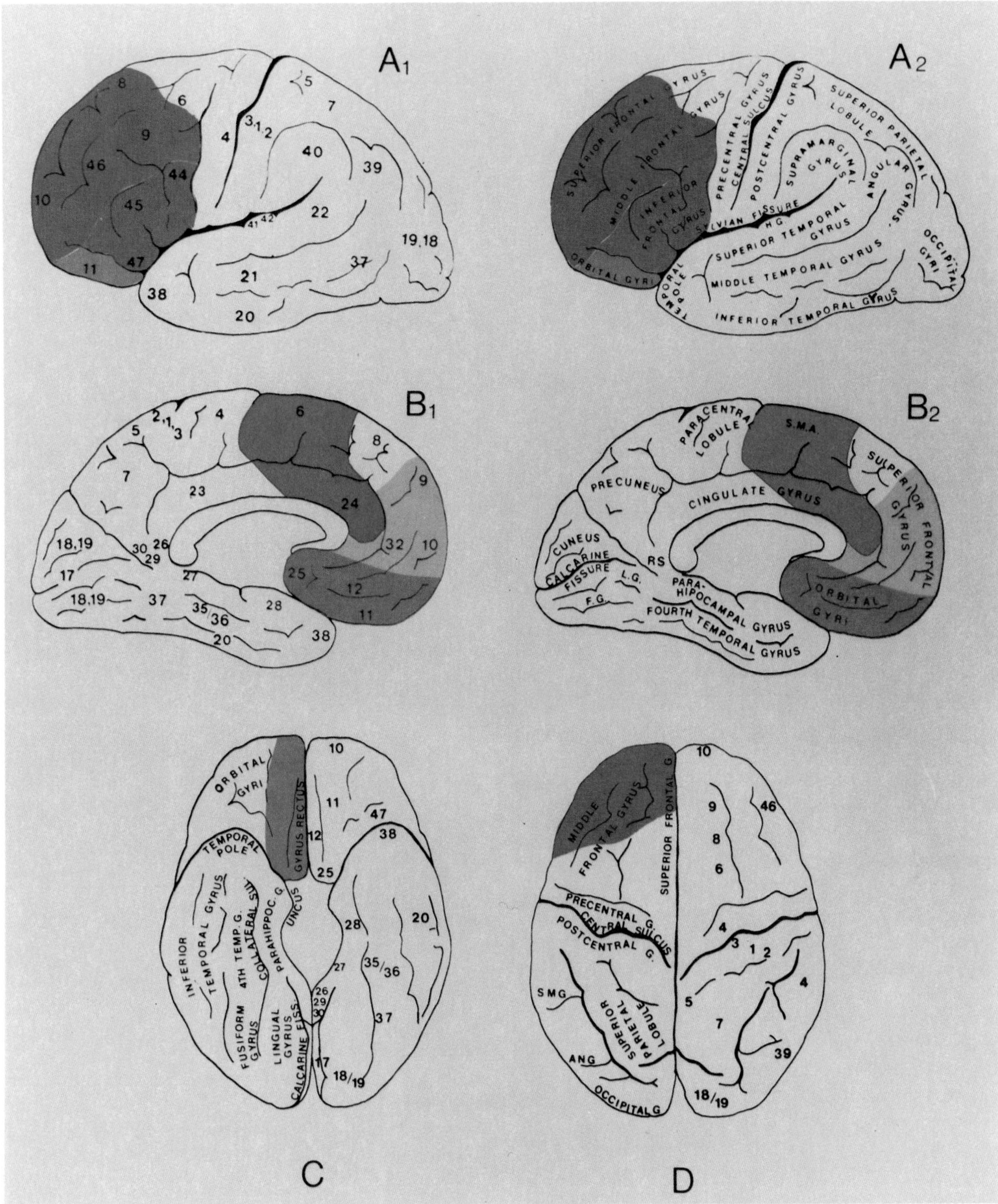

Figure 3–13. Major subdivisions of the frontal lobe: the frontal operculum, formed by areas 44, 45, and 47 (shown in red); the superior mesial region, formed by the mesial aspect of area 6 and the anterior part of the cingulate gyrus (area 24) (shown in green); the inferior mesial region, formed by the basal forebrain and the orbital cortices (areas 11, 12, and 25) (shown in dark yellow); and the lateral prefrontal region, formed by the lateral aspects of areas 8, 9, 46, and 10 (shown in purple). The ventromedial frontal lobe is comprised by the orbital region (shown in dark yellow) and the lower mesial (area 32 and the mesial aspect of areas 10 and 9) cortices (shown in light yellow). Numbers corresponding to Brodmann's cytoarchitectonic areas are depicted on *A1*, *B1*, and the right side (left hemisphere) of *C* and the right side (right hemisphere) of *D*, and standard gyri names are shown on corresponding *A2*, *B2*, and the left side of *C* and *D*. Lateral (*A1* and *A2*), mesial (*B1* and *B2*), inferior (*C*), and superior (*D*) views are represented.

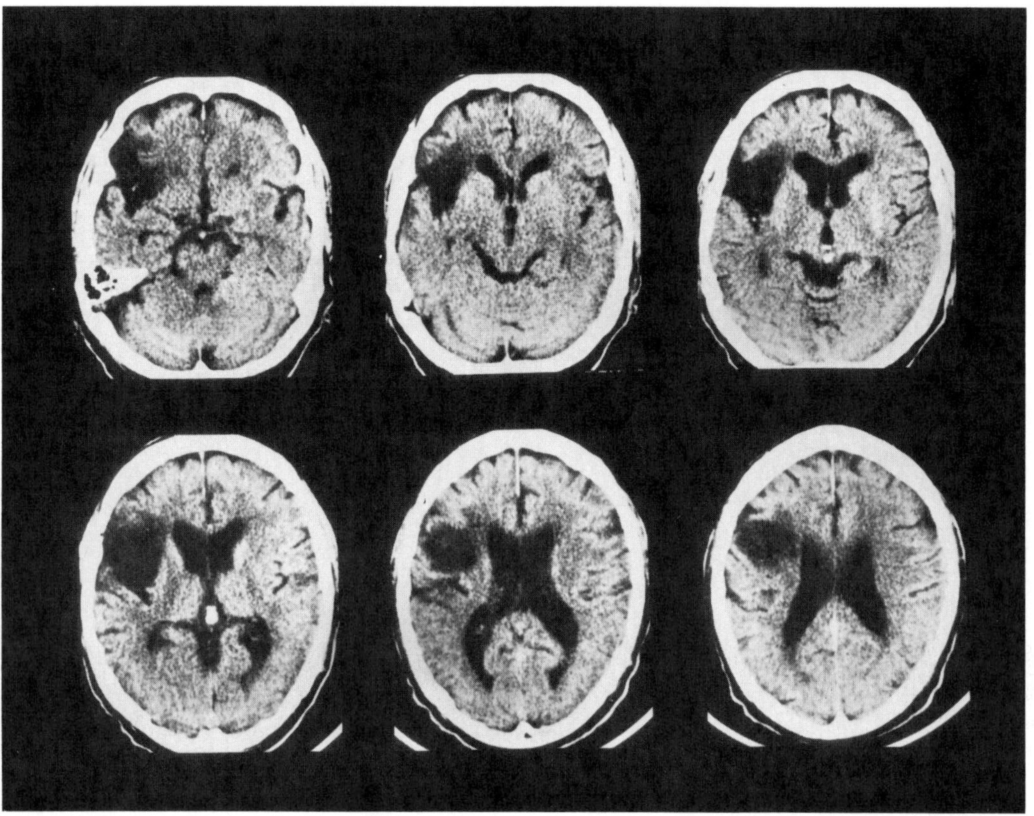

Figure 3–14. Computed tomography (CT) scan of a 76-year-old, right-handed man who developed Broca's aphasia after a left frontal infarction. The lesion, showing as a well-defined area of low density, is squarely in the heart of "Broca's area" (i.e., the frontal opercular region formed by areas 44 and 45).

Superior Mesial Region

The superior mesial aspect of the frontal lobes comprises a set of structures that are critical for the initiation of movement and emotional expression. The supplementary motor area (the mesial aspect of area 6) and anterior cingulate (area 24) cortices are especially important (Figure 3–13). Lesions in this region produce a syndrome of *akinetic mutism* (Damasio and Van Hoesen 1983), in which the patient makes no effort to communicate, either verbally or by gesture, and maintains an empty, noncommunicative facial expression. Movements are limited to tracking of moving targets with the eyes and body and arm movements connected with daily necessities such as eating, pulling up bedclothes, and going to the bathroom. Otherwise, the patient will not move or speak. The mutism can be distinguished from aphasia by the fact that in the latter condition, patients will invariably exhibit an intent to communicate (i.e., they will show frustration at their inability to speak, and will seek compensatory strategies, such as gesturing or writing). By contrast, the patient with akinetic mutism will appear content to lie motionless and silent, regardless of the examiner's reasonable queries. Figure 3–15 depicts a lesion in a patient with akinetic mutism.

There does not appear to be a significant difference in the profile of akinetic mutism as a function of side of lesion; left- and right-sided lesions lead to more or less equivalent defects. However, the defects will be more severe, and will persist longer, with bilateral lesions. Patients with unilateral lesions may recover within a few weeks.

Inferior Mesial Region

Inferiorly, the mesial aspect of the frontal lobes can be subdivided into the orbital region, which includes areas 11 and 12, and the basal forebrain,

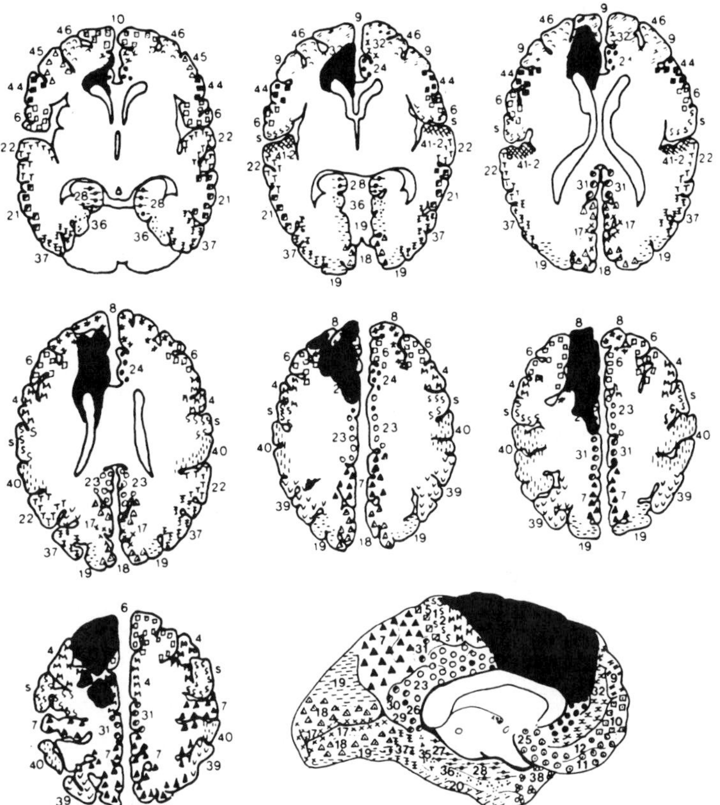

Figure 3–15. Depiction of the lesion in a 40-year-old, right-handed man, marked in black on transverse templates and on the mesial brain. The lesion is in the left hemisphere and involves the mesial aspect of area 6 and the anterior part of the cingulate gyrus (area 24). Initially, the man had severe akinetic mutism, but by 3 months after onset he demonstrated excellent recovery.

which forms the most posterior extension of the inferior mesial region (Figure 3–13). The neuropsychological correlates of these two regions are quite different, and each sector is reviewed in turn below.

Basal forebrain. The basal forebrain comprises a set of bilateral paramidline gray nuclei that includes the septal nuclei, the diagonal band of Broca, the nucleus accumbens, and the substantia innominata. Lesions to this area, commonly caused by the rupture of aneurysms located in the anterior communicating artery or in the anterior cerebral artery, cause a distinctive neuropsychological syndrome in which memory defects figure most prominently (Alexander and Freedman 1983; Damasio et al. 1985b; Damasio et al. 1989c; Volpe and Hirst 1983). An example of this type of presentation is shown in Figure 3–16. The amnesic profile of basal forebrain patients has several intriguing features. It is characterized by an impairment in the integration of modal stimuli, so that patients are able to learn and recall separate aspects of entities and events, but cannot associate those aspects into an integrated memory. They may, for example, learn the name of a person, that person's face, and various associated information such as personality traits; however, when attempting to recall the target individual, they will not bring this information together, but will assign the individual the wrong name or the wrong personality traits. This modal mismatching defect affects the retrograde compartment as well.

Another frequent manifestation in basal forebrain patients is the proclivity for confabulation. The fabrications have a dreamlike quality and occur spontaneously (i.e., they are not prompted by the need to fill gaps of missing information in attempt-

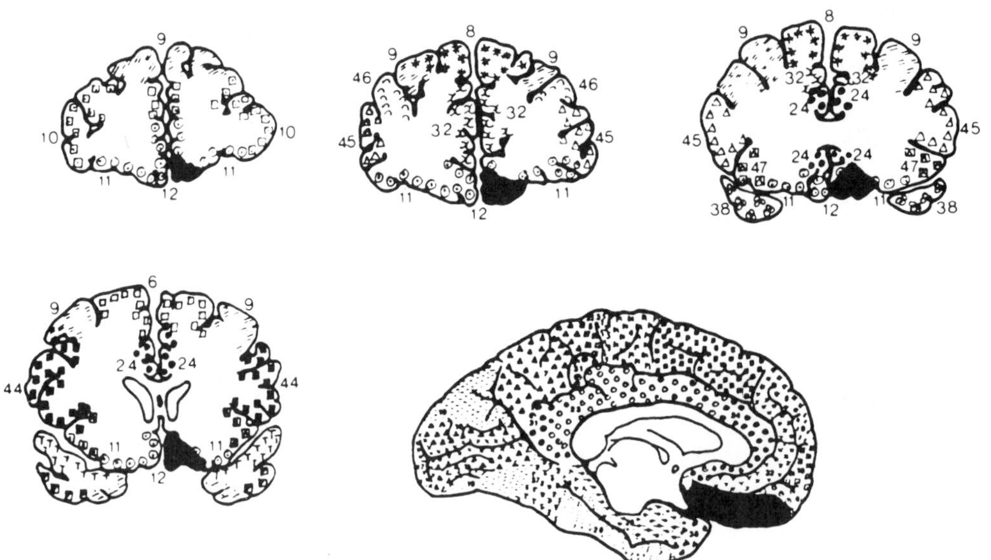

Figure 3–16. Depiction of the lesion in a 32-year-old, right-handed man, who suffered rupture of an anterior communicating artery aneurysm. The lesion, shown in black on coronal sections (left hemisphere on the right) and on the mesial aspect of the hemisphere, involves the left gyrus rectus and the left basal forebrain. The man had a distinctive amnesic syndrome, with confabulation and both anterograde and retrograde deficits.

ing to respond to an examiner's questions). In some instances, the internal experience of the patient may even include fantasies that are not recognized as such; for example, the patient will not be capable of distinguishing reality from nonreality in their own recall (Damasio et al. 1985b, 1989c). The memory defects of basal forebrain patients can persist well into the chronic phase of recovery, so that even after many years patients will continue to manifest learning and recall deficits and a tendency to confabulate. In the chronic phase, however, patients usually gain some insight into their difficulties, and they learn to mistrust their own recall and cross-check their memories against an external source.

Orbital region. The orbital and lower mesial frontal cortices (including cytoarchitectonic fields 11, 12, 25, 32, and the mesial aspect of fields 10 and 9; see Figure 3–13) form the ventromedial frontal lobe, and a number of important neuropsychological correlates have been established for this region. Patients with ventromedial damage, provided the lesion does not extend into the basal forebrain, do not generally develop memory disturbances. In fact, such patients are remarkably free of conventional neuropsychological defects. Patient E. V. R., initially described by Eslinger and Damasio (1985), is prototypical (see Figure 3–17). Findings from E. V. R., together with observations in several other similar patients (e.g., Ackerly and Benton 1948; Brickner 1934, 1936; Hebb and Penfield 1940), have revealed that ventromedial frontal damage causes a severe disruption of social conduct, including defects in planning, judgment, and decision making, although there may be little or nothing deficient in formal neuropsychological testing (e.g., Stuss and Benson 1986). E. V. R., for example, retained superior intellectual and memory capacities following bilateral frontal lobe resection for removal of an orbitofrontal meningioma; however, his social conduct after surgery was marked by numerous instances of inappropriate behavior, disastrous judgment, and impaired interpersonal relationships. The importance of these developments in patient E. V. R. is underscored by the fact that he had been virtually flawless in these domains before his brain damage; he had been a model citizen, with a sound marriage and good standing in his community and in his profession.

Other patients have recently been described, in whom a severe defect in social conduct followed bilateral ventromedial frontal lobe lesions (Ander-

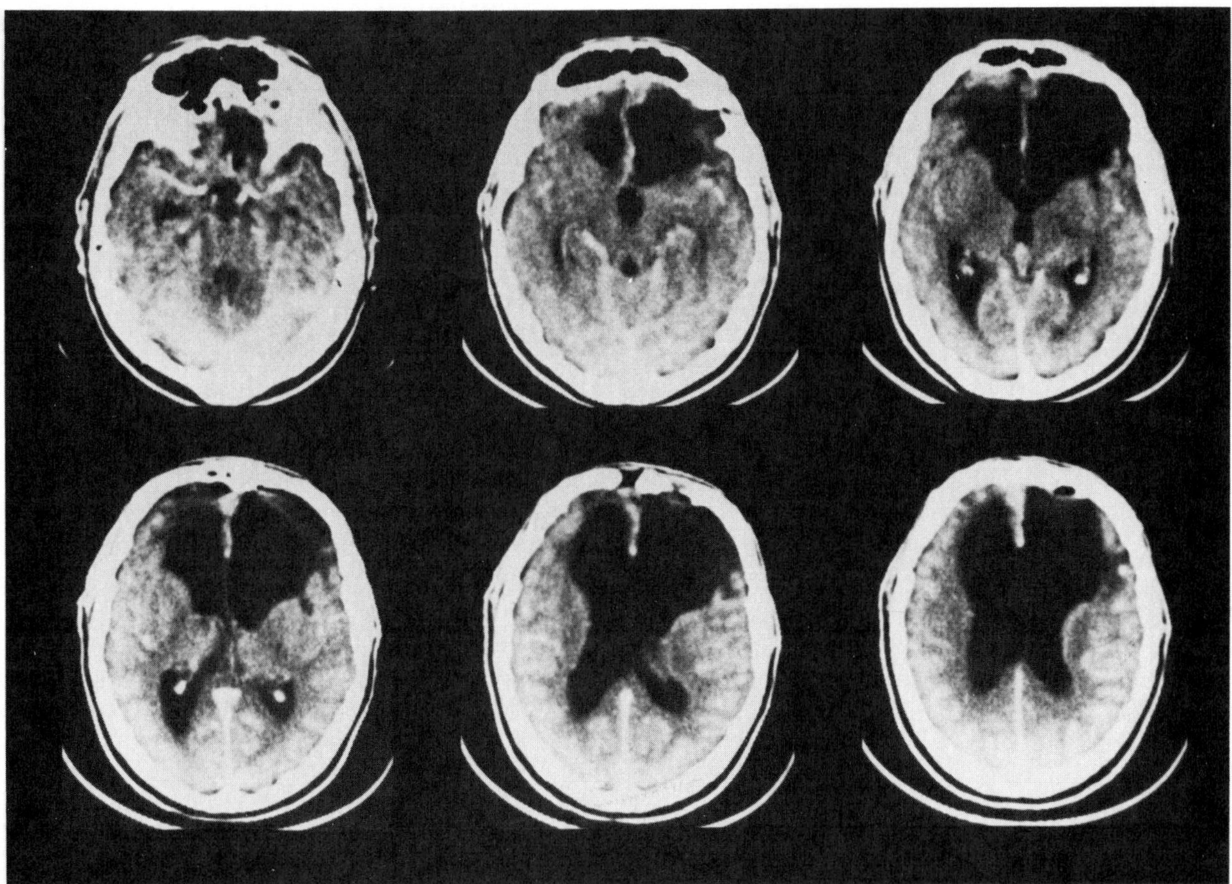

Figure 3–17. Computed tomography (CT) scan of a 44-year-old, right-handed man who underwent resection of a large orbitofrontal meningioma. The lesion, showing as an area of low density, comprises bilateral destruction of the orbital and lower mesial frontal cortices. The basal forebrain is spared. The man developed severe changes in personality but did not manifest defects in conventional neuropsychological procedures.

son et al. 1988; Damasio et al. 1989d). As in patient E. V. R., these patients maintained normal or near-normal levels of performance in most standard areas of neuropsychological functioning, including intellect, memory, perception, and language. It is important to emphasize also, that none of these patients suffered from a social conduct disorder before the onset of brain damage, that is, all had normal personality development and normal social behavior before lesion onset. Recently, a theory has been elaborated to account for the somewhat enigmatic neuropsychological profiles of ventromedial damaged patients. In a nutshell, the theory posits that the social conduct disorder arises because the patients have lost the ability to activate somatic states (i.e., "feeling" states) that were learned in connection with reward and punishment (Damasio et al. 1990d, in press). Thus when confronted with social stimulus configurations, the patients cannot access critical guideposts that would normally assist in selection of appropriate and advantageous responses. Preliminary testing of this theory has revealed that ventromedial damaged patients have defective autonomic responses to socially charged stimuli (Damasio et al. 1990d, in press). This finding has several interesting parallels in the literature on psychopathy. For example, psychopathic individuals have defective autonomic responses in situations involving punishment, that is, situations that normally trigger high levels of anxiety and autonomic responsiveness (e.g., Hare 1978). Also, psychopathic patients fail to show normal autonomic conditioning to highly charged emotional stimuli (e.g., Hare and Quinn 1971). In short, the available data indicate a number of similarities between standard psychopathy and the type of social conduct disorder manifest by ventromedial damaged patients, and one might even term the latter condition a kind of *acquired sociopathy*.

Lateral Prefrontal Region

The dorsolateral aspect of the frontal lobes comprises a vast expanse of cortex that occupies cytoarchitectonic areas 8, 9, 46, and 10 (Figure 3–13). The functions of the lateral prefrontal region exclusive of the frontal operculum and other language-related structures discussed above are not well understood. Presumably, this region is involved in higher-order integrative and executive control functions, and damage to this sector has been linked to intellectual deficits (see Stuss and Benson 1986). Another manifestation noted by several investigators is a memory impairment that affects judgments of recency and frequency of events, but not the content of the events. For example, patients fail to remember how often, or how recently, they have experienced a certain stimulus, but they do recognize the stimulus as familiar (e.g., Milner and Petrides 1984; Milner et al. 1985; Smith and Milner 1988). The reverse dissociation (impaired recognition of content but preserved recency and frequency discrimination) has also been reported (Sagar et al. 1990); in this case, the lesion involved the mesial temporal lobes bilaterally, but the lateral frontal cortices were intact.

The dorsolateral frontal cortices have been linked to the verbal regulation of behavior (e.g., Luria 1969), and verbal fluency, as measured by the ability to generate word lists under certain stimulus constraints, is notably impaired in many patients with dorsolateral lesions, especially when those lesions are bilateral or on the left side (e.g., Benton 1968). Unilateral right dorsolateral lesions may impair fluency in the nonverbal domain. For example, patients may lose the capacity to produce designs in a fluent manner (Jones-Gotman and Milner 1977). Finally, deficits on laboratory tests of "executive function," which commonly test the patient's ability to form, maintain, and change cognitive sets, as well as the tendency to perseverate (e.g., the Wisconsin Card Sorting Test), are usually maximal with dorsolateral lesions, although by no means specific (Anderson et al., in press; Milner 1963).

❑ SUBCORTICAL STRUCTURES

Two sets of subcortical structures are considered in the present discussion, namely, the basal ganglia and the thalamus. A summary of some neuropsychological manifestations of damage to these structures is presented in Table 3–5.

Basal Ganglia

The basal ganglia are a set of deep gray nuclear structures, the putamen and caudate. On the left side, lesions to these structures produce a speech and language disturbance that involves a mixture of manifestations that cannot be easily classified according to standard aphasia nomenclature, hence, the pattern has come to be known as *atypical aphasia* (Damasio et al. 1982a; Naeser et al. 1982). Because damage in this region will almost invariably include the anterior limb of the internal capsule, right hemiparesis is a common accompanying manifestation. The aphasia is characterized by speech that is usually fluent, but paraphasic and dysarthric; auditory comprehension is typically poor, and in some cases repetition is impaired. An MRI of a patient with a basal ganglia lesion and atypical aphasia is shown in Figure 3–18.

It has been noted that patients with basal ganglia lesions and atypical aphasia nearly always have lesions that involve the head of the caudate nucleus, together with the putamen and anterior limb of the internal capsule (H. Damasio 1989). Lesions confined to the putamen, or to laterally adjacent structures such as the anterior insula and subjacent white matter, do not produce an aphasic disturbance, although defects in articulation and prosody may be

TABLE 3–5. NEUROPSYCHOLOGICAL MANIFESTATIONS OF SUBCORTICAL LESIONS

Basal ganglia	Atypical aphasia (left-sided lesions); dysarthria; aprosodia
Thalamus	Thalamic aphasia (left-sided lesions); anterograde amnesia with confabulation; retrograde amnesia with temporal gradient; impairments in "executive functions"; attention/concentration defects

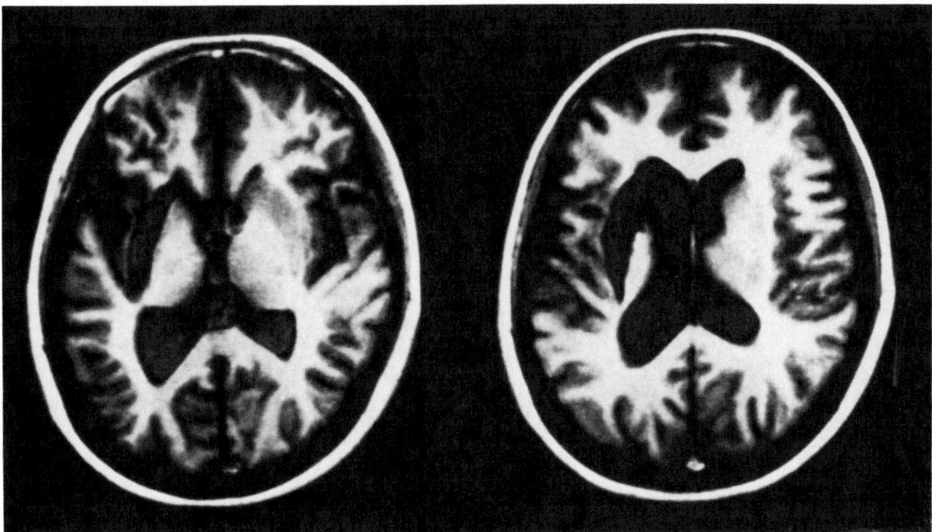

Figure 3–18. T1-weighted magnetic resonance image (MRI) of a 35-year-old, right-handed woman who sustained a subcortical hemorrhage. The lesion, showing as an area of black on these transverse cuts, involves the left basal ganglia, including the head and body of the caudate nucleus, and part of the putamen. The woman had a characteristic "basal ganglia" type aphasia, with marked dysarthria and mixed linguistic impairments.

noted. Other authors (e.g., Alexander 1989), however, have pointed out that in the key reports of aphasia-producing lesions to the basal ganglia (Cappa et al. 1983; Damasio et al. 1982a; Naeser et al. 1982), the patients all had significant damage to white matter structures as well as to basal ganglia involvement. One additional note of importance is that patients with basal ganglia lesions and aphasia tend to show very good recovery (Damasio et al. 1984).

Thalamus

Disturbances of speech and language have been linked to damage in the dominant thalamus (Mohr et al. 1975). The language disorder tends to be primarily a deficit at the semantic level, with prominent word-finding impairment, defective confrontation naming, and semantic paraphasias. This pattern has a number of resemblances to the transcortical aphasias, and it has been linked in particular to damage in anterior thalamic nuclei (Graff-Radford and Damasio 1984; Graff-Radford et al. 1985).

Another well-studied neuropsychological correlate of thalamic lesions is memory impairment. In the setting of chronic alcoholism and the development of Korsakoff's syndrome, such lesions typically involve the dorsomedial nucleus of the thalamus, along with other diencephalic structures such as the mammillary bodies. The amnesic profile associated with such lesions has been extensively investigated (e.g., Butters 1984; Butters and Stuss 1989; Victor et al. 1989). In general, such patients develop a severe anterograde amnesia that covers all forms of declarable information; however, similar to patients such as H. M. and Boswell, learning of perceptuomotor skills is spared. A distinctive feature of patients with Korsakoff's syndrome is their tendency to confabulate when asked direct questions regarding recent memory (e.g., Victor et al. 1989).

Individuals with diencephalic amnesia generally show some defect in the retrograde compartment. The impairment, however, typically shows a temporal gradient, so that recall and recognition improve steadily with increasing distance between the present and the time of initial learning, that is, more remote memories are retrieved more successfully (e.g., Cohen and Squire 1981). Another feature that is relatively common among patients with diencephalic amnesia is a disturbance of problem solving, together with other characteristics reminiscent of "frontal lobe" defects (e.g., Butters and Stuss 1989).

Thalamic lesions occurring as a consequence of stroke can also produce significant amnesia (Graff-Radford et al. 1985). Recent observations have indicated that the memory impairment is most severe when the lesions are anterior and bilateral (Graff-Radford et al. 1990b). Such lesions, which may interfere with hippocampal-related neural systems such as the mammillothalamic tract and with amygdala-related systems such as the ventroamygdalofugal pathway, produce an amnesic profile characterized by severe anterograde amnesia which spares nondeclarative learning, and a retrograde defect which is temporally graded. Posterior thalamic lesions, even when bilateral, were not associated with significant or lasting amnesia (Graff-Radford et al. 1990b).

❑ CONCLUSIONS

Understanding the salient neuropsychological correlates of variously placed cerebral lesions is of obvious importance for the accurate diagnosis and effective management of patients who suffer brain injury. Another consideration, of no less importance, is the relevance of such understanding for the development of theoretical formulations regarding brain-behavior relationships (A. R. Damasio 1989). As our understanding advances, it becomes increasingly important to appreciate the significance of both sides of the brain-behavior equation and to realize that no approach that emphasizes one side to the exclusion of the other can be ultimately successful.

❑ REFERENCES

Ackerly SS, Benton AL: Report of a case of bilateral frontal lobe defect. Research Publication of the Association for Research in Nervous and Mental Disease 27:479–504, 1948

Alexander MP: Clinical-anatomical correlations of aphasia following predominantly subcortical lesions, in Handbook of Neuropsychology, Vol 2. Edited by Boller F, Grafman J. Amsterdam, Elsevier, 1989, pp 47–66

Alexander MP, Freedman M: Amnesia after anterior communicating artery rupture. Neurology 33 (suppl 2):104, 1983

Anderson SW, Tranel D: Awareness of disease states following cerebral infarction, dementia, and head trauma: standardized assessment. The Clinical Neuropsychologist 3:327–339, 1989

Anderson SW, Damasio H, Tranel D, et al: Neuropsychological correlates of bilateral frontal lobe lesions in humans. Society for Neuroscience Abstracts 14:1288, 1988

Anderson SW, Damasio H, Robin DA, et al: Neuropsychological and psychoacoustic effects of bilateral lesions in human auditory cortex. Society for Neuroscience Abstracts 16:580, 1990a

Anderson SW, Damasio H, Tranel D: Neuropsychological impairments associated with lesions caused by tumor or stroke. Arch Neurol 47:397–405, 1990b

Anderson SW, Damasio H, Jones RD, et al: Wisconsin Card Sorting Test performance as a measure of frontal lobe damage. J Clin Exp Neuropsychol (in press)

Babinski J: Contribution a l'etude des troubles mentaux dans l'hemiplegie organique cerebrale (agnosognosie). Rev Neurol 27:845–847, 1914

Bauer RM, Rubens A: Agnosia, in Clinical Neuropsychology, 2nd Edition. Edited by Heilman KM, Valenstein E. New York, Oxford University Press, 1985, pp 187–241

Benson DF: Aphasia, Alexia, and Agraphia. London, Churchill Livingstone, 1979

Benson DF: Classical syndromes of aphasia, in Handbook of Neuropsychology, Vol 1. Edited by Boller F, Grafman J. Amsterdam, Elsevier, 1989, pp 267–280

Benson DF, Brown J, Tomlinson EB: Varieties of alexia. Neurology 21:951–957, 1971

Benson DF, Sheremata WA, Bouchard R, et al: Conduction aphasia: a clinicopathological study. Arch Neurol 28: 339–346, 1973

Benton AL: Differential behavioral effects in frontal lobe disease. Neuropsychologia 6:53–60, 1968

Benton AL: Visuoperceptual, visuospatial, and visuoconstructive disorders, in Clinical Neuropsychology, 2nd Edition. Edited by Heilman KM, Valenstein E. New York, Oxford University Press, 1985, pp 151–186

Benton AL: Neuropsychology: Past, present, and future, in Handbook of Neuropsychology, Vol 1. Edited by Boller F, Grafman J. Amsterdam, Elsevier, 1988, pp 1–27

Benton AL: Facial recognition 1990. Cortex 26:491–499, 1990

Benton AL, Tranel D: Visuoperceptual, visuospatial, and visuoconstructive disorders, in Clinial Neuropsychology, 3rd Edition. Edited by Heilman KM, Valenstein E. New York, Oxford University Press (in press)

Bisiach E, Luzzatti C: Unilateral neglect of representation space. Cortex 14:129–133, 1978

Brickner RM: An interpretation of frontal lobe function based upon the study of a case of partial bilateral frontal lobectomy. Research Publication of the Association for Research in Nervous and Mental Disease 13:259–351, 1934

Brickner RM: The Intellectual Functions of the Frontal Lobes: Study Based Upon Observation of a Man After Partial Bilateral Frontal Lobectomy. New York, Macmillan, 1936

Bruyer R, Laterre C, Seron X, et al: A case of prosopagnosia with some preserved covert remembrance of familiar faces. Brain Cogn 2:257–284, 1983

Butters N: Alcoholic Korsakoff's syndrome: an update. Semin Neurol 4:226–244, 1984

Butters N, Stuss DT: Diencephalic amnesia, in Handbook

of Neuropsychology, Vol 3. Edited by Boller F, Grafman J. Amsterdam, Elsevier, 1989, pp 107–148

Cappa SF, Cavalotti G, Guidotti M, et al: Subcortical aphasia: two clinical-CT scan correlation studies. Cortex 19: 227–241, 1983

Caselli RJ: Rediscovering tactile agnosia. Mayo Clin Proc 66:129–142, 1991

Cohen NJ, Squire LR: Retrograde amnesia and remote memory impairment. Neuropsychologia 19:337–356, 1981

Corbetta M, Miezin FM, Dobmeyer S, et al: Attentional modulation of neural processing of shape, color, and velocity in humans. Science 248:1556–1559, 1990

Corkin S: Tactually guided maze learning in man: effects of unilateral cortical excisions and bilateral hippocampal lesions. Neuropsychologia 3:339–351, 1965

Corkin S: Acquisition of motor skill after bilateral medial temporal-lobe excision. Neuropsychologia 6:255–264, 1968

Corkin S: Lasting consequences of bilateral medial temporal lobectomy: clinical course and experimental findings in HM. Semin Neurol 4:249–259, 1984

Damasio AR: Disorders of complex visual processing: agnosias, achromatopsia, Balint's syndrome, and related difficulties of orientation and construction, in Principles of Behavioral Neurology. Edited by Mesulam M-M. Philadelphia, PA, FA Davis, 1985, pp 259–288

Damasio AR: Time-locked multiregional retroactivation: a systems-level proposal for the neural substrates of recall and recognition. Cognition 33:25–62, 1989

Damasio AR: Category-related recognition defects as a clue to the neural substrates of knowledge. Trends Neurosci 13:95–98, 1990

Damasio AR, Benton AL: Impairment of hand movements under visual guidance. Neurology 29:170–174, 1979

Damasio AR, Damasio H: Anatomical basis of pure alexia. Neurology 33:1573–1583, 1983

Damasio AR, Van Hoesen GW: Emotional disturbances associated with focal lesions of the limbic frontal lobe, in Neuropsychology of Human Emotion. Edited by Heilman KM, Satz P. New York, Guilford, 1983, pp 85–110

Damasio AR, Yamada T, Damasio H, et al: Central achromatopsia: behavioral, anatomical, and physiologic aspects. Neurology 30:1064–1071, 1980

Damasio AR, Damasio H, Rizzo M, et al: Aphasia with lesions in the basal ganglia and internal capsule. Arch Neurol 39:15–20, 1982a

Damasio AR, Damasio H, Van Hoesen GW: Prosopagnosia: anatomic basis and behavioral mechanisms. Neurology 32:331–341, 1982b

Damasio AR, Eslinger P, Damasio H, et al: Multimodal amnesic syndrome following bilateral temporal and basal forebrain damage. Arch Neurol 42:252–259, 1985a

Damasio AR, Graff-Radford NR, Eslinger PJ, et al: Amnesia following basal forebrain lesions. Arch Neurol 42:263–271, 1985b

Damasio AR, Damasio H, Tranel D, et al: Additional neural and cognitive evidence in patient DRB. Society for Neuroscience Abstracts 13:1452, 1987

Damasio AR, Tranel D, Damasio H: "Deep" prosopagnosia: a new form of acquired face recognition defect caused by left hemisphere damage. Neurology 38 (suppl 1):172, 1988

Damasio AR, Damasio H, Tranel D, et al: Effects of selective visual cortex lesions in humans. Paper presented at the 12th annual meeting of the European Neurological Association and 21st annual meeting of the European Brain and Behaviour Society, Turin, Italy, September 1989a

Damasio AR, Tranel D, Damasio H: Disorders of visual recognition, in Handbook of Neuropsychology, Vol 2. Edited by Boller F, Grafman J. Amsterdam, Elsevier, 1989b, pp 317–332

Damasio AR, Tranel D, Damasio H: Amnesia caused by herpes simplex encephalitis, infarctions in basal forebrain, Alzheimer's disease, and anoxia, in Handbook of Neuropsychology, Vol 3. Edited by Boller F, Grafman J. Amsterdam, Elsevier, 1989c, pp 149–166

Damasio AR, Tranel D, Damasio H: Recognition of complex social configurations is impaired by frontal lobe lesions. J Clin Exp Neuropsychol 11:55, 1989d

Damasio AR, Damasio H, Tranel D: Impairments of visual recognition as clues to the processes of categorization and memory, in Signal and Sense: Local and Global Order in Perceptual Maps. Edited by Edelman GM, Gall WE, Cowan WM. New York, Wiley-Liss, 1990a, pp 451–473

Damasio AR, Tranel D, Damasio H: Face agnosia and the neural substrates of memory. Ann Rev Neurosci 13:89–109, 1990b

Damasio AR, Tranel D, Damasio H: Music and the brain. Paper presented at the 42nd annual meeting of the American Academy of Neurology, Miami, FL, April/May 1990c

Damasio AR, Tranel D, Damasio H: Individuals with sociopathic behavior caused by frontal damage fail to respond autonomically to social stimuli. Behav Brain Res 41:81–94, 1990d

Damasio AR, Damasio H, Tranel D, et al: Neural regionalization of knowledge access: preliminary evidence, in Cold Spring Harbor Symposia on Qualitative Biology, Vol LV. Cold Spring Harbor, NY, Cold Spring Harbor Laboratory Press, 1990e, pp 1039–1047

Damasio AR, Tranel D, Damasio H: Somatic markers and the guidance of behavior: theory and preliminary testing, in Frontal Lobe Function and Dysfunction. Edited by Levin HS, Eisenberg HM, Benton AL. New York, Oxford University Press (in press)

Damasio H: Neuroimaging contributions to the understanding of aphasia, in Handbook of Neuropsychology, Vol 2. Edited by Boller F, Grafman J. Amsterdam, Elsevier, 1989, pp 3–46

Damasio H, Damasio AR: The anatomical basis of conduction aphasia. Brain 103:337–350, 1980

Damasio H, Damasio AR: Lesion Analysis in Neuropsychology. New York, Oxford University Press, 1989

Damasio H, Damasio AR: The neural basis of memory, language and behavioral guidance: advances with the lesion method in humans. Semin Neurosci 2:277–286, 1990

Damasio H, Eslinger P, Adams HP: Aphasia following

basal ganglia lesions: new evidence. Semin Neurol 4: 151–161, 1984

Damasio H, Kuljis RO, Yuh W, et al: Visualization of the modular and laminar organization of the human cerebral cortex in vivo with magnetic resonance. Society for Neuroscience Abstracts 16: 287, 1990

Davidoff JB, Donnelly N: Object superiority: a comparison of complete and part probes. Acta Psychol (in press)

Davidoff J, Landis T: Recognition of unfamiliar faces in prosopagnosia. Neuropsychologia 28:1143–1161, 1990

De Renzi E: Prosopagnosia in two patients with CT scan evidence of damage confined to the right hemisphere. Neuropsychologia 24:385–389, 1986

Eslinger PJ, Damasio AR: Severe disturbance of higher cognition after bilateral frontal lobe ablation: patient EVR. Neurology 35:1731–1741, 1985

Eslinger PJ, Damasio AR: Preserved motor learning in Alzheimer's disease: implications for anatomy and behavior. J Neurosci 6:3006–3009, 1986

Farah MJ: The neuropsychology of mental imagery, in Handbook of Neuropsychology, Vol 2. Edited by Boller F, Grafman J. Amsterdam, Elsevier, 1989, pp 395–413

Farah MJ, Hammond KM, Mehta Z, et al: Category-specificity and modality-specificity in semantic memory. Neuropsychologia 27:193–200, 1989

Frisk V, Milner B: The relationship of working memory to the immediate recall of stories following unilateral temporal or frontal lobectomy. Neuropsychologia 28: 121–135, 1990

Gabrieli JDE, Cohen NJ, Corkin S: The impaired learning of semantic knowledge following bilateral medial temporal-lobe resection. Brain Cogn 7:157–177, 1988

Geschwind N: Disconnexion syndromes in animals and man. Brain 88:237–294, 585–644, 1965

Girotti F, Milanese C, Casazza M, et al: Oculomotor disturbances in Balint's syndrome: anatomoclinical findings and electro-oculographic analysis in a case. Cortex 8:603–614, 1982

Graff-Radford NR, Damasio H: Disturbances of speech and language associated with thalamic dysfunction. Semin Neurol 4:162–168, 1984

Graff-Radford NR, Damasio H, Yamada T, et al: Nonhemorrhagic thalamic infarctions: clinical, neurophysiological and electrophysiological findings in four anatomical groups defined by CT. Brain 108:485–516, 1985

Graff-Radford NR, Damasio AR, Hyman BT, et al: Progressive aphasia in a patient with Pick's disease: a neuropsychological, radiologic, and anatomic study. Neurology 40:620–626, 1990a

Graff-Radford NR, Tranel D, Van Hoesen GW, et al: Diencephalic amnesia. Brain 113:1–25, 1990b

Greenblatt SH: Alexia without agraphia or hemianopia: anatomical analysis of an autopsied case. Brain 96:307–316, 1973

Greenblatt SH: Localization of lesions in alexia, in Localization in Neuropsychology. Edited by Kertesz A. New York, Academic, 1983, pp 323–356

Haist F, Squire LR, Damasio AR: Extensive retrograde amnesia in two severely amnesic patients on tests of familiarity and name completion ability. Society for Neuroscience Abstracts 16:287, 1990

Hare RD: Electrodermal and cardiovascular correlates of psychopathy, in Psychopathic Behavior: Approaches to Research. Edited by Hare RD, Schalling D. New York, Wiley, 1978, pp 107–143

Hare RD, Quinn MJ: Psychopathy and autonomic conditioning. J Abnormal Psychol 77:223–235, 1971

Hart J, Berndt RS, Caramazza A: Category-specific naming deficit following cerebral infarction. Nature 316: 439–440, 1985

Hebb DO, Penfield W: Human behavior after extensive bilateral removals from the frontal lobes. Archives of Neurology and Psychiatry 44:421–438, 1940

Heilman KM, Wilder BJ, Malzone WF: Anomic aphasia following anterior temporal lobectomy. Transactions of the American Neurological Association 97:291–293, 1972

Heilman KM, Valenstein E, Watson RT: Localization of neglect, in Localization in Neuropsychology. Edited by Kertesz A. New York, Academic, 1983, pp 471–492

Heilman KM, Watson RT, Valenstein E: Neglect and related disorders, in Clinical Neuropsychology, 2nd Edition. Edited by Heilman KM, Valenstein E. New York, Oxford University Press, 1985, pp 243–293

Hermann BP, Wyler AR: Effects of anterior temporal lobectomy on language function: a controlled study. Ann Neurol 23:585–588, 1988

Horel JA: The neuroanatomy of amnesia: a critique of the hippocampal memory hypothesis. Brain 101:403–445, 1978

Hubel DH, Livingstone MS: Segregation of form, color, and stereopsis in primate area 18. J Neurosci 7:3378–3415, 1987

Hyman BT, Damasio AR, Van Hoesen GW, et al: Alzheimer's disease: cell specific pathology isolates the hippocampal formation. Science 225:1168–1170, 1984

Hyman BT, Tranel D: Hemianesthesia and aphasia: an anatomical and behavioral study. Arch Neurol 46:816–819, 1989

Jones-Gotman M, Milner B: Design fluency: the invention of nonsense drawings after focal cortical lesions. Neuropsychologia 15:653–674, 1977

Landis T, Cummings JL, Christen L, et al: Are unilateral right posterior cerebral lesions sufficient to cause prosopagnosia? Clinical and radiological findings in six additional patients. Cortex 22:243–252, 1986

Lee GP, Meador KJ, Smith JR, et al: Clinical case report: preserved crossmodal association following bilateral amygdalotomy in man. Int J Neurosci 40:47–55, 1988

Levy J: Regulation and generation of perception in the asymmetric brain, in Brain Circuits and Functions of the Mind. Edited by Trevarthen C. Cambridge, Cambridge University Press, 1990, pp 231–246

Lissauer H: Ein Fall von Seelenblindheit nebst einem Beitrag zur Theorie derselben. Arch Psychiatr Nervenkr 21:22–70, 1890

Livingstone MS, Hubel DH: Anatomy and physiology of a color system in the primate visual cortex. J Neurosci 4:309–356, 1984

Livingstone MS, Hubel DH: Psychological evidence for

separate channels for the perception of form, color, movement, and depth. J Neurosci 7:3416–3468, 1987

Livingstone MS, Hubel DH: Segregation of form, color, movement, and depth: anatomy, physiology, and perception. Science 240:740–749, 1988

Lueck CJ, Zeki S, Friston KJ, et al: The color centre in the cerebral cortex of man. Nature 340:386–389, 1989

Luria AR: Frontal lobe syndromes, in Handbook of Clinical Neurology, Vol 2. Edited by Vinken PG, Bruyn GW. North Holland, Amsterdam, 1969, pp 725–757

McCarthy RA, Warrington EK: Evidence for modality-specific meaning systems in the brain. Nature 334:428–430, 1988

Meadows JC: Disturbed perception of colors associated with localized cerebral lesions. Brain 97:615–632, 1974a

Meadows JC: The anatomical basis of prosopagnosia. J Neurol Neurosurg Psychiatry 37:489–501, 1974b

Miceli G, Giustolisi L, Caramazza A: The interaction of lexical and non-lexical processing mechanisms: evidence from anomia. Cortex 27:57–80, 1991

Michel F, Perenin MT, Sieroff E: Prosopagnosie sans hemianopsie apres lesion unilaterale occipito-temporale droite. Revue Neurologique 142:545–549, 1986

Mickel SF, Gabrieli JDE, Rosen TJ, et al: Mirror tracing: preserved learning in patients with global amnesia and some patients with Alzheimer's disease. Society for Neuroscience Abstracts 12:20, 1986

Milner B: Effects of different brain lesions on card sorting: the role of the frontal lobes. Arch Neurol 9:90–100, 1963

Milner B: Visual recognition and recall after right temporal-lobe excision in man. Neuropsychologia 6:191–209, 1968

Milner B: Disorders of learning and memory after temporal lobe lesions in man. Clin Neurosurg 19:421–446, 1972

Milner B, Petrides M: Behavioural effects of frontal-lobe lesions in man. Trends Neurosci 7:403–407, 1984

Milner B, Petrides M, Smith ML: Frontal lobes and the temporal organization of memory. Human Neurobiol 4:137–142, 1985

Mishkin M: Memory in monkeys severely impaired by combined but not separate removal of amygdala and hippocampus. Nature 273:297–298, 1978

Mohr JP, Watters WC, Duncan GW: Thalamic hemorrhage and aphasia. Brain Lang 2:3–17, 1975

Mohr JP, Pessin MS, Finkelstein S, et al: Broca aphasia: pathologic and clinical aspects. Neurology 28:311–324, 1978

Murray EA: Representational memory in nonhuman primates, in Neurobiology of Comparative Cognition. Edited by Kesner RP, Olton DS. Hillsdale, NJ, Lawrence Erlbaum Associates, 1990, pp 127–155

Murray EA, Mishkin M: Severe tactual as well as visual memory deficits follow combined removal of the amygdala and hippocampus in monkeys. J Neurosci 4:2565–2580, 1984

Murray EA, Mishkin M: Amygdalectomy impairs cross-modal association in monkeys. Science 228:604–606, 1985

Murray EA, Mishkin M: Visual recognition in monkeys following rhinal cortical ablations combined with either amygdalectomy or hippocampectomy. J Neurosci 6:1991–2003, 1986

Murray EA, Gaffan D, Mishkin M: Role of the amygdala and hippocampus in visual-visual associative memory in rhesus monkeys. Society for Neuroscience Abstracts 14:2, 1988

Naeser MA, Alexander MP, Helm-Estabrooks N, et al: Aphasia with predominantly subcortical lesion sites. Arch Neurol 39:2–14, 1982

Newcombe F: The processing of visual information in prosopagnosia and acquired dyslexia: functional versus physiological interpretation, in Research in Psychology and Medicine. Edited by Osborne DJ, Bruneberg MM, Eiser JR. London, Academic, 1979, pp 315–322

Newcombe F, Ratcliff G: Disorders of visuospatial analysis, in Handbook of Neuropsychology, Vol 2. Edited by Boller F, Grafman J. Amsterdam, Elsevier, 1989, pp 333–356

Penfield W, Roberts L: Speech and Brain Mechanisms. Princeton, NJ, Princeton University Press, 1959

Rapcsak SZ, Kaszniak AW, Rubens AB: Anomia for facial expressions: evidence for a category specific visual-verbal disconnection syndrome. Neuropsychologia 27: 1031–1041, 1989

Rizzo M: Astereopsis, in Handbook of Neuropsychology, Vol 2. Edited by Boller F, Grafman J. Amsterdam, Elsevier, 1989, pp 415–427

Rizzo M, Hurtig R: Looking but not seeing: attention, perception, and eye movements in simultanagnosia. Neurology 37:1642–1648, 1987

Robin DA, Tranel D, Damasio H: Auditory perception of temporal and spectral events in patients with focal left and right cerebral lesions. Brain Lang 39:539–555, 1990

Rosch E, Mervis CB, Gray WD, et al: Basic objects in natural categories. Cognitive Psychology 8:382–439, 1976

Ross ED: The aprosodias: functional-anatomic organization of the affective components of language in the right hemisphere. Arch Neurol 38:561–569, 1981

Rubens AB: Transcortical motor aphasia, in Studies in Neurolinguistics, Vol 1. Edited by Whitaker H, Whitaker HA. New York, Academic, 1976, pp 293–303

Sagar HJ, Gabrieli JDE, Sullivan EV, et al: Recency and frequency discrimination in the amnesic patient HM. Brain 113:581–602, 1990

Schiff HB, Alexander MP, Naeser MA, et al: Aphemia: clinic-anatomic correlations. Arch Neurol 40:720–727, 1983

Scoville WB, Milner B: Loss of recent memory after bilateral hippocampal lesions. J Neurol Neurosurg Psychiatry 20:11–21, 1957

Semenza C, Zettin M: Generating proper names: a case of selective inability. Cognitive Neuropsychology 5:711–721, 1988

Semenza C, Zettin M: Evidence from aphasia for the role of proper names as pure referring expressions. Nature 342:678–679, 1989

Sergent J, Villemure J-G: Prosopagnosia in a right hemispherectomized patient. Brain 112:975–995, 1989

Smith ML, Milner B: Estimation of frequency of occurrence of abstract designs after frontal or temporal lobectomy. Neuropsychologia 26:297–306, 1988

Smith ML, Milner B: Right hippocampal impairment in

the recall of spatial location: encoding deficit or rapid forgetting? Neuropsychologia 27:71–81, 1989

Stafiniak P, Saykin AJ, Sperling MR, et al: Acute naming deficits following dominant temporal lobectomy: prediction by age at first risk for seizures. Neurology 40: 1509–1512, 1990

Stuss DT, Benson DF: The Frontal Lobes. New York, Raven, 1986

Teuber H-L: Alteration of perception and memory in man: reflections on methods, in Analysis of Behavioral Change. Edited by Weiskrantz L. New York, Harper & Row, 1968

Tranel D: Dissociated verbal and nonverbal retrieval and learning following left anterior temporal damage. Brain Cogn 15:187–200, 1991a

Tranel D: What has been rediscovered in "Rediscovering tactile agnosia"? Mayo Clin Proc 66:210–214, 1991b

Tranel D, Hyman BT: Neuropsychological correlates of bilateral amygdala damage. Arch Neurol 47:349–355, 1990

Tranel D, Damasio AR, Damasio H: Intact recognition of facial expression, gender, and age in patients with impaired recognition of face identity. Neurology 38:690–696, 1988

Van Essen CD, Maunsell JHR: Hierarchical organization and functional streams in the visual cortex. Trends Neurosci 6:370–375, 1983

Van Hoesen GW, Damasio AR: Neural correlates of cognitive impairment in Alzheimer's disease, in Handbook of Physiology: Higher Functions of the Nervous System. Edited by Mountcastle V, Plum F. Bethesda, MD, American Physiological Society, 1987, pp 871–898

Van Hoesen GW, Hyman BT, Damasio AR: Cell-specific pathology in neural systems of the temporal lobe in Alzheimer's disease, in Progress in Brain Research. Edited by Swaab D. Amsterdam, Elsevier, 1986, pp 361–375

Van Lancker D, Kreiman J: Unfamiliar voice discrimination and familiar voice recognition are independent and unordered abilities. Neuropsychologia 25:829–834, 1988

Van Lancker D, Cummings J, Kreiman J, et al: Phonagnosia: a dissociation between familiar and unfamiliar voices. Cortex 24:195–209, 1988

Van Lancker D, Kreiman J, Cummings J: Voice perception deficits: neuroanatomical correlates of phonagnosia. J Clin Exp Neuropsychol 11:665–674, 1989

Victor M, Agamanolis D: Amnesia due to lesions confined to the hippocampus: a clinical-pathologic study. Journal of Cognitive Neuroscience 2:246–257, 1990

Victor M, Adams RD, Collins GH: The Wernicke-Korsakoff Syndrome and Related Neurologic Disorders Due to Alcoholism and Malnutrition, 2nd Edition. Philadelphia, PA, FA Davis, 1989

Vignolo LA: Auditory agnosia. Philos Trans R Soc Lond [Biol] 298:49–57, 1982

Volpe BT, Hirst W: Amnesia following the rupture and repair of an anterior communicating artery aneurysm. J Neurol Neurosurg Psychiatry 46:704–709, 1983

Warrington EK, McCarthy RA: Categories of knowledge: further fractionations and an attempted integration. Brain 110:1273–1296, 1987

Warrington EK, Shallice T: Category specific semantic impairments. Brain 107:829–854, 1984

Weintraub S, Mesulam M-M: Neglect: hemispheric specialization, behavioral components and anatomical correlates, in Handbook of Neuropsychology, Vol 2. Edited by Boller F, Grafman J. Amsterdam, Elsevier, 1989, pp 357–374

Young AW, Newcombe F, Hellawell D, et al: Implicit access to semantic information. Brain Cogn 11:186–209, 1989

Zeki SM: Colour coding in rhesus monkey prestriate cortex. Brain Res 53:422–427, 1973

Zihl J, Von Cramon Z, Mai N: Selective disturbances of movement vision after bilateral brain damage. Brain 106:313–340, 1983

Zola-Morgan S, Squire LR: Memory impairment in monkeys following lesions of hippocampus. Behav Neurosci 100:165–170, 1986

Zola-Morgan S, Squire LR, Amaral DG: Human amnesia and the medial temporal region: enduring memory impairment following a bilateral lesions limited to field CA1 of the hippocampus. J Neurosci 6:2950–2967, 1986

Zola-Morgan S, Squire LR, Amaral DG: Amnesia following medial temporal lobe damage in monkeys: the importance of the hippocampus and adjacent cortical regions. Society for Neuroscience Abstracts 14:1043, 1988

Zola-Morgan S, Squire LR, Amaral DG, et al: Lesions of perirhinal and parahippocampal cortex that spare the amygdala and hippocampal formation produce severe memory impairment. J Neurosci 9:4355–4370, 1989

Section II

Neuropsychiatric Assessment

Chapter

4

Bedside Neuropsychiatry: Eliciting the Clinical Phenomena of Neuropsychiatric Illness

Fred Ovsiew, M.D.

> Unless we take pains to be accurate in our examinations as to the question propounded, our observations will be of little value. The investigator who simply asks leading questions . . . is not accumulating "facts," but is "organising confusion." He will make errors enough without adopting a clumsy plan of investigating which renders blundering certain.
>
> John Hughlings-Jackson (1880–1881)

THIS CHAPTER IS DESIGNED to provide the neuropsychiatric clinician with a scheme for gathering data at the bedside. To this end, in this chapter I review the tools offered by history taking and examination for discovering the contribution of cerebral dysfunction to psychological abnormality. It is my belief that the data available at the bedside are rich and that they are the touchstone for the data gathered elsewhere: when they are incomplete or ignored, error ensues and the patient suffers.

A catalog of the full range of psychopathology is not within the scope of this chapter. Nor is classical neurological examination, which, as Hertzig and Birch (1966) noted many years ago, is a sensitive instrument for detecting dysfunction in the primary sensory and motor areas of the brain (and of course the spinal cord and peripheral nerves), but not for

The author thanks Jeffrey Cummings, M.D., and Philip Gorelick, M.D., for their helpful critiques and Professor W. Alwyn Lishman for his critique and for his example and encouragement.

the investigation of the areas of the brain more involved in complex behavior. Moreover, the links between psychopathological phenomena and their anatomic or physiological substrates are not fully discussed herein. Several writers have offered comprehensive discussions of the "regional affiliations" of psychopathological states (Damasio and Damasio 1989; Lishman 1987). The narrow focus of this chapter is how to use elements of the history and techniques of the examination to reveal the contribution of organic cerebral disease to psychopathology.

In contrast to traditional presentations of similar material, the discussion in this chapter is not divided into "physical" and "mental" examinations. (Is the inference of affect from facial expression "physical" or "mental"? Does asking the patient to tap on his knee turn the assessment of attention from "mental" to "physical"?) At the risk of idiosyncrasy I have reconceptualized the examination to a limited degree. The presentation of the examination is based on the functions it is meant to probe. But the reader must supplement the neuropsychiatric material herein with the standard elements of the neurological and psychiatric assessments. A dropped reflex in a cancer patient with delirium may be the pointer to meningeal carcinomatosis; the epileptic patient's childhood may give the clues to his religious beliefs. For that matter, palpation of the thyroid may yield the explanation for depression. In neuropsychiatry, everything counts.

❑ TAKING THE HISTORY

Obtaining a history is an active process on the part of the interviewer, who must have in mind a matrix to be filled in with information. The excuse, "The patient is a poor historian," has no place in neuropsychiatry. The examiner must realize that he or she (and not the patient) is the historian, responsible for gathering information from all necessary sources and forming a coherent narrative. Discovering that the patient is unable to give an adequate account of his or her life and illness should prompt, first, a search for other informants, and, second, a search for an explanation of the incapacity.

Birth history. The neuropsychiatric history begins even before birth. Maternal illness in pregnancy and the process of labor and delivery must be reviewed with an eye to untoward events associated with fetal maldevelopment. The neuropsychiatrist must inquire about maternal illness, bleeding, and substance abuse during pregnancy; the course of labor; and fetal distress at birth and in the immediate postnatal period. Such complications are associated with neurological signs at birth, although these signs may be subtle and not apparent on the ordinary examination of the newborn (Prechtl 1967). An association of obstetric complications with schizophrenia and autism seems well established (Lewis 1989). Whether obstetric problems are the cause of brain maldevelopment or merely a marker of a developmental process gone awry is, however, unknown (Paneth 1986).

Developmental history. At times the historian can gather information from the first few seconds of extrauterine life, for example when Apgar scores are available in hospital records. More commonly, the examiner must rely on parental recollection of milestones: the age at which the child crawled, walked, spoke words, spoke sentences, went to school, and so on. Parents may be able to compare the patient to a "control" sibling. The infant's temperament (e.g., active, cuddly, or fussy) may give clues to persisting traits. School performance is an important marker of both the intellectual and the social competence of the child, and often it is the only information available about premorbid intellectual level. Childhood illness, including febrile convulsions, head injury, and central nervous system infection, is sometimes the precursor of adult neuropsychiatric disorder.

Handedness. At the bedside, the simplest and most obvious indicator of cerebral dominance is handedness. Numerous questionnaires are available, although their psychometric properties leave something to be desired (Bryden 1977; McMeekan and Lishman 1975). Fortunately, a few very simple inquiries yield information that has an excellent correlation with behavioral observation. Asking the patient which hand he or she uses to write, throw, draw, and use a scissors or toothbrush (Bryden 1977) serves well to establish handedness. Although for research purposes most investigators consider handedness a dimensional rather than categorical variable, many clinicians think of it as a dichotomous variable: strongly dextral or not strongly dextral. With some nonverbal patients (severely mentally retarded patients, for example), throwing a ball or a crumpled piece of paper to the patient allows a simple examination for handedness. The "torque test" of drawing circles (Demarest and Demarest

1980), the examination of the angle formed by the opposed thumb and little finger (Metzig et al. 1975, 1976), and the observation of handwriting posture (Levy and Reid 1976) have their advocates as ways to establish cerebral dominance beyond simple handedness.

History of ictal events. Many sorts of spells or attacks occur in neuropsychiatric patients, and taking the history of a paroxysmal event has certain requirements regardless of the nature of the event. Ounsted et al. (1987) have argued that attacks of many types—ranging from a sneeze through orgasm to the epileptic seizure—share characteristics because they represent the nervous system's "going absolute." The clinician must be concerned with the phases of the paroxysm, starting with a prodrome, then the aura, then the remainder of the ictus (the aura being the onset or core of the ictus), and finally the aftermath. For any attack disorder, it must be determined how frequent and how stereotyped the events are. Rapidity of onset and offset; disturbance of consciousness or of language; the occurrence of autochthonous sensations, ideas, and emotions and of lateralized motor dysfunction; the purposefulness and coordination of actions; memory for the spell; and the duration of the recovery period must be ascertained. I begin the seizure inquiry by asking if the patient has just one sort of spell or more than one. This reduces confusion for the patient who has both partial and generalized seizures, and not a few patients with pseudoseizures will say in nearly so many words that they have epileptic spells and then the other sort that happens when they are upset.

Prodromal phases of epileptic attacks were formerly well known when epileptic individuals lived in colonies and were under observation as they "built up" to a seizure. It has been demonstrated systematically that adverse mood changes commonly occur on the days preceding a seizure (Blanchet and Frommer 1986). Remarkably little is understood of the mechanism of such prodromes to seizures. Prodromes occur in migraine as well, as Sacks (1971) has described.

Hermann et al. (1982) reported that patients with fear as a part of the seizure ictus were at greater risk for psychopathology. This claim is given added plausibility by a comparable finding in an animal model (Griffith et al. 1987). Taylor and Lochery (1987) showed that the nature of the aura in complex partial epilepsy is correlated with age at onset, IQ, laterality, and the nature of the temporal lobe pathology.

History of head injury. Discerning the role of cerebral dysfunction in posttraumatic states is a common diagnostic challenge. The length of the anterograde amnesia—from the moment of trauma to the recovery of the capacity for consecutive memory—can be learned either from the patient or from hospital records. The patient can say what the last memories before the accident are; from last memory to injury is the period of retrograde amnesia. The length of these intervals and the duration of coma are correlated with the severity of brain damage (Lishman 1987). Usually posttraumatic amnesia is the best indicator. The nature of the trauma, including its psychosocial setting, should be learned; at times the most important fact about a head injury is the reckless behavior that produced it.

Alcohol and drug use. Various neurotoxins are in widespread use in our society. Cocaine is currently popular (Mody et al. 1988); alcohol is an old favorite (Lishman 1990). The substance abuse history must be taken from all patients. Questions about vocational, family, and medical impairment attributable to abuse; shame and guilt over abuse and efforts to control it; morning or secret drinking; blackouts; and other familiar issues help the clinician identify pathological behavior in this sphere.

History of mild cognitive impairment. The clinical features of substantial and progressive intellectual impairment—dementia—are well known and are reviewed authoritatively in Chapters 25 and 26 and elsewhere (Lishman 1987). One commonly encounters patients with mild, chronic, stable, global cognitive disturbance not meeting the criteria for a diagnosis of dementia; no doubt the most frequent condition giving rise to this state is traumatic brain injury. Lezak (1978) stressed the patients' experience of perplexity, distractibility, and fatigue in mild and severe brain injury. In my experience, some cognitive symptoms reported by patients are so characteristic as to be diagnostic of organic illness. Other features, such as the tendency to emotional lability and irritability, are characteristic of but not specific to organic states. The following examples illustrate such near-pathognomonic cognitive symptoms.

Before the resection of an arteriovenous malformation, a successful businesswoman had been accustomed to reading the newspaper carefully over breakfast. Afterward, she soon discovered that though she was able to read the newspaper and absorb its import adequately, she was not able to do so while eating breakfast. She could do only one thing at a time. Another patient was said by his wife to have become a "sequential thinker." This loss of the capacity for divided attention is highly characteristic of mild cerebral disease. In a related way, distractibility is heightened, and automatic tasks become ones requiring attention and effort. A patient's digit span was found to be defective. She asked if the window could be closed, because the traffic noise was bothering her. The examiner had not noticed the noise, but with the window closed the patient's digit span was normal. Such deficits are common in more severely impaired patients as well, but are masked by more florid deficits. These symptoms were clearly described and experimentally demonstrated many years ago (Brodal 1973; Chapman and Wolff 1958; Chapman et al. 1958); but in our passion for localization, some of them, being dependent on the bulk of disease in the hemispheres but independent of its location, have been forgotten.

Appetitive functions. Appetitive functions refer to sleep, eating, and sexual interest and performance. Disturbed sleep is common among patients with mental disorders of any origin, as well as in the general population. In a search for clues to organic factors, the clinician inquires about the pattern of disturbance: the early waking of depressive illness, nighttime wakings related to pain or nocturnal myoclonus, the excessive daytime sleepiness of narcolepsy and sleep apnea, sleep attacks in narcolepsy, and the periodic excessive somnolence of the Kleine-Levin syndrome and related disorders. Some neuropsychiatrists take an interest in the patient's dream life; loss of dreaming has been reported in association with cerebral disease (Greenberg and Farah 1986). Similarly, in regard to appetite, patterns of abnormal eating behavior can be recognized beyond the anorexia of depressive illness and so-called anorexia of anorexia nervosa: the hyperphagia of hypothalamic disease, in which food exerts an irresistible attraction; the mouthing and eating of nonfood objects in bilateral amygdaline disease (the Klüver-Bucy syndrome); and the impulsive stuffing of food into the mouth in frontal disease.

Sexual interest and performance are commonly disturbed in brain disease, but often the clinician's inquiry does not extend to these matters. Perhaps this is from delicacy; perhaps our patients seem to have more important worries—seem so to us, that is, not necessarily to them. Helping a patient discuss these matters can be a great relief to the patient even if nothing further is done, and often more can be done. Once the subject is broached, the details of abnormal sexual performance can usually be elicited without great difficulty, and its nature can be related to the known physiology of sexual function (Boller and Frank 1982). Sexual interest (libido) is, in my view, more difficult to elucidate. Only a skilled interviewer can find his or her way through the maze of defenses, and tentatively at that. That said, hyposexuality does seem to be a recognizable feature of epilepsy, although its mechanism is still subject to controversy (Toone et al. 1989). A change in a person's habitual sexual interests, either quantitative or qualitative, occurring de novo in adult life, may bespeak organic disease (Miller et al. 1986).

Aggression. Aggressive behavior is a common and exceptionally distressing consequence of brain dysfunction. It is also alarmingly widespread in contexts where brain disease is absent (Dietz 1987). Patterns of aggressive behavior in brain disease have been described and related to the locus of injury (Bear 1989; Ovsiew and Yudofsky, in press), and epileptic violence has been clearly described (Fenwick 1989). Features of aggressive behavior such as its onset and offset; the patient's mental state and especially clarity of consciousness during the violent period; his (and it is usually males in question) capacity for planned, coordinated, and well-organized action as displayed in the act; his regret or otherwise afterward; and any associated symptoms may yield clues to the contribution of cerebral dysfunction to the behavior.

Personality change. Changes in sexual preference with onset in adult life have already been mentioned (above) as pointers to organic mental disorder. Persisting alterations in or exaggerations of other personality traits, if not related to an abnormal affective state or psychosis, may be important indicators of the development of cerebral disease. A particular set of changes in personality traits is said to be distinctive in temporal lobe epilepsy. These include the development of mystical or religious interests, a shorter temper, and hyposexuality. Whether these traits are related to epilepsy, to the temporal lobe injury underlying epilepsy, or merely to psychopathology remains controversial (Bear et al. 1989).

Occupational history. The relationship of occupational hazards to illness is an entire medical specialty, and an outline for the elicitation of relevant information has been prepared (Occupational and Environmental Health Committee of the American Lung Association of San Diego and Imperial Counties 1983). Exposures to heavy metals or volatile hydrocarbons and repeated blows to the head in boxers are examples of occupational causes of neuropsychiatric illness. Apart from etiological information, the clinician needs to know about the patient's work in order to gauge premorbid capacities and to assess disability.

Family history. Genetic contributors to many neuropsychiatric illnesses are well delineated (e.g., in Huntington's disease); in others the contribution is probable but the mechanism less clear (e.g., in Tourette's syndrome). In epilepsy, there appears to be genetic transmission of a seizure threshold, so that even with a known cerebral insult the family history of epilepsy influences whether seizures occur (Engel 1989). Inquiring about the family history of neuropsychiatric illness relative by relative, even constructing a family tree with the assistance of collateral informants, reveals more relevant information than probes such as "Is there any mental illness in the family?"

❑ EXAMINING THE PATIENT

The British neurologist Henry Miller (1975) referred to psychiatry as "neurology without physical signs" (p. 462). Geoffrey Lloyd (1983) called psychosomatics "medicine without signs" (p. 539). Neuropsychiatry can be considered "psychiatry with signs." The neuropsychiatric examination seeks signs of cerebral dysfunction. Unfortunately, few investigators have discussed such signs with scientific rigor: the sensitivity and specificity of many findings are unknown, even for signs that are routine or traditional in the clinical examination. As a result, too often the clinical examination proceeds by ritual. The clinician who asks the patient with right-hemisphere stroke to interpret proverbs but not to copy figures or asks him to remember three words but not three shapes is bowing to tradition and ignoring the physiology of the brain disease. Sometimes clinicians attempt to elicit not signs of brain disease but so-called positive signs of nonorganic states. Vibratory sensation that shows lateralized deficit on the sternum is an example. These signs are of limited use, not because they are uncommon in hysteria, but because suggestibility is common in organic mental states as well (Gould et al. 1986). They cannot be recommended for differential diagnosis.

The following discussion focuses on the scientific basis for inference from the clinician's observations in the examination room to encourage the thoughtful use of probes guided by specific hypotheses about brain dysfunction.

General Appearance

Asymmetry. Abnormal development of a hemisphere may be betrayed by slight differences in the size of the thumbs or thumbnails. Occasionally this can be a lateralizing sign in epilepsy. Penfield and Robertson (1943) pointed out that a postcentral location of cortical lesions causing asymmetry is characteristic.

Minor physical anomalies. The adult neuropsychiatrist bringing a developmental perspective to the bedside hopes to elicit information that reveals something about the patient's fetal life. Such signs do exist; Table 4–1 lists such minor physical anomalies.

These physical anomalies are stable through childhood and presumably into adulthood. The clinician wishing to use them as diagnostic signs must be cautious, however, because they may occur in subjects with no neuropsychiatric illness. No individual anomaly, except perhaps head circumference (Steg and Rapoport 1975), has a correlation with psychopathology. The cutoff scores for abnormality have varied somewhat in various investigations, but by consensus a finding of four or more anomalies is a pointer to deviant development. The deviation can be confidently traced to the first 4 months of fetal life, and a correlation with both paternal psychopathology and obstetric complications suggests that either genetic or traumatic factors can give rise to the disturbance of gestation (Firestone and Peters 1983; Quinn and Rapoport 1974). Presumably the relationship of the anomalies to the brain disorder lies in a subtle disturbance of cerebral development occurring at the same period of gestation.

Such abnormalities have been shown to correlate with the presence of schizophrenia, especially with early onset of illness and poor premorbid functioning (Green et al. 1989; Gualtieri et al. 1982; Guy

TABLE 4–1. MINOR PHYSICAL ANOMALIES

Head
- Head circumference outside the normal range (normal male: 21"–23"; normal female: 20.5"–22.5")
- Fine "electric" hair (won't comb down)
- More than one hair whorl
- Abnormal epicanthic folds of the eyes
- Hypertelorism or hypotelorism
- Low-set ears (entirely below plane of the pupils)
- Malformed or asymmetric ears
- High palate
- Furrowed tongue

Hands and feet
- Curved fifth finger (clinodactyly)
- Single palmar crease (as is seen in Down's syndrome)
- Wide gap between the first and second toes
- Partial syndactyly of the toes
- Third toe longer than second toe

et al. 1983); autism (Gualtieri et al. 1982; Steg and Rapoport 1975); impulsive, hyperactive, and aggressive behavior in male children (Fogel et al. 1985; Gualtieri et al. 1982; Quinn and Rapoport 1974) and perhaps inhibitedness in female children (Fogel et al. 1985); and recidivistic criminal violence (Kandel et al. 1989). Fogel et al. (1985) went so far as to say that in boys the central nervous system deficit marked by these anomalies seems "almost to be a necessary but not sufficient condition for hyperactive behavior" (p. 554). In another study (Quinn and Rapoport 1974), however, both minor physical anomalies and neurological soft signs were correlated to hyperactivity, but not to each other; the inference was of more than one pathway to the clinical phenomenon.

Olfaction

Assessment of olfaction is often omitted by examiners, "cranial nerves II through XII" being reported as normal. But abnormalities of the sense of smell are not infrequent among neuropsychiatric patients and can be of functional importance and diagnostic significance. Hyposmia or anosmia can be detected in Alzheimer's disease, Parkinson's disease, normal aging, schizophrenia, multiple sclerosis, subfrontal tumor, and traumatic brain injury (Eslinger et al. 1982; Harrison and Pearson 1989; Pinching 1977). The most common cause of hyposmia, however, is local disease of the nasal mucosa, and the examiner must exclude this before regarding a finding as neuropsychiatrically significant.

Two technical issues confront the examining physician: what test odor to use and what to regard as an abnormal response. Pinching (1977) provided a modern assessment of the first issue. It is well known that stimuli that cause trigeminal irritation (e.g., ammonia) are not suitable for testing the integrity of the olfactory pathways proper. Floral and musk odors provide the greatest sensitivity. I use scented lip balm in raspberry and cherry "flavors"; these are simple and strong, and the containers do not break in my medical bag, as the small bottle of oil of cloves I once favored did (with long-lasting results). With regard to the second issue, it is known that the pathways for olfactory recognition differ from those for olfactory detection. In lesions of the temporal lobe, detection thresholds are raised, but those for recognition of the characteristics of the odor are unaffected (Rausch and Serafetinides 1975). Conversely, in lesions of prefrontal cortex, detection is intact but recognition and discrimination are affected (Potter and Butters 1980). However, bedside testing may not have the power to make this distinction between detection and recognition, especially because the odors most sensitive in revealing altered detection thresholds are difficult for even healthy subjects to identify (Pinching 1977). Probably, the examiner needs to settle for asking the patient whether the stimulus is detected, regardless of the patient's capacity to name or describe the stimulus. More sophisticated equipment is available for clinical use (Moore-Gillon 1987).

The Eyes

Pupils, corneas, and irises. The dilated pupils of anticholinergic toxicity may be a clue to the cause of delirium, the small pupils of opiate intoxication to substance abuse. Argyll Robertson pupils—bilaterally small, irregular, and reactive to accommodation but not light—are still a characteristic accompaniment of neurosyphilis in the antibiotic era (Luxon et al. 1979).

A Kayser-Fleischer ring is invariably present when Wilson's disease affects the brain, with the possible rare exception of the patient with coexisting bilateral annulus senilis (Scheinberg et al. 1986). This brownish-green discoloration of the cornea begins at the limbus, at 12 o'clock then 6 o'clock, spreading from each location medially and laterally until a complete ring is formed. Because a Kayser-Fleischer ring can be difficult to discern in patients with dark irises, slit-lamp examination should supplement bedside inspection (Marsden 1987; Walshe 1986).

Some years ago, Korein (1981) reported that pale (blue, green, gray, or hazel) irises were more common among patients with dystonia than among control subjects. Because eye color depends on melatonin, and because the pathway for synthesis of melatonin shares enzymes with that for dopamine, it is plausible that eye color provides an indicator of central monoamine status. The observation has not been confirmed (Lang et al. 1982).

Visual fields. Two applications of this standard test to neuropsychiatric problems can be mentioned. First, localization of lesions to the temporal lobe by bedside examination can be difficult. It is established that when lesions disrupt the white matter of the temporal lobe, a congruent homonymous upper quadrantanopsia or even a full homonymous hemianopsia can result from involvement of Meyer's loop, the portion of the optic radiation that dips into the temporal lobe (Falconer and Wilson 1958). Second, delirium from posterior cerebral or right middle cerebral artery infarction has been described; in such cases, physical signs of stroke may be scant, and a metabolic encephalopathy may be assumed, but hemianopsia is a regular accompaniment (Caplan et al. 1986; Devinsky et al. 1988). It can obviously be difficult to establish the field cut in an agitated, confused patient, but it should be sought in every case of delirium of unknown cause.

Blinking. The normal response to regular 1-per-second tapping on the glabella (with the examiner behind the patient so that the striking finger is not within the patient's visual field) is blinking to the first few taps, then habituation and no blinking. The normal spontaneous blink rate, in the most careful study of healthy subjects at various ages, was shown to increase through childhood, but it was found stable in adulthood at a rate of about 16 ± 8 (Zametkin et al. 1979). In a review of the literature, Karson (1988) suggested considering "about 20" blinks per minute as normal.

In 1978 Stevens drew attention to abnormalities of blinking in schizophrenic patients (and reminded us that Kraepelin, among other early investigators, had already commented on them). She found high spontaneous rates of blinking, paroxysms of rapid rhythmic blinking during episodes of abnormal behavior, and abnormal responses to glabellar tap. On glabellar tap, Stevens's patients either failed to blink, produced a shower of blinks, or failed to habituate. Although her patients were drug free, few were neuroleptic naive, so she could not distinguish between an abnormality intrinsic to schizophrenia and a tardive dyskinesia. This finding has been confirmed by others (Helms and Godwin 1985; Karson 1979) and can be confirmed by any examiner seeing schizophrenic patients.

The matter is of particular interest because the rate of spontaneous blinking is quite insensitive to peripheral stimuli (ambient light, humidity, and even deafferentation of the fifth nerve) but seems to be under dopaminergic control (Karson 1983). This is shown by the clinical finding that blink rate is low in parkinsonism and increases with effective levodopa (L-dopa) treatment (Karson et al. 1984) and by the laboratory finding that blink rate is inversely correlated with monoamine oxidase level (Freed et al. 1980). Thus the blink rate provides a simple, quantitative measure of central dopamine activity. The elevated rates can sometimes be astronomic, and the paroxysms of blinking or blepharospasm provoked by glabellar tap can be quite impressive. Failure to habituate to glabellar tap is seen in parkinsonism as well and is called Myerson's sign.

Eye movements. In the same report, Stevens (1978) called attention to early observations by Kraepelin and others of abnormal eye movements in psychotic patients. These are often given inferential descriptions in clinical practice ("he's looking at the voices"), but it is a useful discipline to attempt a phenomenologic description ("he shows unexplained episodic lateral glances"). Stevens noted gaze abnormalities, abnormality in eye contact with the examiner (e.g., fixed staring or no eye contact), impaired convergence movements, and irregular smooth pursuit movements (the sort of movements generated when the patient follows the examiner's finger with the eyes).

The latter observations can be compared to the laboratory investigations of abnormal smooth pursuit movements in psychotic patients. This abnormality is thought to be a trait variable under genetic control and related to abnormal attentional function and vulnerability to psychosis. Unfortunately these laboratory investigations do not include comparisons to simple bedside tests of smooth pursuit eye movements, comparisons that might reveal the sensitivity and specificity of the bedside finding.

Elucidating the abnormalities of eye movement

in neuropsychiatric patients requires the separate examination of voluntary eye movements without fixation ("look to the left"), generation of saccades to a target ("look at my finger, now at my fist"), and smooth pursuit movement ("follow my finger"). Early failure of vertical saccades, with intact function of the lower motor neuron, is the hallmark of progressive supranuclear palsy. The finding is of impaired voluntary eye movements, but the patient is still able to generate full upgaze and downgaze when fixing his or her eyes on a still target while the examiner moves the patient's head up and down (the doll's eye maneuver). Slowed or hypometric saccades are a feature of Huntington's disease. An internuclear ophthalmoplegia may reveal an illness marked by vague sensory symptoms to be multiple sclerosis. Palsies of eye movement in a confused patient may indicate Wernicke's encephalopathy. In head-eye synkinesia, the patient automatically moves the head along with the eyes in shifting gaze. This sign has been demonstrated in schizophrenia (Kolada and Pitman 1983) and is seen in dementia.

Apraxia of gaze is, like other apraxias, a failure of voluntary movement with the preserved capacity for spontaneous movement, in this case horizontal or vertical gaze. It is a feature of Balint's syndrome (De Renzi 1985). So-called apraxia of eye opening is probably an extrapyramidal disorder of lid movement (Lepore and Duvoisin 1985). The status of apraxia of eye closure is more complicated; in at least some cases, a supranuclear motor disorder affects other bulbar musculature and the designation *apraxia* is inappropriate (Ross Russell 1980). In some cases, there is a link to impersistence (discussed below) (Fisher 1956).

Facial Movement

Dissociated facial paresis. The presence of a double dissociation in the realm of facial movement demonstrates that emotional movements and volitional ones are separately organized (Monrad-Krohn 1924; Wilson 1924). A paresis seen in movements to command ("show me your teeth") is sometimes overcome in spontaneous smiling (still counted as spontaneous if elicited by a joke); this indicates disease in pyramidal pathways. The inverse phenomenon—normal movement to command but asymmetry of spontaneous emotional movements—is seen with disease in thalamus (Bogousslavsky et al. 1988; Graff-Radford et al. 1984), temporal lobe (Remillard et al. 1977); striatum and internal capsule (Trosch et al. 1990); and premotor cortex (Laplane et al. 1976). Damasio and Maurer (1978) reported the occurrence of this sign in autism and argued that it indicated disease in limbic regions. The sign has lateralizing value in temporal lobe epilepsy (Remillard et al. 1977).

Facial expression. The "omega sign" and Verraguth's folds are long-recognized facial signs of depressive illness (Figure 4–1) (Greden et al. 1985). Many brain diseases can be recognized by characteristic facial appearances (e.g., Wilson's disease and myotonic dystrophy); some of these appearances are presented photographically in Spillane's *Atlas* (1975).

Speech

Dysarthria. The disorders of articulation are difficult to describe, although often easy to recognize when heard. In pyramidal disorders, the speech output is slow, strained, and slurred in articulation.

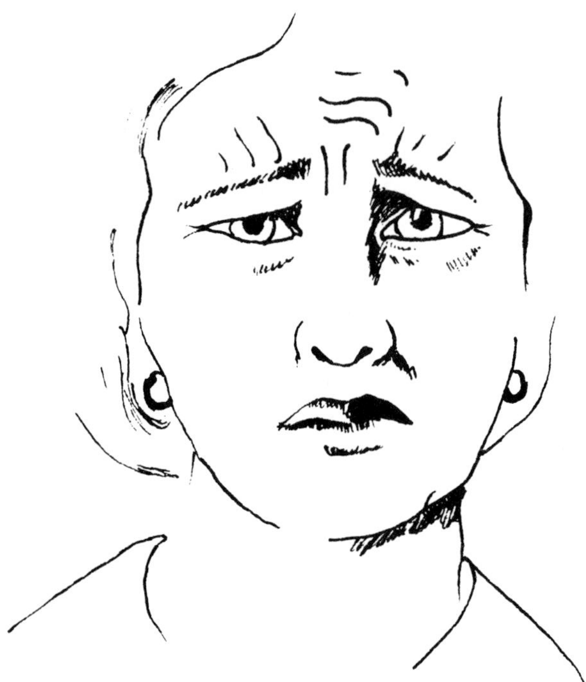

Figure 4–1. The omega sign is the Ω-shaped pattern of wrinkles between and above the eyebrows. Verraguth's folds are the wrinkles sloping medially above the eyebrows. (Adapted from Greden et al. 1985. Used with permission.)

Often accompanying the speech disorder are the other features of pseudobulbar palsy, including dysphagia, drooling, and a disturbance of the expression of emotions. Usually the causative lesions are bilateral, although the onset of the disorder may be after an acute unilateral lesion, the lesion of the opposite hemisphere having preexisted the new lesion. Unilateral lesions of the left motor cortex and frontal operculum can cause dysarthria (discussed below). Bulbar, or flaccid, dysarthria is marked by breathiness and nasality, with impaired articulation present as well. Signs of lower motor neuron involvement can be found in the bulbar musculature. The lesion is in the lower brain stem. Scanning speech is a characteristic sign of disease of the cerebellum and its connections; the speech output is irregular in rate with equalization of the stress on the syllables. In extrapyramidal disorders and in depression, speech is hypophonic and monotonous, often tailing off with longer phrases.

Darley et al. (1975) described in detail a scheme for examination of the motor aspects of speech. It begins with the assessment of the elements of speech production (e.g., facial musculature, tongue, and palate) at rest and during voluntary movement. The patient is asked to produce the vowel *ah* steadily for as long as possible; the performance is assessed for voice quality, duration, pitch, steadiness, and loudness. Production of strings of individual consonants (*puh-puh-puh-puh* and so on) and alternated consonants (*puh-tuh-kuh-puh-tuh-kuh*) is assessed for rate and rhythm. Extended utterances are also examined to observe the effects of fatigue and context.

Stuttering. Stuttering, or stammering, of the common developmental sort is familiar to everyone's ear. The rhythm of speech is disturbed by the repetition, prolongation, or arrest of sounds. The cause of this disorder is unknown, despite extensive research and a multiplicity of hypotheses.

Acquired stuttering is unusual but has been carefully studied. In one report (Helm et al. 1978), acquired stuttering seemed to differ from the developmental variety in occurring on any syllable in a word (not just initial syllables) and on grammatical words as well as substantives. Anxiety and the secondary signs of a struggle to speak (e.g., grimacing), common in developmental stuttering, were absent in the acquired form. These investigators found that visuospatial function and motor rhythm were concomitantly disturbed. Bilateral hemisphere disease was the regular substrate. Another group of investigators (Ludlow et al. 1987) stressed the rapid-fire quality of the speech. Oral motor control was disturbed as was rapid sequential finger movement. In this series of cases, disease lay in deep structures or white matter in either hemisphere; bilateral disease was rare.

Dysprosody. In 1947, the Scandinavian neurologist Monrad-Krohn described dysprosody or "altered melody of language" in a patient with a wartime missile injury of the left frontotemporal region. She was a noncombatant; in fact she had never been out of her small Norwegian town. She showed aphasic troubles, mild right-sided signs, and slight personality change. Most strikingly, her speech pattern had changed, so that she sounded like a German when she spoke her native Norwegian. One can imagine how unwelcome this particular symptom was. Whitty (1964) elaborated on this phenomenon under the name *dysprosody of speech*; he reviewed the literature and reported a case with a well-circumscribed left frontal lesion. In this case, mild dysarthric and dysphasic features resolved, leaving an apparent German accent in an Englishwoman.

Later, Heilman and colleagues (Heilman et al. 1975; Tucker et al. 1977) and Ross and Mesulam (1979) reported cases in which right-hemisphere lesions led to loss of the affective elements of speech. Analysis of the cases led to recognition of syndromes of loss of prosody in expression and of impaired decoding of prosodic information. Ross (1981) later schematized these syndromes—the "aprosodias"—as mirror images of left-hemisphere aphasic syndromes. This apparently simplistic classification has been surprisingly successful (Gorelick and Ross 1987), although it has been criticized on methodological grounds by investigators who found prominent involvement of basal ganglia in disturbances of both prosodic comprehension and prosodic expression (Cancelliere and Kertesz 1990).

It is clear that two different phenomena have been discussed under similar names. The examiner confronted with a patient who has a disturbance of prosody in spontaneous speech of course looks for the features of dysarthria and aphasia. However, the aprosodias discussed by Ross (1981) present differently. There is no disturbance of propositional language; often the dysfunction seems to be in mood or social relatedness. Thus the early report by Ross and Mesulam (1979) included a teacher who could no longer discipline her class; examination proved that she could not produce the only tone of voice that elementary school students respond to. If such is suspected, or if right-hemisphere signs mandate the search for the neighborhood sign of disturbed affective prosody, the examiner must listen to spontaneous speech for prosodic elements; ask the patient to produce statements in various emotional tones (e.g., anger, sadness, surprise, and joy); produce such emotional phrasings himself or herself, using a neutral sentence ("I am going to the store") while turning his or her face away from the patient, and ask the patient to identify the emotion; and ask the patient to reproduce an emotional phrasing the examiner has generated. It can be seen that this duplicates the structure of the examination for disorders of propositional language.

Echolalia. In this phenomenon, another person's speech is repeated by the patient in an automatic fashion, that is, without communicative intent or effect. Because often this speech is that of the examiner, the phenomenon is immediately apparent without specific elicitation and is said to be related to the patient's rapport with the examiner (Ford 1989). However, at times the repetition is of other verbalization in the environment; for example, patients may repeat words overheard from the corridor or the television. Sometimes the patient repeats only the last portion of what he hears, beginning with a natural break in the utterance. Sometimes grammatical corrections are made, when the examiner deliberately utters a grammatically incorrect sentence. Sometimes the patient makes pronoun reversals (e.g., "I" for "you"), altering the sentence in a grammatically appropriate way. In these ways, the phenomenon demonstrates the intactness of syntactic operations. The completion phenomenon may be seen: the patient automatically completes a well-known phrase uttered by the examiner. "Roses are red," says the examiner; "roses are red, violets are blue," responds the patient. Speaking to the patient in a foreign language can elicit obviously automatic echolalic speech (Lecours et al. 1983).

The anatomic and psychopathological associations of echolalia have been reviewed (Ford 1989; Stengel 1947). Its occurrence in transcortical aphasia marks the intactness of primary language areas in the frontal and temporal lobes, with syntax thus unimpaired but disconnected from control by other cerebral functions. Autism, Tourette's syndrome, and disorders of the startle reaction are other underlying disorders. Echolalia also can be seen in catatonic states, whether of clear-cut organic or idiopathic origin. It also occurs as a normal phenomenon in the learning of language in infancy (Lecours et al. 1983).

Palilalia. This phenomenon is the automatic repetition of the patient's own final word or phrase, the voice tailing off in volume and festinant in rate. It can occur separately from echolalia or other disturbances of speech. It seems to be related to bilateral disease of the basal ganglia (Boller et al. 1973), although general paresis and epilepsy with a supplementary motor area focus have been implicated as well (Alajouanine et al. 1959; Critchley 1927; Geschwind 1964).

Blurting. I have seen a few patients whose speech output was marked by "blurting": the impulsive uttering of a stereotyped or simple response, with no aphasic or echolalic features. For example, an elderly woman had recurrent falls. Examination demonstrated limitation of downgaze and mild symmetrical briskness of tendon jerks. She had no evident cognitive abnormality on bedside testing. When questioned, she often replied "yes, yes" or "no, no" even before the questioner finished speaking and regardless of her intended answer to the question. She could then correct herself easily and give the reply she wished to give. She was unable to explain the behavior. The diagnosis in this case seemed to be progressive supranuclear palsy. This patient and others I have seen share evidence of disease in the frontostriatal circuit. The phenomenon seems to be related to echolalia and palilalia, as well as to the impulsive but not stereotyped utterances of patients with frontal disease.

Mutism. Although the term *mutism* may be used to refer to the "loss of the ability to vocalize" (Cummings et al. 1983, p. 255), perhaps it should be reserved for the situation "in which a person does not speak and does not make any attempt at spoken communication despite preservation of an adequate level of consciousness" (Departments of Psychiatry and Child Psychiatry, The Institute of Psychiatry, and The Maudsley Hospital, London 1987, p. 33). Clearly the first order of business in examining an alert patient who does not speak is to discover whether the disorder is due to elementary sensorimotor abnormalities involving the apparatus of speech. These local disturbances can be recognized by examining phonation, articulation, and nonspeech movements of the relevant musculature (e.g., swallowing and coughing).

If an elementary disorder is not at fault, the examination proceeds to a search for specific disturbances of verbal communication. It is necessary to determine whether the patient makes any spontaneous attempt at communication through means other than speech. Does the patient gesture? Can he or she write, or if hemiplegic can he or she write with the nondominant hand? Can he or she arrange letters presented in plastic form (cut-out paper letters or letters from a child's set of spelling toys), or if familiar with sign-language can he or she sign?

A wide variety of disorders can produce mutism (Altshuler et al. 1988). Some patients with lesions restricted to the lower primary motor cortex and the adjacent frontal operculum have a disorder that begins with mutism then recovers through severe dysarthria without agrammatism. This disorder has gone by many names (including the *cortical dysarthria* discussed above); a more recent term is *aphemia* (Schiff et al. 1983). Lesions involving additional surrounding territory may produce language impairment proper; this has been termed a *small Broca's aphasia* (Alexander 1989). In transcortical motor aphasia there is a prominent disturbance of spontaneous speech, occasionally beginning as mutism (Alexander 1989). Damasio and Van Hoesen (1983) described in detail a patient with a lesion in the dominant supplementary motor area; after recovery the patient reported that she lacked the urge to speak. Such a disturbance of verbal communication must be distinguished from a more global disorder of the initiation of activity. At its extreme the latter is the state of akinetic mutism.

Abnormalities of Movement

Weakness. The findings associated with lesions of the pyramidal tracts, spinal cord, peripheral nerves, and muscles are described in texts of neurology (Duus 1989). Greater awareness of the findings in nonpyramidal syndromes may help the clinician recognize disease outside the primary motor regions. Caplan et al. (1990) described the features of a nonpyramidal hemimotor syndrome with caudate lesions. Patients show clumsiness and decreased spontaneous use of the affected limbs; associated movements are decreased as well. What appears on initial testing to be paresis proves to be a slow development of full strength; if coaxed and given time, the patient shows mild weakness at worst. Freund and Hummelsheim (1985) explored the motor consequences of lesions of the premotor cortex. They observed a decrease in spontaneous use of the arm and attributed it to a failure of postural fixation; when supported, the arm showed at worst mild slowing of finger movements. The defect in elevation and abduction of the arm was best demonstrated by asking the patient to swing the arms in a windmill movement. Movement rapidly decomposed when such coordination was required. Pyramidal signs (e.g., increased tendon jerks, Babinski reflex, and spasticity) may be absent in patients with these findings. Stressed gait (e.g., walking heel-to-toe or on the outer aspects of the feet) may reveal a mild asymmetry in patients without other signs.

Akinesia. Akinesia has several aspects: delay in the initiation of movement, slowness in the execution of movement, and special difficulty with complex movements (Marsden 1986). The disturbance is conveniently examined by requiring the patient to perform a repeated action, such as tapping thumb to forefinger, or two actions at once. A decrement in amplitude or freezing in the midst of the act is observed. When established, akinesia is unmistakable in the patient's visage and demeanor, and in the way he or she sits motionlessly and has trouble rising from the chair. A distinction between parkinsonian akinesia and depressive psychomotor retardation is not easy to make, but the associated features of tremor, rigidity, and postural instability are generally absent in depressive illness (Rogers et al. 1987).

Agitation. Properly used, the term *agitation* refers to an increased amount of motor activity accompanying a dysphoric mood. Agitation is an important finding in confusional states, but not by any means a universal one. The term *delirium* is reserved by some for a confusional state (or "acute organic reaction") in which agitation and abnormal perceptual experiences are prominent. Why certain etiologies of confusion (e.g., alcohol withdrawal, hypoxemia, the postictal twilight state, and infarction in the territory of the posterior cerebral artery) commonly produce agitation and others do not is virtually unstudied. A hypothesis about preferential involvement of limbic brain regions is irresistible but entirely speculative.

Other states of overactivity can be distinguished. Akathisia is discussed below. Hyperactivity in childhood has been extensively studied and seems, at least when severe, to be linked to brain dysfunction and developmental disorder (Taylor 1986). Elderly patients with dementia often wander (Burns et al. 1990b), as do postictal epileptic patients sometimes; this is so-called poriomania (Mayeux et al. 1979).

Akathisia. Motor restlessness accompanied by an urge to move but not by abnormal mood is referred to as *akathisia.* The difficulty of eliciting the account of subjective restlessness from a psychotic patient is well known, but the importance of recognizing akathisia and distinguishing it from anxious or psychotic agitation has been stressed by several authors (Ball 1985; Van Putten 1975). Complaints specifically referable to the legs are far more characteristic of akathisia than of anxiety (Braude et al. 1983). In addition, the objective manifestations of akathisia are characteristic (Braude et al. 1983; Gibb and Lees 1986). Although by derivation akathisia refers to an inability to sit, its manifestations are most prominent when the patient attempts to stand still. When required to do so, the patient shifts weight from foot to foot, producing a "marching in place" appearance. Seated, the patient may shuffle or tap his feet or repeatedly cross his legs. When the disorder is severe, the recumbent patient may show myoclonic jerks or a coarse tremor of the legs. Rarely, akathisia may be unilateral (Carrazana et al. 1989; Hermesh and Munitz 1990). Persistent and tardive forms have been described.

Hypertonicity. Three forms of increased muscle tone concern the neuropsychiatrist: spasticity, rigidity, and paratonia. In spasticity, tone is increased in flexors in the upper extremity, extensors in the lower, but not in the antagonists. The hypertonicity shows the characteristic of an increase in resistance followed by an immediate decrease (the clasp-knife phenomenon) and is dependent on the velocity of the passive movement. This is the typical hemiplegic pattern of hemisphere stroke, universally called *pyramidal,* which indicates a lesion actually not in the pyramidal tract but in the corticoreticulospinal tract (Brodal 1981; Burke and Lance 1986). In rigidity, tone is increased in both agonists and antagonists throughout the range of motion, thus the term *lead-pipe* rigidity; the increase is not velocity dependent. This is the characteristic hypertonicity of extrapyramidal disease. In paratonia, or *Gegenhalten,* increased tone is erratic and is dependent on the intensity of the imposed movement, that is, it is oppositional. This pattern of hypertonicity is characteristically related to extensive brain dysfunction. It should be noted that a "cogwheel" feel to increased muscle tone is not intrinsic to the hypertonicity. It has been shown that the cogwheeling in parkinsonism is imparted by tremor superimposed on rigidity; specifically, it is not the rest tremor of parkinsonism but the commonly associated postural tremor that is felt (Findley et al. 1981). This phenomenon gives rise to what I believe is a common error. In delirium and dementia, the paratonia of diffuse brain dysfunction is mistaken for rigidity when the examiner feels cogwheeling, which actually indicates the additional presence of a tremor, common in delirium (see below).

Dystonia. Dystonia refers to "sustained muscle contractions, frequently causing twisting and repetitive movements, or abnormal postures" (Fahn et al. 1987, p. 335). The contractions may be generalized or focal. Typically the dystonic arm hyperpronates, with a flexed wrist and extended fingers; the dystonic lower extremity shows an inverted foot with plantar flexion. A number of syndromes of focal dystonia are well recognized, such as torticollis, writer's cramp, and blepharospasm with jaw and mouth movements (Meige syndrome). A dystonic pattern of particular interest is oculogyric crisis, in which there is forced deviation of the eyes sometimes accompanied by forced thinking or other psychological disturbance (Leigh et al. 1987; Owens 1990). It is characteristic of dystonic movements to worsen with voluntary action and to be evoked only by very specific action patterns. Especially in an early stage or mild form of the illness, this can produce apparently bizarre symptoms, such as a patient who cannot walk because of twisting feet and legs but who is able to run, or a patient who can do everything with his hands except write. Adding to the oddness is the frequent capacity of the patient to reduce the involuntary movement by using sensory tricks (*le geste antagoniste*). In torticollis, for example, the neck contractions that are violent enough to break restraining devices may yield to the patient's simply touching his chin with his own finger. Eliciting a history of such tricks or observing the patient's use of them is diagnostic.

Dystonia, including oculogyric crisis, can occur as an acute or tardive effect of dopamine blockade

(Fitzgerald and Jankovic 1989; Owens 1990). The speculation by Owens (1990) that psychiatrists see as much dystonia as neurologists strikes me as accurate, and the psychiatrist should note that only very rarely are dystonic postures hysterical (Lesser and Fahn 1978).

Tremor. All tremors are rhythmic, regular, oscillating movements around a joint. Three major forms of tremor are distinguished. In rest tremor, the movement is present distally when the limb is supported and relaxed; action reduces the intensity of the tremor. The frequency is usually low, about 4–8 cycles/second. This is the well-known tremor of parkinsonism. Because the amplitude of the tremor diminishes with action, rest tremor is usually less disabling than it might appear. In postural tremor, the outstretched limb oscillates. At times this can be better visualized by placing a piece of paper over the outstretched hand. Several forms of postural tremor have been distinguished, of varying frequencies and amplitudes. Postural tremor is produced by anxiety, certain drugs (e.g., caffeine, lithium, steroids, and adrenergic agonists for asthma), and the disease hereditary essential tremor. A coarse, irregular, rapid postural tremor is frequently seen in metabolic encephalopathy (Plum and Posner 1980). In intention tremor, the active limb oscillates more prominently as the limb approaches its target during goal-directed movements. This is seen in disease of the cerebellum and its connections. It is more properly considered a form of dysmetria than a tremor (Young 1986). If physical maneuvers produce a change of tremor frequency (as opposed to amplitude), as when the tremulous extremity adopts the frequency of a repetitive action (e.g., finger tapping of the opposite extremity), hysteria should be suspected (Koller et al. 1989). Repeated drawings of a spiral give a record of the patient's tremor over time.

Chorea. Choreatic movements are "brief, random, sudden, rapid, arrhythmic, involuntary movements" (Padberg and Bruyn 1986, p. 549), which dance over the patient's body. The patient may incorporate these movements into purposeful ones, in an effort to hide the chorea when it is mild. As with dystonia, chorea may become more evident when elicited by gait or other activity. Predominantly proximal movements, large in amplitude and violent in force, are called *ballistic.* Usually ballism is unilateral and due to lesions in the subthalamic nucleus, but it can be bilateral (Lodder and Baard 1981), and lesions elsewhere in the basal ganglia can be culpable (Dewey and Jankovic 1989).

The differential diagnosis of chorea is wide (Padberg and Bruyn 1986). Only a few notes are offered here. Late-onset abnormal movements due to antipsychotic drugs—tardive dyskinesia—are usually choreatic and predominantly involve oral and facial musculature. Occasionally the movements are somewhat asymmetric (Altshuler et al. 1988). Whether these movements are in fact due to the drugs, or rather to characteristics of the underlying illness, is not entirely settled; probably disease-related factors have been understated (Waddington and Crow 1988). In the setting of psychosis, the clinician must not assume that chorea is tardive dyskinesia but must consider a differential diagnosis of diseases that can produce both chorea and psychosis (e.g., Wilson's disease, systemic lupus erythematosus, Huntington's disease, and Fahr's syndrome) (Hyde et al. 1991). Anticonvulsants and antidepressants can also produce abnormal movements (Fann et al. 1976); and not all antidopaminergic drugs are antipsychotic agents, so the clinician must inquire about use of metoclopramide and prochlorperazine (Lang 1990).

The prevalence of oral chorea in the elderly without either psychiatric illness or a history of dopamine-blocker treatment has been controversial (Marsden 1985). Many elderly dyskinetic patients are edentulous. Koller (1983) reported differences between edentulous dyskinesia and tardive dyskinesia. In his patients with edentulous dyskinesia, abnormal movements of the upper face and limbs were absent, and the tongue lay still in the mouth; tongue protrusion was unimpaired. In contrast, vermicular (wormlike) movements of the tongue inside the mouth are prominent in tardive dyskinesia, and patients are often unable to maintain the tongue protruded. Limb chorea is an inconstant feature. Interestingly, tardive dyskinesia can occur in a phantom limb (Jankovic and Glass 1985).

Myoclonus. This term refers to a complex set of abnormal movements that share suddenness as a key characteristic. The forms of myoclonus are too varied to review here, and the reader is referred to several excellent discussions (Hallett and Ravits 1986; Marsden et al. 1982). Certain forms of myoclonus are within normal experience: the sneeze and jerk that awaken one just as one drifts off to sleep (the hypnic jerk) are myoclonic phenomena. In distinguishing myoclonus from other abnormal movements (Marsden et al. 1982), we note that myoclonus does not show the continuous, dancelike flow of movement that characterizes chorea. When myoclonus is rhythmic, it differs from tremor in having an interval between individual movements, a "square wave" rather than a "sine wave." The distinction of myoclonus from tic is partly based on subjective features: the individual with a tic reports a wish to move, a sense of relief after the movement, and the ability to delay the movement (albeit at the cost of increasing subjective tension). Also, tics can be more complex and stereotyped than myoclonic jerks.

For the most part, myoclonus is recognized from the patient's description (e.g., in the epileptic patient who describes increasing myoclonus prodromally to seizures) or by observation. More subtle assessment requires specialized electrophysiological evaluation, with an electromyogram (EMG) time-locked to the electroencephalogram (EEG). Three maneuvers on examination are worth noting. First, some myoclonus is stimulus sensitive; stimulation such as a tap with the reflex hammer evokes a myoclonic jerk. In this situation, somatosensory-evoked potentials are often abnormal; it is presumed that an abnormally excitable cortical region is giving rise to a fragment of epilepsy. Second, other forms of myoclonus are evoked by action, notably postanoxic myoclonus responsive to serotonin agonists. Third, abnormal startle reactions can be related to myoclonus. This point deserves fuller exploration.

Wilkens et al. (1986) reviewed the physiology of the normal reaction to sudden unexpected auditory stimuli. The clinician produces this with a hand clap outside the patient's field of vision. The reflex invariably involves eye blink. The muscle jerks are most intense cranially, tapering caudally, and occur predominantly in flexor muscles. A rare, usually familial disorder in which this reflex is disturbed is called *hyperekplexia*; it features hyperreflexia, hypertonicity, and abnormal gait in infancy; myoclonus; and an exaggerated startle, frequently causing falls (Andermann and Andermann 1984). Abnormal startle reactions are also seen in Tourette's syndrome; some epilepsies (Wilkens et al. 1986); certain culture-bound syndromes, such as Latah and the "jumping Frenchmen of Maine" (Simons 1980, 1983); and certain diffuse cerebral disorders such as magnesium deficiency, Tay-Sachs disease, and Creutzfeldt-Jakob disease.

Tic. Some of the key features of tics have been described above in differentiating them from myoclonus. Tics are sudden jerks, sometimes simple (such as a blink or a grunt) but sometimes as complex as a well-organized voluntary movement (such as repeatedly touching an object or speaking a word) (Jankovic 1987; Lees 1985). In addition to the subjective features noted above, tics differ from many other abnormal movements in persisting during sleep. (Some myoclonic disorders can as well, and so can epilepsia partialis continua.) Despite the quasi-voluntary quality of some tics, electrophysiological evidence shows that tics differ from identical movements produced voluntarily by the same person in lacking the readiness potential (*Bereitschaftpotential*) that normally precedes a voluntary movement (Obeso et al. 1981).

Stereotypy and mannerism. Lees (1988) offered the following definition of stereotypy: "purposeless, rhythmic, repetitive movements carried out at the expense of all other motor activity for long periods of time" (p. 258). In schizophrenia, a delusional idea associated with such abnormal movements can sometimes, but not always, be elicited (Jones 1965). Similar abnormal movements are seen in autism and in congenital blindness and severe mental retardation, but not in blindness or brain damage that is acquired late (Ridley and Baker 1982). Amphetamine intoxication is a well-recognized cause of stereotypy, known in this setting as *punding* (a Swedish word introduced during a Scandinavian epidemic of amphetamine abuse). Ridley and Baker (1982) provided an extended review of the biology and psychology of stereotypy.

Manneristic movements are purposeful movements carried out in a bizarre way. Lees (1988) suggested that they result from the incorporation of stereotypies into goal-directed movements. He suggested that the "repugnant ludicrous antics" of schizophrenic patients are the expression of manneristic disturbance of simple behaviors such as eating or shaking hands (Lees 1985, p. 124). It is certainly true that mannerism at times makes the diagnosis of schizophrenia evident from across the room, but the cause and mechanism of the disorder must be considered unknown.

Asterixis. Repeated momentary loss of postural tone produces a flapping movement of the outstretched hands (asterixis) originally described in the context of liver failure. It has subsequently been recognized to occur in many or all states of metabolic encephalopathy and in all muscle groups. Young and Shahani (1986) recommended eliciting it by asking the patient to dorsiflex the index fingers for 30 seconds while the hands and arms are outstretched, with the patient watching to ensure maximum voluntary contraction. This test demonstrates the nature of asterixis as a disorder of the maintenance of posture. Physiologically, it is the inverse of multifocal myoclonus: the EMG shows brief silence on the background of sustained discharge (Young and Shahani 1986). The coarse tremor of delirium is a slower version of asterixis. Bilateral asterixis is a very valuable sign because it points unmistakably to a toxic-metabolic confusional state; to my knowledge asterixis has never been described in the "functional" psychoses and is thus pathognomonic for organic states. Rarely, asterixis is unilateral and reflects a lesion of contralateral thalamic, parietal, or medial frontal structures (Young and Shahani 1986).

Catatonia. Catatonia, the syndrome described by Kahlbaum in the last century and incorporated into the concept of dementia praecox by Kraepelin, has now been shown to occur in a wide variety of organic states as well as in the classic "functional" psychoses (see Rogers 1991). Catatonia can be defined broadly as abnormality of movement or muscle tone associated with psychosis (Fisher 1989a) or more narrowly as "at least one motor sign (catalepsy, posturing, or waxy flexibility) in combination with at least one sign of psycho-social withdrawal or excitement and/or bizarre repetitious movement (mutism, negativism, impulsiveness, grimacing, stereotypies, mannerisms, command automatism, echopraxia/echolalia or verbigeration)" (Barnes et al. 1986, p. 991). Manschreck (1986) offered a catalog of these phenomena and their definitions. Such signs are common in severe mental disorder (Rogers 1985). Cataleptic postures or waxy flexibility can be distinguished phenomenologically from other disorders of muscle tone (see above), but are of uncertain anatomic and physiologic mechanism. Manschreck (1986) showed an association of motor abnormality with thought disorder and argued that a disorder of attention is the unifying theme. It is worthy of special mention that neuroleptics can induce catatonia as an isolated phenomenon or as an early feature of the neuroleptic malignant syndrome.

Synkinesia. Normal movement requires that certain unintentional movements take place along with intended ones. The absence of these, such as loss of arm swing with walking, provides signs in the general neurological examination. Excessive synkinesia also occurs in a variety of states (Zulch and Muller 1969).

Schott and Wyke (1977) reviewed the differential diagnosis and pathophysiology of states in which there occur bimanual synkinesias, that is, movements in which one hand obligatorily mirrors the movements of the other. Mild degrees of such movements have been taken to be a soft sign of cerebral dysmaturation (Buchanan and Heinrichs 1989). This is easily observed by asking the patient to touch, in turn, repeatedly, the fingers to the thumb of one hand with the arms outstretched; along with watching the active hand for fine motor coordination, the examiner watches the contralateral hand for mirror movements.

Primitive Reflexes

An extensive literature has grown up about curious reflexes such as the grasp, suck, snout, and palmomental (Table 4–2). This literature was critically, not to say polemically, reviewed by Landau (1989) under the rubric of neuromythology. The received wisdom is that these are reflexes brought about by cortical disease, especially frontal, which disinhibits primitive reflexes (Paulson and Gottlieb 1968). There is considerable doubt that all such reflexes are of pathological significance. For example, Jacobs and Grossman (1980) found that the palmomental reflex could be elicited in more than 20% of healthy subjects in their 30s and 40s and in more than 50% of those in their 90s; the snout could be found in more than 30% of subjects over age 60. Similarly, Koller et al. (1982) found the snout in more than 50% of healthy elderly subjects. It seems fair to say that a reflex present in more than half of healthy people lacks semiologic value.

Still, the possibility remains that some combination of such reflexes, or some specific characteristic of them (such as unilaterality or vigor), may be of diagnostic use. In one study (Benassi et al. 1990), if only severely abnormal reflexes were considered, a combination of any two of them gave a specificity for dementia of 97% (but a sensitivity of only 44%). If less severely abnormal reflexes were considered, three or more or them were required to yield a specificity over 90% (with a sensitivity of 88%). Re-

TABLE 4–2. PRIMITIVE REFLEXES

Reflex	*Stimulus*	*Abnormal response*
Suck	Examiner's knuckle between patient's lips	Any sucking motion
Snout	Minimal pressure of examiner's finger on patient's lips, then drawing away	Puckering of lips
Grasp	Stroking of patient's palm toward fingers while patient is distracted	Flexion of fingers
Avoidance	Same as grasp	Extension of wrist and fingers
Palmomental	Noxious stroking of thenar eminence	Contraction of ipsilateral mentalis muscle
Nuchocephalic	Shoulders of standing patient briskly turned while eyes are closed	Head remains in original position
Self-grasping	Guiding patient's hand toward opposite forearm and allowing fingers to stroke ulna	Grasps own limb

flexes with a short-lasting, nonprominent response were individually of no utility, and in particular the snout, palmomental, and glabellar reflexes were common among control subjects. The grasp and suck reflexes were of greater individual specificity; though of low sensitivity, at least in Alzheimer's disease (Fox et al. 1989), they may be of more significance. This community-based study, however, compared dementia patients with healthy subjects. How the reflexes would fare given a tougher test—say, comparing dementia with depression in the elderly—is unknown.

The localizing value of these reflexes is also incompletely understood. Landau (1989) stated that all primitive reflexes indicate widespread cerebral dysfunction with relative sparing of the primary motor cortex. Brodal (1981), however, linked the grasp reflex quite specifically with disease of the contralateral supplementary motor area. To consider them all equally as frontal release reflexes would seem to go beyond the available evidence. Some less familiar reflexes, such as the nuchocephalic (Jenkyn et al. 1975), avoidance (Denny-Brown 1958), and self-grasping (Ropper 1982), may prove to be relatively specific and of localizing value. But overall these reflexes have probably been given too much weight in the neuropsychiatric examination, and some, such as the snout and palmomental, are useless when taken alone.

"Soft Signs"

Under this rubric is grouped a variegated set of findings taken to demonstrate impairment in sensorimotor integration and motor control. *Soft* is interpreted by some as referring to the nonlocalizing nature of these signs, by some as referring to their dependence on maturation, and by others as betraying their unreliable and therefore semiologically invalid character. Unfortunately, because studies of these signs have not used the same test batteries, comparisons from one study to another are not always easy. The topic was recently reviewed (Buchanan and Heinrichs 1989; Heinrichs and Buchanan 1988; Merriam et al. 1990; Tupper 1987).

A sign presumably related to high-level integration of sensation is graphesthesia: the examiner traces numbers on the patient's hand, and the patient must read the numbers with the eyes closed. Many indicators of defective control of complex motor activity have been proposed (Manschreck 1983). The bedside examiner can seek mild clumsiness by asking the patient to tap the hand and the foot or perform other rapid alternating movements; motor inhibition by looking for mirror movements, discussed above; and motor control on tests of perseveration and reciprocal action programs, discussed below.

Most studies have sought soft signs in schizophrenic patients. It may be that in schizophrenia right-hand agraphesthesia indicates a predominant left-hemisphere abnormality (Torrey 1980). Defective motor control has been linked to thought disorder (Manschreck 1983; Manschreck 1986) and prefrontal signs to negative symptoms (Merriam et al. 1990). A few studies (Gardner et al. 1987; Quitkin et al. 1976) have looked for soft signs in the varied population of patients with character disorders with positive results. A specific link to the development of obsessive-compulsive disorder has been reported (Hollander et al. 1990).

In approaching severely ill patients with whatever psychiatric diagnosis, the neuropsychiatrically informed examiner looks not just for the obvious signs (e.g., a unilateral extensor plantar reflex), but the subtle ones as well. These subtle ones (the soft signs) have been strongly linked to aspects of brain dysfunction that have clinical relevance, even being present where the computed tomography (CT) scan is negative (Lucas et al. 1989), and their subtlety is not reason enough to ignore them (Szatmari and Taylor 1984).

Signs of Callosal Disconnection

Most of the remarkable effects of callosal disconnection have been demonstrated in laboratory experiments using cases of surgical section of the callosum and techniques not available to the bedside diagnostician, notably tachistoscopic presentation of stimuli to one hemisphere at a time. However, Bogen (1985) showed that many of the crucial elements of the disconnection syndrome can be found by simple maneuvers, although these signs may be obscured by the damage to medial frontal lobes seen with naturally occurring lesions such as anterior cerebral artery stroke or frontal glioma.

The history often discloses features typical of disconnection, including dissociative phenomena (e.g., between what the patient is saying and what the left hand is doing). Most remarkably the patient reports behavioral conflict between the hands or merely a sense that the left hand behaves in an alien fashion. (There are states other than callosal section in which the alien hand sign occurs [Goldberg et al. 1981; Riley et al. 1990]. The levitation of the parietal hand [Denny-Brown et al. 1952; Mori and Yamadori 1989], however, is probably a different phenomenon.) On examination, the patient shows an inability to name odors presented to the right nostril. (Bogen [1985] called this a "verbal anosmia," but *olfactory anomia* would be the preferable term.) In visual field testing, a hemianopsia appears to be present in each hemifield alternately, opposite to the hand the patient uses to point to stimuli (i.e., when the patient uses the right hand, he responds only to stimuli in the right hemifield, and using the left only to the left).

An apraxia of the left hand can be shown by the usual testing maneuvers. Because verbal information processed in the left hemisphere cannot be transferred to the right and because the right hemisphere has limited capacity to understand spoken commands, the patient is not able to produce appropriate responses with the left hand to spoken commands. Similarly, writing with the left hand is impossible. These features were stressed in the deconnection syndrome reported by Geschwind and Kaplan (1962) in the article that initiated the modern era of clinical disconnection studies. For reciprocal reasons, the right hand shows a constructional disorder.

The patient has an anomia for unseen objects felt with the left hand. If the examiner places one of the patient's hands (again unseen) into a given posture, the patient is unable to match the posture with the other hand. Similarly the patient cannot touch with the left thumb the finger of left hand corresponding to the finger of the right hand touched by the examiner, and vice versa.

Orientation

Disorientation is the shibboleth of the nonneuropsychiatrist's cognitive examination. *Disoriented* means *organic* in common parlance. The neuropsychiatrist recognizes the shortcomings of this approach. They are twofold. First, many patients have organic cognitive disorders without disorientation. This goes without saying for focal cognitive disorders such as alexia or constructional disorder. But even in the syndromes of delirium and dementia—the syndromes of global cognitive failure—disorientation is far from invariable. For example, in his personal series of 74 cases of acute organic reaction Cutting (1980) found that only 36% were disoriented to the year, 43% to the month, and 34% to the name of the hospital. By contrast, 85% had abnormalities of mood, and 46% had abnormal beliefs. Therefore, disorientation, although a helpful pointer to the presence of delirium, is not as sensitive an indicator as many believe.

Second, disorientation is a very nonspecific indicator. The neuropsychology of disorientation is not well elucidated (Daniel et al. 1987), but clearly it is possible for a patient to be unable to give the date or place because of an impairment in attention, memory, language, or content of thought. The neuropsychiatrist probes these mechanisms by the use of more specific tasks.

The pattern of disorientation can have diagnostic significance. Disorientation to place can carry an entirely different significance from disorientation to date, as discussed below. Delirious disorientation has been distinguished from delusional disorientation in Jacksonian terms by Levin (1951, 1956), who pointed out that the delirious patient mistakes the unfamiliar for the familiar—reducing the novel to the automatic—as when he reports that the hospital is a factory where he formerly worked. By contrast the schizophrenic patient mistakes the familiar for the unfamiliar, as when he locates himself on Mars.

Attention

Even though the field of attention is a growth point in both experimental psychology and clinical neuropsychiatry (Geschwind 1982), the relationship of clinical work to the enormous scientific literature on attention is tenuous, and the doctor (as Bellak [1979] said in another connection) is left to work out what to do until the scientist comes.

Full alertness with normal attention lies at one end of a continuum; at the other end is coma. The position of the patient along this path can be assessed by observing the reaction to a graded series of probes: entering the room, speaking the patient's name, touching the patient without speaking, shouting, and so on through painful stimulation. The proper recording of the response is by specific notation of the probe and the reaction ("makes no response to examiner's entrance but orients to his voice; speaks only when shaken by the shoulder").

Deficits occur in the capacity to maintain attention to external stimuli (vigilance), the capacity to attend consistently to internal stimuli (concentration), and the capacity to shift attention from one stimulus to another. Vigilance can be assessed by the patient's capacity to perform a continuous performance task; such tasks have been extensively used in the psychological laboratory. A bedside adaptation, the "A" test, has been developed (Strub and Black 1988). The patient is presented with a string of letters, one per second, and is required to signal at each occurrence of the letter *A*. A single error of omission or of commission is considered abnormal. Concentration can be assessed by the patients capacity to recite the numbers from *20* to *1*, or to give the days of the week or the months of the year in reverse order. A pathognomonic error is to begin to give the ordinary forward order: "20, 19, 18, 17, 18 . . ." This amounts to a failure to inhibit the intrusion of the more familiar set.

Digit span is a classical psychological test of attention, easily performed at the bedside. The examiner recites strings of numbers, slowly, clearly, and without phrasing into chunks. The patient is required to repeat them immediately. Subsequently, the patient can be asked to repeat strings of digits after reversing them in his head. The normal forward digit span is usually considered to be a minimum of five. The backward digit span may depend on visuospatial processing as well as attention (Black 1986).

A patient whose digit span fluctuated in relation to environmental distraction has already been mentioned. Spontaneous fluctuations of attention are characteristic of confusional states.

Neglect. The patient who pays no attention to the left side of his or her body and the left side of space is one of the most dramatic phenomena in neuropsychiatry. The phenomena of hemineglect have been extensively investigated (Heilman et al. 1985). The bedside clinician can readily identify such patients; they entirely ignore one half of space, leaving their left arm out of the sleeve of their gown, the left side of their breakfast uneaten, and so on. Milder degrees of neglect can be recognized using a line bisection task (patients must place an *X* at the midpoint of a line drawn by the examiner) or a cancellation task (in which patients cross out letters or other items for which they must search on a page) (Figure 4–2). Mesulam (1981) constructed a useful network theory in which parietal cortex, frontal cortex, and cingulate cortex interact to allow attention to the opposite side of space; lesions produce distinguishable contralateral sensory neglect, directional hypokinesia, and reduction in motivational value respectively. Thus Daffner et al. (1990) described a patient whose capacity for spatial exploration in the left hemispace was reduced after a right frontal infarction, as shown by failure on a letter-cancellation task, despite the absence of sensory abnormality. After a subsequent right parietal lesion, visual and auditory extinction on the left emerged

Figure 4–2. Mesulam's letter-cancellation task. The patient must spot all the examples of a given letter in the random array and cross them out. (Reprinted from Mesulam M-M: Principles of Behavioral Neurology. Philadelphia, PA, FA Davis, 1985. Used with permission.)

and the exploratory defect was emphasized. Neglect has been shown to be a transient feature after right-hemisphere stroke, usually disappearing after a few months (Hier et al. 1983).

Posner et al. (1988) argued that right-sided hemineglect is a feature of schizophrenia and linked this to a detailed theory of the pathophysiology of schizophrenia (Early et al. 1989). The methods that they used to demonstrate neglect are not applicable at the bedside, but in their view the right-hand agraphesthesia found among schizophrenic patients (see above) is a clinical manifestation of the disengage deficit—the inability to detach attention from ipsilateral hemispace—that results, in schizophrenia, from left cingulate dysfunction. Voeller and Heilman (1988) found left neglect on a letter-cancellation task in children with attention-deficit disorder.

A curious phenomenon with a kinship to neglect was identified by Bogousslavsky and Regli (1988) as "response-to-next-patient stimulation." They found that patients with right-hemisphere stroke, when examined in a hospital room with several beds, sometimes continued responding to the doctor even after he or she had moved on to the next patient. All their patients had left neglect and anosognosia. The link of this phenomenon to neglect, unawareness of deficit, and perseveration remains to be clarified.

Hypermetamorphosis. Wernicke (Klüver and Bucy 1939) coined the term *hypermetamorphosis* to refer to an excessive and automatic attention to environmental stimuli. Klüver and Bucy (1937) demonstrated this phenomenon in monkeys with bilateral temporal lobectomy; it can be seen in the human Klüver-Bucy syndrome as well (Poeck 1985a). In a personal case, an elderly man presented to the hospital with serial seizures. On awakening he showed a postictal twilight state. During this time, he compulsively attended to elements of the environment and kept up a remarkable running commentary on them: "You're wearing a tie, there's a picture on the wall," and so on. EEG showed bilateral posterior temporal spike foci. Perhaps this was an audible version of the Schneiderian first-rank symptom of voices carrying on a running commentary; perhaps the Schneiderian symptom also reflects hypermetamorphosis and bitemporal dysfunction.

Memory

A reader of the contemporary neuropsychological literature (see Chapter 15 and Mayes 1988) is aware of the poverty of our bedside testing of memory. The ordinary bedside testing of verbal memory can be done briefly and validly, as Kopelman (1986) has shown. Not all tests are of equal power, however. Recall of paragraph-length material after a 45-minute delay may be ideal, but recall of a name and address after several minutes is simple and satisfactory (Katzman et al. 1983; Kopelman 1986). Similar testing of figural memory at the bedside is also easily done. For example, Weintraub and Mesulam's three-words/three-shapes test (1985) compares verbal and figural memory side-by-side in a quick and simple fashion. Weintraub and Mesulam usefully provided lists of words and shapes, including foils for testing recognition memory along with free recall. I sometimes ask patients to recall the three directions I just pointed (using not-easily-verbalized directions, i.e., off at a diagonal, rather than up or down).

This testing of verbal and nonverbal short-term memory, however, does not cover all the memory subroutines that have been identified by neuropsychologists. Whether remote memory can be validly assessed at the bedside is uncertain. The examiner may not be able to construct probes that he or she knows the correct responses to (e.g., "What elementary school did you go to?"), and matching items for difficulty between patients is probably out of reach. Under extraordinary circumstances, such as during an episode of transient global amnesia, a few examiners have been able to define the retrograde limits of remote memory loss (Caplan 1985). For ordinary bedside purposes, a rough estimate of normal or abnormal remote memory may be all we can attain.

And what of the other important memory subsystems? Can we briefly and validly, without specialized materials, make assessments of memory for source and temporal context, functions especially impaired in frontal lobe lesions? Patients with frontal amnesia show relative sparing of recognition memory as compared with memory tested by free recall. Many of us believe we can spot this disparity at the bedside, but can we show our reliability and validity in doing so? Can we assess procedural memory, as for example the learning of a motor task? Developing and validating bedside methods for these domains is a task for the future.

Language and Praxis

Aphasia. Because the subject of language disorders is treated at length in Chapter 13, only brief attention is given to examination of language here. A full account of the scheme for examination of language would require a history of the proposals for classification of aphasia; this is beyond the scope of this chapter and, moreover, largely obviated by the near-consensus that has formed around the scheme codified in the Boston Diagnostic Aphasia Examination (BDAE; Goodglass and Kaplan 1983). Discussions of aphasic disorders from this perspective are offered by Albert et al. (1981) and Benson (1979); valuable alternative perspectives are presented by Lecours et al. (1983) and by Luria and Hutton (1977). In this chapter I review only the scheme of six main areas of language function that the clinician examines.

1. *Spontaneous speech.* For research purposes standard stimuli have been used to elicit spontaneous speech (Goodglass and Kaplan 1983), but of course the clinician has ample opportunity to hear the patient speak during the routine clinical interview. Nonetheless, it is essential to

listen for a period with an ear to language abnormalities. One may not hear what one does not specifically listen for. One listens first for fluency, which refers to several characteristics of speech: its melody, its effortfulness, its rate, and the length of phrases (normal being three to five words). Second, one listens for errors, both of syntax and of word-choice (lexicon). Agrammatism, emptiness, and paraphasic errors can be noted.

2. *Repetition.* As Geschwind (personal communication, December 1981) pointed out, the existence of disorders in which repetition is specifically spared or impaired offers proof that the brain is not organized according to common sense. Why should there be patients who are virtually unable to speak spontaneously yet able to repeat the examiner's complicated phrases without difficulty? (Indeed they may do so automatically, when repetition is not being tested; see echolalia above.) And why should it be that some patients speak and understand speech more or less adequately but generate progressively more outlandish phrases when they attempt to repeat? At any rate, it is important to test repetition separately by offering the patient phrases of increasing length and grammatical complexity. For example, one may start with single words, continue with simple phrases, then invert the phrases into questions, and then make up phrases of grammatical "function" words ("no ifs, ands, or buts" has become traditional).
3. *Naming.* One has already listened for paraphasic errors in the course of the patient's spontaneous speech. Ordinarily more detailed testing by confrontation naming can be simply performed using items at hand: a watch and its parts; parts of the body; items of clothing (e.g., shirt, sleeve, button, and cuff); and so on. Naming is dependent on the frequency of the target word in the vocabulary, so testing must use less frequently named items to detect mild but clinically meaningful deficits. Occasionally alternative methods are required, as with the blind patient (or the patient with either optic aphasia or visual agnosia), for whom tactile naming can be employed. Also one can ask the patient to name items from their description ("What is the vehicle that travels underwater?"; "What do you call the four-legged animal that barks?"). The examiner should be aware that occasionally patients have extraordinary domain-specific dissociations in naming ability; for example, the ability to name vegetables may be intact but the ability to name animals devastated (Humphreys and Riddoch 1987). This remarkable phenomenon (category-specific anomia) has been the source of useful theorizing and is probably often missed at the bedside (Damasio 1990).
4. *Comprehension.* Preferably the output demands are minimized in testing comprehension, so motor responses should not be required (point to the ceiling and so on). Asking yes-no questions of progressive difficulty (e.g., "Am I wearing a hat?"; "Is there a tree in the room?"; "Does lunch come before dinner?"; or "Is ice cream hotter than coffee?") is simple and is systematized in the BDAE. Patients with anterior aphasia often have mild disorders of comprehension of syntactically complex material. This can be observed by asking patients to interpret sentences using the passive voice and similarly difficult constructions. ("The lion was killed by the tiger. Which animal was dead?")
5. *Reading.* Reading comprehension can conveniently be tested by offering the same stimuli as were used orally, and the examiner may wish to have cards on hand with preprinted questions. Reading skills are by no means universal in the population, and before settling on the presence of an alexia one must establish the patient's premorbid level of attainment. It is widely known that alexia can be present with no other abnormality of language (alexia without agraphia). A developmental syndrome of hyperlexia has been described (Huttenlocher and Huttenlocher 1973).
6. *Writing.* This is most conveniently tested by asking the patient to write spontaneously a short paragraph about his illness or being in the hospital. Caplan (1990) suggested having this done while the patient is in the waiting room. Because agraphia is a constant accompaniment of aphasic syndromes, the writing sample is a good screening test of language function (always assuming premorbid literacy), and may reveal visuopractic problems as well. It is a particularly nice test in revealing confusional states; Chédru and Geschwind (1972a, 1972b) showed that writing is highly sensitive to disturbance in this setting. Similarly, agraphic errors can be seen in writing samples of patients with Alzheimer's disease earlier in the course than aphasic errors

in spontaneous speech (Faber-Langendoen et al. 1988; Horner et al. 1988). Hypergraphia is not an aphasic disorder, but it has drawn interest in relation to temporal lobe disease, perhaps especially right temporal lobe epilepsy (Trimble 1986).

Ideomotor apraxia. An incapacity to perform skilled movements in the absence of elementary sensory or motor dysfunction that explains the defect is known as *apraxia*. Limb-kinetic apraxia amounts to a nonpyramidal clumsiness (Freund and Hummelsheim 1985). Ideational apraxia is discussed below. Ideomotor apraxia is discussed here because of its close relationship to language disorders.

Two important forms of ideomotor apraxia are oral apraxia and the left-hand apraxia seen with right hemiparesis from left-hemisphere lesions. These are revealed by requiring the patient to perform learned movements to command. If Geschwind's disconnection hypothesis of the origin of apraxia is correct (Heilman and Rothi 1985), performance in imitation of the examiner does not test the same pathway from verbal input to motor engram as performance to command. In any event it is clearly an easier task. This means that in the presence of auditory comprehension difficulties, the presence of apraxia is hard to establish.

Heilman and colleagues (Heilman and Rothi 1985) suggested that ideomotor apraxia is the result either of a dominant parietal lesion damaging the site of storage of motor engrams, or of a lesion, either callosal or dominant hemispheric, disconnecting these engrams from the motor cortex. For oral apraxia, suitable tests are "Show me how you would blow out a match" or "How do you lick a postage stamp?" For limb apraxia, the patient should demonstrate waving goodbye, thumbing a ride, using a hammer or comb or toothbrush, and the like. It is often said that responses in which the patient uses a body part in lieu of the pantomimed object are defective responses. Thus if the patient continues to use his fingers as the comb despite instruction to pretend he is holding a comb, the body part as object (BPO) response is taken as parapraxic. The evidence in support of this is scanty, and the notion may be erroneous (Duffy and Duffy 1989). What is certain is that here, as elsewhere in the cognitive examination, errors are more telling than simple failures and the patient who shows how to hammer with a flat palm is unequivocally apraxic.

Visuospatial Function

Visuospatial analysis. Abnormalities of visual memory and emotional prosody have already been mentioned as signs of right-hemisphere dysfunction. The traditional probe for impairment in regard to spatial relations is drawing and copying tasks. Copying a Greek cross, intersecting pentagons, a figure from the Bender-Gestalt test, or the figures in Mesulam's three-shapes test, or drawing a clock face serves as a suitable screen; more subtle abnormality may be sought using the Rey Complex Figure (Figure 4–3). It must be recognized, however, that copying performance is impaired by both left- and right-sided lesions, although differently. The complexity of the Rey Complex Figure offers the opportunity to assess not only the final performance but also the patient's strategy. Kaplan and her colleagues (Milberg et al. 1986) suggested having the patient change color of ink several times during the copying process so as to show in the resultant drawing the steps taken to produce it. Most simply, the difference between a piecemeal approach (the patient slavishly copies element by element) and a gestalt approach (the patient grasps the major structures, such as the large rectangle) can be noted, with the former suggestive of right-sided disease. Neglect of the left side of the figure is likewise strongly suggestive of right-hemisphere disease (see Chapter 5).

What about the patient who for motor reasons cannot undertake a copying task? Other tasks probe visuospatial analysis without the same output demand, for example facial recognition (Benton 1990). The anatomy and neuropsychology of prosopagnosia have been extensively analyzed (Damasio et al.

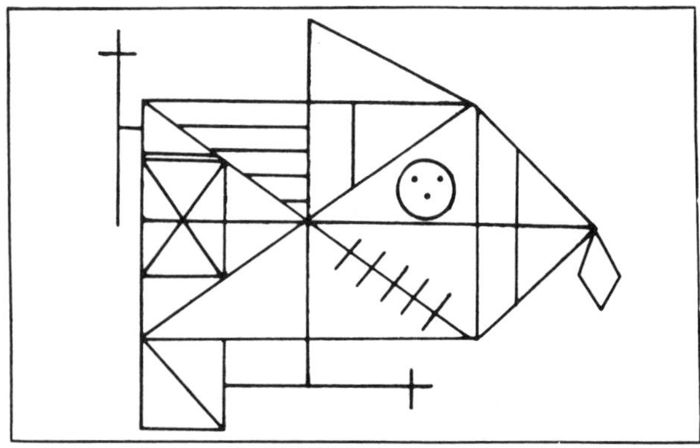

Figure 4–3. The Rey Complex Figure.

1982; Farah 1990). At the bedside, the patient can be asked to identify the pictures of several famous people. Elements of other neuropsychological instruments can be used as well (e.g., in asking the patient to discern overlapping figures or identify objects photographed from noncanonical views). Even if vision is impaired, it is possible to test related functions by topographic skills; "If I go from Chicago to New York, is the Atlantic Ocean in front of me, behind me, to my left or right?" is the sort of probe one may use. Of course, such skills are not universal in the general population, and caution must be used in interpreting the results. Isolated defects of topographic skill have been described (Habib and Sirigu 1987), but usually when one observes a patient having difficulty finding his way to his hospital room the impairment is only one element of a much broader right-hemisphere or bilateral dysfunction. Patients who lack other obvious deficits but with delusional intensity mistake their location have been described under the terms "reduplicative paramnesia" (Pick 1903), "disorientation for place" (Fisher 1982), and "délire spatial" (spatial delusion) (Vighetto et al. 1985); in fact, these patients generally do have cognitive dysfunction of the sort just described, including disturbance of nonverbal memory. One such patient I saw insisted that he was in his own house, thanked me for bringing all the doctors to visit him at home, and explained that he kept iv poles and the like at home in case he needed them.

Disordered reaching. Rarely, patients are unable to guide the movements of the hand and arm by vision (Damasio and Benton 1979). This phenomenon, known as *optic ataxia*, is seen with apraxia of voluntary gaze and an impairment of the simultaneous perception of multiple objects (simultanagnosia) (Farah 1990) as part of Balint's syndrome. If the patient's ordinary act of reaching under visual guidance is seen to be disturbed, movement without visual guidance must be examined, for example by observing the patient (with the patient's eyes closed) dressing, pointing to parts of his own body, or reaching with the right hand to grasp the outstretched left thumb (and vice versa).

Visual agnosia. The relative importance of perceptual processes in the agnosias has been debated; certainly in many cases (the apperceptive agnosias) subtle defects of visual processing can be found (Farah 1990). The bedside clinician can look for evidence of relatively intact elementary sensory processing (e.g., in the visual realm, copying of a picture may be preserved). But although the patient's language is intact (e.g., he is able to name the object in the picture from a description), his capacity to recognize the object—either by naming it or by using it—is strikingly abnormal. Damasio (1985) described the examination for agnosia in detail and pointed out that only if the defect in visual analysis is early in the course of processing (visual "apperceptive" as opposed to "associative" agnosia) will the patient complain of unclear vision.

The Form of Thought

Thought disorder. Thought disorder in functional psychosis has been the subject of much study, and descriptive terms for its features—poverty of speech, pressure of speech, derailment, tangentiality, incoherence, and so on—have been carefully defined (Andreasen 1979). Cutting and Murphy (1988) usefully differentiated between an intrinsic thinking disturbance (including loose associations, concreteness, overinclusiveness, and illogicality); a disorder of the expression of thought (including disturbed pragmatics of language); and a deficit in real-world knowledge (which can produce odd conversational interchange). They argued that the distinctive pattern of schizophrenic thought is suggestive of right-hemisphere dysfunction. Many authors have noted the similarity between the negative features of thought disorder and the characteristics of the frontal lobe syndrome. Cutting (1987) contrasted the positive features of thought disorder in schizophrenia with the thinking process of delirious patients. The latter were prominently illogical or slowed and impoverished in output; more distinctively, the delirious patients gave occasional irrelevant replies amid competent responses. Levin (1956) discussed this contrast as well. The form of thought in mentally retarded and dementia patients has not been well described.

Confabulation. The confabulating patient fabricates material in response to the examiner's queries and may tell tales spontaneously as well. Although this disorder is linked with amnesia and many mistakenly believe it to be tantamount to Korsakoff's syndrome, the neuropsychiatrist recognizes that severe or elaborate confabulation betokens disease outside memory systems, particularly the failure of self-monitoring characteristic of frontal disease. This mechanism has been demonstrated in systematic studies (Shapiro et al. 1981; Stuss et al. 1978).

Akin to confabulation is a phenomenon Geschwind (1982) called "wild paraphasia." He offered the example of a patient who names an iv pole a Christmas tree decoration. Here again the failure lies not within language systems but in the cerebral apparatus for self-monitoring. In this case, disruption of attention in a confusional state is the usual setting.

Vorbeireden. *Vorbeireden,* the German name for the symptom of approximate answers, is the defining feature of the Ganser state (Cutting 1990). The patient's responses show that he understands the questions, but the lack of knowledge implied by the mistaken replies is implausible: the patient reports that a horse has three legs. This is certainly a rare phenomenon.

The narrative process in the interview setting. It is correctly said that in psychiatry the entire interview is the examination. What conclusions can the neuropsychiatrist draw from the way the patient tells his story?

This question was perhaps first addressed by Freud (1905). In a footnote in the Dora case, he referred to a patient taken by others to have hysterical symptoms. When she recounted her story, he noticed the absence of the amnesias he had come to consider characteristic of hysteria. He immediately instituted a careful physical examination (as one would expect from a neurologist of his distinction) and made a diagnosis of tabes. Whatever the characteristics of hysterical discourse (this is not the focus here), we are led to consider that the very process of narration may be disturbed by cerebral disease.

This subject has recently come under study with regard to patients with right-hemisphere disease (Delis et al. 1983; Joanette et al. 1986; Van Lancker and Kempler 1987; Wapner et al. 1981). Despite the adequacy of their lexical and syntactic performance, such patients have deficits in the capacity to tell a story, recognize the point of a joke, or understand metaphor and idiom. Words and sentences are normal, but paragraphs are not. Wapner et al. (1981) offered a qualitative description of the discourse of right-hemisphere patients: these patients rarely give "I don't know" responses, rather they contrive some answer even if implausible; they fail to draw appropriate inferences, especially from emotional data, so that incongruity is not recognized; and the sense of humor is impaired. In what measure these deficits are of right-hemisphere origin, as opposed to frontal origin or due to brain injury of whatever location, remains to be fully worked out. The research is cited here to emphasize the value of open-ended inquiries ("What brings you to the hospital?") with attention to the patient's discourse taken as a whole as a sign of cerebral function.

The Content of Thought

Recent studies have demonstrated that the nature of psychotic ideation and experience does not readily differentiate organic psychoses from "functional" psychoses. (Of course, the neuropsychiatrist is more than inclined to believe that idiopathic schizophrenia and affective illness are also the consequence of brain dysfunction, as yet poorly understood. For example, Trimble [1991] argued that the nuclear syndrome of schizophrenia is a localizing sign, pointing to left-sided limbic lesions.) Johnstone et al. (1988) and Feinstein and Ron (1990) showed that "first-rank" symptoms of schizophrenia occur in psychoses accompanying diagnosable brain disease, as Schneider (1974) must have recognized when he indicated that they held pathognomonic significance when "present in a non-organic psychosis" (p. 44). As a rule, psychotic states related to deep brain lesions (e.g., in basal ganglion disease) resemble idiopathic schizophrenia more closely than those seen with cortical disease (Cummings 1985). But, as Cutting (1990) mordantly noted, it is bootless to refer to a psychosis as "schizophrenia-like" when the only proper reply is to ask, "What *is* schizophrenia like?" Disorders of identification such as Capgras's and Fregoli's syndromes may suggest right-hemisphere dysfunction (Joseph et al. 1990). However, this is not always so; functional psychosis without discoverable organic underpinnings or organic states without focal features may be diagnosed.

With increasing cognitive impairment, the complexity of delusions is reduced (Burns et al. 1990a; Cummings 1985). Often the delusional ideas in dementia have an ad hoc quality: a purse is misplaced, and the delusion arises that someone is stealing personal items. Delusions or hallucinations in Alzheimer's disease may be a marker of a more severe or rapidly progressive process (Lopez et al. 1991). When delusions or hallucinations occur in a patient with dementia, the clinician must exclude a supervening toxic-metabolic encephalopathy. Cutting (1987) pointed out that themes of "imminent misadventure to others" and "bizarre happenings in the immediate vicinity" characterize the delusions in delirium as against those in acute schizophrenic psychosis. In his series of delirious patients, first-rank symptoms were uncommon.

Visual hallucinations have correctly been taken as suggestive of organic states, especially if auditory hallucinations are absent, but it must be recalled that visual hallucinations are common in idiopathic schizophrenia (Bracha et al. 1989). Visual hallucinations without other psychopathology, usually in the presence of ocular disease with visual loss, are also common, especially among the elderly (Gold and Rabins 1989); visual hallucinations in a hemifield blind from cerebral disease are well known and not necessarily associated with other psychopathology. Vivid, elaborate, and well-formed visual hallucinations, often crepuscular (so-called peduncular hallucinosis), may occur with disease in the upper brain stem (Caplan 1980). Hallucinations in the other sensory modalities may have specific regional associations (e.g., olfactory hallucinations with temporal lobe pathology). Some of the abnormal experiences that are well known in temporal lobe epilepsy–the elaborate mental state described by Hughlings-Jackson, including déjà vu, jamais vu, metamorphopsia, and the like (see Gloor et al. 1982)—may occur in affective disorders as well (Silberman et al. 1985).

Emotion and Its Display

Mood and its disorders are discussed from a neuropsychiatric perspective in Chapter 14. For the most part, the assessment of emotion and its modulation are performed by the clinician as a natural part of the observation of the patient during the examination. In addition, the examiner asks questions about the patient's emotional experience. There is no substitute for extended and sensitive conversation.

Pathological laughter and crying are defined not only by the lack of congruent inner experience but also by the elicitation of the behavior by nonemotional stimuli (such as waving a hand before the patients face) and by the all-or-none character of the response (Poeck 1985b). One must distinguish this sign—usually representing lesions of the descending tracts modulating brain stem centers—from the affective dyscontrol, with lability and shallowness, that occurs in frontal disease or dementia. This latter finding, also called *emotionalism,* was studied by House et al. (1989), who took its defining characteristics to be an increase in the amount of tearfulness (or, more rarely, laughter) and the sudden, unexpected, and uncontrollable quality of the tears. They found it to be common, associated with cognitive impairment, and related to left frontal and temporal lesions; but it was not dissociated from the patient's emotional experience or situation. Ross and Stewart (1987) usefully suggested that pathological affect may screen a major depressive syndrome. Thus faced with pathological affect the examiner should seek not only the signs of pseudobulbar palsy but also the symptoms and signs of melancholia.

Apathy is the absence or quantitative reduction of affect. It differs from depression; even the slowed, unexpressive depressed patient reports unpleasant emotional experience if carefully questioned. Euphoria, a persistent and unreasonable sense of well-being without the elevated mental and motor rate of a manic state, is often alluded to in connection with multiple sclerosis. Actually it is unusual, and when it occurs it almost always signals substantial cognitive impairment.

There are a few other ways to assess emotionality. One is the exploration of prosody discussed above. Another is assessing the patient's capacity to recognize emotion in faces or scenes; neuropsychological instruments for this purpose have been developed and can be applied in a limited way to the bedside setting.

The Initiation and Organization of Action

Perseveration. Perseveration refers to the continuation into present activity of elements of previous actions. Luria (1965) referred to inertia in psychological processes and argued that pathological inertia took two forms. In efferent perseveration, the patient can initiate the switch to a new motor program, but elements of the prior task intrude into the newly required behavior. In contrast, a central or cortical form of perseveration leads to disturbance of the action program itself; there is a general aspontaneity, and the patient cannot switch from one program to another.

Luria (1965) devised a number of bedside tasks to probe the programming of action and to reveal perseveration. In the simplest of motor tasks, the patient is asked to form alternately a ring and a fist with his hand. Luria noted that in the most characteristic form of abnormality the patient perseverates on one position or the other, even while correctly saying aloud "ring—fist—ring—fist." This is the disconnection of action from verbal mediation that Luria regarded as the essence of frontal dysfunction (Luria and Homskaya 1963). A similar task, but one of greater difficulty, is to alternate from fist to edge of hand to palm, or the patient can be asked to alternate repeatedly from outstretched left fist and right palm to outstretched right fist and left palm.

If similar tasks are posed to the patient in the graphomotor sphere, a permanent record of the patient's performance results. Simply obtaining a writing sample often elicits perseveration. In Figure 4–4, a patient's response to the request to write a note to a family member is shown. She looked at the upper line, wondered aloud why she kept repeating things, and produced the lower line. Other tasks include asking for repeated sequences of two crosses and a circle or three triangles and two squares.

Sandson and Albert (1987) systematically investigated perseveration using categories rather similar to Luria's but a different terminology. In recurrent perseveration, a prior response occurs in the context of a new set (demand for action); in confrontation naming, word-list generation, and comparable nonverbal tasks, old elements recur when the task is changed. Every examiner has had the experience of having a patient name a "pen" correctly, then call the point a "pen," the watch a "pen," and so on. In stuck-in-set perseveration, the patient maintains a category or set inappropriately, demonstrating a disorder of conceptual shifting or flexibility. The task posed by Sandson and Albert involved asking the patient to shift from responding with a circle or square to specified stimuli to responding with a square or circle to those stimuli (i.e., to reverse the response). Others have used tasks of reciprocal action programs. For example, the patient is asked to point with one finger when the examiner points with two, and vice versa. I sometimes ask the patient to tap once when I tap twice, and vice versa; I do this immediately after employing a go/no-go tapping task (see below), thus complicating the demand for the use of a new response strategy. Continuous perseveration, in Sandson and Albert's terminology (1987), entails continuation or prolongation of response without cessation. This may be tested by asking the patient to produce repeated loops or the letters *m* and *n* (in cursive script).

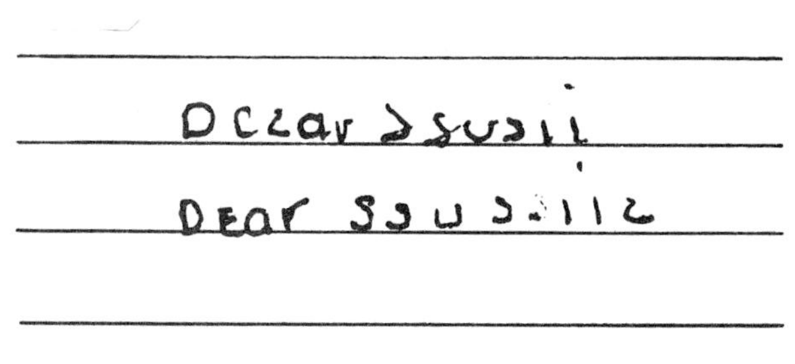

Figure 4–4. A case of perseveration in writing. The patient was asked to write a note to a family member. Self-cuing by language was ineffective in reducing perseveration.

Luria (1965) believed that efferent perseveration indicates disease in frontal plus basal ganglionic regions, whereas central perseveration is a pointer to frontal disease alone. In fact, perseveration can be seen in disease of a wide variety of brain regions, but when related to disease outside frontal regions it is characteristically limited to a specific modality of processing or response. For example, a patient with disease in temporoparietal language areas may make recurrent perseverative errors on language testing. Sandson and Albert (1987) claimed that continuous perseveration is related to nondominant hemisphere disease. The pervasiveness of perseveration in frontal disease was discussed in detail by Goldberg and Bilder (1987). Levin (1955) discussed perseveration in terms of the concepts of Hughlings-Jackson. Fisher (1989b) pointed out that perseverative activity in a broad sense is one of the important general principles of cerebral dysfunction; it occurs in confusional states, dementia, ideational apraxia, and transient global amnesia—from Fisher's point of view, whenever the brain is working sufficiently poorly in generating effective new action programs.

Disinhibition. The loss of the capacity for planful action leaves the patient with organic cerebral disease prey to impulses. For the most part, the clinician learns about such deficits from the history. In my opinion, the sort of question often used to examine "judgment" ("What would you do if you found a stamped, addressed envelope in the street?") is not useful. Anyone who has examined a sociopathic patient has observed the disconnection between words and actions that makes it a worthless inquiry. Indeed, Eslinger and Damasio (1985) argued that in frontal disease this disconnection is the characteristic feature of impulsivity.

Usually, but not always, the structuring effect of the interview and examination prevents display of impulsive behavior. One middle-aged patient, being interviewed in his wife's presence, took advantage of this examiner's attention to the wife's account to remove the chewing gum from his mouth and carefully place it underneath the radiator cover. Few formal tests demonstrate this functional defect. One that may is the performance of a go/no-go task. Such tasks are commonly used to explore the effects of frontal lesions in animals. A human experiment was described by Drewe (1975).

A simple bedside adaptation is a tapping task in which the patient is instructed to tap for one stimulus and to refrain for another: "When I tap once I want you to tap twice; when I tap twice you do nothing at all." After a practice trial, a single error of commission represents a failure. Leimkuhler and Mesulam (1985) showed the test's validity as a sign of medial frontal dysfunction in one case. (By contrast, delayed alternation tasks, characteristically impaired in dorsolateral frontal lesions in animals, do not seem to be specifically useful as clinical tests [Chorover and Cole 1966].)

Ideational apraxia. This phenomenon is usually described along with ideomotor apraxia under the rubric of left-hemisphere disorders. Rarely, focal lesions produce ideational apraxia, but far more often it occurs in association with confusional states or severe dementia and represents a global disorder of the organization of behavior. (The focal lesions implicated have been callosal, left parietal, and biparietal [Heilman and Rothi 1985].) The phenomenon is the incapacity to carry out a sequential or ordered set of actions toward a unitary goal. For example, the patient may be able to carry out the individual acts involved in preparing a letter to be sent—folding the letter, placing it in the envelope, sealing the envelope—but not be able to do them in the proper order to produce a useful result. In my experience, when patients fail to pantomime such sequences it is often unclear whether comprehension and attention are adequate; when they fail with real objects it is in the setting of global cognitive impairment. Asking the patient to describe a sequence ("How do you change a flat tire?" or "How do you cook a chicken?") has not been a useful probe; failures may depend on many mechanisms, including the disorders of narration described above.

Abulia. Adams and Fisher (Fisher 1984) resurrected the old term *abulia* to describe the slowness and loss of spontaneity in cerebral disease, of which the extreme case is akinetic mutism. Whereas apathy is in the emotional sphere, abulia is in the sphere of action: a pathological absence. In its less severe (Fisher [1984] called it "minor") form, the phenomena include slowness, delays before response, laconic speech, and a reduction in initiative and effort, perhaps with the patient performing only one of a series of requested actions. Fisher (1968) used the term *intermittent interruption of behavior* to describe a transient but repeated lack of response of this sort. At times even severe abulia can be overcome by stimuli that elicit automatic responses. This is the basis of the telephone test, in which the clinician whose hospital patient is making no response to queries goes to a nearby room and phones the patient, who may astonishingly be capable of having a conversation on the telephone (L. R. Caplan, personal communication, 1983). A patient of mine who replied to no more than one question out of a dozen, not even to inquiries as simple as the place or her name, was glad to recite a whole stanza of the *Rubaiyat* of Omar Khayyam, her favorite poem.

It is convenient here to consider tests of verbal fluency, although these tasks reflect capacity in several areas other than spontaneity. Generating lists of words by categories—"Name all the animals you can think of, or all the modes of transportation, or items one might buy in a supermarket"—requires sustained attention to a task and the ability to organize an effective search of memory as well as intact language and, of course, a certain amount of real-world knowledge. Quantitative scoring—the BDAE data suggest 12 animals in 1 minute as a cutoff for normal performance (Goodglass and Kaplan 1983)—is only part of the story. The examiner also must assess the strategy the patient applies. Normally, a patient names all the animals that come to mind from one class, say barnyard animals, then switches to another class, say jungle animals. One patient of mine, an engineer, named "antelope, bear, cat, dog, elephant . . .," a quite exceptional alphabetic strategy. The patient with a disorder of spontaneity and flexible attention has trouble picking a productive strategy and switching it when necessary.

Impersistence. Some patients fail to cooperate during the examination. One such apparent failure has been discussed as paratonia: when you overhear an examiner testing muscle tone repeating with exasperation to the patient, "Just relax," you know the patient has paratonia. A transient or constant lack of response has just been discussed as abulia. A related phenomenon is motor impersistence. Fisher (1956) first described the incapacity of certain patients to sustain activities they were quite capable of beginning. The patient with impersistence peeks when asked to do tasks requiring the eyes to be closed or gaze to be averted. Maintaining eyelid closure, tongue protrusion, mouth opening, and lateral gaze to the left may be the tasks most sensitive to this incapacity (Jenkyn et al. 1977; Kertesz et al. 1985). In most but not all studies, impersistence has been a pointer to right-hemisphere disease (De Renzi et al. 1986; Jenkyn et al. 1977; Joynt et al. 1962; Kertesz et al. 1985).

Utilization behavior. Lhermitte et al. (1986) described new signs in frontal disease. In imitation behavior, the patient imitates the gestures and behavior of the examiner even if asked to stop. This is taken to be a deliberate, not an automatic or reflex, response; patients explain that they feel they have to imitate. The authors differentiated this phenomenon from echopraxia, which is taken to be automatic, without voluntary mediation.

The phenomenon is explained within a framework of understanding the frontal lobes as providing a capacity for individual autonomy; with dysfunction of the frontal system, a state of environmental dependency is produced. As this worsens, not only is there imitation of social behavior but also a similar pseudovoluntary use of objects in the physical environment, which the authors called "utilization behavior"; for example, seeing a pitcher and a glass, the patient pours and drinks water as if it were required of him. Lhermitte described an extraordinary experiment (Lhermitte 1986; Shallice et al. 1989) involving taking patients with frontal lobe injury to natural settings (e.g., Lhermitte's apartment) and watching them fall prey to what they took to be the demands of the locales (e.g., inspecting every painting in the room when the word *museum* was uttered).

Echopraxia has been described in a variety of conditions, including Tourette's syndrome, schizophrenia, and dementia (Lees 1985). Unfortunately, the descriptions of the patient's understanding of what they are doing may not be sufficient to be sure that echopraxia differs from what Lhermitte et al. (1986) described as imitation behavior. Still, the general point that frontal patients are intensely dependent on the environment for the organization and regulation of their behavior is an important one and has been made by many authors. The clinician examining a patient in a highly artificial setting, such as a hospital room, must consider the generalizability of his findings. For example, a patient in a rehabilitation hospital after traumatic brain injury was judged to be doing well and allowed to have a pass to go across the street to buy cigarettes. When he got outside and saw a bus on the street, he jumped on and took the bus to where it was going. This point bears also on the ecological validity of neuropsychological assessment, which may underestimate patients' difficulties because of the structure provided by the test situation itself.

Awareness of Deficit

The patient who lacks awareness of a deficit obvious to everyone else is a common phenomenon in neuropsychiatry, one with important implications for treatment. The striking state of anosognosia in right-parietal lesions with denial of a left hemiparesis is well recognized, but the phenomenon has a much wider reach. A range of states occurs, from minimization of the gravity of the deficit to denial of its impact to bizarre denial of ownership of the affected body part. For example, psychotic patients regularly are unaware of the pathological nature of their perceptions and beliefs and resent attempts to intervene (Amador et al. 1991). It is common for the patient with Alzheimer's disease to lack awareness of the reason his or her spouse is bringing him or her to see the doctor. It is not unusual for a patient to be unaware of a hemianopsia, but he or she may recognize it when it is pointed out. The possible mechanisms of these states have been reviewed extensively (Levine 1990; McGlynn and Schacter 1989). The bedside examiner should repeatedly explore with the patient his understanding of the nature of his symptoms.

Psychological Management in the Neuropsychiatric Examination

In neuropsychiatry—as in all of medicine—the diagnostic evaluation is also part of the psychological treatment. The interest shown by the examiner, the rapport formed with the patient and the family, and the laying on of hands all form the basis of subsequent treatment and must be attended to from the beginning of the consultation.

A common difficulty for beginners is how to introduce the formal cognitive inquiry. All too often one hears the examiner apologize for the silly but routine questions he or she is about to ask. (One never hears a cardiologist apologize for the silly but routine instrument he or she is about to apply to the patient's precordium.) This is rarely the best way to gain the patient's full cooperation and best effort. Most of the time patients report symptoms that can lead naturally—that is, naturally from the patient's point of view—to a cognitive examination. For example, a patient with depressive symptoms may report trouble concentrating. If the examiner then says, "Let me ask you some questions to check your concentration," the patient is more likely to collaborate and less likely to be offended. At this point nearly any tasks can be introduced.

At what point in the interview should this be done? If the initial few minutes of the patient's talk gives reason to suspect substantial cognitive difficulty, one may wish to do at least some of the testing promptly. Not all of the cognitive examination needs to be done at once, although many examiners do things this way (presumably because it is easier to keep matters straight in their own minds). But fatigue is well known to be an important factor in the cognitive performance of many patients, and long examinations may not elicit their best performances. Caplan (1978) pointed out that variability in performance is characteristic of patients with cerebral lesions and that perseveration may lead to drastic declines as tasks proceed. For this reason short snatches of probing may yield new perspectives on a patient's capacities. This may also help avoid the catastrophic reaction that ensues when a patient's capacities are exceeded. This reaction of agitation and disorganization, described by Goldstein (1952; see also Reinhold 1953), is usefully diagnostic of organic disease but certainly counterproductive for emotional rapport. Furthermore, for a time after such a reaction the patient is incapable of tasks that are otherwise within his capacities, so the data subsequently collected are limited in their significance.

Who should be present for the diagnostic inquiry? Often it is necessary to interview ancillary informants to gather a neuropsychiatric history. Not infrequently one discovers that a family member has misjudged the nature or severity of the patient's impairment. This error, usually in the direction of minimizing the deficit, may be referred to in many ways; I am inclined to call it loyalty. I usually test the patient in front of the family to reveal the difficulties in a way that allows consensual validation and mutual discussion. Needless to say, this often requires tact and occasionally requires breaking off the examination, but it has proven its worth as a technique.

❑ CONCLUSIONS

The complete examination is a figment. No practical examination can include all possible elements, and if it did it would be mindless. The expert clinician is constantly generating hypotheses and constructing an examination to confirm or refute them (Caplan 1990). The diagnostician as historian is constantly aiming at writing the patient's biography: how did *this* person arrive at *this* predicament at *this* time? Needless to say, this is a far more complex endeavor than attaching a DSM-III-R (American Psychiatric Association 1987) label to a case. Diagnosis in neuropsychiatry does not mean the search only for etiology, nor only for localization, nor only for functional capacity. It means the construction of a pathophysiological and psychopathological formulation from cause to effect, from etiologic factor to symptomatic complaint or performance. The formulation of a pathogenetic mechanism that leads from cause—in genetic endowment, perinatal injury, acquired illness, or environmental provision—to effect—the symptoms and signs we have reviewed—is a paragraph, not a phrase, and provides a rational framework for intervention in each of these domains.

Still, the evaluation cannot be free-form; systematic assessment of major areas of functioning, whether there are pointers to abnormality or not, is required. For example, for every patient a screen for cognitive abnormality is necessary. Several inves-

TABLE 4–3. SCREENING TESTS FOR COGNITIVE IMPAIRMENT

Mini-Mental State Exam

Maximum score	
5	What is the (year)(season)(date)(day)(month)?
5	Where are we: (state)(county)(town)(hospital)(floor)?
3	Name three objects: 1 second to say each. Then ask the patient all three after you have said them. Give 1 point for each correct answer. Then repeat them until he learns all three. Count trials and record.
5	Serial 7s. 1 point for each correct. Stop after five answers. Alternatively spell *world* backward.
3	Ask for the three objects repeated above. Give 1 point for each correct.
2	Name a pencil, and a watch.
1	Repeat the following: "No ifs, ands, or buts."
3	Follow a 3-stage command: "Take a paper in your right hand, fold it in half, and put it on the floor."
1	Read and obey the following: "CLOSE YOUR EYES."
1	Write a sentence.
1	Copy a design: intersecting pentagons, each side about 1 inch.

Orientation-Memory-Concentration Test

Items		*Maximum error*	*Score*		*Weight*		
1	What year is it now?	1	____	×	4	=	____
2	What month is it now?	1	____	×	3	=	____
Memory phrase	Repeat this phrase after me: John Brown, 42 Market St., Chicago	1	____	×	3	=	____
3	About what time is it (within 1 hour)?						
4	Count backwards from 20 to 1.	2	____	×	2	=	____
5	Say the months in reverse order.	2	____	×	2	=	____
6	Repeat the memory phrase.	5	____	×	2	=	____

Sources. Mini-Mental State Exam reprinted from Folstein MF, Folstein SE, McHugh PR: Mini-Mental State: a practical method for grading the cognitive state of patients for the clinician. J Psychiatr Res 12:189–198, 1975. Used with permission. Orientation-Memory-Concentration Test reprinted from Katzman R, Brown T, Fuld P, et al: Validation of a short orientation-memory-concentration test of cognitive impairment. Am J Psychiatry 140:734–739, 1983. Used with permission.

tigators have developed brief screening tests of cognitive functioning. Some of these, including the well-known Mini-Mental State Exam (Folstein et al. 1975) (Table 4–3), were reviewed by Nelson et al. (1986). Katzman et al. (1983) offered a particularly simple and well-validated screening examination for dementia (Table 4–3). Jenkyn et al. (1977) validated a screening battery (Table 4–4) that includes both physical maneuvers and cognitive tasks. These batteries are most useful for the recognition of diffuse intellectual decline, such as in Alzheimer's disease. They provide repeatable, quantifiable measures that can be noted in the patients record.

As this chapter has shown, however, many areas not included in such cognitive screening approaches are relevant to the recognition of cerebral disease in patients with psychopathology. Historical

TABLE 4–4. ITEMS FOR A SCREENING BATTERY FOR DIFFUSE CEREBRAL DYSFUNCTION, SELECTED BY VIRTUE OF FALSE-NEGATIVE RATES LESS THAN 60%

Nuchocephalic reflex
Glabellar blink
Suck
Upgaze
Downgaze
Visual tracking
Lateral gaze impersistence
Paratonia of both arms
Paratonia of both legs
Limb placement
Accurate spelling of *world* in reverse
Accurate order of past presidents in reverse
Accurate recall of three items over time with distraction

Source. Jenkyn et al. 1977.

indicators, focal areas of cognitive dysfunction, physical signs, and the patient's behavior and discourse taken as a whole can be reviewed for clues to pathogenesis. In the cognitive examination, not only the quantitative but also the qualitative aspects of performance—the nature of errors, the choice of strategies are revealing. With growing expertise, the examiner can go beyond screening and toward formulation as discussed above. I trust that the information in this chapter is helpful in that enterprise.

❑ REFERENCES

Alajouanine TH, Castaigne P, Sabouraud O, et al: Palilalie paroxystique et vocalisations itératives au cours de crises épileptiques par lésion intéressant l'aire motrice supplémentaire. Rev Neurol 101:685–697, 1959

Albert ML, Goodglass H, Helm HA, et al: Clinical Aspects of Dysphasia. Vienna, Springer-Verlag, 1981

Alexander MP: Frontal lobes and language. Brain Lang 37:656–691, 1989

Altshuler LL, Cummings JL, Bartzokis G, et al: Lateral asymmetries of tardive dyskinesia in schizophrenia. Biol Psychiatry 24:83–86, 1988

Amador XF, Strauss DH, Yale SA, et al: Awareness of illness in schizophrenia. Schizophr Bull 17:113–132, 1991

American Psychiatric Association: Diagnostic and Statistical Manual of Mental Disorders, 3rd Edition, Revised. Washington, DC, American Psychiatric Association, 1987

Andermann F, Andermann E: Startle disease, or hyperekplexia. Ann Neurol 16:367–368, 1984

Andreasen NC: Thought, language, and communication disorders. Arch Gen Psychiatry 36:1315–1321, 1979

Ball R: Drug-induced akathisia: a review. J R Soc Med 78:748–752, 1985

Barnes MP, Saunders M, Walls TJ: The syndrome of Karl Ludwig Kahlbaum. J Neurol Neurosurg Psychiatry 49: 991–996, 1986

Bear D: Hierarchical neural regulation of aggression: some predictable patterns of violence, in Current Approaches to the Prediction of Violence. Edited by Brizer DA, Crowner M. Washington, DC, American Psychiatric Press, 1989, pp 85–99

Bear D, Hermann B, Fogel B: Interictal behavior syndrome in temporal lobe epilepsy: the views of three experts. Journal of Neuropsychiatry and Clinical Neurosciences 1:308–318, 1989

Bellak L: The schizophrenic syndrome: what the clinician can do until the scientist comes, in Disorders of the Schizophrenic Syndrome. Edited by Bellak L. New York, Basic Books, 1979, pp 589–590

Benassi G, D'Alessandro R, Gallassi R, et al: Neurological examination in subjects over 65 years: an epidemiological survey. Neuroepidemiology 9:27–38, 1990

Benson DF: Aphasia, Alexia, and Agraphia. New York, Churchill Livingstone, 1979

Benton A: Facial recognition 1990. Cortex 26:491–499, 1990

Black FW: Digit repetition in brain-damaged adults: clinical and theoretical implications. J Clin Psychol 42:770–782, 1986

Blanchet P, Frommer GP: Mood change preceeding epileptic seizures. J Nerv Ment Dis 174:471–476, 1986

Bogen JE: The callosal syndromes, In Clinical Neuropsychology, 2nd Edition. Edited by Heilman KM, Valenstein E. New York, Oxford University Press, 1985, pp 295–338

Bogousslavsky J, Regli F: Response-to-next-patient-stimulation: a right hemisphere syndrome. Neurology 38: 1225–1227, 1988

Bogousslavsky J, Regli F, Uske A: Thalamic infarcts: clinical syndromes, etiology, and prognosis. Neurology 38: 837–848, 1988

Boller F, Frank E: Sexual Dysfunction in Neurological Disorders: Diagnosis, Management, and Rehabilitation. New York, Raven, 1982

Boller F, Boller M, Denes G, et al: Familial palilalia. Neurology 23:1117–1125, 1973

Bracha HS, Wolkowitz OM, Lohr JB, et al: High prevalence of visual hallucination in research subjects with chronic schizophrenia. Am J Psychiatry 146:526–528, 1989

Braude WM, Barnes TRE, Gore SM: Clinical characteristics of akathisia: a systematic investigation of acute psychiatric inpatient admissions. Br J Psychiatry 143:139–150, 1983

Brodal A: Self-observations and neuro-anatomical considerations after a stroke. Brain 96:675–694, 1973

Brodal A: Neurological Anatomy in Relation to Clinical Medicine, 3rd Edition. New York, Oxford University Press, 1981

Bryden MP: Measuring handedness with questionnaires. Neuropsychologia 15:617–624, 1977

Buchanan RW, Heinrichs DW: The Neurological Evaluation Scale (NES): a structured instrument for the assessment of neurological signs in schizophrenia. Psychiatry Res 27:335–350, 1989

Burke D, Lance JW: Function and dysfunction of the myotatic unit, in Diseases of the Nervous System: Clinical Neurobiology. Edited by Asbury AK, McKhann GM, McDonald WI. Philadelphia, PA, WB Saunders, 1986, 336–351

Burns A, Jacoby R, Levy R: Psychiatric phenomena in Alzheimer's disease, I: disorders of thought content. Br J Psychiatry 157:72–76, 1990a

Burns A, Jacoby R, Levy R: Psychiatric phenomena in Alzheimer's disease, IV: disorders of behavior. Br J Psychiatry 157:86–94, 1990b

Cancelliere AEB, Kertesz A: Lesion localization in acquired deficits of emotional expression and comprehension. Brain Cogn 13:133–147, 1990

Caplan LR: Variability of perceptual function: the sensory cortex as a "categorizer" and "deducer." Brain Lang 6:1–13, 1978

Caplan LR: "Top of the basilar" syndrome. Neurology 30:72–79, 1980

Caplan LR: Transient global amnesia, in Handbook of Clinical Neurology, Vol 45. Edited by Frederiks JAM. Amsterdam, Elsevier, 1985, 205–218

Caplan LR: The Effective Clinical Neurologist. Cambridge, Blackwell, 1990

Caplan LR, Kelly M, Kase CS, et al: Infarcts of the inferior division of the right middle cerebral artery: mirror image of Wernicke's aphasia. Neurology 36:1015–1020, 1986

Caplan LR, Schmahmann JD, Kase CS, et al: Caudate infarcts. Arch Neurol 47:133–143, 1990

Carrazana E, Rossitch E, Martinez J: Unilateral "akathisia" in a patient with AIDS and a toxoplasmosis subthalamic abscess. Neurology 39:449–450, 1989

Chapman L, Wolff HG: Disease of the neopallium and impairment of the highest integrative functions. Med Clin North Am 42:677–689, 1958

Chapman L, Thetford WN, Berlin L, et al: Highest integrative functions in man during stress. Brain and Human Behavior 36:491–534, 1958

Chédru F, Geschwind N: Disorders of higher cortical functions in acute confusional states. Cortex 8:395–411, 1972a

Chédru F, Geschwind N: Writing disturbances in acute confusional states. Neuropsychologia 10:343–353, 1972b

Chorover SL, Cole M: Delayed alternation performance in patients with cerebral lesions. Neuropsychologia 4: 1–7, 1966

Critchley M: On palilalia. Journal of Neurology and Psychopathology 8:23–31, 1927

Cummings JL: Organic delusions: phenomenology, anatomical correlations, and review. Br J Psychiatry 146: 184–197, 1985

Cummings JL, Benson DF, Houlihan JP, et al: Mutism: loss of neocortical and limbic vocalization. J Nerv Ment Dis 171:255–259, 1983

Cutting J: Physical illness and psychosis. Br J Psychiatry 136:109–119, 1980

Cutting J: The phenomenology of acute organic psychosis: comparison with acute schizophrenia. Br J Psychiatry 151:324–332, 1987

Cutting J: The Right Cerebral Hemisphere and Psychiatric Disorders. Oxford, Oxford University Press, 1990

Cutting J, Murphy D: Schizophrenic thought disorder: a psychological and organic interpretation. Br J Psychiatry 152:310–319, 1988

Daffner KR, Ahern GL, Weintraub S, et al: Dissociated neglect behavior following sequential strokes in the right hemisphere. Neurology 28:97–101, 1990

Damasio AR: Disorders of complex visual processing: agnosias, achromatopsia, Balint's syndrome, and related difficulties of orientation and construction, in Principles of Behavioral Neurology. Edited by Mesulam M-M. Philadelphia, PA, FA Davis, 1985, pp 259–288

Damasio AR: Category-related recognition defects as a clue to the neural substrates of knowledge. Trends Neurosci 13:95–98, 1990

Damasio AR, Benton AL: Impairment of hand movements under visual guidance. Neurology 29:170–178, 1979

Damasio AR, Maurer RG: A neurological model for childhood autism. Arch Neurol 35:777–786, 1978

Damasio AR, Van Hoesen G: Emotional disturbances associated with focal lesions of the limbic frontal lobe, in Neuropsychology of Human Emotion. Edited by Heilman KM, Satz P. New York, Guilford, 1983, pp 85–110

Damasio AR, Damasio H, Van Hoesen GW: Prosopagnosia: anatomic basis and behavioral mechanisms. Neurology 32:331–341, 1982

Damasio H, Damasio AR: Lesion Analysis in Neuropsychology. New York, Oxford University Press, 1989

Daniel WF, Crovitz HF, Weiner RD: Neuropsychological aspects of disorientation. Cortex 23:169–187, 1987

Darley FL, Aronson AE, Brown JR: Motor Speech Disorders. Philadelphia, PA, WB Saunders, 1975

De Renzi E: Disorders of spatial orientation, in Handbook of Clinical Neurology, Vol 45: Clinical Neuropsychology. Edited by Frederiks JAM. Amsterdam, Elsevier, 1985, pp 405–422

De Renzi E, Gentilini M, Bazolli M: Eyelid movement disorders and motor impersistence in acute hemisphere disease. Neurology 36:414–418, 1986

Delis DC, Wapner W, Gardner H, et al: The contribution of the right hemisphere to the organization of paragraphs. Cortex 19:43–50, 1983

Demarest J, Demarest L: Does the "torque test" measure cerebral dominance in adults? Percept Mot Skills 50: 155–158, 1980

Denny-Brown D: The nature of apraxia. J Nerv Ment Dis 126:9–32, 1958

Denny-Brown D, Meyer JS, Horenstein S: The significance of perceptual rivalry resulting from parietal lesion. Brain 75:433–471, 1952

Departments of Psychiatry and Child Psychiatry, The Institute of Psychiatry, and The Maudsley Hospital, London: Psychiatric Examination: Notes on Eliciting and Recording Clinical Information in Psychiatric Patients, 2nd Edition. Oxford, Oxford University Press, 1987

Devinsky O, Bear D, Volpe BT: Confusional states following posterior cerebral artery infarction. Arch Neurol 45:160–163, 1988

Dewey RB, Jankovic J: Hemiballism-hemichorea: clinical and pharmacologic findings in 21 patients. Arch Neurol 46:862–867, 1989

Dietz PE: Patterns in human violence, in American Psychiatric Association Annual Review, Vol 6. Edited by Hales RE, Frances AJ. Washington, DC, American Psychiatric Press, 1987, pp 465–490

Drewe EA: Go-no go learning after frontal lobe lesions in humans. Cortex 11:8–16, 1975

Duffy RJ, Duffy JR: An investigation of Body Part as Object (BPO) responses in normal and brain-damaged adults. Brain and Cognition 10:220–236, 1989

Duus P: Topical Diagnosis in Neurology. New York, Thieme, 1989

Early TS, Posner MI, Reiman EM, et al: Hyperactivity of the left striato-pallidal projection, I: lower level theory. Psychiatric Developments 2:85–108, 1989

Engel J: Seizures and Epilepsy. Philadelphia, PA, FA Davis, 1989

Eslinger PJ, Damasio AR: Severe disturbance of higher cognition after bilateral frontal lobe ablation: patient EVR. Neurology 35:1731–1741, 1985

Eslinger PJ, Damasio AR, Van Hoesen GW: Olfactory dysfunction in man: anatomical and behavioral aspects. Brain and Cognition 1:259–285, 1982

Faber-Langendoen K, Morris JC, Knesevich JW, et al: Aphasia in senile dementia of the Alzheimer type. Neurology 23:365–370, 1988

Fahn S, Marsden CD, Calne DB: Classification and investigation of dystonia, in Movement Disorders, 2nd Edition. Edited by Marsden CD, Fahn S. London, Butterworths, 1987, pp 332–358

Falconer MA, Wilson JL: Visual field changes following anterior temporal lobectomy: their significance in relation to "Meyer's loop" of the optic radiation. Brain 81:1–14, 1958

Fann WE, Sullivan JL, Richman BW: Dyskinesias associated with tricyclic antidepressants. Br J Psychiatry 128: 490–493, 1976

Farah MJ: Visual Agnosia: Disorders of Object Recognition and What They Tell Us about Normal Vision. Cambridge, MA, MIT Press, 1990

Feinstein A, Ron MA: Psychosis associated with demonstrable brain disease. Psychol Med 20:793–803, 1990

Fenwick P: The nature and management of aggression in epilepsy. Journal of Neuropsychiatry and Clinical Neuroscience 1:418–425, 1989

Findley LJ, Gresty MA, Halmagyi GM: Tremor, the cogwheel phenomenon and clonus in Parkinson's disease. J Neurol Neurosurg Psychiatry 44:534–546, 1981

Firestone P, Peters S: Minor physical anomalies and behavior in children: a review. J Autism Dev Disord 13: 411–425, 1983

Fisher CM: Intermittent interruption of behavior. Transactions of the American Neurological Association 93: 209–210, 1968

Fisher CM: Disorientation for place. Arch Neurol 39:33–36, 1982

Fisher CM: Abulia minor vs agitated behavior. Clin Neurosurg 31:9–31, 1984

Fisher CM: "Catatonia" due to disulfiram toxicity. Arch Neurol 46:798–804, 1989a

Fisher CM: Neurologic fragments, II: remarks on anosognosia, confabulation, memory, and other topics; and an appendix on self-observation. Neurology 39:127–132, 1989b

Fisher M: Left hemiplegia and motor impersistence. J Nerv Ment Dis 123:201–218, 1956

Fitzgerald PM, Jankovic J: Tardive oculogyric crises. Neurology 39:1434–1437, 1989

Fogel CA, Mednick SA, Michelsen N: Hyperactive behavior and minor physical anomalies. Acta Psychiatr Scand 72:551–556, 1985

Folstein MF, Folstein SE, McHugh PR: Mini-Mental State: a practical method for grading the cognitive state of patients for the clinician. J Psychiatr Res 12:189–198, 1975

Ford RA: The psychopathology of echophenomena. Psychol Med 19:627–635, 1989

Fox JH, Bennett DA, Heyworth JA, et al: Primitive reflexes. Neurology 39:1001–1002, 1989

Freed WJ, Kleinman JE, Karson CN, et al:. Eye-blink rates and platelet monoamine oxidase activity in chronic schizophrenic patients. Biol Psychiatry 15:329–332, 1980

Freud S: Fragment of an analysis of a case of hysteria, in Standard Edition of the Complete Psychological Works of Sigmund Freud, Vol 7. Edited by Strachey J. London, Hogarth, 1905, pp 3–122

Freund H-J, Hummelsheim H: Lesions of premotor cortex in man. Brain 108:697–733, 1985

Gardner D, Lucas PB, Cowdry RW: Soft sign neurological abnormalities in borderline personality disorder and normal control subjects. J Nerv Ment Dis 175:177–180, 1987

Geschwind N: Non-aphasic disorders of speech. Int J Neurol 4:207–214, 1964

Geschwind N: Disorders of attention: a frontier in neuropsychology. Philos Trans R Soc Lond [Biol] 298:173–185, 1982

Geschwind N, Kaplan E: A human cerebral deconnection syndrome: a preliminary report. Neurology 12:675–685, 1962

Gibb WRG, Lees AJ: The clinical phenomenon of akathisia. J Neurol Neurosurg Psychiatry 49:861–866, 1986

Gloor P, Olivier A, Quesny LF, et al: The role of the limbic system in experiential phenomena of temporal lobe epilepsy. Ann Neurol 12:129–140, 1982

Gold K, Rabins PV: Isolated visual hallucinations and the Charles Bonnet syndrome: a review of the literature and presentation of six cases. Compr Psychiatry 30:90–98, 1989

Goldberg E, Bilder RM: The frontal lobes and hierarchical organization of cognitive control, in The Frontal Lobes Revisited. Edited by Perecman E. Hillsdale, NJ, Lawrence Erlbaum, 1987, pp 159–187

Goldberg G, Mayer NH, Toglia JU: Medial frontal cortex infarction and the alien hand sign. Arch Neurol 38:683–686, 1981

Goldstein K: The effect of brain damage on the personality. Psychiatry 15:245–260, 1952

Goodglass H, Kaplan E: The Assessment of Aphasia and Related Disorders, 2nd Edition. Philadelphia, PA, Lea & Febiger, 1983

Gorelick PB, Ross ED: The aprosodias: further functional-anatomical evidence for the organisation of affective language in the right hemisphere. J Neurol Neurosurg Psychiatry 50:553–560, 1987

Gould R, Miller BL, Goldber MA, et al: The validity of hysterical signs and symptoms. J Nerv Ment Dis 174: 593–597, 1986

Graff-Radford NR, Eslinger PJ, Damasio AR, et al: Nonhemorrhagic infarction of the thalamus: behavioral, anatomic, and physiologic correlates. Neurology 34:14–23, 1984

Greden JF, Genero N, Price HL: Agitation-increased electromyogram activity in the corrugator muscle region: a possible explanation of the "omega sign"? Am J Psychiatry 142:348–351, 1985

Green MF, Satz P, Gaier DJ, et al: Minor physical anomalies in schizophrenia. Schizophr Bull 15:91–99, 1989

Greenberg MS, Farah MJ: The laterality of dreaming. Brain Cogn 5:307–321, 1986

Griffith N, Engel Jr J, Bandler R: Ictal and enduring interictal disturbances in emotional behaviour in an animal model of temporal lobe epilepsy. Brain Res 400:360–364, 1987

Gualtieri CT, Adams A, Shen CD, et al: Minor physical anomalies in alcoholic and schizophrenic adults and hyperactive and autistic children. Am J Psychiatry 139: 640–643, 1982

Guy JD, Majorski LV, Wallace CJ, et al: The incidence of minor physical anomalies in adult male schizophrenics. Schizophr Bull 9:571–582, 1983

Habib M, Sirigu A: Pure topographical disorientation: a definition and anatomical basis. Cortex 23:73–85, 1987

Hallett M, Ravits J: Involuntary movements, in Diseases

of the Nervous System: Clinical Neurobiology. Edited by Asbury AK, McKhann GM, McDonald WI. Philadelphia, PA, WB Saunders, 1986, pp 452–460

Harrison PJ, Pearson RCA: Olfaction and psychiatry. Br J Psychiatry 155:822–828, 1989

Heilman KM, Rothi LJG: Apraxia, in Clinical Neuropsychology, 2nd Edition. Edited by Heilman KM, Valenstein E. New York, Oxford University Press, 1985, pp 131–150

Heilman KM, Scholes R, Watson RT: Auditory affective agnosia: disturbed comprehension of affective speech. J Neurol Neurosurg Psychiatry 38:69–72, 1975

Heilman KM, Watson RT, Valenstein E: Neglect and related disorders, in Clinical Neuropsychology, 2nd Edition. Edited by Heilman KM, Valenstein E. New York, Oxford University Press, 1985, pp 243–293

Heinrichs DW, Buchanan RW: Significance and meaning of neurological signs in schizophrenia. Am J Psychiatry 145:11–18, 1988

Helm NA, Butler RB, Benson DF: Acquired stuttering. Neurology 28:1159–1165, 1978

Helms PM, Godwin CD: Abnormalities of blink rate in psychoses: a preliminary report. Biol Psychiatry 20: 103–106, 1985

Hermann BP, Dikmen S, Schwartz MS, et al: Interictal psychopathology in patients with ictal fear: a quantitative investigation. Neurology 32:7–11, 1982

Hermesh H, Munitz H: Unilateral neuroleptic-induced akathisia. Clin Neuropharmacol 13:253–258, 1990

Hertzig ME, Birch HG: Neurologic organization in psychiatrically disturbed adolescent girls. Arch Gen Psychiatry 15:590–598, 1966

Hier DB, Mondlock J, Caplan LR: Recovery of behavioral abnormalities after right hemisphere stroke. Neurology 33:345–350, 1983

Hollander E, Schiffman E, Cohen B, et al: Signs of central nervous system dysfunction in obsessive-compulsive disorder. Arch Gen Psychiatry 47:27–32, 1990

Horner J, Heyman A, Dawson D, et al: The relationship of agraphia to the severity of dementia in Alzheimer's disease. Arch Neurol 45:760–763, 1988

House A, Dennis M, Molyneux A, et al: Emotionalism after stroke. Br Med J 298:991–994, 1989

Hughlings-Jackson J: On right- or left-sided spasm at the onset of epileptic paroxysms, and on crude sensation warnings and elaborate mental states. Brain 3:192–206, 1880–1881

Humphreys GW, Riddoch MJ: On telling your fruit from your vegetables: a consideration of category-specific deficits after brain damage. Trends Neurosci 10:145–148, 1987

Huttenlocher PR, Huttenlocher J: A study of children with hyperlexia. Neurology 23:1107–1116, 1973

Hyde TM, Hotson JR, Kleinman JE: Differential diagnosis of choreiform tardive dyskinesia. Journal of Neuropsychiatry and Clinical Neurosciences 3:255–268, 1991

Jacobs L, Grossman MD: Three primitive reflexes in normal adults. Neurology 30:184–188, 1980

Jankovic J: The neurology of tics, in Movement Disorders, 2nd Edition. Edited by Marsden CD, Rahn S. London, Butterworths, 1987, pp 383–405

Jankovic J, Glass JP: Metoclopramide-induced phantom dyskinesia. Neurology 35:432–435, 1985

Jenkyn LR, Walsh DB, Walsh BT, et al: The nuchocephalic reflex. J Neurol Neurosurg Psychiatry 38:561–566, 1975

Jenkyn LR, Walsh DB, Culver CM, et al: Clinical signs in diffuse cerebral dysfunction. J Neurol Neurosurg Psychiatry 40:956–966, 1977

Joanette Y, Goulet P, Ska B, et al: Informative content of narrative discourse in right-brain-damaged right-handers. Brain Lang 29:81–105, 1986

Johnstone EC, Cooling NJ, Frith CD, et al: Phenomenology of organic and functional psychoses and the overlap between them. Br J Psychiatry 153:770–776, 1988

Jones IH: Observations on schizophrenic stereotypes. Compr Psychiatry 6:323–335, 1965

Joseph AB, O'Leary DH, Wheeler HG: Bilateral atrophy of the frontal and temporal lobes in schizophrenic patients with Capgras syndrome: a case-control study using computed tomography. J Clin Psychiatry 51:322–325, 1990

Joynt RJ, Benton AL, Fogel ML: Behavioral and pathological correlates of motor impersistence. Neurology 12: 876–881, 1962

Kandel E, Brennan PA, Mednick SA, et al: Minor physical anomalies and recidivistic adult criminal behavior. Acta Psychiatr Scand 79:103–107, 1989

Karson CN: Oculomotor signs in a psychiatric population: a preliminary report. Am J Psychiatry 136:1057–1060, 1979

Karson CN: Spontaneous eye-blink rates and dopaminergic systems. Brain 106:643–653, 1983

Karson CN: Physiology of normal and abnormal blinking, in Advances in Neurology, Vol 49: Facial Dyskinesias. Edited by Jankovic J, Tolosa E. New York, Raven, 1988, pp 25–37

Karson CN, Burns RS, PA LeWitt, et al: Blink rates and disorders of movement. Neurology 34:677–678, 1984

Katzman R, Brown T, Fuld P, et al: Validation of a short orientation-memory-concentration test of cognitive impairment. Am J Psychiatry 140:734–739, 1983

Kertesz A, Nicholson I, Cancelliere A, et al: Motor impersistence: a right-hemisphere syndrome. Neurology 35:662–666, 1985

Klüver H, Bucy PC: Psychic blindness and other symptoms following bilateral temporal lobectomy in rhesus monkeys. Am J Physiol 119:352–353, 1937

Klüver H, Bucy PC: Preliminary analysis of functions of the temporal lobes in monkeys. Archives of Neurology and Psychiatry 42:979–1000, 1939

Kolada SJ, Pitman RK: Eye-head synkinesia in schizophrenic adults during a repetitive visual search task. Biol Psychiatry 18:675–684, 1983

Koller WC: Edentulous orodyskinesia. Neurology 13:97–99, 1983

Koller WC, Glatt S, Wilson RS, et al: Primitive reflexes and cognitive function in the elderly. Ann Neurol 12: 302–304, 1982

Koller W, Lang A, Vetere-Overfield B, et al: Psychogenic tremors. Neurol 39:1094–1099, 1989

Kopelman MD: Clinical tests of memory. Br J Psychiatry 148:517–525, 1986

Korein J: Iris pigmentation (melanin) in idiopathic dystonic syndromes including torticollis. Ann Neurol 10: 53–55, 1981

Landau WM: Reflex dementia: disinhibited primitive thinking. Neurology 39:133–137, 1989

Lang AE: Clinical differences between metoclopramide- and antipsychotic-induced tardive dyskinesias. Can J Neurol Sci 17:137–139, 1990
Lang AE, Ellis C, Kingon H, et al: Iris pigmentation in idiopathic dystonia. Ann Neurol 12:585–586, 1982
Laplane D, Orgogozo JM, Meininger V, et al: Paralysie faciale avec dissociation automatic-volontaire inverse par lesion frontale: son origine corticale: ses relations avec l'A.M.S. Rev Neurol 132:725–734, 1976
Lecours AR, Lhermitte F, Bryans B: Aphasiology. London, Balliere Tindall, 1983
Lees AJ: Tics and Related Disorders. Edinburgh, Churchill Livingstone, 1985
Lees AJ: Facial mannerisms and tics, in Facial Dyskineasias (Advances in Neurology Series, Vol 49). New York, Raven, 1988, pp 255–261
Leigh RJ, Foley JM, Remler BF, et al: Oculogyric crisis: a syndrome of thought disorder and ocular deviation. Ann Neurol 22:13–17, 1987
Leimkuhler ME, Mesulam M-M: Reversible go-no go deficits in a case of frontal lobe tumor. Ann Neurol 18:617–619, 1985
Lepore FE, Duvoisin RC: "Apraxia" of eyelid opening: an involuntary levator inhibition. Neurology 35:423–427, 1985
Lesser RP, Fahn S: Dystonia: a disorder often misdiagnosed as a conversion reaction. Am J Psychiatry 135: 349–352, 1978
Levin M: Delirium: a gap in psychiatric teaching. Am J Psychiatry 107:689–694, 1951
Levin M: Perseveration at various levels of complexity, with comments on delirium. Archives of Neurology and Psychiatry 73:439–444, 1955
Levin M: Thinking disturbances in delirium. Archives of Neurology and Psychiatry 75:62–66, 1956
Levine DN: Unawareness of visual and sensorimotor defects: a hypothesis. Brain Cogn 13:233–281, 1990
Levy J, Reid M: Variations in writing posture and cerebral organization. Science 194:614–615, 1976
Lewis SW: Congenital risk factors for schizophrenia. Psychol Med 19:5–13, 1989
Lezak MD: Subtle sequelae of brain damage: perplexity, distractibility, and fatigue. Am J Phys Med 57:9–15, 1978
Lhermitte F: Human autonomy and the frontal lobes, II: patient behavior in complex and social situations: the "environmental dependency syndrome." Ann Neurol 19:335–343, 1986
Lhermitte F, Pillon B, Serdaru M: Human autonomy and the frontal lobes, I: imitation and utilization behavior: a neuropsychological study of 75 patients. Ann Neurol 19:326–334, 1986
Lishman WA: Organic Psychiatry: The Psychological Consequences of Cerebral Disorder, 2nd Edition. Oxford, Blackwell, 1987
Lishman WA: Alcohol and the brain. Br J Psychiatry 156: 635–644, 1990
Lloyd G: Medicine without signs. Br Med J 287:539–542, 1983
Lodder J, Baard WC: Paraballism caused by bilateral hemorrhagic infarction in basal ganglia. Neurology 31:484–486, 1981
Lopez OL, Becker JT, Brenner RP, et al: Alzheimer's disease with delusions and hallucinations: neuropsychological and electroencephalographic correlates. Neurology 41:906–912, 1991
Lucas PB, Gardner DL, Cowdry RW, et al: Cerebral structure in borderline personality disorder. Psychiatry Res 27:111–115, 1989
Ludlow CL, Rosenberg J, Salazar A, et al: Site of penetrating brain lesions causing chronic acquired stuttering. Ann Neurol 22:60–66, 1987
Luria AR: Two kinds of motor perseveration in massive injury of the frontal lobes. Brain 88:1–10, 1965
Luria AR, Homskaya ED: Le trouble du role régulateur du langage au cours des lésions du lobe frontal. Neuropsychologia 1:9–26, 1963
Luria AR, Hutton JT: A modern assessment of the basic forms of aphasia. Brain Lang 4:129–151, 1977
Luxon L, Lees AJ, Greenwood RJ: Neurosyphilis today. Lancet 1:90–93, 1979
McGlynn SM, Schacter DL: Unawareness of deficits in neuropsychological syndromes. J Clin Exp Neuropsychol 11:143–205, 1989
McMeekan ERL, Lishman WA: Retest reliabilities and interrelationship of the Annett Hand Preference Questionnaire and the Edinburgh Handedness Inventory. Br J Psychol 66:53–59, 1975
Manschreck TC: Psychopathology of motor behavior in schizophrenia. Progress in Experimental Personality Research 12:53–99, 1983
Manschreck TC: Motor abnormalities in schizophrenia, in Handbook of Schizophrenia, Vol I: The Neurology of Schizophrenia. Edited by Nasrallah HA, Weinberger DR. Amsterdam, Elsevier, 1986, pp 65–96
Marsden CD: Is tardive dyskinesia a unique disorder? in Dyskinesia Research and Treatment. Edited by Casey T, Chase T, Christensen P, et al. Berlin, Springer-Verlag, 1985, pp 64–71
Marsden CD: Basal ganglia and motor dysfunction, in Diseases of the Nervous System: Clinical Neurobiology. Edited by Asbury AK, McKhann GM, McDonald WI. Philadelphia, PA, WB Saunders, 1986, pp 394–400
Marsden CD: Wilson's disease. Q J Med 65:959–966, 1987
Marsden CD, Hallett M, Fahn S: The nosology and pathophysiology of myoclonus, in Movement Disorders. Edited by Marsden CD, Fahn S. London, Butterworth Scientific, 1982, pp 196–248
Mayes AR: Human Organic Memory Disorders. Cambridge, Cambridge University Press, 1988
Mayeux R, Alexander MP, Benson DF, et al: Poriomania. Neurology 29:1616–1619, 1979
Merriam AE, Kay SR, Opler LA, et al: Neurological signs and the positive-negative dimension in schizophrenia. Biol Psychiatry 28:181–192, 1990
Mesulam M-M: A cortical network for directed attention and unilateral neglect. Ann Neurol 10:309–325, 1981
Mesulam M-M: Principles of Behavioral Neurology. Philadelphia, PA, FA Davis, 1985
Metzig E, Rosenberg S, Ast M: Lateral asymmetry in patients with nervous and mental disease: a preliminary study. Neuropsychobiology 1:197–202, 1975
Metzig E, Rosenberg S, Ast M, et al: Bipolar manic-depressives and unipolar depressives distinguished by tests of lateral asymmetry. Biol Psychiatry 11:313–323, 1976
Milberg WP, Hebben N, Kaplan E: The Boston Process Approach to neuropsychological assessment, in Neu-

ropsychological Assessment of Neuropsychiatric Disorders. Edited by Grant I, Adams KM. New York, Oxford University Press, 1986, pp 65–86

Miller BL, Cummings JL, McIntyre H, et al: Hypersexuality or altered sexual preference following brain injury. J Neurol Neurosurg Psychiatry 49:867–873, 1986

Miller H: Psychiatry—medicine or magic? in Contemporary Psychiatry: Selected Reviews from the British Journal of Hospital Medicine. Edited by Silverstone T, Barraclough B. Ashford, England, Headley, 1975, pp 462–466

Mody CK, Miller BL, McIntyre HB, et al: Neurologic complications of cocaine abuse. Neurology 38:1189–1193, 1988

Monrad-Krohn GH: On the dissociation of voluntary and emotional innervation in facial paresis of central origin. Brain 47:22–35, 1924

Monrad-Krohn GH: Dysprosody or altered "melody of language." Brain 70:405–415, 1947

Moore-Gillon V: Testing the sense of smell. Br Med J 294: 793–794, 1987

Mori E, Yamadori A: Rejection behaviour: a human homologue of the abnormal behaviour of Denny-Brown and Chambers' monkey with bilateral parietal ablation. J Neurol Neurosurg Psychiatry 52:1250–1266, 1989

Nelson A, Fogel BS, Faust D: Bedside cognitive screening instruments: a critical assessment. J Nerv Ment Dis 174: 73–83, 1986

Obeso JA, Rothwell JC, Marsden CD: Simple tics in Gilles de la Tourette's syndrome are not prefaced by a normal premovement EEG potential. J Neurol Neurosurg Psychiatry 44:735–738, 1981

Occupational and Environmental Health Committee of the American Lung Association of San Diego and Imperial Counties: Taking the occupational history. Ann Intern Med 99:641–651, 1983

Ounsted C, Lindsay J, Richards P: Temporal Lobe Epilepsy 1948–1986: A Biographical Study. Oxford, Blackwell Scientific, 1987

Ovsiew F, Yudofsky SC: Agression: a neuropsychiatric perspective, in Rage, Power, and Aggression. Edited by Roose SP. New Haven, CT, Yale University Press (in press)

Owens DGC: Dystonia: a potential psychiatric pitfall. Br J Psychiatry 156:620–634, 1990

Padberg GW, Bruyn GW: Choreadifferential diagnosis, in Handbook of Clinical Neurology, Vol 5: Extrapyramidal Disorders. Edited by Vinken PJ, Bruyn GW, Klawans HL. Amsterdam, Elsevier, 1986, pp 549–564

Paneth N: Birth and the origins of cerebral palsy. N Engl J Med 315:124–126, 1986

Paulson G, Gottleib G: Development reflexes: the reappearance of foetal and neonatal reflexes in aged patients. Brain 91:37–52, 1968

Penfield W, Robertson JSM: Growth asymmetry due to lesions of the postcentral cerebral cortex. Arch Neurol Psychiatry 50:405–430, 1943

Pick A: Clinical studies, III: on reduplicative paramnesia. Brain 26:260–267, 1903

Pinching AJ: Clinical testing of olfaction reassessed. Brain 100:377–388, 1977

Plum F, Posner JB: The Diagnosis of Stupor and Coma, 3rd Edition. Philadelphia, PA, FA Davis, 1980

Poeck K: The Klüver-Bucy syndrome in man, in Handbook of Clinical Neurology, Vol 45: Clinical Neuropsychology. Edited by Frederiks JAM. Amsterdam, Elsevier, 1985a, pp 257–263

Poeck K: Pathological laughter and crying, in Handbook of Clinical Neurology, Vol 45: Clinical Neuropsychology. Edited by Frederiks JAM. Amsterdam, Elsevier, 1985b, pp 219–225

Posner MI, Early TS, Reiman E, et al: Asymmetries in hemispheric control of attention in schizophrenia. Arch Gen Psychiatry 45:814–821, 1988

Potter H, Butters N: An assessment of olfactory deficits in patients with damage to prefrontal cortex. Neuropsychologia 18:621–628, 1980

Prechtl HFR: Neurological sequelae of prenatal and perinatal complications. Br Med J 4:763–767, 1967

Quinn PO, Rapoport JL: Minor physical anomalies and neurologic status in hyperactive boys. Pediatrics 53: 742–747, 1974

Quitkin F, Rifkin A, Klein DF: Neurologic soft signs in schizophrenia and character disorders. Arch Gen Psychiatry 33:845–853, 1976

Rausch R, Serafetinides EA: Specific alterations of olfactory function in humans with temporal lobe lesions. Nature 255:557–558, 1975

Reinhold M: Human behaviour reactions to organic cerebral disease. J Ment Sci 99:130–135, 1953

Remillard GM, Andermann F, Rhi-Sausi A, et al: Facial asymmetry in patients with temporal lobe epilepsy: a clinical sign useful in the lateralization of temporal epileptogenic foci. Neurology 27:109–114, 1977

Ridley RM, Baker HF: Stereotypy in monkeys and humans. Psychol Med 12:61–72, 1982

Riley DE, Lang AE, Lewis A, et al: Cortico-basal ganglionic degeneration. Neurology 40:1203–1212, 1990

Rogers D: The motor disorders of severe psychiatric illness: a conflict of paradigms. Br J Psychiatry 147:221–232, 1985

Rogers D: Catatonia: a contemporary approach. Journal of Neuropsychiatry and Clinical Neurosciences 3:334–340, 1991

Rogers D, Lees AJ, Smith E, et al: Bradyphrenia in parkinson's disease and psychomotor retardation in depressive illness. Brain 110:761–776, 1987

Ropper AH: Self-grasping: a focal neurological sign. Ann Neurol 12:575–577, 1982

Ross ED: The aprosodias: functional-anatomic organization of the affective components of language in the right hemisphere. Arch Neurol 38:561–569, 1981

Ross ED, Mesulam M-M: Dominant language functions of the right hemisphere? Arch Neurol 36:144–148, 1979

Ross ED, Stewart RS: Pathological display of affect in patients with depression and right frontal brain damage: an alternative mechanism. J Nerv Ment Dis 175:165–172, 1987

Ross Russell RW: Supranuclear palsy of eyelid closure. Brain 103:71–82, 1980

Sacks O: Migraine: evolution of a common disorder. London, Faber and Faber, 1971

Sandson J, Albert ML: Perseveration in behavioral neurology. Neurology 37:1736–1741, 1987

Scheinberg IH, Sternlieb I, Walshe JM: Wilson's disease and Kayser-Fleischer rings. Ann Neurol 19:613–614, 1986

Schiff HB, Alexander MP, Naeser MA, et al: Aphemia: clinical-anatomic correlations. Arch Neurol 40:720–727, 1983

Schneider K: Primary and secondary symptoms in schizophrenia, in Themes and Variations in European Psychiatry: An Anthology. Edited by Hirsch SR, Shepherd M. Bristol, England, John Wright & Sons, 1974, pp 40–44

Schott GD, Wyke MA: Obligatory bimanual associated movements: report of a non-familial case in an otherwise normal left-handed boy. J Neurol Sci 33:301–312, 1977

Shallice T, Burgess PW, Schon F, et al: The origins of utilization behavior. Brain 112:1587–1598, 1989

Shapiro BE, Alexander MP, Gardner H, et al: Mechanisms of confabulation. Neurology 31:1070–1076, 1981

Silberman EK, Post RM, Nurnberger J, et al: Transient sensory, cognitive and affective phenomena in affective illness: a comparison with complex partial epilepsy. Br J Psychiatry 146:81–89, 1985

Simons RC: The resolution of the Latah paradox. J Nerv Ment Dis 168:195–206, 1980

Simons RC: Latah II: problems with a purely symbolic interpretation: a reply to Michael Kenny. J Nerv Ment Dis 171:168–175, 1983

Spillane JD: An Atlas of Clinical Neurology, 2nd Edition. London, Oxford University Press, 1975

Steg JP, Rapoport JL: Minor physical anomalies in normal, neurotic, learning disabled, and severely disturbed children. Journal of Autism and Childhood Schizophrenia 5:299–307, 1975

Stengel E: A clinical and psychological study of echo-reactions. Journal of Mental Science 93:27–41, 1947

Stevens JR: Eye blink and schizophrenia: psychosis or tardive dyskinesia. Am J Psychiatry 135:223–226, 1978

Strub RL, Black FW: The bedside mental status examination, in Handbook of Neuropsychology, Vol I. Edited by Boller F, Grafman J. Amsterdam, Elsevier, 1988, pp 29–46

Stuss DT, Alexander MP, Lieberman A, et al: An extraordinary form of confabulation. Neurology 28:1166–1172, 1978

Szatmari P, Taylor DC: The neurological examination in child psychiatry: a review of its uses. Can J Psychiatry 29:155–162, 1984

Taylor DC, Lochery M: Temporal lobe epilpsy: origin and significance of simple and complex auras. J Neurol Neurosurg Psychiatry 50:673–681, 1987

Taylor EA: Childhood hyperactivity. Br J Psychiatry 149: 562–573, 1986

Toone BK, Edeh J, Nanjee MN, et al: Hyposexuality and epilepsy: a community survey of hormonal and behavioural changes in male epileptics. Psychol Med 19: 937–943, 1989

Torrey EF: Neurological abnormalities in schizophrenic patients. Biol Psychiatry 15:381–388, 1980

Trimble MR: Hypergraphia, in Aspects of Epilepsy and Psychiatry. Edited by Trimble MR, Bolwig TG. Chichester, England, John Wiley, 1986, 75–87

Trimble MR: Can schizophrenia be localized? Journal of Neuropsychiatry and Clinical Neurosciences 3:89–94, 1991

Trosch RM, Sze G, Brass LM, et al: Emotional facial paresis with striatocapsular infarction. J Neurol Sci 98:195–201, 1990

Tucker DM, Watson RT, Heilman KM: Discrimination and evocation of affectively intoned speech in patients with right parietal disease. Neurology 27:947–950, 1977

Tupper DE (ed): Soft Neurological Signs. Orlando, FL, Grune & Stratton, 1987

Van Lancker DR, Kempler D: Comprehension of familiar phrases by left- but not by right-hemisphere damaged patients. Brain Lang 32:265–277, 1987

Van Putten T: The many faces of akathisia. Compr Psychiatry 16:43–47, 1975

Vighetto A, Henry E, Garde P, et al: Le délire spatial: une manifestation des lésions de l'hémisphère mineur. Rev Neurol 141:476–481, 1985

Voeller KKS, Heilman KM: Attention deficit disorder in children: a neglect syndrome? Neurology 38:806–808, 1988

Waddington JL, Crow TJ: Abnormal involuntary movements and psychosis in the preneuroleptic era and in unmedicated patients: implications for the concept of tardive dyskinesia, in Tardive Dyskinesia: Biological Mechanisms and Clinical Aspects. Edited by Wolf ME, Mosnaim AD. Washington, DC, American Psychiatric Press, 1988, pp 51–66

Walshe JM: Wilson's disease, in Handbook of Clinical Neurology, Vol 49: Extrapyramidal Disorders. Edited by Vinken PJ, Bruyn GW, Klawans HL. Amsterdam, Elsevier, 1986, pp 223–238

Wapner W, Hamby S, Gardner H: The role of the right hemisphere in the apprehension of complex linguistic materials. Brain Lang 14:15–33, 1981

Weintraub S, Mesulam M-M: Mental state assessment of young and elderly adults in behavioral neurology, in Principles of Behavioral Neurology. Edited by Mesulam M-M. Philadelphia, PA, FA Davis, 1985, pp 71–123

Whitty CWM: Cortical dysarthria and dysprosody of speech. J Neurol Neurosurg Psychiatry 27:507–510, 1964

Wilkens DE, Hallett M, Wess MM: Audiogenic startle reflex of man and its relationship to startle syndromes: a review. Brain 109:561–573, 1986

Wilson SAK: Some problems in neurology, No 11: pathological laughing and crying. Journal of Neurology and Psychopathology 4:299–333, 1924

Young RR: Tremor, in Diseases of the Nervous System: Clinical Neurobiology. Edited by Asbury AK, McKhann GM, McDonald WI. Philadelphia, PA, WB Saunders, 1986, pp 434–451

Young RR, Shahani BT: Asterixis: one type of negative myoclonus, in Myoclonus (Advances in Neurology Series, Vol 43). Edited by Fahn S. New York, Raven, 1986, pp 137–156

Zametkin AJ, Stevens JR, Pittman R: Ontogeny of spontaneous blinking and of habituation of the blink reflex. Ann Neurol 5:453–457, 1979

Zulch KJ, Muller N: Associated movements in man, in Handbook of Clinical Neurology, Vol 1. Edited by Vinken PJ, Bruyn GW. Amsterdam, North-Holland Publishing, 1969, pp 404–426

Chapter

5

The Neuropsychological Evaluation

Diane B. Howieson, Ph.D.
Muriel D. Lezak, Ph.D.

NEUROPSYCHOLOGICAL EVALUATIONS have been used since the 1940s for the diagnosis of acquired or congenital problems presumed to be a result of brain disease or trauma (Hebb 1942; Teuber 1948). The neuropsychologist assesses brain function inferred from an individual's cognitive, sensory, motor, emotional, or social behavior. During the early history of neuropsychology, these assessments were often the most direct measure of brain integrity in persons without localizing neurological signs and symptoms and with problems confined to higher mental functions. Neuropsychological measures still are useful diagnostic indicators of brain dysfunction for many conditions and will remain the major diagnostic modality for some (Eisenberg and Levin 1989; Jernigan and Hesselink 1987; Mapov 1988). However, diagnosis of brain damage has become increasingly accurate in recent decades as a result of improved visualization of brain structure by computed tomography (CT), magnetic resonance imaging (MRI), and angiography (Theodore 1988). These developments have allowed a shift in the focus of neuropsychological assessment from the diagnosis of possible brain damage to a better understanding of specific brain-behavior relationships and of the psychosocial consequences of brain damage.

❑ WHEN A NEUROPSYCHOLOGICAL EVALUATION IS INDICATED

Patients referred to a neuropsychologist for assessment may be classified into one of three groups. The first and probably largest group consists of patients with known brain damage. The more common brain disorders are cerebrovascular disorders, head injury, hydrocephalus, Alzheimer's disease, Parkinson's disease, multiple sclerosis, Huntington's chorea, tumors, seizures, and infections. A neuropsychological evaluation can be useful in defining the nature and severity of resulting functional problems. The assessment provides information about the patient's cognition, personality characteristics, social behavior, emotional status, and adjustment to limitations. The individual's potential for independent living and productive activity can be derived from these data. Information about the patient's behavioral strengths and weaknesses can be used for treatment planning, vocational training, competency determination, and counseling for both patients and their families (Acker 1989; Newcombe 1987). For example, a 52-year-old real estate agent had a left-hemisphere stroke producing mild aphasia and right-sided hemiparesis. A neuropsychological examination several months later showed that she had good language comprehension and reading skills, mild word-finding problems, mild visuospatial deficits, and moderate impairment in verbal memory. Like many patients with strokes (Niemi et al. 1988; Parikh and Robinson 1987; Robinson and Price 1982), she was also depressed. Information from the examination was used to make decisions about the likelihood of returning successfully to her previous job, for planning rehabilitation and strategies to help her compensate for persistent cognitive deficits, for recommendations regarding treatment of her depression, and for family counseling.

The second group of patients referred to a neuropsychologist consists of persons with a known risk factor for brain damage in whom a change in behavior might be the result of such disease or injury to the brain. In these cases a neuropsychological evaluation might be used both to provide evidence of brain dysfunction and to describe the nature and severity of problems. For example, a 34-year-old office manager was involved in an automobile accident, receiving a blow to the head that produced a loss of consciousness for several minutes and no apparent further complications except some bruises and sore muscles. On returning to work after 1 week, she found that she was unable to keep up with the demands of her job. After several weeks of on-the-job difficulties she was sent to a neuropsychologist for evaluation of possible brain damage from the accident. The examiner looked for evidence of problems with divided attention, sustained concentration and mental tracking, and memory, all of which are common findings in the weeks or months after mild head injury (Alves and Jane 1985; Binder 1986; Gronwall and Sampson 1974; Russell 1974). The woman was advised that these problems frequently occur after head injury and that she was likely to experience considerable improvement during the next month or two. She was given recommendations about how to structure her work activities to minimize both these difficulties and the equally common problem of fatigue. A repeat examination was scheduled for 3 months after the injury to see if these predictions held true and to assess her adjustment and possible need for further counseling or other treatment.

Many medical conditions can affect brain function (Tarter et al. 1988). Brain function can be disrupted by systemic illnesses: endocrinopathies; metabolic and electrolyte disturbances; diseases of the kidney, liver, and pancreas; nutritional deficiencies; toxins; and conditions producing decreased blood supply to the brain (e.g., trauma, vascular disorders, cardiac disease, pulmonary disease, anemia, carbon monoxide, and complications of anesthesia or surgery). Age and health habits must also be taken into consideration when evaluating a person's behavioral alterations because they affect the probability of cerebral disorder (Dubois et al. 1990; Heaton et al. 1986; Kolb 1989). In addition, many medicines can disrupt cognition through their subtle effects on alertness, attention, and memory (Cope 1988; Schmidt 1986).

In the last group, brain disease or trauma often is suspected based on the observation of a change in a person's behavior without an identifiable etiology; that is, the patient has no known risk factors for brain damage, and this diagnosis is being considered on the basis of exclusion of other diagnoses. Frequently psychiatrists are asked to evaluate an adult with no previous psychiatric history who has had an uncharacteristic change in behavior or personality and for whom no obvious sources of current emotional distress can be identified. An explanation is sought because behavior patterns and personality are relatively stable characteristics of adults. The list of differential diagnoses is long and may include a wide variety of brain disorders that range from metabolic disturbance, vitamin deficiency, endocrine disorder, and heavy metal poisoning to neoplasm, infection, and multiple small strokes. The psychiatric literature contains numerous examples of individuals who were being treated for psychiatric illness before it was discovered that they had brain disease, such as a frontal lobe tumor (Berg 1988; Kaszniak et al. 1985; Lesser 1985; Price and Mesulam 1985).

The most common application of the neuropsychological evaluation of adults without obvious risk factors for brain damage is in the early detection of progressive dementia, such as dementia of the Alzheimer type (Botwinick et al. 1986; Cutler et al. 1985;

Huff et al. 1987; LaRue and Jarvik 1987; Vitaliano et al. 1984). Most persons have symptoms associated with dementia for at least 1 year before they see a health care provider because the problems initially are minor and easily attributed to factors such as aging or recent emotional stress. The progression of these symptoms is insidious, and people have "good" as well as "bad" days during the early course of this illness. Neuropsychological assessment is useful in evaluating whether problems noted by the family or the individual are age related, attributable to other factors such as depression, or suggestive of an early dementing illness. During the past decade, human immunodeficiency virus (HIV) infection and the complications of drug abuse have been added as conditions that can produce an insidious dementia in younger persons (Goethe et al. 1989; Kovner et al. 1989; Van Gorp et al. 1989).

Another condition that produces no clinical clues for brain damage except for a change in behavior is the so-called silent stroke. Without obvious sensory, motor, or speech problems, a stroke may go undetected yet produce a persistent change in behavior or abilities. A series of small strokes can produce an insidious dementia. Environmental toxins comprise another class of hidden conditions that present general patterns of neuropsychological impairment (Freed and Kandel 1988; Ryan et al. 1988; Weiss 1983).

In such cases, with no known etiology to explain mental deterioration, a search for possible risk factors or other evidence for brain disease is conducted through history taking, physical examination, laboratory tests, and interviews with the patient's family or close associates. If a structural lesion such as a tumor, hydrocephalus, or brain infection is suspected, the diagnostic workup should include CT and MRI visualization of the brain. If this search proves negative, a diagnostic neuropsychological study might be useful.

The neuropsychological examination of persons with or without known risk factors for brain damage is diagnostically useful if a meaningful pattern of deficits is found. A "meaningful" pattern would be one that is relative specific to one, or only a few, diagnoses, such as a pattern of cognitive disruption suggestive of a focal brain lesion. For example, an examination was conducted on a man with HIV infection who had a 2-week history of "feeling odd." He became easily lost, even in familiar settings, and complained of an inability to perform a task as simple as making his sheets "fit the bed." He said that he could not read because he was unable to follow a line consistently across the page. He had stopped working as a barber after giving a poor haircut. He had no established symptoms of his infection. Although he was known to have an appropriate reactive depression related to his infection, his complaints were atypical for depression. A neuropsychological evaluation showed that he had severe and circumscribed visuospatial and constructional deficits, a pattern of cognitive deficits usually associated with right parietal dysfunction. A subsequent MRI scan showed white matter disease involving a large area of the right parietal lobe and several small areas elsewhere in the right hemisphere. A biopsy confirmed the diagnosis of multifocal progressive leukoencephalopathy.

Neuropsychological signs and symptoms that are possible indicators of a pathological brain process are presented in Table 5–1. Positive neuropsychological diagnoses are much more likely to be made when risk factors for brain dysfunction exist or signs and symptoms of brain dysfunction are observed than when neuropsychological diagnoses are considered solely on the basis of exclusion of other diagnoses.

One of the greatest challenges for a neuropsychologist is to assess whether psychiatric patients have evidence of an underlying brain disorder. Many psychiatric patients without neurological disease have cognitive disruption and behavioral or emotional aberrations that also occur in patients with brain damage (Frith and Done 1988; Taylor and Abrams 1987). Anxiety and depression often impair concentration and memory and may also slow thinking (Kaszniak et al. 1985; Levin 1984; McAllister 1981; Mayes 1988; Stromgren 1977). Numerous studies (Heaton et al. 1978; Lenzer 1980) have shown that neuropsychological test scores alone often fail to discriminate between patients with schizophrenia and those with brain damage. Although neuropsychological assessment provides a measure of the type and degree of cognitive disorder, it often cannot specify the etiology of the disturbance. In the absence of known or suspected brain injury, a patient with known psychiatric illness and nonspecific cognitive impairment is most likely experiencing cognitive disruption on the basis of the psychiatric illness. On the other hand, an adult patient previously functioning well and with no history of psychiatric illness or recent stress would be suspect for brain disease.

TABLE 5–1. NEUROPSYCHOLOGICAL SIGNS AND SYMPTOMS THAT ARE POSSIBLE INDICATORS OF A PATHOLOGICAL BRAIN PROCESS

Functional class	*Symptoms and signs*
Speech and language	Dysarthria Dysfluency Marked change in amount of speech output Paraphasias Word-finding problems
Academic skills	Alterations in reading, writing, frequent letter or number reversals, calculating, and number abilities
Thinking	Perseveration of speech Simplified or confused mental racking, reasoning, and concept formation
Motor	Weakness or clumsiness, particularly if lateralized Impaired fine motor coordination (e.g., changes in handwriting) Apraxias Perseveration of action components
Memory[a]	Impaired recent memory for verbal or visuospatial material or both Disorientation
Perception	Diplopia or visual field alterations Inattention (usually left-sided) Somatosensory alterations (particularly if lateralized) Inability to recognize familiar stimuli (agnosia)
Visuospatial abilities	Diminished ability to perform manual skills (e.g., mechanical repairs and sewing) Spatial disorientation Left-right disorientation Impaired spatial judgment (e.g., distances angulation)
Emotions[b]	Diminished emotional control with temper outburst and antisocial behavior Diminished empathy or interest in interpersonal relationships Affective changes Irritability without evident precipitating factors Personality change
Comportment[b]	Altered appetites and appetitive activities Altered grooming habits (excessive fastidiousness and carelessness) Hyper- or hypoactivity Social inappropriateness

[a]Many emotionally disturbed persons complain of memory deficits, which most typically reflect the person's self-preoccupation, distractibility or anxiety rather than a dysfunctional brain. Thus memory complaints in themselves do not necessarily warrant neuropsychological evaluation.

[b]Some of these changes are most likely to be neuropsychologically relevant in the absence of depression, although they can also be mistaken for depression.

❑ THE ROLE OF THE REFERRING PSYCHIATRIST

The referring psychiatrist has the tasks of selection of patients who might benefit from an evaluation, preparation of the patient, and formulating referral questions that best define the needed neuropsychological information. A valid evaluation depends on obtaining the patient's best performance. It usually is impossible to obtain satisfactory evaluations of patients who are uncooperative, fatigued, actively psychotic, seriously depressed, or highly anxious. For example, seriously depressed patients may resemble patients with mild dementia by their poor performance on cognitive tests, and the evaluation may underestimate the individual's full potential (Caine 1986; Marcopulos 1989; Wells 1979). Whenever possible such patients should be referred after there has been clinical improvement, when the results may be more representative of the patient's true ability uncontaminated by performance factors.

Preparation of the patient for the evaluation is important to obtain the patient's cooperation and alleviate unnecessary anxiety (Lezak 1983). The patient should understand the purpose and nature of the evaluation. The explanation usually includes a statement that the evaluation is requested to assess how the brain is functioning by looking at activities that the brain controls such as mental abilities. In most cases patients should know that the purpose of the evaluation is to look for mental and emotional strengths as well as weaknesses to assist with counseling and planning.

The more explicit the referral question is, the more likely it is that the evaluation will be conducted to provide useful information. The referral question should include

- Identifying information about the patient
- The reasons why the evaluation is requested
- A description of the problem to be assessed
- Pertinent history

The neuropsychological evaluation will be designed differently for a referral question asking whether the patient is a candidate for psychotherapy compared with an evaluation requested for a personal injury lawsuit. Many referrals seek behavioral descriptions, such as "Does this man who has multiple sclerosis show evidence of cognitive deficits?" Other referral questions may be framed around treatment recommendations for patient management, counseling, and educational or vocational planning.

❑ THE ASSESSMENT PROCESS

Interview and observation are the chief means by which neuropsychological evaluations are conducted. The interview provides the basis of the evaluation (Christensen 1979; Luria 1980). The main purposes are to elicit the patient's and family's complaints, understand the circumstances in which these problems occur, and evaluate the patient's attitude toward these problems. Understanding the range of the patient's complaints, as well as which ones the patient views as most troublesome, contribute to the framework on which the assessment and recommendations are based.

The presenting problems and the patient's attitude toward them may also provide important diagnostic information. Patients with certain neuropsychological conditions lack awareness of their problems or diminish the significance of them. Many patients with right-hemisphere stroke, Alzheimer's disease, and frontal lobe damage are unaware of or unable to appreciate the problems resulting from their brain injury. In its extreme form, some right-hemisphere stroke patients with hemiplegia are unable to comprehend that the left side of their body is part of them, let alone that they cannot use it. In a more muted form, many dementia patients attribute their memory problems to aging and minimize its significance. Conversely, patients, families, or caregivers sometime attribute problems to brain damage when a careful history suggests otherwise. It is not rare for patients to be referred for neuropsychological evaluations of persistent sequelae of head injury when there is no temporal relationship between the onset of current symptoms and the head injury.

The interview provides an opportunity to observe the patient's appearance, speech, motor abilities, and to evaluate affect, appropriateness of behavior, orientation, insight, and judgment. The interview can provide information about the patient's premorbid intellectual ability and personality, occupational and school background, social situation, and ability to use leisure time.

The tests used by neuropsychologists are simply standardized observation tools that, in many instances, have the added advantage of providing normative data that aid in interpreting the observations. Various assessment approaches are available, but they all have in common the goals of determining whether the patient shows evidence of brain dysfunction and of identifying the nature of problems detected. The two main approaches are individually tailored examinations and fixed assessment procedures. The former approach is often referred to as *hypothesis testing* because test selection is based on hypotheses about the etiology and nature of the brain dysfunction from information acquired before and during the assessment (Kaplan 1988).

Using this approach, information is obtained about the individual's medical and psychological background and about the patient's activities from the individual and other knowledgeable sources. Hypotheses regarding neuropsychological deficits are generated and tested. For example, the case may involve an individual known to have had a heart attack who sustained brief and unremarked hypoxia. The family reports that the individual has appeared depressed because he sits all day without showing an interest in other people or activities. Several hypotheses could be generated from this information to explain the behavior. The patient may indeed be depressed. Alternatively, the individual may have inertia secondary to cerebral damage. The examiner may decide to include tests that are relatively unstructured and require the patient's initiation and de novo organization. Other hypotheses that might be considered and tested include that the patient is confused and unable to respond to the situations that the family describe or that the patient has serious memory difficulties that interfere with his intention to initiate or maintain ongoing activities.

The more information that can be gained before the assessment procedure begins, the more efficiently specific hypotheses can be generated. Moreover, hypothesis testing continues throughout the assessment. When a problem is observed on a particular test, new hypotheses are generated or old ones are modified as to the nature of the observed problem. Typically the examination focuses on problem areas, while briefly screening other areas that appear to be relatively intact. When detailed information about residual competencies is required, as for developing a remediation program, the focus may be expanded to assess areas of strength.

A second approach to neuropsychological testing is to use a fixed battery of tests (Boll 1981; Reitan and Wolfson 1985). This approach involves examining the same range of cognitive and behavioral functioning in every individual. It is analogous to a physician conducting a standard physical examination on all patients. These fixed battery examinations frequently last from 6 to 8 hours. The advantage of fixed batteries is that the patient has a fairly broad-based examination. The consistency of the administration procedures and wide range of data make batteries useful for research purposes. However, this fixed approach does not focus on specific areas of difficulty. Time may be wasted in testing areas of cognition or sensorimotor functioning that are not problems, and subtle problems can be overlooked. Moreover, aspects of neuropsychological functioning not included in a fixed battery will not be examined.

Cognitive performance is only one aspect of an assessment. A full evaluation of the individual assesses emotional and social characteristics as well. Many patients with brain injury have changes in personality, mood, or ability to control emotional states (Lishman 1987). In some cases these changes may be secondary to cognitive impairment. Right-hemisphere stroke patients may show impaired processing of emotional material and complex social situations, which leads to interpersonal problems (Lezak 1979). Although the history and observers' reports will inform the examiner of changes in these characteristics, current emotional status and personality can also be evaluated by standard psychological tests. Performance by brain-injured populations on some of these tests have shown patterned alternations of personality and emotional status (Lezak et al. 1990; Robinson et al. 1984).

A recent development has been the use of computers for testing purposes (Adams and Brown 1986; Lezak 1988b). This new technology offers the possibility of obtaining test results under highly standardized conditions with minimal time expenditure by the examiner. Computers also have timing and scoring features and can plot data graphically. In addition, computer programs are available in some cases for interpreting test responses. The revision of the Minnesota Multiphasic Personality Inventory (MMPI; Hathaway and McKinley 1951)—the MMPI-2 (Butcher et al. 1989)—is available with computer scoring and, if purchased separately, interpretation (Butcher 1989). Computerized interpretations of the MMPI-2 and other tests presumably provide the most common interpretations of test patterns but are not applicable to every case, especially for individuals with brain damage. Therefore, they should be used only as a source of hypotheses about individuals to be confirmed or negated by data from other sources.

Although many adults with brain injury can tolerate responding to the computer format, and some may even enjoy it, these methods lose important information about the way the individual approaches cognitive tasks or why errors are made unless the examiner monitors the process (Lezak, in press). Some patients with brain damage are impulsive, and others overly cautious; either factor could greatly alter a test score without providing information about the particular function that is the object of investigation.

❑ THE NATURE OF NEUROPSYCHOLOGICAL TESTS

An important component of neuropsychological evaluations is psychological testing in which an individual's cognitive, and often emotional, status and executive functioning are assessed. Neuropsychological assessment differs from psychological assessment in its basic assumptions. The latter compares the individual's responses with normative data from a sample of people from the population at large taking the same test (Anastasi 1988). The neuropsychological assessment of adults relies on comparisons between the patient's present level of functioning and the known or estimated level of premorbid functioning (Lezak 1986).

Two types of standardized neuropsychological tests are available. Some tests are constructed of cognitive or sensorimotor tasks that can be accomplished by all intact adults within the culture. They are designed so that all individuals are expected to be able to perform the task, and thus failure to do so may be interpreted as impairment. Examples of this approach include many aphasia tests of basic language skills. Anyone from English-speaking, Western cultural backgrounds would be expected to name, describe, and demonstrate the use of common objects as tested by the Porch Index of Communicative Ability (PICA; Porch 1983). The Dementia Rating Scale (DRS; Mattis 1988) is based on the assumption that adults will be able to perform most of the cognitive tasks used in this test. The manual specifies the small number of errors considered "normal."

Many tests are constructed without the expectation that neuropsychologically intact persons will obtain a near perfect score. In fact, most tests of abilities are designed with the expectation that only very few persons will obtain a perfect score and that most scores will cluster in a middle range. For these tests, scores are reported as a continuous variable. The scores of many persons taking the test can be plotted as a distribution curve. Most scores on tests of complex learned behaviors fall into a characteristic bell-shaped curve called a *normal distribution curve* (Figure 5–1). The statistical descriptors of the curve are the "mean" or average of all scores, the degree of spread of scores about the mean expressed as the "standard deviation," and the "range" or highest to lowest scores obtained.

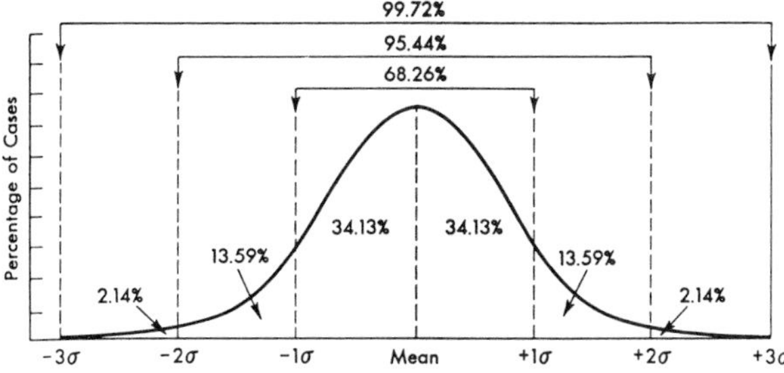

Figure 5–1. A normal distribution curve showing the percentage of cases between −1 standard deviation (−σ) and +1 standard deviation (+σ). The average range is defined as −0.6 to +0.6 standard deviations or 25th to 75th percentile. (Reprinted from Anastasi A: Psychological Testing, 6th Edition. New York, Macmillan, 1988, p 77. Copyright 1988 Macmillan Publishing Co. Used with permission.)

Most cognitive functions, as well as other behaviors, vary from individual to individual and also within the same individual at different times. This variability also has the characteristics of a normal curve, as in Figure 5–1. Because of the normal variability of a score, any single score can be considered only as representative of a range and must not be taken as a precise value. For example, a score at the 75th percentile (the equivalent of a scaled score of 12 on a Wechsler Intelligence Scale [WIS; Wechsler 1944, 1955, 1981] subtest) must be understood as likely representing a range of scores from the 50th to the 90th percentile. For this reason many neuropsychologists are reluctant to report scores, but rather describe their findings in terms of ability levels.

An individual's score is compared with the normative data, often by calculating a standard or *z* score, which describes the individual's performance in terms of standard deviations from the mean. Using this calculation, scores within ±0.6 standard deviations are considered average because 50% of the normative sample scored within this range. Moreover, *z* scores are used to describe the probability that a deviant response occurs by chance or because of an impairment. A performance in the below-average direction that is greater than 2 standard deviations from the mean usually is described as "impaired" because 97.8% of the normative sample taking the test achieved better scores.

Some test makers recommend "cutoff" scores to evaluate certain test performances. The cutoff scores represent those exceeded by most neuropsychologically intact persons; scores below the cutoff point are typically achieved by persons suffering impairment in the relevant abilities. Cutoff scores usually are derived on the basis of the distribution of scores of a healthy control sample. The threshold for "normal" is typically set at 1.5 standard deviations below the mean to include the top 95% of the control sample. One difficulty with many fixed cutoff scores is that they are not based on normative samples that are fully appropriate for the individual being studied. For example, calculation of the cutoff score may not have taken into account the individual's level of intelligence. A score that is satisfactory for a person of average ability may be unsatisfactory for a person of superior ability. Or the cutoff score may derive from a biased sample, such as unselected psychiatric patients, in which brain impairment occurs more frequently than in a "normal" control group. Cutoff scores work best on tests of abilities normally expected in all adults, such as basic language or motor skills.

Psychological tests should be constructed to have both reliability and validity (Anastasi 1988). The reliability of a test refers to the consistency of test results when given to the same individual at different times or with different sets of equivalent items. As perfect reliability cannot be achieved for any test, each individual score represents a range of variability, which narrows to the degree that the test's reliability approaches the ideal (Anastasi 1988). Tests have validity when they measure what they purport to measure. If a test is designed to measure attention disorders, then patient groups known to have attention deficits should perform more poorly on the test than persons from the population at large. Tests also should be constructed with large normative samples of individuals with similar demographic characteristics, particularly for age and education (Gade et al. 1985; Heaton et al. 1986; Prigatano and Parsons 1976). For example, the Wechsler Adult Intelligence Scale-Revised (WAIS-R; Wechsler 1981) has normative data of 1,880 individuals stratified for age, sex, race, geographic region, occupation, and education according to United States Census information. Most tests have much smaller normative samples in the range of 30 to 200 individuals.

Some psychological tests detect subtle deficits better than others. A simple signal detection test of attention, such as crossing out all of the letter *A*'s on a page, is a less sensitive test of attention than a divided attention task, such as crossing out all *A*'s and *C*'s. Tests of concentration and new learning are more sensitive than many other cognitive tests at reflecting brain damage because a wide variety of brain disorders can easily disrupt performance on them. However, other factors such as depression, anxiety, medicine side effects, and low energy level due to systemic illness may also disrupt cognition on these sensitive tests. Therefore, they are sensitive to cognitive disruption but not specific to one type of cognitive disturbance, such as brain damage. The specificity of a test in indicating a disorder depends on the overlap in distribution of scores between persons who are intact and those who have the disorder (Figure 5–2). The less overlap there is, the more diagnostic the test result will be. A test that is highly specific, such as the Token Test (Boller and Vignolo 1966; De Renzi and Vignolo 1962), which assesses language comprehension, produces few abnormal test results in nonaphasic persons or false-positive cases. Many neuropsychological tests offer a tradeoff between sensitivity and specificity.

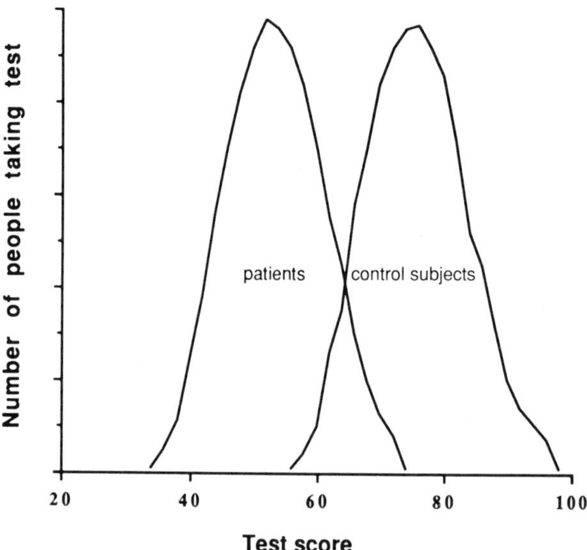

Figure 5–2. Distribution of hypothetical test scores by a control group and a patient group. In this case, scores between 56 and 74 occurred in both groups. The smaller the area of overlapping curves, the higher the test specificity.

Test selection involves a careful consideration of which tests are most likely to provide useful information. Results from any testing can yield false-positive or false-negative information. Interpretation of neuropsychological tests involves consideration by experienced clinicians of response patterns in the light of meaningful patterns and inconsistencies.

Indications of brain dysfunction come from qualitative features of the patient's performance as well as from test scores (Pankratz and Taplin 1982; Walsh 1985). There are many reasons for failing a test, and a poor score does not tell the means to the end (Walsh 1987). Occasionally a patient gives a "far-out" response to a question. The wise examiner who asks the patient to repeat the question often finds that the patient has misunderstood the question or instruction rather than lacked the ability to produce a correct response. Some features of behavioral disturbance show up best in the manner in which the patient approaches the testing situation or behaves with the examiner. Patients with brain injury are prone to problems with short attention span, distractibility, impulsiveness, poor self-monitoring, disorganization, irritability, perplexity, and suspiciousness. A sensitive and knowledgeable examiner can distinguish these factors from simple cognitive incompetence.

INTERPRETATION PRINCIPLES AND CAUTIONS

The interpretation of test data is based on performance expectations for each individual patient, which require that deviations from expectation be evaluated in terms of known deficit patterns (Lezak 1983, 1986). Most people perform within a statistically definable range on cognitive tests, and this range of performance levels is considered to be characteristic of them. Deviations below this expected range raise the question of an impairment. A person may have scores in the high-average range on many tests and low-average performance in one functional area. Figure 5–3 presents scores achieved by a 91-year-old former artist referred by her family for evaluation of whether her gradual functional decline was related to aging or to a progressive dementia. Her performance, expressed in *z* scores, was compared to neuropsychologically intact persons of her age and educational background. As can be seen, her performance was deficient on memory tests and confrontational naming. Deviations this large could not be assumed to be within expectation for her age group. The impaired performance and history were interpreted as supporting a diagnosis of mild dementia.

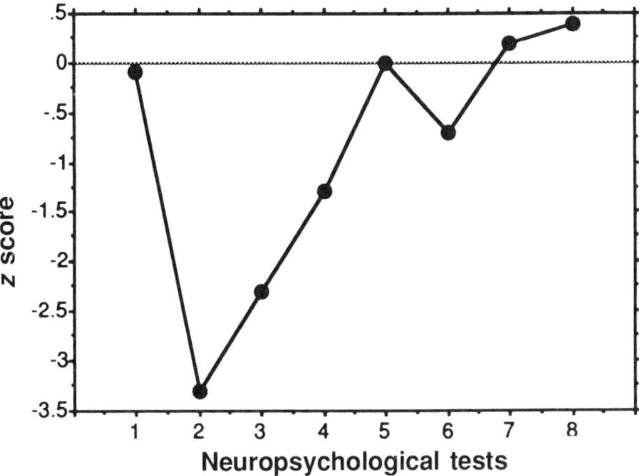

Figure 5–3. Performance (expressed as *z* scores) by a 91-year-old woman with mild dementia of the Alzheimer type on eight neuropsychological tests. 1 = information; 2 = verbal memory; 3 = visuospatial memory; 4 = naming; 5 = comprehension; 6 = verbal reasoning; 7 = visual reasoning; 8 = constructional praxis.

The assumptions of deficit measurement are valid in most cases, although outliers do exist who show an unusual variability on cognitive tasks (Matarazzo and Prifitera 1989). Multiple measures on similar tasks increase the reliability of findings. If someone has a deviant score on a task, performance on other tasks requiring the same skills will show whether the deviant finding persists across tasks. If so, the finding is considered reliable. If the deviant performance is not found using similar tasks, either the finding was spurious or the additional tasks varied in important features that avoided the patient's problem area. These possibilities can be examined further. The need for multiple measures of many cognitive functions explains why neuropsychological examinations are often lengthy.

Interpretation of test performances also must take into account demographic variables. When estimating the premorbid ability levels necessary for making intraindividual comparisons, the examiner must consider the patients' educational and occupational background, sex, and race along with their level of test performance. The more severely impaired patients are, the more unlikely it is that their performance will reach premorbid levels on any of the tests, thus increasing the examiner's reliance on demographic and historical data to estimate premorbid functioning (Crawford et al. 1989; Karzmark et al. 1985). Some tests, such as recognition vocabulary and fund of information, are fairly resistant to disruption by brain damage and may offer the best estimates of premorbid ability (Baddeley et al. 1988; Crawford et al. 1988).

For meaningful interpretations of neuropsychological test performance, examiners must rely on many tests and search for a response pattern that makes neuropsychological sense. Because there are few pathognomonic findings in neuropsychology, or most other branches of medical sciences for that matter (Sox et al. 1988), response patterns can often suggest several diagnoses. For example, a performance pattern including slowed thinking and mild impairment of concentration and memory is a nonspecific finding associated with several conditions:

very mild dementia, a mild post concussion syndrome, mild toxic encephalopathy, multiple sclerosis, depression, or fatigue, to name a few. Other patterns may be highly specific for certain conditions. The findings of left-sided neglect and visuospatial impairment are highly suggestive of brain dysfunction and specifically occur with right-hemisphere damage. For many neuropsychological conditions, typical patterns of deficits are known, and the examiner evaluates the patient's performances in light of these known patterns for a possible match.

The quality of a neuropsychological evaluation depends on many factors. In general, consumers of neuropsychological services must beware of conclusions from evaluations in which test scores alone (i.e., without information from history, interview, and observations of examination behavior) are used to make diagnostic decisions and in which dogmatic statements are made without strongly supportive evidence. It also is important to remember that neuropsychological tests do not measure brain damage. Rather, the finding of impaired mental functioning *implies* an underlying brain disorder; that is, poor performance on neuropsychological tests does not necessarily mean that the patient has brain damage; other possible interpretations may exist.

❑ THE MAJOR TEST CATEGORIES

In this section we present a brief review of tests used for assessment of major areas of cognition and personality. Many useful neuropsychological tests are not described in this summary. (For a relatively complete review, see Lezak, in press.)

Intellectual Ability

The most commonly used sets of tests of general intellectual function of adults are contained in one or another version of the WIS. These batteries of brief tests, often referred to as *subtests*, provide scores on various cognitive tasks covering a range of skills. Each version was originally developed as an "intelligence" test to predict academic and vocational performance of neurologically intact adults by giving an "IQ" score: an intelligence quotient score based on the mean performance on the tests in this battery. Table 5–2 lists the traditional interpretations of IQ scores. The entire battery of 11 tests is frequently among those tests included in a neuropsychological examination. The tests were designed to assess relatively distinct areas of cognition, such as arithmetic, abstract thinking, and visuospatial organization, and thus are differentially sensitive to dysfunction of various areas of the brain. Therefore, the WIS is often used to screen for specific areas of cognitive deficits. When given to neuropsychologically impaired persons, the summary IQ scores can be very misleading because they will be affected by specific cognitive deficits yet in themselves provide no clue to the nature of contributing brain disorder(s) (Lezak 1988a).

TABLE 5–2. INTELLIGENCE CLASSIFICATIONS

IQ	*Classification*
130 and above	Very superior
120–129	Superior
110–119	High average
90–109	Average
80–89	Low average
70–79	Borderline
69 and below	Mentally retarded

For example, a patient with a visuoperceptual deficit consisting of an inability to recognize familiar objects would have difficulty performing the Picture Completion subtest, which requires the identification of missing features in line drawings of familiar objects. It is possible that such a patient would perform well on other tests in the Wechsler battery, but a summation of all the scores would both hide the important data and be lower than the other test scores in the battery would warrant. Therefore, neuropsychologists attend to the pattern of the WIS scores rather than a score representing the summed or average performance on all the tests in the battery.

In some cases neuropsychologists have used discrepancies between summed scores on what is called the Verbal Scale of the WIS (i.e., Verbal IQ) and summed scores on the so-called Performance Scale (i.e., Performance IQ) to indicate a specific area of cognitive deficit. The procedure has developed because there is a tendency for left-hemisphere lesions to produce a relatively depressed Verbal IQ score, whereas both right-hemisphere lesions and diffuse damage (as in dementing conditions) produce a depressed Performance IQ score. Even this amount of summation can mask important data (Bornstein 1983; Grossman 1983; Larrabee 1986). In the example above, impaired performance on one test would not be likely to produce sufficient relative lowering of the Performance IQ to reveal the cognitive deficit. Moreover, the Arithmetic and Digit Span tests of the Verbal Scale do not measure only verbal functions, and only three of the Performance Scale measures involve motor response: one (Picture Completion) calls for a purely verbal response. Therefore, it is important to use and interpret these tests discretely. Each test raw score is converted into a "scaled score," a form of standard score based on the distribution of scores of the normative sample. The Wechsler manuals provide tables for converting test raw scores into scaled scores based on individual age groups ranging from 16–17 years to 70–74 years. The age-graded scaled scores represent the degree of variation of the individual's score from the mean of the normative sample in that age group and as such are the most relevant for neuropsychological purposes. Differences among age-graded scaled scores for the individual tests are examined for meaningful discrepancies.

The equivalent tests for assessing children are the Wechsler Intelligence Scale for Children-Revised (WISC-R; Wechsler 1974) and the newly revised Wechsler Intelligence Scale for Children–Third Edition (WISC-III; Wechsler 1991). They contain subtests similar to the WAIS-R, but appropriate for children 6–16 years old.

Language

Lesions to the hemisphere dominant for speech and language, which is the left hemisphere in 95%–97% of right-handers and 60%–70% of left-handers (Corballis 1983; Strauss and Goldsmith 1987), can produce any of a variety of disorders of symbol formulation and use (i.e., the aphasias). Although many aphasiologists argue against attempting to classify all patients into one of the standard aphasia syndromes because of individual differences, aphasic patients tend to be grouped according to whether the main disorder is in language comprehension (receptive aphasia), expression (expressive aphasia), repetition (conduction aphasia), or naming (anomic aphasia). Many comprehensive language assessment tests are available. Comprehensive aphasia test batteries are best administered by speech pathologists or other clinicians with special training in this field. These batteries usually include measures of spontaneous speech, speech comprehension, repetition, naming, reading, and writing.

Test selection may be based on whether the information is to be used for diagnostic, prognostic, or rehabilitation purposes. For example, the Boston Diagnostic Aphasia Examination (BDAE; Goodglass and Kaplan 1983) might be selected as an aid for treatment planning because of its wide scope and sensitivity to different aphasic characteristics. The PICA best measures treatment progress because of its sensitivity to small changes in performance. A useful brief examination is the Aphasia Language Performance Scales (ALPS; Keenan and Brassell 1975), an approximately 30-minute examination that provides measures of listening, talking, reading, and writing.

Attention and Mental Tracking

A frequent consequence of brain injury is slowed thinking and impaired ability for focused behavior (Gronwall and Sampson 1974). In addition, damage to the brain stem or diffuse damage involving the cerebral hemispheres can produce various attentional deficits. Many neuropsychological assessments will include measures of these abilities. The Wechsler scales contain several. The Digit Span subtest measures attention span or short-term memory for numbers by assessing forward digit repetition. The task also measures backward digit repetition, which is a more demanding task requiring concentration and mental tracking. It is not uncommon for patients with brain damage, even those who are severly impaired, to perform poorly only on the backward repetition portion of this test. Because Digits Forward and Digits Backward measure different functions, assessment data for each should be given separately. The Digit Symbol subtest also requires concentration and both motor and mental speed for successful performance: the patient must code numbers into symbols accurately and rapidly. Persons with attentional disorders may also perform poorly on the Arithmetic test despite good mathematical skills. Because the problems are presented orally, good attention and concentration are required for retaining lengthy statements while performing the mental calculations.

Another commonly used measure of concentration and mental tracking is the Trail Making Test (Armitage 1946). In part A of this test, the patient is asked to draw rapidly and accurately a line connecting in sequence a random display of numbered circles on a page. The level of difficulty is increased in part B by having the patient again sequence a random display of circles, this time containing both numbers and letters, requiring the patient to go from *1* to *A* to *2* to *B* to *3*, and so forth (Figure 5–4). It examines concentration, visual scanning, and flexibility in shifting cognitive sets. This test is among those that are most sensitive to the presence of brain injury (Crockett et al. 1988; Spreen and Benton 1965; van Zomeren and Brouwer 1990). However, it shares with other highly sensitive tests vulnerability to many other kinds of deficits, among which are diminished visual acuity and motor slowing, which could be due to peripheral factors such as nerve damage or joint disease. It is also sensitive to educational deprivation and cannot be used with persons not accustomed to the alphabet as Western countries know it.

In cases of subtle brain injury, assessment sensitivity can be increased by selecting a more difficult measure of concentration and mental tracking, such as the Paced Auditory Serial Addition Test (PASAT; Gronwall 1977; Gronwall and Sampson 1974). The patient is required to add consecutive pairs of numbers rapidly under an interference condition. As numbers are presented at a fixed rate, the patient must always add the last two numbers presented and ignore the number that represents the last summation. For example, if the numbers "*3-5-2-7*" are presented, the patient must respond "*8*" after the number *5*, and then "*7*" after the number *2*, and then "*9*." It is a difficult task because of the strong tendency to add the last number presented to the last summation. The level of difficulty can be heightened by speeding up the rate of presentation of numbers.

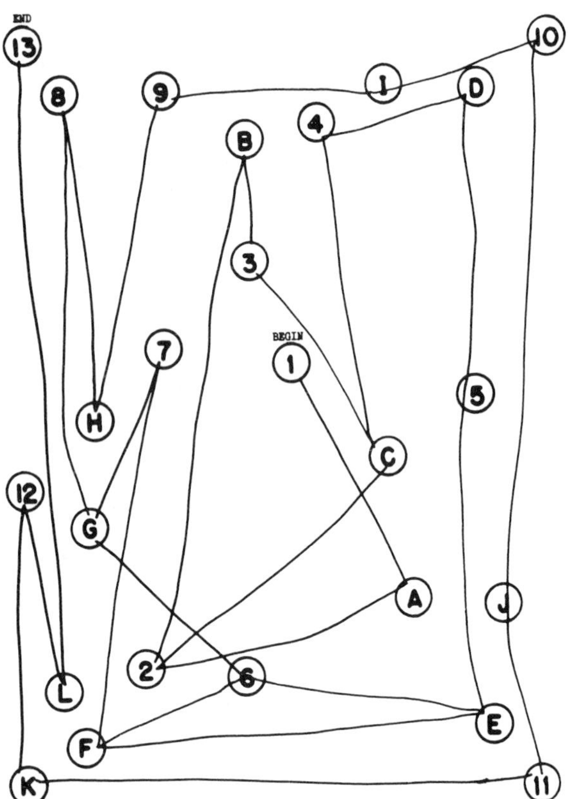

Figure 5–4. Trail Making Test (Armitage 1946) part B performance by a 61-year-old man with normal-pressure hydrocephalus. Two type of errors are demonstrated: erroneous sequencing (*1→A→2→C*) and failure to alternate between numbers and letters (*D→5→E→F*).

Memory

Memory is another cognitive function that is often impaired by brain injury. Many diffuse brain injuries produce general impairments in abilities for new learning and retention. Many focal brain injuries also produce memory impairments, with left-hemisphere lesions most likely to produce primarily verbal memory deficits, whereas visuospatial memory impairments tend to be associated with right-hemisphere lesions (Milner 1978; Ojemann and Dodrill 1985). Memory impairment often is a prominent feature of herpes encephalitis, hypoxia, closed head injury, and neurological degenerative diseases such as multiple sclerosis and early stages of Alzheimer's disease (Kapur 1988; Mayes 1988). Several conditions produce amnesic syndromes in which memory impairment is paramount. These conditions include Huntington's chorea, Korsakoff's syndrome, and some anoxic conditions (Butters et al. 1976; Parkin et al. 1987).

In most cases of brain injury, memory for information learned before the injury is relatively preserved compared with new learning. For this reason many patients with memory impairment will perform relatively well on tests of fund of information or recall of remote events. However, amnesic disorders can produce a retrograde amnesia extending back weeks, months, or years before the onset of the injury. The retrograde amnesia of Huntington's chorea or Korsakoff's syndrome can extend to decades (Butters and Miliotis 1985; Cermak 1982). However, in extremely rare cases a patient will have a retrograde amnesia without significant anterograde amnesia, that is, when new learning ability remains intact (Goldberg 1981; Kapur et al. 1986; Roman-Campos et al. 1980). Most cases of isolated retrograde amnesia or amnesia for personal identity are of a psychogenic etiology.

The Wechsler Memory Scale-Revised (WMS-R; Wechsler 1987) is the most commonly used set of tests of new learning and retention in the United States. This battery is composed of various subtests measuring free recall or recognition of both verbal and visuospatial material. In addition, the WMS-R includes measures of recall of personal information and attention, concentration, and mental tracking. The original version of the test (Wechsler 1945) lacked the sensitivity of the recently revised version because it failed to include the most difficult memory condition, delayed recall of newly learned information (Prigatano 1978). Several of the subtests of the revised version provide measures of both immediate and delayed (approximately 30-minute) recall.

Other memory tests frequently used include word-list learning tasks, such as the Rey Auditory Verbal Learning Test (Lezak 1983; Rey 1964) or the California Verbal Learning Test (Delis et al. 1986, 1987) and visuospatial tasks, such as the Rey Complex Figure Test (Baser and Ruff 1987; Delbecq-Derouesne and Beauvois 1989; Osterrieth 1944; Rey 1941). When patients are unable to produce verbal responses or use their preferred hand for producing drawings, recognition memory tests requiring a simple "yes" or "no" response are useful. These recognition tests include the Continuous Recognition Memory Test (Hannay and Levin 1989; Trahan et al. 1986), the Continuous Visual Memory Test (Trahan and Larrabee 1988), and the Recognition Memory Test (Warrington 1984).

Perception

Perception arising from any of the sensory modalities can be affected by brain disease. Perceptional inattention (sometimes called *neglect*) is one of the major perceptual syndromes because of its frequency in association with focal brain damage (Bisiach and Vallar 1988; Heilman et al. 1987; Posner 1988). This phenomenon involves diminished or absent awareness of stimuli in one side of personal space by a patient with an intact sensory system. Unilateral inattention is often most prominent after acute-onset brain injury such as stroke. Most commonly seen is left-sided inattention associated with right-hemisphere stroke.

Several techniques can be used to elicit unilateral inattention. Visual inattention can be assessed using a Line Bisection Test (Schenkenberg et al. 1980), in which the patient is asked to bisect a series of lines on a page, or a cancellation task requiring the patient to cross out a designated symbol distributed among other similar symbols on a page (Bisiach and Vallar 1988; Gauthier et al. 1985; Mesulam 1985). A popular tactile inattention test is the Face-Hand Test (Berg et al. 1987; Smith 1983). The patient is instructed to indicate with the eyes closed whether points on the face (cheeks) or hands are touched by the examiner. Each side is touched singly and then in combination with the other side, such as left cheek and right hand. The patient should have no difficulty reporting a single point of stimulation. Failure to report stimulation to one side when both sides are stimulated is referred to as tactile inattention or double simultaneous extinction.

The most commonly used forms of perceptual tests assess perceptual discrimination among similar stimuli. These visual tests may include discrimination of geometric forms, angulation, color, faces, or familiar objects (Lezak 1983; McCarthy and Warrington 1990; Newcombe and Ratcliff 1989; Tranel et al. 1987). Some perceptual tasks examine the patient's ability for perceptual synthesis. The Hooper Visual Organization Test (Hooper 1958) presents line drawings of familiar objects in fragmented, disarranged pieces and ask for the name of each object. Many of these tests also can be administered in tactile version (Craig 1985; Van Lancker et al. 1989; Varney 1986). Frequently used tactile tests include form recognition and letter or number recognition (Reitan and Wolfson 1985).

Another important area of perceptual assessment is recognition of familiar visual stimuli. Although the syndromes are rare and often occur independently of one another, a brain injury can produce an inability to recognize visually familiar objects (visual object agnosia) or faces (prosopagnosia) (Benson 1989; Damasio et al. 1989). Recognition assessment typically involves asking the patient to give the name of real objects or of representations of objects, sometimes in a masked or distorted form. The WIS includes a perceptual task in which the patient is asked to identify missing features of line drawings of familiar objects.

Some patients with brain injury have difficulty discriminating sounds even when there are no primary auditory deficits and no aphasia. Therefore tests have been devised to measure the ability to discriminate speech sounds (Benton et al. 1983; Halstead 1947) and nonsymbolic sound patterns (Seashore et al. 1960). Impaired discrimination of speech tends to be associated with left temporal lobe lesions, whereas poor comprehension of nonsymbolic sounds such as sirens, bells, and doors closing seems to be associated with right temporal lobe lesions (Gordon 1974; Milner 1971). In interpreting patients' performances on certain tests involving auditory discrimination, the examiner must be sensitive to the possible effects of attentional deficits because low scores on these tests can result from a constricted auditory span or compromised ability to concentrate. The potential for misinterpretation of examination findings is always present and one of the reasons that valid neuropsychological assessment requires knowledgeable and experienced examiners.

Praxis

Many aphasic patients have at least one form of apraxia. Their inability to perform the required sequence of motor activities is not based on motor weakness. Rather, the deficit is in planning and carrying out the required activities (De Renzi et al. 1983; Haaland and Flaherty 1984; Jason 1990). Tests of praxis measure the patient's ability to reproduce learned movements of the face or limbs. These learned movements can include the use of objects (usually pantomime use of objects), gestures, or sequences of movements demonstrated by the examiner (Christensen 1979).

Constructional Ability

Although constructional problems were once considered a form of apraxia, analysis has shown that the underlying deficits involve impaired appreciation of one or more aspects of spatial relationships, including distortions in perspective, angulation, size, and distance judgment or difficulty appreciating or integrating details. Therefore, unlike apraxias, the problem is not an inability to draw lines or assemble constructions, but rather misperceptions and misjudgments involving spatial relationship or the fine-grained characteristics of a percept. Neuropsychological assessments may include any of a number of measures of visuospatial processing. Patients may be asked to copy geometric designs, such as the Rey Complex Figure (Rey 1964) presented in Figure 5–5 or one of the alternate forms (Loring et al. 1988; K. J. Meador, H. S. Taylor, D.W., unpublished observations, January 1990; Taylor 1979). The WIS battery includes constructional tasks involving

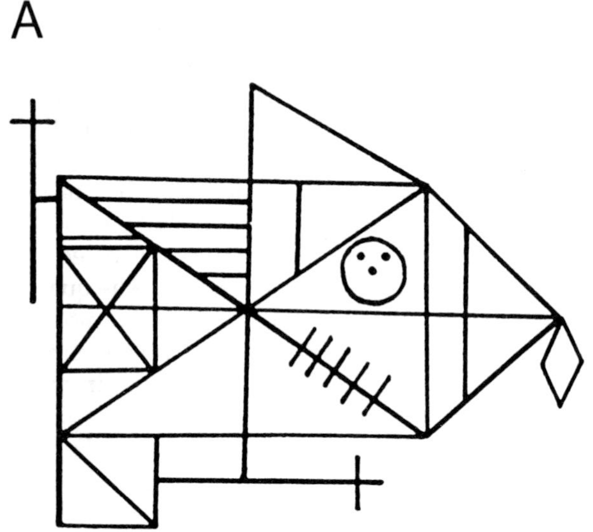

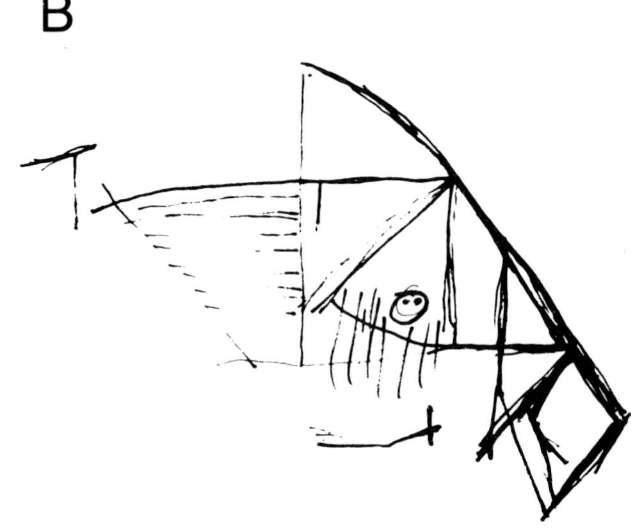

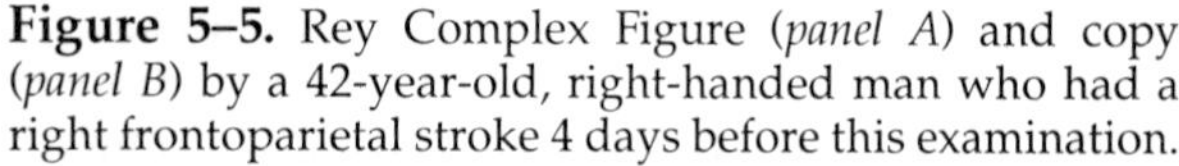
Figure 5–5. Rey Complex Figure (*panel A*) and copy (*panel B*) by a 42-year-old, right-handed man who had a right frontoparietal stroke 4 days before this examination. The copy shows the patient's neglect of the left and lower portions of the figure, a strong perseverative tendency, as well as visuospatial fragmentation.

reconstructing designs with blocks and assembling puzzle pieces (Wechsler 1944, 1955, 1981). Lesions of the posterior cerebral cortex cause the greatest difficulty with constructions, with right-hemisphere lesions producing greater deficits than left-hemisphere lesions.

Conceptual Functions

Tests of concept formation measure aspects of thinking including reasoning, abstraction, and problem solving. Conceptual dysfunction tends to occur with serious brain injury regardless of site. Most neuropsychological tests require intactness of simple conceptual functioning. For example, reasoning skills are required for the successful performance of most WIS tests: Comprehension assesses commonsense verbal reasoning and interpretation of proverbs, Picture Completion requires perceptual reasoning, Similarities measures ability to make verbal abstractions by asking for similarities between objects or concepts, Arithmetic involves arithmetic problem solving, Picture Arrangement examines sequential reasoning for thematic pictures, and Block Design and Object Assembly test visuospatial analysis and problem solving of block designs and puzzles.

Other commonly used tests of concept formation include the Category Test (Halstead 1947) and the Wisconsin Card Sorting (WCS) Test (Berg 1948; Grant and Berg 1948). These tests measure concept formation, hypothesis testing, problem solving, and flexibility of thinking. The Category Test presents patterns of stimuli and requires the patient to figure out a principle or concept that is true for each item within a set based on feedback about the correctness of each response. The patient is told that the correct principle may be the same or different among the six different sets. For example, the correct principle in one set is position (first, second, and so on) of the stimulus on the page, whereas for another it is the number of items on the page.

The WCS is similar to the Category Test in requiring the patient to figure out a principle that is true for items within a set. The examiner changes the correct principle as the test proceeds without warning the patient. Therefore, the patient must realize that a shift in principles has occurred and act accordingly.

Tests of conceptualization and reasoning illustrate some of the interpretation problems inherent in most neuropsychological tests because they require complex mental activity. Thus patients with recent memory disorders and those who are highly distractible may be able to solve the conceptual problems presented by these tests but fail because of inability to keep the correct solution in mind. Here again, it is important that the examiner go beyond the score alone to evaluate the patient's overall performance.

Executive Functions

Executive functions include abilities to formulate a goal, make plans, and effectively carry out goal-directed plans and to monitor and self-correct spontaneously and reliably (Lezak 1982). These are difficult tasks for many patients with frontal lobe or diffuse brain injuries (Luria 1980). Yet they are essential for most adult responsible and socially appropriate conduct. Tasks that best assess executive functions are tests of planning and/or open-ended tests that permit the patient to decide when the task is complete. One type of test that requires planning is a maze. The patient must plan an exit to the maze, which involves foresight to minimize trial-and-error behavior. The Bender-Gestalt (Bender 1938), an old favorite neuropsychological test, requires foresight to arrange nine drawings on a single page so that space is well used. Other tasks that rely heavily on planning for successful completion are multistep tasks requiring decision making or priority setting. Few neuropsychological tests are designed specifically to assess this aspect of behavior, yet many complex tasks depend on this analysis.

One example of a priority-setting task is the Twenty Questions Test, which is known as a popular game. In the test version (Laine and Butters 1982), the patient is shown an array of 42 drawings of familiar objects and told to identify the one the examiner is thinking of by asking only "yes-or-no" questions. The goal is to identify the specified objects with as few questions as possible. The quality of the questions varies according to the number of objects it includes or excludes as a possible target. Many patients with frontal lobe injury begin questioning with low-priority questions or even by asking whether the target is a specific object. Frontal lobe patients also can have difficulty with the conceptual requirement of the test because high-priority questions are more abstract.

Inertia presents one of the most difficult assessment problems for neuropsychologists because there are few open-ended tests that measure initiation or ability to carry out purposeful behavior. By their very nature, most tests are structured and require little initiation by the patient (Lezak 1982). Examples of less structured tests include the Tinkertoy Test, in which patients decide what to build and how to design it (Bayless et al. 1989; Lezak 1982), and free drawing tests, in which patients are requested to draw a bicycle or house. Because there are few rules, patients must choose their level of productivity.

Motor Functions

Neuropsychological tests can supplement the neurological examination of motor functions by providing standardized measures of motor activities. Normative data have been acquired for commonly measured functions such as grip strength and finger tapping (Bornstein 1985). More complex tests of fine motor coordination include tests that require patients to rapidly place pegs in holes, such as the Grooved Pegboard Test (Baser and Ruff 1987; Bornstein 1985; Matthews and Haaland 1979) and the Purdue Pegboard Test (Purdue Research Foundation 1948; see also, Agnew et al. 1988). These tests examine absolute performance as well as comparing the preferred hand against the nonpreferred hand to measure the possibility of lateralized motor deficit and comparing the performance of one hand to that of two as a measure of bilateral integration.

Personality and Emotional Status

Numerous questionnaires have been developed to measure symptoms of physical and emotional distress of patient's with neurological or medical problems (Lezak 1989). As an example, the Neurobehavioral Rating Scale (Levin et al. 1987) is an examiner-rated measure of problems commonly associated with head trauma.

Many tests originally devised as measures of psychological distress or psychiatric illness have been used with brain-injured persons. The revised version of the Symptom Check List-90 (SCL-90-R; Derogatis 1983) is a self-report of symptoms associated with psychiatric disorders when they occur at high-frequency levels. MMPI (Hathaway and McKinley 1951; Welsh and Dahlstrom 1956) has been used extensively with brain-injured patients (Chelune et al. 1986; Dahlstrom et al. 1975; Mueller and Girace 1988). The recently revised version—MMPI-2—(Butcher and Pope 1990; Butcher et al. 1989), contains the same basic clinical scales with deletions of a small percentage of the items and new normative data. The small changes in test items would not be expected to produce substantial changes in clinical profiles, but information about the effects of the new normative data is lacking because of the recency of the revision.

In general, persons with brain damage tend to have elevated MMPI profiles, which may reflect the relatively frequent incidence of emotional disturbance in these patients (Filskov and Leli 1981), their accurate reporting of symptoms and deficits (Lezak 1983), or their compromised ability to read or understand the test questions. Elevations in the Hypochondriasis (Hs), Hysteria (Hy), and Schizophrenia (Sc) scales are common because many "neurological" symptoms appear on these scales (Alfano et al. 1990). The interpretation of MMPI data for persons with brain damage must take into account the contributions of neurological symptoms, emotional reactions to brain injury, and premorbid personality.

Many attempts have been made to use the MMPI to differentiate diagnoses of psychiatric and neurological illness. Results generally have been unsatisfactory, probably because of the extreme variety of brain injury and their associated problems (Alfano et al. 1990; Gass et al., in press; Lezak 1983; Mueller and Girace 1988). The MMPI also has been an inefficient instrument for localizing cerebral lesions (Lezak 1983).

Neuropsychologists are asked frequently to evaluate "psychological overlay" or functional complaints. This diagnostic problem occurs because some individuals may be financially motivated to establish injuries related to work or accidents for which financial compensation may be sought. In addition, some individuals receive emotional or social rewards for invalidism, leading to malingering and functional disabilities. It is difficult to establish with complete certainty that a person's complaints are functional. To add to the complexity of the diagnosis, patients with established brain injury sometimes embellish their symptoms, wittingly or unwittingly, so that the range of problems represents a combination of true deficits and exaggeration. The clinician usually must search for a combination of factors that would support or discredit a functional diagnosis. General factors include evidence of inconsistency in history, report of symptoms, or test performance; the individual's emotional predisposition; the probability of secondary gain; and the patient's emotional reactions to their complaints, such as the classic *la belle indifference.*

Psychological tests may be helpful in establishing evidence of exaggeration of symptoms. The MMPI validity scales (L, F, and K) provide information about the patient's cooperativeness while taking this test and the likelihood that symptoms are exaggerated. In cognitively intact persons, the strongest sign of exaggerated symptoms would be an elevated F scale, which contains items that fewer than 10% of the normative population endorsed. Typically, when persons desire to appear worse off than they truly are ("fake bad"), the F scale is highly elevated, and the L and K scales are at or slightly below the mean (Graham 1987). However, a high F scale also occurs when patients have difficulty comprehending items or appreciating the validity of their responses because of brain damage.

Because people faking brain damage tend to exaggerate poor performance on testing, another useful diagnostic approach has been the Symptom Validity Test (Pankratz 1979). The fundamental procedure is that patient's complaints are examined by forcing a response to a simple, two-alternative problem. Using many trials, the examiner can calculate the likelihood that the performance deviates from chance. Because extreme exaggeration of complaints is common for malingerers, results sometimes indicate that patients are performing statistically below chance on the task, thereby suggesting that they are deliberately giving erroneous responses. Patients may perform at chance levels for many reasons other than deliberate falsification, which, by contrast, does not lead to straightforward interpretation. The Portland Digit Recognition Test (Binder and Willis 1990) is offered as a validity test for examining memory complaints in which the patient indicates recall of a short series of numbers using a forced-choice, two-item recognition task.

❑ SPECIAL ASSESSMENT TOOLS

Batteries

Many examiners use a preferred battery of tests in evaluating patients. In these cases the neuropsychologist develops considerable skill and familiarity in the use of a preselected set of tests. The WIS battery of tests, described earlier, is commonly used for this purpose.

Of the commercial batteries designed for neuropsychological evaluations, by far the most popular in the United States is the Halstead-Reitan Battery. This battery was designed to assess frontal lobe disorders by W. C. Halstead (1947) and subsequently used by R. Reitan (1969), who added some tests and recommended this battery as a diagnostic test for all kinds of brain damage. The tests include the Category Test, described above; the Tactual Performance Test, a tactile visuospatial performance and memory test; the Rhythm Test, a nonverbal auditory perception test; Speech Sounds Perception Test, a phoneme discrimination test; the Finger Tapping Test, a motor speed test; the Trail Making Test, described above; a shortened version of Wepman's Aphasia Screening Test, which Wepman later rejected as inadequate (see Snow 1987); a sensory examination; and a measure of grip strength. Most examiners administer this battery with one of the forms of the WIS, WMS, and MMPI.

One of the newest batteries offered as an all-purpose set of examination techniques is the Luria-Nebraska Neuropsychological Battery (Golden et al. 1978, 1980). It has generated great controversy because of its many psychometric flaws (Adams 1984; Lezak 1988b; Stambrook 1983). It derives its name from the takeover of test items used by the late Russian neurologist and neuropsychologist A. R. Luria (1980) and described by A-L. Christensen (1979). However, neither Luria nor Christensen advocated the use of a fixed battery. The examiner must be extremely cautious about drawing conclusions based on the scores and indices of this battery (Lezak 1983).

Examinations designed to address specific diagnostic questions are available. Several dementia examinations have been devised. The Mattis Dementia Rating Scale (Mattis 1976, 1988) contains items assessing attention, initiation and/or perseveration, construction, conceptualization, and memory and is useful in distinguishing dementia from cognitive decline associated with aging.

Screening Tests

Many clinicians would like to have a brief, reliable screening examination with good sensitivity for brain damage of unknown etiology or where it is only suspected. However, there is a tradeoff between the amount of information obtained in an assessment and its actual usefulness in the detection of brain dysfunction. Brief examinations are often too restricted in range or too simple to be sensitive to subtle or circumscribed areas of dysfunction. The commonly used Mini-Mental State Exam (MMSE; Folstein et al. 1975) contains only 11 simple tasks. It is useful for examining patients with global confusion or poor memory. However, many patients with brain injury, such as those with stroke, mild to moderate head injury, and even early dementia, perform adequately on this examination. (Auerbach and Faibish 1989; Beatty and Goodkin 1990; Naugle and Kauczak 1989).

As screening examinations become lengthier and contain more difficult items their usefulness improves. An example of an expanded examination that has proven useful for screening is the Neurobehavioral Cognitive Status Examination (NCSE; Kiernan et al. 1987; Mysiw et al. 1989; Schwamm et al. 1987). This examination takes approximately 30 minutes and contains reasonably difficult items of attention; language comprehension, repetition, and naming; constructional ability; memory; calculations; reasoning; and judgment, which together make it fairly sensitive. The NCSE is a screening examination however and not a substitute for a thorough neuropsychological examination. It may be used to acquire information to decide whether further evaluation is warranted. As with any screening examination, intact performance does not exclude the possibility of brain dysfunction.

Figure 5–6 presents the NCSE profile of a 42-year-old alcoholic man with several past occasions of blows to the head causing brief loss of consciousness. The screening examination was used as part of his evaluation as an inpatient when he had been sober for 6 days. The test shows that he had difficulty with attention (repeating digits forward) and constructions (reconstructing designs with tiles) and that he performed other tasks within expectation. These findings are consistent with the known effects of alcoholism on cognition, and past blows to the head may not have contributed to his impairments. Cognitive impairment is reversible in some patients with alcoholism (Brandt et al. 1983; Jenkins and Parsons 1980), and a full neuropsychological evaluation was recommended if the patient remained sober for at least 3 months.

Competency

A cognitive competency determination usually is based on a specialized interview in which patients' ability to handle financial matters and/or make decisions regarding their well-being is assessed by asking questions about their personal situation. The patients' understanding of their personal needs is more relevant to a competency determination than a score on a formal test. Nevertheless, the Cognitive Competency Test (Wang et al. 1987) is a useful component of a competency examination of patients with brain injury because it evaluates cognitive skills that are required to maintain safe and independent living. The test samples a wide range of cognitive skills varying from overlearned, basic living skills (e.g., understanding change and counting change) to memory, abstract problem solving, and safety judgment. However, it omits areas that also need to be assessed such as awareness of personal needs and basic current events.

❑ TREATMENT AND PLANNING

Examination findings provide information about an individual's strengths and weaknesses necessary for formulating treatment interventions. Clinical interventions vary according to each individual's specific needs. Many patients with brain damage have primary or secondary emotional problems for which psychotherapy or counseling may seem advisable. However, patients with brain damage frequently have problems that compromise their capacity to use such treatment. Foremost among these problems are cognitive rigidity, which may limit the patient's adaptability, and defective learning, which may restrict his or her ability to acquire new attitudes, understanding, or interpersonal skills. Therefore, neuropsychological evaluations provide important information about treatment strategies. The evaluation is also frequently used for consideration of a person's ability for independence in society and for estimating educational or vocational potential.

❑ WHO IS QUALIFIED

The field of neuropsychology is enriched by the diversity of areas of expertise of those interested in the study of brain-behavior relationships. Professionals in this field come from backgrounds in psychology, psychiatry, neurology, neurosurgery, and language pathology to name only a few. In psychology alone professionals come from backgrounds in clinical, cognitive, developmental, and physiological psychology.

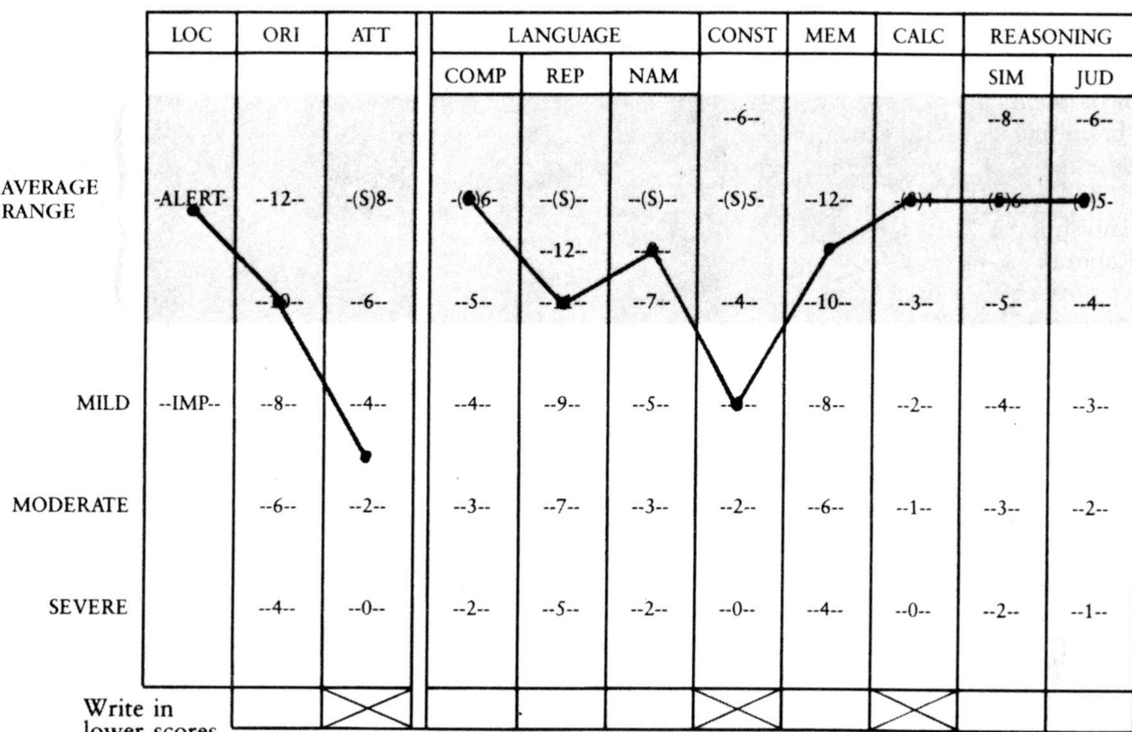

Figure 5–6. The Neurobehavioral Cognitive Status Examination (NCSE) performance profile of a 42-year-old alcoholic man, showing mild deficits on attention and constructional tasks. LOC = level of consciousness; ORI= orientation; ATT = attention; COMP = comprehension; REP = repetition; NAM = naming; CONST = construction; MEM = memory; CALC = calculations; SIM = similarities; JUD = judgment; (S) = screening item; IMP = impaired. (Reprinted from Northern California Neurobehavioral Group: Test Booklet for the Neurobehavioral Cognitive Status Examination. Fairfax, CA, 1988. Copyright 1988, The Northern California Neurobehavioral Group, Inc. Used with permission.)

Professionals qualified to provide clinical evaluations have both expertise in brain-behaviors relationships and skills in diagnostic assessment and counseling (Bornstein 1988a, 1988b). There are a growing number of qualified neuropsychologists and a recently established recognition of proficiency in this subspecialty area by the American Board of Professional Psychology's award of Diploma in Clinical Neuropsychology (Bieliauskas and Matthews 1987).

❑ REFERENCES

Acker MB: A review of the ecological validity of neuropsychological tests, in The Neuropsychology of Everyday Life: Assessment and Basic Competencies. Edited by Tupper DE, Cicerone KD. Boston, Kluver, 1989, pp 19–55

Adams KM: Luria left in the lurch: unfulfilled promises are not valid tests. Journal of Clinical Neuropsychology 6:455–465, 1984

Adams KM, Brown GG: The role of the computer in neuropsychological assessment, in Neuropsychological Assessment of Neuropsychiatric Disorders. Edited by Grant I, Adams KM. New York, Oxford University Press, 1986, pp 87–99

Agnew J, Bolla-Wilson K, Kawas CH, et al: Purdue Pegboard age and sex norms for people 40 years old and older. Developmental Neuropsychology 4:29–36, 1988

Alfano DP, Finlayson AJ, Stearns GM, et al: The MMPI and neurologic dysfunction: profile configuration and analysis. Clinical Neuropsychologist 4:69–79, 1990

Alves WM, Jane JA: Mild brain injury: damage and outcome, in Central Nervous System Trauma: Status Report—1985. Edited by Becker DP, Povlishock JT. Washington, DC, National Institutes of Health, 1985, pp 255–270

Anastasi A: Psychological Testing, 6th Edition. New York, Macmillan, 1988

Armitage SG: An analysis of certain psychological tests used for the evaluation of brain injury. Psychological Monographs (No 277) 60:1–48, 1946

Auerbach VS, Faibish GM: Mini-Mental State Examination: diagnostic limitations in a hospital setting (abstract). J Clin Exp Neuropsychol 11:75, 1989

Baddeley A, Emslie H, Nimmo-Smith I: Estimating premorbid intelligence (abstract). J Clin Exp Neuropsychol 10:326, 1988

Baser CA, Ruff RM: Construct validity of the San Diego Neuropsychological Test Battery. Archives of Clinical Neuropsychology 2:13–32, 1987

Bayless JD, Varney NR, Roberts RJ: Tinker Toy Test performance and vocational outcome in patients with closed head injuries. J Clin Exp Neuropsychol 11:913–917, 1989

Beatty WW, Goodkin DE: Screening for cognitive impairment in multiple sclerosis. Archives of Neurology 47: 297–301, 1990

Bender L: A visual motor gestalt test and its clinical use. American Orthopsychiatric Association Research Monographs (No 3):1–8, 1938

Benson DF: Disorders of visual gnosis, in Neuropsychology of Visual Perception. Edited by Brown JW. New York, IRBN, 1989, pp 59–76

Benton AL, Hamsher K deS, Varney NR, et al: Contributions to Neuropsychological Assessment. New York, Oxford University Press, 1983

Berg EA: A simple objective test for measuring flexibility in thinking. J Gen Psychol 39:15–22, 1948

Berg G, Edwards DR, Danzinger WL, et al: Longitudinal change in three brief assessments of SDAT. J Am Geriatr Soc 35:205–212, 1987

Berg RA: Cancer, in Medical Neuropsychology. Edited by Tarter RE, Van Thiel DH, Edwards KL. New York, Plenum, 1988, pp 265–290

Bieliauskas LA, Matthews CG: American Board of Clinical Neuropsychology: Policies and Procedures. The Clinical Neuropsychologist 1:21–28, 1987

Binder LM: Persisting symptoms after mild head injury: a review of postconcussive syndrome. J Clin Exp Neuropsychol 8:323–346, 1986

Binder LM, Willis SC: Assessment of motivation after compensable minor head trauma (abstract). J Clin Exp Neuropsychol 12:45, 1990

Bisiach E, Vallar G: Hemineglect in humans, in Handbook of Neuropsychology, Vol 1. Edited by Boller F, Grafman J, Rizzolatti G, et al. Amsterdam, Elsevier, 1988, pp 195–222

Boll TJ: The Halstead-Reitan Neuropsychology Battery, in Handbook of Clinical Neuropsychology. Edited by Filskov SB, Boll TJ. New York, Wiley-Intersciences, 1981, pp 577–607

Boller F, Vignolo LA: Latent sensory aphasia in hemisphere-damaged patients: an experimental study with the Token Test. Brain 89:815–831, 1966

Bornstein RA: Verbal IQ-Performance IQ discrepancies on the Wechsler Adult Intelligence Scale-Revised in patients with unilateral or bilateral cerebral dysfunction. J Consult Clin Psychol 51:779–780, 1983

Bornstein RA: Normative data on selected neuropsychological measures from a nonclinical sample. J Clin Psychol 41:651–659, 1985

Bornstein RA: Entry into clinical neuropsychology: graduate, undergraduate, and beyond. Clinical Neuropsychologist 2:213–220, 1988a

Bornstein RA: Reports of the Division 40 Task Force on Education, Accreditation, and Credentialing. Clinical Neuropsychologist 2:25–29, 1988b

Botwinick J, Storandt M, Berg L: A longitudinal, behavioral study of senile dementia of the Alzheimer type. Arch Neurol 43:1124–1127, 1986

Brandt J, Butters N, Ryan C, et al: Cognitive loss and recovery in long-term alcohol abusers. Arch Gen Psychiatry 40:435–442, 1983

Butcher JN: User's Guide for the MMPI-2 Minnesota Report: Adult Clinical System. Minneapolis, MN, National Computer Systems, 1989

Butcher JN, Pope KS: MMPI-2: a practical guide to clinical, psychometric, and ethical issues. Independent Practitioner 10:20–25, 1990

Butcher JN, Dahlstrom WG, Graham JR, et al: Minnesota Multiphasic Personality Inventory (MMPI-2): Manual for Administration and Scoring. Minneapolis, MN, University of Minnesota, 1989

Butters J, Miliotis P: Amnesic disorders, in Clinical Neuropsychology, 2nd Edition. Edited by Heilman KM, Valenstein E. New York, Oxford University Press, 1985, pp 403–451

Butters N, Tarlow S, Cermak LS, et al: A comparison of the information processing deficits of patients with Huntington's Chorea and Korsakoff's syndrome. Cortex 12:134–144, 1976

Caine ED: The neuropsychology of depression: the pseudodementia syndrome, in Neuropsychological Assessment of Neuropsychiatric Disorders. New York, Oxford University Press, 1986, 221–243

Cermak LS (ed): Human Memory and Amnesia. Hillsdale, NJ, Laurence Erlbaum Associates, 1982

Chelune GJ, Ferguson W, Moehle K: The role of standard cognitive and personality tests in neuropsychological assessment, in Clinical Application of Neuropsychological Test Batteries. Edited by Incagnoli T, Goldstein G, Golden CJ. New York, Plenum, 1986, pp 75–119

Christensen A-L: Luria's Neuropsychological Investigation: Test Manual, 2nd Edition. Copenhagen, Munksgaard, 1979

Cope DN: Neuropharmacology and brain damage, in Neuropsychological Rehabilitation. Edited by Christensen A-L, Uzzell B. Boston, MA, Kluver Academic, 1988, pp 19–38

Corballis MC: Human Laterality. New York, Academic, 1983

Craig JC: Tactile pattern perception and its perturbations. J Acoust Soc Am 77:238–246, 1985

Crawford JR, Parker DM, Besson JAO: Estimation of premorbid intelligence in organic conditions. Br J Psychiatry 153:178–181, 1988

Crawford JR, Stewart LE, Cochrane RHB, et al: Estimating premorbid IQ from demographic variables: regression equations derived from a UK sample. Br J Clin Psychol 280:275–278, 1989

Crockett D, Tallman K, Hurwitz T, et al: Neuropsychological performance in psychiatric patients with or without documented brain dysfunction. Int J Neurosci 41:71–79, 1988

Cutler NR, Haxby JV, Duara R, et al: Clinical history, brain metabolism, and neuropsychological function in Alzheimer's disease. Ann Neurol 18:298–309, 1985

Dahlstrom WG, Welsh GS, Dahlstrom LE: An MMPI Handbook, Vol 1: Clinical Interpretation, Revised. Minneapolis, MN, University of Minnesota, 1975

Damasio AR, Tranel D, Damasio H: Disorders of visual recognition, in Handbook of Neuropsychology, Vol 2. Edited by Boller F, Grafman J. Amsterdam, Elsevier, 1989, pp 317–332

Delbecq-Derouesne J, Beauvois M-F: Memory processes and aging: a defect of automatic rather than controlled processes. Archives of Gerontology and Geriatrics Supplement 1:121–150, 1989

Delis DC, Kramer JH, Kaplan E, et al: California Verbal Learning Test. San Antonio, TX, Psychological Corporation, 1986

Delis DC, Kramer JH, Kaplan E, et al: California Verbal Learning Test, Form II (Research Edition). San Antonio, TX, Psychological Corporation, 1987

De Renzi E, Vignolo LA: The Token Test: a sensitive test to detect disturbances in aphasics. Brain 85:665–678, 1962

De Renzi E, Faglioni P, Lodesani M, et al: Performance of left brain-damaged patients on imitation of single movements and motor sequences. Cortex 19:333–343, 1983

Derogatis LR: Symptom Checklist-90, Revised (SCL-90-R). Towson, MD, Clinical Psychometric Research, 1983

Dubois B, Pillon B, Sternic N, et al: Age-induced cognitive deficit in Parksinson's disease. Neurology 40:38–41, 1990

Eisenberg HM, Levin HS: Computed tomography and magnetic resonance imaging in mild to moderate head injury, in Mild Head Injury. Edited by Levin HS, Eisenberg HM, Benton AL. New York, Oxford University Press, 1989, pp 133–141

Filskov SB, Leli DA: Assessment of the individual in neuropsychological practice, in Handbook of Clinical Neuropsychology. Edited by Filskov SB, Boll TJ. New York, Wiley, 1981, pp 545–576

Folstein MF, Folstein SE, McHugh PR: Mini-Mental State: A practical method for grading the cognitive state of patients for the clinician. J Psychiatr Res 12:189–198, 1975

Freed DM, Kandel E: Long-term occupational exposure and the diagnosis of dementia. Neurotoxicology 9:391–400, 1988

Frith CD, Done DJ: Towards a neuropsychology of schizophrenia. Br J Psychiatry 153:437–443, 1988

Gade A, Mortensen EL, Udensen H, et al: On the importance of control data and background variables in the evaluation of neuropsychological aspects of brain functioning, in Neurobehavioral Methods in Occupational and Environmental Health (Environmental Health Series). Copenhagen, World Health Organization, 1985, pp 91–96

Gass CS, Russell EW, Hamilton RA: Accuracy of MMPI-based inferences regarding memory and concentration in closed-head-trauma patients. Psychological Assessment: A Journal of Consulting and Clinical Psychology (in press)

Gauthier L, Gauthier S, Joanette Y: Visual neglect in left, right, and bilateral Parkinsonians (abstract). J Clin Exp Neuropsychol 7:145, 1985

Goethe KE, Mitchell JE, Marshall DW, et al: Neuropsychological and neurological function of human immunodeficiency virus seropositive asymptomatic individuals. Arch Neurol 46:129–133, 1989

Goldberg E: Retrograde amnesia: possible role of mesencephalic reticular activation in long-term memory. Science 213:1392–1394, 1981

Golden CJ, Hammeke TA, Purisch AD: Diagnostic validity of a standardized neuropsychological battery derived from Luria's neuropsychological tests. J Consult Clin Psychol 46:1258–1265, 1978

Golden CJ, Hammeke TA, Purisch AD: Manual for the Luria-Nebraska Neuropsychological Battery. Los Angeles, CA, Western Psychological Services, 1980

Goodglass H, Kaplan E: Assessment of Aphasia and Related Disorders, 2nd Edition. Philadelphia, PA, Lea and Febiger, 1983

Gordon HW: Auditory specialization of the right and left hemispheres, in Hemispheric Disconnection and Cerebral Function. Edited by Kinsbourne M, Smith WL. Springfield, IL, Charles C Thomas, 1974

Graham JR: The MMPI: A Practical Guide, 2nd Edition. New York, Oxford University Press, 1987

Grant DA, Berg EA: A behavioral analysis of degree of reinforcement and ease of shifting to new responses on a Weigl-type card-sorting problem. J Exp Psychol 38:404–411, 1948

Gronwall DMA: Paced Auditory Serial-Addition Task: a measure of recovery from concussion. Percept Mot Skills 44:367–373, 1977

Gronwall DMA, Sampson H: The psychological effects of concussion. Auckland, New Zealand, University Press, 1974

Grossman FM: Percentage of WAIS-R standardization sample obtaining verbal-performance discrepancies. J Consult Clin Psychol 51:641–642, 1983

Haaland KY, Flaherty D: The different types of limb apraxia made by patients with left vs. right hemisphere damage. Brain Cogn 3:370–384, 1984

Halstead WC: Brain and Intelligence. Chicago, IL, University of Chicago Press, 1947

Hannay HC, Levin HS: Visual continuous recognition memory in normal and closed head-injured adolescents. J Clin Exp Neuropsychol 11:444–460, 1989

Hathaway SR, McKinley JC: The Minnesota Multiphasic Personality Inventory Manual (Revised). New York, Psychological Corporation, 1951

Heaton RK, Baade LE, Johnson KL: Neuropsychological test results associated with psychiatric disorders in adults. Psychol Bull 85:141–162, 1978

Heaton RK, Grant I, Matthews CG: Differences in neuropsychological test performance associated with age, education, and sex, in Neuropsychological Assessment of Neuropsychiatric Disorders. Edited by Grant I,

Adams KM. New York, Oxford University Press, 1986, pp 100–120

Hebb DO: The effect of early and late brain injury upon test scores, and the nature of normal adult intelligence. Proceedings of the American Philosophical Society 85: 275–292, 1942

Heilman KM, Bowers D, Valenstein E, et al: Hemispace and hemispatial neglect, in Neurophysiological and Neuropsychological Aspects of Spatial Neglect. Edited by Jeannerod M. Amsterdam, Elsevier Science, 1987, pp 115–150

Hooper HE: The Hooper Visual Organization Test. Los Angeles, CA, Western Psychological Services, 1958

Huff FJ, Growdon JH, Corkin S, et al: Age at onset and rate of progression of Alzheimer's disease. J Am Geriatr Soc 35:27–30, 1987

Jason GW: Disorders of motor function following cortical lesions: review and theoretical considerations, in Cerebral Control of Speech and Limb Movements. Edited by Hammond GR. Amsterdam, Elsevier, 1990, pp 141–168

Jenkins RL, Parsons OA: Recovery of cognitive abilities in male alcoholics, in Currents in Alcoholism. Edited by Galanter M. New York, Grune & Stratton, 1980, pp 229–237

Jernigan TL, Hesselink JR: Human brain-imaging: basic principles and applications in psychiatry, in Psychiatry, Vol 3. Edited by Michels R, Cavenar JO. Philadelphia, PA, JB Lippincott, 1987, Chapter 51

Kaplan E: A process approach to neuropsychological assessment, in Clinical Neuropsychological and Brain Function: Research, Measurement, and Practice. Edited by Boll T, Bryant BK. Washington, DC, American Psychological Association, 1988, pp 125–167

Kapur N: Memory Disorders in Clinical Practice. London, Butterworth, 1988

Kapur N, Heath P, Meudell P, et al: Amnesia can facilitate memory performance: evidence from a patient with dissociated retrograde amnesia. Neuropsychologia 24: 215–221, 1986

Karzmark P, Heaton RK, Grant I, et al: Use of demographic variables to predict full scale IQ: A replication and extension. J Clin Exp Neuropsychol 7:412–420, 1985

Kaszniak AW, Sadeh M, Stern LZ: Differentiating depression from organic brain syndromes in older age, in Depression in the Elderly: An Interdisciplinary Approach. Edited by Chaisson-Stewart GM. New York, Wiley, 1985, pp 161–189

Keenan JS, Brassell EG: Aphasia Language Performance Scales. Murfreesboro, TN, Pinnacle Press, 1975

Kiernan RJ, Mueller J, Langston JW, et al: The Neurobehavioral Cognitive Status Examination: a brief but differentiated approach to cognitive assessment. Ann Intern Med 107:481–485, 1987

Kolb B: Preoperative events and brain damage: a commentary, in Preoperative Events: Their Effects on Behavior Following Brain Damage. Edited by Schulkin J. New York, Erlbaum, 1989, pp 305–311

Kovner R, Perecman E, Lazar W, et al: Relation of personality and attentional factors to cognitive deficits in human immunodeficiency virus-infected subjects. Arch Neurol 46:274–277, 1989

Laine M, Butters N: A preliminary study of problem solving strategies of detoxified long-term alcoholics. Drug Alcohol Depend 10:235–242, 1982

Larrabee GJ: Another look at VIQ-PIQ scores and unilateral brain damage. Int J Neurosci 29:141–148, 1986

LaRue A, Jarvik LR: Cognitive function and prediction of dementia in old age. Int J Aging Hum Dev 25:79–89, 1987

Lenzer I: Halstead-Reitan Test Battery: problem of differential diagnosis. Percept Mot Skills 50:611–630, 1980

Lesser RP: Psychogenic seizures, in Recent Advances in Epilepsy. Edited by Pedley TA, Meldrum BS. New York, Churchill Livingstone, 1985, pp 273–293

Levin HS, Grafman J, Eisenberg, HM (eds): Neurobehavioral Recovery from Head injury. New York, Oxford University Press, 1987

Levin S: Frontal lobe dysfunctions in schizophrenia, II. Journal of Psychiatry 18:57–72, 1984

Lezak MD: Behavioral concomitants of configurational disorganization. Paper presented at the seventh annual meeting of the International Neuropsychological Society, New York, February 1979

Lezak MD: The problem of assessing executive functions. International Journal of Psychology 17:281–297, 1982

Lezak MD: Neuropsychological Assessment, 2nd Edition. New York, Oxford University Press, 1983

Lezak MD: An individualized approach to neuropsychological assessment, in Clinical Neuropsychology. Edited by Logue PE, Schear JM. Springfield, IL, CC Thomas, 1986, pp 29–49

Lezak MD: IQ: R.I.P. J Clin Exp Neuropsychol 10:351–361, 1988a

Lezak MD: Neuropsychological tests and assessment techniques, in Handbook of Neuropsychology. Edited by Boller F, Grafman J, Rizzolatti G, et al. Amsterdam, Elsevier, 1988b, pp 47–68

Lezak MD: Assessment of psychosocial dysfunctions resulting from head trauma, in Assessment of the Behavioral Consequences of Head Trauma, Vol 7: Frontiers of Clinical Neuroscience. Edited by Lezak MD. New York, Alan R Liss, 1989, pp 113–144

Lezak MD: Neuropsychological Assessment, 3rd Edition. New York, Oxford University Press (in press)

Lezak MD, Witham R, Bourdette D: Emotional impact of cognitive inefficiencies in multiple sclerosis (abstract). J Clin Exp Neuropsychol 12:50, 1990

Lishman WA: Organic Psychiatry, 2nd Edition. Oxford, England, Blackwell Scientific, 1987

Loring DW, Lee GP, Meador KJ: Revising the Rey-Osterrieth: rating right hemisphere recall. Archives of Clinical Neuropsychology 3:239–247, 1988

Luria AR: Higher Cortical Functions in Man, 2nd Edition. New York, Basic Books, 1980

McAllister TW: Cognitive functioning in the affective disorders. Compr Psychiatry 22:572–586, 1981

McCarthy RA, Warrington EK: Cognitive Neuropsychology: A Clinical Introduction. San Diego, CA, Academic, 1990

Mapov RL: Testing to detect brain damage; an alternative to what may no longer be useful. J Clin Exp Neuropsychol 10:271–278, 1988

Marcopulos BA: Pseudodementia, dementia, and depression: test differentiation, in Testing Older Adults: A Reference Guide for Geropsychological Assessments. Edited by Hunt T, Lindley CJ. Austin, TX, Pro-ed, 1989, pp 70–91

Matarazzo JD, Prifitera A: Subtest scatter and premorbid intelligence: lessons from the WAIS-R standardization sample. J Consult Clin Psychol 1:186–191, 1989

Matthews CG, Haaland KY: The effect of symptom duration on cognitive and motor performance in parkinsonism. Neurology 29:951–956, 1979

Mattis S: Mental status examination for organic mental syndrome in the elderly patient, in Geriatric Psychiatry. Edited by Bellak L, Karasu TB. New York, Grune & Stratton, 1976, pp 77–121

Mattis S: Dementia Rating Scale (DRS) Manual. Odessa, FL, Psychological Assessment Resources, 1988

Mayes AR: Human Organic Memory Disorders. New York, Cambridge University Press, 1988

Mesulam M: Principles of Behavioral Neurology. Philadelphia, PA, FA Davis, 1985

Milner B: Interhemispheric differences in the localization of psychological processes in man. Br Med Bull 27:272–277, 1971

Milner B: Clues to the cerebral organization of memory, in Cerebral Correlates of Conscious Experience (INSERM Symposium No. 6). Edited by Buser PA, Rougeul-Buser A. Amsterdam, Elsevier/North Holland Biomedical, 1978, pp 139–153

Mueller SR, Girace M: Use and misuse of the MMPI, a reconsideration. Psychol Rep 63:483–491, 1988

Mysiw WJ, Beegan JG, Gatens PF: Prospective cognitive assessment of stroke patients before inpatient rehabilitation: the relationship of the Neurobehavioral Cognitive Status Examination to functional improvement. Am J Phys Med Rehabil 68:168–171, 1989

Naugle RI, Kauczak K: Limitations of the Mini-Mental State Examination. Cleve Clin J Med 56:277–281, 1989

Newcombe F: Psychometric and behavioral evidence: scope, limitations, and ecological validity, in Neurobehavioral Recovery from Head Injury. Edited by Levin HS, Grafman J, Eisenberg HM. New York, Oxford University Press, 1987, pp 129–145

Newcombe F, Ratcliff G: Disorders of visuospatial analysis, in Handbook of Neuropsychology, Vol 2. Edited by Boller F, Grafman J. Amsterdam, Elsevier, 1989, pp 333–356

Niemi M-L, Laaksonen R, Kotila M, et al: Quality of life 4 years after stroke. Stroke 19:1101–1107, 1988

Northern California Neurobehavioral Group: Test Booklet for the Neurobehavioral Cognitive Status Examination. Fairfax, CA, 1988

Ojemann GA, Dodrill CB: Verbal memory deficits after left temporal lobectomy for epilepsy. J Neurosurg 62: 101–107, 1985

Osterrieth PA: Le test de copie d'une figure complex. Archives de Psychologie 30:206–356, 1944

Pankratz L: Symptom validity testing and symptom retraining: procedures for the assessment and treatment of functional sensory deficits. J Consult Clin Psychol 47:409–410, 1979

Pankratz LD, Taplin JD: Issues in psychological assessment, in Critical Issues, Developments, and Trends in Professional Psychology. Edited by McNamara JR, Barclay AG. New York, Praeger, 1982, pp 115–151

Parikh RM, Robinson RG: Mood and cognitive disorders following stroke, in Animal Models of Dementia. Edited by Coyle JT. New York, Alan R Liss, 1987, pp 103–135

Parkin AJ, Miller J, Vincent R: Multiple neuropsychological deficits due to anoxic encephalopathy: a case study. Cortex 23:655–665, 1987

Porch BE: Porch Index of Communicative Ability Manual. Palo Alto, CA, Consulting Psychologists, 1983

Posner MI: Structures and functions of selective attention, in Clinical Neuropsychology and Brain Function: Research, Measurement, and Practice. Edited by Boll T, Bryan BK. Washington, DC, American Psychological Association, 1988, pp 169–202

Price BH, Mesulam M: Psychiatric manifestations of right hemisphere infarctions. J Nerv Ment Dis 173:610–614, 1985

Prigatano GP: Wechsler Memory Scale: a selective review of the literature. J Clin Psychol 34:816–832, 1978

Prigatano GP, Parsons OA: Relationship of age and education to Halstead test performance in different patient populations. J Consult Clin Psychol 44:527–533, 1976

Purdue Research Foundation. Examiner's Manual for the Purdue Pegboard. Chicago, IL, Science Research Associates, 1948

Reitan RM: Manual for the Administration of Neuropsychological Test Batteries for Adults and Children. Indianapolis, IN, Author, 1969

Reitan RM, Wolfson D: The Halstead-Reitan Neuropsychological Test Battery: Theory and Clinical Interpretation. Tucson, AZ, Neuropsychology Press, 1985

Rey A: L'examen psychologique dans les cas d'encephalopathie traumatique. Archives de Psychologie 28:286–139, 1941

Rey A: L'examen clinique en psychologie. Paris, Presses Universitaires de France, 1964

Robinson RG, Price TR: Post-stroke depressive disorders: a follow-up study of 103 patients. Stroke 13:635–640, 1982

Robinson RG, Kubos KL, Starr LB, et al: Mood disorders in stroke patients. Importance of location of lesion. Brain 107:81–93, 1984

Roman-Campos G, Poser CM, Wood FB: Persistent retrograde memory deficit after transient global amnesia. Cortex 16:509–518, 1980

Russell WR: Recovery after minor head injury (letter). Lancet 2:1315, 1974

Ryan CM, Morrow LA, Hodgson M: Cacosmia and neurobehavioral dysfunction associated with occupational exposure to mixtures of organic solvents. Am J Psychiatry 145:1442–1445, 1988

Schenkenberg T, Bradford DC, Ajax ET: Line bisection and unilateral visual neglect in patients with neurologic impairment. Neurology 30:509–517, 1980

Schmidt D: Toxicity of anti-epileptic drugs, in Recent Advances in Epilepsy (No 3). Edited by Pedley TA, Meldrum. New York, Churchill Livingstone, 1986, pp 211–232

Schwamm LH, Van Dyke C, Kiernan RJ, et al: The Neurobehavioral Cognitive Status Examination: comparison with the Cognitive Capacity Screening Examination and the Mini-Mental State Examination in a neurosurgical population. Ann Intern Med 107:486–491, 1987

Seashore CE, Lewis D, Saetveit DL: Seashore Measures of Musical Talents, Revised Edition. New York, Psychological Corporation, 1960

Smith A: Clinical psychological practice and principles of neuropsychological assessment, in Handbook of Clinical Psychology: Theory, Research and Practice. Edited by Walker CE. Homewood, IL, Dorsey, 1983, pp 445–500

Snow WG: Aphasia Screening Test performance in patients with lateralized brain damage. J Clin Psychol 43:266–271, 1987

Sox HC, Blatt MA, Higgins MC, et al: Medical Decision Making. Boston, MA, Butterworths, 1988

Spreen O, Benton AL: Comparative studies of some neuropsychological tests for cerebral damage. J Nerv Ment Dis 140:323–333, 1965

Stambrook M: The Luria-Nebraska neuropsychological battery: a promise that may be partly fulfilled. Journal of Clinical Neuropsychology 5:247–269, 1983

Strauss E, Goldsmith SM: Lateral preferences and performance on non-verbal laterality tests in a normal population. Cortex 23:495–503, 1987

Stromgren LS: The influence of depression on memory. Acta Psychiatr Scand 56:109–128, 1977

Tarter RE, Van Thiel DH, Edwards KL: Medical Neuropsychology. New York, Plenum, 1988

Taylor LB: Psychological assessment of neurosurgical patients, in Functional Neurosurgery. Edited by Rasmussen T, Marino R. New York, Raven, 1979, pp 165–180

Taylor MA, Abrams R: Cognitive impairment patterns in schizophrenia and affective disorder. J Neurol Neurosurg Psychiatry 50:895–899, 1987

Teuber H-L: Neuropsychology, in Recent Advances in Diagnostic Psychological Testing. Edited by Harrower MR. Springfield, IL, CC Thomas, 1948, pp 30–52

Theodore WH: Clinical neuroimaging, in Frontiers of Neuroscience, Vol 4. Edited by Theodore WH. New York, Alan R Liss, 1988

Trahan DE, Larrabee GJ: Continuous Visual Memory Test. Odessa, FL, Psychological Assessment Resources, 1988

Trahan DE, Larrabee GJ, Levin HS: Age-related differences in recognition memory for pictures. Exp Aging Res 12:147–150, 1986

Tranel D, Damasio AR, Damasio H: Covert discrimination of familiar stimuli other than faces in patients with visual recognition impairments caused by occipitotemporal damage. Society for Neuroscience Abstracts 13:1453, 1987

Van Gorp WG, Miller EN, Satz P, et al: Neuropsychological performance in HIV-1 immunocompromised patients. J Clin Exp Neuropsychol 11:763–773, 1989

Van Lancker DR, Dreiman J, Cummings J: Voice perception deficits: neuroanatomical correlates of phonagnosia. J Clin Exp Neuropsychol 11:665–674, 1989

van Zomeren AH, Brouwer WH: Assessment of attention, in Principles and Practice of Neuropsychological Assessment. Edited by Crawford J, McKinlay W, Parker D. London, Taylor & Francis, 1990

Varney NR: Somesthesis, in Experimental Techniques in Human Neuropsychology. Edited by Hannay HJ. New York, Oxford University Press, 1986, pp 212–237

Vitaliano PP, Breen AR, Albert MS, et al: Memory, attention, and functional status in community-residing Alzheimer type dementia patients and optimally healthy aged individuals. J Gerontol 39:58–64, 1984

Walsh KW: Understanding Brain Damage. Edinburgh, Churchill Livingstone, 1985

Walsh KW: Neuropsychology, 2nd Edition. Edinburgh, Churchill Livingstone, 1987

Wang PL, Ennis KE, Copland SL: CCT: Cognitive Competency Test Manual. Toronto, Ontario, Department of Psychology, Mount Sinai Hospital, 1987

Warrington EK: Recognition Memory Test. Windsor, England, NFER-Nelson, 1984

Wechsler D: The Measurement of Adult Intelligence, 3rd Edition. Baltimore, MA, Williams & Wilkins, 1944

Wechsler D: A standardized memory scale for clinical use. J Psychol 19:87–95, 1945

Wechsler D: WAIS Manual. New York, Psychological Corporation, 1955

Wechsler D: WISC-R Manual: Wechsler Intelligence Scale for Children-Revised. New York, Psychological Corporation, 1974

Wechsler D: WAIS-R Manual. New York, Psychological Corporation, 1981

Wechsler D: Wechsler Memory Scale-Revised Manual. San Antonio, TX, Psychological Corporation, 1987

Wechsler D: WISC-III Manual: Wechsler Intelligence Scale for Children-Third Edition. New York, Psychological Corporation, 1991

Weiss B: Behavioral toxicology and environmental health science. Am Psychol 38:1174–1187, 1983

Wells CE: Pseudodementia. Am J Psychiatry 136:895–900, 1979

Welsh GS, Dahlstrom WG (eds): Basic Readings on the MMPI in Psychology and Medicine. Minneapolis, MN, University of Minnesota Press, 1956

Chapter

6

Electrodiagnostic Techniques in Neuropsychiatry

Thomas C. Neylan, M.D.
Charles F. Reynolds III, M.D.
David J. Kupfer, M.D.

IN THE LAST 15 YEARS there has been an extraordinary growth in technique for imaging brain anatomy. Computed tomography (CT) and magnetic resonance imaging (MRI) have perhaps overshadowed electrodiagnostic techniques in clinical neuropsychiatry. However, as Niedermeyer (1990) suggested, clinicians must avoid overreliance on brain morphology for diagnosis. Electrophysiological techniques are powerful and perhaps underutilized for measuring brain dysfunction that might otherwise be missed with CT or MRI. They complement imaging techniques by providing a noninvasive measure of physiology.

Historically, electrophysiological techniques were used by neuropsychiatrists to rule out epilepsy and gross brain pathology. However, advances in computer analysis have led to an expanded clinical role for electrodiagnostic tests. Electrophysiology continues to be a powerful research tool in the exploration of the biologic substrate for neuropsychiatric disorders. In this chapter we provide a broad overview of the clinical and research uses of electrophysiological tests.

❑ ELECTROENCEPHALOGRAPHY

History With Respect to Neuropsychiatry

The electroencephalogram (EEG) was first discovered in England by Richard Caton (1875) (Table 6–1), who demonstrated that oscillating electrical

This work was supported in part by Grants MH 00295 (to CFR: RSA), MH37869 (to CFR), MH30915 (to DJK), and AG06836 (to CFR).

TABLE 6–1. HISTORY OF ELECTROENCEPHALOGRAPHY IN NEUROPSYCHIATRY

1791	Galvani experiments with frog nerve preparations and speculates that nervous tissue has intrinsic electrical activity.
1848	Dubois-Reyinond discovers the action potential of nerve tissue.
1875	Richard Caton discovers the electroencephalogram (EEG) in animals. He shows that the brain is electrically active at rest and that sensory stimulation evokes cortical potential changes.
1912	Kaufman reports abnormal EEG discharges in experimentally induced epilepsy in animals.
1929	Hans Berger presents the first human EEG study.
1935	Biggs and colleagues describe the spike and wave discharge in human epilepsy.

Source. Adapted from Brazier 1986.

potentials could be detected by electrodes placed on the cerebral cortex of animal brains (Brazier 1986). Caton demonstrated that the cerebral cortex had a baseline or tonic level of electrical activity and that phasic electrical activity could be evoked in response to sensory stimulation. In 1912, Kaufman (in Russia) discovered abnormal EEG discharges in experimentally induced epilepsy in animals. Years later, the use of the EEG in humans was pioneered in Germany by the work of Hans Berger (1929). In his original report, he described the posterior alpha rhythm and its disappearance with eye opening. Soon thereafter, the spike and wave discharges were described in epileptic patients, heralding the rapid growth of the field of epileptology (Gibbs et al. 1935) and the wide use of EEG in clinical practice.

Theoretical Overview of What EEG Actually Measures

The electrical signal detected by the electroencephalograph is the final summation of a multitude of potentials generated by the cerebral cortex. The structural organization of the cerebral cortex can be conceptualized as a mosaic of vertical columns with apical dendrites oriented toward the surface and axons projecting to deeper structures (Fenton 1989). Thus the signal detected by the scalp electrode is predominated by the excitatory and inhibitory postsynaptic potentials on dendrites and neuronal cell bodies, and not the deeper axon action potentials (Goff et al. 1978; Goldensohn 1979). The superficial cortical layers are influenced by projections from the thalamus, which in turn receive input from the reticular activating system. Thus the cortical EEG is regulated by brain stem structures controlling arousal and sleep. For example, during waking, the brisk tonic activity of the reticular activating system leads to the desynchronization of the cortical EEG. At sleep onset, the thalamocortical rhythms are unmasked and synchronized, leading to a slower, higher-amplitude signal (Andersen and Andersson 1968; Fenton 1989).

Although brain potentials may range in frequency from 0.1 to 1,000 Hz (Niedermeyer 1990; Rodin et al. 1971), the EEG has an upper frequency range of approximately 70 Hz. This range is subdivided into frequency bands defined as beta (Hz >13), alpha (8–13 Hz), theta (4–7 Hz), and delta (≤ 3.0 Hz) (Figure 6–1). Large areas of cortex may fire in relative synchrony when the brain is at rest. Therefore, frequencies such as the alpha rhythm are better detected than high frequencies, which are highly asynchronous and attenuated by transmission through the skull and scalp (Cooper et al. 1965).

Overview of Clinical EEG

The routine EEG is performed when the subject is awake and at rest. Activation procedures such as hyperventilation and photic stimulation may be used to elicit abnormal activity. Sleep deprivation can increase the sensitivity for detecting epileptiform activity. The electrode placement generally follows the standard 10–20 montage (Jasper 1958). Special leads electrodes such as nasopharyngeal or ethmoid electrodes may be used to increase sensitivity or further enhance localization of abnormal discharges.

The most prevalent method of analysis of the EEG in the clinical setting remains visual analysis by the electroencephalographer. The record is first examined for focal abnormalities, epileptiform activity, paroxysmal activity, asymmetries, and artifact. The human visual association cortex remains far superior to any computer method of detection of epileptiform or paroxysmal activity. After this, the background activity is quantified with respect

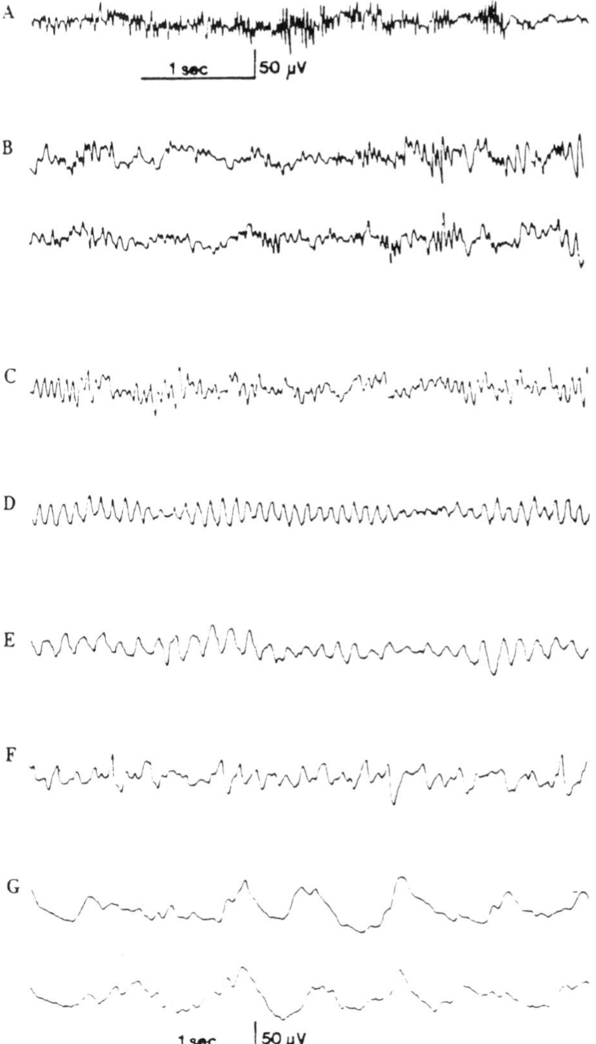

Figure 6–1. The electroencephalographic frequencies. *A*, fast activity, around 30–35 per second: fast beta range. *B*, mixed activity with beta waves in the 20–25 per second range. *C*, mixed activity with beta waves in the 14–18 per second range. *D*, alpha rhythm, 9 per second. *E*, theta rhythm 5–6 per second. *F*, mixed delta and theta activity, mainly in the 2.5–5 per second range. *G*, predominant delta activity, mostly in the 1–1.5 per second range. (Reprinted from Niedermeyer E: Introduction to electroencephalography, in The Epilepsies: Diagnosis and Management. Baltimore, MD, Urban & Schwarzenberg, 1990, pp 35–49. Used with permission.)

to frequency and amplitude. It is perhaps this aspect of EEG analysis that holds the most promise in electrophysiological research in neuropsychiatry. Because there are no specific waveforms seen in neuropsychiatric disorders, electrophysiological differentiation of patients from control subjects may be obtainable only by demonstrating a quantitative difference between the two groups (Shagass 1977).

The EEG is a nonspecific indicator of cerebral function. Any pathophysiological insult to the central nervous system can result in alterations in electrophysiology. Thus with few exceptions (Table 6–2), the EEG does little in providing a precise diagnosis. EEG abnormalities are most pronounced with acute injuries of the outer cortex. Disorders that affect deep brain structures or result in a chronic indolent loss of neurons may show little to no EEG changes (Fenton 1989).

A listener sitting outside a football stadium, who cannot see the activity inside, may be able to make some reasonable guesses about the course of the game based on hearing the fluctuating roar of the crowd. This vantage point does not allow the listener to fully understand the details of the game, let alone what individual conversations may be taking place between the coach and players. Similarly, the scalp EEG electrode can detect the fluctuating tonic activity of millions of neurons, allowing the electroencephalographer to make some broad assumptions about the functioning of the brain. However, this technique is not sensitive to the exquisite detail that is needed to appreciate neural activity associated with cognitive processes or mood states.

Epilepsy and Epileptiform Activity

The most important use of EEG continues to be in the diagnosis of seizure disorders. No other brain abnormality has an electrophysiological pattern as distinctive as epilepsy (Duffy 1988). Epilepsy is found in approximately 0.4%–1.0% of adults in the general population (Zielinsky 1988). Spikes, defined as a potential with a duration of less than 70 milliseconds (msec); sharp waves (70–200 msec); and polyspikes, frequently followed by a slow wave, are often seen interictally in epilepsy patients (Aminoff 1986; Goodin and Aminoff 1984). The study of the behavioral consequences of epilepsy has a rich history (Hill 1964; Reynolds 1989) and is discussed in detail in Chapter 17 of this volume.

Epileptiform activity is found in 1%–10% of the nonepileptic general population (Zivin and Marsan 1968). It is occasionally seen in nonepileptic patients who are on antidepressant or antipsychotic medications (Fenton 1989). More frequently, nonepileptic

TABLE 6–2. ELECTROENCEPHALOGRAPHIC (EEG) FINDINGS IN A SAMPLE OF NEUROPSYCHIATRIC DISORDERS

Disorder	*EEG findings*
Epilepsy	Focal and generalized spikes, sharp waves, polyspikes, and spike-wave complexes
Delirium	Generalized slowing and irregular high-voltage delta activity
Encephalitis	Background slowing, diffuse epileptiform activity, and periodic lateralized epileptiform discharges (PLEDs)
Barbiturate or benzodiazepine intoxication	Background slowing and diffuse superimposed beta activity
Tumor or infarction	Focal slowing at border of infarction or tumor and necrotic tissue is electrically silent
Aging	Generalized slowing of alpha rhythm, diffuse theta and delta activity, decline of low-voltage beta activity, and focal delta activity in temporal areas
Dementia	Accelerated development of EEG changes of normal aging, paroxysmal bifrontal delta activity, and asymmetry between hemispheres
Creutzfeldt-Jakob disease and subacute sclerosing panencephalitis	Periodic complexes
Uremic or hepatic encephalopathy	Triphasic waves

Source. Adapted from Fenton 1989.

patients may have paroxysmal EEG activity during sedative-hypnotic withdrawal states. This illustrates the importance of the clinical maxim: "Treat the patient, not the EEG."

Aging, Dementia, and Delirium

The background alpha rhythm changes very little with normal aging (Visser 1985) and is extremely useful in longitudinal studies. A drop of 1 Hz over a short period of time may indicate a significant encephalopathic process, even though the alpha rhythm remains in the normal range (Pro and Wells 1977). Low-voltage beta activity increases in adults up to age 60 and declines thereafter. Mild diffuse slowing is found in approximately 20% of healthy individuals over the age of 75. Focal delta activity, particularly in the anterior temporal areas, is seen in 30%–40% of the healthy population over the age of 60 (Fenton 1989).

The EEG is useful in the study and diagnosis of cognitive disorders. For example, EEG slowing has been found to be correlated with the severity of dementia (Fenton 1986) and the number of senile plaques (Deisenhammer and Jellinger 1974) in Alzheimer's disease. Similarly, the severity of delirium has been found to be correlated with EEG abnormalities (Romano and Engel 1944). The EEG is a valuable tool in hospital psychiatry in that it can help distinguish a mild delirium from major depression.

Schizophrenia

Schizophrenia has been chosen as an example of the use of EEGs in the study of neuropsychiatric disorders. Although there are no specific EEG findings in schizophrenia, most studies do show that schizophrenic patients have more abnormalities than do control subjects. Abnormal EEGs have been described in up to 80% of schizophrenic patients, although studies with adequate control subjects have reported a much lower rate (McKenna et al. 1985). Several studies (Abrams and Taylor 1979; Nasrallah 1986) have documented EEG asymmetries, particularly in the left hemisphere. The lack of a family history of schizophrenia is associated with an increased likelihood of an abnormal EEG in schizophrenic patients (Kendler and Hays 1982). Although an abnormal EEG may be a predictor for drug resistance to neuroleptic medications (Itil 1982), its principal clinical use in schizophrenia is as a screening tool for gross neuropathology or seizure disorder.

Screening EEGs

The routine use of screening EEGs in psychiatric patients remains controversial. Unsuspected abnormal EEGs have been found in approximately 20% of psychiatric patients (Struve 1976, 1984). However, it remains unclear as to how significant the abnormal EEG is in redirecting treatment choices or in improving clinical outcome. A retrospective study of 698 psychiatric inpatients (Warner et al. 1990) found that a screening EEG altered the clinical diagnosis in only 1.7% of cases.

Quantitative EEG

Spectral analysis is a computer-based method of analyzing the EEG frequency spectrum over time (Bickford et al. 1973). It allows for the determination of the relative predominance or power of any frequency band. It takes advantage of the analytic power of the computer and its ability to translate an enormous quantity of background EEG frequency data into concise parameters by a method called the *fast Fourier transform* (Press et al. 1986). The correlation between the spectra of contralateral or adjacent leads provides a measure of EEG coherence. A subtle neuropathological process may be detected only from observing a change in coherence or relative EEG power of specific frequency bands. For example, analysis of EEG spectra and coherence could distinguish patients with Alzheimer's disease from those with multi-infarct dementia, as well as from control subjects (Leuchter and Walter 1989; Leuchter et al. 1987). Further, quantitative EEG analysis has advantages over conventional EEG in confirming the diagnosis of delirium (Leuchter and Jacobson 1991).

Brain Mapping

Brain mapping, or functional brain imaging, combines the qualitative analysis of EEG data to a spatial dimension in the form of topographical mapping (Duffy et al. 1979). The marketing success of brain mapping has perhaps outpaced its known clinical applications. Brain mapping devices, which were commercially unavailable in 1984, were produced by 17 different manufacturers by 1987 (Duffy 1989). Although the earliest devices were developed in the 1950s (Walter and Shipton 1951), the wider use of brain mapping awaited the availability of compact powerful computers needed to analyze the enormous quantity of data.

The electroencephalographer makes a visual inspection of the background EEG rhythm. However, it is impossible to appreciate or analyze, unaided, the time-dependent changes in frequency content, particularly when there are multiple leads. Brain mapping devices can analyze the mean frequency content and assign it a visual analogue, such as color, allowing the formation of a topographical map. It effectively makes the enormous amount of data contained in a typical electrophysiological recording more accessible.

Other forms of EEG-derived data can be condensed into a topographical map. For example, derivative statistics such as the coefficient of variation can be topographically mapped, giving the neurophysiologist an immediate visual impression of the variability of spectral content (Duffy 1986). Electrophysiological data from multiple subjects can be summarized into a consolidated group map. Group maps of various patient groups and control subjects can be visually and statistically compared (Rosse et al. 1987). Finally, maps demonstrating the functional activation of electrical activity secondary to performing specific neuropsychological tasks can be compared to maps of the resting state (Gruzelier and Liddiard 1989).

Brain mapping has been used in clinical research to examine if patients with psychiatric disorders can be distinguished electrophysiologically from control subjects. For example, several studies (Guenther et al. 1986; Morihisa et al. 1983; Morstyn et al. 1983) have shown that schizophrenic patients have more delta activity, particularly over the frontal cortex, compared with control subjects. Subsequent studies that controlled for eye movement artifact (e.g., Karson et al. 1987) replicated the finding of increased diffuse delta activity in schizophrenic patients but failed to find a tendency for frontal localization. Preliminary findings with dementia have shown a significant difference in power between presenile-onset and senile-onset patients;

whereas little difference is seen between young and old control subjects (Gueguen et al. 1989). Multiple reports have noted increased delta activity in intoxication, delirium, and dementia (Figure 6–2). A recent American Psychiatric Association task force report (American Psychiatric Association 1991) concluded that quantitative EEG had its greatest utility in disorders with slow-wave abnormalities, although its advantage over conventional EEG is modest.

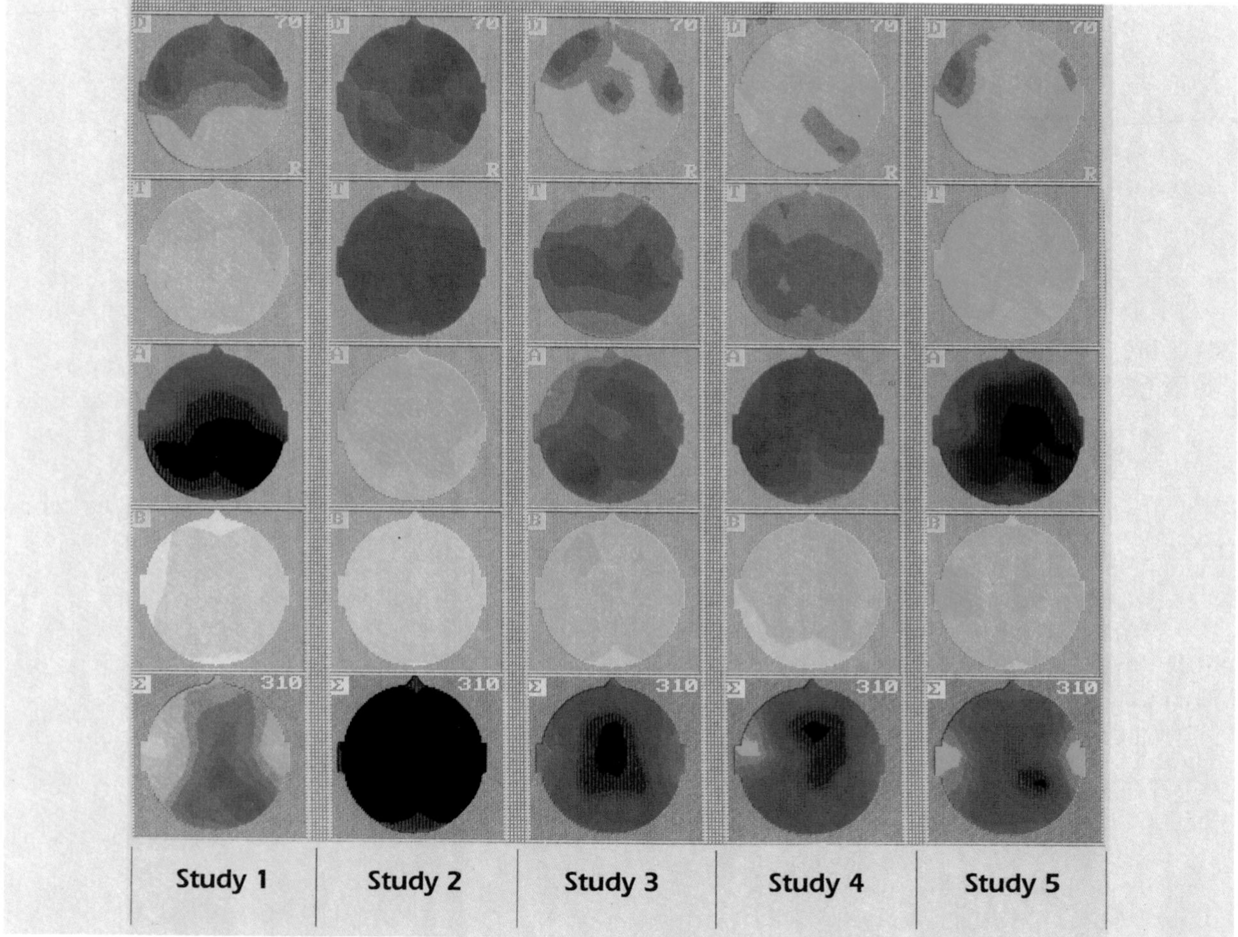

Figure 6–2. This series of maps shows the evolution of a delirium in a 76-year-old woman. The maps represent a series of five electroencephalograms (EEGs). Study 1 shows a baseline for the patient before receiving treatment for bipolar depression. Because of erratic medication compliance, the patient developed acute lithium toxicity (lithium level > 2.0) and was hospitalized for management of delirium. Study 2 shows her brain electrical activity during the acute phase of her lithium-related delirium. Studies 3, 4, and 5, each obtained between 1 and 3 days after the previous study, correlate with the gradual resolution of a delirium and show the patient's brain electrical activity shifting from lower-frequency bands to a normal distribution, comparable to her baseline state. These maps represent "relative power," that is, the percentage of brain electrical activity in each of the four major frequency bands (from *top* to *bottom*: delta, theta, alpha, and beta). The color grade, from white to black, represents the gradient from minimal to maximal relative power. The *bottom row* represents the summary of power in each study. Thus in the baseline study, the patient has a high concentration of EEG power in the alpha band, with most of the power in the delta band (*top row*) concentrated in the frontal regions and probably representing eye movement artifact. In study 2, there is a dramatic shift of the patient's brain electrical activity to the delta and theta bands. The activity gradually shifts to higher frequencies in subsequent studies as the delirium resolves. For all of these maps, the head is represented as viewed from above, with frontal regions at the *top* of each map. (From A. F. Leuchter, University of California, Los Angeles, Neuropsychiatric Institute and Hospital, Los Angeles, California.)

Another potential use of EEG topography is to determine if particular psychoactive drugs produce a characteristic profile (Itil and Itil 1986). Although the fact that psychotropic drugs can affect the EEG has been known since 1933 (Berger 1933), the search for specific drug-related EEG patterns did not begin until the 1950s (Saletu 1989). The advent of EEG mapping has greatly accelerated this work. For example, imipramine causes a decrease in alpha power and an increase in delta activity in the posterior regions. In contrast, diazepam decreases delta activity in the posterior regions and increases beta activity in the vertex and frontal regions (Saletu et al. 1987). Although these reports are intriguing, to date no drug has been found to have a specific EEG signature. At present, pharmacological EEG studies are useful only as a research tool.

❑ MAGNETOENCEPHALOGRAPHY

Magnetoencephalography (MEG) is the recording of the magnetic fields generated by intraneuronal electric current. The "right-hand rule" of electromagnetism is that magnetic fields occur at right angles to the direction of current flow (Zimmerman 1983). Thus the MEG signal, which is a billionfold weaker than the earth's magnetic field (Reeve et al. 1989), can be conceptualized as the magnetic counterpart to the EEG or evoked potential (EP) signal. MEG naturally complements EEG and has potential advantages in localization and a broader range in frequency resolution (Cuffin and Cohen 1979; Rose et al. 1987). For example, MEG is more accurate in detecting deep-brain sources and can detect tangential current sources such as from neurons in the sulci whose axial orientation is parallel to the scalp (Reite et al. 1989). Perhaps its greatest promise is to accurately detect the neuronal sources of known EEG and EP signals (Reeve et al. 1989; Reite et al. 1989). The models that link magnetic topography to the source of the electromagnetic activity remain to be validated. The principal disadvantage of MEG is that the magnetometer must contend with a low signal-to-noise ratio necessitating the use of expensive shielding from ambient magnetic noise. Recordings can take several hours to perform and require considerable cooperation from patients. At present, MEG is principally an experimental tool.

❑ POLYSOMNOGRAPHY

History With Respect to Neuropsychiatry

The interest in sleep for neuropsychiatrists began with a fascination with dreams. (For an excellent review see Mendelson 1987.) In 1868, Griesinger speculated that dreams were occurring when sleeping subjects had eye movements. Freud (1895) suggested that dreaming was associated with profound relaxation to prevent the physical expression of dreams. Eight years after the first published human EEG study, the first all-night EEG study showed that sleep comprised discrete stages (Loomis et al. 1937). Finally, in 1953, Aserinsky and Kleitman discovered and electrographically characterized rapid-eye-movement (REM) sleep. Since that time there has been a tremendous growth in sleep research as well as the emergence of the field of sleep medicine. Perhaps the most important result of this development has been the recognition that symptoms of insomnia and excessive sleepiness have broad differential diagnoses and warrant a thorough assessment (see Chapter 18).

Overview of What Polysomnography Measures

Normal sleep consists of recurring 70- to 120-minute cycles of non-rapid-eye-movement (NREM) and REM sleep characterized polysomnographically by the EEG, the electrooculogram (EOG), and the electromyogram (EMG) (Rechtschaffen and Kales 1968). Typically, sleep progresses from wakefulness through the 4 stages of NREM sleep until the onset of the first REM period. The length of the first NREM period is referred to as *REM latency*—an important variable in diagnosing narcolepsy and in research studies of major depression.

During wakefulness, the EEG is characterized by low-voltage fast activity consisting of a mix of alpha (8–13 Hz) and beta (>13 Hz) frequencies. Stage 1 of NREM sleep is a transitional stage between wakefulness and sleep during which the predominant alpha rhythm disappears, giving way to the slower theta (4–7 Hz) frequencies. Tonic EMG activity decreases, and the eyes move in a slow rolling pattern (Figure 6–3). Stage 2 is characterized by a background theta rhythm and the episodic appearance of sleep spindles (brief bursts of 12–14 Hz activity) and K complexes (a K complex is a single high-amplitude, slow-frequency electronegative wave followed by a single electropositive wave).

Muscle tone remains diminished and eye movements are rare (Figure 6–4). Stages 3 and 4, also called slow-wave or delta sleep, are defined as epochs of sleep consisting of more than 20% and 50%, respectively, of high-amplitude activity in the delta band (0.5–3.0 Hz). Muscle tone is nearly atonic and eye movements are absent (Figure 6–5). REM sleep is characterized by a low-amplitude, mixed frequency EEG, rapid eye movements, and absent muscle tone (Figure 6–6).

The term *polysomnography* is progressively becoming ambiguous. The physiological variables that can be measured during all-night recordings are numerous (Table 6–3). A thorough polysomnographic study provides data on sleep continuity, sleep architecture, REM physiology, sleep-related respiratory impairment, oxygen desaturation, cardiac arrhythmias, and periodic movements. Additional measures may include nocturnal penile tumescence, temperature, and infrared video monitoring. Polysomnography remains the principal diagnostic tool in the field of sleep medicine.

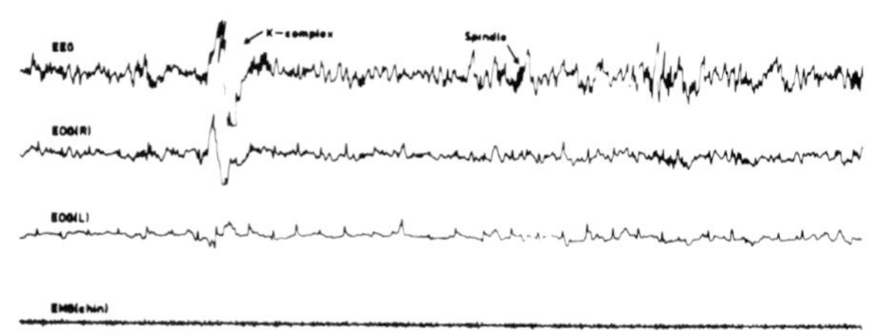

Figure 6–4. Stage 2 non-rapid-eye-movement (NREM) sleep in a 32-year-old man. The electroencephalogram (EEG) shows characteristic phasic events: K complexes and spindles. Slow eye movements have disappeared from the right (R) and left (L) electrooculograms (EOGs), which now reflect largely brain rather than eye potentials. The chin electromyogram (EMG) is lower than in wakefulness, but not atonic as in rapid-eye-movement (REM) sleep. As stage 2 deepens, the incidence of delta activity (0.5–3 Hz) gradually increases until the subject is considered to be in slow-wave sleep (stages 3 and 4). (Reprinted from Reynolds CF, Kupfer DJ: Sleep disorders, in the American Psychiatric Press Textbook of Psychiatry. Edited by Talbott JA, Hales RE, Yudofsky SC. Washington, DC, American Psychiatric Press, 1988, pp 737–752. Used with permission.)

Polysomnography in Evaluation of Chronic Insomnia

The routine use of polysomnography in the evaluation of chronic insomnia is controversial. For practical, economic, and scientific reasons the pro forma use of polysomnography is not warranted. However, several studies have shown that polysomnography yields important diagnostic information in 49%–65% of chronic insomnia patients that was not discernible from a thorough clinical assessment (Edinger et al. 1989; Jacobs et al. 1988). Several investigators (e.g., Aldrich 1990; Perez-Guerra 1990; Regestein 1988) have commented that it is not clear that the additional information yielded by polysomnography favorably alters clinical outcome. Field studies examining this question are currently under way.

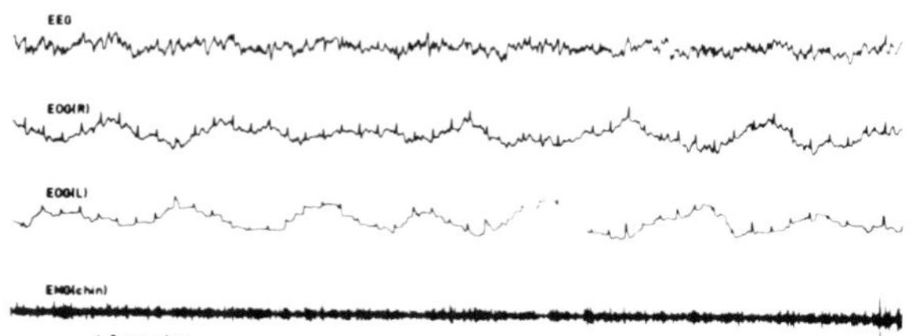

Figure 6–3. Stage 1 non-rapid-eye-movement (NREM) sleep in a 32-year-old man. The electroencephalogram (EEG) shows mixed theta (4–7 Hz) and beta (14–18 Hz) activity, with less than 50% alpha (8–13 Hz) activity. The right (R) and left (L) electrooculograms (EOGs) show slow eye movements, and the chin electromyogram (EMG) displays a gradual decrease in activity during this transitional period from wakefulness to "true" sleep (i.e., stage 2). (Reprinted from Reynolds CF, Kupfer DJ: Sleep disorders, in the American Psychaitric Press Textbook of Psychiatry. Edited by Talbott JA, Hales RE, Yudofsky SC. Washington, DC, American Psychiatric Press, 1988, pp 737–752. Used with permission.)

Polysomnography in the Evaluation of Hypersomnia

Although a much larger percentage of the population complains of insomnia, over half of those patients referred for formal sleep studies have symptoms of hypersomnolence (Coleman et al. 1982). Approximately 4%–5% of the general population complain of excessive sleepiness (Bixler et al. 1979). Hypersomnolence is clinically more alarming than insomnia because of the higher degree of psychosocial impairment, as well as the high rate of automobile and occupational accidents (Guilleminault and Carskadon 1977; Mitler et al. 1988; Roth et al. 1989). The routine use of polysomnography in the evaluation of hypersomnolent patients is well justified

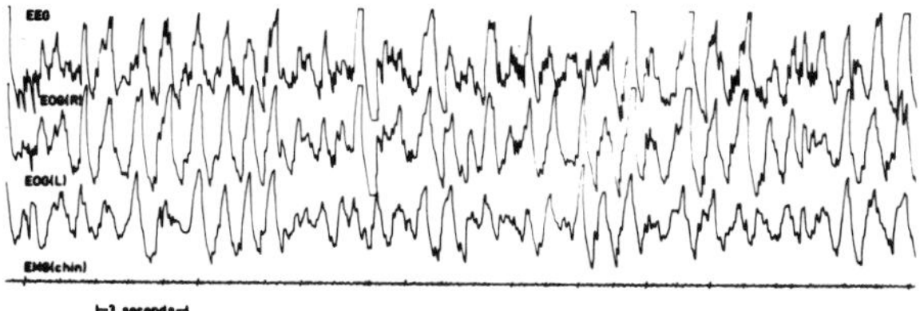

Figure 6–5. Stage 4 non-rapid-eye-movement (NREM) sleep (slow-wave sleep) in a 31-year-old man. The electroencephalogram (EEG) shows at least a 50% incidence of high-amplitude delta activity (75–200 μV, 0.5–3 Hz). Similar activity is also "seen" by the right (R) and left (L) electrooculogram (EOG) electrodes. The chin electromyogram (EMG) shows very little tonic activity. Arousal thresholds are greatest now. Stage 3 is basically similar, but with lower overall incidence of delta activity (20%–50% of the epoch). (Reprinted from Reynolds CF, Kupfer DJ: Sleep disorders, in the American Psychiatric Press Textbook of Psychiatry. Edited by Talbott JA, Hales RE, Yudofsky SC. Washington, DC, American Psychiatric Press, 1988, pp 737–752. Used with permission.)

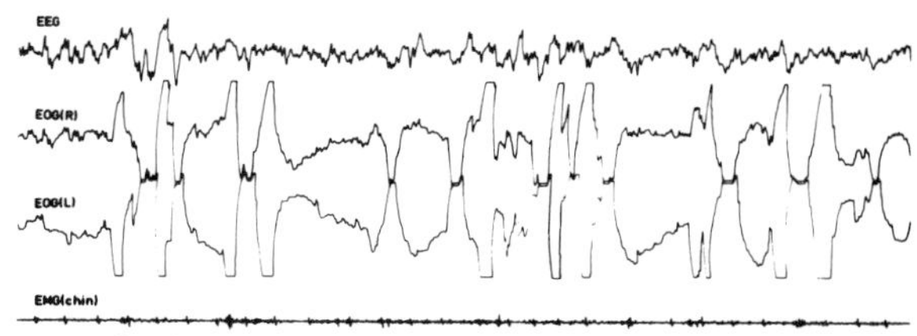

Figure 6–6. Rapid-eye-movement (REM) sleep in a 32-year-old man. The electroencephalogram (EEG) shows low-voltage, desynchronized (i.e., variable frequency) activity, similar to wakefulness (hence the frequent designation of REM sleep as "paradoxical" sleep), whereas the right (R) and left (L) electrooculograms (EOGs) show the highly characteristic binocularly conjugate rapid eye movements and the chin electromyogram (EMG) reflects inhibition of muscle tone. (Reprinted from Reynolds CF, Kupfer DJ: Sleep disorders, in the American Psychaitric Press Textbook of Psychiatry. Edited by Talbott JA, Hales RE, Yudofsky SC. Washington, DC, American Psychiatric Press, 1988, pp 737–752. Used with permission.)

given the high incidence of sleep apnea and narcolepsy in this group (Coleman et al. 1982).

The Multiple Sleep Latency Test (MSLT; Carskadon et al. 1986) is the most objective and valid measure of excessive sleepiness. Other measures such as the Stanford Sleepiness Scale (Hoddes et al. 1973) and the Maintenance of Wakefulness Test (Mitler et al. 1982) are less reliable. In the MSLT, the patient is given the opportunity to fall asleep in a darkened room for five 20-minute periods in 2-hour intervals across the patient's usual period of wakefulness. The average latency to sleep onset, measured polysomnographically, is a direct measure of the propensity to fall asleep. Multiple studies have shown that an average sleep latency of less than 5 minutes indicates a pathological degree of sleepiness associated with a high rate of intrusive sleep episodes during the wake period and decrements in work performance (Carskadon et al. 1981; Dement et al. 1978; Nicholson and Stone 1986). The detection of sleep-onset REM periods in the MSLT has become a cornerstone in the diagnosis of narcolepsy (Mitler 1982).

❑ EVOKED POTENTIALS

The earliest studies of EEG demonstrated that sensory stimuli provoked a measurable electrophysiological response (Caton 1875). This allowed a more refined and noninvasive method of mapping the sensory cortex in contrast to earlier ablation techniques (Brazier 1986). Detailed study of these evoked responses was limited by the fact that they involve potentials in the 0.1–10 μV range, whereas the amplitude of the background EEG ranges from 10 to 100 μV. This was overcome in part by the development of the technique of signal averaging, in which the potentials elicited from repeated stimulation were superimposed by computer analysis. Signal averaging enhances the stimulus-specific response, or EP, and causes the background activity to average to zero (Knight 1985).

Signal averaging quickly led to the characterization of the somatosensory, visual, and brain stem auditory EPs. These potentials have well-defined positive and negative peaks and occur within the first 50 msec after the stimulus. They represent the electrical activity of the primary neural pathway from sensory receptor to the cortex (Rosse et al. 1987). The clinical utility of the primary sensory EPs are well established. In short, they are useful for determining that the neuroanatomy of the sensory pathways is intact. Structural damage (e.g., as may result from multiple sclerosis) or functional impairment (e.g., as from delirium [Trzepacz et al. 1989]) will result in abnormal primary sensory EPs.

The middle (50–250 msec) and late (250–500 msec) potentials are of particular interest in neuropsychiatry in that they represent higher cognitive

TABLE 6–3. PHYSIOLOGICAL VARIABLES FREQUENTLY MEASURED DURING POLYSOMNOGRAPHY

Physiological variable	*Utility*
Electroencephalogram (EEG)	Defines sleep stage; multiple leads may be used to diagnose sleep-associated seizures
Electrooculogram (EOG)	Detects eye movements; helpful in defining stage 1 and rapid-eye-movement (REM) sleep and in detecting eye movement artifact in the EEG signal
Electromyogram (EMG): submentalis	Demonstrates muscle atonia seen in REM sleep
EMG: anterior tibialis	Demonstrates periodic leg movements (nocturnal myoclonus)
EMG: intercostal and diaphragm	Demonstrates respiratory effort
Thoracic or abdominal strain gauge	Demonstrates respiratory effort
Esophageal pressure balloon	Demonstrates respiratory effort
Throat microphone	Detects airflow and snoring
Nasal or oral thermistors	Detects nasal and oral airflow (sleep apnea)
Oximetry	Measures oxygen saturation
Transcutaneous carbon dioxide monitor	Measures carbon dioxide content
Electrocardiogram	Detects cardiac rate and arrhythmias
Video camera	Documents sleeping position and presence of abnormal movements
Penile strain gauges	Monitors nocturnal penile tumescence
Esophageal pH probe	Detects gastroesophageal reflux

processes. Cognitions take place in milliseconds and often manifest electrophysiologically in high-frequency cortical activity (Knight 1985). These high frequencies are poorly resolved by surface EEG electrodes (Pfurtscheller and Cooper 1975). EP recordings therefore have advantages in the study of information processing. There are multiple middle and late potentials studied in neuropsychiatry. Several are named in reference to the experimental condition that elicits the response, such as the contingent negative variation and selective attention effect, whereas others are named for their electrophysiological characteristics, such as the P300 (positive wave 300 msec).

The contingent negative variation (CNV), often referred to as the *readiness potential,* is a negative potential that occurs after a warning stimulus alerts the subject that a second stimulus demanding a response is forthcoming (Fenwick 1989). It represents a preparation or priming of the cortex to facilitate an expected activity. Some studies have found an association between CNV characteristics and personality traits (Howard et al. 1982).

The P300 potential has received the greatest attention in neuropsychiatric electrophysiology. It is elicited when a subject correctly identifies a rare stimulus presented sequentially with other nontarget stimuli. Most studies have reported changes in latency and amplitude associated with different patient groups. The evidence to date suggests that the source of this potential is in temporal limbic structures (Halgren et al. 1986).

Multiple studies have found that schizophrenic patients have abnormal P300 potentials. The most consistent finding is a reduction in amplitude (Levit et al. 1973; Roth et al. 1980) (Figure 6–7). Pfefferbaum et al. (1989) found that P300 abnormalities were evident in both medicated and drug-free patients and were associated with negative symptoms. Of interest, Kutcher et al. (1987) found that P300 abnormalities were prevalent in patients with borderline personality disorder and could distinguish them from those of patients with other personality disorders but not from those of schizophrenic patients.

These findings, which are not unique to schizophrenia, have been linked to deficits in cognition. For example, EP studies of information processing using the P300 response (e.g., Grillon et al. 1990) have shown that schizophrenic patients have difficulties in screening out distracting stimuli. This is strong support for the hypothesis that schizophrenic patients have impaired sensorimotor gating or filtering of internal and external stimuli (Braff and Geyer 1990; McGhie and Chapman 1961). P300 abnormalities in schizophrenic patients have been found to be correlated with left fissure of Sylvius enlargement and CT scan, as well as with positive symptoms (McCarley et al. 1989). Additional studies are needed to validate the correlational data so far obtained and to clarify inconsistencies in the reported findings.

Middle and late EPs may provide important insights to the physiology of attention, categorization, and filtering of sensory stimuli. However, unlike the earlier peaks, they are more prone to experimental artifact. Motivation, level of consciousness, medications, sensory acuity, and movement artifact all can confound the data (Rosse et al. 1989). Studies currently under way are examining EP patterns in genetic studies of first-degree relatives of patients with neuropsychiatric disorders.

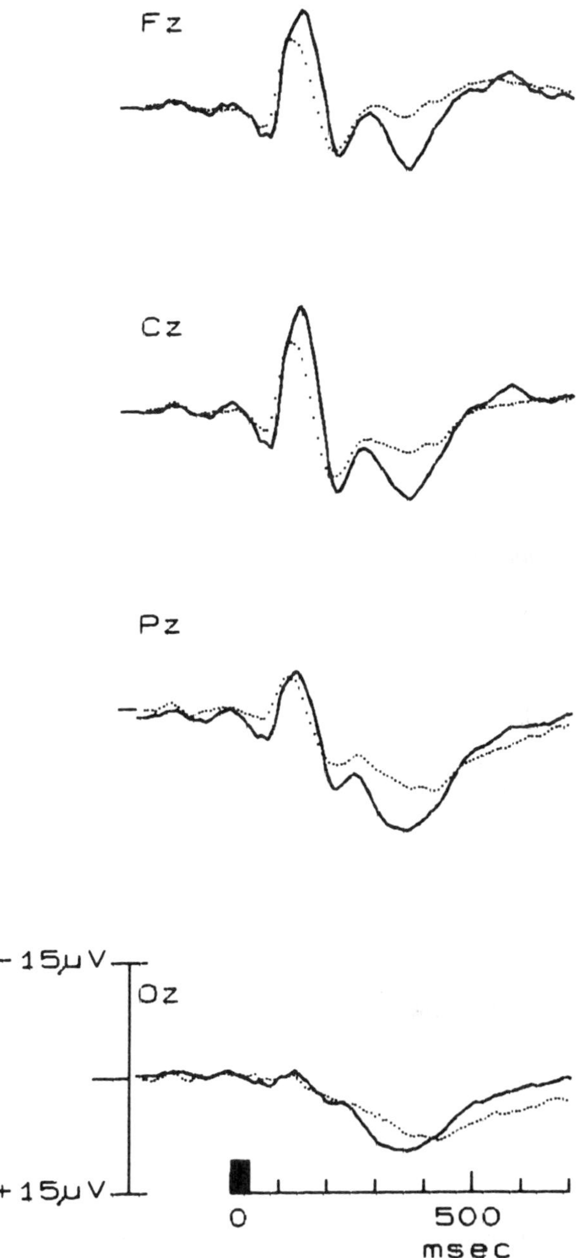

Figure 6–7. Event-related potentials (ERPs) of a group of 19 control subjects (*solid line*) overlaid with a group of 26 outpatients with schizophrenia. The data represent the grand mean ERP at midline electrodes in response to an infrequent auditory tone that the subject counts silently. Positivity is drawn downward. Thus P300 is the large positive wave appearing at approximately 300 milliseconds (msec) and is significantly larger in the control subjects than in the patients. P300 is most prominent at the midline parietal (Pz) electrode. Fz = midline frontal; Cz = central midline; Oz = midline occipital. (From S. R. Steinhauer, Department of Veterans Affairs Medical Center; University of Pittsburgh School of Medicine, Pittsburgh, Pennsylvania.)

❑ ELECTRODERMAL ACTIVITY

The conductance of electricity through skin is dependent on sweat gland activity, which in turn is controlled by the sympathetic nervous system (Rosse et al. 1987). However, other factors may influence electrodermal activity such as skin thickness and the number of sweat glands (Venables and Christie 1973). Measuring skin conductance therefore provides an indirect and relatively crude measure of arousal. Decreased electrodermal activity has been found in antisocial adolescents (Raine and Venables

1984). In one of the few prospective studies, Raine et al. (1990) found that low arousal, as measured by electrodermal activity, predicted future criminal behavior. This supports a theory that criminality is associated with decreased central and autonomic arousal (Eysenck 1977).

❑ CONCLUSIONS

Neuropsychiatric electrophysiology continues to be a powerful clinical and research tool. It remains one of the few noninvasive probes of brain function. The future advances in this field will likely come from computer quantitative analysis of EEG, polysomnographic, or EP data obtained from well-defined clinical populations and well-selected control groups. The clinical applicability of quantitative EEG and EP techniques holds much promise, but has yet to be firmly established.

❑ REFERENCES

Abrams R, Taylor MA: Laboratory studies in the validation of psychiatric diagnoses, in Hemisphere Asymmetries of Function in Psychopathology. Edited by Gruzelier JH, Flor-Henry P. New York, Elsevier/North-Holland Biomedical, 1979, pp 363–372

Aldrich MS: Polysomnographic assessment of insomnia. Sleep 13:188–189, 1990

American Psychiatric Association Task Force on Quantitative Electrophysiologic Assessment: Quantitative electroencephalography: a report on the present state of computerized EEG techniques. Am J Psychiatry 148: 961–964, 1991

Aminoff MJ: Electroencephalography: general principles and clinical applications, in Electrodiagnosis in Clinical Neurology. Edited by Aminoff MJ. New York, Churchill Livingstone, 1986, pp 21–75

Andersen P, Andersson SA: Physiologic Basis of the Alpha Rhythm. New York, Appleton-Century-Crofts, 1968

Aserinsky E, Kleitman N: Regularly occurring periods of eye motility and concomitant phenomena during sleep. Science 118:273–274, 1953

Berger H: Uber das Elektrenkephalogramm des Menschen. Archives Psychiatrik Nervenkrankheiten 87:527–570, 1929

Berger H: Uber das Elektroencephalogramm des Menschen, VIII: Mitteilung. Archives Psychiatrik Nervenkrankheiten 101:452–469, 1933

Bickford RG, Brimmer J, Berger L: Application of a Compressed Spectral Array in Clinical EEG. New York, Raven, 1973

Bixler EO, Kales A, Soldatos CR, et al: Prevalence of sleep disorders in the Los Angeles metropolitan area. Am J Psychiatry 136:1257–1262, 1979

Braff DL, Geyer MA: Sensorimotor gating and schizophrenia. Arch Gen Psychiatry 47:181–188, 1990

Brazier MAB: The emergence of electrophysiology as an aid to neurology, in Electrodiagnosis in Clinical Neurology. Edited by Aminoff MJ. New York, Churchill Livingstone, 1986, pp 1–19

Carskadon MA, Harvey K, Dement WC: Sleep loss in young adolescents. Sleep 4:299–312, 1981

Carskadon MA, Dement WC, Mitler MM, et al: Guidelines for the Multiple Sleep Latency Test (MSLT): a standard measure of sleepiness. Sleep 9:519–524, 1986

Caton R: The electric currents of the brain. Br Med J 2:278, 1875

Coleman RM, Roffwarg HP, Kennedy SJ, et al: Sleep-wake disorders based on a polysomnographic diagnosis: a national cooperative study. JAMA 247:997–1003, 1982

Cooper R, Winter AL, Crow HJ, et al: Comparison of subcortical, cortical and scalp activity using chronically indwelling electrodes in man. Electroencephalogr Clin Neurophysiol 18:217–228, 1965

Cuffin BN, Cohen D: Comparison of the magnetoencephalogram and electroencephalogram. Electroencephalogr Clin Neurophysiol 47:132–146, 1979

Deisenhammer E, Jellinger K: EEG in senile dementia. Electroencephalogr Clin Neurophysiol 36:91, 1974

Dement WC, Carskadon MA, Richardson GS: Excessive daytime sleepiness in the sleep apnea syndrome, in Sleep Apnea Syndromes. Edited by Guilleminault C, Dement WC. New York, Alan R Liss, 1978, pp 23–46

Duffy FH: Topographic Mapping of Brain Electrical Activity. Boston, MA, Butterworths, 1986

Duffy FH: Issues facing the clinical use of brain electrical activity mapping, in Functional Brain Imaging. Edited by Pfurtscheller G, Lopes da Silva FH. Toronto, Ontario, Hans Huber, 1988, pp 149–160

Duffy FH: Topographic mapping of brain electrical activity: clinical applications and issues, in Topographic Brain Mapping of EEG and Evoked Potentials. Edited by Maurer K. Berlin, Springer-Verlag, 1989, pp 19–52

Duffy FH, Burchfiel IL, Lombroso CT: Brain electrical activity mapping (BEAM): a method for extending the clinical utility of EEG and evoked potential data. Ann Neurol 5:309–332, 1979

Edinger JD, Hoelscher TJ, Webb MD, et al: Polysomnographic assessment of DIMS: empirical evaluation of its diagnostic value. Sleep 12:315–322, 1989

Eysenck HJ: Crime and Personality. St Albans, England, Paladin Frogmore, 1977

Fenton GW: The electrophysiology of Alzheimer's disease. Br Med Bull 42:29–33, 1986

Fenton GW: The EEG in neuropsychiatry, in The Bridge Between Neurology and Psychiatry. Edited by Reynolds EH, Trimble MR. Edinburgh, Churchill Livingstone, 1989, pp 302–333

Fenwick P: The significance of a seizure, in The Bridge Between Neurology and Psychiatry. Edited by Reynolds EH, Trimble MR. Edinburgh, Churchill Livingstone, 1989, pp 247–262

Freud S: Project for a scientific psychology (1895), in The Origins of Psychoanalysis: Letters to Wilhelm Fliess, Drafts and Notes, 1887–1902. Edited by Bonaparte M, Freud A, Kres E. New York, Basic Books, 1954, p 400

Gibbs FA, Davis H, Lennox WG: The electroencephalogram in epilepsy and in conditions of impaired consciousness. Archives of Neurology and Psychiatry 34: 1133–1135, 1935

Goff WR, Allison T, Vaughan HG: The functional neuroanatomy of event-related potentials, in Event-Related Brain Potentials in Man. Edited by Callaway E, Tueting P, Koslow SH. New York, Academic, 1978, pp 1–79

Goldensohn ES: Neurophysiologic substrates of EEG activity, in Current Practice of Electroencephalography. New York, Raven, 1979, pp 421–439

Goodin DS, Aminoff MJ: Does the interictal EEG have a role in the diagnosis of epilepsy? Lancet 1:837, 1984

Griesinger W: Berliner medicinisch-psychologische Gesellschaft. Archives Psychiatrik Nervenkrankheiten 1: 200–204, 1868

Grillon C, Courchesne E, Ameli R, et al: Increased distractibility in schizophrenic patients. Arch Gen Psychiatry 47:171–179, 1990

Gruzelier J, Liddiard D: The neuropsychology of schizophrenia in the context of topographical mapping of electrocortical activity, in Topographic Brain Mapping of EEG and Evoked Potentials. Edited by Maurer K. Berlin, Springer-Verlag, 1989, pp 421–437

Gueguen B, Etevenon P, Plancon D, et al: EEG mapping in pathological aging and dementia: utility for diagnosis and therapeutic evaluation, in Topographic Brain Mapping of EEG and Evoked Potentials. Edited by Maurer Berlin, Springer-Verlag, 1989, pp 219–225

Guenther W, Breitling D, Banquet JP, et al: EEG mapping of left hemisphere dysfunction during motor performance in schizophrenia. Biol Psychiatry 21:249–262, 1986

Guilleminault C, Carskadon M: Relationship between sleep disorders and daytime complaints, in Sleep 1976. Edited by Koeller WP, Oevin PW. Basel, Karger, 1977, pp 95–100

Halgren E, Stapleton JM, Smith M, et al: Generators of the human scalp P3, in Frontiers of Clinical Science. Edited by Cracco R, Bodis-Wollner B. New York, Alan R Liss, 1986, pp 269–284

Hill D: The bridge between neurology and psychiatry. Lancet 1:509–514, 1964

Hoddes E, Zarcone VP, Smythe H, et al: Quantification of sleepiness: a new approach. Psychophysiology 10:431–436, 1973

Howard R, Fenton G, Fenwick P: Event-Related Brain Potentials and Personality in Psychopathology: A Pavlovian Approach (Research Studies Press). Chichester, England, Wiley, 1982

Itil TM: The use of electroencephalography in the practice of psychiatry. Psychosomatics 23:799–813, 1982

Itil TM, Itil KZ: The significance of pharmacodynamic measurement in the assessment of bioavailability and bioequivalence of psychotropic drugs using CEEG and dynamic brain mapping. J Clin Psychiatry 47 (suppl): 20–27, 1986

Jacobs EA, Reynolds CF, Kupfer DJ, et al: The role of polysomnography in the differential diagnosis of chronic insomnia. Am J Psychiatry 145:346–349, 1988

Jasper HH: The ten-twenty electrode system of the International Federation. Electroencephalogr Clin Neurophysiol 10:371–375, 1958

Karson CN, Coppola R, Moiihisa JM, et al: Computed electroencephalographic activity mapping in schizophrenia. Arch Gen Psychiatry 44:514–517, 1987

Kaufman PY: Electrical phenomenon in cerebral cortex (Russian). Obzory Psikhiatrii Nevrologii Eksperirnental'noi Psikhologii 7–8:403, 1912

Kendler KS, Hays P: Familial and sporadic schizophrenia: a symptomatic, prognostic and EEG comparison. Am J Psychiatry 139:1557–1562, 1982

Knight RT: Electrophysiology in behavioral neurology, in Principles of Behavioral Neurology. Edited by Mesulam M-M. Philadelphia, PA, FA Davis, 1985, pp 327–346

Kutcher SP, Blackwood DHR, St Clair D, et al: Auditory P300 in borderline personality disorder and schizophrenia. Arch Gen Psychiatry 44:645–650, 1987

Leuchter AF, Jacobson SA: Quantitative measurement of brain electrical activity in delirium. International Psychogeriatrics 3:203–223, 1991

Leuchter AF, Walter DO: Diagnosis and assessment of dementia using functional brain imaging. International Psychogeriatrics 1:63–72, 1989

Leuchter AF, Spar JE, Walter DO, et al: Electroencephalographic spectra and coherence in the diagnosis of Alzheimer's type and multi-infarct dementia. Arch Gen Psychiatry 44:993–998, 1987

Levit AL, Sutton S, Zubin J: Evoked potential correlates of information processing in psychiatric patients. Psychol Med 3:487–494, 1973

Loomis AL, Harvey EN, Hobart GA: Cerebral states during sleep, as studied by human brain potentials. J Exp Psychol 21:127–144, 1937

McCarley RW, Faux SF, Shenton M, et al: CT abnormalities in schizophrenia: a preliminary study of their correlations with P300/P200 electrophysiological features and positive/negative symptoms. Arch Gen Psychiatry 46:698–708, 1989

McGhie A, Chapman J: Disorders of attention and perception in early schizophrenia. Br J Med Psychol 34:103–116, 1961

McKenna PJ, Kane JM, Parrish K: Psychotic syndromes in epilepsy. Am J Psychiatry 142:895–904, 1985

Mendelson W: Human Sleep: Research and Clinical Care. New York, Plenum, 1987

Mitler MM: The multiple sleep latency test as an evaluation for excessive somnolence, in Disorders of Sleeping and Waking: Indications and Techniques. Edited by Guilleminault C. Menlo Park, CA, Addison-Wesley, 1982, pp 145–153

Mitler MM, Gujavarty KS, Browman CP: Maintenance of Wakefulness Test: a polysomnographic technique for evaluating treatment efficacy in patients with excessive somnolence. Electroencephalogr Clin Neurophysiol 53:658–661, 1982

Mitler MM, Carskadon MA, Czeisler CA, et al: Catastrophes, sleep, and public policy: consensus report. Sleep 11:100–109, 1988

Morihisa JM, Duffy FH, Wyatt RJ: Brain electrical activity mapping in schizophrenic patients. Arch Gen Psychiatry 40:719–728, 1983

Morstyn R, Duffy FH, McCarley RW: Altered topography of EEG spectral content in schizophrenia. Electroencephalogr Clin Neurophysiol 38:263–271, 1983

Nasrallah HA: Is schizophrenia a left hemisphere disease? in Can Schizophrenia Be Localized in the Brain? Edited by Andreasen NC. Washington, DC, American Psychiatric Press, 1986, pp 55–74

Nicholson AN, Stone BM: Impaired performance and the tendency to sleep. Eur J Clin Pharmacol 30:27–32, 1986

Niedermeyer E: Introduction to electroencephalography, in The Epilepsies: Diagnosis and Management. Baltimore, MD, Urban & Schwarzenberg, 1990, pp 35–49

Perez-Guerra F: Nothing new about insomnia. Sleep 13:189–190, 1990

Pfefferbaum A, Ford JM, White PM, et al: P3 in schizophrenia is affected by stimulus modality, response requirements, medication status, and negative symptoms. Arch Gen Psychiatry 46:1035–1044, 1989

Pfurtscheller G, Cooper R: Frequency dependence of the transmission of the EEG from cortex to scalp. Electroencephalogr Clin Neurophysiol 38:93–96, 1975

Press WH, Flannery BP, Teukolsky SA, et al: Numerical Recipes: The Art of Scientific Computing. New York, Cambridge University Press, 1986

Pro JD, Wells CE: The use of the electroencephalogram in the diagnosis of delirium. Diseases of the Nervous System 38:804–808, 1977

Raine A, Venables PH: Electrodermal nonresponding, antisocial behavior, and schizoid tendencies in adolescents. Psychophysiology 21:424–433, 1984

Raine A, Venables PH, Williams M: Relationships between central and autonomic measures of arousal at age 15 years and criminality at age 24 years. Arch Gen Psychiatry 47:1003–1007, 1990

Rechtschaffen A, Kales A: A Manual of Standardized Terminology, Techniques, and Scoring System for Sleep Stages of Human Subjects. Bethesda, MD, U. S. Department of Health, Education, and Welfare, Public Health Service, 1968

Reeve A, Rose DF, Weinberger DR: Magnetoencephalography: applications in psychiatry. Arch Gen Psychiatry 46:573–576, 1989

Regestein QR: Polysomnography in the diagnosis of chronic insomnia. Am J Psychiatry 145:1483, 1988

Reite M, Teale P, Goldstein L, et al: Late auditory magnetic sources may differ in the left hemisphere of schizophrenic patients. Arch Gen Psychiatry 46:565–572, 1989

Reynolds EH: Epilepsy and mental illness, in The Bridge Between Neurology and Psychiatry. Edited by Reynolds EH, Trimble MR. Edinburgh, Churchill Livingstone, 1989, pp 231–246

Reynolds CF, Kupfer DJ: Sleep disorders, in American Psychiatric Press Textbook of Psychiatry. Edited by Talbott JA, Hales RE, Yudofsky SC. Washington, DC, American Psychiatric Press, 1988, pp 737–752

Rodin E, Onuma T, Wasson S, et al: Neurophysiological mechanism involved in grand mal seizures induced by metrazol and megimide. Electroencephalogr Clin Neurophysiol 30:62–72, 1971

Romano J, Engel CL: Delirium, I: electroencephalographic data. Archives of Neurology and Psychiatry 51:356–377, 1944

Rose DF, Smith PD, Sato S: Magnetoencephalography and epilepsy research. Science 238:329–335, 1987

Rosse RB, Owen CM, Morihisa JM: Brain imaging and laboratory testing in neuropsychiatry, in The American Psychiatric Press Textbook of Neuropsychiatry. Edited by Hales RE, Yudofsky SC. Washington, DC, American Psychiatric Press, 1987, pp 17–39

Rosse RB, Warden DL, Morihisa IM: Applied Electrophysiology, in Comprehensive Textbook of Psychiatry, 5th Edition. Edited by Kaplan HI, Sadock BJ. Baltimore, MD, Williams & Wilkins, 1989, pp 74–85

Roth T, Roehrs T, Carskadon M, et al: Daytime sleepiness and alertness, in Principles and Practices of Sleep Medicine. Edited by Kryger MH, Roth T, Dement WC. Philadelphia, PA, WB Saunders, 1989, pp 14–23

Roth WT, Horvath TB, Pfefferbaum A, et al: Event related potentials in schizophrenics. Electroencephalogr Clin Neurophysiol 48:127–139, 1980

Saletu B: EEG imaging of brain activity in clinical psychopharmacology, in Topographic Brain Mapping of EEG and Evoked Potentials. Edited by Maurer K. Berlin, Springer-Verlag, 1989, pp 482–506

Saletu B, Anderer P, Kinsperger K, et al: Topographic brain mapping of EEG in neuropsychopharmacology, II: clinical applications (pharmaco-EEG imaging). Methods Find Exp Clin Pharmacol 9:385–408, 1987

Shagass C: Twisted thoughts, twisted brain waves? in Psychopathology and Brain Dysfunction. Edited by Shagass C, Gershon S, Friedhoff AJ. New York, Raven, 1977, pp 353–378

Struve FA: The necessity and value of screening routine EEG in psychiatric patients: a preliminary report on the issues of referrals. Clin Electroencephalogr 7:115–130, 1976

Struve FA: Selective referral versus routine screening of clinical EEG assessment of psychiatric inpatients. Psychiatr Med 1:317–343, 1984

Trzepacz PT, Sclabassi RJ, Van Thiel DH: Delirium: a subcortical phenomenon? Journal of Neuropsychiatry and Clinical Neurosciences 1:283–290, 1989

Venables PH, Christie MJ: Mechanisms, instrumentation, recording techniques, and quantification of responses, in Electrodermal Activity in Psychological Research. Edited by Prokasky WF, Raskin DC. Orlando, FL, Academic, 1973

Visser SL: EEG and evoked potentials in the diagnosis of dementia, in Senile Dementia of the Alzheimer Type. Edited by Traber J, Gispen WH. Berlin, Springer, 1985, pp 102–116

Walter WG, Shipton HW: A new topographic display system. Electroencephalogr Clin Neurophysiol 3:281–292, 1951

Warner MD, Boutros NN, Peabody CA: Usefulness of screening EEGs in a psychiatric inpatient population. J Clin Psychiatry 51:363–364, 1990

Zielinsky JJ: Epidemiology, in A Textbook of Epilepsy, 3rd Edition. Edited by Laidlaw J, Richens A. Edinburgh, Churchill-Livingstone, 1988, pp 21–48

Zimmerman JE: Magnetic quantities, units, materials, and measurements, in Biomagnetism: An Interdisciplinary Approach. Edited by Williamson SJ, Romani GL, Kaufman L et al. New York, Plenum, 1983, pp 17–42

Zivin L, Marsan CA: Incidence and prognostic significance of "epileptiform" activity in the EEG of nonepileptic subjects. Brain 91:751–779, 1968

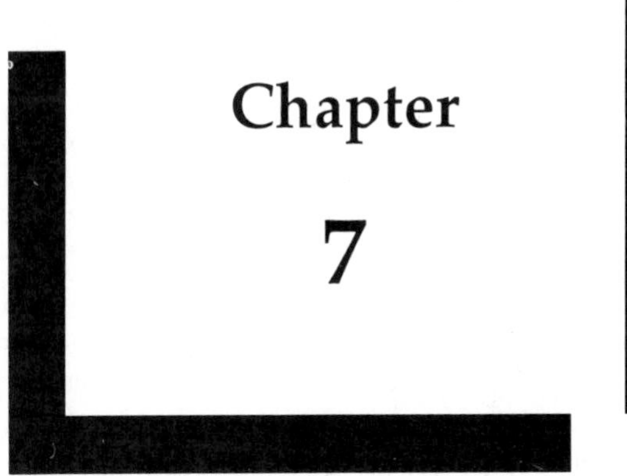

Brain Imaging in Neuropsychiatry

David G. Daniel, M.D.
Jeffrey R. Zigun, M.D.
Daniel R. Weinberger, M.D.

IN THE DECADES SINCE the initial demonstration of the anatomic contours of the living brain with pneumoencephalography (Dandy 1919) and the pioneering measurement of whole brain cerebral blood flow (CBF) (Kety et al. 1948), increasingly incisive imaging techniques have revolutionized clinical research and practice in neuropsychiatry by providing noninvasive methods of direct study of the anatomy, physiology, and biochemistry of the living brain. The prediction by nonpsychiatric investigators who use these techniques that their greatest utility will ultimately occur in psychiatry reflects their suitability to the task of establishing physiological and anatomic concomitants of behavioral and cognitive disorders that may have especially subtle pathophysiology. Already, convincing findings have emerged suggesting that these techniques are indeed capable of associating disorders of behavior and cognition with identifiable neurobiological pathology.

At the current state of their evolution, the primary relevance of brain imaging techniques to psychiatry is as research tools. Clinically they currently are most useful for ruling out nonpsychiatric etiologies of behavioral disorders including space occupying lesions, vascular disease, and degenerative processes. At this time, there are no brain imaging findings that are pathognomonic or even strongly suggestive of a diagnosis of any primary psychiatric disorder. Relatively few neuroimaging findings in psychiatry have been consistently replicated and as a rule must be considered tentative. However, the field is evolving rapidly, and this situation may change in the near future. Evidence is accumulating, for example, for a clinically useful role for functional imaging in the differential diagnosis and early detection of several dementing illnesses.

Use of in vivo structural brain imaging techniques in neuropsychiatric research has advanced through pneumoencephalography (Jacobi and Winkler 1927) to computed tomography (CT) (Johnstone et al. 1976) and most recently to magnetic resonance imaging (MRI). The latter provides the best resolution of any currently available in vivo technology for examining brain structure or function. The impact of these technologies is illustrated by the fact that enlargement in the size of the cerebral ventricles in many patients with primary psychiatric diagnoses, as measured in vivo, has emerged as perhaps the most frequently replicated finding in the entire field of psychiatric research. Neurofunctional imaging systems currently in relatively widespread use in psychiatric research range from relatively inexpensive and labor-unintensive devices designed for two-dimensional measurement of regional cerebral blood flow (rCBF) and electrical activity (electroencephalography [EEG]) to progressively more sophisticated tomographic techniques such as single photon emission computed tomography (SPECT) and positron-emission tomography (PET). In this chapter we summarize the methods, research findings, and potential clinical applications of currently available tools for anatomic and functional brain imaging. EEG is discussed separately, in Chapter 6.

❑ IN VIVO STRUCTURAL BRAIN IMAGING

Method

Before Hounsfield's introduction of CT scanning in 1973, existing modalities for imaging the brain (i.e., skull X rays and pneumoencephalography [PEG]) involved a simple geometric projection of X rays onto roentgenographic film to create a two-dimensional representation. Structural imaging now involves three-dimensional representation in the form of slices. The methods of the two primary techniques of obtaining structural brain images (CT and MRI) are threefold: 1) a device is used to pass energy through (CT) or excite nuclei (MRI) in tissue, 2) a detector device measures energy which passes through (CT) or is given off by tissue (MRI), and 3) a computer model is used to reconstruct a three-dimensional image of the tissue in the form of slices.

CT scanning. Like classical radiological procedures, CT scanning exploits the fact that tissues of differing electron density differentially absorb X rays. Transaxially oriented slices (i.e., the plane oriented perpendicularly to the longitudinal axis) are generated by having a collimated X-ray source rotate around and pass thin beams of radiation through the body while detectors are arrayed to detect nonabsorbed X rays on the opposite side. A computer then applies a mathematical algorithm to create slices from multiple linear X-ray projections (Fullerton and Potter 1988). Image enhancement can be obtained with electron dense iodinated contrast materials to provide greater distinction of lesions that involve abnormal vascular structures or a disruption of the blood-brain barrier.

MRI scanning. MRI is a nonradiological technique that exploits electromagnetic phenomena in biological tissues to generate images (Keller 1990). Atoms with unpaired nucleons, that is having an odd numbers of protons or neutrons (e.g., hydrogen, 1; carbon, 13; fluorine, 19; sodium, 23; and phosphorus, 31), exhibit net magnetization and behave as infinitesimally small dipoles. In the natural state, the random distribution of dipoles in tissue results in no net magnetic direction. MRI scanners use a strong magnetic field (0.15–2.0 teslas; tens of thousands of times greater than the earth's magnetic field) to artificially align the magnetic dipoles so that one net direction is created. After the dipoles are aligned in the magnet, they are briefly exposed to short-wave radiofrequencies. For each type of atom at a given magnetic field strength there is a unique radiofrequency (the Larmour frequency) at which nuclei absorb energy and move to an excited state. The nuclei are then allowed to relax back to their original aligned state in the magnetic field. During relaxation, absorbed excitation energy is released in the form of radio wave signals, which are then measured and computer processed to create an image. It is the "resonance" of the magnetic nuclei going from relaxed to excited state and then back to the relaxed state that gives MRI its name.

Traditionally, MRI images are described as T1, T2, or proton density "weighted." The degree to which a scan depicts attributes of one of these variables is determined by the timing and strength of the radiofrequency excitation (pulse sequences). "T1 relaxation time" is the constant describing the time after excitation when 63% of magnetization returns to the longitudinal axis (in the direction of the externally applied field). "T2 relaxation time" is the constant describing the time after radiofrequency excitation when 63% of net magnetization is lost in the transverse plane (perpendicular to the magnetic field). T1 relaxation times involve energy loss due to local environment "spin-lattice interactions," whereas T2 relaxation represents loss due to dephasing from "spin-spin interactions" between nuclei. T1 times are always longer than T2 times. Proton-weighted scans are based on the number of protons in tissues. T1- and proton-density–weighted scans are best at defining anatomy and showing gray/white matter differences, whereas T2-weighted scans are best at revealing subtle pathological changes. In T1- and proton-density–weighted MRI scans, cerebrospinal fluid (CSF) appears black and parenchyma appears gray or white. In T2-weighted scans, CSF appears white. T2-weighted scans are the ones associated with the "unidentified bright objects" (UBOs) described in more detail below.

Gadolinium DTPA is the first MRI contrast-enhancing agent approved for use in the United States (Niendorf et al. 1990). This paramagnetic agent enhances proton relaxation by altering the local magnetic environment and thus relaxation times. Because this agent does not normally cross the blood-brain barrier, only pathological changes that disrupt the barrier will lead to tissue enhancement. Recently, using contrast agents and special pulse sequence techniques, it has become possible to image the cerebral vasculature with quality comparable to angiograms without the risks associated with these invasive radiological procedures (Ross et al. 1989).

In addition to depiction of brain anatomy, MRI technology can also provide information about brain chemistry. Magnetic resonance spectroscopy (MRS) uses the same principles of nuclear magnetic resonance found in the organic chemistry laboratory (Bottomley 1989). This technology can measure quantities of atoms such as phosphorus-31, protons (H1), carbon-13, and fluorine-19. Phosphorus spectroscopy enables measurement of inorganic phosphate, phosphocreatine, adenosine triphosphate (ATP), phosphomonoesters (PMEs), and phosphodiesters (PDEs). ATP measures can help assess energy utilization, whereas the ratio of PME to PDE provides information on cell membrane stability. Proton spectroscopy allows for measurement of lactic acid in the brain, which can provide an index of anaerobic metabolism. Proton spectroscopy can also be used to assess glutamate, aspartate, and γ-aminobutyric acid (GABA) concentrations. Carbon-13–labeled compounds and fluorine-19–labeled compounds may enable this technology to be used to assess the distribution of pharmacological agents in the brain.

Principles of Research Design

In vivo structural brain imaging research seeks to compare anatomic structural parameters such as size, shape, and tissue characteristics between control subjects and patients with various behavioral or cognitive disorders. Crucial issues in study design are proper matching of patients and control subjects, standardization of image acquisition and measurement techniques within studies and across investigators, and enhancement of anatomic boundaries for image analysis.

All study designs must take into account the normal variability of the brain as well as nonpathological trait and state factors that affect these measures. In comparing control subjects and patients, state- and trait-related factors that may affect brain structure should be as carefully controlled as possible. Age and gender have very important effects on brain size (Bridge et al. 1985; Haug 1977; Meese et al. 1980; Zatz et al. 1982). Women tend to have smaller brain and ventricular volume than do men (Haug 1977). Atrophy and increasing ventricular size are associated with aging in control subjects (Meese et al. 1980; Zatz et al. 1982). Brain size increases with height and weight (Lankenau et al. 1985). Water balance, hormonal state, lipid stores, and other state factors may also influence structural measures (Kreig et al. 1987).

Even with carefully controlled comparisons, the distribution of the patients' measurements often overlaps with that of control subjects, but it is shifted toward the abnormal end of the spectrum. Thus it may appear that only a minority of patients with a certain disorder have abnormal structural measurements compared with control subjects. This pattern of findings has been widely interpreted to signify that the abnormality in question may be a "marker" for an etiologically distinct subtype of the disorder. However, an alternative interpretation is that due to nonspecific variability in brain morphology, anatomic neuropathological deviations that are actually general characteristics of the disease may be misinterpreted as only being found in a subgroup (Daniel and Weinberger 1991). Thus the ideal control subject for a patient with a given disorder would be the same patient without the disorder. The closest known way to approximate such a control subject is with monozygotic twins discordant for the disorder. As discussed below, studies of monozygotic twin pairs discordant for schizophrenia, for example, suggest that experimental designs that define abnormal measurements by where they fall in relationship to a frequency distribution of control subjects may underestimate the prevalence of neurobiological deviance.

Poor image resolution resulting in indistinct anatomic boundaries, particularly on earlier generation CT scans, hindered accurate and reliable measurements. Inconsistent findings among researchers have also resulted from differences in measurement techniques. Approaches to enhancing anatomic boundaries include magnification, contrast enhancement, color coding, and automated edge detection based on optical density gradients. Volume may be calculated as the sum of cylindrical area measurements from adjacent slices. For more complex shapes (e.g., gyri), analog scales tend to be used, although shape analysis techniques have also been employed (Casanova et al. 1990).

Research Findings

Organic mental disorders. Structural imaging investigations of dementia have attempted to elucidate structural-functional relationships and to define characteristic etiology-specific anatomic abnormalities that might assist in clinical differential diagnosis. Thus far, no pathognomonic anatomic changes detectable in vivo have been identified for any psychiatric disorders except those secondary to neoplasms, vascular disease, or specific neurological diseases such as multiple sclerosis (MS). Neurodegenerative disorders such as Alzheimer's disease typically show pronounced generalized atrophy and ventriculomegaly. In Pick's disease the atrophy may be relatively more severe in the frontal and anterior temporal lobes. Multiple small infarcts are associated with one of the two most common dementias, multi-infarct dementia. T2-weighted MRI scans are superior to CT in depicting such infarctions, which may be subtle (Erkinjuntti et al. 1987). However, for primary dementing disorders, overlap in findings between age-matched control subjects and patients is considerable, especially early in the course of disease when differential diagnosis is most difficult. A more sensitive intraindividual indicator would be changes in a patient's scan over time.

Although early attempts to use T1, T2, and proton measures in differential diagnosis have produced inconsistent findings, MRS appears more promising. Brown et al. (1989) were able to differentiate senile dementia, Alzheimer type (SDAT), from control subjects and multi-infarct dementia by measuring the ratio of phosphocreatine to inorganic orthophosphate in temporoparietal and frontal regions (increased in multi-infarct dementia) and the ratio of phosphomonoester to phosphodiesters (elevated in SDAT). The first ratio identified 100% of multi-infarct dementia patients and 92% of SDAT patients; the latter ratio correctly identified all multi-infarct dementia and mislabeled only 1 out of 17 SDAT patients.

Structural imaging findings are consistent with postmortem neuropathology in some movement disorders with prominent psychiatric manifestations. In Huntington's disease bilateral atrophy of the head of the caudate nucleus and associated loss of the normal shape of the frontal horns of the lateral ventricles are common findings, particularly later in the course of the disorder. In contrast no consistently replicated findings have been associated with tardive dyskinesia, which also presents with choreiform movements. In Parkinson's disease, MRI often reveals narrowing of the pars compacta of the substantia nigra (Braffman et al. 1988). Decreased T2-weighted intensity related to iron deposition has also been reported (Drayer 1987). MRI is also useful in detecting and monitoring iron and copper deposition in hemochromatosis and Wilson's disease, respectively. In hemiballismus the MRI may detect contralateral infarction of the subthalamic nucleus.

MRI has significantly contributed to the diagnosis and monitoring of MS (Kelly et al. 1983). Before the advent of MRI, laboratory evaluation focused on CSF studies and sensory-evoked potentials. Although CT scans occasionally show hypodense old demyelinated plaques, T2-weighted MRI scans reveal not only clinically expected lesions but also previously unrecognized small areas of demyelination that may or may not evolve into plaques (Figure 7–1). Correlations of the extent of pathology and functional impairment have been reported (Rao et al. 1989) but are still preliminary. The presence of many apparently clinically silent lesions has raised interesting questions about the relationship of demyelination and plaques to clinical manifestations in this illness (Willoughby et al. 1989).

In general, attempts to correlate measures of ventricular size, atrophy, tissue density, and signal hyperintensity on MRI with cognitive deficits in organic mental disorders appear promising but have, to date, yielded less robust relationships than expected (Bondareff et al. 1988). Because of the normal interindividual variation that occurs in these measures, correlations between time-related intraindi-

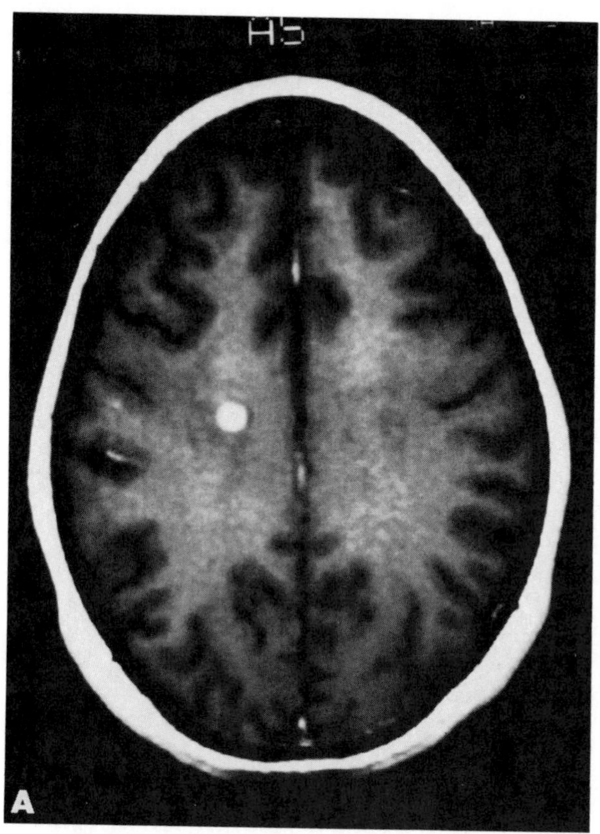

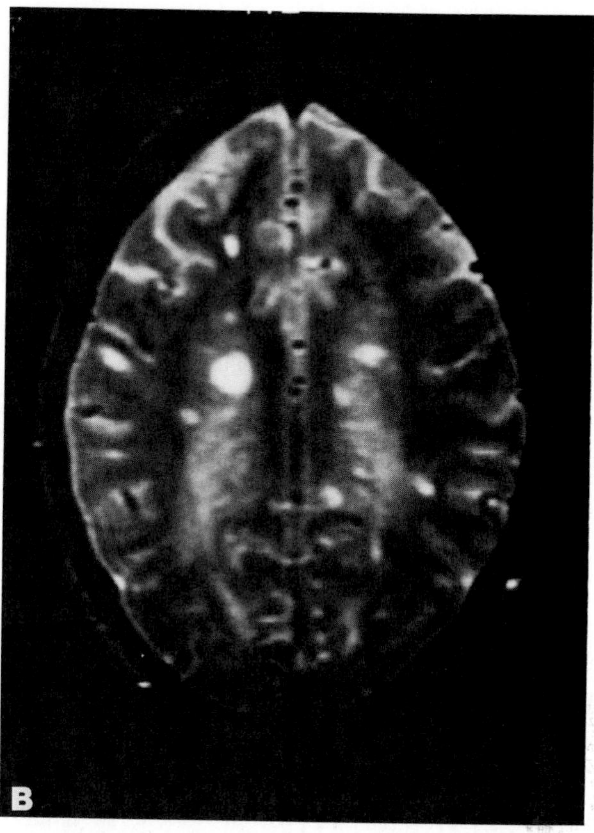

Figure 7–1. T1-weighted (*panel A*) and T2-weighted (*panel B*) magnetic resonance imaging (MRI) transaxial views of the same subject illustrating demyelination secondary to multiple sclerosis. T1-weighted scans are superior for defining anatomy and differentiating gray and white matter, whereas T2-weighted scans better illustrate subtle pathological changes.

vidual changes in cognitive and structural measures might be a more sensitive measure.

Before the advent of CT scanning there was no radiological technique to indicate the presence of ischemic cerebrovascular disease. On a CT scan, ischemic parenchymal change is noticeable as a decrease in tissue density, usually after a 5- to 10-day delay. T2-weighted MRI scanning has the advantage of showing ischemic changes within hours of an event. This is because MRI detects the early subtle changes in tissue properties associated with tissue anoxia. In CT scanning of intracerebral hemorrhage, extravasated blood is seen acutely as a collection of increased density that then resolves to become isodense with surrounding brain tissue and eventually hypodense. MRI scans, especially with gadolinium contrast, can also depict bleeding early in the evolution of pathological events, although it may not differentiate hemorrhage from edema as clearly as CT scanning can.

Large tumors can be identified by PEG or angiography based on mass effect or increased vascularization. As demonstrated in Figure 7–2, CT and MRI have improved greatly on the clinical information that can be obtained, particularly in identifying smaller masses. For tumor detection the order of increasing sensitivity is unenhanced CT, enhanced CT, T2-weighted MRI, and gadolinium-contrasted MRI. T2-weighted images depict edematous pathological changes by highlighting areas in which water leaks out of normal tissue. Therefore, differentiating tumor and edema can be difficult in some cases with T2-weighted MRI images. Gadolinium enhancement for MRI is especially helpful for extraaxial tumors (meningioma and neuroma). Metastatic lesions with punctate disruptions of the blood-brain

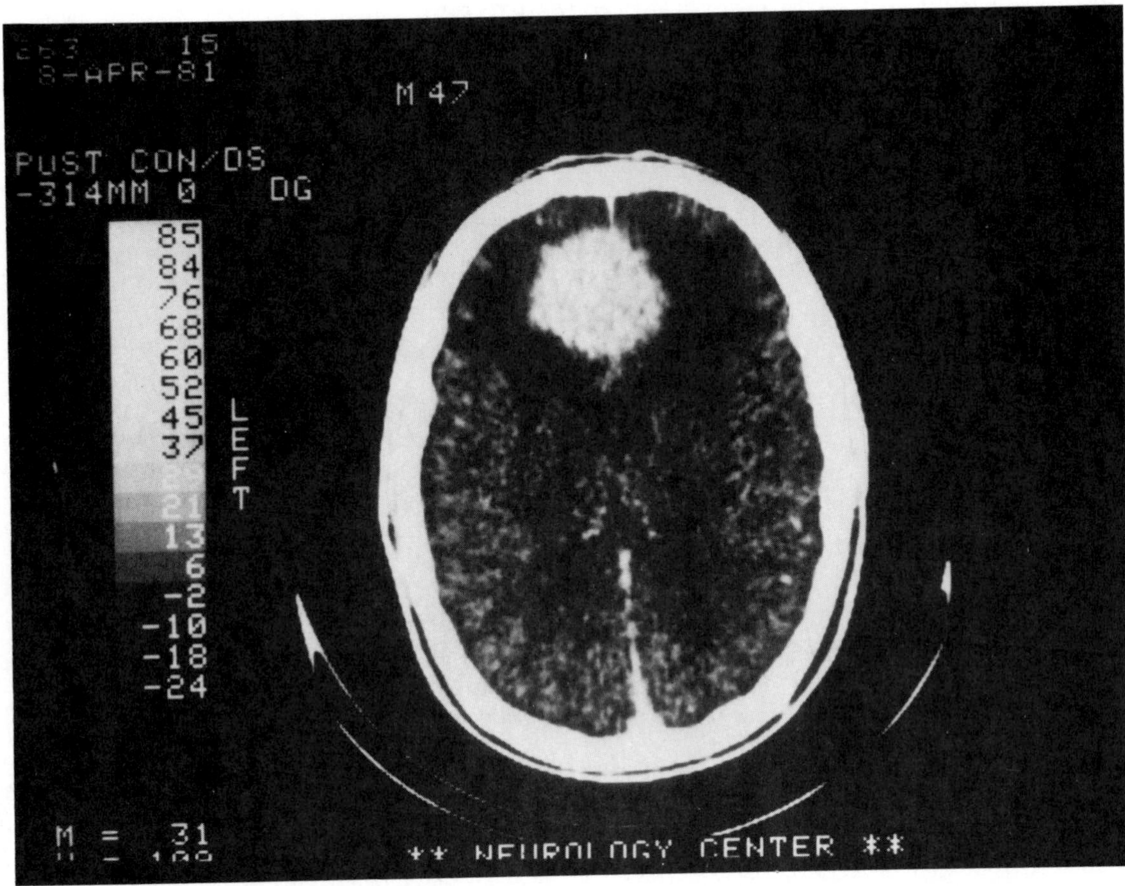

Figure 7–2. Computed tomography (CT) scan illustrating contrast-enhancing meningioma in the frontal lobes of a male adult who presented with a depressive syndrome.

barrier are more noticeable with contrast-enhanced CT or MRI.

In seizure disorders due to mass lesions (e.g., vascular malformations or tumors), CT or MRI scanning provides additional information about the size and location of pathology. However, most patients with epilepsy have more subtle pathology, often of the anteromedial temporal lobe. Localization of such pathology is possible in many cases using MRI. This is particularly important for patients whose seizures do not respond to medication and who are referred for neurosurgical treatment. Discrete structural lesions or increased intensity on T2-weighted MRI scans that reflect sclerotic changes is seen in many of these patients (Jack et al. 1990).

Schizophrenia. In vivo brain changes in schizophrenia were first noted in PEG studies in the 1920s (Jacobi and Winkler 1927). Within several years of the development of CT scanning, the first report of brain changes in schizophrenia was published (Johnstone et al. 1976). Over the course of the last 15 years, hundreds of studies have been conducted. The following observations have been made about changes in the brains of patients with schizophrenia compared with those of control subjects (Zigun and Weinberger, in press):

- Enlargement of the lateral ventricles
- Enlargement of the third ventricle
- Dilatation of cortical sulci
- Thinning of cerebellar folia
- Reversal of normal cerebral asymmetries
- Changes in brain density
- Changes in corpus callosum size and shape

- Changes in thalamic size
- Changes in temporal lobe structures

Of these observations, lateral and third ventricular enlargement, dilatation of cortical sulci, and changes in temporal lobe structures have been consistently replicated. The others are less clearly demonstrated.

Increased size of the lateral ventricles was the first and most consistently noted brain change in patients with schizophrenia. It is important to appreciate that the "ventriculomegaly" described in the neuropsychiatric literature is smaller than the amount of ventricular enlargement indicated when a neuroradiologist makes a clinical diagnosis. Data from numerous studies suggest the following about lateral ventriculomegaly in patients with schizophrenia:

- With the use of adequately matched control subjects, a slight increase in lateral ventricular volume occurs in almost all patients. This is best demonstrated in studies of monozygotic twins discordant for schizophrenia (Reveley et al. 1982; Suddath et al. 1990). Even when the affected twin had "normal-sized" ventricles, the well co-twin had even smaller ventricles (Figure 7–3).
- The increase in ventricular volume is not due to pharmacotherapy, probably predates the emergence of symptoms, and does not change much over time. Pneumoencephalographic studies in the preneuroleptic era found the same type of changes described in modern studies. "First-break" studies (Iacono et al. 1988; Weinberger et al. 1982) and follow-up (Illowsky et al. 1988) studies suggested that there is no further increase in ventricular volume over the course of illness in most patients even though the clinical course of the illness varies.
- Various neuropsychological and neurochemical deficits are associated in some studies with increases in ventricular size, as well as poor pre-

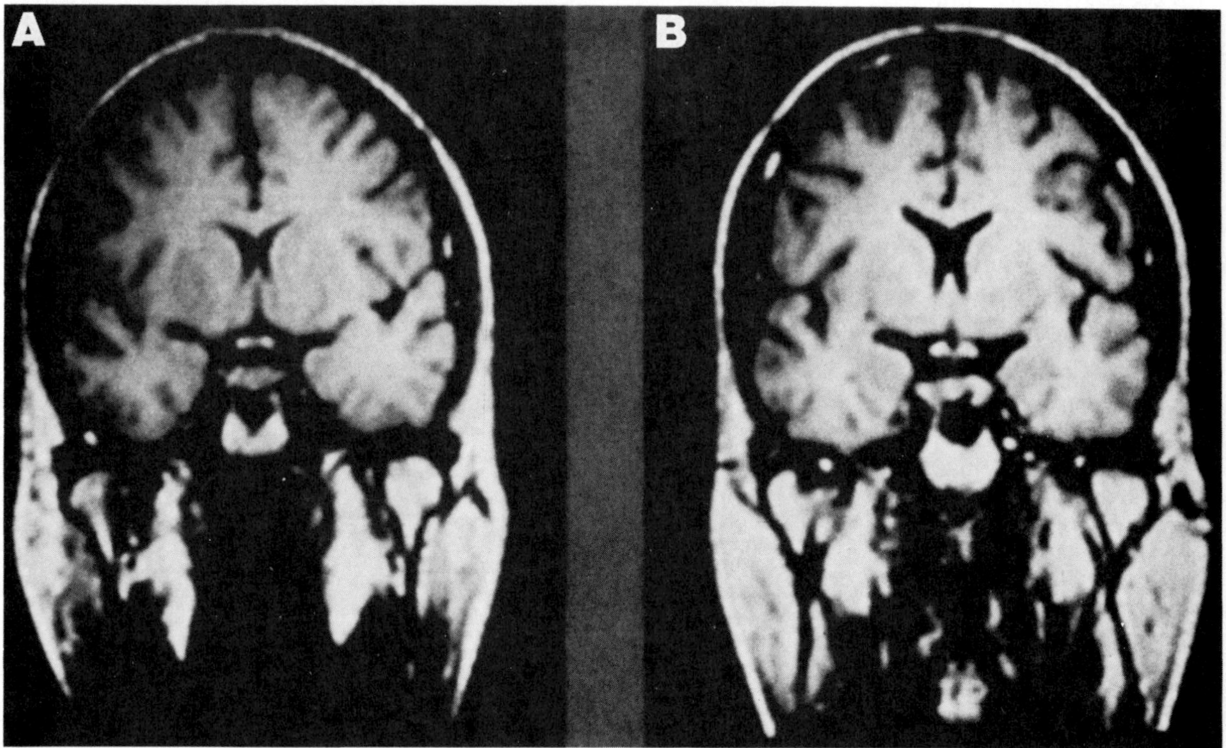

Figure 7–3. Magnetic resonance imaging (MRI) coronal views from a set of monozygotic twins discordant for schizophrenia showing subtle enlargement of the lateral ventricles in the affected twin (*panel B*) compared with the unaffected twin (*panel A*). Note that the size of the ventricles of the affected twin fall within the range that is commonly considered "normal."

morbid psychosocial functioning, suggesting that the process underlying the psychopathology is related to brain dysfunction (Shelton and Weinberger 1986).

Recent advances in MRI technology and image analysis systems have allowed for more sophisticated measurement of small structures. In particular, in vivo MRI studies of the temporal lobes have been conducted to verify reports of changes in postmortem tissues (Falkai et al. 1988). Decreases in the size of the hippocampus have been reported by several groups including a study with monozygotic twins discordant for schizophrenia (Suddath et al. 1990). There have also been reports of increases in the size of the temporal horns and decreases in the volume of temporal lobe tissue (Bogerts et al. 1990; Johnstone et al. 1989; Suddath et al. 1990).

Despite the information these findings have contributed to our understanding of pathological processes in schizophrenia, they do not represent criteria by which a diagnosis can be made. The great variation in the size of brain structures in control subjects is such that although more schizophrenic patients than control subjects may have larger ventricles, there are many such patients with ventricles smaller than those of control subjects. In a review (Daniel et al. in press) of all English-language studies in which individual data points of ventricle-to-brain ratio in schizophrenic patients were published, the distribution of schizophrenic patients was found to overlap with that of control subjects (although shifted upward toward the abnormal end). This finding appears to be true for the other structural differences described as well.

Mood disorders. Studies of structural changes in patients with unipolar depression have almost as many negative as positive reports using CT or MRI. Findings of enlarged ventricles in depressed patients are also complicated by a correlation with length of illness, which is not the case with schizophrenic patients. Further, unlike the first-break studies in the schizophrenia literature, there have not been findings of changes in patients on first presentation for depression compared with age-matched control subjects (Iacono et al. 1988). As with studies of unipolar patients, some reports have claimed an increase in ventricular size in bipolar patients compared with control subjects, whereas others have not (Dewan et al. 1988).

In contrast to conflicting reports about structural changes, MRI studies have indicated a greater incidence of T2-weighted, high-intensity (i.e., bright areas on the scan) lesions in affective disorders. Compared with control subjects, an elderly depressed population referred for electroconvulsive therapy (ECT) was found to have an increased frequency of high-signal, white matter lesions in T2-weighted images (Coffey et al. 1988, 1990). This apparent "leukoencephalopathy" has also been reported in adult bipolar patients (Dupont et al. 1990; Swayze et al. 1990). Although these lesions suggest that structural changes are present in some patients with mood disorders, they are not a consistent or specific finding. In fact, high-signal, white matter lesions (so-called UBOs) occur in older control subjects with no apparent neuropsychiatric compromise and have been observed in a patient with first-break schizophrenia (Figure 7–4). Although these

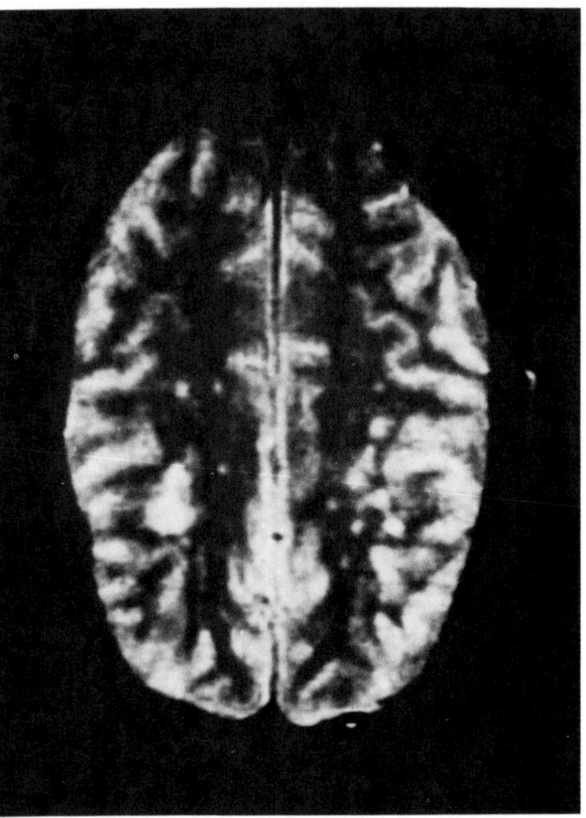

Figure 7–4. T2-weighted magnetic resonance imaging (MRI) transaxial view of a patient during the initial hospitalization for schizophrenia illustrating high-intensity lesions in the white matter.

most common functional imaging parameters currently studied in neuropsychiatry are the local cerebral metabolic rate of glucose (LCMRglu), rCBF, and the density and binding affinity of neuroreceptors. Also, there is growing interest in quantification of the activity of enzymes, synthesis of proteins using labeled amino acids, and the metabolism of neurotransmitters.

The metabolic rate of glucose (currently the most widely measured parameter of cerebral function) reflects the extent to which regions of the brain are working or failing to work, but doesn't explain the etiology of the dysfunction. Because neuronal metabolism is greatest at the synapse, this measure is highly linked to the degree of neuronal information transfer taking place. The metabolic rate of the primary cerebral energy substrate (glucose) is ascertained either by tagging a glucose analog (deoxyglucose) with the positron-emitting radionuclide fluorine-18 or by tagging glucose itself with carbon-11. Distribution of these compounds as measured by PET camera systems provides superb spatial resolution and anatomic detail. Radio-tagged deoxyglucose compounds are ideal for studying metabolism because physiologically they behave identically to glucose until after they have entered the cell. Subsequent to phosphorylation they become trapped intracellularly where they emit radioactive particles suitable for imaging.

Measurement of rCBF is of interest not because it provides information about the vasculature, but because it is normally tightly coupled with and therefore is an indirect indicator of glucose metabolism. Radiotracers widely used in the measurement of rCBF by PET include intravenously injected oxgen-15 water and inhaled $C^{15}O$ or $^{15}O_2$, intravenously injected technetium-99m HMPAO, technetium-99m ECD, I-123 N-isopropyl-p-iodoamphetamine (iodine-123 IMP), and iodine-123 HIPDM for static SPECT studies, and inhaled xenon-133 and xenon-127 for dynamic SPECT and nontomographic rCBF measurement.

Evidence suggestive of disordered neurotransmitter activity in many psychiatric disorders has generated enormous interest in quantification of receptor binding in vivo. This is accomplished by PET or SPECT measurement of the location of an injected radioactively labeled specific receptor ligand. Quantification is still somewhat uncertain because complex kinetic models must be applied to explain the distribution, redistribution, and nonspecific binding of the compound. Most commonly used receptor ligands are tagged with fluorine-18 or carbon-11 (as in the case of PET) or with iodine-123 (as in the case of SPECT) and provide for measurement of dopamine, serotonin, opiate, benzodiazepines, and muscarinic receptors, as well as of receptors for a number of other neurochemical systems. Carbon-11–labeled drugs such as chlorpromazine have been used to trace the fate of psychotropic medications in the brain (Comar et al. 1979). In addition, tracers such as [^{18}F]dopa now permit localization and quantification of presynaptic dopamine metabolism. (For a partial listing of PET and SPECT tracers, see Tables 7–1 and 7–2, respectively.)

Linking Tracer Distribution to Neurofunction

All quantitative functional imaging techniques require valid kinetic models linking the distribution and behavior of the tracer in the brain to brain function. Ideally, these models require tracers that 1) physiologically behave indistinguishably from the natural substrate; 2) are highly extracted across the blood-brain barrier whereas any peripheral metabolites are not; 3) are highly specific for the receptor or neurochemical parameter of interest, or in the case of a CBF tracer distributed like blood; and 4) emit photons of high enough energy to resist pro-

TABLE 7–1. POSITRON-EMISSION TOMOGRAPHY (PET) TRACERS

Glucose metabolism	**Dopamine receptors**
[^{18}F]deoxyglucose	[^{11}C]methylspiperone
[^{11}C]glucose	[^{11}C]raclopride
Protein synthesis	[^{11}C]SCH 23390
[^{11}C]methionine, -leucine, and -valine	[^{18}F]haloperidol
[^{18}F]tyrosine	[^{11}C]nomifensine
Benzodiazepine receptors	**Dopamine metabolism**
[^{11}C]R015-1788	[^{18}F]dopa
[^{11}C]flunitrazepam	**Monoamine oxidase**
Serotonin receptors	[^{11}C]deprenyl
[^{11}C]methylbromo lysergide	[^{11}C]clorgyline
[^{11}C]cyclofoxy	**Muscarinic receptors**
Blood flow	[^{11}C]dexetimide
CO_2^{15}	[^{11}C]methylscopolamine
H_2O^{15}	**Opiate receptors**
[^{13}N]ammonia	[^{11}C]carfentanil
[^{11}C]methane	[^{11}C]ketanseri

TABLE 7–2. SINGLE PHOTON EMISSION COMPUTED TOMOGRAPHY (SPECT) TRACERS

Blood flow	**Dopamine receptors**
^{133}Xe	[^{77}Br]spiperone
^{99m}Tc HMPAO, ^{99m} ECD	[^{123}I]spiperone
[^{123}I]IMP, [^{123}I]HIPDM	[^{123}I]sulpiride
Cholinergic receptors	[^{123}I]BZP
[^{123}I]QNB	[^{123}I]BZM
[^{123}I]dexetimide	[^{123}I]SCH 23392
Benzodiazepine receptors	**Amino acids**
[^{123}I]Ro16-0154	[^{123}I]α-methyltyrosine
Serotonergic receptors	**Norepinephrine systems**
[^{123}I]lysergide	[^{123}I]DHTP
[^{123}I]bromolysergide	**Other**
[^{123}I]ritanserin	[^{123}I]MK-801

nounced attenuation and scattering by tissue that they can be counted by extracranial detectors.

The in vivo behavior of most tracers can be loosely characterized as static or dynamic in nature. Static tracers become fixed in the brain and continuously emit radiation, permitting imaging to proceed for a period during which there is no change in the distribution of the tracer. Static tracers (e.g., technetium-99m HMPAO, [^{11}C]methylspiperone, and [^{123}I]sulpiride) are used to image receptor distribution and density, neuronal uptake sites for various biologically important substrates, and relative distribution of rCBF and glucose metabolism. Dynamic models rely on measurements of the rate of change in radioactivity in a specific brain region to characterize the underlying physiological kinetic process. This technique is used to quantitate rCBF and the intensity with which receptors bind neurotransmitters.

Techniques for Imaging Tracer Distribution

Two-dimensional rCBF measurement. The nontomographic two-dimensional (2-D) rCBF technique has been the most extensively used in vivo neurophysiological research technique in psychiatry other than EEG, but it is being rapidly supplanted by tomographic techniques such as PET and SPECT. Although 2-D rCBF is not a brain imaging technique, per se, its data may be presented as a 2-D brain image. The contemporary noninvasive 2-D xenon-133 inhalation technique uses xenon-133 as the rCBF tracer and calculates rCBF on the basis of the rate of disappearance of radioactive emissions after saturation of the brain with the tracer. Radioactivity is measured over various brain regions by arrays of cylindrical extracranial detectors. The xenon-133 inhalation rCBF technique has relatively modest start-up and operating costs and uses an inexpensive, relatively long-lived isotope that can be manufactured in a central location and shipped to users. However, the xenon-133 rCBF method suffers from substantial technical limitations including poor spatial resolution, inability to image subcortical structures, and necessity for a relatively long period of extracranial recording.

Tomographic techniques such as SPECT and PET, although moderately and extremely more expensive and labor intensive, respectively, offer substantial advantages including 1) three-dimensional imaging, 2) improved resolution, and 3) the capacity to radioactively label a number of biologically important compounds.

PET. PET is currently the most sophisticated and expensive and has the highest resolution of any in vivo functional imaging technique. Although transverse section imaging with photons was described in 1962, the first positron computed tomograph was not developed until 1975 (Phelps et al. 1982). Currently, PET is limited to relatively few academic centers because the half-life of the radionuclides used to label tracers is so brief that a local cyclotron is required. A PET image is reconstructed in the following way. A positron-emitting radionuclide label is attached to a molecule of biological interest and is injected into the body. An emitted positron travels approximately 1–2 mm before colliding with an electron, resulting in an "annihilation reaction" in which two gamma rays are emitted at 180° degrees from each other. A high degree of spatial resolution (2–6 mm) is attained using a fixed ring of extracranial detectors individually coded to photomultiplier tubes. The detectors are programmed to detect emissions that are paired at 180°. The resulting "rays," which characterize a line on which the annihilation reaction occurred, are mathematically reconstructed into the images of the distribution of the tracer. Factors significantly limiting PET resolution include the distance the positron must travel before the annihilation event occurs, problems in the mechanical coupling of photomultiplier tubes to scintillation detectors, efficiency, speed and light output limitations with current detectors, registering of false coincidences, and statistical uncertainty in reconstruction resulting from the limited number of coincidence detections (Brownell et al. 1982).

SPECT. Unlike PET, SPECT uses single photon emitting radionuclides as tracers rather than relying on positron emitters to produce pairs of photons. Theoretically, this offers an advantage in resolution because no information about the location of the tracer is sacrificed by the distance the positron must travel before the annihilation reaction. However, with current technology, coincidence detection with PET and the considerably higher photon energy of the emissions lead to superior resolution compared with SPECT (less than 5 mm and 8 mm in-plane resolution, for PET and SPECT, respectively). Reconstruction of single photon emissions for SPECT is further compromised by inadequately validated models for correcting attenuation and scatter effects. However, this is likely to be corrected in the near future. In this regard, it is often incorrectly stated that SPECT is not "quantitative." There is nothing intrinsically less quantitative about SPECT compared with PET. Both methods require attenuation and scatter correction algorithms for quantitative imaging.

SPECT has the potential for relatively widespread use compared with the limited distribution of PET scanning systems. This is primarily because single photon emitting compounds have relatively long physical half-lives and thus can be manufactured in one site and transported to distant sites, saving the costs of a cyclotron and extensive radiopharmaceutical staff associated with PET. The hardware associated with SPECT varies from relatively inexpensive "single-head" rotating gamma camera systems to moderately priced (i.e., $700,000) dedicated-head systems. Dedicated-head systems are preferable because their enhanced sensitivity may permit dynamic imaging and because resolution of rotating gamma camera systems is often limited by the distance separating the camera from the head. The single photon emitting tracers described in Table 7–2 may be used for the same types of rCBF, substrate analog, and neurotransmitter studies as positron-emitting tracers. However, compared with PET, radioactive tagging with the relatively larger single photon emitting nuclides, such as iodine-123, is more likely to interfere with the chemical activity of the tagged molecule.

❑ RESEARCH

Despite the rapid proliferation of functional imaging research in the past decade, relatively few findings in neuropsychiatry have been independently verified. This is in part due to methodological inconsistencies and the restriction of PET research to a relatively small number of specialized academic centers. However, the number of PET centers is increasing, and SPECT investigations of the neurophysiology of psychiatric disorders are expected to mushroom in the future because of the lower expense and wide availability of this technique.

Principles of Research Design

Characterization of abnormalities in neurophysiology and neurochemistry underlying psychiatric disorders requires carefully controlled comparison to the cerebral function of control subjects. Because a number of factors other than illness can vary the usual landscape of cerebral function, patients and control subjects must be carefully matched for a multitude of state and trait factors. Examples of state-related factors that ideally should be carefully controlled at the time of scanning include sensorimotor activity, emotional state, level of arousal, autonomic activity, focus of cognitive activity, and medication status. The normal cerebral landscape at rest with the eyes closed exhibits relatively greater flow in the frontal areas of the brain, a phenomenon that has been referred to as a *hyperfrontal pattern*. An absence of sensory stimulation tends to diminish global rCBF and metabolism and accentuates the hyperfrontal pattern. However, rCBF and metabolism are quite sensitive to even mild sensory stimulation. For example, opening the eyes or turning on a light may cause marked occipital lobe activation. Normally, even subtle motor activity increases rCBF and glucose metabolism in the motor cortex of the contralateral hemisphere. The emotional state of the patient, particularly the level of anxiety, may alter patterns of cerebral activity in numerous ways.

Because the subjective experience of the resting state varies enormously between individuals, many investigators prefer to image during some type of sensory, motor, or cognitive stimulation that is more likely to be experienced in a common way across individuals. Moreover, sensorimotor and cognitive activation during imaging may increase the sensitivity for detecting subtle abnormalities of cerebral sensorimotor and cognitive systems in a manner analogous to the increased sensitivity of an electrocardiogram performed during treadmill exercise compared with that during rest. Paradigms have been designed to link cognitive tasks with activation of specific anatomic areas such as the Wisconsin Card Sorting Test (WCS; Heaton 1985) with the prefrontal cortex (PFC) and Raven's Progressive Matrices (Court 1977) with the parietal cortex.

Examples of trait factors that may alter the normal cerebral landscape include age, sex, and laterality of cerebral function. Some groups have reported a gradual decline in global CBF and glucose metabolism and diminution of the hyperfrontal pattern in normal aging (Matsuda et al. 1984; Shaw et al. 1984). Other groups have found no age effect or found that it disappears with cognitive challenge (Gur et al. 1987) or can be attributed to parallel changes in cerebral volume (Yoshii et al. 1988). Globally increased glucose metabolism (Baxter et al. 1987) and globally increased and more symmetrical rCBF have been reported in female patients compared with male patients (Rodriguez et al. 1988). Right- and left-handed persons may show differential laterality patterns of both cognitive and motor cerebral activation.

Research Findings

Organic mental disorders. The most replicated neuropsychiatric functional imaging findings are in disorders with relatively well-defined neuropathological or electrophysiological correlates, such as some forms of dementia and epilepsy. Both SPECT and PET have shown preliminary indications of adjunctive utility in the differential diagnosis of dementias (Figure 7–5). The decreased brain activity associated with cognitive deficits in dementia may be manifest in many ways, including decrements in rCBF, glucose metabolism, and neurotransmitter activity.

The patterns of distribution of these deficits appear to vary by illness. In Alzheimer's disease, extensive symmetrical parietal cortical deficits in uptake of the SPECT rCBF tracer iodine-123 IMP have been consistently observed (Cohen et al. 1986; Jagust et al. 1987; Johnson et al. 1987; Mueller et al. 1986) and appear to correlate with cognitive deficits. Among patients with Alzheimer's disease, the [^{18}F]-fluorodeoxyglucose (FDG) PET method has shown cerebral glucose metabolism to be globally reduced compared with that of age-matched control subjects. The deficits are typically most pronounced in the parietal cortex, followed by the temporal and to a lesser extent frontal cortices (Hoffman et al. 1989) and, unlike age-related findings in control subjects, persist after correction for cerebral atrophy and volume. Hypometabolic findings seem to be most pronounced in presenile-onset cases (Small et al. 1989) and correlate with cognitive deficits. In patients with mild memory dysfunction who later developed Alzheimer's disease, the ratio of glucose metabolic activity between the parietal lobe and caudate was significantly reduced before the development of absolute deficits in parietotemporal metabolism (Kuhl et al. 1987).

In another study of the very early stages of Alzheimer's disease, Haxby et al. (1990) found lateralized asymmetries in the association cortex that progressed as the dementia worsened longitudinally and predicted lateralizing neuropsychological deficits. In vivo imaging of muscarinic acetylcholine receptors may also be useful in the differential diagnosis of dementia with early indications using SPECT suggestive of relative diminished density of muscarinic acetylcholine receptors in the posterior temporal-inferior parietal area (Weinberger et al. 1991).

In Pick's disease and clinically related frontal dementia syndromes, deficits in rCBF, glucose metabolism, and muscarinic acetylcholine receptor density are suggestive of a lesion that is proportionately more anteriorly located than that seen in Alzheimer's disease. These findings mirror the characteristic pattern of cerebral atrophy. Multi-infarct dementia typically produces an irregular topographic pattern of rCBF and metabolic deficits. Although disparate functional imaging findings have been reported in depressive disorders (Chabrol et al. 1986; Sackeim et al. 1990; Silfverskiöld 1989), the so-called pseudodementia sometimes associated with major depression is not associated with a consistent pattern of metabolic or rCBF deficits. In Huntington's disease diminished caudate glucose metabolism is characteristic, but cortical metabolism is only slightly diminished, even in early cases.

In Parkinson's disease, progressive supranuclear palsy, and striatal-nigral degeneration, neuropathological findings are predominantly subcortical with relative sparing of the cortex, yet the most prominent functional imaging finding is hypometabolism of the frontal cortex, possibly because of loss of normal afferent activity. Moreover, deficits

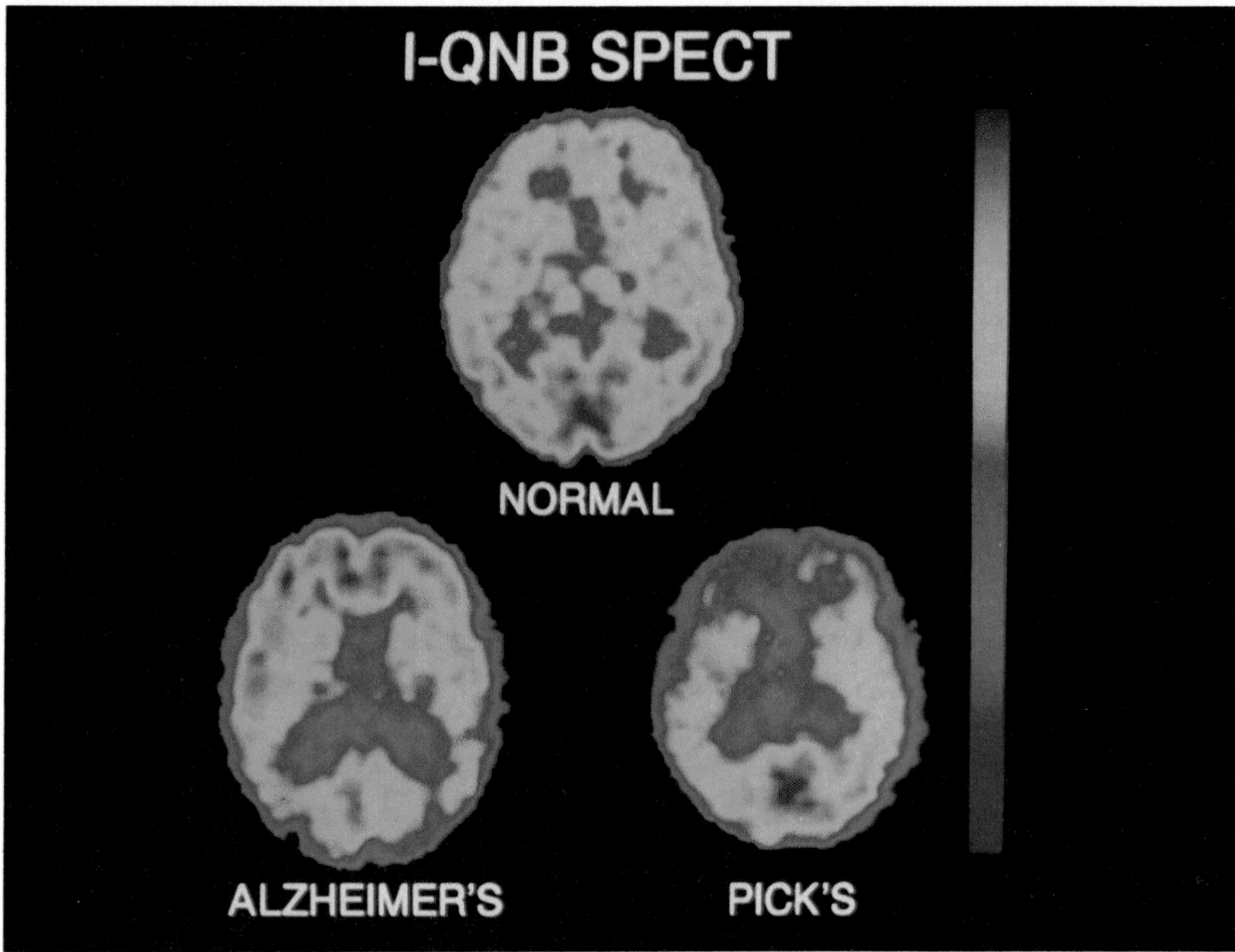

Figure 7–5. Iodine-123–labeled 3-quinuclidinyl-4-iodobenzilate ([^{123}I]QNB [I-QNB; *in figure*]) single photon emission computed tomography (SPECT) scans of a control subject (normal) and patients with clinical diagnoses of Alzheimer's disease and Pick's disease. [^{123}I]QNB labels muscarinic acetylcholine receptors. The color scale is keyed to percentage receptor occupancy with warmer colors corresponding to greater relative receptor occupancy. Note the relatively posterior temporoparietal pattern of defects in the patient with Alzheimer's disease and the predominantly frontal anterior temporal pattern of defects in the patient with Pick's disease.

in striatal dopamine formation and storage (Leenders et al. 1988) and in density of dopamine receptors in the caudate (Nahmias et al. 1985) have also been reported. Sporadic reports of parkinsonian patients with dementia having metabolic or rCBF deficits similar to the parietotemporal pattern seen in Alzheimer's disease may reflect comorbidity of the two disorders. Investigations of metabolic activity and rCBF in the striatum where dopaminergic deficits are thought to be most pronounced have not yielded consistent findings, nor have attempts to correlate striatal metabolism with clinical motor function in Parkinson's disease. In Parkinson's disease metabolic deficits have generally not been correctable by levodopa (L-dopa), suggesting that the metabolic deficits are not state dependent on dopaminergic neurotransmitter levels.

Seizure disorders have been associated with a number of rCBF and metabolic patterns both ictally and interictally that may aid in localization of focal abnormalities (Figure 7–6) even when the EEG findings are inconclusive (Theodore et al. 1983). In the ictal state, rCBF and metabolism are increased at the site from which the seizure originates and then

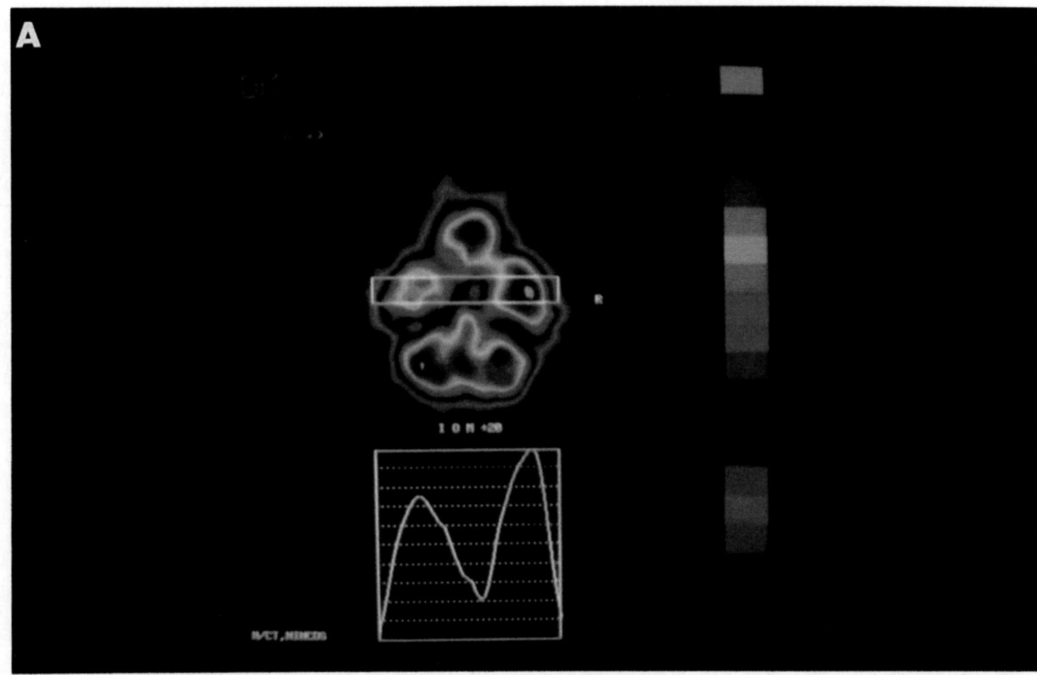

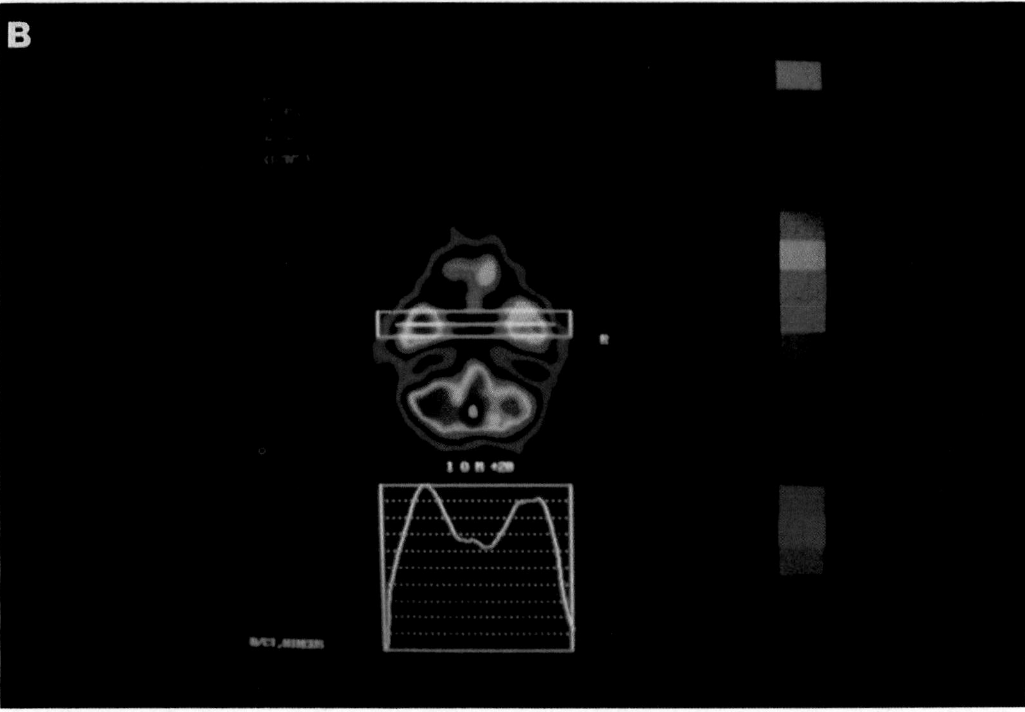

Figure 7–6. Interictal [^{18}F]fluorodeoxyglucose (FDG) positron-emission tomography (PET) scan illustrating a hypometabolic area of 23% in the left temporal region of a patient with partial complex seizures confirmed by mid-temporal epileptiform discharges seen on electroencephalography (*panel A*). In contrast, an ictal PET scan from the same patient illustrates hypermetabolic activity of 9% in the left temporal region (*panel B*). The color scale is keyed to the glucose utilization rate with the warmer colors indicating relatively higher rates of glucose utilization. (Courtesy of W.H. Theodore and associates, National Institute of Neurological Diseases and Strokes, Bethesda, Maryland.)

propagate outward. Interictally the seizure focus usually shows deficits in rCBF and metabolism. These findings help in localization of epileptogenic foci for surgical excision and alleviate the need for implantation of depth electrodes.

Schizophrenia. The most commonly examined issues in PET studies of schizophrenia to date are 1) global, anteroposterior, and lateralizing patterns of cerebral rCBF and metabolism and 2) dopamine, subtype 2 (D_2), receptor affinity and density.

Studies of rCBF and glucose metabolic patterns in schizophrenia have provided inconsistent findings in large part because of variations in patient experience and state. However, when imaging is performed during performance of a cognitive task that activates the prefrontal cortex of normal controls, deficits in prefrontal cortex rCBF and metabolism in schizophrenic patients are identified much more consistently (Figure 7–7). For example, in a recent study of 10 pairs of monozygotic twin pairs discordant for schizophrenia (Berman et al., in press). the ill twin demonstrated less PFC rCBF activation than the well twin in 10 of 10 cases, suggesting that metabolic hypofrontality in schizophrenia is at least partially nongenetic in origin and is a consistent finding when interindividual variation is properly controlled for.

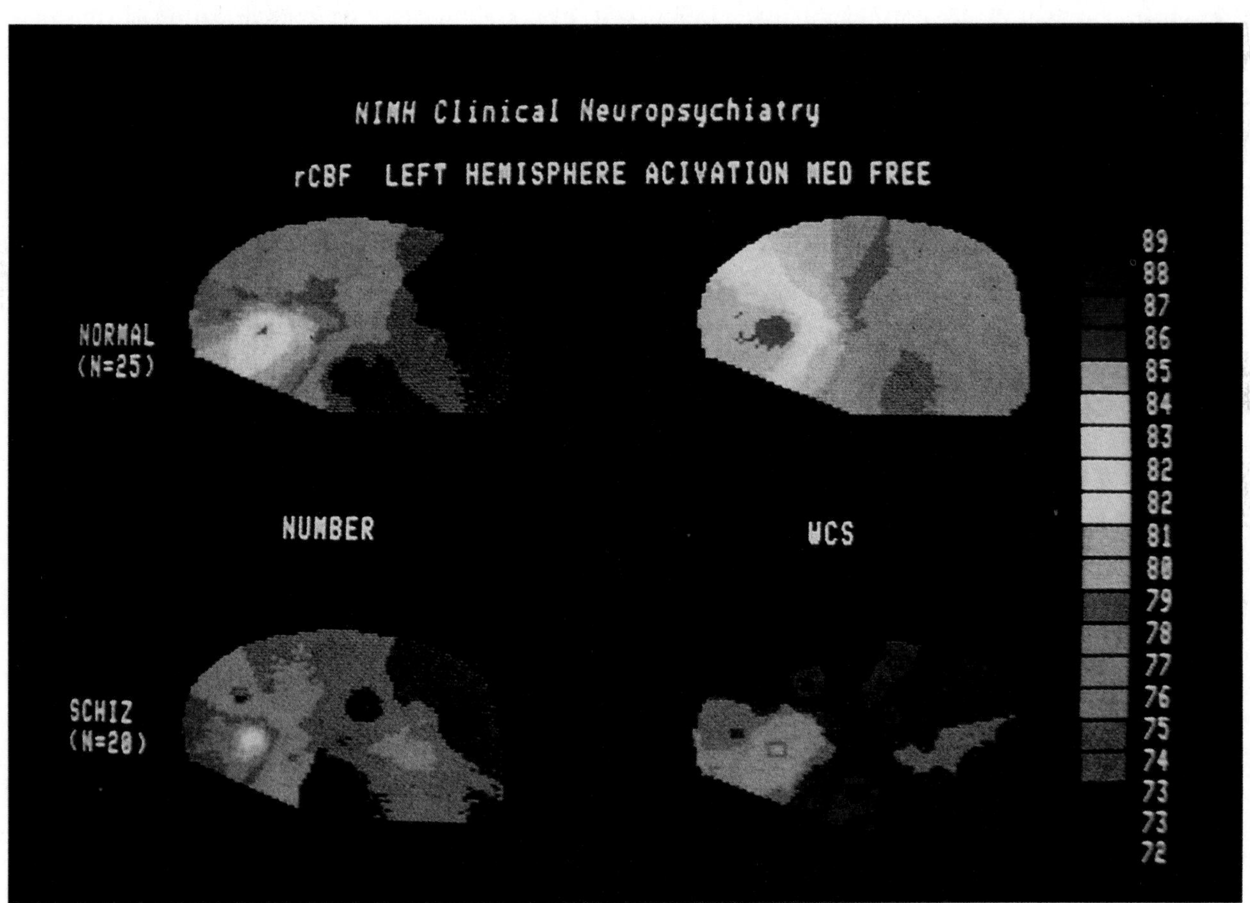

Figure 7–7. Composite topographic gray-matter group mean regional cerebral blood flow (rCBF) maps illustrating lateral views of the cerebral cortex with the anterior pole pointing to the left. The color scale is keyed to rCBF with warmer colors indicating higher flow. The upper panels illustrate activation of rCBF in the prefrontal cortex (PFC) in control subjects (normal) during performance of a prefrontal-linked cognitive task (*right*) compared to a control task (*left*). The *lower panels* indicate lack of PFC activation in schizophrenic patients. WCS = Wisconsin Card Sorting Test (Heaton 1985).

There are inconsistent reports of an elevated ratio of left-hemisphere to right-hemisphere rCBF and metabolism in schizophrenia. The weight of evidence does not support globally decreased rCBF or metabolism in schizophrenia. Attempts to link clinical phenomenology in schizophrenia and PET findings have not been replicated with consistency. Preliminary evidence suggests that metabolic hypofrontality and lower global metabolism may be associated with deficit syndromes (Volkow et al. 1987). The evidence across techniques for a neuroleptic effect on rCBF and cerebral glucose metabolism is contradictory and inconclusive. Figure 7–8 illustrates changes in basal ganglia metabolism with neuroleptics.

The dopamine hypothesis of the pathophysiology of schizophrenia has generated considerable interest in the measurement of dopamine receptor density (B_{max}) and affinity (K_d) in schizophrenia, particularly in patients not previously exposed to the potentially receptor-altering activity of neuroleptics. Figure 7–9 illustrates the use of PET to map the distribution of dopamine, subtype 1 (D_1), and D_2 receptors in the brain (Farde et al. 1989). Although Wong et al. (1986) found two- to threefold higher dopamine receptor density in the caudate of a group of drug-naive patients with schizophrenia, such changes were not detected in several other reports (Farde et al. 1990; Herold et al. 1985; Martinot et al. 1990). An unconfirmed report suggested relatively higher B_{max} values in the left than in the right putamen in schizophrenic patients but not in control subjects (Farde et al. 1990).

Mood disorders. There are few consistent independently verified findings in mood disorders, both due to the modest number of investigations and variation in methodology. One PET finding in mood disorders that has been independently replicated is reduced generalized global metabolism, possibly greatest in the left frontal cortex (Baxter et al. 1989; Martinot et al. 1990). The cyclic nature of most affective disorders permits each subject to serve as his or her own control for possible differentiation of the pathophysiology of euthymic, depressive, and manic states. For example, using PET, mood-dependent variations have been reported in left-right prefrontal asymmetry of glucose metabolism and in

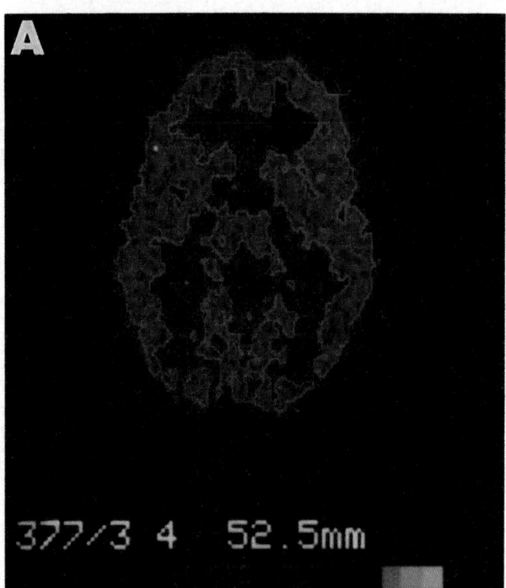

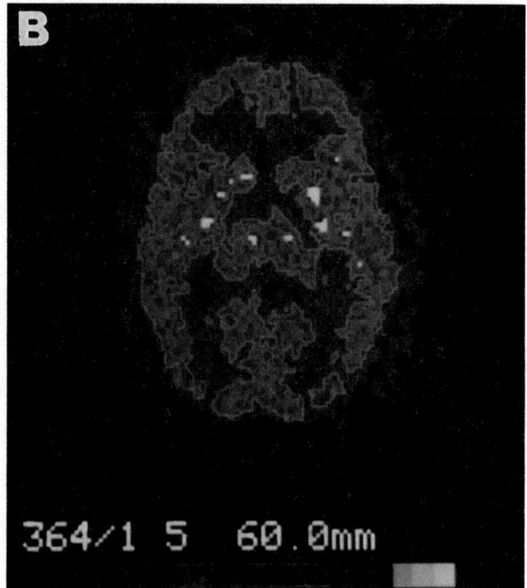

Figure 7–8. [^{18}F]fluorodeoxyglucose (FDG) positron-emission tomography (PET) scan at the level of the caudate-putamen in a drug-free schizophrenic patient (*panel A*) and the same patient after chronic treatment with neuroleptic (fluphenazine) (*panel B*). The color scale is keyed to glucose metabolic activity with the warmer colors indicating relatively higher activity. Note the increase in metabolic activity in the caudate and putamen nuclei after chronic neuroleptic treatment. (Courtesy of D. Pickar and associates, National Institute of Mental Health, Bethesda, Maryland.)

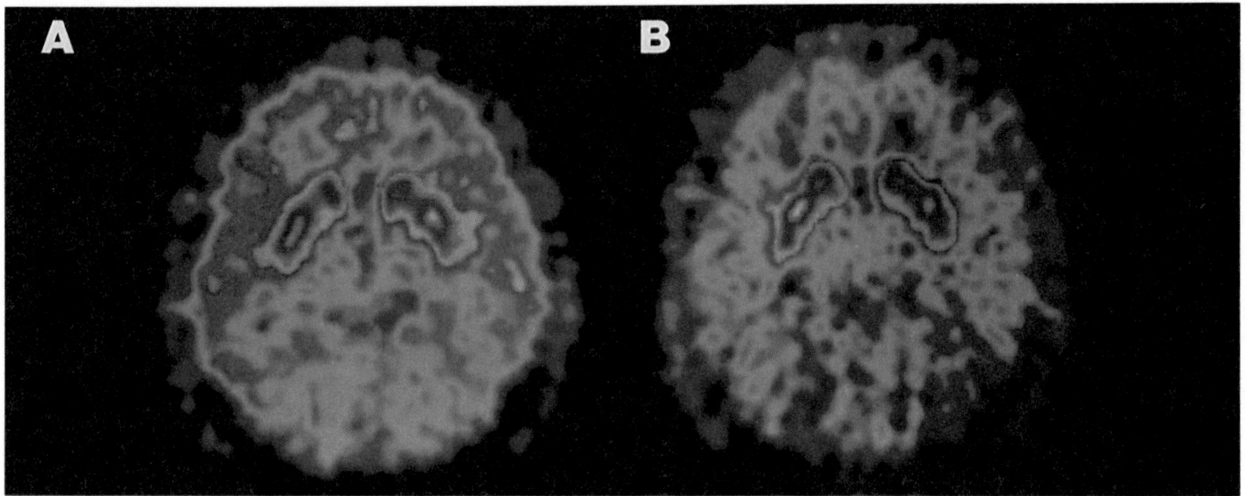

Figure 7–9. Positron-emission tomography (PET) scan at the level of the caudate-putamen after injection of 100 MBq [^{11}C]SCH23390 (*panel A*) and 100 MBq [^{11}C]raclopride (*panel B*) in a patient with schizophrenia. [^{11}C]SCH23390 (*panel A*) labels dopamine, subtype 1 (D_1), receptors, whereas, [^{11}C]raclopride (*panel B*) labels dopamine, subtype 2 (D_2), receptors. The color scale is keyed to percent receptor occupancy with the warmer colors indicating relatively higher occupancy. In both scans the caudate and putamen nuclei are prominently labeled. (Courtesy of L. Farde and associates, Karolinska Institute, Stockholm.)

cortical levels of amino acids (Kishimoto et al. 1987; Martinot et al. 1990). The potential of PET for in vivo measurement of neurotransmitter-receptor binding in mood disorders has only barely been broached. In an early application of this technique in stroke patients, the ratio of ipsilateral to contralateral serotonin receptor, subtype 2, binding predicted the severity of depressive symptoms in patients with left-hemispheric lesions (Mayberg et al. 1988).

Other psychiatric disorders. Anticipatory anxiety and lactate-induced panic are robustly associated with bilateral increases in activity of the anterior temporal poles (Nordahl et al. 1990; Reiman et al. 1986, 1989a, 1989b). In obsessive-compulsive disorder findings of elevated metabolism in both the caudate nucleus (Baxter et al. 1988; Swedo et al. 1989) and frontal orbital cortex (Baxter et al. 1988; Nordahl et al. 1989; Swedo et al. 1989) may explain why surgical procedures that disconnect the prefrontal cortex from the caudate (i.e., leukotomy) sometimes are clinically effective for these patients.

Functional imaging investigations of other neuropsychiatric disorders including transient global amnesia, Down's syndrome, autism, Tourette's syndrome, eating disorders, drug abuse, and alcoholism have been performed but for the most part have not received independent verification and are considered inconclusive.

Summary of Clinical Applications

When should a psychiatrist order a functional imaging scan? At present there is no accepted clinical indication for performing either a 2-D rCBF, SPECT, or PET scan on the brain. Furthermore, although rCBF and cerebral glucose metabolism findings in epilepsy, Alzheimer's disease, and Huntington's disease are as close to clinically useful findings as have yet emerged, the frequency of false positives and false negatives has not yet been firmly established.

❑ CONCLUSIONS

Dramatic technologies for the noninvasive study of the anatomy and biochemistry of the living human brain now exist. These techniques are tailored to the task of associating disorders of behavior and cognition with identifiable neurobiological pathology. The primary applicability of these techniques (at their current state of evolution) is as a research tool.

However, ultimately, as methodological limitations are overcome and a sufficient data base is accumulated, their clinical applicability will likely increase. Currently, the primary clinical usefulness of available imaging techniques is to rule out nonpsychiatric etiologies of behavioral and cognitive disorders. This is accomplished with MRI and CT.

❑ REFERENCES

Baxter LR, Mazziotta JC, Phelps ME, et al: Cerebral glucose metabolic rates in normal human females versus normal males. Psychiatry Res 21:237–245, 1987

Baxter LR, Swartz JM, Mazziotta JC: Cerebral glucose metabolic rates in nondepressed patients with obsessive-compulsive disorder. Am J Psychiatry 145:1560–1563, 1988

Baxter LR, Swartz JM, Phelps ME, et al: Reduction of prefrontal cortex glucose metabolism common in three types of depression. Arch Gen Psychiatry 46:243–250, 1989

Berman KF, Torrey EF, Daniel DG, et al: Regional cerebral blood flow in monozygotic twins discordant and concordant for schizophrenia. Arch Gen Psychiatry (in press)

Besson JAO: Magnetic resonance imaging and its applications in neuropsychiatry. Br J Pscyhiatry 157 (suppl 9):25–37, 1990

Bogerts B, Ashtari M, DeGreef G, et al: Reduced temporal limbic structure volumes on magnetic resonance images in first episode schizophrenia. Psychiatry Res 35: 1–3, 1990

Bondareff W, Raval J, Colletti PM, et al: Quantative magnetic resonance imaging (MRI) and severity of dementia in Alzheimer's disease. Am J Psychiatry 145:853–858, 1988

Bottomley PA: Human in vivo NMR spectroscopy in diagnostic medicine: clinical tool or research probe? Radiology 170:1–15, 1989

Braffman BH, Grossman RI, Goldberg HI, et al: MR imaging of Parkinson's disease with spin-echo and gradient-echo sequences. American Journal of Neuroradiology 9:1093–1099, 1988

Bridge TP, Parker ES, Ingraham L, et al: Gender effects seen in the cerebral ventricular/brain ratio (VBR). Biol Psychiatry 20:1132–1136, 1985

Brown GG, Levine SR, Gorell JM, et al: In vivo 31 P NMR profiles of Alzheimer's disease and multiple subcortical infarct dementia. Neurology 39:1423–1427, 1989

Brownell GL, Budinger TF, Lauterbur PC, et al: Positron tomography and nuclear magnetic resonance imaging. Science 215:619–626, 1982

Casanova MF, Godberg TE, Suddath RL, et al: Quantitative shape analysis of the temporal and prefrontal lobes of schizophrenic patients: a magnetic resonance imaging study. Journal of Neuropsychiatry and Clinical Neurosciences 2:363–372, 1990

Chabrol H, Barrere M, Gwell A, et al: Hyperfrontality of cerebral blood flow in depressed adolescents. Am J Psychiatry 143:263–264, 1986

Coffey CE, Figiel GS, Djang WT, et al: Leukoencephalopathy in elderly depressed patients referred for ECT. Biol Psychiatry 24:143–161, 1988

Coffey CE, Figiel GS, Djang WT, et al: Subcortical hyperintensity on magnetic resonance imaging: a comparison of normal and depressed elderly subjects. Am J Psychiatry 147:187–189, 1990

Cohen MB, Graham LS, Lake R, et al: Diagnosis of Alzheimer's disease and multiple infarct dementia by tomographic imaging of iodine-123 IMP. J Nucl Med 27:769–774, 1986

Comar D, Zarifian E, Verhas M, et al: Brain distribution and kinetics of 11-C-Chlorpromazine in schizophrenics: positron emission tomography studies. Psychiatry Res 1:23–29, 1979

Court JH: Researcher's Bibliography for Raven's Progressive Matrices and Mill Hall Vocabulary Scales, 4th Edition. Bedford Park, Australia, Flinders University of South Australia, 1977

Dandy WE: Roentgenography of the brain after injection of air into the spinal cord. Ann Surg 70:397–403, 1919

Daniel DG, Weinberger DR: Ex multi uno: a case for neurobiological homogeneity in schizophrenia, in Advances in Neuropsychiatry and Psychopharmacology, Vol I: Schizophrenia Research. Edited by Tamminga CA, Schulz SC. New York, Raven, 1991, pp 227–235

Daniel DG, Goldberg TE, Gibbons R, et al: Lack of a bimodal distribution of ventricular size in schizophrenia: a Gaussian mixture analysis of 1056 cases and controls. Biol Psychiatry, (in press)

Dewan MJ, Haldipur CV, Lane EE, et al: Bipolar affective disorder, I: comprehensive quantitative computed tomography. Acta Psychiatr Scand 77:670–676, 1988

Dolan RJ, Mitchell J, Wakeling A: Structural brain changes in patients with anorexia nervosa. Psychol Med 18:349–353, 1988

Drayer BP: Magnetic resonance imaging and brain iron: implications in the diagnosis and pathochemistry of movement disorders and dementia. Barrow Neurological Initiative Quarterly 3:15–30, 1987

Dupont Rm, Jernigan Tl, Butters N, et al: Subcortical abnormalities detected in bipolar affective disorder using magnetic resonance imaging. Arch Gen Psychiatry 47: 55–60, 1990

Erkinjuntti T, Ketonen L, Sulkava R, et al: Do white matter changes on MRI and CT differentiate vascular dementia from Alzheimer's disease. J Neurol Neurosurg Psychiatry 50:37–42, 1987

Falkai P, Bogerts B, Rozumek M: Limbic pathology in schizophrenia: the entorhinal region: a morphometric study. Biol Psychiatry 24:515–521, 1988

Farde L, Wiesel FA, Nordstrom A-L, et al: D1- and D2-dopamine receptor occupancy during treatment with conventional and atypical neuroleptics. Psychopharmacology 99:S28–S31, 1989

Farde L, Wiesel F-A, Stone-Elander S, et al: D2 dopamine receptors in neuroleptic-naive schizophrenic patients: a positron emission tomography study with [C11] raclopride. Arch Gen Psychiatry 47:213–219, 1990

Fullerton GD, Potter JL: Computed tomography, in Textbook of Diagnostic Imaging. Edited by Putman CE, Ravin CE. Philadelphia, PA, WB Saunders, 1988, pp 47–60

Gur RC, Gur RE, Obrist WD, et al: Age in regional cerebral blood flow at rest and during cognitive activity. Arch Gen Psychiatry 44:617–621, 1987

Haug G: Age and sex dependence of the size of normal ventricles on computed tomography. Neuroradiology 14:201–204, 1977

Haxby JV, Grady CL, Coss E: Longitudinal study of cerebral metabolic asymmetries in associated neuropsychological patterns in early dementia of the Alzheimer's type. Arch Neurol 47:753–760, 1990

Heaton R: Wisconsin Card Sorting Test. Odessa, TX, Psychological Assessment Resources, 1985

Herold S, Leenders KL, Turton DR, et al: Dopamine receptor binding in schizophrenic patients as measured with [C11] methylspiperone and PET. J Cereb Blood Flow Metab 5 (suppl 1):S191–S192, 1985

Hoffman GW, Ellinwood EH, Rockwell WJK, et al: Cerebral atrophy in anorexia nervosa: a pilot study. Biol Psychiatry 26:321–324, 1989

Hoffman JM, Guze BH, Baxter LR, et al: 18F Fluorodeoxyglucose (FDG) and positron emission tomography (PET) in aging and dementia. Eur Neurol 29 (suppl 3):16–24, 1989

Hounsfield GN: Computerized transverse axial scanning (tomography), I: description of system. Br J Radiol 46: 1016–1022, 1973

Iacono WG, Smith GN, Moreau M, et al: Ventricular and sulcal size at the onset of psychosis. Am J Psychiatry 145:820–824, 1988

Illowsky BP, Juliano DM, Bigelow LB, et al: Stability of CT scan findings in schizophrenia: results of an 8 year follow-up study. J Neurol Neurosurg Psychiatry 51: 209–213, 1988

Jack CR, Sharbrough FW, Twomey CK, et al: Temporal lobe seizures: lateralization with MR volume measurements of the hippocampal formation. Radiology 175: 423–429, 1990

Jacobi W, Winkler H: Encephalographische studien an chronisch schizophrenen. Archiv für Psychiatrie und Nervenkrankheiten 81:299–332, 1927

Jagust WJ, Buddinger TF, Reed BR: Diagnosis of dementia with single photon emission computed tomography. Arch Neurol 44:258–262, 1987

Johnson KA, Mueller St, Walshe TM, et al: Cerebral perfusion imaging in Alzheimer's disease: use of single photon emission computed tomography and iofetamine hydrochloride I-123. Arch Neurol 44:165–168, 1987

Johnstone EC, Crow TJ, Frith CD, et al: Cererbral ventricular size and cognitive impairment in chronic schizophrenia. Lancet 2:924–926, 1976

Johnstone EC, Owens DGC, Crow TJ, et al: Temporal lobe structure as determined by nuclear magnetic resonance in schizophrenia and bipolar affective disorder. Journal of Neurology, Neurosurgery, and Psychiatry 52:736–741, 1989

Keller PJ: Basic Principles of Magnetic Resonance Imaging. Milwaukee, WI, General Electric, 1990

Kelly GR, Jackson JA, Leake DR, et al: CT versus NMR imaging of multiple sclerosis. American Journal of Neuroradiology 4:1136, 1983

Kety SS, Woodford RB, Harmel MH, et al: Cerebral blood flow in metabolism in schizophrenia: effects of barbiturate seminarcosis, insulin, and electroshock. Am J Psychiatry 104:765–770, 1948

Kishimoto H, Takazu O, Ohno S, et al: C11-glucose metabolism in manic and depressed patients. Psychiatry Res 22:81–88, 1987

Kreig JC, Lauer C, Pirke KM: Hormonal and metabolic mechanisms in the development of cerebral pseudoatrophy in eating disorders. Psychosom Med 48:176–180, 1987

Kuhl DE, Small GW, Riege WH, et al: Cerebral metabolic patterns before the diagnosis of probable Alzheimer's disease. J Cereb Blood Flow Metab 7:S406, 1987

Lankenau H, Swigar ME, Bhimani S, et al: Cranial CT scans in eating disorder patients and controls. Compr Psychiatry 26:136–147, 1985

Leenders KL, Frackowiak RS, Lees AJ: Steele-Richardson-Olszewski syndrome: brain energy metabolism, blood flow and fluorodopa uptake measured by positron emission tomography. Brain 111 (part 3):615–630, 1988

Martinot J-L, Peron-Magnan P, Huret JD, et al: Striatal D2 dopaminergic receptors assessed with positron emission tomography [76Br] bromospiperone in untreated schizophrenic patients. Am J Psychiatry 147:44–50, 1990

Matsuda H, Maeda T, Masato Y, et al: Age-matched normal values in topographic maps for regional cerebral blood flow measurements by xenon-133 inhalation. Stroke 15:336–342, 1984

Mayberg HS, Robinson RG, Wong MD, et al: PET imaging of cortical S2 serotonin receptors after stroke: lateralized changes and relationship to depression. Am J Psychiatry 145:937–943, 1988

Meese W, Kluge W, Grumme T, et al: CT evaluation of CSF spaces of healthy persons. Neuroradiology 19:131–136, 1980

Mueller SP, Johnson KA, Hamil D, et al: Assessment of I-123 IMP SPECT in mild/moderate Alzheimer's disease. J Nucl Med 27:889, 1986

Nahmias C, Garnett ES, Firnau G, et al: Striatal dopamine distribution in parkinsonian patients during life. J Neurol Sci 69:223–230, 1985

Niendorf HP, Dinger JC, Haustein J, et al: Tolerance of Gd-DTPA: clinical experience, in Contrast Media in MRI. Edited by Dinger JC, Bydder G, Bucheler E, et al. Berlin, Medicom, 1990, pp 31–39

Nordahl TE, Benkelfat C, Semple WE, et al: Cerebral glucose metabolic rates in obsessive-compulsive disorder. Neuropsychopharmacology 2:23–28, 1989

Nordahl TE, Semple WE, Gross M, et al: Cerebral glucose metabolic differences in patients with panic disorder. Neuropsychopharmacology 3:261–272, 1990

Phelps ME, Mazziotta JC, Huang S-C: Study of cerebral function with positron computed tomography. J Cereb Blood Flow Metab 2:113–162, 1982

Rao SM, Leo GJ, Houghton VM, et al: Correlation of magnetic resonance imaging with neuropsychological testing in multiple sclerosis. Neurology 39:161–166, 1989

Reiman EM, Faichle ME, Robins E, et al: The application of positron emission tomography to the study of panic disorder. Am J Psychiatry 143:469–477, 1986

Reiman EM, Fusselman MJ, Fox PT, et al: Neuroanatomical correlates of anticipatory anxiety. Science 243:1071–1074, 1989a

Reiman EM, Raichle ME, Robins E, et al: Neuroanatomical correlates of lactate-induced anxiety attack. Arch Gen Psychiatry 46:493–500, 1989b

Reveley Am, Reveley MA, Clifford CA, et al: Cerebral ventricular size in twins discordant for schizophrenia. Lancet 1:540–541, 1982

Rodriguez G, Warkentin S, Risberg J, et al: Sex differences in cerebral blood flow. J Cereb Blood Flow Metab 8: 783–789, 1988

Ross JS, Masaryk TJ, Modic MT, et al: Magnetic resonance angiography of the extracranial carotid arteries and intracranial vessels: a review. Neurology 39:1369–1376, 1989

Sackeim HA, Prohovnik I, Moeller JR, et al: Regional cerebral blood flow in mood disorders, I: comparison of major depressives and normal controls at rest. Arch Gen Psychiatry 47:60–70, 1990

Shaw TG, Mortel KF, Meyue JS, et al: Cerebral blood flow changes in benign aging and cerebral vascular disease. Neurology 34:855–862, 1984

Shelton RC, Weinberger DR: X-ray computerized tomography studies in schizophrenia: a review and synthesis, in Handbook of Schizophrenia. Edited by Nasrallah HA, Weinberger DR. Amsterdam, Elsevier Science, 1986, pp 207–250

Silfverskiöld P, Risberg J: Regional cerebral blood flow in depression and mania. Arch Gen Psychiatry 46:253–259, 1989

Small GW, Kuhl DE, Riege WH, et al: Cerebral glucose metabolic patterns in Alzheimer's disease: effect of gender and age at dementia onset. Arch Gen Psychiatry 46:527–532, 1989

Suddath RL, Christison GW, Torrey EF, et al: Anatomical abnormalities in the brains of monozygotic twins discordant for schizophrenia. N Engl J Med 322:789–794, 1990

Swayze VW, Andreasen NC, Alliger RJ, et al: Structural brain abnormalities in bipolar affective disorder. Arch Gen Psychiarty 47:1054–1059, 1990

Swedo SE, Schapiro MB, Grady CL, et al: Cerebral glucose metabolism in childhood onset obsessive-compulsive disorder. Arch Gen Psychiatry 46:518–523, 1989

Theodore WH, Newmark ME, Sato S, et al: [18F]Fluorodeoxyglucose positron emisssion tomography in refractory partial seizures. Ann Neurol 14:429–437, 1983

Volkow ND, Wolf AP, Gelder PV, et al: Phenomenological correlates of metabolic activity in 18 patients with chronic schizophrenia. Am J Psychiatry 144:151–158, 1987

Weinberger DR: Brain disease and psychiatric illness: when should a psychiatrist order a CAT scan? Am J Psychiatry 141:1521–1527, 1984

Weinberger DR, DeLisi LE, Perman G, et al: Computed tomography scans in schizophreniform disorder and other acute psychiatric patients. Arch Gen Psychiatry 39:778–783, 1982

Weinberger DR, Gibson R, Coppola R, et al: The distribution of cerebral muscarinic acetyl-choline receptors in vivo in patients with dementia: a controlled study with I-123 QNB and SPECT. Arch Neurol 48:169–176, 1991

Willoughby EW, Grochowski E, Li DKB, et al: Serial magnetic resonance scanning in multiple sclerosis: a second prospective study in relapsing patients. Ann Neurol 25:43–49, 1989

Wong DF, Wagner HN, Tone LE, et al: Positron emission tomography reveals elevated D2 dopamine receptors in drug naive schizophrenics. Science 234:1558–1562, 1986

Yoshii F, Barker WW, Chang JY, et al: Sensitivity of cerebral glucose metabolism to age, gender, brain volume, brain atrophy, and cerebrovascular risk factors. J Cereb Blood Flow Metab 8:654–661, 1988

Zatz LM, Jernigan TL, Ahumada AJ: Changes on computed cranial tomography with aging: intracranial fluid volume. American Journal of Neuroradiology 3: 1–11 1982

Zigun JR, Weinberger DRW: In vivo studies of brain morphology in schizophrenia, in New Biological Vistas on Schizophrenia. Edited by Lindenmayerand J-P, Stanley RK. New York, Brunner/Mazel (in press)

Chapter

8

Epidemiology and Genetics of Neuropsychiatric Disorders

Dolores Malaspina, M.D.
H. Matthew Quitkin, A.B.
Charles A. Kaufmann, M.D.

FROM THE TIME OF HIPPOCRATES, clinicians have suspected roles for both exogenous and endogenous factors in the etiology of disease (Lyons and Petrucelli 1987). During the past century, the powerful techniques of epidemiology and genetics have enabled us to identify specific environmental and hereditary contributions to illness. In this chapter we focus on the application of these disciplines to the study of neuropsychiatric disorders.

The authors express their thanks to Megan Harris. This work was supported in part by an National Institute of Mental Health Schizophrenia Academic Award K07MH00824 (to DM), a Physician Scientist Award K11MH00682 (to CAK), a Stanley Scholar Award (to HMQ), and by the WM Keck Foundation.

❑ INTRODUCTION

Epidemiological Studies

Epidemiology is based on the fundamental assumption that factors causal to human disease can be identified through the systematic examination of different populations, or of subgroups within a population, in different places or at different times (Hennekens and Buring 1987). Epidemiological research may be viewed as directed at a series of questions: What is the frequency of a disorder? Are there subgroups in which the disorder is more frequent? What specific risk factors are associated with the disorder? Are these risk factors consistently and specifically related to the disorder? Does exposure to these factors precede the development of disease? A variety of epidemiological strategies have been developed to address these questions (Table 8–1).

Measures of Disease Frequency

Measures of disease frequency serve as the basis for formulating and testing etiologic hypotheses because they permit a comparison of frequencies between different populations or among individuals within a population with particular exposures or characteristics. The two measures of disease frequency used most often are prevalence and incidence. Prevalence refers to the number of existing cases of a disease at a given point in time, as a proportion of the total population. Incidence refers to the number of new cases of a disease during a given period of time, as a proportion of the total population at risk. The two measures are interrelated: prevalence of a disease depends on both its incidence and duration. One can compare two populations with and without a factor suspected of contributing to the development of disease through the calculation of the ratio of disease frequency in the two populations; this is known as the *relative risk.*

Descriptive Studies

Correlational studies of populations and descriptive studies of single individuals or groups of individuals also contribute to formulating etiologic hypotheses by demonstrating a statistical association between exposure to specific risk factors and occurrence of disease. Hypotheses regarding risk factors may emerge from studying various characteristics of affected individuals (e.g., gender, age, and birth cohort), their place of residence, or the timing of their exposure. Descriptive studies, however, cannot be used to test etiologic hypotheses: they lack adequate comparison groups, making it difficult to determine the specificity of exposure to the disease, and they are cross-sectional, making it difficult to determine the temporal relationship between an exposure and the development of disease.

Analytic Studies

Etiologic hypotheses may be tested through various analytic strategies. These include case-control studies that compare exposure to a risk factor in individuals with a disease ("cases") with that in appropriate control subjects, as well as cohort studies that (retrospectively or prospectively) follow up groups of exposed individuals for development of disease.

Genetic Studies

Genetic research may be considered the subset of epidemiological research concerned with the contribution of inherited factors to the development of disease. It, too, may be conceptualized as directed at a series of questions: Is the disorder familial? Is it inherited? What is being inherited in the disorder (i.e., what constitutes predisposition to the disorder and what are the earliest manifestations of such predisposition)? What additional ("epigenetic") variables increase or decrease the chances of genetically predisposed individuals developing the disorder? How is the disorder inherited? Where, and what, are the abnormal genes conferring genetic risk? What are the molecular, and ultimately the pathological, consequences of these abnormal genes? Various genetic strategies have been developed to address these questions (Table 8–2).

TABLE 8–1. THE EPIDEMIOLOGY OF NEUROPSYCHIATRIC DISORDERS—QUESTIONS AND STRATEGIES

Question	*Strategy*
What is the frequency of a disorder? Are there subgroups in which the disorder is more frequent?	Measures of disease frequency
What specific risk factors are associated with the disorder?	Descriptive studies
Are these risk factors consistently and specifically related to the disorder? Does exposure to these factors precede development of disease?	Analytic studies

TABLE 8–2. THE GENETICS OF NEUROPSYCHIATRIC DISORDERS—QUESTIONS AND STRATEGIES

Question	*Strategy*
Is the disorder familial?	Family studies
Is it inherited?	Twin studies Adoption studies
What is being inherited in the disorder? What "epigenetic" factors influence development of the disorder?	High-risk studies
How is the disorder inherited?	Segregation analysis Pedigree analysis
Where is (are) the abnormal gene(s)?	Linkage analysis
What is the abnormal gene? What is its molecular and pathological effect?	Molecular approaches

Family, Twin, and Adoption Studies

Family studies are a specific type of relative risk study. They can demonstrate an elevated risk for an illness in first-degree relatives of an affected individual compared with that in the general population (Table 8–3), but cannot distinguish if this elevated risk is due primarily to shared genetic or environmental factors. Other strategies, including twin and adoption studies, can further resolve the genetic contribution to the etiology of a disorder.

Although exposed to the same familial environment, monozygotic (MZ) and dizygotic (DZ) twin pairs differ in their genetic endowment (sharing 100% and 50% of their genes, respectively). When genetic factors are important in etiology, the MZ and DZ co-twins of probands will differ in their risk for the disorder. One can measure the heritability of a disorder by comparing the relative concordance rates for MZ and DZ twins. Heritability refers to the proportion of variability that can be attributed to genetic, as opposed to environmental and stochastic, factors.

Adoption studies are particularly useful in research of psychiatric disorders, for which cultural vertical transmission might allow for familial clustering of behaviors. Four varieties of adoption studies have been applied: 1) the adoptee study, 2) the cross-fostering study, 3) the adoptee's family study, and 4) the study of MZ twins reared apart. The adoptee study method compares offspring separated from their affected mothers at birth with the adopted-away offspring of control mothers. This can be considered a special form of cohort study. Cross-fostering studies contrast rates of illness among adoptees with biologic parents without illness, reared by both affected and unaffected adoptive parents. In the adoptee's family study method, the biologic relatives of affected adoptees are matched to the biologic relatives of control adoptees, and their rates of illness are compared. Such studies are examples of the case-control paradigm.

High-Risk Studies

The high-risk approach represents another form of cohort study. Individuals at genetic risk for a disorder (e.g., those with affected parents) are followed prospectively, from early in life through the period of maximum risk for the disorder (Watt et al. 1984). This strategy permits the identification of features that are of primary pathogenic significance to the disorder, in contrast to those that are secondary to the illness or to its treatment. Moreover, by contrasting characteristics of at-risk individuals who go on to develop the disorder with characteristics of those who do not, this strategy allows for the identification of additional genetic and environmental influences that contribute to disease expression.

Identifying the Mode of Inheritance

Even when family, twin, and adoption studies suggest a role for genetic factors, they say nothing of

TABLE 8–3. RELATIVE RISK FOR NEUROPSYCHIATRIC DISORDERS

Disease	*Population prevalence per 100,000*	*Morbid risk in first-degree relatives (%)*	*Relative risk*
Gerstmann-Straüssler syndrome	0.01	50	5,000,000
Acute intermittent porphyria	2	50	25,000
Metachromatic leukodystrophy	2.5	25–50	20,000
Myotonic dystrophy	5.5	50	9,090
Narcolepsy	10–100	30–50	5,000
Huntington's disease	19	50	2,630
Lesch-Nyhan syndrome	10	25	2,500
Wilson's disease	10	25	2,500
Pick's disease	24	17	708
Tourette's syndrome	28.7	3.6	125
Parkinson's disease	133	8.3	62.4
Bipolar disorder	500	8	16
Schizophrenia	900	12.8	14.2
Dyslexia	5,000–10,000	45	9.0
Epilepsy	1,700	4.1	2.4
Alzheimer's disease	7,700	14.4	1.90

what, or even how many, genes are involved. Single-gene mutations produce more than 3,000 "monogenic" disorders, many of which affect mental functioning (McKusick 1983). These are inherited in a Mendelian dominant, recessive, or sex-linked manner. Nonetheless, any one monogenic disorder is rare, and common diseases are likely to be "polygenic," representing the combined small effects of many genes. Polygenic models have viewed diseases like diabetes, atherosclerosis, or cleft lip (palate) as quasicontinuous or threshold characteristics (Reich et al. 1975). Even with genetic liability, environmental influences may be necessary for an illness to be expressed. Monogenic and polygenic transmission can be viewed as limiting cases of a general multifactorial transmission model that provides for the joint effects of a single major gene (or a few major genes), polygenic background, environmental influences (both intergenerational cultural factors and sporadic factors), and their interaction on inheritance.

Recently, sophisticated research strategies, such as segregation analysis and pedigree analysis, have allowed direct comparison of monogenic and polygenic models. Segregation analysis compares the distribution of illness observed in family members to that predicted by a given genetic hypothesis and provides estimates of gene frequency and penetrance. Its power is limited because it treats each family as a separate observation but assumes the same genetic disorder is present in all families (Kidd 1981).

Pedigree analysis, on the other hand, examines more relationships within a given pedigree, identifying affected individuals over several generations. It is less likely to result in a Type II error, failing to support a particular genetic model because of etiologic heterogeneity, but more likely to result in a Type I error, because an individual pedigree may manifest an idiosyncratic form of the disorder (Elston and Stewart 1971; Goldin et al. 1981). Examination of multiplex sibships in which two or more sibs are affected represents a compromise approach between segregation and pedigree analysis (Anderson et al. 1981; Morton and Mi 1968).

There are some conditions, such as recessive or intermediate disorders with low heterozygote penetrance, under which segregation analysis is relatively insensitive to major loci. Linkage analysis, however, may be able to both detect and localize important disease genes under these conditions (Goldin et al. 1984). Linkage analysis is a powerful technique for finding the chromosomal location of major genes in diseases with clear-cut inheritance patterns, including dominant disorders like Huntington's disease (HD) (Gusella et al. 1983) and recessive disorders like spinal muscular atrophy (Brzustowicz et al. 1990). Linkage analysis has set the stage for the ultimate isolation of pathogenic proteins underlying other Mendelian disorders:

dystrophin in muscular dystrophy of the Duchenne type (Brown and Hoffman 1988) and cystic fibrosis transmembrane conductance regulator in cystic fibrosis (Riordan et al. 1989). Given its success in uncovering the bases of such relatively rare, albeit "simple" Mendelian disorders, linkage analysis has recently been directed toward more common, but "complex" disorders like autoimmune, cardiovascular, neoplastic, neurological, and psychiatric diseases.

Complex Disorders

The application of linkage analysis to complex disorders presents certain challenges (Table 8–4). These may include 1) an unknown mode of inheritance; 2) incomplete penetrance, wherein additional environmental factors may be necessary for the final expression of even genetic forms of the disorder; 3) epistasis, where the disorder may result from the interaction of several major genes; 4) variable expression, in which a single form of the disorder may have several phenotypic expressions; 5) diagnostic instability, such that a subject's affection status may change over time; and 6) etiologic heterogeneity, under which an ordinarily genetic syndrome may have sporadic (environmentally produced) forms, known as *phenocopies,* as well as a variety of genetic forms resulting from disruption in a number of different genes, a condition known as "nonallelic heterogeneity." Clinical and statistical approaches to the linkage analysis of complex disorders exist for offsetting these uncertainties (Kaufmann and Malaspina, in press).

Linkage Analyses

Linkage studies are used to find the chromosomal locations of genes (or loci) involved in transmitting a disorder. They are based on establishing, within pedigrees, the coinheritance of the disorder with identifiable genetic markers of known chromosomal location. Mendel's second law (the law of independent assortment) (Cavalli-Sforza and Bodmer 1971) implies that the disease gene, and hence the disorder, will not be consistently coinherited with a marker allele derived from a different chromosome. Moreover, even if the disease and marker alleles originally lie on the same parental chromosome (i.e., are "syntenic"), they may become separated during gametogenesis through the process of "recombination" or "crossing-over," wherein genetic material on homologous chromosomes is exchanged (Figure 8–1). These rearranged chromosomes are ultimately passed on to the offspring. The probability of a disease and marker allele recombining depends on their distance from one another. In fact, the frequency with which the two alleles recombine (the recombination rate, θ) can be used as a measure of the distance between their respective loci: 1% recombination is synonymous with a genetic distance of 1 centimorgan (cM) and roughly corresponds to a physical distance of 10^6 base pairs (bp) of DNA.

If disease and marker alleles lie nearby one another, crossing-over will only rarely occur and parental gametes will be overrepresented. The disease and marker loci are then said to be "linked." Statistical support for linkage is obtained by examining the cosegregation of disease and marker phenotypes within a pedigree and determining the probability (likelihood, Z) of achieving the observed distribution of phenotypes given. Z is calculated as a function of the recombination fraction, θ, which ranges from 0.00 to 0.50 (the latter representing no linkage). One may then calculate the odds ratio (defined as the ratio $Z[\theta]/Z[\theta = 0.50]$), that is, the relative likelihood of there being linkage versus no linkage. By convention, the odds ratio is expressed as its base$_{10}$ logarithm (known as the *lod score*) so that linkage data from several pedigrees can be pooled and their respective contributions added to obtain a combined probability of linkage. Also, by convention, when the lod score at the best estimate of θ (defined as that estimate that yields the highest lod score) is greater than +3, linkage is confirmed; when it is less than −2, linkage is rejected.

It is worth emphasizing that linkage refers to the two loci and not to their associated alleles; although crossing-over may be rare and certain allele pairs may be disproportionately represented within any given pedigree, recombination does occasionally occur and eventually results in an even distri-

TABLE 8–4. COMPLEX DISORDERS—CHALLENGES FOR LINKAGE ANALYSIS

Unknown mode of inheritance
Incomplete penetrance
Epistasis
Variable expression
Diagnostic instability
Etiologic heterogeneity

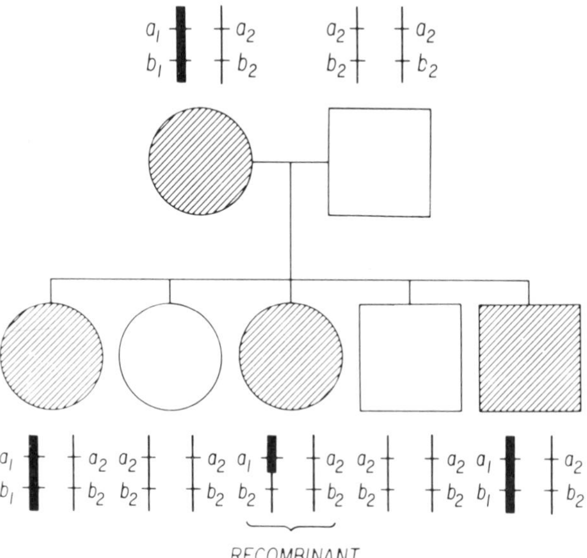

Figure 8–1. Genetic linkage and recombination. Depicted is a hypothetical family (circles = females; squares = males) segregating for an autosomal dominant disease. The disease locus A (containing either the defective allele [a_1] or its normal counterpart [a_2]) lies close to a polymorphic marker locus B (containing marker alleles b_1 and b_2). The mother is affected with the disease (closed symbol) and is heterozygous at both the disease and marker loci. The father is unaffected (open symbol) and is homozygous at both loci. Because the disease and marker loci are genetically linked (i.e., they lie nearby one another), crossing-over rarely occurs between them. Most children who inherit the disease allele (a_1) will also receive the b_1 allele from their mother. Occasionally, a recombination event will occur in the mother, and she will transfer a chromosome bearing the b_2 marker allele along with the disease allele (as has occurred in the daughter labelled "recombinant"). (Reprinted from Rieder RO, Kaufmann CA: Genetics, in The American Psychiatric Press Textbook of Psychiatry. Edited by Talbott JA, Hales RE, Yudofsky SC. Washington, DC, American Psychiatric Press, 1988, pp 33–65. Used with permission.)

bution of allele combinations within the population at large. Thus linkage of two loci does not necessarily imply an association of specific disease and marker phenotypes in the general population. An exception to this occurs when disease and marker loci lie so near one another that it takes many generations for the allele combinations to equilibrate (e.g., if the two loci are separated by 1 cM, it will take 69 generations, or about 2,000 years, for the frequency of an allele combination to go halfway to its equilibrium value) (Ott 1985).

Linkage analysis depends on the ability to distinguish marker alleles inherited from one parent from those inherited from the other. To do this consistently, marker loci must be polymorphic, that is, they must harbor a number of allelic variants. A variety of polymorphic markers now exist, including restriction fragment length polymorphisms (RFLPs) (Botstein et al. 1980) (Figure 8–2), minisatellite sequences (Jefferys et al. 1985), variable number tandem repeat (VNTR) sequences (Nakamura et al. 1987), and CA repeat sequences (Weber and May 1989).

Linkage analyses may be conveniently grouped into those involving anonymous markers, favored locus markers, and candidate genes. Anonymous markers, usually derived from noncoding DNA sequences, demonstrate significant polymorphism. When systematically drawn from throughout the genome, they may confirm linkage between a disorder and specific chromosomal regions. Conversely, they may reject linkage to these regions, thereby contributing to an "exclusion map" for the disorder. Markers from several regions may be examined concurrently; such a simultaneous search of the genome may detect multiple loci contributing to the disorder under epistasis. A major disadvantage of the anonymous marker approach is that it is undirected: at least 150 different markers must be examined to ensure that one lies within 10 cM of a major disease locus.

The favored locus approach narrows the search for linkage by examining markers derived from specific regions: portions of chromosomes involved in cytogenetic abnormalities associated with the disorder. Chromosomal translocations and deletions have provided important leads for linkage analyses of several neuropsychiatric disorders, including muscular dystrophy of the Duchenne type, Alzheimer's disease (AD), schizophrenia, and bipolar disorder.

Candidate genes offer the most focussed approach. Hypothesis-dependent candidate genes (those nominated by neurobiological clues to disease pathogenesis) and hypothesis-independent candidate genes (those put forward without regard to pathogenic hypotheses) may be explored. An etiologic role for the candidate gene or nearby regions of the genome can be excluded with as little as one or a few recombinants. A disadvantage of the candidate gene approach is that these markers are not very polymorphic, as they are necessarily derived from coding regions of the genome. Moreover, this

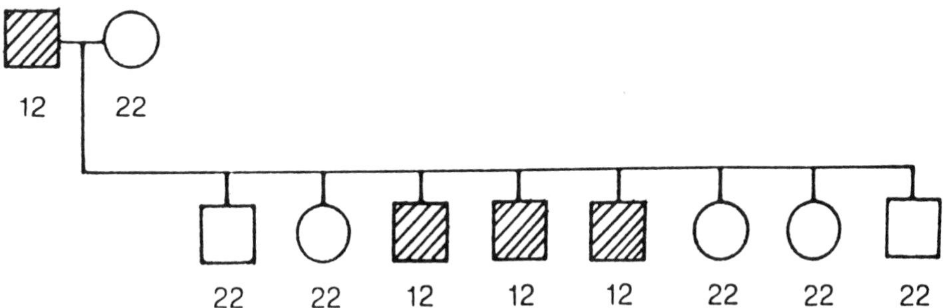

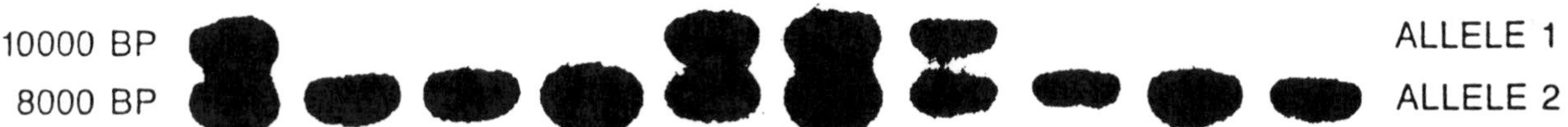

Figure 8–2. Coinheritance of a disease and a restriction fragment length polymorphism (RFLP). Depicted is a hypothetical family segregating an autosomal dominant disease (circles = females; squares = males; closed symbols = affected with the disease; open symbols = unaffected). There is an RFLP at the marker locus, resulting in two alleles, designated 1 (10,000 base pairs [bp]) and 2 (8,000 bp). The affected father and three affected sons all carry one copy of each allele. The unaffected mother and offspring have two copies of the normal allele. (Adapted from Gilliam et al. 1989.)

approach is so focussed that it provides only limited information for an exclusion map.

Molecular Approaches

Once linkage analysis has implicated a particular chromosomal region in the etiology of a disorder, various molecular genetic approaches exist for identifying the disease gene and its pathological consequences. Thus markers in linkage disequilibrium with, and thus in close proximity to, the disease gene may be identified. Genetic markers flanking the disease gene may also be recognized, thereby defining the minimal genetic region containing the disease gene. Overlapping cytogenetic anomalies producing the disease may then narrow this minimal genetic region. When the region has been narrowed to less than 10^6 bp, physical cloning strategies may be invoked, including pulse-field gel electrophoresis, yeast artificial chromosomes, and chromosome walking, hopping, and jumping. Ultimately, "open-reading frames" of DNA, corresponding to the genes themselves, may be found (e.g., through the recognition of so-called CpG islands that bound them). Physiologically important genes may then be distinguished by phylogenetic conservation, and those relevant to disease pathogenesis may be recognized through appropriate anatomic distribution of their corresponding messenger RNAs (mRNAs). Specific molecular abnormalities (e.g., insertions, deletions, and base substitutions) within the disease gene may then be discovered using single-strand conformational changes seen on denaturing gels, through the appearance of novel restriction endonuclease cleavage sites, or by direct DNA sequencing. The pathological consequences of the disease mutation may be determined by introducing the normal or disease gene into appropriate in vitro and in vivo model systems (Kimura et al. 1989; Rich et al. 1990).

In the following sections, we discuss epidemiological and genetic studies of selected neuropsychiatric illnesses. For didactic purposes, we have chosen disorders affecting diverse functions of the nervous system and displaying diverse degrees of heritability, modes of inheritance, and molecular mechanisms. We have followed the organization of Baraitser (1990), dividing these disorders into those affecting the basal ganglia, those occurring in childhood, those resulting in dementia, those associated with seizures, those involving muscle, and others.

❑ BASAL GANGLIA DISEASE

Huntington's Disease

HD is a disorder characterized by progressive dementia and chorea. Age at onset is usually between 25 and 50 years: earlier presentation is often associated with a severe course and premonitory psychiatric disturbances. The dementia of HD is remarkable for poor cognitive ability generally; a lack of language disorder or other focal cortical deficits suggests subcortical pathology (Lishman 1987). Choreic movements consist of randomly timed and irregularly distributed jerks, grimaces, and twitches. In cases of very early onset, chorea may be replaced by akinesia and rigidity (the so-called Westphal variant). Psychiatric symptoms may include a change in personality, paranoia, psychosis, or depression. In one survey (Folstein et al. 1983), affective disturbance antedated the diagnosis of HD by 2 to 20 years. Suicide is common, accounting for 7% of deaths among unhospitalized patients (Reed and Chandler 1958).

Computed tomography (CT) scans of HD patients show dilated ventricles and atrophy of the caudate nucleus, with loss of the convex bulging of the nucleus into the frontal horn of the lateral ventricle. Neuropathological examination reveals significant damage to the caudate nucleus, putamen, and globus pallidus, in a pattern consistent with the destruction of glutamate-receptive neurons. This suggests an excitotoxic model for cell loss in the disease (Coyle and Schwarcz 1976).

Epidemiological studies. The prevalence of HD was 19/100,000 among persons in Minnesota dying after the age of 40 (Heston and Mastri 1977).

Family studies. The age at onset of HD is variable and appears to depend on the parental origin of the disease gene. Thus many early-onset cases inherit the HD gene from their father (and may demonstrate "anticipation," i.e., a significantly earlier age at onset than their father [Ridley et al. 1988]), whereas many late-onset cases inherit the gene from their mother. This "parental origin effect" has been attributed to maternally inherited extrachromosomal factors. It may also be explained by genomic imprinting, whereby a gene is differentially methylated (and therefore expressed) depending on whether it passed through the maternal or paternal germline (Reik 1988).

High-risk studies. The amplitude of the somatosensory-evoked potential was diminished in 22 individuals at (50%) risk for HD compared with 22 hospitalized neurotic patients (Josiassen et al. 1988). Attempts to differentiate individuals who may go on to develop HD with oculomotor screening tests have proven less successful (Collewijn et al. 1988). The availability of DNA markers linked to the HD gene (see below) has allowed a comparison of asymptomatic individuals at high (96%) and low (4%) risk for having inherited the disease gene. In one study (Jason et al. 1988), 5 out of 7 high-risk subjects, but none of 3 low-risk subjects, showed neuropsychological impairments in frontal and parietal lobe functioning ($P = 0.08$); subjects were at least 12 years younger than their affected parents were at symptom onset, suggesting that these impairments may be present years before the appearance of overt neurological dysfunction. In a second study (Hayden et al. 1987), all 8 high-risk subjects showed reductions in caudate glucose utilization on positron-emission tomography (PET) scan that was 1 to 2 standard deviations below the mean value of age-matched control subjects; 3 out of 8 subjects had utilization more than 2 standard deviations below the control mean. Of note, 1 out of 5 presumably low-risk subjects had diminished glucose utilization, suggesting that a recombination had occurred between the DNA marker and the HD gene in this individual.

Mode of inheritance. An autosomal dominant mode of inheritance for HD is suggested by family studies: affected individuals usually have an affected parent. Conversely, approximately one-half of the offspring of affected parents are themselves affected. Formal testing of this mode of inheritance by segregation analysis is complicated: the variable age at onset that characterizes the disease prevents unambiguous identification of gene carriers. Elston et al. (1980) performed a segregation analysis on data from 11 HD families comprising 430 individuals and one large seven-generation kindred of 559 individuals. Age at onset was assumed to be normally distributed. A dominant mode of inheritance fit both data sets; both Mendelian recessive and environmental hypotheses were rejected.

Linkage analysis. The gene underlying HD was assigned to the short arm of chromosome 4 by demonstrating close linkage (lod score = 8.53 at $\theta = 0.00$) to the anonymous DNA marker D4S10 in a large Venezuelan kindred and a smaller American kindred (Gusella et al. 1983). Extension of these findings to pedigrees from throughout the world provided strong evidence against nonallelic heterogeneity in this disorder (combined lod score > 80!) (Haines et al. 1986). Variability in phenotypic expression appears to characterize HD families linked to D4S10. In one family, affected individuals over three generations show a 50-year variation in age at onset (16–67); in a second family, cerebellar signs accompanied chorea and dementia: CT and magnetic resonance imaging (MRI) revealed olivopontocerebellar atrophy along with striatal atrophy (Sax et al. 1989). A third family was described with long-tract signs but no chorea; autopsy showed prominent involvement of the brain stem and spinal cord, but only mild striatal atrophy given the duration of illness (Zweig et al. 1989). Phenotypic variations within families may represent unlinked autosomal modifying loci that influence HD gene expression; variations across families may represent different allelic genes at the HD locus.

Molecular approaches. The HD gene maps 4 cM distal to the D4S10 (G8) marker in the terminal 4p16.3 subband of chromosome 4. D4S10 and a novel marker, D4S90 (D5), lying even more distal on chromosome 4, may flank the HD gene (Youngman et al. 1989). Linkage disequilibrium between the HD gene and markers D4S95 and D4S98 also suggests that the gene lies proximal to D4S90 (Snell et al. 1989). It is currently estimated that the 2–3 megabase (Mb) region surrounding the HD locus contains 50 or more candidate genes: novel cloning strategies, such as "exon trapping" (Duyk et al. 1990) promise to reveal the identity of these candidates quickly. Two such candidates, 385 and IT7, corresponding to mRNAs expressed in the brain, have been identified recently: studies are currently under way to establish whether differences in the size and/or abundance of their respective transcripts characterize postmortem brain material from HD patients (Thompson et al. 1990).

Although the HD gene has yet to be isolated, the availability of several new highly polymorphic multiallele RFLPs in the vicinity of the HD gene allow for preclinical diagnosis (MacDonald et al. 1989). In one study (Misra et al. 1988), 37% of adults at high risk for HD had appropriate pedigree structures for presymptomatic testing; it was estimated that fetal exclusion tests could be performed in approximately 80% of at-risk pregnancies. The availability of markers linked to the HD locus allow for the study of nonfamilial, as well as familial, HD. Thus genotyping of the entirely asymptomatic extended family of an individual with typical HD (onset at age 36) revealed that several healthy siblings shared one or the other or both of the patient's haplotypes; this is consistent with the patient harboring a new mutation (Wolff et al. 1989).

Lesch-Nyhan Syndrome

Lesch-Nyhan (LN) syndrome results from deficient purine nucleotide synthesis. It is an X-linked "genetically lethal" disorder. The clinical diagnosis of LN is based on developmental delay, spastic movements, postural tremors, and retardation in a male child after the first year of life. Later there are self-mutilation, seizures, severe neurological abnormalities, and impaired renal function. The most curious symptom evidenced in LN is self-mutilation, particularly biting of the lips, mouth, and fingers, and head banging. There is no effective treatment for the central nervous system (CNS) damage, and death usually ensues in the second or third decade from infection and renal failure.

Biochemically, there is an elevated uric acid level from the deficient enzyme hypoxanthine-guanine phosphoribosyltransferase (HPRT) (EC 2.4.2.8). Those with a partial deficiency do not incur the CNS abnormalities, but they do acquire early adulthood gouty arthritis and uric acid renal stones. These are treatable with allopurinol, a xanthine oxidase inhibitor. LN is a potential candidate for somatic cell gene therapy.

Epidemiological studies. The prevalance of LN is 10/100,000 males. Male LN patients have carrier mothers in more than two-thirds of cases. A female LN patient was described by Ogasawara et al. (1989). She had a de novo gametic event, a microdeletion in the maternally derived HPRT, with nonrandom inactivation of the genetically normal paternal X chromosome.

Molecular approaches. The gene for HPRT has been cloned and characterized. It is encoded as a single-structural gene localized to Xq26-27. The LN syndrome has been found to be a heterogeneous group that includes frequent de novo mutations. Affected males usually have unique genetic backgrounds and have not inherited a common founder chromosome (Gibbs et al. 1989; Igarashi et al. 1989; Wilson et al. 1986). The HPRT locus is apparently quite vulnerable to mutation. The mutations at the site include base substitutions, deletions, single-base insertions, and RNA splicing errors. The HPRT locus has been used extensively to study mammalian mutation and reversion events.

Parkinson's Disease

Parkinson's disease (PD) is a progressive movement disorder characterized by tremor, rigidity, bradykinesia, and postural changes. It may be associated with a variety of psychiatric syndromes including cognitive and affective disturbances, personality changes, and psychosis (Lishman 1987).

Structural brain imaging in patients with PD has revealed ventricular enlargement and cortical atrophy greater than that seen in age-matched control subjects (Sroka et al. 1981). Neuropathological changes primarily include a loss of pigmented (dopaminergic) neurons in the zona compacta of the substantia nigra. Other neurons, such as those in the locus coeruleus and nucleus basalis of Meynert, may also be affected.

Epidemiological studies. The prevalence of PD has been estimated as 133/100,000; the average age at onset is 63 years (Bekkelund et al. 1989). The incidence of the disorder has been reported as 11/100,000 person years (Hofman et al. 1989a). Studies of temporal trends in incidence in the nonindustrialized community of Rochester, Minnesota (Schoenberg 1987), suggested virtually no change over the previous 35 years.

In the United States, death rates for PD suggest that race (white greater than black), sex (male greater than female), and geography (north greater than south) are independent risk factors for the disease, perhaps reflecting an etiologic role for some environmental agent (Kurtzke and Goldberg 1988). In a cross-sectional survey in Israel (Goldsmith et al. 1990), spatial clustering of PD was found in three adjacent kibbutzim (prevalence 2.2%) and was felt to represent a common environmental factor (such as agricultural chemicals or drinking water). Temporal clustering of PD has also been noted in six families with the disease: mean difference in time at onset in different generations was 4.6 years, whereas mean difference in age at onset in children and parents was 25.2 years, suggesting an environmental cause (Calne et al. 1987). 1-Methyl-4-phenyl-1,2,3,6-tetradhyropyridine (MPTP) represents an environmental neurotoxin known to cause PD in man and primates (Marsden and Jenner 1987). Population studies also suggest increased risk for PD in individuals born in the years of influenza pandemics between 1890 and 1930, suggesting that intrauterine influenza might predispose to PD, perhaps through depleting neurons in the developing substantia nigra (Mattock et al. 1988).

In North America and Europe, early-onset PD appears to be associated with rural residence, perhaps reflecting exposure to pesticides, well water, or wood pulp (Tanner 1989). A case-control study of 57 patients with PD and 122 age-matched control subjects (Hertzmann et al. 1990) suggested that increased risk was conferred by exposure to paraquat and decreased risk by exposure to tobacco (relative risk 0.6) (see also Barbeau et al. 1987; Ho et al. 1989; Hofman et al. 1989a). Similarly a study of 106 patients with PD and spouse control subjects suggested increased risk with exposure to pesticides and decreased risk with early-life vitamin E intake (Golbe et al. 1990a). Increased risk (relative risk 21) has also been described with high blood mercury levels (Ngim and Devathasan 1989).

Family studies. Since the time of Gowers (1903), the observation that patients with PD frequently have affected relatives has suggested a role for genetic factors in the disease. Martin et al. (1973) examined aggregation of illness among the first-, second-, and third-degree relatives of patients with PD compared with the relatives of spouse control subjects; 26.8% of probands and 14.8% of control subjects reported at least one affected relative. The greatest risk was for the relatives of young probands (8.3% of the sibs of probands aged 35–44 were affected versus 1.4% of the sibs of probands aged 65–74). That younger-onset probands have a more familiar form of PD, however, has not been universally found (Marttila and Rinne 1988), and young and older forms of the disorder may not be clinically or pathologically distinguished. Young-onset PD should be distinguished from juvenile PD (onset before age 21), which is invariably familial (Quinn et al. 1987; Yokochi et al. 1984). Of interest, PD may be three times more common among the relatives of AD probands than among control subjects, suggesting etiological overlap between these disorders (Hofman et al. 1989b). Increased frequency of PD among the first-degree relatives of patients with lymphoreticular malignancies compared with the relatives of hospital control subjects (relative risk 3.0), suggests a shared genetic susceptibility, perhaps through immune dysfunction (Grufferman et al. 1989).

Twin studies. MZ concordance rates are only slightly higher than DZ rates for both narrowly defined PD and broadly defined PD (including typical PD, possible PD, atypical PD, and isolated dementia, the latter added to allow for cases of diffuse Lewy body disease, which may only present with dementia and which bears an uncertain etiologic relation to PD) (W. G. Johnson et al. 1990; Ward et al. 1983). Similarly, the prevalence of PD in twins is similar to that in the general population (Marttila et al. 1988). Twin studies have been limited by uncertainty regarding the affection status of "asymptomatic" co-twins. Thus the prevalence of asymptomatic Lewy body disease in populations over the age of 60 may be high (perhaps ten times that of overt disease). Similarly, 80% of basal ganglia dopamine may need to be lost before symptoms of PD become overt. Of interest, such subclinical loss may be demonstrable with PET scanning, suggesting a more sensitive means than clinical examination for evaluating co-twins (W. G. Johnson et al. 1990).

Mode of inheritance. PD may prove to be etiologically heterogeneous. Apparent autosomal dominant inheritance with reduced penetrance is found in some families (Farrer et al. 1989; Golbe et al. 1990b), although the presence of atypical features, such as cerebellar signs, has suggested that some of these families may be segregating olivopontocerebellar atrophy. Autosomal recessive inheritance may characterize juvenile-onset PD (Yamamura et al. 1973). Furthermore, maternal inheritance, suggesting a mitochondrial gene, may characterize others (W. G. Johnson et al. 1990). Martin et al. (1973) suggested a multifactorial polygenic mode of inheritance: this model is consistent with the observation that the risk for an individual to develop familial PD increases with the number of affected individuals in his or her family.

Tourette's Syndrome

Tourette's syndrome (TS) is a disorder characterized by multiple motor and vocal tics, varying in anatomic location, type, number, and frequency. Most TS patients have an onset of illness before age 15, with a mean age of onset of 6.7 years. Clinical samples of patients with TS suggest a male to female ratio of 3:1; nonclinical samples suggest a ratio closer to unity. With respect to symptomatology, age at onset, and sex ratio, as well as clinical course and treatment response, TS appears to lie on a continuum with other tic disorders (Shapiro and Shapiro 1989).

Macroscopic structural lesions have not been demonstrated by CT or MRI, nor have characteristic neuropathological changes been seen at autopsy. Preliminary results of functional brain imaging with PET suggest decreased glucose utilization in the basal ganglia (compare with HD, see below).

Epidemiological studies. The prevalence of TS has been reported as 28.7/100,000 school children (Caine et al. 1988). Estimates for the prevalence of transient and chronic motor tic disorders, which are probably formes fruste of TS, vary from 4% to 28% for boys and from 4% to 20% for girls.

In a case series of 31 TS patients (Leckman et al. 1990), perinatal histories were compiled to identify epigenetic risk factors associated with tic severity: severity of maternal life stress during pregnancy, gender of the child, and severe nausea and/or vomiting during the first trimester were significantly associated with tic severity.

Family studies. The familial nature of TS was described by Gilles de la Tourette himself in 1885 when he observed that mild cases of the disorder occurred in the same families as more classic cases (Baraitser 1990). Eisenberg et al. (1959) first demonstrated familial aggregation. The risk of TS in the first- and second-degree relatives of patients with TS is 3.6% (Zausmer and Dewey 1987). The TS spectrum may include chronic motor tics and, in at least some pedigrees, transient tic disorder (Kurlan et al. 1988). Seventy-nine percent of TS patients have at least one family member with motor or vocal tics; 10% have relatives with marked obsessive-compulsive behavior (Jankovic and Rohaidy 1987). Comings and Comings (1987) described 11 pedigrees in which an index patient with TS had first- or second-degree relatives with obsessive-compulsive disorder or agoraphobia with panic attacks. Conversely, there is a significantly increased rate of tics among patients with obsessive-compulsive disorder and their relatives (Pitman et al. 1987).

Twin studies. In a systematically conducted twin study using strict diagnostic criteria, the MZ concordance was 53%, and the DZ concordance was 8%, suggesting a role for genetic factors in the disorder (Price et al. 1985). Nonetheless, it has been suggested that many cases of TS are not genetic in origin but phenocopies (Comings et al. 1984).

Adoption studies. TS has been described in triplets reared apart from early infancy, again emphasizing the importance of genetic factors underlying the disease (Segal et al. 1990).

Mode of inheritance. A large Mennonite kindred has been described in which 54 of 159 members had TS or chronic motor tics and in which these phenotypes demonstrated an autosomal dominant mode of transmission (Kurlan et al. 1987). Pauls et al. (1990) conducted a formal segregation analysis of TS in a large multigenerational kindred. The analysis was consistent with an autosomal dominant mode of inheritance under three definitions of affection (TS alone, TS or chronic tics, and TS or chronic tics or obsessive-compulsive disorder), with homozygous/heterozygous penetrances of 0.99/0.99 (males) and 0.70/0.70 (females).

Linkage analysis. Pairwise linkage analysis in an extended pedigree between TS and 140 anonymous marker loci comprising 30% of the genome failed to identify a linked marker (Pauls et al. 1990). A second study examining 122 markers comprising 65% of the genome (Heutink et al. 1990) also failed to identify a linked marker. Given an important role for dopamine in the pathophysiology of TS, Gelernter et al. (1990) have recently examined the gene for the dopamine, subtype 2 (D_2), receptor as a candidate gene for the disorder. They were able to exclude linkage between the receptor gene and nearby markers on chromosome 11q and TS, using both narrow and broad definitions of affection status.

Molecular approaches. Comings et al. (1986) reported a family in which six members with varying manifestations of TS all had the balanced translocation 7q22:18q22. Subsequently, linkage analysis has excluded all of chromosome 18 in 9 extended families comprising 380 individuals (74 affected) when TS plus tics were regarded as the affected phenotype (Heutink et al. 1990).

Wilson's Disease

In 1912, Wilson described "a familial nervous disease associated with cirrhosis of the liver" (p. 1). Patients with the disease that bears his name (also known as *hepatolenticular degeneration*) present with the triad of neuropsychiatric deterioration, liver dysfunction (chronic active hepatitis or cirrhosis), and Kayser-Fleischer rings of the cornea. Renal impairment may also be present. Neurological features include either spasticity, rigidity, dysarthria, and dysphagia or a flapping tremor of the wrist and shoulder. Psychiatric manifestations are frequent and variable, ranging from poor school performance through behavioral disturbances (including aggressiveness and childishness) to mood disturbances and frank psychosis (Rosenberg 1986).

A deficiency in circulating ceruloplasmin underlies the disorder (Scheinberg and Gitlin 1952). This appears to be due to impairment in the incorporation of copper into newly synthesized ceruloplasmin and not in the synthesis of the apoenzyme itself. Ceruloplasmin levels may be < 20 mg/dl; incorporation of radiolabeled copper-64 (^{64}Cu) into ceruloplasmin may be reduced, and both circulating non-ceruloplasmin-bound copper and urinary copper excretion may be increased. Brain deposits of copper may be widespread but especially affect the basal ganglia. Deposition appears to be greater in glia than in neurons. Liver dysfunction also may be associated with accumulation of copper, whereas golden-brown Kayser-Fleischer rings, visible bilaterally near the limbus on slit lamp examination, reflect granule deposition on the inner surface of the cornea in Descemet's membrane.

Epidemiological studies. The disorder has a prevalence of 10/100,000. Onset may be as early as 4 years or as late as the fifth decade. Presentation of the disease appears to partly depend on age at onset. Thus patients with an early age at onset are more likely to present with hepatic, rather than neuropsychiatric, signs (Cox et al. 1972). Nonetheless, many patients with signs of intellectual deterioration and movement disorder may present before age 10.

Family studies. Sibs affected with Wilson's disease (WD) have been described by several investigators (Bearn 1960; Bickel et al. 1957; Walshe 1967). High rates of consanguinity, for example among Indian and Arab patients, suggest autosomal recessive inheritance (Dastur et al. 1967; Passwell et al. 1977).

High-risk studies. Sibs of patients with WD are at 25% risk for developing the disorder. Because most families are complete by the time the diagnosis is made in the first sib, this information is mostly helpful in directing secondary prevention. Early recognition of biochemical evidence of illness in at-risk individuals may allow for treatment to begin with dietary copper restriction and penicillamine before overt disease can develop.

Mode of inheritance. In their study of 28 Canadian families, Cox et al. (1972) suggested that WD is heterogeneous, with three different identifiable forms. In a rare, German-Mennonite "atypical form," heterozygotes show about 50% of the normal level of ceruloplasmin. In the two "typical" forms, heterozygotes have normal ceruloplasmin levels but reduced incorporation of radiolabeled ^{64}Cu into the protein. These forms can be further divided into "juvenile" and "Slavic" types. The former, occurring in Western Europeans and several other ethnic groups, has onset before age 16, and as previously mentioned frequently presents with hepatic manifestations. The latter, occurring among Eastern Europeans, occurs later and is characterized by neuropsychiatric signs.

Linkage analysis. Frydman et al. (1985) investigated linkage between WD and 27 autosomal markers in a large inbred Israeli-Arab pedigree with affected members in two generations. They found a lod score of 3.21 at $\theta = 0.06$ with the chromosome 13 marker esterase D. Combining these results with those of a second unrelated 10-member sibship gave a lod score of 4.55 at $\theta = 0.04$. Bonne-Tamir et al. (1986) confirmed this linkage in two unrelated Druze kindreds, reporting a maximum lod score of 5.49 at $\theta = 0.03$. Subsequent study with DNA markers on chromosome 13 placed the WD locus distal to esterase D (Bonne-Tamir et al. 1986).

Molecular approaches. Czaja et al. (1987) demonstrated reduced ceruloplasmin gene transcription (44% of that of control subjects) in 4 patients with WD.

❑ DEGENERATIVE ILLNESSES OF CHILDHOOD

Acute Intermittent Porphyria

Acute intermittent porphyria (AIP) is a relapsing, remitting disorder resulting from reduced activity of the heme-synthesizing enzyme porphobilinogen deaminase (EC 4.3.1.8). It may appear at any age from puberty onward, most commonly in the third decade. Clinical features include acute abdominal pain, or pain in the limbs or back, frequently accompanied by nausea, vomiting, and headache. Patients often develop a predominantly motor neuropathy; weakness or muscle wasting may persist after the attack. Seizures occur in about one-fifth of patients. Psychiatric manifestations, including personality changes, depression, psychosis, or delirium, occur in one-quarter to three-quarters of cases. Attacks may be precipitated by a number of porphyrinogenic drugs, such as amitriptyline, barbiturates, carbamazepine, methyldopa, phenytoin, and sulfonamides (Lishman 1987).

Attacks are associated with increased urinary excretion of porphyrin precursors like δ-aminolevulinic acid and porphobilinogen. Porphyrins are endogenous ligands for the mitochondrial-associated benzodiazepine receptor, alterations in this molecule perhaps accounting for the neuropsychiatric manifestations of this disorder (Verma et al. 1987).

Epidemiological studies. AIP occurs with low prevalence, perhaps 2/100,000, in all ethnic groups. The prevalence is especially high (100/100,000) in northern Sweden (Waldenstrom 1956). These figures may underestimate the rates of latent AIP: some individuals with reduced enzyme activity (apparent in cultured lymphocytes or erythrocytes) appear unaffected; others show periodic increases in urine porphyrin precursor excretion in the absence of clinical symptoms (Waldenstrom 1956). AIP may thus be described as associated with reduced penetrance. In addition, the disorder appears to be characterized by etiologic heterogeneity, manifested by variations in enzyme activity and enzyme immunoreactivity between pedigrees (McKusick 1988).

Mode of inheritance. Unlike most other enzymopathies, which are inherited as recessive traits, AIP is inherited as an autosomal dominant disorder (most enzymes are not so rate limiting as to critically affect a metabolic pathway when their activity is reduced 50%) (Sassa 1974).

Linkage analysis. The gene for porphobilinogen deaminase has been localized to the region 11q23.2 to 11qter (de Verneuil et al. 1982). An *Msp*I RFLP within the porphobilinogen deaminase gene is highly polymorphic and has been shown to be tightly linked (lod score 3.14 at $\theta = 0.00$) to the AIP locus

(Llewellyn et al. 1987). This polymorphism appears to offer better carrier detection than enzyme activity levels in suitable families.

Molecular approaches. Allelic variations in the structural gene for porphobilinogen deaminase have been examined in 165 AIP heterozygotes from 92 unrelated families. Different mutations were seen, providing a molecular basis for the clinical heterogeneity previously described (Desnick et al. 1985; Grandchamp et al. 1990).

Metachromatic Leukodystrophy

Metachromatic leukodystrophy (MCL) refers to diffuse demyelination secondary to a deficiency in the enzyme arylsulfatase A (ASA) (EC 3.1.6.1); the enzyme defect leads to the accumulation of metachromatic lipids (cerebroside sulfate) in the peripheral and central white matter and in peripheral organs. Some rarer cases may result from multiple sulfatase deficiencies. Five clinical types are described: late-infantile, juvenile, adult, variant, and pseudo ASA deficiency. Psychosis can be the first manifestation in the adult type (Alves et al. 1986; Cerizza et al. 1987; Finelli 1985; Skomer et al. 1983).

The infantile type presents at age 1–2 years with irritability and decreased motor tone (floppiness) that progresses to motor hypertonicity. Electroencephalography (EEG) shows marked cerebral slowing, and electromyography (EMG) shows peripheral nerve involvement. Spasticity and myoclonic jerks become prominent as the illness progresses. The juvenile-onset type presents between the ages of 3 and 21 years. Gait disturbance and movement disorders are seen concomitant with behavior problems and subtle mental deterioration. The adult-onset MCL manifests after the second decade but is not clearly demarcated from the juvenile form. Presentation can include personality changes and intellectual deterioration, and it must be considered in the etiology of psychotic and dementing disorders, especially presenile dementia. It can also begin in very late life. The CNS process can be detected by white matter changes on CT and MRI.

Three percent of the general population are homozygous for a pseudo ASA gene. They are clinically normal and do not have MCL, despite having low ASA levels. This ASA variant can catabolize sulfatide. These clinically normal, pseudodeficient individuals may sometimes carry the MCL gene heterozygously. These forms need to be considered in genetic counseling (Baldinger et al. 1987). Pseudo ASA deficiency has been found in psychiatric patients, although any causal relationship is quite speculative. Two of 295 psychiatric and neurological patients studied by Herska et al. (1987) and 13 of 99 patients with chronic psychiatric disorders evaluated by Galbraith et al. (1989) had ASA deficiency, with the normal allele and intact enzyme kinetic features.

Atypical MCL cases have been described, including a sibling pair with low ASA and myotonic seizures (Grasso et al. 1989) and a case of adult-onset MCL without psychiatric symptoms (Klemm and Conzelmann 1989).

Epidemiological studies. The incidence of the late-infantile type of MCL is 2.5/100,000 (Gustavson and Hagberg 1971).

Family studies. Usually within a family the clinical picture is comparable, yet intrafamilial variation in clinical expression in MCL, as in other lysosomal storage diseases, can occur. This can include dissimilarity in age at onset, severity, and neurological involvement. The variation may be secondary to genetic heterogeneity or related to nongenotypic factors (Zlotogora 1987). MCL siblings with identical biochemical profiles and dramatically different clinical courses have been described (Clark et al. 1989).

Mode of inheritance. MCL has both dominant and recessive forms. Some family studies have supported dominant forms of MCL. In a study by Kohn et al. (1988), MCL heterozygotes showed normal neurological and EEG examinations, but had impaired performance in tests involving spatial and constructional components. The presence of an autosomal recessive form of MCL is suggested by the proportion of affected siblings suffering from the juvenile type (Schutta et al. 1966).

Molecular approaches. The ASA locus on chromosome 22q is polymorphic: at least 4–5 alleles exist besides the normal ASA, the 2–3 deficiency alleles, and the pseudodeficiency allele. Stein et al. (1981) have cloned and sequenced a full-length complementary DNA (cDNA) for human ASA. It contains 507 residues with three potential *N*-glycosylation sites. The pseudo ASA deficient enzyme lacks a glycosylation site but it has sufficient residual activity to function (Ameen et al. 1990). In addition to

ASA, the lysosomal catabolism of sulfatide requires a specific sphingolipid activator protein, SAP 1. A mutation in the SAP 1 gene is a less frequent cause of MCL. Four potential SAP proteins are coded for by one gene on chromosome 10; defects in this gene also have been found in Gaucher disease (Zhang et al. 1990).

Prenatal diagnosis is based on demonstration of reduced ASA in the fetus by either amniocentesis or by chorionic villi sampling. Presymptomatic diagnosis can be made in apparently unaffected families by reduced ASA enzyme activity and diminished nerve conduction velocity.

Intervention studies are currently under way in MCL. Bone marrow transplantation in a patient with late-infantile MCL having the characteristically low ASA level prevented the expected CNS deterioration (Krivit et al. 1987).

❑ DEMENTIA

Alzheimer's Disease

AD accounts for about 70% of dementia. It usually begins after age 45, with a progressive clinical course leading to death. It is a clinical diagnosis of exclusion and can be detected with certainty only at autopsy. Many of the present epidemiological studies have been based only on presumed clinical diagnosis.

Personality changes usually precede neurological findings in AD. As the illness progresses, Babinski reflex, rigid limbs, frontal release findings, and seizures can appear. Laboratory examination is uninformative, and neuroimaging may reveal only cortical atrophy and ventriculomegaly. Degeneration is marked in the hippocampal formation of the temporal lobe and in the temporo-parieto-occipital association cortex. Primary motor and sensory areas are relatively spared.

The specific pathological phenomena are neurofibrillary tangles, senile plaques, and granulovacuolar degeneration. Subcortical structures are also affected. There is a loss of acetylcholinergic neurotransmitter cells from the nucleus basalis of Meynert (Whitehouse et al. 1981) that project widely to the cerebral cortex, hippocampus, and limbic formation. This loss of cholinergic axons underlies the cognitive deficits of AD (Coyle et al. 1983), and the decrement of the enzyme choline acetyltransferase (EC 2.3.1.6) correlates with the extent of dementia. It has recently been theorized that the neuronal degeneration in AD triggers compensatory mechanisms promoting neuronal growth and leading to further plaque formation and pathological changes (Crutcher et al. 1991).

AD is considered to be a disease process and not the normal process of brain aging. Age at onset of less than 60 years distinguishes presenile from senile dementia, although this is debatable. The neuropathology is the same, although population studies suggest that the presenile group has more language dysfunction and a more rapid clinical course (Seltzer and Sherwin 1983).

Epidemiological studies. Approximately 10% of the population over age 65 and 45% of those over 85 are affected with AD. Theories implicated in its etiology include genetic mechanisms, viral infection, metal intoxication (notably aluminum), head trauma, and others. A review of the published prevalence of dementia found that the actual rates differed across studies and by methodology but that the rate doubled every 5.1 years. AD is said to be more common among women, whereas multi-infarct dementia is more common among men (Jorm et al. 1987).

Family studies. Epidemiological studies reveal an increased prevalence of dementia in the family members of AD patients. The estimates of increased risk are variable and may be small: 10%–14.4% for parents and 3.8%–13.9% for siblings (Amaducci et al. 1986; Constantinidis et al. 1962; Heston and Mastri 1977; Heston et al. 1981; Heyman et al. 1983; Whalley et al. 1982).

Life table studies that adjust for non-AD deaths find the risk of AD may be as high as 50% in family members by age 90 and only 10% in control subjects (Breitner et al. 1986; Huff et al. 1988; Mohs et al. 1987). These analyses support a common autosomal gene for AD with an age-dependent penetrance. However, Farrer et al. (1989), who also factored in diagnostic uncertainties, found a risk of only 24% to first-degree relatives by age 93 and of 16% to control subjects by age 90.

These and other estimates of the increase in AD risk to family members vary widely. Family studies in AD have been well reviewed by St. George-Hyslop et al. (1989). Family studies are hindered by the late age at onset, because individuals can die from other conditions or develop a dementia from a different etiology. The increased family prevalence of AD may occur predominantly in the early-onset group (Heston 1981), although such cases just may be more easily ascertained and both early- and late-onset cases often occur within a single family.

Presumably, there are both familial and sporadic forms of AD. Even in families showing an autosomal dominant mode of inheritance, the penetrance is likely to be incomplete. The relative contribution of genetic and environmental factors to the development of AD is unknown. Familial AD may be extremely common or unusual, with the possibility that apparent familial AD results from shared exposure to environmental factors.

Twin studies. A large twin study of AD is currently under way, but only a small number of twin studies have been published (Cook et al. 1981; Embry and Bruyland 1985; Jarvik et al. 1980; Nee et al. 1987). The concordance rates, thus far, are similar in MZ and DZ pairs (about 40%) with some pairs having quite disparate ages at onset. These twin studies support a large environmental influence on the etiology of AD.

Linkage analysis. The occurrence of neuropathological changes indicative of AD in individuals with Down's syndrome directed a search for an AD locus on chromosome 21. This chromosome also contains the locus for the amyloid precursor protein (APP), the precursor of amyloid, itself a major constituent of the senile plaques of AD. St. George-Hyslop et al. (1987) first reported evidence for an AD gene linked to the pericentromeric region of chromosome 21 (Figure 8–3). Three groups also found linkage to chromosome 21 in certain pedigrees (David and Lucotte 1988; Goate et al. 1989; Van Broeckhoven et al. 1988), although linkage was not found in pedigrees evaluated by Schellenberg et al. (1988) or in a separate set of pedigrees evaluated by both Roses et al. (1988) and Pericak-Vance et al. (1988). Of interest, the AD locus on chromosome 21 appears to be close to, but not colocalized with, the APP locus in some families (Tanzi et al. 1987). Yet, Hardy and associates (Goate et al. 1991) identified a mutation in the APP gene that cosegregated with AD in two unrelated chromosome 21 linked, early-onset families (Figure 8–4). This supports, but does not prove, a role for this abnormality and amyloid deposition in at least some families with AD. The positive linkage represented only a portion of families with familial AD, implying genetic heterogeneity.

Although no second locus has been confirmed for AD, Schellenberg et al. (1987) initially described an association of familial AD with the apolipoprotein (APO) C2 allele on chromosome 19. Recently, in a preliminary communication (Pericak-Vance et al. 1990), 32 families with predominantly late-onset AD have demonstrated linkage to two chromosome 19 markers (BCL3 and ATP1AC) by the affected pedigree method; multipoint linkage gave a lod score of 4.38 in analysis that only considered ill individuals as affected.

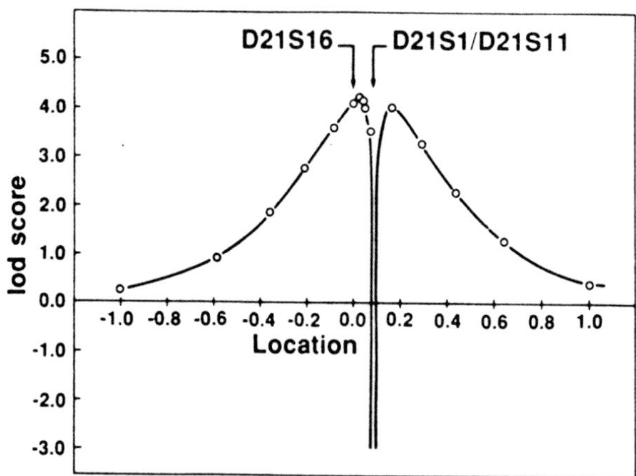

Figure 8–3. Linkage analysis of Alzheimer's disease (AD). Lod scores have been calculated for various locations (in Morgans) of the gene for AD relative to fixed positions for the two chromosome 21 anonymous marker loci, D21S16 and D21S1/D21S11. Composite data are shown for four pedigrees segregating AD. Two maxima are seen, with lod scores of 4.25 and 4.06, respectively; both scores are greater than the critical value of +3 suggesting linkage. (Reprinted from St. George-Hyslop PH, Tanzi RE, Polinsky RJ, et al: The genetic defect causing familial Alzheimer's disease maps on chromosome 21. Science 235:885–890, 1987. Copyright 1987 by AAAS. Used with permission.)

Molecular approaches. As noted, the APP gene, coding for the precursor to β-amyloid, has been considered as a candidate gene for familial AD. It has been unclear if the amyloid deposition characteristic of AD is a secondary response to neuronal degeneration or of primary pathogenic significance. Although it is not abnormal in all AD patients, the cloning and characterization of APP may allow the identification of other abnormal genes (Schellenberg et al. 1989). These genes may participate in coding or controlling mechanisms for APP or other proteins involved in AD.

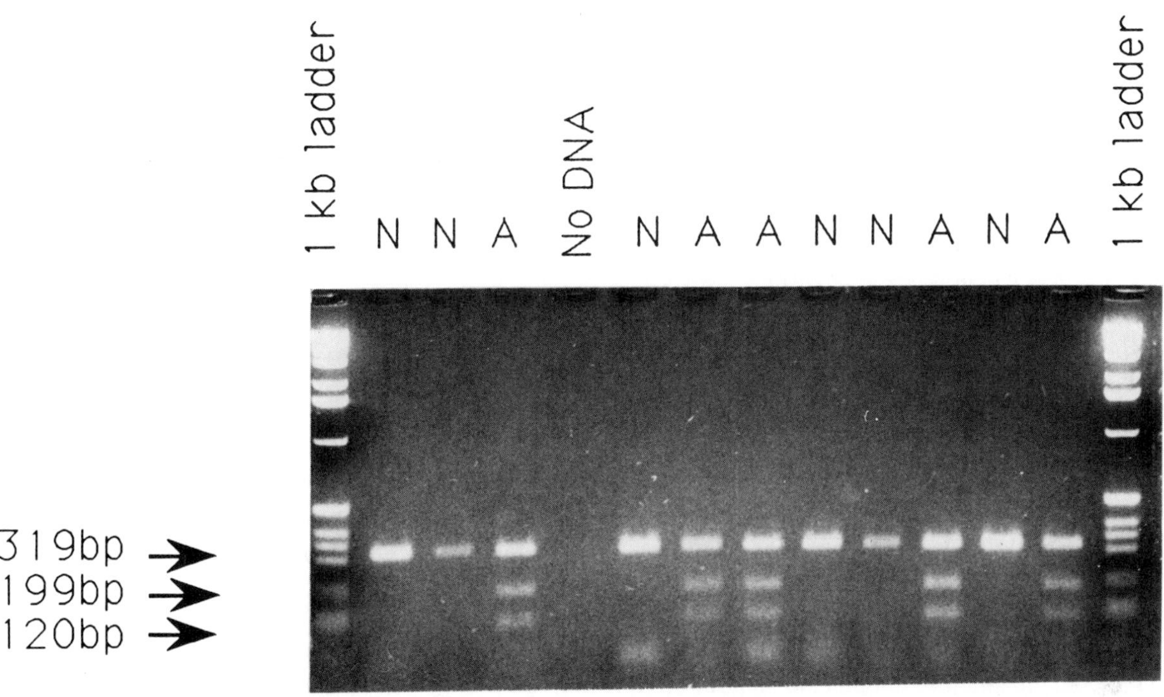

Figure 8–4. Missense mutation in the amyloid precursor protein (APP) gene and Alzheimer's disease (AD). A single base pair (bp) (C→T) mutation at bp 2149 within exon 17 of the APP results in the creation of a novel cleavage site for the restriction endonuclease *Bcl*I. This polymorphism has been visualized by ethidium bromide staining of polymerase chain reaction (PCR)-amplified, *Bcl*I-digested DNA from the vicinity of exon 17. Individuals unaffected (N) with AD are homozygous for the normal (319 bp) allele, whereas affected individuals (A) are heterozygous, with one copy of the normal allele and one copy of the mutated allele (appearing as two smaller fragments of 199 bp and 120 bp). The term *Kb ladder* refers to size markers run with the samples. Linkage analysis suggests that AD is linked to the missense mutation in one multiplex family segregating an early-onset form of the disease (maximum lod score 3.37 at $\theta = 0.00$). The finding of the *Bcl*I restriction site in a second family with AD, as well as the failure to find the site in any of 200 normal chromosomes, suggests that the missense mutation may be not only a genetic marker for AD but of pathogenic significance in the disorder. (Reprinted from Goate A, Chartier-Harlin MC, Mullan M, et al: Segregation of a missense mutation in the amyloid precursor protein gene with familial Alzheimer's disease. Nature 349:704–706, 1991. Used with permission.)

Gerstmann-Straüssler Syndrome

Gerstmann-Straüssler syndrome (GSS) is a rare and unusual neurodegenerative disorder that can be transmitted horizontally, like an infectious disease, and vertically, like a genetic disease. Patients initially present with dementia or ataxia and follow an ingravescent course to death within 1–10 years. Neuropathological examination reveals neuronal vacuolation, astrocytic gliosis, and deposition of amyloid plaques.

Epidemiological studies. The exact prevalence of GSS is unknown but is estimated to be between 0.001 and 0.01/100,000.

Molecular approaches. As an infectious disease, GSS can be transmitted to subhuman primates and rodents via intracerebral inoculation. In this regard, the disorder resembles other "slow" or "unconventional" virus infections of the CNS like Creutzfeldt-Jakob disease and kuru in man and scrapie in sheep and goats. Infectivity is associated with a 27- to 30-kilodalton protein known as the *scrapie prion protein* (PrP^{Sc}). Antibodies to PrP^{Sc} react with the previously mentioned amyloid plaques. Of interest, PrP^{Sc} appears to be encoded, not by a packaged (i.e., virus-related) nucleic acid, but by a host mRNA. The host translation product corresponding to this mRNA is a 33- to 35-kilodalton protein (PrP^{C}), differing from PrP^{Sc} in posttranslational processing (Westaway et al. 1989).

As a genetic disease, GSS (as well as a familial form of Creutzfeldt-Jakob disease) demonstrates autosomal dominant transmission. The human PrP gene is located on the short arm of chromosome 20. Hsiao et al. (1989) reported that the human PrP locus is tightly linked to GSS in two extended pedigrees segregating the disorder (maximum lod score 3.26 at $\theta = 0.00$). Of note, all 3 affected individuals in these two families demonstrated what appears to be a novel single-base mutation in codon 102 of the PrP open reading frame, resulting is a proline to leucine amino acid change in the PrP protein. This mutation was not seen in 8 unaffected relatives of these 3 individuals who had lived beyond the age of risk for the disease. It was also not seen in a random sample of 100 unrelated white individuals. The amino acid substitutions in the two affected families probably arose independently, suggesting that the proline to leucine change may be more than just a linked marker for GSS but of primary pathogenic significance to disease development; that is, the amino acid substitution might account for the appearance of the abnormal isoform of the PrP protein in familial GSS. A similar mechanism might account for sporadic forms of prion disease like Creutzfeldt-Jakob disease. Thus, stochastic events in a single cell might result in the conversion of PrP^{C} to PrP^{Sc}, with then infectious PrP^{Sc}-containing prions spreading to neighboring cells (Westaway et al. 1989).

Pick's Disease

Pick's disease refers to a progressive dementia primarily involving the frontal and temporal lobes. Macroscopically, these lobes show bilateral atrophy. The ventricles are dilated. Microscopically, neurons are lost and replaced by glia. Neurons may contain so-called Pick's bodies: cytoplasmic basophilic inclusions made up of cytoskeletal elements that bind antibodies to neurotubules and neurofilaments. Neurofibrillary tangles and senile plaques, in abundance in AD, are no more prevalent than in age-matched control subjects. Neurochemically, the neocortical cholinergic deficit that characterizes AD is not seen (Wood et al. 1983). Despite these differences, Pick's disease and AD are difficult to distinguish on clinical grounds (Morris et al. 1984).

Epidemiological studies. Heston and Mastri (1977) reported on the prevalence of autopsy-confirmed Pick's disease in Minnesota among persons dying after age 40. The rate of 24/100,000 deaths should be compared with a rate of 70/100,000 for AD. Men may be at higher risk for Pick's disease than for AD; this may be another way in which these disorders differ (Heston et al. 1987).

Family studies. Up to 1974, there had been 16 pedigrees published in which more than one member had histologically proven Pick's disease (Constantinidis 1978). Heston et al. (1987) assessed 488 relatives of 18 probands with neuropathological evidence of Pick's disease by interview and medical record review. Fifteen secondary cases of dementia were identified among the relatives; neuropathological findings in the 3 relatives who were autopsied were comparable to those in probands. The overall risk for first-degree relatives was 17% by age 75. The risk for second-degree relatives was about half that of first-degree relatives at specific ages. This discrepancy in risk between first- and second-degree relatives is consistent with some contribution of genetic factors to etiology.

High-risk studies. Groen and Endtz (1982) reported on a 6 generation pedigree with 25 members receiving clinical diagnoses of Pick's disease (autopsy proven in 14). Twelve members at high risk for the disease (but clinically well) were assessed by CT scan and EEG. Frontal atrophy was demonstrated in 4 subjects, 2 of whom subsequently went on to develop the disease.

Mode of inheritance. Dominant pedigrees have been described by Malamud and Waggoner (1943) and Keddie (1967). Three additional pedigrees showing dominant inheritance were reported by Sim and Bale (1973). Constantinidis (1969) discussed a pedigree in which two cousins, the offspring of two brothers who married two (unrelated) sisters, were affected. The parents were unaffected, with the distribution of affected individuals consistent with a recessive mode of inheritance.

Schizophrenia

Schizophrenia refers to a group of serious psychiatric disorders characterized by "positive" (psychotic) symptoms, "negative" (deficit) symptoms, early onset, and a chronic deteriorating course. It is a common and particularly crippling syndrome: the lifetime morbid risk for schizophrenia is 0.9% (Gottesman and Shields 1982). Most patients are initially affected in young adulthood; 50% go on to experience some disability throughout their lives, and an additional 25% never recover and require lifelong care.

The genetic contribution to schizophrenia was recognized by early investigators, such as Bleuler (1911), who noted that relatives of patients were often tainted by hereditary mental disease. Other nonaffective psychoses, schizoaffective disorder, and schizotypal and paranoid personality disorders also aggregate in the biological relatives of schizophrenic probands (Baron et al. 1981, 1983; Kendler and Gruenberg 1984; Kendler et al. 1981; Kety et al. 1975). It is not clear, however, what inherited factor predisposes to schizophrenia. In addition to the so-called schizophrenia spectrum disorders, other candidates include positive symptoms, negative symptoms, attentional and preattentional psychophysiological abnormalities, a latent trait predisposing to both schizophrenia and eye movement dysfunctions, and soft neurological signs.

Family studies. Beginning with the pioneering work of Rudin (1916), Kallmann (1946), and others in the Berlin school, over 20 family risk studies have examined the incidence of schizophrenia in relatives of affected individuals. These studies have consistently demonstrated an elevated morbid risk for schizophrenia in the first-degree relatives of schizophrenic probands (parents, mean 5.6%; sibs, 10.1%; and children, 12.8%), compared with that for the general population (0.9%), suggesting that schizophrenia is familial (Gottesman and Shields 1982).

Although schizophrenia and other psychotic illnesses, like bipolar disorder, tend to "breed true" (Odegaard 1963; Rosenthal 1970), the incidence of both disorders is higher in the families of schizophrenic probands (Rosenthal 1970). Similarly, the incidence of other psychotic disorders (e.g, schizoaffective disorder, paranoid disorder, and atypical psychosis) is increased among the relatives of schizophrenic probands (Kendler et al. 1985), suggesting a genetic predisposition to psychosis itself.

Attentional dysfunction has long been thought to be a central feature of schizophrenia (Kraepelin 1919). Deficits on the Continuous Performance Task (CPT; see Kornetsky and Orzack 1978) are estimated to exist in approximately 40% of schizophrenic patients, whereas similar deficits, when found, exist at a lower rate in other psychiatric patients (Kornetsky and Orzack 1978; Nuechterlein and Dawson 1984; Walker 1981). These CPT deficits appear to be trait related, possibly as phenotypic expressions of genetic vulnerability factors to schizophrenia.

A failure to show suppression of the 50 millisecond (msec) preattentional component of the auditory-evoked potential in a conditioning testing paradigm has been implicated as a genetic vulnerability marker (Siegel et al. 1984). Several reports (Adler et al. 1982, 1985; Baker et al. 1987; Franks et al. 1983; Freedman et al. 1983; Siegel et al. 1984) have suggested that this abnormality is trait related in schizophrenia and occurs at a higher rate in schizophrenic patients and their first-degree relatives compared with other psychiatric patients or control subjects.

A majority (85%) of patients with chronic schizophrenia and about 50% of those with acute schizophrenia exhibit abnormalities in smooth pursuit eye movements (SPEM) (Holzman et al. 1973, 1974, 1988; Klein et al. 1976), in contrast to a base rate in the normal population of about 6%–8%. Approximately 50% of the first-degree relatives of schizophrenic patients also exhibit SPEM disruption (Holzman 1987; Holzman and Levy 1977; Iacono 1982; Kuechenmeister et al. 1977), suggesting that it may serve as a genetic marker for schizophrenia or represent the variable expression of an underlying "latent trait" (Matthysse et al. 1986). There are numerous reports of increased neurological soft signs in schizophrenic patients (Quitkin et al. 1976; Torrey 1980). These have also been found elevated in first-degree family members of patients (Kinney et al. 1986; Rieder and Nichols 1979).

Twin studies. The heritability of schizophrenia is supported by twin study data. MZ and DZ co-twins of probands with schizophrenia differ in their risk for the disorder with weighted mean probandwise concordances of 59.2% and 15.2%, respectively (Kendler 1986). Environmental factors might account for the existence of the discordant MZ twins. Kidd (1978) estimated that up to 25% of cases of schizophrenia may represent phenocopies. Fischer (1971), however, studied the offspring of discordant MZ twins and found equivalent risks for schizophrenia (9.6% and 12.9%), again emphasizing the heritability of schizophrenia.

Adoption studies. The adoptee study method (Heston 1966; Rosenthal et al. 1968; Tienari et al.

1983) revealed a significant increase in schizophrenia in the offspring of schizophrenic mothers separated at birth compared with the offspring of control mothers. A cross-fostering study found equivalent low rates of severe psychiatric illness among adoptees with healthy biologic parents, whether they were reared by adoptive parents with schizophrenia or those without (Wender et al. 1974). The adoptee's family study method, employed by Kety et al. (1975), found that schizophrenia and related disorders were more common among the biologic relatives of 34 schizophrenic adoptees than among the biologic relatives of matched control adoptees. The rates for these disorders did not differentiate the adoptive relatives of either adoptee group, being low in both. Finally, two studies of MZ twins reared apart (Gottesman and Shields 1982) have shown high pairwise concordance for schizophrenia, providing further evidence for a genetic component in the etiology of this disorder.

High-risk studies. CPT abnormalities have identified individuals at risk for schizophrenia (Asarnow and MacCrimmon 1978; Erlenmeyer-Kimling and Cornblatt 1987; Nuechterlein 1983). Interestingly, a form of these deficits has also been found in non-psychotic subjects who have schizotypal features (Golden and Meehl 1979) suggesting that CPT may be a marker of core deficits associated with schizophrenia-related disorders.

Mode of inheritance. An entire array of genetic models has been proposed for schizophrenia. Although a dominant gene has been considered (Book 1953; Slater 1958; Slater and Cowie 1971; Zerbin-Rudin 1967), the reproductive disadvantage of schizophrenia (Larson and Nyman 1973) would seem to strongly select against this mode of inheritance.

A recessive monogenic model predicts that the incidence of schizophrenia among the offspring of two schizophrenic parents would be comparable to the probandwise concordance for MZ twins, and this is, in fact, what has been observed (Kringlen 1978). Similarly, a recessive model could allow for the maintenance of the abnormal gene in the population despite reduced reproductive fitness of those with the illness. Recessive models have been examined by Rudin (1916), Garrone (1962), Elston and Campbell (1970), and Stewart et al. (1980).

Sex-linked models have been proposed (DeLisi and Crow 1989) based on gender differences in the clinical presentation of the illness (later onset and more benign course in women) and the increased incidence of psychosis in those with sex chromosome aneuploidies.

Oligogenic models were initially proposed by Karlsson (1972), who suggested a two-locus hypothesis for the inheritance of schizophrenia. Matthysse et al. (1979) postulated an intermediate oligogenic model considering a small number of genes with disproportionately large effects on phenotype. More recently, Risch (1990a, 1990b) has suggested that a two- to three-locus epistasis model provides for the pattern of recurrence risk observed among individuals varying in degree of relatedness to schizophrenic probands.

Polygenic models are also compatible with the sharp drop in risk for schizophrenia as one moves from MZ twins, to siblings and offspring, and then to second- and third-degree relatives. They can also account for the observed increase in risk of schizophrenia in relatives with increasing severity in the proband (Gottesman and Shields 1982) and with greater numbers of other affected relatives (Odegaard 1972; but see Essen-Moller 1977).

Formal studies comparing monogenic and polygenic models have included both segregation (Carter and Chung 1980; Debray et al. 1978; Risch and Baron 1984; Tsuang et al. 1982) and pedigree analyses (Elston et al. 1978). On balance these analyses have produced inconclusive results regarding the mode of inheritance of schizophrenia.

Linkage analysis. Following up on initial suggestions (Turner 1979) of linkage between schizophrenia spectrum disorders and the human leukocyte antigen (HLA) region on chromosome 6p in 6 informative pedigrees, McGuffin et al. (1983) excluded linkage between Present State Examination (PSE; Wing et al. 1974) diagnosed schizophrenia and the HLA region, as well as markers Gc (chromosome 4q) and Gm (chromosome 14q) in 11 informative families segregating the disorder. Chada et al. (1986) and Goldin et al. (1987) likewise excluded linkage to the HLA locus in a total of 18 nuclear families containing at least two members with Research Diagnostic Criteria (RDC; Spitzer et al. 1978) diagnosed schizophrenia. Finally, Andrew et al. (1987), examining 20 phenotypic markers in 20 pedigrees, found no evidence supportive of linkage between schizophrenia or spectrum disorders and various blood group components and HLA.

Molecular approaches. A large number of cytogenetic anomalies have been associated with schizophrenia (for a review see DeLisi et al. 1988). Aschauer et al. (1989), following up on a translocation 2;18 associated with the disorder, reported linkage (maximum lod score 2.34) between DSM-III (American Psychiatric Association 1980) diagnosed schizophrenia and markers on chromosome 2 in four pedigrees. They invoked nonallelic heterogeneity in two additional families to explain their excluding linkage (lod score –2.79). Nonetheless, the overall lod score (–0.45 at $\theta = 0$) was inconclusive. More recently, W. Byerley and colleagues (personal communication, November 1990) have excluded linkage between schizophrenia and a VNTR marker in the vicinity of the 2;18 breakpoint in 6 pedigrees (lod score –5.88 at $\theta = 0$).

Chromosome 5q has been widely investigated as the location of a potential major susceptibility locus for schizophrenia after a report (Bassett et al. 1988) of an uncle and nephew pair with neuroleptic-responsive DSM-III-R (American Psychiatric Association 1987) schizophrenia and a partial trisomy of chromosome 5. A third family member with a balanced translocation involving the trisomic region was phenotypically normal. Sherrington et al. (1988) examined five Icelandic and two English pedigrees and found linkage of 5q to schizophrenia, spectrum disorder, and various other psychiatric disorders ("fringe diagnoses"). These fringe diagnoses included alcoholism, major and minor depressive disorders, and anxiety disorders. Counterintuitively, lod scores increased as affection status was broadened, achieving a maximal lod score of 6.49 for affection, which was considered to be schizophrenia plus spectrum disorder plus the fringe diagnoses.

Several subsequent groups (Aschauer et al. 1990; Detera-Wadleigh et al. 1989; Kaufmann et al. 1989; Kennedy et al. 1989; St. Clair et al. 1989), however, have failed to replicate this initial linkage finding. Furthermore, they found that the strongest evidence against linkage was achieved with the broadest definition of affection, in direct contrast to the finding by Sherrington et al. (1988).

DeLisi and Crow (1989) reported on a study of eight families and excluded linkage to four areas of the X chromosome. They are currently examining markers from the pseudoautosomal regions of the sex chromosomes in suitable families.

Candidates genes have also been examined for linkage to schizophrenia. The regulatory gene, homeobox 2 (chromosome 17p), appears not to be linked to the schizophrenia locus in a Swedish isolate. Similarly, the neurochemical gene tyrosine hydroxylase (TH [11p]) was excluded in these pedigrees (Kennedy et al. 1989), whereas a 13 cM region around the gene for the D_2 receptor (11q) was also excluded (Moises et al. 1991). Recently, the gene for a schizophrenia-associated synaptic antigen, EP10 (chromosome 17), has been excluded in these pedigrees (Kennedy et al. 1991). An earlier study (Feder et al. 1985) had excluded the candidate neurochemical gene, pro-opiomelanocortin (2p23) in other families segregating schizophrenia.

The elucidation of the genetics of schizophrenia, a complex disorder, poses certain challenges. Although the contribution of heritable factors has long been suspected, recent advances in population, molecular, and statistical genetics may reveal the chromosomal location and identity of these factors.

❑ EPILEPSY

Epilepsy was already identified as a familial disease in ancient Greece. A seizure is an abnormal discharge of brain neurons: epilepsy refers to repeated seizures without an acute precipitant. The hypoxia associated with protracted and severe uncontrolled seizures can result in profound neurological sequelae, but before the onset of epilepsy (and when seizures are well controlled) affected individuals usually are unimpaired.

Seizures can be classified by etiology. In secondary epilepsy there is a preceding neurological insult, and in primary (idiopathic) epilepsy there are no known precipitants. Seizures also may be divided by clinical or EEG manifestations into partial or generalized. These etiologically distinct seizure types vary in age at onset, prognosis, and (most likely) their recurrence risk within families (Hauser et al. 1983). Idiopathic seizures, for example, are thought to be more heritable than secondary seizures.

Seizures and EEG abnormalities can be induced in susceptible individuals by photic stimuli, hyperventilation, and certain medications. Such seizures might result from a defect in control in the systems that maintain the optimal state of excitement of neurons; these systems include neural inhibition, inactivation of excitatory neurons, feedback loops maintaining homeostasis, and other mechanisms. The affectation status of individuals at risk for a seizure disorder has become less well defined as subclinical forms of the disorder have come to be identified with EEG recording techniques.

Epidemiological studies. The reported incidence and prevalence of epilepsy varies greatly depending on the means of ascertainment; most series include only patients who have been evaluated at medical facilities. Moreover, underreporting of family history is common, because successfully treated patients may not reveal the condition to family members, because epilepsy remits, and because stigma is associated with the disorder.

The cumulative incidence of any seizure is 12.4%. The cumulative risk of repeated seizures increases with age, with estimates of 0.7% by age 10, 1.7% by age 40, and 4.1% by age 80. Febrile convulsions are sometimes placed in a separate category from other epilepsies, although they may be a risk factor for those epilepsies. The cumulative incidence of febrile seizures in childhood has been reported as 2.3%; many early-onset patients have a spontaneous remission by age 10, because there in an increase of the seizure threshold with maturation. Estimates of those with febrile convulsions who go on to have epilepsy vary from 2% to 22% (Harrison and Taylor 1976; Nelson and Ellenberg 1978), with most studies finding a two- to sixfold increase above the population rates.

A trend toward an increased risk of epilepsy in males may be explained by their higher incidence of seizures secondary to head trauma. Alternatively, there may be an interaction of genetic factors with such secondary precipitants (Evans 1962; Jennett 1982). There seems to be racial variation in the expression of convulsions, with differences in diet, exposures to toxins, or other exogenous factors possibly explaining this divergence.

Family studies. A variety of Mendelian genetic disorders are known to result in seizures. These are often, but not always, associated with mental retardation and have notable physical manifestations. Most of these syndromes are quite rare and are unlikely to account for most of the genetic predisposition to seizures that has been repeatedly observed in large studies.

Summarizing data across many studies, Vandenberg et al. (1986) found a recurrence risk for epilepsy of 4.1% in the parents and siblings of probands with idiopathic epilepsy, a rate comparable to the risk (2.4%–4.5%) to offspring of epileptic patients (Janz and Beck-Managetta 1982). An earlier age at onset predicts an increased family recurrence (Eisner et al. 1959). This may indicate greater genetic loading so that the disorder requires less exposure to an environmental precipitant to become manifest. A higher risk of seizures is found in the offspring of affected women than of affected men, supporting the existence of a maternally derived influence (a mitochondrial gene, genomic imprinting of a susceptibility gene, or an intrauterine or early childhood exposure) (Ottman 1990).

There is genetic variation and high heritability of characteristics of the human EEG. Furthermore, there is an increased risk for certain EEG patterns (generalized spike and wave abnormalities) in epilepsy families (Doose and Gerken 1972; Metrakos and Metrakos 1961). Although these EEG findings are increased by as much as fivefold in siblings of epilepsy patients, they have not yet been shown to increase their risk of epilepsy.

The partial epilepsies are considered less familial than the generalized epilepsies. Thus the prevalence of a family history of seizures for partial epilepsy is two-thirds that for generalized seizures (Eisner et al. 1959; Lennox and Lennox 1960; Tsuboi and Endo 1977). As reviewed by Ottman (1989), although the partial epilepsies are less familial, complex partial (also called temporal lobe and psychomotor) seizures are only slightly less familial than other types of epilepsy. It is unclear whether family recurrence risk is increased in individuals with multiple versus few seizures.

The offspring of epileptic mothers have an increase in febrile seizures (Janz and Beck-Managetta 1982). Febrile convulsions further increase the risk of epilepsy both to probands and to other family members. Juvenile myoclonic epilepsy is fairly specifically transmitted in families, with its incidence in family members increased some twentyfold over population rates.

Twin studies. There have been many twin studies in epilepsy. Early studies were reviewed by Anderson et al. (1989), who found MZ concordance rates of 58% and DZ rates of 11%. Reduced penetrance is suggested by these low rates of MZ concordance. Even lower concordance has been found when the affected discordant MZ twin has had brain damage (Lennox and Jolly 1954), suggesting the presence of phenocopies.

It is noteworthy that, although DZ twins have different EEGs, the EEGs of MZ twins are as similar as those taken from the same individual on separate occasions, even when the twins are reared apart (Lykken et al. 1982).

Values for twin concordance rates for epilepsy approximate the twin concordance rates for febrile seizures. Heritability estimates (71% for females and 78% for males) indicate that many individuals with febrile seizures have developed them on a genetic basis (Tsuboi 1989).

Mode of inheritance. There is an acknowledged heterogeneity in epilepsies that makes genetic modelling difficult. Thus for example, plasma amino acid studies have identified elevation in plasma glutamic acid levels in a subgroup of patients with epilepsy and their families (Janjua et al. 1989).

Autosomal dominant models with reduced penetrance have been suggested for epilepsy, especially when the diagnosis includes the presence of an abnormal EEG. In general the family data best conform to a polygenic multifactorial model, wherein an undetermined number of genetic and environmental variables contribute to the expression of the illness. Segregation analysis of juvenile myoclonic epilepsy fits a two-locus dominant-recessive model when subclinical EEG abnormalities are included as part of the affected phenotype (Greenberg et al. 1989; Janz 1989).

Linkage analysis. HLA associations to epilepsy have been reported but are inconsistent, possibly because of etiologic heterogeneity (for a review see Durner et al. 1989). Presently, linkage analyses are under way with large informative pedigrees. Ultimately, such studies may identify genes that control or modify neural excitability, and may trace the developmental and regional expression of their gene products.

❑ MUSCLE DISORDERS

Myotonic Dystrophy

Myotonic dystrophy (MD) is a neurological condition consisting of muscle wasting and weakness in combination with "myotonia": the delayed relaxation of skeletal muscle after voluntary contraction. It is of particular psychiatric interest because of its frequent association with mental disorder. Atrophy and weakness are selective and symmetric, affecting the face and neck, the muscles of mastication, and the distal arms and legs. Associated features may include cataract, frontal baldness, testicular atrophy in males, menstrual irregularities or infertility in females, and electrocardiographic and immunoglobulin abnormalities (Lishman 1987).

Psychiatric difficulties include impairment in intellect, both mental retardation from birth (40%) and deterioration in level of functioning during school years (20%) (Maas and Paterson 1937). Personality abnormalities, including reduced initiative and social deterioration, may be even more common than defective intelligence (Thomasen 1948).

Various CNS measurements may be affected by the disease. Thus over 50% of patients show EEG abnormalities, with slowing and sharp-wave activity. Likewise, ventricular enlargement has been seen on air encephalography and may increase with progression of the disease (Refsum et al. 1967). In one autopsy series (Rosman and Kakulas 1966), three of four patients had disordered cortical architecture associated with microscopic heterotopias indicative of an arrest in cortical neuron migration during embryogenesis.

Epidemiological studies. The prevalence for MD has been estimated at 5.5/100,000 (Grimm 1975; Mostacciuolo et al. 1987). Of interest, congenital forms of MD have been observed, and almost invariably are associated with an affected mother (51 out of 54 cases), suggesting some maternal intrauterine influence (Harper 1975). Also of interest, it would appear that the inheritance of MD displays "anticipation" (i.e., with each succeeding generation, the onset of MD appears to be earlier and its form more severe [Howeler et al. 1989]). For the noncongenital form of MD, the average age at onset is in the third decade.

Mode of inheritance. The disorder appears to be inherited as an autosomal dominant condition: in one series (Thomasen 1948), all probands had an affected parent. Although the risk to offspring of an affected parent is theoretically 50%, late-onset and reduced penetrance account for a lower empirical risk. Thus the risk of severe illness to offspring of primiparous affected mothers is 9%; the risk to offspring of multiparous affected mothers with a neonatally severely affected infant is 29% (Glanz and Fraser 1984). Detection of gene carriers makes genetic counseling difficult: as many as 18% of asymptomatic first-degree relatives of affected individuals were found, through EMG or slit lamp examination, to have subclinical forms of the disease (Harper 1973). Similarly, formal segregation analysis suggests that classifying individuals with minor clinical features as affected results in the best fit-to-observed data (Mostacciuolo et al. 1987).

Linkage analysis. The MD disease locus has been linked to the loci for APO C2, APO E, muscle-type creatine kinase (CKMM), peptidase D, and to the anonymous marker locus D19S19 (Bartlett et al. 1987; Bird et al. 1987; Brunner et al. 1989). All five loci have been localized to the chromosomal region 19qcen to 19q13.2. Linkage disequilibrium has been demonstrated for the APO C2 gene and MD, suggesting that the two loci are very near each other (MacKenzie et al. 1989). At present it is thought that APO C2 and D19S19 lie proximal to the MD locus, that CKMM lies nearest MD, and that another locus, D19S51, lies distal to MD (K. Johnson et al. 1989, 1990). The recognition of markers flanking the MD locus defines for the first time the genetic interval into which the MD mutation must map. Of interest, not only has linkage analysis defined the region containing the MD gene, it has also suggested that MD may be genetically distinct from other (clinically similar) myotonias, like myotonia congenita (Koch et al. 1989).

Molecular approaches. Linkage analysis has also excluded a number of muscle-related candidate genes from involvement in MD. These include the poliovirus-sensitivity gene (Siddique et al. 1988), the protein kinase C γ gene (Johnson et al. 1988), and the ryanodine receptor gene (MacKenzie et al. 1990).

❑ OTHER DISORDERS

Bipolar Disorder

Bipolar, or manic-depressive, disorder refers to an episodic disturbance in mood alternately characterized by mania (elevated or irritable mood, increased psychomotor activity, distractibility, diminished need for sleep, and often psychosis) and depression (dysphoric mood, diminished psychomotor activity, decreased concentration, sleep and appetite disturbance, and frequently suicidality). Subgroups of bipolar disorder, differing in the severity of disturbance during the manic phase and designated as bipolar I and II, have been identified (Dunner et al. 1976).

Various biological abnormalities have been described in bipolar disorder, ranging from alterations in lateralized brain functions to changes in brain biogenic amines (for a review see Goodwin and Jamison 1990). No consistent neuropathological changes have been identified (Jeste et al. 1988).

Epidemiological studies. Estimates of the general population risk (prevalence) of bipolar disorder have ranged from 0.1% to 1.1% with a mean of 0.5%. The population risk for unipolar depression is higher, with values ranging from 3.4% to 18.0%, with a mean of 6.2% (Tsuang and Faraone 1990). It would appear that the risk for mood disorders has increased over time: this seems to be due to a "period effect" (i.e., the effect of some exogenous pathogenic factor over a limited period of time [Lavori et al. 1986]). The risk of bipolar disorder in women is approximately equal to that in men, whereas the risk of unipolar disorder in women is about twice that in men (Weissman et al. 1988). Patients with bipolar illness seem to be overrepresented in the upper social and educational classes: this may reflect certain personality and behavioral patterns (e.g., heightened productivity) associated with a rise in social position in the relatives of bipolar probands (Goodwin and Jamison 1990).

Family studies. Recent double-blind, controlled family studies (Gershon et al. 1982; Tsuang et al. 1985) have compared the morbid risk of bipolar disorder in the first-degree relatives of bipolar probands with that in the relatives of nonbipolar probands. These studies suggest that the risk to the former group ranges from 3.9% to 8.0%, whereas the risk to the latter group ranges from 0.2% to 0.5%. Morbid risk appears to be especially elevated for the relatives of "early-onset" (i.e., those with onset in childhood) probands (Strober et al. 1988); this cannot be attributed to the period effect mentioned above (Tsuang and Faraone 1990). In addition to bipolar disorder, a number of other psychiatric conditions aggregate in the relatives of bipolar probands including bipolar II disorder (patients with major depression who have had hypomania but not mania); unipolar, cyclothymic, and schizoaffective disorders; and suicide. Some studies have suggested that alcoholism is also part of the bipolar disorder spectrum; others have not (for a review see Gershon 1990).

Twin studies. Ten twin studies of mood disorders conducted since 1928 have suggested increased concordance rates in MZ pairs (58%–74%) compared with same-sex DZ pairs (17%–29%) (for a review see Tsuang and Faraone 1990). A relative scarcity of unipolar-bipolar pairs argues against these disorders being genotypically identical, although the existence of some of these pairs suggests some relationship between the two disorders. In addition to supporting a major role (51% of the variance) for genetic factors in the development of mood disorders, these twin studies have also suggested an important role (42% of the variance) for shared environmental factors in disease pathogenesis.

Adoption studies. Similarly, two methodologically sound adoption studies (Mendlewicz and Rainer 1977; Wender et al. 1986) of the biological relatives of bipolar probands and control subjects have suggested an important role for genetic factors. Bipolar probands' relatives were at increased risk for bipolar disorder, unipolar disorder, and schizoaffective disorder, further clarifying the boundaries of the bipolar spectrum. The strongest findings among biological relatives appear to be for completed suicide: the rate among relatives of bipolar adoptees may be as much as 15 times the rate among relatives of control adoptees (Wender et al. 1986). Of interest, several environmental factors in the adoptive family appear to predict the development of mood disorders: parental alcohol problems for male adoptees and other parental psychiatric problems and parental death before the adoptee reaches age 19 for female adoptees (Cadoret et al. 1985).

High-risk studies. High-risk children of bipolar parents appear to have greater degrees of aggressiveness, obsessionality, and affective expression than age-matched control subjects (for a review see Goodwin and Jamison 1990). Cognitive deficits, especially on performance subtests of the Wechsler Intelligence Scale for Children-Revised (WISC-R; Wechsler 1974), suggestive of right-hemisphere dysfunction and reminiscent of deficits seen in adult bipolar patients, have also been found in high-risk children (Kestenbaum 1979).

Mode of inheritance. The absence of male-to-male transmission of bipolar disorder in some families has suggested a dominant X-linked form of the disease (Winokur et al. 1969). Risch et al. (1986) suggested that as many as one-third of bipolar patients may have this X-linked subtype. Segregation analyses have not provided convincing support for either single major locus or polygenetic-multifactorial transmission of bipolar disorder (Tsuang and Faraone 1990). Such analyses have assumed that major depression and bipolar disorder are mild and severe forms of the same disorder. For monogenic transmission these might represent allelic variants at the same locus; for polygenetic transmission these might represent different thresholds on the same continuum of liability to illness. These analyses have been confounded by a secular increase in the rate of affective illness over the past three generations (the aforementioned period effect) and limited by incomplete penetrance and possible nonallelic genetic heterogeneity (Goldin et al. 1984).

Linkage analysis. Linkage analyses of bipolar disorder have included anonymous marker studies, implicating chromosome 11p15; favored locus studies, implicating chromosome Xq28; and candidate gene studies, arguing against the tyrosine hydroxylase and D_2 receptor genes. Egeland et al. (1987) reported linkage between bipolar I and related disorders (bipolar II disorder; schizoaffective disorder, bipolar type; and unipolar major depression) and the chromosome 11 *HRAS1* oncogene in 19 of 81 members of an extended Old Order Amish pedigree (maximum lod score 4.08 at $\theta = 0.00$, penetrance = 0.85). They also suggested possible linkage between a bipolar locus and the *INS* locus (3 cM from *HRAS1*). Multipoint linkage suggested lod score >3.0 at all positions within 30 cM of *INS-HRAS1*.

Other studies (Detera-Wadleigh et al. 1987; Hodgkinson et al. 1987) have excluded linkage between a major locus for bipolar disorder and these chromosome 11 markers. Kelsoe et al. (1989) reevaluated the original Egeland report with the following changes: new onset of mood disorder in 2 members of the original pedigree, additional genotype data on 10 previously incompletely typed members of the original pedigree, new genotype data on 6 individuals in a newly included sibship (the "left" extension), and new genotype data on 31 additional relatives (the "right" extension). Linkage was excluded to the chromosome 11 markers in these 118 pedigree members (lod score [at $\theta = 0.00$] –9.31 for *HRAS1*) (Figure 8–5). Possible explanations for discrepancies between the Egeland and Kelsoe reports include nonallelic heterogeneity (even in relative population isolates), frequent phenocopies (or their occurrence in critical parts of the pedigree), and Type I errors (owing to the large number of genetic models that the Egeland study tested).

Turning to X chromosome studies, Baron et al.

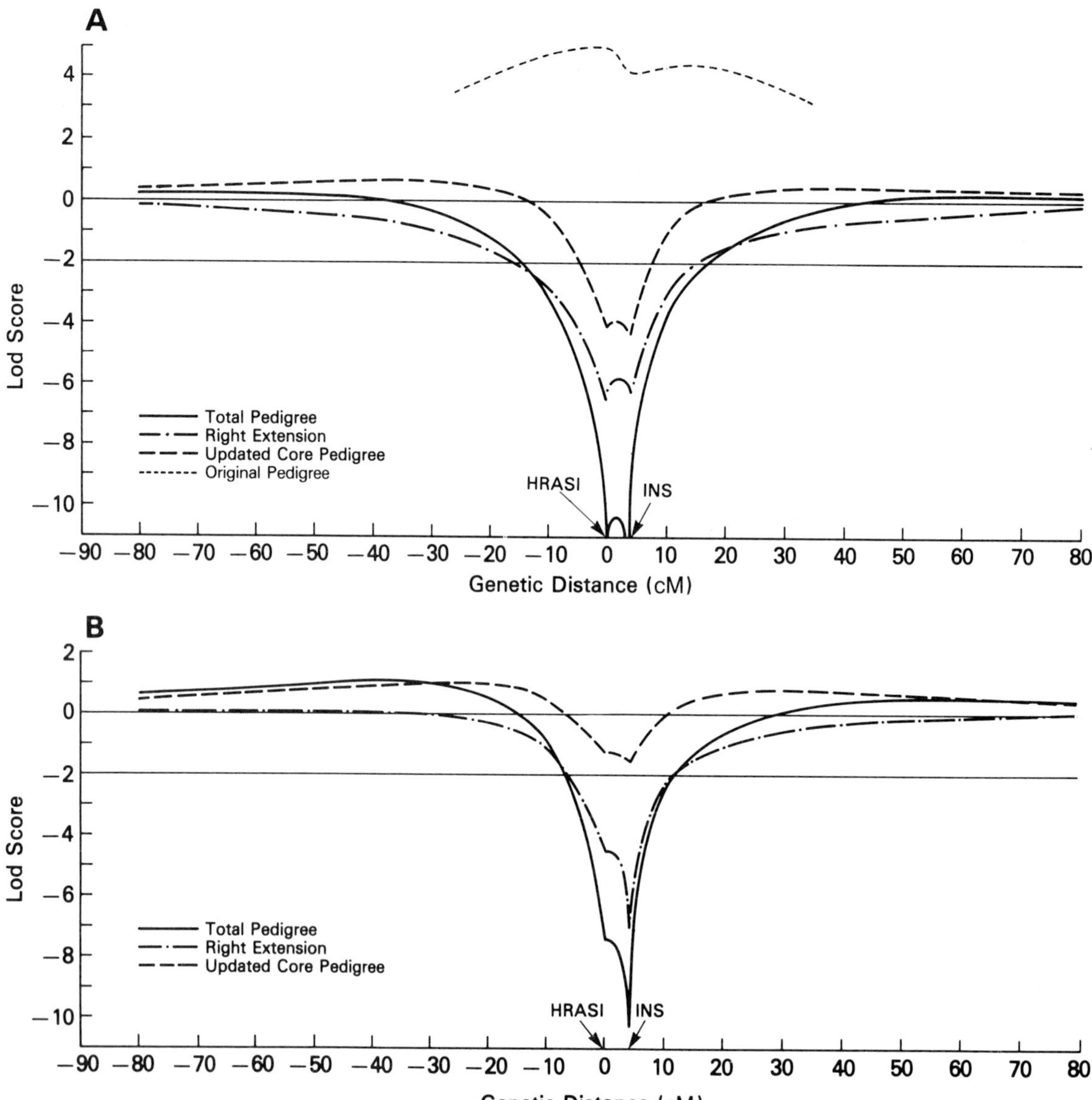

Figure 8–5. Linkage analysis of bipolar disorder: effects of pedigree extension and rediagnosis. Lod scores have been calculated for various locations (genetic distance; in centimorgans [cM]) of the gene for bipolar disorder relative to fixed positions for two chromosome 11 marker loci, *HRAS1* and *INS,* in an extended Old Order Amish pedigree. *Panel A* refers to narrow criteria (RDC diagnosed bipolar disorder, major affective disorder, and schizoaffective disorder) for the affected phenotype; *panel B* refers to broad criteria (clinically diagnosed bipolar disorder, recurrent unipolar major affective disorder, and schizoaffective disorder) for the affected phenotype. An earlier linkage analysis with 81 individuals (referred to as the "original pedigree") resulted in a maximum (two-point) lod score of 4.08 (at θ = 0.00) between bipolar disorder and *HRAS1,* and a (multipoint) lod score of approximately 5 using both *HRAS1* and *INS.* Completing the genotyping in members of the original pedigree, extending the pedigree to include 120 individuals, and updating the diagnosis on two members of the original pedigree who had become affected after the original study resulted in a precipitous drop in the lod score (minimum two-point lod score with *HRAS1* of −9.31 at θ = 0.00). Thus reanalysis suggests that this pedigree no longer confirms, and in fact excludes, linkage between bipolar disorder and this region of chromosome 11 (11p15). RDC = Research Diagnostic Criteria (Spitzer et al. 1978). (Reprinted from Kelsoe JR, Ginns EI, Egeland JA, et al: Re-evaluation of the linkage relationship between chromosome 11p and the gene for bipolar affective disorder in the Old Order Amish. Nature 342:238–243, 1989. Used with permission.)

(1987) reported strong evidence for linkage between bipolar disorder and two Xq phenotypic markers (red-green color vision and G6PD deficiency) in Israeli-Jewish pedigrees (maximum lod score 9.17 at $\theta = 0.00$). This finding was especially apparent in non-Ashkenazic families and has been corroborated recently using genotypic (RFLP) markers (T. C. Gilliam, personal communication, June 1990). Furthermore, Mendlewicz et al. (1987) provided weaker evidence for linkage between bipolar disorder and a more centromeric X chromosome locus, the hemophilia B (Factor IX) locus (maximum lod score 3.10 at $\theta = 0.11$). One explanation for disparate locations in the two X chromosome studies is that the confidence intervals associated with these two linkage findings are so wide that they may implicate the same locus. X-linked manic depressive disease appears to be a severe form of the illness, with early age at onset, a predominance of the bipolar form, and recurrent unipolar depression (Baron et al. 1990).

Molecular approaches. Linkage studies have looked at tyrosine hydroxylase (TH) as a candidate gene for bipolar disorder: it is both neurochemically plausible, because it is the rate-limiting enzyme in catecholamine synthesis, and cytologically plausible, because it is in the same chromosomal region of 11p as *HRAS1* and *INS*. Because TH is farther from the bipolar disorder locus than *HRAS1*, it would appear that it is not the bipolar disorder gene. Candidate gene studies have also looked at the D_2 receptor gene: it is both neurochemically plausible, because elevations in D_2 receptor density have been seen antemortem in patients with bipolar disorder on PET scans, and cytologically plausible, because chromosomal rearrangements (balanced translocations) involving the region of the D_2 receptor gene on chromosome 11q have been associated with mood disorders in two separate pedigrees (St. Clair et al. 1990). Preliminary linkage evidence argues against the D_2 receptor gene as the bipolar disorder gene.

Dyslexia

Dyslexia refers to what are undoubtedly a group of disorders characterized by significant deficits in reading and written language skills in children. The acquisition of these skills is inconsistent with a child's age, educational exposure, and apparent intellectual potential (Vandenberg et al. 1986).

Neurobiological research has suggested that abnormalities in hemispheric lateralization may underlie dyslexia. When brains have been examined for asymmetries, structures normally larger in the left hemisphere (the planum temporale and fissure of Sylvius) were symmetrical, suggesting arrested left-hemisphere growth. Neuropathological studies have found dysplasias and ectopias preferentially involving the left inferior frontal gyrus and posterior temporoparietal region, areas implicated in expressive and receptive language (Shepherd et al. 1989).

Epidemiological studies. Estimates of dyslexia typically range from 5% to 10% of schoolchildren (Benton and Pearl 1978). Three to four males are affected for every female (Vandenberg et al. 1986).

Family studies. That reading disability aggregates in families was noted as early as 1907 (Stephenson 1907). Subsequently, numerous reports of dyslexia in several generations of extended pedigrees appeared (Finucci 1978; Marshall and Ferguson 1939). In one series (Zahalkova et al. 1972), family members of 45% (29 of 65) of reading-disabled probands had secondary cases of dyslexia. Male relatives of affected individuals appear to be affected more often than do female relatives (Wolf 1967). Systematic comparisons of the families of 125 dyslexic probands with those of 125 control subjects were made in the Colorado Family Reading Study (De Fries et al. 1978). A variety of deficits (e.g., in both reading recognition and reading comprehension) in the parents and siblings of probands conclusively demonstrated the familial nature of the disorder.

Twin studies. Concordance rates for dyslexia in MZ twin pairs have ranged from 84% to 100%; rates in these studies in same-sex DZ twin pairs have ranged from 21% to 29% (Bakwin 1973; Hermann and Norrie 1958). These results suggest that genetic factors are both necessary and insufficient to account for the etiology of reading disability.

Mode of inheritance. In an extensive (but nonblinded) study of the families of 116 dyslexic probands, Hallgren (1950) found evidence to support an autosomal dominant mode of inheritance: a probable direct line of descent through three generations was seen in 29 families and at least one affected parent was present in 83% of cases. Conversely, the absence of consanguinity in these families argued against recessive inheritance. Statistical analyses of families in which one parent was affected (80% of families) gave Mendelian ratios for males consistent with single-gene effects; results for females did not fit such a hypothesis. These data were felt to be compatible with gender-related differences in disease penetrance, with the illness affecting or being diagnosed less frequently in females (Hallgren 1950). Later analyses of Hallgren's data were felt to be consistent with autosomal dominant inheritance with reduced penetrance in males but essentially autosomal recessive inheritance in females (Sladen 1970). Similarly, formal segregation analysis of the Colorado Family Reading Study was consistent with autosomal recessive inheritance in the families of female probands (Lewitter et al. 1980).

Other authors (e.g., Finucci 1978) have contended that the variation in severity of illness between individuals and the unequal distribution in illness between the sexes is consistent with a polygenic mode of inheritance. Thus segregation analyses of all families, as well as the families of male probands, in the Colorado Family Reading Study rejected all single-gene hypotheses (Lewitter et al. 1980).

Explanations of discrepancies in genetic models have focussed on etiologic heterogeneity (Lewitter et al. 1980). Ingram (1970) suggested that there are three forms of the disorder, characterized by visuospatial difficulties, speech-sound difficulties, or both. Boder (1971) also suggested three forms, each distinguished by characteristic spelling errors.

Linkage analysis. Further support for genetic heterogeneity in dyslexia (as well as a potential chromosomal location for one form) has come from linkage analysis. Smith et al. (1983) examined 9 pedigrees comprising 84 individuals, of whom 50 were affected. All pedigrees were identified through male probands. Linkage was excluded to 21 conventional markers; linkage to variations in banding patterns (heteromorphisms) on chromosome 15, however, was confirmed, with a maximum lod score of 3.24 at $\theta = 0.13$. One pedigree showed a very large negative lod score (-1.89 at $\theta = 0.05$). Although a formal test of nonallelic heterogeneity was not significant, this finding was suggestive of a different genetic form of disorder in this family.

Narcolepsy

Narcolepsy probably results from a defect in the rapid-eye-movement (REM)-inhibiting mechanisms of sleep, although it is at times mistakenly considered to be a psychological phenomenon. Onset can be at any age but peaks in young adulthood or late adolescence: 85% of cases begin before age 25. Narcolepsy that includes cataplexy is classic narcolepsy. Hallmark features of narcolepsy are irresistible excessive daytime sleepiness and polysomnographic EEG evidence of abnormal REM sleep. Other phenomena include onset of REM within 10 minutes of sleep initiation that precipitates hypnagogic hallucinations, sleep paralysis, and cataplexy. Much less frequently there are blackouts with automatic behaviors. Abnormalities in brain monoaminergic and cholinergic functioning have been implicated in the pathophysiology of narcolepsy.

Epidemiological studies. The prevalence of narcolepsy varies from 10/100,000 to 100/100,000 in the United States and Europe to 160/100,000 in Japan and 0.2/100,000 in Israel. The frequency of narcolepsy varies greatly and correlates with the geographical variation of the incidence of HLA-DR2. Twenty percent of unaffected Britons carry this particular HLA (Kramer et al. 1987), and only 11%–12% of Israelis yet 34% of the Japanese population display this HLA type.

Family studies. There is strong familial clustering of narcolepsy: 30%–50% of affected probands have an affected relative (Baraitser and Parkes 1978; Yoss and Daly 1957). The clinical expression of the disorder can vary markedly, however, even within the same family.

Mode of inheritance. The inheritance of narcolepsy is probably dominant with variable penetrance. Concordant identical twins are rare in the literature, (Douglass et al. 1989; Montplaisir and Poirier 1987) and nongenetic factors likely play a major role in the expression of narcolepsy. Onset follows an illness or psychological factor in about one-half of patients (Passouant and Billiard 1976), although this association may be coincidental.

Linkage analysis. Nearly 100% of narcoleptic individuals have HLA-DR2, except among blacks, almost all of whom have LA-DQw1 (Langdon et al. 1984; Neely et al. 1987; Parkes et al. 1986). These chromosome 6p antigens are part of the major histocompatibility complex, essential to cell recognition and the organization of immune responses. The association of these HLA types and narcolepsy is among the highest known for HLA-linked syndromes.

Molecular approaches. The HLA-DR2, Dw2 gene has been cloned (Uryu et al. 1989); no difference in sequence between narcoleptic and normal individuals has been found. This indicates that narcolepsy is not the result of a mutation at this site; it is possible, however, that the narcolepsy gene lies near the HLA-D region in linkage disequilibrium with it.

❑ CONCLUSIONS

In this chapter we have focussed on identifying the environmental and hereditary factors that contribute to neuropsychiatric disease. As is apparent, these factors often act in concert to produce a given disorder. Nonetheless, the role of environmental factors is large in some illnesses, like PD, and smaller in others, like HD. Traditionally, epidemiology has focussed on exogenous influences and genetics on endogenous influences. In reality, the fields often overlap and genetic epidemiology is merely a discipline within epidemiology.

In defining environmental effects on disease, epidemiology proceeds in a stepwise manner. First, it establishes an association between exposure to a particular factor and development of the disease. Next, it determines whether this association is valid or the consequence of chance, bias, or confounds through the introduction of suitable control subjects and "blinds." Finally, it judges whether this association represents a cause-effect relationship by means of its magnitude, consistency, and biological plausibility (Hennekens and Buring 1987).

Likewise, genetic studies proceed to uncover heritable effects, first by establishing the association of familial and genetic "exposure" to the disease and then by validating this association, again with appropriate control subjects and "blinds." Subsequently, genetic studies specify the genes mediating these effects by one of two paths, colloquially known as "forward" and "reverse" genetics. With some disorders, the abnormal gene product (e.g., a defective enzyme) may be known, and the disease gene coding for that product thereby may be isolated. This is the case with "inborn errors of metabolism" like LN, WD, AIP, and MCL.

For other disorders (the majority considered in this chapter), the abnormal gene product is unknown and may be coded for by any of the estimated 50,000 genes that contribute to CNS function. In these disorders, the search for the disease gene begins with establishing its chromosomal location. The gene may then be isolated through the rapidly evolving techniques of molecular genetics. Once again, in accord with Koch's postulates (1912) (now extended to genetic illnesses), a causal role for the gene in the etiopathogenesis of the disorder requires its specific and consistent association with the disorder, its biological plausibility, and, ideally, its ability to transmit the disorder. The last postulate may be achieved through the creation of an abnormal (cellular) phenotype following the introduction of the disease gene or the reversal of the abnormal phenotype with the introduction of the normal allele. These criteria have been realized for the shiverer mutation in the mouse and for the cystic fibrosis mutation in man (Kimura et al. 1989; Rich et al. 1990).

The confirmed and postulated chromosomal locations of the disorders discussed in this chapter, arrived at through these alternative paths, are shown in Figure 8–6.

The "reverse" genetic approach has been particularly successful with so-called simple disorders (i.e., those with a known mode of inheritance, complete penetrance, consistent expression, and etiologic homogeneity). As we have seen, a number of the disorders discussed in this chapter lack one or more of these features, and may be referred to as "complex" disorders. A preliminary categorization of neuropsychiatric diseases into simple and complex disorders is provided in Table 8–5.

TABLE 8–5. SIMPLE AND COMPLEX NEUROPSYCHIATRIC DISORDERS

Simple
- Acute intermittent porphyria
- Gerstmann-Straüssler syndrome
- Huntington's disease
- Lesch-Nyhan syndrome
- Metachromatic leukodystrophy
- Myotonic dystrophy
- Narcolepsy
- Wilson's disease

Complex
- Alzheimer's disease
- Bipolar disorder
- Dyslexia
- Epilepsy
- Parkinson's disease
- Pick's disease
- Schizophrenia
- Tourette's syndrome

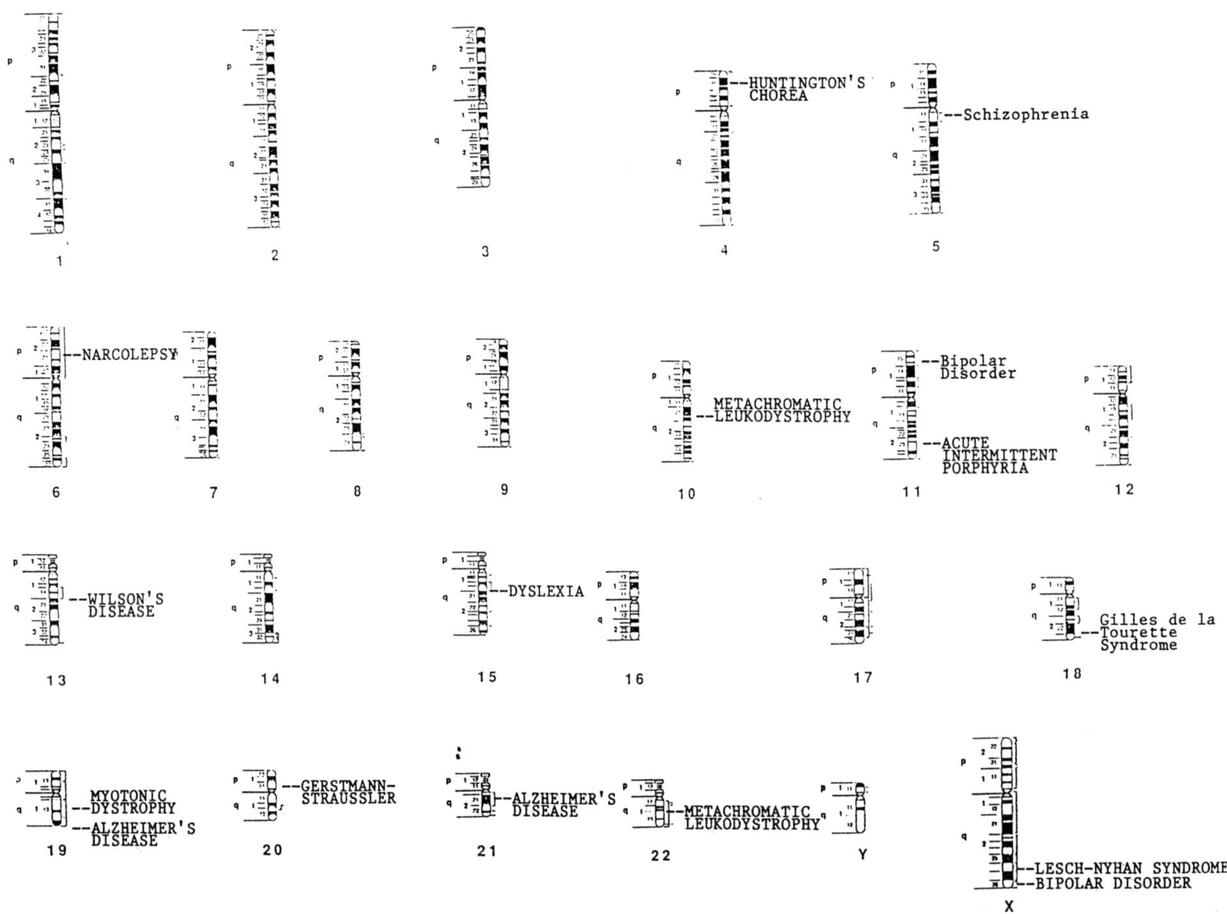

Figure 8–6. Morbid neuroanatomy of the human genome. Shown are the approximate chromosomal locations of genes contributing to the various neuropsychiatric disorders discussed in the text. Known gene mutations and replicated linkage findings are shown in all uppercase letters. Suspected gene locations and unreplicated linkage findings are shown in upper- and lowercase letters. (Adapted from McKusick 1988.)

Simple disorders appear to be caused by single-gene mutations, inherited in either an autosomal dominant, recessive, or X-linked manner (as with HD, WD, and LN, respectively). Complex disorders may result from a few major (oligo)genes (as has been postulated for schizophrenia) or from the combined effects of many (poly)genes (as has been proposed for PD).

Similarly, complex disorders are characterized by incomplete penetrance, with the concordance rate for MZ twins perhaps representing an upper boundary. The advent of sophisticated structural and functional imaging techniques, however, may extend this boundary upward, as subclinical forms of disease (so-called endophenotypes) are identified. This seems to be the case with PET and PD, through which subthreshold loss of dopaminergic neurons may be visualized.

Both simple and complex disorders may demonstrate variable expression. Thus simple disorders like AIP may vary in the presence or absence of neuropsychiatric symptoms. In other simple disorders, like HD and WD, whether and which neuropsychiatric symptoms are present depends on the age of the affected individual. This may reflect (nonallelic) etiologic heterogeneity, with different forms of the disorder having both different presentations and different ages at onset (as may be the case with WD). Disorders arising from a single locus, however, may still demonstrate varying phenotypes. Thus variable expression appears to characterize HD families linked to D4S10. This may result from allelic variants at the disease locus or from the effect of distant modifying gene loci. Alternatively, it may reflect the interaction of a fixed molecular lesion with a brain in various states of maturation (e.g., both WD and MCL often present with psychosis when onset is in the third decade) (Weinberger 1987).

Variable expression may be characterized as one genotype resulting in several phenotypes. Conversely, one phenotype may derive from several genotypes. This is the case with etiologic heterogeneity. The phenotype may be symptomatological or pathophysiological. Thus psychosis may be an heritable clinical feature common to both schizophrenia and bipolar disorder. Likewise, parkinsonism may be a heritable syndrome common to both PD and AD. Finally, TS may share a common pathophysiology with obsessive-compulsive disorder, both perhaps resulting from the asynchronous activation of corticostriatothalamocortical "minicircuits" (Leckman et al. 1991). In the limiting case, etiologic heterogeneity can refer to molecular heterogeneity within a disease gene. Thus a variety of molecular abnormalities, including point mutations, deletions, and insertions, may arise (often through new mutations) in LN.

It is clear that abnormalities in single autosomal or sex genes cannot account for the full presentation of simple and complex disorders. There may be mitochondrial genes at work in some forms of HD, PD, and epilepsy, perhaps affecting age at onset or penetrance. Nonetheless, the establishment of linkage between disease and major loci contributing to pathogenesis has become the holy grail of neuropsychiatric genetics. To date, a variety of potential linkages have been discovered: some (e.g, chromosome 4 in HD and chromosome 13 in WD) have been well replicated; others (e.g., chromosome 11 in bipolar disorder) have not. Only with replication can these preliminary findings be considered valid.

Once linkage has been established, the full armamentarium of modern molecular biology may be brought to bear on isolating disease genes. We can expect that this new knowledge will radically alter existing nosologies as genotype-phenotype associations are clarified. For example, a 3 bp deletion resulting in the loss of a phenylalanine residue at codon 508 of the cystic fibrosis transmembrane conductance regulator is found in approximately 70% of cystic fibrosis chromosomes and may predict a subtype of the disorder associated with early onset and pancreatic insufficiency.

After 25 centuries, we have come full circle: from identifying diseases and suspecting environmental and hereditary factors in their development, to ultimately specifying those factors and redefining the diseases themselves. We hope that this new knowledge will not only shed light on pathogenesis but suggest fundamental approaches to the prevention and treatment of these disabling afflictions.

❑ REFERENCES

Adler LE, Pachtman E, Franks RD, et al: Neurophysiological evidence for a defect in neuronal mechanisms involved in sensory gating in schizophrenia. Biol Psychiatry 16:640–654, 1982

Adler LE, Waldo MC, Freedman R: Neuropsychologic studies of sensory gating in schizophrenia: comparison of auditory and visual responses. Biol Psychiatry 20: 1284–1296, 1985

Alves D, Pieres MM, Guimaraes A, et al: Four cases of metachromatic leukodystrophy in a family: clinical, biochemical and neuropathological studies. J Neurol Neurosurg Psychiatry 49:1417–22, 1986

Amaducci LA, Fratiglioni L, Rocca WA, et al: Risk factors for clinically diagnosed Alzheimer's disease: a case study of an Italian population. Neurology 36:922–931, 1986

Ameen M, Lazzarino DA, Kelly BM, et al: Deficient glycosylation of arylsulfatase A in pseudoarylsulfatase A deficiency. Mol Cell Biochem 92(2):117–127, 1990

American Psychiatric Association: Diagnostic and Statistical Manual of Mental Disorders, 3rd Edition. Washington, DC, American Psychiatric Association, 1980

American Psychiatric Association: Diagnostic and Statistical Manual of Mental Disorders, 3rd Edition, Revised. Washington, DC, American Psychiatric Association, 1987

Anderson VE, Chern MM, Schwanebeck E: Multiplex families and the problem of heterogeneity, in Genetic Research Strategies for Psychobiology and Psychiatry. Edited by Gershon ES, Matthysse S, Breakefield XO, et al. Pacific Grove, CA, Boxwood, 1981, pp 341–351

Anderson VE, Wilcox KJJ, Rich SS, et al: Twin studies in epilepsy, in Genetics of the Epilepsies. Edited by Beck-Mannagetta G, Anderson VE, Doose H, et al. Berlin, Springer-Verlag, 1989, pp 145–155

Andrew B, Watt DC, Gillespie C, et al: A study of genetic linkage in schizophrenia. Psychol Med 17:363–370, 1987

Asarnow RF, MacCrimmon DJ: Residual performance deficit in clinically remitted schizophrenics: a marker of schizophrenia? J Abnorm Psychol 87:597–608, 1978

Aschauer H, Aschauer-Treiber G, Cloninger CR, et al: Heterogeneity of schizophrenia: preliminary evidence for multiple genetic loci. Schizophrenia Research 2:39–51, 1989

Aschauer HN, Aschauer-Treiber G, Isenberg KE, et al: No evidence for linkage between chromosome 5 markers and schizophrenia. Hum Hered 40:109–115, 1990

Baker N, Adler LE, Franks RD, et al: Neurophysiological assessment of sensory gating in psychiatric inpatients: comparison between schizophrenia and other diagnoses. Biol Psychiatry 22:603–617, 1987

Bakwin H: Reading disability in twins. Dev Med Child Neurol 15:184–187, 1973

Baldinger S, Piermont ME, Wenger DA: Pseudodeficiency of aralysulfatase A: a counseling dilemma. Clin Genet 31(2):70–76, 1987

Baraitser M: The Genetics of Neurological Disorders, 2nd Edition. New York, Oxford Medical, 1990

Baraitser M, Parkes JO: Genetic study of narcoleptic syndrome. J Med Genet 15:254–59, 1978

Barbeau A, Roy M, Bernier G, et al: Ecogenetics of Parkinson's disease: prevalence and environmental aspects in rural areas. Can J Neurol Sci 14:36–41, 1987

Baron M, Asnis L, Gruen R: The Schedule for Schizotypal Personalities (SSP): a diagnostic interview for schizotypal features. Psychiatry Res 4:213–228, 1981

Baron M, Asnis L, Gruen R: Plasma amine oxidase and genetic vulnerability to schizophrenia. Arch Gen Psychiatry 40:275–279, 1983

Baron M, Risch N, Hamburger R, et al: Genetic linkage between X-chromosome markers and bipolar affective disorder. Nature 326:289–292, 1987

Baron M, Hamburger R, Sandkuyl LA, et al: The impact of phenotypic variation on genetic analysis: application to X-linkage in manic depressive illness. Acta Psychiatr Scand 82:196–203, 1990

Bartlett RJ, Pericak-Vance MA, Yamadka L, et al: A new probe for the diagnosis of myotonic muscular dystrophy. Science 235:1648–1650, 1987

Bassett AS, Jones B, McGillivray BC, et al: Partial trisomy chromosome 5 cosegregating with schizophrenia. Lancet 1:799–801, 1988

Bearn AG: A genetical analysis of thirty families with Wilson's disease (hepatolenticular degeneration). Ann Hum Genet 24:33–43, 1960

Bekkelund SI, Selseth B, Mellgren SI: Parkinson's disease in a population group in northern Norway. Tidsskr Nor Laegeforen 109:561–563, 1989

Benton AL, Pearl D: Dyslexia: An Appraisal of Current Knowledge. New York, Oxford University Press, 1978

Bickel H, Neale FC, Hall G: A clinical and biochemical study of hepatolenticular degeneration (Wilson's disease). Q J Med 26:527–558, 1957

Bird TD, Boehnke M, Schellenberg G, et al: The use of apolipoprotein CII as a genetic marker for myotonic dystrophy. Arch Neurol 44:273–275, 1987

Bleuler E: Dementia Praecox or the Group of Schizophrenias. Leipzig, Deuticke, 1911

Boder E: Developmental dyslexia: prevailing diagnostic concepts and a new diagnostic approach through patterns of reading and spelling, in Progress in Learning Disabilities, Vol 2. Edited by Myklebust HR. New York, Grune & Stratton, 1971, pp 663–687

Bonne-Tamir B, Farrer LA, Frydman M, et al: Evidence for linkage between Wilson disease and esterase D in three kindreds: detection of linkage for an autosomal recessive disorder by the family study method. Genet Epidemiol 3:201–209, 1986

Book JA: A genetic and psychiatric investigation of a north Swedish population with special regard to schizophrenia and mental deficiency. Acta Genet 4:1–139, 1953

Botstein D, White RL, Skolnick M, et al: Construction of a genetic linkage map using restriction fragment length polymorphisms. Am J Hum Genet 32:314–331, 1980

Breitner JCS, Murphey EA, Folstein MF: Familial aggregation of Alzheimer dementia, II: clinical genetic implications of age dependent onset. J Psychiatr Res 20: 45–55, 1986

Brown RH Jr, Hoffman EP: Molecular biology of Duchenne muscular dystrophy. Trends Neurosci 11:480–484, 1988

Brunner HG, Korneluk RG, Coerwinkel-Driessen M, et al: Myotonic dystrophy is closely linked to the gene for muscle-type creatine kinase (CKMM). Hum Genet 81: 308–310, 1989

Brzustowicz LM, Lehner T, Castilla LH, et al: Genetic mapping of chronic childhood-onset spinal muscular atrophy to chromosome 5q11.2-13.3. Nature 344:540–541, 1990

Cadoret RJ, O'Gorman TW, Heywood E, et al: Genetic and environmental factors in major depression. J Affect Disord 9:155–164, 1985

Caine ED, McBride MC, Chiverton P, et al: Tourette's syndrome in Monroe County school children. Neurology 38:472–475, 1988

Calne S, Schoenberg B, Martin W, et al: Familial Parkinson's disease: possible role of environmental factors. Can J Neurol Sci 14:303–305, 1987

Carter CL, Chung CS: Segregation analysis of schizophrenia under a mixed genetic model. Hum Hered 30:350–356, 1980

Cavalli-Sforza LL, Bodmer WF: The Genetics of Human Populations. San Francisco, CA, Freeman, 1971

Cerizza M, Nemni R, Tamma F: Adult metachromatic leukodystrophy: an underdiagnosed disease. J Neurolog Neurosurg Psychiatry 50:1710–1712, 1987

Chada R, Kulhara P, Singh T, et al: HLA antigens in schizophrenia: a family study. Br J Psychiatry 149:612–615, 1986

Clark J, Skomorowski MA, Chang PL: Marked clinical difference between 2 sibs affected with juvenile MRA. Am J Med Genet 33:10–13, 1989

Collewijn H, Went LN, Tamminga EP, et al: Oculomotor defects in patients with Huntington's disease and their offspring. J Neurol Sci 86(2–3):307–320, 1988

Comings DE, Comings BG: Hereditary agoraphobia and obsessive-compulsive behaviour in relatives of patients with Gilles de la Tourette's syndrome. Br J Psychiatry 151:195–199, 1987

Comings DE, Comings BG, Devor EJ, et al: Detection of major gene of Gilles de la Tourette syndrome. Am J Hum Genet 36:586–600, 1984

Comings DE, et al: Evidence the Tourette syndrome gene is at 18q22.1 (abstract). 7th International Congress of Human Genetics, Berlin, Part II, 620, 1986

Constantinidis J: Forme hereditaire de la maladie de Pick sans lesions neutronales specifiques. Acta Neurologica Psychiatrica Hellen 8:226–232, 1969

Constantinidis J: Is Alzheimer's disease a major form of senile dementia? clinical, anatomical and genetic data, in Alzheimer's Disease: Senile Dementia and Related

Disorders, Vol 7: Ageing. Edited by Katzman R, Terry RD, Bick KL. New York, Raven, 1978, pp 15–25

Constantinidis J, Garrone G, de Ajuriaguerra: L'Heridte des demences de l'age avance. Encephale 51:301–344, 1962

Cook RH, Schneck SA, Clark DB: Twins with Alzheimer's disease. Arch Neurol 38:300–301, 1981

Cox DW, Fraser FC, Sass-Kortsak A: A genetic study of Wilson's disease: evidence for heterogeneity. Am J Hum Genet 24:646–666, 1972

Coyle JT, Schwarcz R: Lesion of striatal neurons with kainic acid provides a model for Huntington's chorea. Nature (London) 263:244–246, 1976

Coyle JT, Price DL, Delong MR: Alzheimer's disease: a disorder of the cholinergic innervation of cortex. Science 219:1184–1190, 1983

Crutcher KA, Neaderhauser J, Schmidt P, et al: Neurite outgrowth on postmortem human brain chryostat sections: studies of non-Alzheimer's and Alzheimer's tissue. Exp Neurol 114:228–236, 1991

Czaja MJ, Weiner FR, Schwarzenberg SJ, et al: Molecular studies of ceruloplasmin deficiency in Wilson's disease. J Clin Invest 80:1200–1204, 1987

Dastur DK, Manghani DK, Wadia NH: Wilson's disease in India, in Progress in Neurogenetics. Edited by Barbeau A, Brunette JR. Amsterdam, Excerpta Medical, 1967, pp 615–21

David F, Lucotte G: Cosegregation between D21S11 EcoR1 alleles and the FAD gene in a pedigree. Alzheimer Dis Assoc Dis 2:287, 1988

De Fries J, Singer S, Foch T, et al: Familial nature of reading disability. Br J Psychiatry 132:361–367, 1978

Debray Q, Caillard V, Stewart J: Schizophrenia: a study of genetic models and some of their implications. Neuropsychobiol 4:257–269, 1978

DeLisi LE, Crow TJ: Evidence for a sex chromosome locus for schizophrenia. Schizophr Bull 15:431–440, 1989

DeLisi LE, Reiss AL, White BJ, et al: Cytogenetic studies of males with schizophrenia: screening for the fragile X chromosome and other chromosomal abnormalities. Schizophrenia Research 1:277–281, 1988

Desnick RJ, Ostasiewicz LT, Tishler PA, et al: Acute intermittent porphyria: characterization of a novel mutation in the structural gene for porphobilinogen deaminase—demonstration of noncatalytic enzyme intermediates stabilized by bound substrate. J Clin Invest 76:865–874, 1985

Detera-Wadleigh SD, Berrettini WH, Goldin LR, et al: Close linkage of c-Harvey-ras-1 and the insulin gene to affective disorder is ruled out in three North American pedigrees. Nature 325:806–808, 1987

Detera-Wadleigh SD, Goldin LR, Sherrington R, et al: Exclusion of linkage to 5q11-13 in families with schizophrenia and other psychiatric disorders. Nature 340: 391–393, 1989

de Verneuil H, Phung N, Nordmann Y, et al: Assignment of human uroporphyrinogen I synthase locus to region 11qter by gene dosage effect. Hum Genet 60:212–213, 1982

Doose H, Gerken H: On the genetics of EEG anomalies in childhood. Neuropaediatre 4(2):162–171, 1972

Douglass AB, Harris L, Pazderka F: Monozygotic twins concordant for the narcoleptic syndrome. Neurology 39:149–141, 1989

Dunner DL, Gershon ES, Goodwin FK: Heritable factors in the severity of affective illness. Biol Psychiatry 11:31–42, 1976

Durner M, Zingsem DA, Greenberg T, et al: HLA and epilepsy, in Genetics of the Epilepsies. Edited by Beck-Managetta G, Anderson VE, Doose H, et al. New York, Springer-Verlag, 1989, pp 156–161

Duyk GM, Kim S, Pritchard C, et al: Isolation of Huntington disease candidate genes by Exon Trapping. Am J Hum Genet 47 (suppl):A249, 1990

Egeland JA, Gerhard DS, Pauls DL, et al: Bipolar affective disorders linked to DNA markers on chromosome 11. Nature 325:783–787, 1987

Eisenberg L, Ascher E, Kanner L: A clinical study of Gilles de la Tourettes's disease (Maladie des tics) in children. Am J Psychiatry 115:715–723, 1959

Eisner V, Pauli LL, Livingston S: Heredity aspects of epilepsy. Johns Hopkins Hospital Bulletin 105:245–271, 1959

Elston RC, Campbell MA: Schizophrenia: evidence for the major gene hypothesis. Behav Genet 1:3–10, 1970

Elston RC, Stewart J: A general model for the genetic analysis of pedigree data. Hum Hered 21:523–542, 1971

Elston RC, Namboodiri KK, Spence MA, et al: A genetic study of schizophrenic pedigrees, II: one-locus hypotheses. Neuropsychobiology 4:193–206, 1978

Elston RC, Pericak-Vance MA, Meyers DA, et al: Pedigree analysis of Huntington disease allowing for variable age of onset. Am J Hum Genet 32:142A, 1980

Embry C, Bruyland S: Presumed Alzheimer's disease beginning at different ages in two twins. J Am Geriatr Soc 33:61–62, 1985

Erlenmeyer-Kimling LE, Cornblatt B: The New York High Risk Project: a follow-up report. Schizophr Bull 13:451, 1987

Essen-Moller E: Evidence for polygenic inheritance in schizophrenia. Acta Psychiatr Scand 55:202–207, 1977

Evans JH: Post traumatic epilepsy. Neurology 12:665–674, 1962

Farrer LA, O'Sullivan DM, Cupples A, et al: Assessment of genetic risk for Alzheimer's disease among first-degree relatives. Ann Neurol 25:485–493, 1989

Feder J, Gurling HMD, Darby J: DNA restriction fragment analysis of the proopiomelanocortin gene in schizophrenia. Am J Hum Genet 37:286–294, 1985

Finelli PF: Metachromatic leukodystrophy manifesting as a schizophrenic disorder: computed tomographic correlation. Ann Neurol 18:94–95, 1985

Finucci JM: Genetic considerations in dyslexia, in Progress in Learning Disabilities, Vol 4. Edited by Myklebust HR. New York, Grune & Stratton, 1978, pp 41–63

Fischer M: Psychoses in the offspring of schizophrenic monozygotic twins and their normal co-twins. Br J Psychiatry 118:43–52, 1971

Folstein SE, Abbott MH, Chase GA, et al: The association of affective disorder with Huntington's disease in a case series and in families. Psychol Med 13:537–542, 1983

Franks RD, Adler LE, Waldo ME, et al: Neurophysiological studies of sensory gating in mania: comparison with schizophrenia. Biol Psychiatry 18:989–1005, 1983

Freedman R, Adler LE, Waldo ME, et al: Neurophysiological evidence for a defect in inhibitory pathways:

comparison of medicated and drug-free patients. Biol Psychiatry 18:537–551, 1983

Frydman M, Bonne-Tamir B, Farrer LA, et al: Assignment of the gene for Wilson disease to chromosome 13: linkage to esterase D locus. Proc Natl Acad Sci U S A 82: 1819–1821, 1985

Galbraith DA, Gordon BA, Feleki V, et al: Metachromatic leukodystrophy in hospitalized adult psychiatric patients resistent to drug treatment. Can J Psychiatry 34: 299–302, 1989

Garrone G: Etude statistique et genetique de la schizophrenie a Geneve de 1901 a 1950. J Genet Hum 11:89–219, 1962

Gelernter J, Pakstis AJ, Pauls DL, et al: Gilles de la Tourette syndrome is not linked to the D_2-dopamine receptor. Arch Gen Psychiatry 47:1073–1077, 1990

Gershon E: Genetics, in Manic-Depressive Illness. Edited by Goodwin FK, Jamison KR. New York, Oxford University Press, 1990, pp 373–401

Gershon ES, Hamovit J, Guroff JJ, et al: A family study of schizoaffective, bipolar I, bipolar II, unipolar, and normal control probands. Arch Gen Psychiatry 39:1157–1167, 1982

Gibbs RA, Nguyen P, McBride LJ, et al: Identification of mutations leading to the Lesch-Nyhan syndrome by automated direct DNA sequencing of in vitro amplified cDNA. Proc Natl Acad Sci U S A 86:1919–1923, 1989

Gilliam TC, Freimer NB, Kaufmann CA, et al: Deletion mapping of DNA markers to a region of chromosome 5 that co-segregates with schizophrenia. Genomics 5: 940–944, 1989

Glanz A, Frazer PC: Risk estimates for neonatal myotonic dystrophy. J Med Genet 21:186–188, 1984

Goate AM, Haynes AR, Owen MJ, et al: Predisposing locus for AD on chromosome 21. Lancet 1:352–355, 1989

Goate A, Chartier-Harlin MC, Mullan M, et al: Segregation of a missense mutation in the amyloid precursor protein gene with familial Alzheimer's disease. Nature 349:704–706, 1991

Golbe LI, Farrell TM, Davis PH: Follow-up study of early-life protective and risk factors in Parkinson's disease. Mov Disord 5:66–70, 1990a

Golbe LI, Di Iorio G, Bonavita V, et al: A large kindred with autosomal dominant Parkinson's disease. Ann Neurol 27:276–282, 1990b

Golden RR, Meehl PE: Detection of the schizoid taxon with MMPI indicators. J Abnorm Psychol 88:217–233, 1979

Goldin LR, Kidd KK, Matthysse S, et al: The power of pedigree segregation analysis for traits with incomplete penetrance, in Genetic Research Strategies for Psychobiology and Psychiatry. Edited by Gershon ES, Matthysse S, Breakefield XO, et al. Pacific Grove, CA, Boxwood, 1981, pp 305–317

Goldin LR, Cox NJ, Pauls DL, et al: The detection of major loci by segregation and linkage analysis: a simulation study. Genet Epidemiol 1:285–296, 1984

Goldin LR, DeLisi LE, Gershon ES: Relationship of HLA to schizophrenia in 10 nuclear families. Psychiatry Res 20:69–77, 1987

Goldsmith JR, Herishanu Y, Abarbanel JM, et al: Clustering of Parkinson's disease points to environmental etiology. Arch Environ Health 45(2):88–94, 1990

Goodwin FK, Jamison KR: Manic-Depressive Illness. New York, Oxford University Press, 1990

Gottesman II, Shields J: Schizophrenia: The Epigenetic Puzzle. Cambridge, Cambridge University Press, 1982

Gowers WR: A Manual of Diseases of the Nervous System, 2nd Edition. Philadelphia, PA, Blakiston, 1903

Grandchamp B, Delfau MH, Picat C, et al: Heterogeneity of the molecular defects in acute intermittent porphyria. Am J Hum Genet 47 (suppl):A156, 1990

Grasso A, Fiumara A, Biondi R, et al: On a rare atypical form of MLD. Acta Neurol (Napoli) 11(4):233–238, 1989

Greenberg DA, Delgado-Escueta, Maldonado HH, et al: Segregation analysis of juvenile myoclonic epilepsy, in Genetics of the Epilepsies. Edited by Beck-Managetta G, Anderson VE, Doose H, et al. New York, Springer-Verlag, 1989

Grimm T: The ages of onset and at death in dystrophia myotonica. J Genet Hum 23 (suppl):172, 1975

Groen JJ, Endtz LJ: Pick's disease: hereditary second reexamination of a large family with discussion of other hereditary cases with particular reference to electroencephalography and computerized tomography. Brain 105:443, 1982

Grufferman S, Cohen HJ, Delzell ES, et al: Familial aggregation of multiple myeloma and central nervous system diseases. J Am Geriatr Soc 37:303–309, 1989

Gusella JF, Wexler NS, Conneally PM, et al: A polymorphic DNA marker genetically linked to Huntington's disease. Nature 306:234–238, 1983

Gustavson KH, Hagberg B: The incidence and genetics of metachromatic leukodystrophy in northern Sweden. Acta Paediatr Scand 60:585–590, 1971

Haines J, Tanzi R, Wexler N, et al: No evidence of linkage heterogeneity between Huntington disease (HD) and G8 (D4S10) (abstract). Am J Hum Genet 39:A156, 1986

Hallgren B: Specific dyslexia: A clinical and genetic study. Acta Psychiatr Neurologica Suppl (suppl 65):1–287, 1950

Harper PS: Pre-symptomatic detection and genetic counselling in myotonic dystrophy. Clin Genet 4:134–140, 1973

Harper PS: Congenital myotonic dystrophy in Britain, II: genetic basis. Arch Dis Child 50:514–521, 1975

Harrison RM, Taylor DC: Childhood seizures: a 25-year follow-up social and medical prognosis. Lancet 1:948–951, 1976

Hauser WA, Annegers JF, Anderson VE: Epidemiology and the genetics of epilepsy, in Epilepsy. Edited by Ward AA, Penry JK, Purpura D. New York, Raven, 1983, pp 267–294

Hayden MR, Hewitt J, Stoessl AJ, et al: The combined use of positron emission tomography and DNA polymorphisms for preclinical detection of Huntington's disease. Neurology 37:1441–1447, 1987

Hennekens CH, Buring JE: Epidemiology in Medicine. Boston, MA, Little, Brown, 1987

Hermann K, Norrie E: Is congenital word-blindness an hereditary type of Gerstmann's syndrome? Psychiatria et Neurologia 136:59–73, 1958

Herska M, Moscovich DG, Kalian M, et al: Aryl sulfatase A deficiency in psychiatric and neurologic patients. Am J Med Genet 26(3):629–35, 1987

Hertzmann C, Wiens M, Bowering D, et al: Parkinson's disease: a case-control study of occupational and environmental risk factors. Am J Ind Med 17:349–355, 1990
Heston LL: Psychiatric disorders in foster home reared children of schizophrenic mothers. Br J Psychiatry 112: 819–825, 1966
Heston LL: Genetic studies of dementia: with emphasis on Parkinson's disease and Alzheimer's neuropathology, in The Epidemiology of Dementia. Edited by JA Mortimer, LM Schuman. New York, Oxford University Press, 1981, pp 101–114
Heston LL, Mastri AR: The genetics of Alzheimer's disease: associations with hematologic malignancy and Down syndrome. Arch Gen Psychiatry 34:976–981, 1977
Heston LL, Mastri AR, Anderson E, et al: Dementia of the Alzheimer type: clinical genetics, natural history, and associated conditions. Arch Gen Psychiatry 38:1085–1090, 1981
Heston LL, White JA, Mastri AR: Pick's disease: clinical genetics and natural history. Arch Gen Psychiatry 44: 409–411, 1987
Heutink P, van der Wetering BJM, Breedveld GJ, et al: Study on the heredity of Gilles de la Tourette syndrome. Am J Hum Genet 47 (suppl):A183, 1990
Heyman A, Wilkinson WEE, Hurwitz BJ, et al: Alzheimer's disease: genetic aspects and associated clinical disorder. Ann Neurol 14:507–515, 1983
Ho SC, Woo J, Lee CM: Epidemiologic study of Parkinson's disease in Hong Kong. Neurology 39:1314–1318, 1989
Hodgkinson S, Sherrington R, Gurling H, et al: Molecular genetic evidence for heterogeneity in manic depression. Nature 325:805–806, 1987
Hofman A, Collette HJ, Bartelds AI: Incidence and risk factors of Parkinson's disease in the Netherlands. Neuroepidemiol 8(6):296–299, 1989a
Hofman A, Schulte W, Tanja TA, et al: History of dementia and Parkinson's disease in 1st-degree relatives of patients with Alzheimer's disease. Neurology 39:1589–1592, 1989b
Holzman PS: Recent studies of psychophysiology and schizophrenia. Schizophr Bull 13:49–75, 1987
Holzman PS, Levy DL: Smooth-pursuit eye movements and functional psychoses: a review. Schizophr Bull 3: 15–27, 1977
Holzman PS, Proctor LR, Hughes DW: Eye tracking patterns in schizophrenia. Science 181:179–180, 1973
Holzman PS, Proctor LR, Levy DL, et al: Eye tracking dysfunctions in schizophrenic patients and their relatives. Arch Gen Psychiatry 31:143–151, 1974
Holzman PS, Kringlen E, Matthysse S, et al: A single dominant gene can account for eye tracking dysfunctions and schizophrenia in offspring of discordant twins. Arch Gen Psychiatry 45:641–647, 1988
Howeler CJ, Busch HF, Geraedts JP, et al: Anticipation in myotonic dystrophy: fact or fiction? Brain 112 (Pt 3): 779–797, 1989
Hsiao K, Baker HF, Crow TJ, et al: Linkage of a prion protein missense variant to Gerstmann-Straüssler syndrome. Nature 338:342–345, 1989
Huff FJ, Auerbach J, Chakravarti A, et al: Risk of dementia in relatives of patients with Alzheimer's disease. Neurology 38:786–790, 1988
Iacono WG: Bilateral electrodermal habituation/dishabituation and resting EEG in remitted schizophrenics. J Nerv Ment Dis 170:91–101, 1982
Igarashi T, Minami M, Nisheda Y: Molecular analysis of hypoxanthine guanine phosphoribosyl transferase mutations in 5 unrelated Japanese patients. Acta Paediatr Jpn Overseas Ed 31:303–313, 1989
Ingram TTS: The nature of dyslexia, in Early Experience and Visual Information Processing in Perceptual and Reading Disorder. Edited by Young FA, Lindsley DB. Washington, DC, National Academy of Sciences, 1970, pp 405–444
Janjua NA, Andermann E, Eeg-Olofsson O, et al: Plasma amino acid and genetic studies in epilepsy, in Genetics of the Epilepsies. Edited by Beck-Managetta G, Anderson VE, Doose H, et al. New York, Springer-Verlag, 1989, pp 162–171
Jankovic J, Rohaidy H: Motor, behavioral and pharmacologic findings in Tourette's syndrome. Can J Neurol Sci 14 (3 suppl):541–546, 1987
Janz D: Family studies on the genetics of juvenile myoclonic epilepsy, in Genetics of the Epilepsies. Edited by Beck-Managetta G, Anderson VE, Doose H, et al. New York, Springer-Verlag, 1989, pp 43–52
Janz D, Beck-Managetta G: Epilepsy and neonatal seizures in the offspring of parents with epilepsy, in Genetic Basis of the Epilepsies. Edited by Anderson VE, Hauser WA, Penry JK, et al. New York, Raven, 1982, pp 135–143
Jarvik LF, Ruth V, Matsuyama SS: Organic brain syndrome and aging: a six year follow up of surviving twins. Arch Gen Psychiatry 37:280–286, 1980
Jason GW, Pajurkova EM, Suchowersky O, et al: Presymptomatic neuropsychological impairment in Huntington's disease. Arch Neurol 45:769–773, 1988
Jeffreys AJ, Wilson V, Thien SL: Hypervariable "minisatellite" regions in human DNA. Nature 314:67–73, 1985
Jennett B: Post traumatic epilepsy, in A Textbook of Epilepsy. Edited by Laidlaw J, Richen A. New York, Churchill Livingstone, 1982, pp 146–154
Jeste DV, Lohr JB, Goodwin FK: Neuroanatomical studies of affective disorders: a review and suggestions for further research. Br J Psychiatry 153:444–459, 1988
Johnson KJ, Jones RJ, Spurr N, et al: Linkage relationships of the protein kinase C gamma gene which exclude it as a candidate for myotonic dystrophy. Cytogenet Cell Genet 48:13–15, 1988
Johnson K, Shelbourne P, Davies J, et al: Recombination events that locate myotonic dystrophy distal to APO C2 on 19q. Genomics 5:746–751, 1989
Johnson K, Shelbourne P, Davies J, et al: A new polymorphic probe which defines the region of chromosome 19 containing the myotonic dystrophy locus. Am J Hum Genet 46:1073–1081, 1990
Johnson WG, Hodge SE, Duvoisin R: Twin studies and the genetics of Parkinson's disease—a reappraisal. Mov Disord 5:187–194, 1990
Jorm AF, Korten AE, Henderson AS: The prevalence of dementia: a quantitative integration of the literature. Acta Psychiatr Scand 76:465–479, 1987

Josiassen RC, Shagass C, Roemer RA, et al: A sensory evoked potential comparison of persons "at risk" for Huntington's disease and hospitalized neurotic patients. Int J Psychophysiol 6(4):281–289, 1988

Kallmann FJ: The genetic theory of schizophrenia. Am J Psychiatry 103:309–322, 1946

Karlsson JL: A two-locus hypothesis for inheritance of schizophrenia, in Genetic Factors in Schizophrenia. Edited by Kaplan AR. Springfield, IL, Charles C Thomas, 1972, pp 246–255

Kaufmann CA, Malaspina D: Molecular genetics of schizophrenia, in Molecular Approaches to Neuropsychiatric Disease. Edited by Brosius J, Fremeau RT Jr. New York, Academic (in press)

Kaufmann CA, DeLisi LE, Lehner T, et al: Physical mapping and linkage analysis of a putative susceptibility locus for schizophrenia on chromosome 5q. Schizophr Bull 15:441–452, 1989

Keddie KMG: Presenile dementia, clinically of the Pick's disease variety occurring in a mother and daughter. International Journal of Neuropsychiatry 3:182–187, 1967

Kelsoe JR, Ginns EI, Egeland JA, et al: Re-evaluation of the linkage relationship between chromosome 11p and the gene for bipolar affective disorder in the Old Order Amish. Nature 342:238–243, 1989

Kendler KS: Genetics of schizophrenia, in Psychiatry Update: American Psychiatric Association Annual Review, Vol 5. Edited by Frances AJ, Hales RE. Washington, DC, American Psychiatric Press, 1986, pp 25–41

Kendler KS, Gruenberg AM: An independent analysis of the Copenhagen sample of the Danish adoption study, VI: the pattern of psychiatric illness, as defined by DSM-III in adoptees and relatives. Arch Gen Psychiatry 41:555–564, 1984

Kendler KS, Gruenberg AM, Strauss JS: An independent analysis of the Copenhagen sample of the Danish Adoption Study of Schizophrenia, II: the relationship between schizotypal personality disorder and schizophrenia. Arch Gen Psychiatry 38:982–984, 1981

Kendler KS, Gruenberg AM, Tsuang MT: Psychiatric illness in first-degree relatives of schizophrenic and surgical control patients. Arch Gen Psychiatry 42:770–779, 1985

Kennedy JL, Giuffra LA, Moises HW, et al: Molecular genetic studies of schizophrenia. Schizophr Bull 15: 383–391, 1989

Kennedy JL, Honer WG, Gelernter J, et al: Linkage studies of two new genes of neuropsychiatric interest. Biol Psychiatry 29:57S, 1991

Kestenbaum CJ: Children at risk for manic-depressive illness: possible predictors. Am J Psychiatry 136:1206–1208, 1979

Kety SS, Rosenthal D, Wender PH, et al: Mental illness in the biological and adoptive families of adopted individuals who have become schizophrenic: a preliminary report based on psychiatric interviews, in Genetic Research in Psychiatry. Edited by Fieve RR, Rosenthal D, Brill H. Baltimore, MD, Johns Hopkins University Press, 1975, pp 147–166,

Kidd KK: A genetic perspective on schizophrenia, in The Nature of Schizophrenia: New Approaches to Research and Treatment. Edited by Wynne LC, Cromwell RL, Matthysse S. New York, John Wiley, 1978, pp 70–75

Kidd KK: Genetic models for psychiatric disorders, in Genetic Research Strategies for Psychobiology and Psychiatry. Edited by Gershon ES, Matthysse S, Breakefield XO, et al. Pacific Grove, CA, Boxwood, 1981, pp 369–382

Kimura M, Sato M, Akatsuka A, et al: Restoration of myelin formation by a single type of myelin basic protein in transgenic shiverer mice. Proc Natl Acad Sci U S A 86:5661–5665, 1989

Kinney D, Woods BT, Yurgelun-Todd MA: Neurologic abnormalities in schizophrenic patients and their families. Arch Gen Psychiatry 43:665–668, 1986

Klein RH, Salzman LF, Jones F, et al: Eye tracking in psychiatric patients and their offspring. Psychophysiology 13:186, 1976

Klemm E, Conzelmann E: Adult onset MLD presenting without psychiatric symptoms. J Neurol 236:427–429, 1989

Koch M, Harley H, Sarfarazi M, et al: Myotonia congenita (Thomsen's disease) excluded from the region of the myotonic dystrophy locus on chromosome 19. Hum Genet 82(2):163–166, 1989

Koch R: Gesammelte Werke von Robert Koch. Leipzig, Thieme, 1912

Kohn H, Manowitz P, Miller M, et al: Neuropsychological deficits in obligatory heterozygotes for metachromatic leucodystrophy. Hum Genet 79(1):8–12, 1988

Kornetsky C, Orzack M: Physiological and behavioral correlates of attentional dysfunction in schizophrenic patients. J Psychiatr Res 14:69–79, 1978

Kraepelin E: Dementia Praecox and paraphrenia (1919). Translated by Barclay RM. Edinburgh, Livingstone, 1971

Kramer ER, Dinner DS, Braun WE, et al: HLA-DR2 and narcolepsy. Arch Neurol 44:853–855, 1987

Kringlen E: Adult offspring of two psychotic parents, with special reference to schizophrenia, in The Nature of Schizophrenia. Edited by Wynne LC, Cromwell RL, Matthysse S. New York, John Wiley, 1978, pp 9–24

Krivit W, Lipton ME, Tsai M, et al: Prevention of deterioration in metachromatic leucodystrophy by bone marrow transplantation. Am J Med Sci 249(2):80–85, 1987

Kuechenmeister CA, Linton PH, Mueller TV, et al: Eye tracking in relation to age, sex and illness. Arch Gen Psychiatry 34:578–579, 1977

Kurlan R, Behr J, Medved L, et al: Severity of Tourette's syndrome in one large kindred: implication for determination of disease prevalance rate. Arch Neurol 44: 268–269, 1987

Kurlan R, Behr J, Medved L, et al: Transient tic disorder and the spectrum of Tourette's syndrome. Arch Neurol 45:1200–1201, 1988

Kurtzke JF, Goldberg ID: Parkinsonism death rates by race, sex, and geography. Neurology 38:1558–1561, 1988

Langdon N, Welsa KI, van Dam M, et al: Genetic markers in narcolepsy. Lancet 2:1170–1180, 1984

Larson CA, Nyman GE: Differential fertility in schizophrenia. Acta Psychiatr Scand 49:272–280, 1973

Lavori PW, Klerman GL, Keller MB, et al: Age-period-cohort analysis of secular trends in onset of major depression: findings in siblings of patients with major affective disorder. J Psychiatr Res 21:23–35, 1986

Leckman JF, Dolnansky ES, Hardin MT, et al: Perinatal factors in the expression of Tourette's syndrome: an exploratory study. J Am Acad Child Adolesc Psychiatry 9:220–226, 1990

Leckman JF, Knorr AM, Rasmusson AM, et al: Basal ganglia research and Tourette's syndrome (letter). Trends Neurosci 14:94, 1991

Lennox WG, Jolly DH: Seizures, brain waves and intelligence tests of epileptic twins. Res Publ Assoc Res Nerv Ment Dis 33:325–345, 1954

Lennox WG, Lennox M: Epilepsy and Related Disorders, Vol 1. Boston, MA, Little, Brown, 1960

Lewitter F, De Fries JC, Elston RC: Genetic models of reading disability. Behav Genet 10:9–30, 1980

Lishman WA: Organic Psychiatry: The Psychological Consequences of Cerebral Disorder, 2nd Edition. Oxford, England, Blackwell Scientific, 1987

Llewellyn DH, Elder GH, Kalsheker NA, et al: DNA polymorphism of human porphobilinogen deaminase gene in acute intermittent porphyria. Lancet 2:706–708, 1987

Lykken DT, Tellegen A, Iacono WG: EEG spectra in twins: evidence for a neglected mechanism of genetic determination. Physiol Psychol 10:60–65, 1982

Lyons AS, Petrucelli RJ II: Medicine: An Illustrated History. New York, Harry N Abrams, 1987

Maas O, Paterson AS: Mental changes in families affected by dystrophia myotonica. Lancet 1:21–23, 1937

MacDonald ME, Cheng SV, Zimmer M, et al: Clustering of multiallele DNA markers near the Huntington's disease gene. J Clin Invest 84:1013–1016, 1989

McGuffin P, Festenstein H, Murray R: A family study of HLA antigens and other genetic markers in schizophrenia. Psychol Med 13:31–43, 1983

MacKenzie AE, MacLeod HL, Hunter AG, et al: Linkage analysis of the apolipoprotein C2 gene and myotonic dystrophy on human chromosome 19 reveals linkage disequilibrium in a French Canadian population. Am J Hum Genet 44:140–147, 1989

MacKenzie AE, Korneluk RG, Zorzato F, et al: The human ryanodine receptor gene: its mapping to 19q13.1, placement in a chromosome 19 linkage group, and exclusion as the gene causing myotonic dystrophy. Am J Hum Genet 46:1082–1089, 1990

McKusick V: Mendelian Inheritance in Man, 6th Edition. Baltimore, MD, Johns Hopkins University Press, 1983

McKusick VA: Mendelian Inheritance in Man, 8th Edition. Baltimore, MD, Johns Hopkins University Press, 1988

Malamud N, Waggoner RW: Genelogic and clinico pathologic study of Pick's disease. Archives of Neurology and Psychiatry (Chicago) 50:288–303, 1943

Marsden CD, Jenner PG: The significance of 1-methyl-4-phenyl-1,2,3,6-tetrahydropyridine. Ciba Found Symp 126:239–256, 1987

Marshall W, Ferguson J: Hereditary word blindness as a defect of selective attention. J Nerv Ment Dis 89:164–173, 1939

Martin WE, Young WI, Anderson VE: Parkinson's disease—a genetic study. Brain 96:495–506, 1973

Marttila RJ, Rinne UK: Parkinson's disease and essential tremor in families of patients with early-onset Parkinson's disease. J Neurol Neurosurg Psychiatry 51:429–431, 1988

Marttila RJ, Kaprio J, Koskenvuo M, et al: Parkison's disease in a nationwide twin cohort. Neurology 38:1217–1219, 1988

Matthysse S, Lange K, Wagener DK: Continuous variation caused by genes with graduated effects. Proc Natl Acad Sci U S A 76:2862, 1979

Matthysse S, Holzman PS, Lange K: The genetic transmission of schizophrenia: application of Mendelian latent structure analysis to eye-tracking dysfunctions in schizophrenia and affective disorders. J Psychiatr Res 20:57–65, 1986

Mattock C, Marmot M, Stern G: Could Parkinson's disease follow intra-uterine influenza? a speculative hypothesis. J Neurol Neurosurg Psychiatry 51:753–756, 1988

Mendlewicz J, Rainer JD: Adoption study supporting genetic transmission in manic-depressive illness. Nature 268:327–329, 1977

Mendlewicz J, Simon P, Sevy S, et al: Polymorphic DNA marker on X chromosome and manic depression. Lancet 1:1230–1232, 1987

Metrakos JD, Metrakos K: Genetics of the convulsive disorders, II: genetic and encephalographic studies in centrocephalic epilepsy. Neurology 11:474–483, 1961

Misra VP, Baraitser M, Harding AE: Genetic prediction in Huntington's disease: what are the limitations imposed by pedigree structure? Mov Disord 3:233–236, 1988

Mohs RC, Breitner JCS, Silverman JM, et al: Alzheimer's disease: morbid risk in relatives approximates 50% by age 90. Arch Gen Psychiatry 44:405–408, 1987

Moises HW, Gelernter J, Giuffra LA, et al: No linkage between D_2 dopamine receptor gene region and schizophrenia. Arch Gen Psychiatry 48:643–647, 1991

Montplaisir J, Poirier G: Narcolepsy in monozygotic twins. Neurology 37:1089, 1987

Morris JC, Cole M, Banker BQ, et al: Hereditary dysphasic dementia and the Pick-Alzheimer spectrum. Ann Neurol 16:455–466, 1984

Morton NE, Mi MP: Multiplex families with two or more probands. Am J Hum Genet 20:361–367, 1968

Mostacciuolo ML, Lombardi A, Cambissa V, et al: Population data on benign and severe forms of X-linked muscular dystrophy. Hum Genet 75:217–220, 1987

Nakamura Y, Leppert M, O'Connell P, et al: Variable number of tandem repeat (VNTR) markers for human gene mapping. Science 235:1616–1622, 1987

Nee LE, Eldridge R, Sunderland T, et al: Dementia of the Alzheimer type: clinical and family study of 22 twin pairs. Neurology 37:359–363, 1987

Neely S, Rosenberg R, Spire JP, et al: HLA antigens in narcolepsy. Neurology 37:1858–60, 1987

Nelson K, Ellenberg J: Prognosis in children with febrile seizures. Pediatrics 61:720–722, 1978

Ngim CH, Devathasan G: Epidemiologic study on the association between body burden mercury level and idiopathic Parkinson's disease. Neuroepidemiol 8: 1281–141, 1989

Nuechterlein K: Signal detection in vigilance tasks and behavioral attributes among offspring of schizophrenic mothers and among hyperactive children. J Abnorm Psychol 92:4–28, 1983

Nuechterlein KH, Dawson ME: Information processing and attentional functioning in the developmental course of schizophrenic disorders. Schizophr Bull 10: 160–203, 1984

Odegaard O: The psychiatric disease entities in the light of genetic investigation. Acta Psychiatr Scand 39 (suppl 169):94–104, 1963

Odegaard O: The multifactorial theory of inheritance in predisposition to schizophrenia, in Genetic Factors in Schizophrenia. Edited by Kaplan AR. Springfield, IL, Charles C Thomas, 1972, pp 256–275

Ogasawara N, Stout JT, Goto H, et al: Molecular analysis of a female Lesch-Nyhan patient. J Clin Invest 84:1024–1027, 1989

Ott J: Analysis of Human Genetic Linkage. Baltimore, MD, Johns Hopkins University Press, 1985

Ottman R: Genetics of the partial epilepsies: a review. Epilepsia 30:107–111, 1989

Ottman R: Sex specific recurrence risks and the maternal effect in epilepsy. Am J Hum Genet 47 (suppl):A142, 1990

Parkes JD, Langdon N, Lock C: Narcolepsy and immunity. Br Med J 292:359–360, 1986

Passouant P, Billiard M: The evolution of narcolepsy with age, in Narcolepsy. Edited by Guilleminault C, Dement WC, Passouant P. New York, Spectrum, 1976, pp 179–196

Passwell J, Adam A, Garfinkel D, et al: Heterogeneity of Wilson's disease in Israel. Isr J Med Sci 13:15–19, 1977

Pauls DL, Pakstis AJ, Kurlan R, et al: Segregation and linkage analyses of Tourette's syndrome and related disorders. J Am Acad Child Adolesc Psychiatry 29:195–203, 1990

Pericak-Vance MA, Yamaoka LH, Haynes CS, et al: Genetic linkage studies in Alzheimers disease families. Exp Neurol 102:271–279, 1988

Pericak-Vance MA, Bebout JL, Haynes CA, et al: Linkage studies in familial Alzheimers disease: evidence for chromosome 19 linkage. Am J Hum Genet 47 (suppl): A194, 1990

Pitman RK, Green RC, Jenike MA, et al: Clinical comparison of Tourette's disorder and obsessive-compulsive disorder. Am J Psychiatry 144:1166–1171, 1987

Price RA, Kidd KK, Cohen DJ, et al: A twin study of Tourette syndrome. Arch Gen Psychiatry 42:815–820, 1985

Quinn N, Critchley P, Marsden CD: Young onset Parkinson's disease. Mov Disord 2(2):73–91, 1987

Quitkin F, Rifkin A, Klein D: Neurologic soft signs in schizophrenia and character disorders. Arch Gen Psychiatry 33:845–853, 1976

Reed TE, Chandler JH: Huntington's chorea in Michigan, I: demography and genetics. Am J Hum Genet 10:201–225, 1958

Refsum S, Lonnum A, Sjaastad O, et al: Dystrophia myotonica: repeated pneumoencephalographic studies in ten patients. Neurology 17:345–348, 1967

Reich T, Cloninger CR, Guze S: The multifactorial model of disease transmission, I: description of the model and its use in psychiatry. Br J Psychiatry 127:1–10, 1975

Reik W: Genomic imprinting: a possible mechanism for the parental origin effect in Huntington's chorea. J Med Genet 25:805–808, 1988

Rich DP, Anderson MP, Gregory RJ, et al: Expression of cystic fibrosis transmembrane conductance regulator corrects defective chloride channel regulation in cystic fibrosis airway epithelial cells. Nature 347:358–363, 1990

Ridley RM, Frith CD, Crow TJ, et al: Anticipation in Huntington's disease is inherited through the male line but may originate in the female. J Med Genet 25:589–595, 1988

Rieder RO, Kaufmann CA: Genetics, in The American Psychiatric Press Textbook of Psychiatry. Edited by Talbott JA, Hales RE, Yudofsky SC. Washington, DC, American Psychiatric Press, 1988, pp 33–65

Rieder RO, Nichols PL: Offspring of schizophrenics, III. Arch Gen Psychiatry 36:665–674, 1979

Riordan JR, Rommens JM, Kerem B, et al: Identification of the cystic fibrosis gene: cloning and characterization of complementary DNA. Science 245:1066–1073, 1989

Risch N: Linkage strategies for genetically complex traits, I: multilocus models. Am J Hum Genet 46:222–228, 1990a

Risch N: Genetic linkage and complex diseases, with special reference to psychiatric disorders. Genet Epidemiol 7:3–16, 1990b

Risch N, Baron M: Segregation analysis of schizophrenia and related disorders. Am J Hum Genet 36:1039–1059, 1984

Risch N, Baron M, Mendlewicz J: Assessing the role of X-linked inheritance in bipolar-related major affective disorder. J Psychiatr Res 20:275–288, 1986

Rosenberg RN: Neurogenetics: Principles and Practice. New York, Raven, 1986

Rosenthal D: Genetic Theory and Abnormal Behavior. New York, McGraw-Hill, 1970

Rosenthal D, Wender PH, Kety SS, et al: Schizophrenics' offspring reared in adoptive homes. J Psychiatr Res 6:377–391, 1968

Roses AD, Pericak-Vance MA, Dawson DV, et al: Standard likelihood and sib pair analyses in late onset Alzheimers disease, in Current Communications in Molecular Biology. Edited by Davis P, Finch C. Cold Spring Harbor, NY, Cold Spring Harbor Laboratory, 1988, pp 180–186

Rosman NP, Kakulas BA: Mental deficiency associated with muscular dystrophy: a neuropathological study. Brain 89:769–787, 1966

Rudin E: Zur Vererbung und Neuenstehung der Dementia Praecox. Berlin, Springer Verlag, 1916

Sassa S, Granick S, Bickers DR, et al: A microassay for uroporphyrinogen I synthase, one of three abnormal enzyme activities in acute intermittent porphyria, and its application to the study of the genetics of this disease. Proc Natl Acad Sci U S A 71:732–736, 1974

Sax DS, Bird ED, Gusella JF, et al: Phenotypic variation in 2 Huntington's disease families with linkage to chromosome 4. Neurology 39:1332–1336, 1989

Scheinberg IH, Gitlin D: Deficiency of ceruloplasmin in patients' hepatolenticular degeneration (Wilson's disease). Science 116:484–485, 1952

Schellenberg GD, Deeb SS, Boehnke ML, et al.: Association of apolipoprotein CII allele with familial dementia of the Alzheimer type. Neurogenetics 4:97–108, 1987

Schellenberg GD, Bird TD, Wijsman EM, et al: Absence of linkage of chromosome 21q21 markers to familial Alzheimer's disease. Science 241:1507–1510, 1988

Schellenberg GD, Bird TD, Wijisman EM, et al: The genetics of Alzheimers Disease. Biomed Pharmacother 43:463–468, 1989

Schoenberg BS: Descriptive epidemiology of Parkinson's disease: disease distribution and hypothesis formulation. Adv Neurol 45:277–283, 1987

Schutta HS, Pratt RTC, Metz H, et al: A family study of the late infantile and juvenile forms of metachromatic leucodystrophy. J Med Genet 3:86–90, 1966

Segal NL, Dysken MW, Bouchard TJ, et al: Tourette's disorder in a set of reared-apart triplets: genetic and environmental influences. Am J Psychiatry 147:196–199, 1990

Seltzer B, Sherwin I: A comparison of clinical features in early and late onset primary degenerative dementia: one entity or two? Arch Neurol 40:143–146, 1983

Shapiro AK, Shapiro E: Tic disorders, in The Comprehensive Textbook of Psychiatry, 5th Edition. Edited by Kaplan HI, Sadock BJ. Baltimore, MD, Williams & Wilkins, 1989, pp 1865–1878

Shepherd MJ, Charnow DA, Silver LB: Developmental reading disorder, in Comprehensive Textbook of Psychiatry, 5th Edition. Edited by Kaplan HI, Sadock BJ. Baltimore, MD, Williams & Wilkins 1989, pp 1790–1796

Sherrington R, Brynjolfsson J, Petursson H, et al: Localization of a susceptibility locus for schizophrenia on chromosome 5. Nature 336:164–167, 1988

Siddique T, McKinney R, Hung WY, et al: The poliovirus sensitivity (PVS) gene is on chromosome 19q12-q13.2. Genomics 3(2):156–160, 1988

Siegel C, Waldo M, Minzner G, et al: Deficits in sensory gating in schizophrenic patients and their relatives: evidence obtained with auditory-evoked responses. Arch Gen Psychiatry 41:607–612, 1984

Sim M, Bale RN: Familial pre-senile dementia: the relevance of a histological diagnosis of Pick's disease. Br J Psychiatry 122:671–673, 1973

Skomer C, Stears JU, Austin J: Metachromatic leucodystrophy, XV: adult with focal lesions by computed tomography. Arch Neurol 40:354–5, 1983

Sladen B: Inheritance of dyslexia. Bulletin of the Orton Society 20:30–40, 1970

Slater E: The monogenic theory of schizophrenia. Acta Genetica et Statistica Medica 8:50–56, 1958

Slater E, Cowie V: The Genetics of Mental Disorders. London, Oxford University Press, 1971

Smith S, Kimberling W, Pennington B, et al: Specific reading disability: identification of an inherited form through linkage analysis. Science 219:1345–1347, 1983

Snell RG, Lazarou LP, Youngman S, et al: Linkage disequilibrium in Huntington's disease: an improved localisation for the gene. J Med Genet 26:673–675, 1989

Spitzer RL, Endicott J, Robins E: Research Diagnostic Criteria: rational and reliability. Arch Gen Psychiatry 35: 773–782, 1978

Sroka H, Elizan TS, Yahr MD, et al: Organic mental syndrome and confusional states in Parkinson's disease. Relationship to computerised tomographic signs of cerebral atrophy. Arch Neurol 38:339–342, 1981

St Clair D, Blackwood D, Muir W, et al: No linkage to chromosome 5q11-q13 markers to schizophrenia in Scottish families. Nature 339:305–309, 1989

St Clair D, Blackwood D, Muir W, et al: A balanced autosomal translocation associated in a single large pedigree with multiple cases of major mental illness including schizophrenia and schizoaffective disorder. Lancet 336:13–16, 1990

St George-Hyslop PH, Tanzi RE, Polinsky RJ, et al: The genetic defect causing familial Alzheimer's disease maps on chromosome 21. Science 235:885–890, 1987

St George-Hyslop PH, Myers R, Haines JL, et al: Familial Alzheimer's disease: progress and problems. Neurobiol Aging 10:417–25, 1989

Stein C, Gieselman V, Kreysing J, et al: Cloning and expression of human arylsulfatase A. J Biol Chem 264: 1252–1259, 1981

Stephenson S: Six cases of congenital word blindness affecting three generations of one family. Ophthalmoscope 5:482–484, 1907

Stewart J, Debray Q, Caillard V: Schizophrenia: the testing of genetic models. Am J Hum Genet 32:55–63, 1980

Strober M, Morrell W, Burroughs J, et al: A family study of bipolar I disorder in adolescence: early onset of symptoms linked to increased family loading and lithium resistance. J Affective Disord 15:255–268, 1988

Tanner CM: The role of environmental toxins in the etiology of Parkinson's disease. Trends Neurosci 12(2): 49–54, 1989

Tanzi RE, St George-Hyslop PH, Haines JL, et al: The genetic defect in familial Alzheimer's disease is not tightly linked to the amyloid beta-protein gene. Nature 329:156–157, 1987

Thomasen E: Myotonia: Thomsen's Disease (Myotonia Congenita), Paramyotonia, and Dystrophia Myotonica. Aarhus, Denmark, Universitetsforlaget, 1948

Thompson LM, Plummer S, Altherr M, et al: Isolation and characterization of cDNA clones representing transcripts from the region /f 4p16.3 containing the Huntington disease gene. Am J Hum Genet 47 (suppl):A118, 1990

Tienari P, Lahti I, Naarald M: Biological mothers in the Finnish adoption study: alternative definitions of schizophrenia. Paper presented at the VIIth World Congress of Psychiatry, Vienna, Austria, June 1983

Torrey EF: Neurologic abnormalities in schizophrenic patients. Biol Psychiatry 15:381–387, 1980

Tsuang MT, Faraone SV: The Genetics of Mood Disorders. Baltimore, MD, Johns Hopkins University Press, 1990

Tsuang MT, Bucher KD, Fleming JA: Testing the monogenic theory of schizophrenia: an application of segregation analysis to blind family study data. Br J Psychiatry 140:595–599, 1982

Tsuang MT, Faraone SV, Fleming JA: Familial transmission of major affective disorders: is there evidence supporting the distinction between unipolar and bipolar disorders? Br J Psychiatry 146:268–271, 1985

Tsuboi T: Genetic analysis of febrile convulsions, in Genetics of the Epilepsies. Edited by Beck-Managetta G,

Anderson VE, Doose H, et al. New York, Springer-Verlag, 1989, pp 25–33

Tsuboi T, Endo S: Incidence of seizures and EEG abnormality among offspring of epileptic patients. Hum Genet 36:173–89, 1977

Turner WD: Genetic markers for schizotaxia. Biol Psychiatry 14:177–205, 1979

Uryu N, Maeda M, Nagata Y, et al: No difference in the nucleotide sequence of the DQB B1 domain between narcoleptic and healthy individuals with DR2, DW2. Hum Immunol 24:175–181, 1989

Van Broeckhoven C, van Hul W, Backhoven H, et al: The familial Alzheimer gene is located close to the centromere of chromosome 21. Am J Hum Genet 43:A205, 1988

Vandenberg SG, Singer SM, Pauls DL: The Heredity of Behavior Disorders in Adults and Children. New York, Plenum, 1986

Verma A, Nye JS, Snyder SH: Porphyrins are endogenous ligands for the mitochondrial (peripheral-type) benzodiazepine receptor. Proc Nat Acad Sci U S A 84:2256–2260, 1987

Waldenstrom J: Studies on the incidence and heredity of acute porphyria in Sweden. Acta Genetica et Statistica Medica 6:122–131, 1956

Walker E: Attentional and neuromotor functions of schizophrenics, schizoaffectives, and patients with other affective disorders. Arch Gen Psychiatry 38:1355–1358, 1981

Walshe JM: The physiology of copper in man and its relation to Wilson's disease. Brain 90:149–176, 1967

Ward CD, Duvoisin RC, Ince SE, et al: Parkinson's disease in 65 pairs of twins and in a set of quadruplets. Neurology 33:815–824, 1983

Watt NF, Anthony EJ, Wynne LC, et al: Children at Risk for Schizophrenia: A Longitudinal Perspective. Cambridge, Cambridge University Press, 1984

Weber JL, May PE: Abundant class of human DNA polymorphisms which can be typed using the polymerase chain reaction. Am J Hum Genet 44:388–396, 1989

Wechsler D: WISC-R Manual: Wechsler Intelligence Scale for Children-Revised. New York, Psychological Corporation, 1974

Weinberger DR: Implications of normal brain development for the pathogenesis of schizophrenia. Arch Gen Psychiatry 44:660–669, 1987

Weissman MM, Leaf PJ, Tischler GL, et al: Affective disorders in five United States communities. Psychol Med 18:141–153, 1988

Wender PH, Rosenthal D, Kety SS, et al: Cross-fostering: a research strategy for clarifying the role of genetic and experiential factors in the etiology of schizophrenia. Arch Gen Psychiatry 30:121–128, 1974

Wender PH, Kety SS, Rosenthal D, et al: Psychiatric disorders in the biological and adoptive families of adopted individuals with affective disorders. Arch Gen Psychiatry 43:923–929, 1986

Westaway D, Carlson GA, Prusiner SB: Unraveling prion diseases through molecular genetics. Trends Neurosci 12:221–227, 1989

Whalley LJ, Carothers AD, Collyer S, et al: A study of familial factors in Alzheimer's disease. Br J Psychiatry 140:249–256, 1982

Whitehouse PJ, Price DL, Clark JT, et al: Alzheimer disease: evidence for selective loss of cholinergic neurons in the nucleus basalis. Ann Neurol 10:122–126, 1981

Wilson JM, Stout JT, Palella TD, et al: A molecular survey of hypoxanthine-guanine phosphoribosyltransferase deficiency in man. J Clin Invest 77:188–195, 1986

Wilson SAK: Progressive lenticular degeneration: a familial nervous disease associated with cirrhosis of the liver. Brain 34:295–507, 1912

Wing JK, Cooper JE, Sartorius N: The Measurement and Classification of Psychiatric Symptoms. New York, Cambridge University Press, 1974

Winokur G, Clayton PJ, Reich T: Manic Depressive Illness. St. Louis, MO, CV Mosby, 1969

Wolf C: An experimental investigation of specific language disability. Bulletin of the Orton Society 17:32–38, 1967

Wolff G, Deuschl G, Wienker TF, et al: New mutation to Huntington's disease. J Med Genet 26:18–27, 1989

Wood PL, Nair NP, Etienne P, et al: Lack of cholinergic deficit in the neocortex in Pick's disease. Prog Neuropsychopharmacol Biol Psychiatry 7:725–727, 1983

Yamamura Y, Sobue I, Ando K, et al: Paralysis agitans of early onset with marked diurnal fluctuation of symptoms. Neurology (Minneapolis) 23:239–244, 1973

Yokochi M, Narabayashi H, Iizuka R: Juvenile parkinsonism—some clinical, pharmacological and neuropathological aspects. Adv Neurol 40:407–413, 1984

Yoss RE, Daly DD: Criteria for the diagnosis of the narcoleptic syndrome. Proceedings of the Staff Meeting of the Mayo Clinic 32:320–328, 1957

Youngman S, Sarfarazi M, Bucan M, et al: A new DNA marker (D4S90) is located terminally on the short arm of chromosome 4, close to the Huntington disease gene. Genomics 5:802–809, 1989

Zahalkova M, Vrzal V, Kloboukova E: Genetical investigations in dyslexia. J Med Genet 9:48–52, 1972

Zausmer DM, Dewey ME: Tics and heredity. A study of the relatives of child tiqueurs. Br J Psychiatry 150:628–634, 1987

Zerbin-Rudin E: Endogene Psychosen, in Humangenetik: Ein Kurzes Handbuch. Edited by Becker PE. Stuttgart, Georg Thieme Verlag KG, 1967, pp 446–513

Zhang XL, Rafi MA, Degala G, et al: Mechanism for defective splicing causing a 33 nucleotide insertion in a patient with SAP-1 deficient metachromatic leucodystrophy. Am J Hum Genet 47 (suppl):A172, 1990

Zlotogora J: Intrafamilial variability in lysosomal storage diseases. Am J Med Genet 27:633–638, 1987

Zweig RM, Koven SJ, Hedreen JC, et al: Linkage to the Huntington's disease locus in a family with unusual clinical and pathological features. Ann Neurol 26:78–84, 1989

Section III

Neuropsychiatric Symptomatologies

Chapter

9

Differential Diagnosis in Neuropsychiatry

Richard L. Strub, M.D.
Michael G. Wise, M.D.

WHEN THE BRAIN IS DAMAGED or rendered dysfunctional by chemical imbalances, behavior is often modified. Such organically based behavioral changes constitute the foundation of neuropsychiatry (Cummings 1985). Recognizing and understanding these characteristic symptoms, symptom clusters, and syndromes are the essence of the diagnostic process in neuropsychiatry (Benson and Blumer 1982; Frederiks et al. 1985; Heilman and Valenstein 1985). This diagnostic process is of both theoretical and practical importance. Of theoretical interest is the attempt to understand brain-behavioral relationships; this includes not only the explanation of the specific cognitive symptoms seen in dementia, delirium, and focal brain lesions, but also insights (gained through the study of organically produced affective and delusional disorders) into the neurobiology of classic psychiatric disorders, such as manic depressive illness or schizophrenia (Mesulam 1985a).

We wish to thank Mary Usner for her secretarial assistance in preparing the manuscript.

In a very practical sense, making the correct neuropsychiatric diagnosis can literally be lifesaving. For example, if an examiner cannot differentiate the fluent aphasia produced by a patient with a temporal lobe mass from the psychotic language of a decompensated schizophrenic patient, he is likely to make a serious misdiagnosis. From a broader yet simplistic perspective of patient management, patients with different neuropsychiatric disorders require very different plans of management. The patient with simple dementia can be leisurely evaluated as an outpatient, the patient with a delirium is sick usually from a medical or neurological disorder and must be admitted to the hospital on an acute medical or neuropsychiatric service, and the patient with a restricted behavioral syndrome such as an aphasia or parietal lobe syndrome caused by a focal brain lesion should be seen and evaluated by a neurologist or neurosurgeon. These examples underscore the tremendous practical importance of differential diagnosis in neuropsychiatry.

The diagnostic process itself is no different from that in any other medical specialty. Historical information and examination findings are matched with known syndromes in an effort to establish a clinical diagnosis. In neuropsychiatry, the collection of data must be oriented toward organic disease, and the clinical examination must include an expanded mental status examination that encompasses a comprehensive evaluation of various cognitive functions and common organic behavior signs (e.g., frontal lobe signs) (Folstein et al. 1975; Strub and Black 1985). The diagnostic process involves first, the recognition of the patient's symptoms as organic in origin, and second, the understanding that the specific symptoms and symptom clusters are characteristic of a particular clinical syndrome or cerebral localization (Kertesz 1983; Strub and Black 1988). An experienced examiner can often move quickly from a few symptoms to a clinical diagnosis; however, even for the seasoned neuropsychiatrist, there is really no substitute for a complete history with full mental status and neurological examinations. With this data base the clinician can usually generate a diagnosis either of a general or global neurobehavioral syndrome such as dementia or delirium (organic mental syndrome) or of a specific disease such as Alzheimer's disease or alcoholic Korsakoff's syndrome (organic mental disorder).

Although a neuropsychiatrist is usually concerned with a recent change in behavior secondary to a new brain disease or disorder, there are neuropsychiatric disorders that are the remnants of developmental disorders. For example, the patient with mild mental retardation, dyslexia, or mild autism may have compensated adequately for the disorder until challenged by sufficient stress or a specific demand later in life. At such a point, the congenitally weak neurobiological systems may fail to adjust to the new set of physical (illness) or environmental demands, and clinically significant symptoms can be produced. The true nature of the patient's new behavioral problem is not fully understood until the developmental history is known and the interaction of the congenital problem with the new challenge is untangled.

Differential diagnosis has three levels of specificity in neuropsychiatry (Figure 9–1). The first is the age-old differential between an organic and a nonorganic mental syndrome. The second is the differential among the various organic mental syndromes, and the third and final step is the establishment of a specific diagnosis or identification of a specific organic mental disorder such as Alzheimer's dementia or multi-infarct dementia. This final diagnostic step usually involves the ordering and interpretation of appropriate medical, neurodiagnostic, and psychological tests. In the final diagnostic impression, the examiner must also consider important historical information such as associated medical disease (hypertension, stroke, and thyroid disease), medications, and neurological symptoms (weakness, double vision, headache, episodic phenomena, syncope, and seizure).

Most psychiatrists have greater skill and are more comfortable in analyzing verbal, affective, and interpersonal and interactive data than they are with testing cognitive symptoms. For this reason, we discuss these symptoms at length and include several diagnostic algorithms in this chapter to assist in the organization of the differential diagnostic process.

❑ TYPES AND SPEED OF BEHAVIORAL CHANGE

The rapidity of the onset of behavioral change is a very important element in the differential diagnosis in neuropsychiatry. Behavior changes can occur acutely as in stroke, subacutely as in delirium or, chronically as in dementia. In each of these clinical situations there is a logical decision-making process that will lead the examiner to the correct diagnosis. The decision tree in Figure 9–2 has been developed for evaluating a patient with chronic behavior change. The types of behavioral changes in neuropsychiatry have often been separated into two general categories: cognitive and noncognitive. Examples of each are listed in Table 9–1.

Evaluating patients who have developed changes in noncognitive spheres is often more difficult than evaluating patients who have changes in cognitive function. Noncognitive change is usually subjective and is often primarily psychiatric and not neuropsychiatric. Certain features help the clinician to identify patients who have noncognitive changes secondary to organic disease (such as brain pathology), medical illness, or medications. The first is knowledge of the epidemiology of common psychiatric disorders (Figure 9–3). For example, a 60-year-old man with no prior psychiatric problems who is referred for evaluation for new onset of anxiety, "schizophrenia," or depression needs very close scrutiny. There is a very high likelihood that an organic etiology is responsible for the behavioral change. The second is a careful history. The examiner must have a complete medical history and know

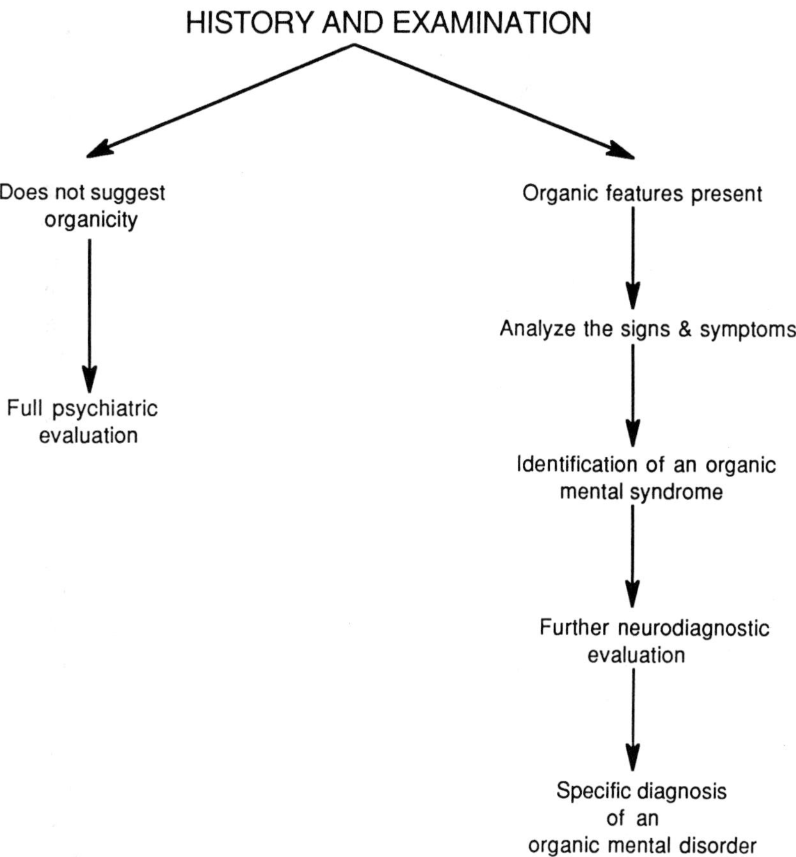

Figure 9–1. Diagnostic process.

all medications, both prescription and nonprescription, that the patient is taking. Third, a careful mental status examination and neurological examination are essential.

❑ SPECIFIC SYMPTOMS AND THEIR GENERAL SIGNIFICANCE IN NEUROPSYCHIATRY

Because most individual symptoms can be produced by a variety of causes and can be seen in different neuropsychiatric conditions (Tables 9–2 and 9–3), one can generate an enormous differential diagnosis for each of the symptoms mentioned in Table 9–1. In this section we discuss these major neuropsychiatric symptoms and allude to their most common causes. Other chapters in this volume expand on these introductory discussions.

Cognitive

Altered level of consciousness. Psychiatric consultation is often sought by members of the medical and surgical services for patients who have experienced what is routinely called "a recent change in mental status." In most instances this means the patient is either lethargic (not as alert as would be expected after surgery or some medical intervention) or agitated and disruptive. In addition to the change in the level of consciousness, such patients often exhibit evidence of an alteration in thought content or what has been called the *content of consciousness.* This change in both level of alertness and content of consciousness produces the clouded consciousness that typifies the confusional behavior seen in delirium (Lipowski 1990).

Any patient who is difficult to arouse or will not remain alert without constant stimulation is quite likely to be physically ill. There are, however,

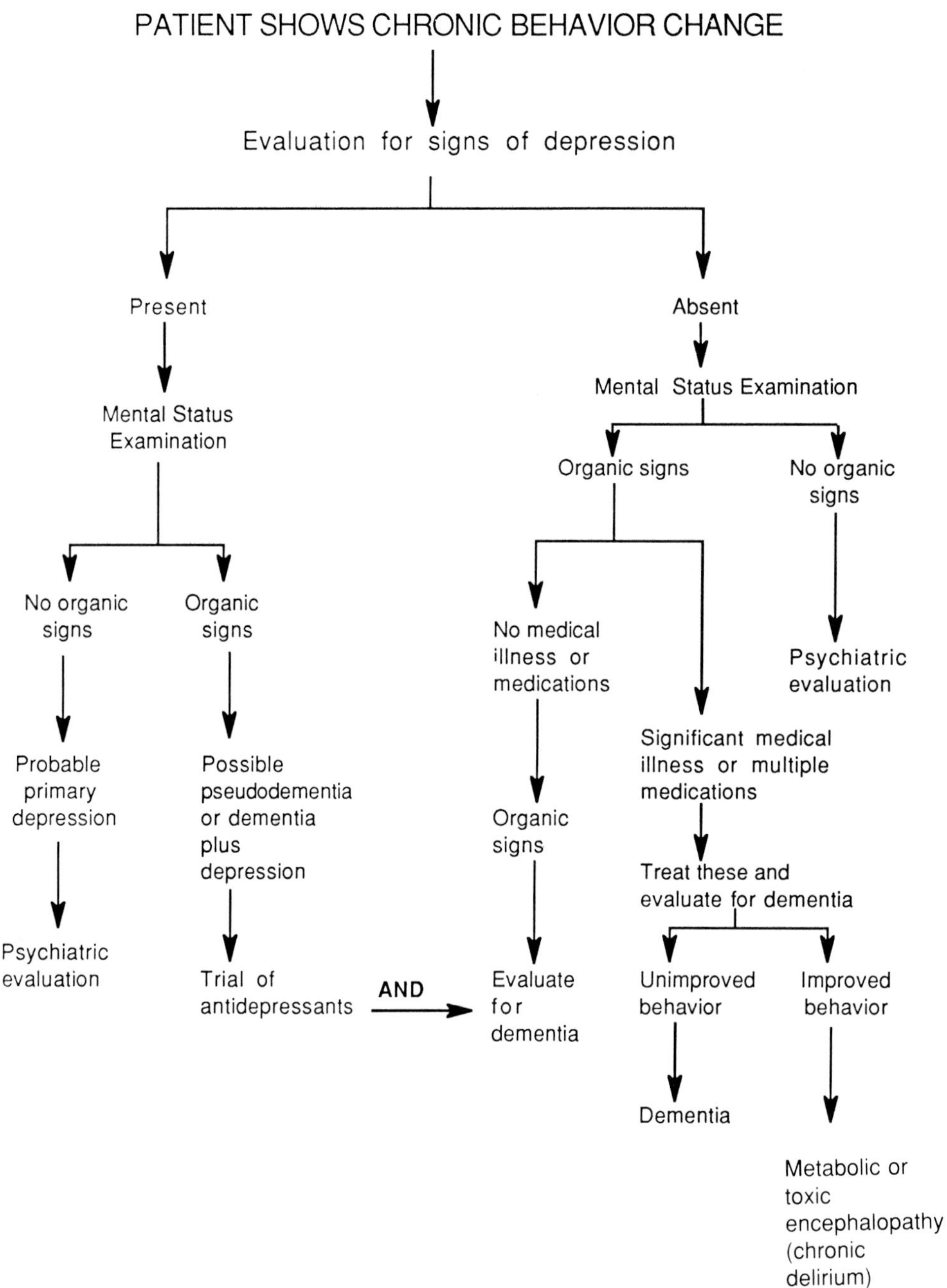

Figure 9–2. Decision tree for chronic behavior change. (Reprinted from Weisberg LA, Strub RL, Garcia CA: Decision Making in Adult Neurology. Toronto, Ontario, Decker, 1987, pp 70–71. Used with permission.)

other clinical situations that may mimic a medically significant decreased level of consciousness. For example, sleepiness, boredom, simple intoxication, or a primary sleep disorder will all produce lethargy at times. In addition, depressed patients with significant psychomotor retardation may be withdrawn and slow to respond; they are, however, rarely confused or lethargic in the sense used here. There are also a few patients who will actually feign unconsciousness, so-called psychogenic unresponsiveness. Such a diagnosis is only entertained after a full medical and neurological evaluation has not yielded

TABLE 9–1. CATEGORIES OF BEHAVIOR CHANGE

Cognitive
Consciousness
Attention
Speech and language
Memory
Disorientation in space

Noncognitive
Affect and mood
Personality (character)
Anxiety
Thought disorder
Hallucination
Aggression
Psychomotor activity

a more plausible explanation. Such patients usually have either a prior psychiatric history or significant current environmental chaos to explain the withdrawal behavior.

Presented with a patient who has a decrease in level of consciousness due to a medical or neurological illness, the clinician must begin the diagnostic processes used in assessing a patient with a delirium or coma. The differential diagnosis includes toxic (medications, alcohol, and illicit drugs) and metabolic disturbances as the most common causes; these patients will have a nonlocalizing neurological examination. Destructive cerebral lesions such as stroke, subdural hematoma, tumor, or abscess will also cause a decreased level of consciousness, but characteristically demonstrate focal neurological findings (Magoun 1963). Meningitis, seizures, and subarachnoid hemorrhage are also diagnostic possibilities. A more extensive discussion on this topic appears in Chapters 11 and 12. There are many excellent references available on the topics of delirium and coma (Plum and Posner 1980).

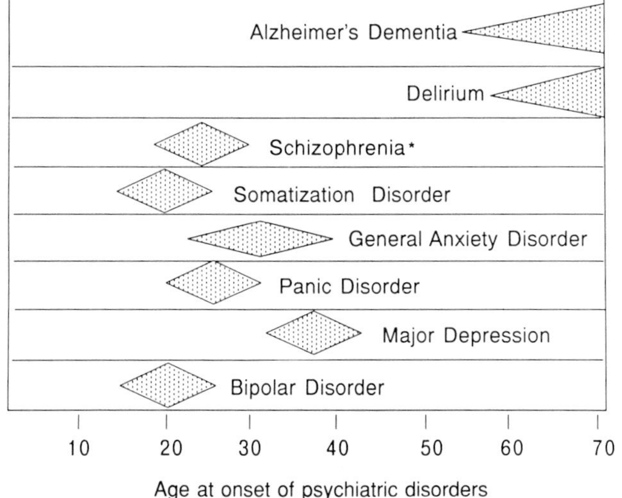

Figure 9–3. Differential diagnosis in neuropsychiatry. *Earlier onset in males

Inattention. The capacity to direct and maintain one's attention while screening out extraneous and irrelevant stimuli is a very basic yet highly complex neuropsychological function (Berlucchi and Rizzolatti 1987; McGhie 1969). Inattention (the breakdown of selective attention) and distractibility are common and clinically very significant neuropsychiatric symptoms. In addition to its clinical importance, inattention can also complicate the entire evaluation process (Mesulam 1985b; Pribram and McGuinness 1975). For example, an inattentive patient will frequently fail tests of memory or calculation on the basis of inattention alone. Caution, therefore, must be used in the interpretation of cognitive failure in the inattentive patient.

As important as it is to recognize that inattention can adversely affect performance on the mental status examination, it is equally important to realize that this symptom is probably the least specific of any symptom in neuropsychiatry. Inattention is seen in conditions as diverse as simple anxiety or fatigue, delirium, dementia, schizophrenia, mania, and focal brain lesions, particularly those localized in the inferior frontal or parietal lobes.

In addition to these conditions in which patients display global inattention, there is a special type of inattention in which patients are inattentive to only half of their body and the extrapersonal space on the same side (Kinsbourne 1970). This syndrome, called *hemiattention* or *hemineglect,* is most frequently manifested as a left hemiattention in a patient who has suffered a right-hemisphere brain lesion (Weinstein and Friedland 1977).

Because of the ubiquitous nature of inattention it stands alone only in indicating the presence of a problem. It must be combined with more specific symptoms before its clinical significance can be fully appreciated.

TABLE 9–2. MEDICATIONS THAT CAUSE BEHAVIORAL CHANGE

Analgesics	**Cardiac drugs**
Meperidine	Captopril
Opiates	Clonidine
Pentazocine	Digitalis
	Disopyramide
Anticholinergic drugs	Lidocaine
Antihistamines	Mexiletine
Antiparkinson drugs	Methyldopa
Benztropine	Propranolol
Biperiden	Reserpine
Antispasmodics	
Atropine/homatropine	**Drug withdrawal**
Belladonna alkaloids	Alcohol
Chlorpheniramine	Barbiturates
Diphenhydramine	Benzodiazepines
Phenothiazines	
(especially thioridazine)	**Sedative-hypnotics**
Promethazine	Barbiturates
Scopolamine	Benzodiazepines
Tricyclic antidepressants	Glutethimide
(especially amitriptyline)	
Trihexyphenidyl	**Sympathomimetics**
	Aminophylline
Anticonvulsant drugs	Amphetamines
Phenobarbital	Cocaine
	Ephedrine
Anti-inflammatory drugs	Phenylephrine
Adrenocorticotropic	Phenylpropanolamine
hormone (ACTH)	Theophylline
Corticosteroids	
	Miscellaneous drugs
Antiparkinsonian drugs	Alcohol
Amantadine	Cimetidine
Bromocriptine	Hallucinogens
Carbidopa	Metoclopramide
Levodopa	Metrizamide
	Yohimbine

Note. Almost any medication that enters the central nervous system has the potential to induce cognitive or noncognitive change. The medications listed in this table do so more frequently.

Speech and language disorders. Because verbal language is the primary means of communication between people, any departure from the patient's accustomed manner of verbal interchange is readily recognized. There are many ways in which verbal communication can change, and each has its own clinical significance neuropsychiatrically. For example, certain patients can have a pure speech disorder (such as stuttering, in which basic language function is normal), whereas others demonstrate a primary language disorder (such as aphasia) (Holland 1984). In a third type of patient, basic speech and language are intact, but changes in timbre, pitch, and speed of delivery may reflect an underlying affective disorder. Table 9–4 lists the general areas of speech and language disorders that are most commonly encountered.

Changes in the affective tone and speed of speech production have always been important symptoms to the psychiatrist. Organic lesions however can produce similar changes. One example is the decreased melodic quality of speech that can occur in patients with a right-hemisphere lesion, particularly a lesion that involves the temporal and parietal lobes. A right temporal lesion can cause patients to produce speech with a flat, almost monotonic or aprosodic character (Young 1983). As part of their overall apathy and psychomotor retarda-

TABLE 9–3. CLINICAL CONDITIONS THAT MAY PRODUCE BEHAVIOR CHANGE

Neurological disease	Medical illness
Infections	Infectious—sepsis
Encephalitis	Toxins
Meningitis	Alcohol and illicit drugs
Brain abscess	Organic compounds
Acquired immunodeficiency syndrome (AIDS)	Metallic poisons
Syphilis	Metabolic disease
Creutzfeldt-Jakob disease	Thyroid
Vascular	Parathyroid
Cerebral vascular accident	Pituitary
Multi-infarct dementia	Adrenal
Large arteriovenous malformations	Immune disorders
Tumors	Systemic lupus erythematosus
Trauma	AIDS
Subdural hematoma	Cancer—indirect effects
Intracerebral hemorrhage	
Frontal and temporal contusions	
General closed head injury	
Hydrocephalus	
Degenerative	
Alzheimer's disease	
Pick's disease	
Huntington's disease	
Demyelinating—multiple sclerosis	

tion, patients with frontal lobe lesions can also demonstrate a speech delivery that is very flat but has greater inflection than that of the patient with a right temporal/parietal lesion.

Dysarthria, another general speech disorder, refers to any alteration in speech production that is caused by a lesion or disease process that interferes with the muscles of articulation. Dysarthria can occur secondarily in disease of the vocal apparatus, in certain neurological disorders, or in a metabolic or toxic condition such as alcohol intoxication. Neurological conditions that can produce dysarthria are legion; anything from parkinsonism, amyotrophic lateral sclerosis, and multiple strokes to myasthenia gravis or oculopharyngeal dystrophy can be responsible. Articulatory disturbances are important to recognize because they frequently signal significant neurological or otolaryngological disease that will require evaluation by the appropriate specialist.

Stuttering (dysfluency) is an interesting condition that is usually a developmental disorder of childhood, but it can appear de novo in adulthood. When stuttering does present in an adult, it is often due to a new brain lesion, such as a stroke, and requires investigation as a sentinel symptom of a potentially serious neurological condition.

Mutism is another fascinating communication disorder. It can be seen in both classic neurological disease such as stroke (akinetic mutism) (Segarra and Angelo 1970) or basal ganglion disease (parkinsonism), as well as in emotional disorders such as

TABLE 9–4. COMMON SPEECH AND LANGUAGE DISORDERS

Change in affective tone

Speech disorders
- Dysarthria
- Stuttering (dysfluency)
- Mutism
- Aprosodia

Language disorders
- Aphasia
- Alexia
- Agraphia
- Schizophrenic language
- Confusional or incoherent language

depression or psychosis. The mute patient, like the catatonic patient, deserves a full neurological evaluation.

The patient who presents with disordered language production presents a very interesting diagnostic challenge to the neuropsychiatrist. Four of the most common conditions that present in this fashion are fluent aphasia, dementia in its middle stage, delirium, and schizophrenia. Each diagnosis carries different clinical and management implications. The neuropsychiatric examiner should have no major difficulty in making a correct diagnosis in these cases if a good history is available and a full mental status is performed.

Clinically, the patient with fluent aphasia (produced by a lesion in the left temporoparietal region) will produce very paraphasic speech with poor syntax and demonstrate poor verbal comprehension. Other mental status testing may reveal other parietal lobe signs (e.g., constructional apraxia) but good visual memory. The history and neurological examination will further restrict the diagnostic possibilities. For example, an older patient with evidence of arteriosclerosis and the onset of acute aphasia most likely had a middle cerebral artery stroke. If, on the other hand, the patient has slowly developed the language disorder and has headaches and papilledema, a brain tumor would be the probable diagnosis.

In patients with dementia, the language disorder develops slowly and is characterized by vagueness in communication with a tendency to speak tangentially and with less precision. In the later stage, there is evidence of a significant aphasia with difficulty finding the proper words, trouble understanding conversation, and production of disjointed phrases with scattered paraphasic words. Comprehension in a patient with dementia, however, is far superior to that of the fluent aphasic patient discussed above.

Delirious patients frequently produce confused and incoherent speech but are not dramatically aphasic. Their speech and language disorder is never the sole presenting complaint but merely an associated feature of the delirium. The difficult case to analyze is the patient whose delirium is due to a focal left-hemisphere lesion where delirium and significant aphasia are present together.

The schizophrenic patient also has a disturbance in language production, but it is rarely confused with the classic organic patterns of aphasia, dementia, or delirium. The paranoia, relative paucity of neologisms (compared with an aphasic patient), excellent comprehension, lack of significant cognitive loss, and lack of altered level of consciousness will usually readily identify the schizophrenic patient.

Language disorders in general are discussed extensively in Chapter 13. However, it is important to emphasize that the appearance of an aphasia (a disorder of comprehension, word choice, or syntax) (Albert et al. 1981; Goodglass and Kaplan 1983; Kertesz 1979), alexia (acquired reading disorder), or agraphia (acquired writing disorder) usually indicates acquired brain damage or dysfunction involving the patient's language dominant hemisphere. Aphasia, alexia, and agraphia are virtually always organic symptoms that should lead the examiner to search for a specific neurological cause. There is an enormous literature on the neurology, neuropsychology, and neurolinguistic aspects of language disorders, but the overwhelmingly practical consideration in these disorders for the neuropsychiatrist is the ability to recognize the disorder and pursue its etiology.

Memory loss. Memory loss is undoubtedly one of the most common symptoms that the neuropsychiatrist is asked to evaluate. This complaint can also be difficult to assess because it has many different causes. Because of the complexity of the differential diagnosis of memory loss, its evaluation serves as an excellent example of the diagnostic process used by the skilled neuropsychiatrist. The algorithm in Figure 9–4 demonstrates the most frequently encountered types of memory loss and the line of investigation that should be followed to arrive at a correct diagnosis. It is important to remember that memory loss can be symptomatic of either a psychogenic or an organic condition. Epidemiological as well as historical information about the patient is very useful when considering the possible diagnoses. In general, the patient under age 40, particularly one with a history of previous or concomitant emotional problems, is likely to have a psychogenic amnesia; whereas the elderly person with progressive memory loss will more frequently be suffering from an organic dementing illness.

The assessment of memory loss is one of the most important clinical skills that the neuropsychiatrist must acquire. Haphazard testing that demonstrates memory problems can often lead to erroneous findings. For example, a patient may be given an improper diagnosis of dementia when the memory problem may actually be due to anxiety or de-

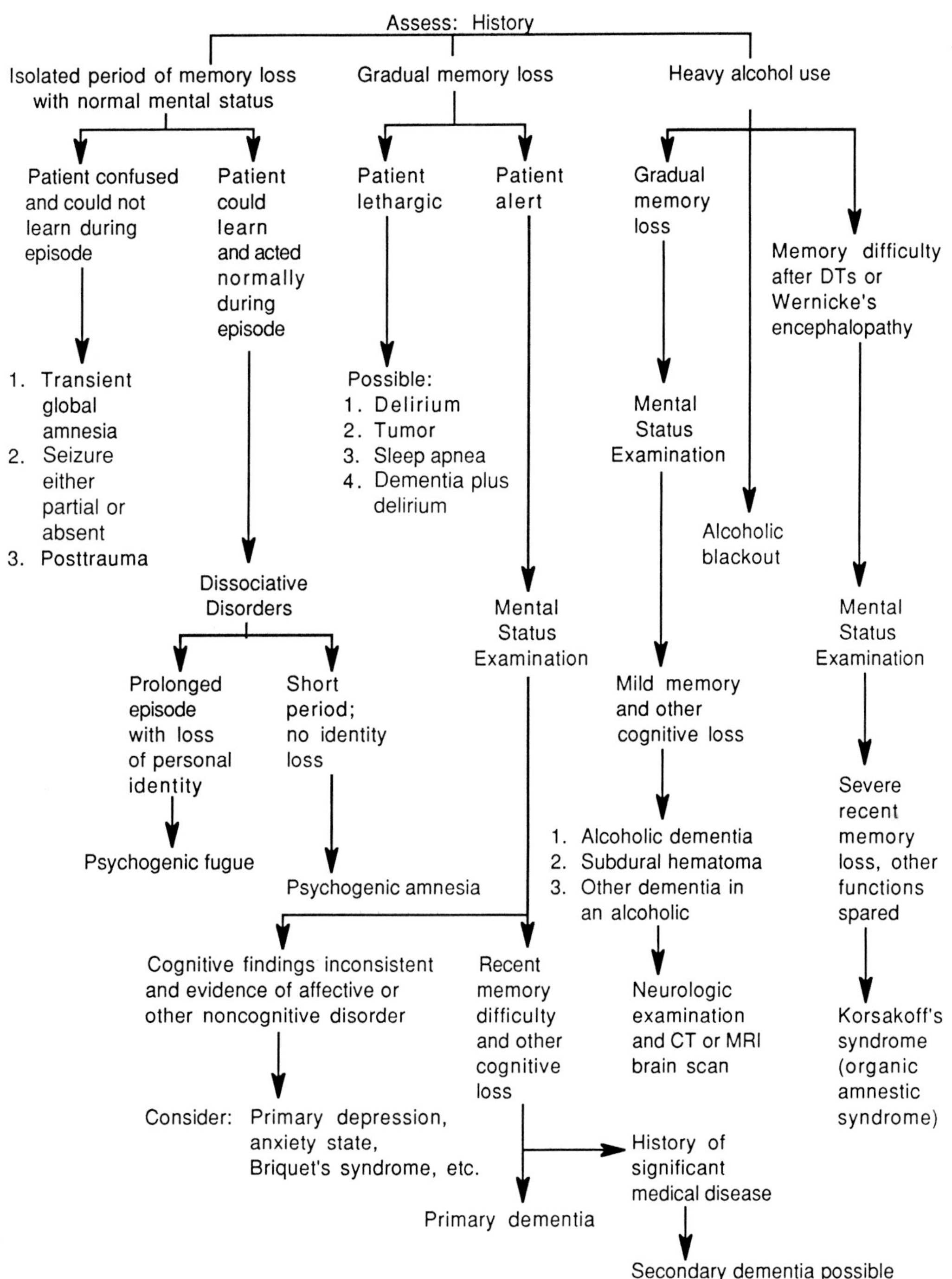

Figure 9–4. Decision tree for memory loss. DT = delirium tremens; CT = computed tomography scan; MRI = magnetic resonance imaging. (Reprinted from Weisberg LA, Strub RL, Garcia CA: Decision Making in Adult Neurology. Toronto, Ontario, Decker, 1987, pp 72–74. Used with permission.)

pression. This is especially true in the elderly patient. A diagnosis is only as good as the data used to make it. There are good discussions on memory testing in this volume (Chapters 4 and 5) and in the works by Strub and Black (1985, 1988), Squire and Butters (1984), and Victor et al. (1989).

Disorientation in space. It is very frightening to become lost or disoriented in one's own environment. Driving to the store and becoming hopelessly lost, being unable to find one's car in a shopping center parking lot, and losing one's way to the bathroom in one's own home are all common clinical examples of geographic disorientation or disorientation in space. Analysis of this symptom reveals that it is far from unitary. There are varied neuropsychological mechanisms by which this single cognitive function, spatial orientation, can be impaired. For example, a man who loses his car in a large parking lot may be perfectly "normal" but was merely preoccupied at the time he parked and failed to note the location. In others, the symptom is not so innocent, such as a woman with mild delirium who, from her clouded consciousness and its attendant muddled thinking, may be disoriented in all spheres and lose her car as a symptom of her disorder. In like fashion, patients with dementia or amnesia may not be able to remember because of their recent memory or new learning deficit.

A totally different type of spatial disorientation occurs in patients with parietal lobe damage (De-Renzi 1985). Such patients have a true geographic disorientation and fail to find their car because of visual spatial disorientation. These patients have visual perception deficits as well as problems integrating visual perception with the location of objects in extrapersonal space. This true spatial disorientation is more common among patients with a lesion in the right parietal lobe but can occur with lesions in other areas of the brain. There is an additional type of spatial disorientation that is seen in patients with hemineglect or hemiattention. These patients usually have right parietal lesions and fail to pay attention to the left side of their environment.

In each of the examples above the geographic disorientation was due to a different neuropsychological mechanism and a different disease process. The ability to analyze a specific symptom and understand its differential diagnosis is a very important skill to develop in neuropsychiatry.

Noncognitive

Affect and mood. Affect is the description of an individual's emotional state at a particular point in time, such as depressed, euphoric, or angry; whereas mood describes an individual's pervasive, sustained emotional state over an extended span of time, such as a week or month. Alteration in mood can occur as a reaction or adjustment to a stressful situation; this is usually classified as an adjustment disorder. Mood alteration can also occur as a result of organic factors. When organic factors such as medications, medical disorders, or neurological disease cause a change in mood, the disorder is classified as an organic mood disorder (according to DSM-III-R criteria [American Psychiatric Association 1987]), or secondary mood disorder. In a study of 755 hospitalized patients seen in psychiatric consultation (Rundell and Wise 1989), 87% of manic patients and 38% of depressed patients warranted a diagnosis of organic mood disorder. When no medical factors are found that explain the mood alteration, the patient is diagnosed with a primary mood disorder, such as major depressive episode, manic episode, or dysthymia.

Medical illness, medications, and neurological disease can cause clinical depression and mania (Goodwin and Jamison 1990). For example, patients who have had strokes are at high risk for depression and may also experience mania. Factors that influence the likelihood of developing a mood disorder include whether the stroke occurs in the right or left hemisphere, the location of the stroke in the hemisphere, and, possibly, the presence of preexisting central nervous system (CNS) pathology (Robinson and Starkstein 1990). Failure to recognize and treat poststroke depression can impact long-term recovery (Parikh et al. 1990). Medical illnesses, such as thyroid disease, can markedly affect mood. A patient with hyperthyroidism may become manic (Lishman 1987) or may become depressed (Gold et al. 1981). Many medications are also implicated as causes for depression, and there are numerous medications that are known to cause mania (Krauthammer and Klerman 1978). The cause-and-effect connection between medications and mood changes is largely based, however, on anecdotal reports and not prospective data. Research in this area is needed. The classic examples of medications that cause depression are reserpine and α-methyldopa (Benson et al. 1983). On the other hand, corticosteroids—particularly when given in high doses, such as after organ transplantation—not uncommonly cause mood elevation and may even cause a manic episode (Rundell and Wise 1989; Wise et al. 1988).

When a patient presents with a mood disorder, a methodical search for causal factors is important. The clinician must gather a thorough history to include prior mood episodes, medications (both over-the-counter and prescribed), drugs (including illicit drugs, alcohol, and caffeine), associated and past medical disorders, and family history of mood disorders. Complete physical, neurological, and mental status examinations, as well as laboratory investigation for abnormalities, are necessary.

Personality change. Any CNS traumatic injury or disease has the potential to cause a change in personality. "Circumscribed brain damage may operate more directly by disruption of cerebral systems upon which the synthesis of the personality depends" (Lishman 1987, p. 160). Diagnostically, this is referred to as an *organic personality syndrome* or *secondary personality syndrome.* Typical injury or lesions associated with personality change are head trauma, partial complex seizures (temporal lobe seizures), CNS tumors, multiple sclerosis, dementia, and strokes. Mild cognitive impairment may or may not be present in secondary personality disorders; global cognitive deficits suggest a diagnosis of dementia (Dian et al. 1990).

Injury to particular regions of the frontal lobes as a result of head trauma or CNS pathology is sometimes associated with characterological change (Blumer and Benson 1975). Lesions in the orbital region of the frontal lobes can cause varying degrees of disinhibition in patients, from mild irritability to outright aggression. Such patients behave inappropriately and exhibit poor impulse control. This behavioral change has been referred to as *pseudopsychopathic.* Lesions to the convex portions of the frontal lobes can cause apathy and abulia. Because of this lack of motivation, the patient is often incorrectly diagnosed as depressed. The patient appears depressed, but is not; thus the term *pseudodepression* has been used (Stuss and Benson 1986).

Personality change caused by partial complex seizures (temporal lobe seizures) is an area of some controversy (Bear and Fedio 1977; Master et al. 1984). The argument that, given sufficient time, poorly treated seizures or subseizure threshold electrical activity in the CNS can change personality has far-reaching implications; these implications are more extensively discussed in Chapter 17. Personality characteristics that have been associated with temporal lobe epilepsy by some investigators include hyposexuality, obsessiveness, overly elaborated conversation, mood variability, hyperreligiosity, hypergraphia, humorlessness, interpersonal "stickiness," easy irritability, paranoia, and "oceanic" philosophical concerns (Bear and Fedio 1977).

The clinician must rely heavily on past history to decide whether the observed behavior is a change from the patient's previous behavior. If the abnormal characterological behavior is new, then the patient is diagnosed as having an organic personality syndrome. History may reveal, however, that the individual has exhibited sociopathic behavior since age 9, long before the alleged injury, and that the current behavior merely typifies his life-long behavior pattern. In other cases, the patient may have incurred mild cognitive or physical deficits as a result of CNS injury or pathology, which may cause mild problems in adjustment, or the patient may exhibit a "personality change" solely as a result of increased stress. Such a patient usually has a history of similar behavioral reactions when faced with stress in other situations. Regardless of the clinical circumstances, a full psychosocial history is a valuable aid to diagnosis.

Anxiety. Anxiety is a ubiquitous phenomenon that occurs in individuals as a normal part of living. When anxiety is excessive and unrealistic, it is often associated with autonomic nervous system and motoric overactivity; cognitive dysfunction, such as difficulties with attention and concentration; and feelings of dread, terror, panic, or apprehension. Such extreme forms of anxiety occur in primary and secondary anxiety disorders and occur concomitantly with other psychiatric disorders. For example, a patient with dementia may become extremely anxious when faced with a difficult task. The patient may abreact and have a "catastrophic reaction" (Goldstein 1942). This reaction does not represent an anxiety disorder, but occurs because of the patient's inability to cope with his or her cognitive dysfunction. Therefore, the examiner must rule out other psychiatric disorders, such as dementia, delirium, psychotic disorders, or mood disorders, before diagnosing an anxiety disorder. Anxiety caused by a specific organic factor is referred to as an *organic anxiety disorder* or *secondary anxiety disorder.*

Secondary anxiety syndromes may be caused by medications, substance abuse (both ingestion and withdrawal), and medical or neurological illnesses (Wise and Taylor 1990). Certain medications (e.g, sympathomimetic agents, the theophyllines, and thyroid) are potentially anxiogenic. Substance abuse can cause anxiety syndromes in two ways. First, some drugs are anxiogenic when ingested in sufficient quantity. This is particularly true of caffeine and other stimulants, such as amphetamines. Second, anxiety typically accompanies withdrawal syndromes, particularly withdrawal from sedative-hypnotic–type drugs and alcohol (Rickels et al. 1990). Medical and neurological disorders sometimes cause pathological anxiety. For example, anxiety may be caused by endocrine conditions (such as pheochromocytoma and thyroid dysfunction) and neurological disorders (such as subarachnoid hemorrhage, tumors in the vicinity of the third ventricle, and seizures) (Lishman 1987).

Medically ill patients with an organic anxiety syndrome can often be differentiated from patients with primary psychiatric disorders or adjustment disorders by careful scrutiny of their histories (Geringer and Stern 1988). A careful mental status examination and past medical and psychiatric history are essential parts of the evaluation. Even though anxiety is commonly seen in patients with medical and neurological disorders, prospective studies, such as those looking at depression in post-stroke patients, are lacking.

Thought disorder. Disordered thinking is reflected in speech, communications, or content of thought, such as thought derailment, ideas of reference, hallucinations, delusions, poverty of thoughts, loosening of associations, and perseveration (Stone 1988). A thought disorder can be seen in organic disorders such as delirium, dementia, and psychoactive substance use, or in primary thought disorders such as schizophrenia, mania, and psychotic depression (Black et al. 1988). The division of thought disorders into a functional-versus-organic dichotomy is no longer realistic; therefore, the terms primary thought disorder (manic episode due to bipolar disorder) and secondary thought disorder (manic episode due to steroids) are used for this discussion.

Certain clinical characteristics in patients suggest a primary thought disorder. Such patients are usually younger, have no related medical illness, no clouding of consciousness, and no disorientation, but they do have a prior psychiatric history, predominantly auditory hallucinations, and ego-syntonic delusions and hallucinations. Patients with a secondary thought disorder usually have an older age at onset, associated medical illness(es) and medication(s), no prior psychiatric history, a fluctuating level of consciousness, disorientation, ego-dystonic hallucinations and delusions, hallucinations that predominantly involve sensory modalities other than hearing, and fleeting, poorly systemized delusional beliefs.

The clinician must use his or her knowledge and collective experience about psychiatric disorders to recognize secondary thought disorders. An obvious example would be an 82-year-old woman referred for evaluation of "new-onset schizophrenia." She would most likely have a delirium, dementia, or possibly some other medically or medication-induced alteration in mental status. With patients who have a thought disorder, there is no substitute for a thorough history, examination, and laboratory investigation.

Hallucinations. A hallucination occurs when the patient perceives a stimulus that does not exist. The hallucinatory perception can be visual, auditory, tactile, olfactory, gustatory, or kinesthetic. Although cultural variation must be taken into account, hallucinations that occur in an awake individual are almost always symptomatic of a pathological process. Auditory hallucinations are more typical of so-called functional patients with psychiatric disorders. The one notable exception is alcoholic hallucinosis—vivid auditory hallucinations that occur in a fully oriented alcoholic patient (Victor and Hope 1958). Hallucinations that involve other sensory modalities are more typically associated with organic disorders. (For a more detailed discussion, see Cummings 1985.)

Auditory hallucinations, unlike visual hallucinations, more typically occur in psychotic psychiatric disorders, such as schizophrenia, mania, or a psychotic depression. For example, auditory hallucinations are reported in 28%–72% of schizophrenic patients (Black et al. 1988). The quality and quantity of the auditory hallucination may help the clinician diagnostically. If the patient reports clearly audible voices that comment on his actions, argue, repeat thoughts, or are deprecatory, the disorder is most likely psychiatric. If the patient reports hearing his name called or other brief, repetitive auditory hallucinations, this may represent an organic etiology, such as partial complex seizures, ear disease, or may be symptomatic of a number of psychiatric disorders, such as borderline personality disorder, somatization disorder, or multiple personality disorder.

Visual hallucinations are more typically associated with organic brain disease, although they can also occur in nonpsychiatric patients with severe recent visual loss and patients with primary psychiatric disorders. Visual hallucinations are associated with ingestion of hallucinogens, delirium, narcolepsy, epilepsy, migraine, brain stem lesions, optic nerve disease, postocular surgery, and vitreous detachment.

Visual hallucinations can also occur in healthy individuals during sensory or sleep deprivation, hypnosis, or sleep (dreams). Patients with schizophrenia, particularly chronic schizophrenia, frequently report visual hallucinations. Individuals who have an affective disorder such as a mania or depression episode will sometimes report visual hallucinations. For example, a psychotically depressed patient sees the "face of the devil" or a manic patient sees the "face of God smiling at me." Patients with other psychiatric disorders such as conversion disorder, somatization disorder, or borderline personality disorder occasionally report visual hallucinations.

Tactile hallucinations occur commonly in patients who have a limb amputation or who are in drug withdrawal delirium. "Phantom limb" sensation, the feeling that the limb is still present, is reported by a majority of amputees. Given time, the amputee's tactile hallucinations diminish and usually disappear (Frederiks 1969). Tactile hallucinations also occur in psychiatric disorders, such as schizophrenia, or in organic disorders, such as delirium and complex partial seizures, or after ingestion of hallucinogens.

Olfactory (smell), gustatory (taste), or kinesthetic (body movement) hallucinations are rare and are most commonly experienced by patients with partial complex seizures (Lishman 1987); however, they are sometimes found in patients with psychiatric or other organic disorders. All three types of hallucinations can be found in patients with somatization disorder and are occasionally reported in patients with psychotic psychiatric disorders. Olfactory and gustatory hallucinations are also found in patients with monosymptomatic hypochondriasis.

Aggression. Anger captures the attention of individuals in the patient's environment faster than any other affective state. Actual aggression or alleged aggressive acts require a very thorough inquiry into past and present history. There is a natural tendency for observers to exaggerate such anxiety-provoking experiences, and a calm examination that elicits exact details is invaluable in the evaluation process.

The evaluation of a patient who has committed a violent act usually reveals one of several scenarios:

1. The patient meets the diagnostic criteria for an antisocial personality disorder; that is, there exists a life-long history of sociopathic behavior and this violent act is one episode among many.
2. The patient commits the aggressive act under the influence of a disinhibiting psychoactive substance. When this occurs, psychoactive substance abuse or dependence must be suspected as a primary diagnosis.
3. The patient had normal impulse control until a CNS event such as head trauma, tumor, encephalitis, or dementia occurred, and the patient's personality changed (Barns et al. 1990; Mark and Erwin 1970). A thorough medical and neurological evaluation is mandatory. (The pharmacological treatment of aggression is discussed in Chapter 29.)
4. The patient has significant psychosocial stressors and "reached the breaking point." Aggressive acts in these patients are usually infrequent, and crisis-oriented psychotherapy is helpful.
5. The patient has a primary or secondary thought disorder and misperceives the environment as threatening. Identification of the reason for the thought disorder and proper treatment is essential.

Aggression does not happen in a vacuum, and a combination of factors is often responsible for the final violent outburst. The clinician must be willing to take the time to sort through the past and recent history, as well as to perform a thorough evaluation. Psychological and neuropsychological testing may aid the clinician in determining the role of personality, cognitive function, and thought patterns in the patient's recent aggressive act.

Psychomotor activity. Psychomotor activity refers to a patient's verbal and nonverbal behavior and includes reaction time, speed of movement, flow of speech, involuntary movements, and handwriting (Lipowski 1990). Psychomotor agitation refers to generalized overactivity, and psychomotor retardation refers to generalized slowing of physical and mental activity. Psychomotor agitation and retardation can occur in organic mental disorders such as delirium and dementia, after psychoactive substance use, and in other psychiatric disorders such as mood disorders. In catatonia, a profound form of psychomotor retardation, the patient may have a severe psychotic depression or encephalitis. The psychomotor behavior is indistinguishable; often only an electroencephalogram (EEG) can differentiate the patient who has the primary psychiatric disorder (normal EEG) from the patient with encephalitis (abnormal EEG) (Wise 1988; see also Chapter 12.)

Certain etiologies tend to give rise to either increased or decreased psychomotor activity. For example, patients who are withdrawing from alcohol or other depressant substances have psychomotor agitation, whereas patients who have a metabolic encephalopathy or an infarction in the territory of the right middle cerebral artery tend to have psychomotor retardation. Some patients with delirium will fluctuate between psychomotor agitation and psychomotor retardation, just as catatonic schizophrenic patients might fluctuate from catatonia to frantic activity (catatonic excitement). Patients with depression can display agitation or can have profound psychomotor retardation. Bipolar, manic patients have increased motor responses, rapid speech, and accelerated mental activity.

Finally, complex partial seizures (psychomotor seizures) typically involve impairment in the level of consciousness and may involve automatisms (repetitive motor movements).

❑ SYNDROME ANALYSIS

Once a decision is made that the patient has organic disease the next step in the differential diagnosis process is to determine whether the patient's symptoms and signs fit a pattern of one of the classic organic mental syndromes. Because many of the remaining chapters of this book discuss these syndromes in more detail, only a sketchy introduction to the diagnostic process involved is presented here.

Global Syndromes

The most common and well-recognized global syndrome is dementia: a syndrome of slowly progressive deterioration in cognitive function with associated alterations in mood and behavior (Cummings and Benson 1983). Dementia is a syndrome with many etiologies and many clinical variations. The most common type of dementia is Alzheimer's disease, a disease that develops over months to years and is characterized, in its earliest stage, by a problem with recent memory (new learning) and mild behavioral abnormalities such as lack of interest in usual activities, an increase in concern about minor physical complaints, and, at times, anxiety or mild depression.

There are other presentations of Alzheimer's disease and it is important for the neuropsychiatrist to be aware of the clinical spectrum. Some patients, particularly young patients with a strong family history of Alzheimer's disease, may initially demonstrate a progressive aphasia. Other cases have been reported with progressive frontal lobe, parietal lobe, and parietal occipital lobe syndromes. Patients with progressive focal cognitive deficits obviously require evaluation for brain tumor and other focal lesions.

Dementia is also seen in patients with multiple strokes (multi-infarct dementia). Such patients typically have a stepwise deterioration in mental status with accompanying neurological signs and symptoms. In its classic form, multi-infarct dementia is relatively easy to diagnose, but there are multi-infarct patients with normal neurological history and examination results consistent with Alzheimer's disease. There is also a large percentage of such patients (15%–20%) who probably have a mixed dementia with Alzheimer's disease and strokes.

There are dementia patients who present predominantly with frontal lobe signs such as Pick's disease, general paresis, Huntington's disease, and normal-pressure hydrocephalus. There are other patients whose symptoms are primarily subcortical, such as those with progressive supranuclear palsy, Huntington's disease, or acquired immunodeficiency syndrome (AIDS). In all of these cases, the basic history is similar: slowly progressive mental change.

Another common global syndrome frequently encountered in a general hospital setting is delirium. The most characteristic symptom cluster for this condition consists of history of short duration, fluctuating course with the examination demonstrating an altered level of consciousness, inattention, and pervasive defects in cognitive function. Patients with delirium tend to ramble and produce disorga-

TABLE 9–5. COMMON FOCAL BEHAVIORAL SYNDROMES AND THEIR LOCALIZATION

Left hemisphere (language dominant)
- Language problems in almost all right-handed patients and a high percentage of left-handed patients (Holland 1984)
  - Anterior (frontal) expressive language difficulty
  - Posterior (parietal) comprehension both written and verbal
- Writing problems
- Constructional problems
- Calculation difficulties
- Right-left disorientation

Right hemisphere (nondominant)
- Constructional problems; frontal and parietal
- Geographic disorientation in the environment; frontal and parietal
- Dressing problem; parietal
- Right-left disorientation; parietal
- Loss of musical ability (primarily carrying melody); temporal
- Language problems in rare right-handed patients and many left-handed patients; all lobes

Frontal lobes (bilateral) (Stuss 1986)
- Impulse and character changes
- Mild memory disturbances

nized language without aphasia, to be slow in their thought processes, and, on specific testing, to show cognitive deficits in many areas (Lipowski 1990).

Focal Syndromes

Patients whose behavioral symptoms are secondary to a focal brain lesion are also neuropsychiatrically important. The brain has a certain degree of regional specialization for cognitive functions; these are discussed extensively in Chapter 3. It is important for the examiner to appreciate this localization and to recognize when the patient's symptoms are indicative of a focal rather than a diffuse process. Table 9–5 lists some of the common symptoms of focal lesions.

Whenever a patient's history and examination suggest a localized brain abnormality, a destructive neurological lesion such as tumor or stroke must be considered. The speed of onset of the deficit is critical in the differential diagnosis. A sudden focal deficit is usually due to a vascular event, although tumors can hemorrhage and give a similar clinical picture. Slowly progressive focal deficits suggest an expanding lesion such as a tumor, but in rare cases these can be symptoms of atypical cases of Alzheimer's disease, Pick's disease, and Creutzfeldt-Jakob disease.

❑ CONCLUSIONS

The diagnostic process in neuropsychiatry is an orderly one in which the examiner combines data gained from history and examination and then matches it with known neuropsychiatric syndromes. In order for this process to yield valid diagnoses the examiner must not only be skilled and comfortable with the aspects of mental status testing that identify these organically based behavioral changes, but also thoroughly familiar with the clinical syndromes. This chapter is intended to help the examiner make that difficult transition from data to diagnosis. The other chapters of this volume will acquaint the reader with the clinical syndromes encountered in a neuropsychiatric practice so that the examiner can successfully carry out the differential diagnostic process.

❑ REFERENCES

Albert ML, Goodglass H, Helm NA, et al: Clinical Aspects of Dysphasia. Vienna, Springer-Verlag, 1981

American Psychiatric Association: Diagnostic and Statistical Manual of Mental Disorders, 3rd Edition, Revised. Washington, DC, American Psychiatric Association, 1987

Barns A, Jacoby R, Levy R: Psychiatric phenomena in Alzheimer's disease, IV: disorders of behavior. Br J Psychiatry 157:86–94, 1990

Bear DM, Fedio P: Quantitative analysis of interictal behavior in temporal lobe epilepsy. Arch Neurol 34:454–467, 1977

Benson DF, Blumer D (eds): Psychiatric Aspects of Neurologic Disease, Vol 2. New York, Grune & Stratton, 1982

Benson D, Peterson LG, Bartay J: Neuropsychiatric manifestations of antihypertensive medications. Psychiatr Med 1:205–214, 1983

Berlucchi G, Rizzolatti G: Special Issue: Selective Visual Attention. Neuropsychologia 25 (no 1A):1–145, 1987

Black DW, Yates WR, Andreasen NC: Schizophrenia, schizophreniform disorder, and delusional (paranoid) disorders, in Textbook of Psychiatry. Edited by Talbott JA, Hales RE, Yudofsky SC. Washington, DC, American Psychiatric Press, 1988, pp 357–402

Blumer D, Benson DF: Personality changes with frontal and temporal lobe lesions, in Psychiatric Aspects of Neurologic Disease. Edited by Benson DF, Blumer D. New York, Grune & Stratton, 1975, pp 151–170

Cummings JL: Clinical Neuropsychiatry. New York, Grune & Stratton, 1985

Cummings JL, Benson DF: Dementia: A Clinical Approach. Woburn, MA, Butterworth, 1983

DeRenzi E.: Disorders of spatial orientation, in Handbook of Clinical Neurology, Vol 1: Clinical Neuropsychology. Edited by Frederiks JAM. Amsterdam, Elsevier, 1985, pp 405–422

Dian L, Cummings JL, Petry S, et al: Personality alterations in multi-infarct dementia. Psychosomatics 31: 415–419, 1990

Folstein MF, Folstein SE, McHugh PR: "Mini-Mental State": a practical method for grading the cognitive state of patients for the clinician. J Psychiatr Res 12:189–198, 1975

Frederiks JAM: Disorders of the body schema, in Handbook of Clinical Neurology, Vol 4. Edited by Vinken PJ, Bruyn GW. Amsterdam, North-Holland Publishing, 1969

Frederiks JAM, Vinken PJ, Bruyn GW, et al: Neurobehavioral disorders, in Handbook of Clinical Neurology, Vol 46. Edited by Vinken PJ, Bruyn GW, Klawans HL. Amsterdam, Elsevier, 1985

Geringer ES, Stern TA: Anxiety and depression in critically ill patients, in Problems in Critical Care. Edited by Wise MG. Philadelphia, PA, JB Lippincott, 1988, pp 35–44

Gold MS, Pottash ALC, Extein I: Hypothyroidism and depression: evidence from complete thyroid function evaluation. JAMA 245:1919–1922, 1981

Goldstein K: After Effects of Brain Injury in War. New York, Grune & Stratton, 1942

Goodglass H, Kaplan E: The Assessment of Aphasia and Related Disorders, 2nd Edition. Philadelphia, PA, Lea & Febiger, 1983

Goodwin FK, Jamison KR: Manic-Depressive Illness. New York, Oxford University Press, New York, 1990

Heilman KM, Valenstein E (eds): Clinical Neuropsychology, 2nd Edition. New York, Oxford University Press, 1985

Holland A (ed): Language Disorders in Adults. San Diego, CA, College Hill Press, 1984

Kertesz A: Aphasia and Associated Disorders: Toxonomy, Localization and Recovery. New York, Grune & Stratton, 1979

Kertesz A: Localization in Neuropsychology. New York, Academic, 1983

Kinsbourne M: The cerebral basis of lateral asymmetries in attention. Acta Psychol 33:193–201, 1970

Krauthammer C, Klerman GL: Secondary mania. Arch Gen Psychiatry 35:1333–1339, 1978

Lipowski ZJ: Delirium: Acute Confusional States. New York, Oxford University Press, 1990

Lishman A: Organic Psychiatry, 2nd Edition. Oxford, England, Blackwell Scientific Publications, 1987

McGhie A: Pathology of Attention. Middlesex, England, Penguin Books, 1969

Magoun HW: The Waking Brain. Springfield, IL, Charles C Thomas, 1963

Mark VH, Erwin FR: Violence and the Brain. New York, Harper & Row, 1970

Master DR, Toone BK, Scott DF: Interictal behavior in temporal lobe epilepsy, in Advances in Epileptology: XVth Epilepsy International Symposium. Edited by Porter RJ, Mattson RH, Ward AA, et al. New York, Raven, 1984, pp 557–565

Mesulam M-M (ed): Principles of Behavioral Neurology. Philadelphia, PA, FA Davis, 1985a

Mesulam M-M: Attention, confusional states, and neglect, in Principles of Behavioral Neurology. Edited by Mesulam M-M. Philadelphia, PA, FA Davis, 1985b, pp 125–140

Parikh RM, Robinson RG, Lipsey JR, et al: The impact of post-stroke depression on recovery in activities of daily living over a 2-year follow-up. Arch Neurol 47:785–789, 1990

Plum F, Posner G: The Diagnosis of Stupor and Coma, 3rd Edition. Philadelphia, PA, FA Davis, 1980

Pribram KH, McGuinness P: Arousal, activation and effort in the control of attention. Psychol Rev 82:116–149, 1975

Rickels K, Schweizer E, Case G, et al: Long-term therapeutic use of benzodiazepines, I: effects of abrupt discontinuation. Arch Gen Psychiatry 47:899–907, 1990

Robinson RG, Starkstein SE: Current research in affective disorders following stroke. Journal of Neuropsychiatry and Clinical Neurosciences 2:1–14, 1990

Rundell JR, Wise MG: Causes of organic mood disorder. Journal of Neuropsychiatry and Clinical Neurosciences 1:398–400, 1989

Segarra JM, Angelo JN: Anatomic Determinants of Behavior Change, in Behavior Change in Cerebrovascular Disease. Edited by Benton AL. New York, Harper & Row, 1970, pp 3–26

Squire LR, Butters N (eds): Neuropsychology of Memory. New York, Guilford, 1984

Stone E (ed): American Psychiatric Glossary, 6th Edition. Washington, DC, American Psychiatric Press, 1988, p 104

Strub RL, Black FW: The Mental Status Examination in Neurology, 2nd Edition. Philadelphia, PA, FA Davis, 1985

Strub RL, Black FW: Neurobehavioral Disorders: A Clinical Approach. Philadelphia, PA, FA Davis, 1988

Stuss DT, Benson DF: The Frontal Lobes. New York, Raven, 1986

Victor M, Hope JM: The phenomenon of auditory hallucinations in chronic alcoholism: a critical evaluation of the status of alcoholic hallucinosis. J Nerv Ment Dis 126:451–481, 1958

Victor M, Adams RD, Collins GH: The Wernicke-Korsakoff Syndrome and Related Neurologic Disorders Due to Alcoholism and Malnutrition, 2nd Edition. Philadelphia, PA, FA Davis, 1989

Weinstein EA, Friedland RP (eds): Hemi-Inattention and Hemispheric Specialization, (Advances in Neurology Series, Vol 18). New York, Raven, 1977

Weisberg LA, Strub RL, Garcia CA: Decision Making in Adult Neurology. Toronto, Ontario, Decker 1987

Wise MG: Delirium, in The American Psychiatric Press Textbook of Neuropsychiatry. Edited by Hales RE, Yudofsky SC. Washington, DC, American Psychiatric Press, 1988, pp 89–105

Wise MG, Taylor SE: Anxiety and mood disorders in medically ill patients. J Clin Psychiatry 51 (suppl):27–32, 1990

Wise MG, Brannan SK, Shanfield SB, et al: Psychiatry aspects of organ transplantation (letter). JAMA 260:3437, 1988

Young AW (ed): Functions of the Right Cerebral Hemisphere. London, Academic, 1983

Chapter 10

Neuropsychiatric Aspects of Pain Management

William G. Brose, M.D.
David Spiegel, M.D.

PAIN IS A COMMON, FRUSTRATING, and treatable problem. Because pain perception is mediated by all of the neural processes that modulate perception, it is a fascinating neuropsychiatric phenomenon.

Prevalence

Approximately one-third of all Americans are estimated to suffer with some form of chronic pain. Back pain, arthritis, headaches, and musculoskeletal disorders, as well as pain due to neurological, cardiac, or oncologic disease combined to affect an estimated 97 million people in 1986 (Bonica 1990). Cancer pain affects approximately one-third of cancer patients with primary disease and two-thirds of those with metastatic disease. The denial of chest pain is a common contributor to mortality from myocardial infarction. The social and economic impact of this suffering is staggering. When the health care costs, indirect costs, lost work, and disability payments due to pain are combined, an estimated $79 billion was lost during 1986 in the United States alone (Bonica 1990).

Cortical Modulation of Pain

Like any other perceptual phenomenon, pain is modulated by attentional processes. Novelty tends to enhance pain perception (as with an acute injury), although overwhelming and serious injury is sometimes accompanied by a surprising absence of pain perception until hours after the injury. This traumatic dissociation has been observed in victims of natural disaster, combat, and motor vehicle accidents (Spiegel et al. 1988).

Pain perception is influenced by state of consciousness. For example, chronic pain tends to be greater during evenings and weekends when people are not distracted by routine activities. It is usually, of course, reduced in sleep but may in fact interfere with sleep; more severe kinds of pain can substantially reduce sleep efficiency. Many of the more potent drugs that treat pain reduce alertness and arousal, an often unwanted side effect or one that can lead to abuse of analgesic medications.

Pain is the ultimate psychosomatic phenomenon. It is composed of both a somatic signal that something is wrong with the body and a message or interpretation of that signal involving attentional, cognitive, affective, and social factors. The limbic system and cortex provide means of modulating pain signals (Melzack 1982), either amplifying them through excessive attention or affective dysregulation, or minimizing them through denial, inattention, relaxation, or attention control techniques. It is well known that many athletes and soldiers sustain serious injuries in the height of sport or combat and are unaware of the injury until someone points out bleeding or swelling. On the other hand, some individuals with comparatively minor physical disturbance report being totally immobilized and demoralized by pain. A single parent with a sarcoma complained of severe unremitting pain that was interlaced with tearful concern about her failure to discuss her terminal prognosis with her adolescent son. When an appropriate meeting was arranged to plan for his future and discuss her fate with him, the pain resolved (Kuhn and Bradnan 1979).

Cognitive Factors Influencing Pain

Attention to pain. Health perception is modulated by the cortex, which enhances or diminishes awareness of incoming signals. Recent neuropsychological and brain imaging research has demonstrated at least three attentional centers that modulate perception: a posterior parieto-occipital orienting system, a focusing system localized to the anterior cingulate gyrus, and an arousal-vigilance system in the right frontal lobe (Posner and Petersen 1990). These systems provide, among other things, for selective attention to incoming stimuli allowing competing stimuli to be relegated to the periphery of awareness.

When Melzack and Wall (1965) postulated the gate control theory of pain, they observed that higher cortical input could inhibit pain signals as well. They cited Pavlov's observation that repeated shocks to dogs eventually failed to elicit pain behavior; that is, the dogs habituated to the painful signals, and this could only be explained as cortical inhibition of pain response. Thus in their model, there is room for descending inhibition of pain via the substantia gelatinosa as well as competitive inhibition at the gate (Melzack 1982; Wall 1972). The original formulation of the gate control theory has been disproven, and extensive revisions of the hypothesis have been provided (Melzack 1982; Wall 1972). The important concept we gain from this theory is the interaction between central processing and perception of noxious stimuli at the periphery.

Meaning. It has been known for half a century that the meaning structure in which pain is embedded influences the intensity of pain. In his classic study, Beecher (1956) noted surprise at how soldiers on the Anzio beachhead, who were quite badly wounded, seemed to require very little in the way of analgesic medication. He examined a set of surgical patients at Massachusetts General Hospital with equal or less serious surgically induced wounds. They demanded far higher levels of analgesic medication than did the combat soldiers. Beecher concluded that this difference was based on a difference in the meaning of the pain. To combat soldiers, the pain was almost welcome as an indication that they were likely to get out of combat alive, whereas to the surgical patients it represented an interference with life and a threat to survival. This means that patients who interpret pain signals as an ominous sign of the worsening of their disease are likely to experience a greater intensity of pain. This hypothesis has been confirmed, for example, among cancer patients. Those who believe the pain represents a worsening of their disease show more pain (Spiegel and Bloom 1983a).

Mood disorders. Bond and Pearson (1969) reported a correlation between neuroticism on the Maudsley Personality Inventory (Eysenck and Eysenck 1964) and pain among patients who had cervical carcinoma. This result was confirmed by Woodforde and Fielding (1970), who reported that cancer patients who sought treatment in a pain clinic were rated as more depressed and having more psychosomatic, gastrointestinal, and hypochondriacal symptoms than cancer patients who did not. Several other studies (Ahles et al. 1983; Derogatis et al. 1983; Lansky et al. 1985; Massie and Holland 1987; Spiegel and Bloom 1983a) have reported that patients with pain score higher on measures of depression, anxiety, and other signs of mood disturbance. In particular, depression and anxiety are noted as frequent concomitants of pain (Blumer and

Heilbronn 1982; Bond 1973; Bond and Pearson 1969; Woodforde and Fielding 1970). This early work implied that patients with psychopathology complained more about pain. Later work suggested that there is an interaction and that perhaps chronic pain amplifies or produces depression (Peetet et al. 1986; Spiegel and Sands 1988).

Depression is the most frequently reported psychiatric diagnosis among chronic pain patients. Reports of depression among chronic pain populations range from 10% to 87% (Dworkin et al. 1990; Pilowski et al. 1977; Reich et al. 1983). The relative severity of the depression observed in chronic pain patients is illustrated by the finding by Katon et al. (1985) that 32% of a sample of 37 pain patients met criteria for major depression and 43% had a past episode of major depression.

Patients with two or more pain conditions have been found to be at elevated risk for major depression, whereas those patients with only one pain condition did not show such an elevated rate of mood disorder in a large sample of health maintenance organization (HMO) patients (Dworkin et al. 1990). Although pain patients referred to psychiatric treatment are clearly selected for a higher prevalence of depression and anxiety (Lansky et al. 1985), there is general agreement in the literature that pain and mood disorder co-occur and therefore that the treatment of pain from a neuropsychiatric point of view must include appropriate treatment of depression and anxiety.

Anxiety is especially a concomitant of acute pain. Like depression it may be an appropriate response to serious trauma through injury or illness. Pain may serve a signal function or be part of an anxious preoccupation as in the case of the woman with the sarcoma cited above. Similarly, anxiety and pain may reinforce one another, producing a snowball effect of escalating and mutually reinforcing central and peripheral symptoms.

❑ NEUROLOGICAL MECHANISMS OF PAIN

The classical teaching of a simple pathway for pain transmission still exists in the minds of many practicing medical professionals. The understated sophistication of a dedicated spinothalamic tract that relayed all pain messages received from peripheral nerves arising on the contralateral side of the body supported the concepts of pain and analgesia prevalent even in the mid to later 1900s. An ever-increasing body of knowledge has now displaced this simple approach to pain transmission. Very complex interactions of many different peripheral and central nervous system structures, from the skin surface to the cerebral cortex, are now known to be involved in the processing of pain. Blockade of any of these pathways and/or antagonism of involved neurotransmitters may now be rationally considered to treat specific pain problems. Presentation of these various treatment options is best preceded by a brief discussion of certain established parts of this complex pathway for pain transmission. Yaksh (1988) summarized the detailed neurophysiological and neuropharmacological findings from 1913 until 1986 in a review that referenced over 700 reports.

Peripheral Sensory Receptors

Each individual can appreciate that when a potentially damaging stimulus is applied to a sensitive area of the body such as the skin, a chain of signals is initiated that results in the identification of the stimulus as painful. Early descriptions of peripheral nerves indicated that they were modality specific and that each class of nerve fiber was responsible for only one sensory modality (Müller 1844). This concept was not supported by anatomical studies of skin surface, which demonstrated that each class of nerve ending is not present in all skin areas. More recent neurophysiological work has established the existence of specific primary afferent nerves for signalling noxious stimulation. These nerves are termed *nociceptors.*

Nociceptors are activated by some form of energy (mechanical, thermal, or chemical) (Figure 10–1). They transduce that energy into an electrical impulse that is conducted through the nerve axon toward the brain. The reflex response and subjective report of pain associated with a noxious stimulus is the result of spinal cord, brain stem, midbrain, and higher cortical processing of signals from the numerous primary afferent nociceptors that were activated by the stimulus. Nociceptors are characterized by 1) high threshold to all naturally occurring stimuli compared with other receptors in the same tissue and 2) progressively augmenting response to repeated or increasingly noxious stimuli (sensitization).

Cutaneous pain sensation. *Mechanosensory* nociceptors respond when the pressure to produce tis-

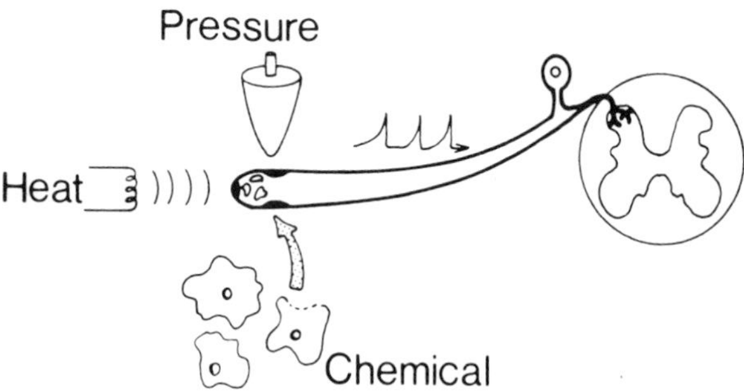

Figure 10–1. Sensitivity range of the polymodal C fiber nociceptor. Available evidence suggests that the terminals are sensitive to direct heat or mechanical distortion. Thus transduction can occur at the terminal. The terminals are also sensitive to chemicals released from damaged cells. In this manner, any tissue cell can serve as an intermediate in the transduction process. In a sense, all tissue cells are "receptors" for injury. (Reprinted from Fields HL: Pain. New York, McGraw-Hill, 1987, p 27. Used with permission.)

sue damage has been achieved. Most of these receptors initiate impulses carried by thinly myelinated fibers (Aδ). The responses increase in proportion to magnitude of the pressure applied. These receptors in the trunk have fairly large receptive fields whereas those in the face have smaller fields.

Thermoreceptive nociceptors respond to normal heating or cooling with sensitivity near 1°C when the temperature is 30°–40°C; they also respond to noxious thermal stimuli with an increasing frequency of discharge. High-frequency discharge can be seen in C fiber afferents after application of intense heat (47°–51°C) to the small receptive fields near these receptors.

Mechanothermal nociceptors are activated by high-intensity heat or pressure sensation. They have small receptive fields and are likely responsible for the "first pain" transmitted by small myelinated Aδ fibers.

Polymodal C fiber nociceptors respond to many different noxious stimuli. These are the most common of all nociceptors. They are activated by pressure, temperature, and chemical stimuli supplied to their small receptive fields.

Skeletal muscle pain. Nociceptors found in skeletal muscle respond to chemical agents that are released locally during muscle contraction. Metabolic by-products alone do not trigger these receptors. There appears to be a need for other algogenic agents, perhaps prostaglandins released during intense muscle contraction, to be present as well.

Cardiac muscle pain. Cardiac muscle afferents are activated by high-intensity mechanical stimulation, heat, and chemical agents. Humoral agents released locally may be responsible for the pain seen with angina. Prostaglandins are released following myocardial hypoxia. Prostaglandins, histamine, bradykinin, or serotonin have all been shown to stimulate these receptors.

Joint pain. Joint nociceptors activated by deformation or expansion within the joint will relay pain messages via Aδ fiber afferents. These receptors also appear to be sensitized by certain chemical substances injected into the joint (e.g., urate crystals, endotoxin, and prostaglandins).

Visceral pain. These nociceptors have not been well identified. Pain is seen in response to mechanical (distension), as well as thermal and chemical, stimuli. These receptors also appear to be sensitized by the presence of certain chemicals (e.g., prostaglandins).

As indicated above, particular nociceptors respond only to particular types of stimuli. Although the exact pathways involved in the transduction of noxious information nociceptors has not yet been elucidated, it appears that the peripheral terminal of the Aδ mechanical nociceptor is likely to function as a receptor (Fields 1987). Whether this is true for other nociceptors remains the subject of speculation. The presence of vesicles in primary nociceptive afferent terminals has been determined by electron microscopy. These vesicles likely provide the substrate for various peripherally active agents.

Substance P (sP) is an undecapeptide found in small-diameter primary afferent neurons. This peptide has been shown to be transmitted to the periphery by these nerves, and stimulation of these primary afferents leads to the release of sP from the distal terminus of the nerve. However, local application of exogenous sP to these nerve terminals does not induce a painful response. It does appear to activate local vasculature to cause extravasation of fluid into the tissues. Other chemicals present in the blood and tissues have been demonstrated to be algesic. Serotonin, histamine, acetylcholine, bradykinin, slow-reacting substance of anaphylaxis (SRS-A), calcitonin-gene–related peptide (CGRP), and potassium all excite primary noxious afferents. At this time the definition of "pain" neuropeptide has not been specified. Prostaglandins alone do not excite pain fibers; however, they do appear to sensitize primary afferents to painful substances.

Direct tissue trauma results in potassium release, synthesis of bradykinin in plasma, and synthesis of prostaglandins in the region of damaged tissue (Figure 10–2; *panel A*). Antidromic impulses in primary nociceptor afferents result in an increase in sP from nerve endings. This is associated with increase in vascular permeability and, in turn, results in marked release of bradykinin. There is also an increase in histamine production from mast cells and an increase in serotonin production from platelets; both of these are capable of powerful activation of nociceptors (Figure 10–2; *panel B*). Histamine release combines with sP release to increase vascular permeability. Local increases in histamine and serotonin, via activation of nociceptors, results in a further increase in sP so that a self-perpetuating cycle can be seen to develop at each region of the nociceptive afferent nerve fiber in the damaged tissue. In surrounding extracellular fluid, increases in histamine and serotonin result in activation of nearby nociceptors, and this is one reason for secondary hyperalgesia (Figure 10–2; *panel C*). Superimposed on all of these events are the effects of increased release of catecholamines from sympathetic nerve endings, which results in sensitization of nociceptors. Evidence from animal models of arthritis and various human data point to the sympathetic postganglionic neuron as being integral in the changes seen in vascular permeability in response to activation of primary afferent nociceptors (Levine et al. 1988).

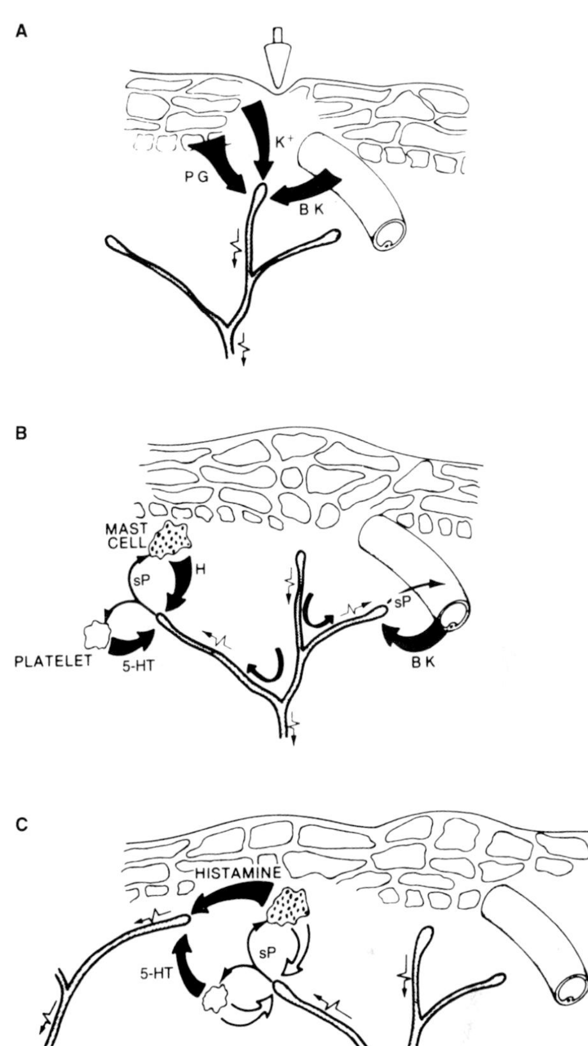

Figure 10–2. Events leading to activation, sensitization, and spread of sensitization of primary afferent nociceptor terminals. *Panel A:* Direct activation by intense pressure and consequent cell damage. Cell damage leads to release of potassium (K^+) and to synthesis of prostaglandins (PG) and bradykinin (BK). PGs increase the sensitivity of the terminal to BK and other pain-producing substances. *Panel B:* Secondary activation. Impulses generated in the stimulated terminal propagate not only to the spinal cord, but into other terminal branches, where they induce the release of peptides, including substance P (sP), which causes vasodilation and neurogenic edema with further accumulation of BK. In addition, sP causes the release of histamine (H) from mast cells and serotonin (5-hydroxytryptamine [5-HT]) from platelets. *Panel C:* Histamine and 5-HT levels rise in the extracellular space, secondarily sensitizing nearby nociceptors. This leads to a gradual spread of hyperalgesia and/or tenderness. (Reprinted from Fields HL: Pain. New York, McGraw-Hill, 1987, p 36. Used with permission.)

Primary Afferent Transmission

After a noxious stimulus has been detected by a nociceptor, the resultant impulse travels away from the point of origin via the primary afferent nerve. The primary afferent nerves that carry pain impulses are almost exclusively unmyelinated C fibers and finely myelinated Aδ fibers. Most C fiber afferents originate from polymodal nociceptors that are activated by mechanical, chemical, and thermal noxious stimuli. The conduction velocity of these C fibers is approximately 1 meter per second (m/s), which likely explains the "slow pain" felt 1–2 seconds after the application of a noxious stimulus (Figure 10–3). The finely myelinated Aδ fibers also transmit pain impulses, but the conduction velocity of these neu-

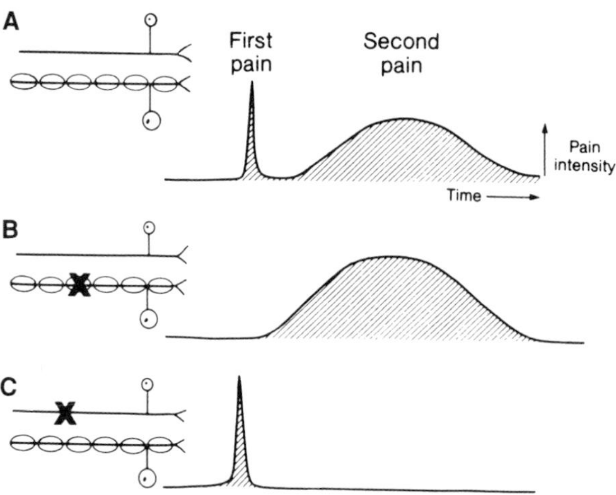

Figure 10–3. First and second pain are carried by two different primary afferent axons (*panel A*). First pain is abolished by selective blockade of myelinated axons (*panel B*) and second pain by blocking C fibers (*panel C*). (Reprinted from Fields HL: Pain. New York, McGraw-Hill, 1987, p 26. Used with permission.)

rons is much faster (12–30 m/s). Aδ fibers are particularly sensitive to stimulation with sharp instruments. In addition, 20%–50% of Aδ fibers respond to heat as well as mechanical stimulation. These fiber types carry the impulses that initially report a noxious stimulus. These primary afferent nociceptors make up the majority of fibers in any peripheral nerve.

Lesion of these peripheral nerves does not necessarily correlate with presence or absence of pain. Although the gate theory of pain promoted by Melzack and Wall (1965) is incomplete, it does explain the pain present with some disease states whose primarily lesion is demyelination of large fiber afferents. The loss of large fiber input in these cases leads to an open gate that allows transmission of all noxious stimuli that might otherwise be blocked by large fiber afferent transmission closing the gate. However, pain is found in Fabry's disease in which selective destruction of small fiber afferents would predict abolition of painful sensation. This is likely explained by altered modulation at high-processing centers. Thus it appears that single balance of large fiber and small fiber activity is far too simplistic a view of pain modulation at the spinal cord level.

Peripheral nerve injuries can also lead to pain. The proposed pathways for such an injury to evoke a pain response include

1. Increased activity in sympathetic fibers near the damaged area
2. Neuroma formation due to sprouting from damaged axons
3. Collaterals sprouting from intact neighboring fibers
4. Changes in dorsal root ganglion cells or in central terminals of damaged axons that have lost part of their dorsal input
5. Stimulation of nociceptive nervi nervorum of peripheral nerves

Spinal Cord Terminals of Primary Afferents

Dorsal and ventral roots. The cell bodies of all somatic primary afferent fibers are in the dorsal root ganglia adjacent to the spinal cord. The only primary afferent cell body outside this position is the trigeminal ganglia, which is the rostral continuation of the dorsal root ganglia. Fibers from the dorsal root are organized within the root according to diameter. The large-diameter afferents enter the spinal cord in the dorsal region of the entry zone whereas the small-diameter afferents enter into the lateral region of the cord. Having entered the spinal cord, the nociceptive primary afferent fibers (Aδ and C fibers) bifurcate into both cephalad- and caudad-projecting branches travelling in the Lissauer's tract (dorsolateral tract). These fibers terminate primarily in the ipsilateral dorsal gray matter, but a small number of the fibers will cross dorsal to the central canal to terminate in the dorsal gray of the contralateral side. The majority of sensory afferents enter the spinal cord through the dorsal root entry zone. However, nonmyelinated C fiber afferents have also been discovered in the ventral root. The clinical relevance of the fibers that cross or those that enter the ventral root is not known. This heterogeneity in the pathway of the primary afferents associated with pain transmission helps explain the incomplete pain relief that is seen after ablation of a unilateral dorsal root entry zone.

Dorsal horn. Once the impulses have entered the spinal cord via the dorsal or ventral roots, they terminate in the ipsilateral dorsal horn of the spinal cord. The dorsal horn is organized into distinct laminae, with specific primary afferent terminals found in individual laminae (Figure 10–4). Aδ fibers terminate primarily in lamina I, in ventral portions in

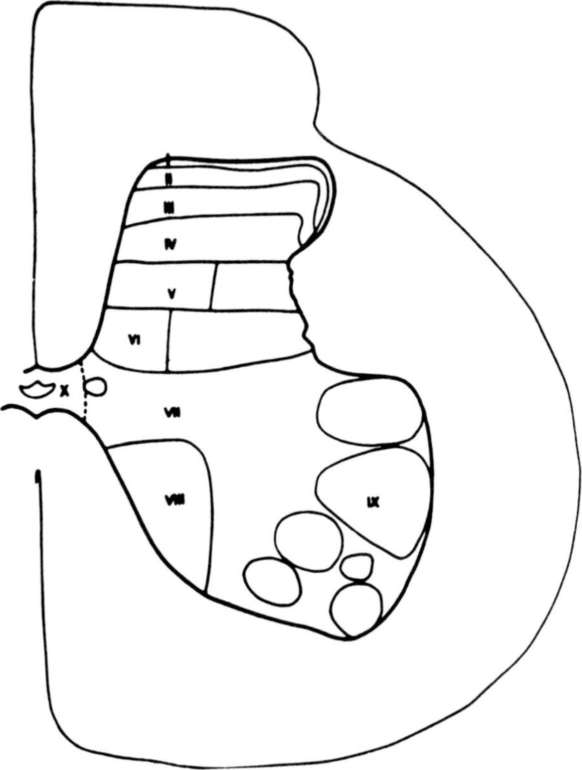

Figure 10–4. Schematic drawing of the lamination of the ventral cell column of the 7th lumbar spinal cord segment in the full-grown cat. (Reprinted from Rexed B: Cytoarchitectonic organization of the spinal cord in the cat. J Comp Neurol 96:415–495, 1952. Used with permission.)

lamina II, and through most of lamina III. Unmyelinated C fibers terminate in lamina II.

Lamina I. Lamina I is a thin superficial layer of neurons that make up the marginal zone. The neurons with cell bodies in lamina I are termed *marginal cells.* These marginal cells receive projections from Aδ and C fiber afferents responsive to noxious mechanical stimuli. In addition, they respond to some polymodal C fiber afferents as well as Aδ temperature impulses. The neurons that respond to Aδ and C fiber noxious stimuli also show response to group III and group IV muscle afferents. This dual response accounts for a convergence of pain impulses from both skin and muscle. These neurons then project to one of several areas: the thalamus by way of the contralateral spinothalamic tracts, the ipsilateral dorsal white matter, or the ipsilateral dorsal gray matter for an area of several segments.

Lamina II. Lamina II is also known as the substantia gelatinosa owing to the clear appearance of this section of spinal matter in comparison with surrounding marginal layer and nucleus proprius. This region has undergone extensive evaluation. The neurons of lamina II act as a modulating center for afferent impulses of small and large fibers that terminate in this region. Afferent input is from noxious stimulation as well as light touch and pressure sensations. The area is densely packed with cells that make extensive synaptic connections with other cells in the area. The axons of most of these cells are short, and only a few of them project to the thalamus through the contralateral-anterolateral columns. The clinical phenomena of selective spinal cord opiate analgesia are mediated through opioid receptors found in lamina II (Yaksh 1988). Stimulation of these receptors leads to inhibition of marginal cell firing in response to primary afferent signals. Similar inhibition has been postulated with other neurochemicals acting on this lamina, but much more work is needed to delineate the complex interactions involved in processing noxious stimuli here.

Laminae III and IV. The nucleus proprius is made up of the neurons located in laminae III and IV. One of the predominant populations of cells in the nucleus proprius responds to Aβ, Aδ, and C fiber input; these are termed wide dynamic range neurons (WDRs). Although the receptive fields of the individual afferents may be quite small, the corresponding WDR has a larger receptive field. Afferent input from closely related somatotopic fields is typically seen on a single WDR, accounting for the somatotopic convergence seen in stimulation of different areas. In addition to somatotopic convergence, there is also evidence that visceral afferents travelling with sympathetic neurons also converge on WDRs. WDRs project throughout the anterolateral funiculus to the thalamus.

The convergence of somatic nociceptive afferents and visceral nociceptive afferents on the same neuron in the dorsal horn likely explains the phenomena of referred pain. The presence of viscero-somatic, muscle-somatic, and viscero-viscero convergence seen in the various laminae of the dorsal horn and the development of fairly large receptive fields in some of these second-order neurons also help to explain some the peculiar characteristics of nonsomatic pain. These are shown schematically in Figure 10–5.

Lamina X (central canal). The central canal has also been identified as receiving input from the Aδ fibers associated with noxious stimulation. These fibers terminate on cells with small receptive fields, like those seen in the marginal zone. The afferents are sensitive to temperature and pinch stimuli. The cells of the central canal are subsequently known to ascend ipsilaterally and contralaterally in the ventrolateral tract to the reticular formation.

Ascending sensory pathways. The second-order neurons that arise in the respective laminae of the dorsal horn of the spinal cord subsequently use several specific routes to carry their messages to higher brain centers (Figure 10–6). The specific routes are characterized as tracts and systems that include the neospinothalamic, paleospinothalamic, and spinoreticular systems and dorsal columns. The names given to these nociceptive pathways are derived from the point of origin and termination of their respective fibers. The spinothalamic and spinoreticular systems represent the most important tracts associated with pain transmission in humans. The fibers from these tracts make up the anterolateral funiculus.

Axons from laminae I, IV, V, VII, and VIII make up the spinothalamic tract. These axons ascend pre-

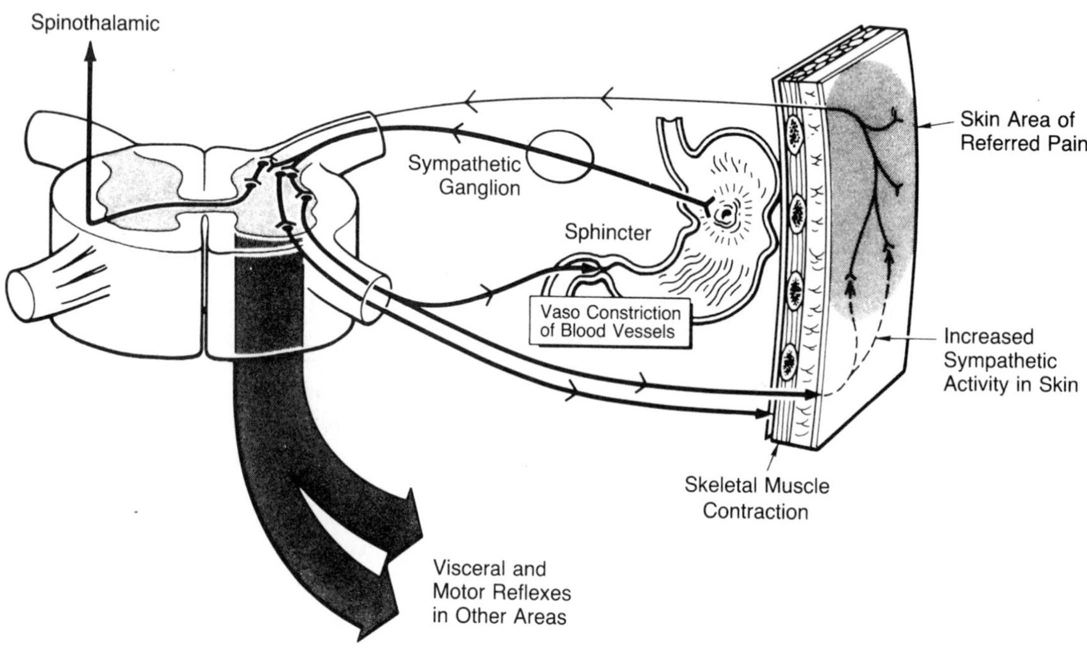

Figure 10–5. Visceral pain: convergence of visceral and somatic nociceptive afferents. Visceral sympathetic afferents converge on the same dorsal horn neuron as do somatic nociceptive afferents. Visceral noxious stimuli are then conveyed, together with somatic noxious stimuli, via the spinothalamic pathways to the brain. Note: 1) Referred pain is felt in the cutaneous area corresponding to the dorsal horn neurons on which visceral afferents converge; this is accompanied by allodynia and hyperalgesia in this skin area. 2) Reflex somatic motor activity results in muscle spasm, which may stimulate parietal peritoneum and initiate somatic noxious input to the dorsal horn. 3) Reflex sympathetic efferent activity may result in spasm of sphincters of viscera over a wide area causing pain remote from the original stimulus. 4) Reflex sympathetic efferent activity may result in visceral ischemia and further noxious stimulation; also, visceral nociceptors may be sensitized by norepinephrine release and microcirculatory changes. 5) Increased sympathetic activity may influence cutaneous nociceptors, which may at least be partly responsible for referred pain. 6) Peripheral visceral afferents branch considerably, causing much overlap in the territory of individual dorsal roots; only a small number of visceral afferent fibers converge on dorsal horn neurons compared with somatic nociceptive fibers. Also, visceral afferents converge on the dorsal horn over a large number of segments. This dull, vague visceral pain is very poorly localized and is often called *deep visceral pain.* (Reprinted from Cousins MJ, Bridenbaugh PO [eds]: Neural Blockade in Clinical Anesthesia and Management of Pain, 2nd Edition. Philadelphia, PA, JB Lippincott, 1988, p 743. Used with permission.)

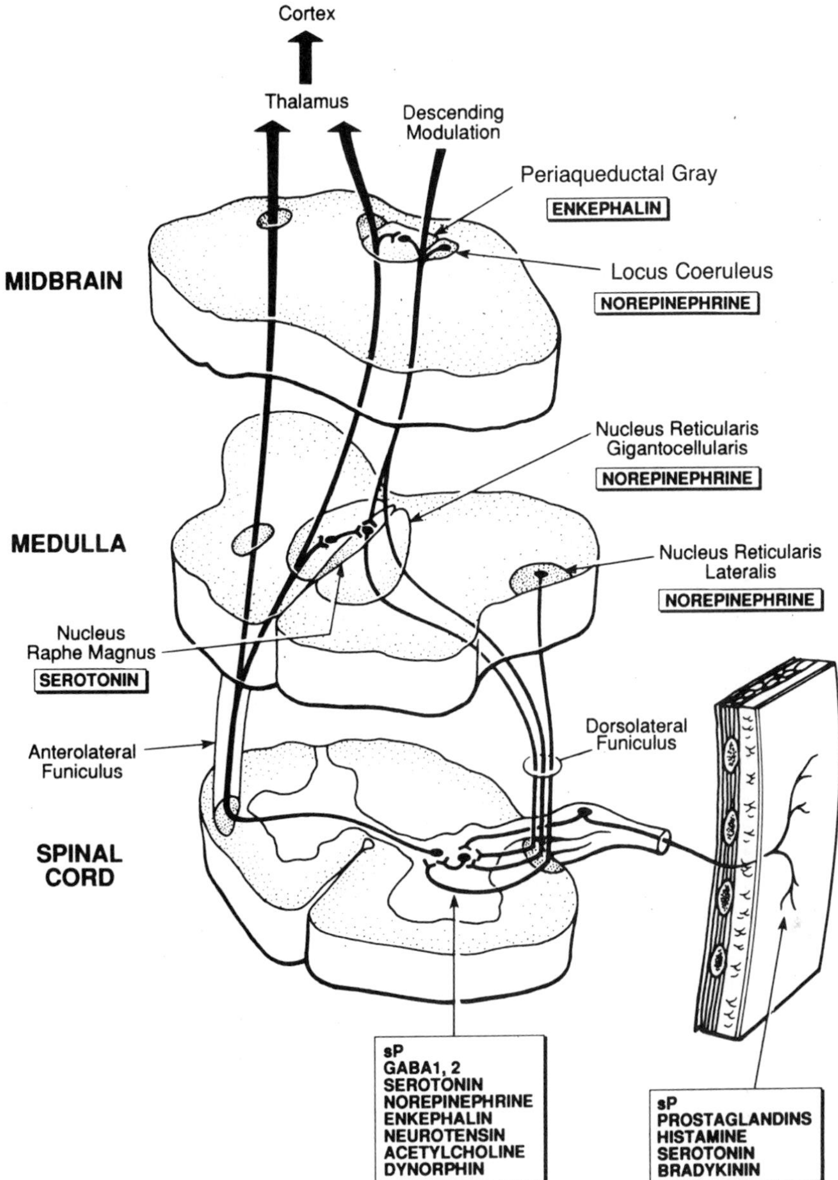

Figure 10–6. Schematic drawing of nociceptive processing, outlining ascending (*left side of diagram*) and descending (*right side of diagram*) pathways. Stimulation of nociceptors in the skin surface leads to impulse generation in the primary afferent. Concomitant with this impulse generation, increased levels of various endogenous algesic agents (substance P [sP], prostaglandins, histamine, serotonin, and bradykinin) are detected near the area of stimulation in the periphery. The noxious impulse is conducted to the dorsal horn or the spinal cord where it is subjected to local factors and descending modulation. The endogenous neurochemical mediators of this interaction at the dorsal horn that have been characterized to date are listed in the figure. Primary nociceptive afferents relay to projection neurons in the dorsal horn that ascend in the anterolateral funiculus to end in the thalamus. En route, collaterals of the projection neurons activate the nucleus reticularis gigantocellularis. Neurons from the nucleus reticularis gigantocellularis project to the thalamus and also activate the periacqueductal gray of the midbrain. Enkephalinergic neurons from the periaqueductal gray and noradrenergic neurons from the nucleus reticularis gigantocellularis activate descending serotonergic neurons of the nucleus raphe magnus. These fibers join with noradrenergic fibers from the locus coeruleus reticularis lateralis to project descending modulatory impulses to the dorsal horn via the dorsolateral funiculus. GABA = γ-aminobutyric acid. (Reprinted from Brose WG, Cousins MJ: Gynecologic pain, in Gynecologic Oncology. Edited by Coppelson M, et al. Edinburgh, Churchill Livingstone [in press]. Used with permission.)

dominantly in the contralateral ventral quadrant of the spinal cord. Crossed fibers predominate, but neuroanatomic studies have indicated that perhaps 25% of all fibers ascend in the ipsilateral ventral quadrant (Yaksh 1988). These spinothalamic fibers subsequently ascend to the thalamus.

Numerous other systems are also involved in the rostral projection of nociceptive information. Important among these other systems would be the dorsal funicular systems and intersegmental systems, which are likely involved in descending inhibitory transmission as well.

Brain stem processing. The brain stem is involved in transmission of all ascending and descending information. Nociceptive afferent fibers relay to projection neurons in the dorsal horn, which ascend in the anterolateral funiculus to end in the thalamus. During the rostral conduction of these impulses, collaterals activate the nucleus reticularis gigantocellularis, which in turn sends projections to the thalamus, as well as to the periaqueductal gray matter (Figure 10–6).

Thalamic relays. Several nuclear groups of the thalamus are associated with the relay of nociceptive afferent impulses (Figure 10–7). Included among these are the posterior nuclear complex, the ventrobasilar complex, and the medial intralaminar nuclear complex. In the thalamus, spinothalamic neurons terminate largely on the ventroposteriolateral and the centromedian nuclei. The ventrobasilar complex also receives input from the dorsal columns. The ventroposteriolateral nucleus projects to areas 1, 2, and 3 of the parietal lobe, but these areas have not been found to be involved with aversive or emotional aspects of nociception. Consequently, it is currently believed that the ventroposteriolateral nucleus is involved with localization of the impulse, rather than its qualitative aspects (Beeson and Chaouch 1987; Willis 1985). The centromedian nucleus is believed to be involved in the qualitative aspects of nociception in that stimulation of this region triggers the unpleasantness associated with tissue damage (Beeson and Chaouch 1987). The projections of the centromedian nucleus are poorly understood at present, but presumably they activate the aversive centers in the limbic system. The nucleus submedius has also been implicated in nociceptive processing, as it receives all of its input from terminals of marginal projection neurons in the spinal cord. However, the physiological functions and connections of this nucleus are unknown.

Cerebral cortex. The somatosensory cortex receives processed input from spinothalamic, spinoreticular, and dorsal column systems, as outlined earlier. The majority of attention has been focused on SII as the principal cortical region involved with the reception and perception of noxious information. The anterior portion of SII receives input from the ventrobasilar thalamus, whereas the posterior portion of SII receives input from the posterior thalamus. Berkley and Palmer (1974) demonstrated that bilateral ablation of the posterior region of SII produces an increase in nociceptive threshold.

Descending modulation. Up to this point the discussion of pain pathways has been limited to the rostral projection of primary noxious stimuli. The failure of a particular painful stimulus to provoke given behavior in different individuals points out the uncoupling of a simple stimulus-response concept of pain processing. The uncoupling of pain stimulus and response is perhaps best identified by observing the absence of pain in some individuals that are injured in battle or in association with a sporting event. One of the primary focuses of research over the past two decades has been to delineate the physiological explanations for these observed differences in pain response. Through this investigation it has become apparent that the discussion of the afferent limb of the pain pathway mandates consideration of the modulating influences on that pain transmission.

Modulation of pain stimuli can occur at many different levels in the pathway. In their proposal of the gate control theory, Melzack and Wall (1965) predicted modulation of small fiber activity by the presence of large fiber activity in the same region of the dorsal horn. Cutaneous activation of large fiber afferents through transcutaneous nerve stimulation supports this peripheral modulation at the dorsal horn. In addition, the stimulation of dorsal columns that mimics the activation of descending inhibition has also been shown to inhibit the discharge of dorsal horn interneuron nociceptors.

Earlier work by Hagbarth and Kerr (1954) demonstrated the existence of descending long-tract systems to modulate spinal evoked activity. Virtually every pathway carrying nociceptive information, including the spinothalamic and spinoreticular tracts, is under modulatory control from supraspinal sys-

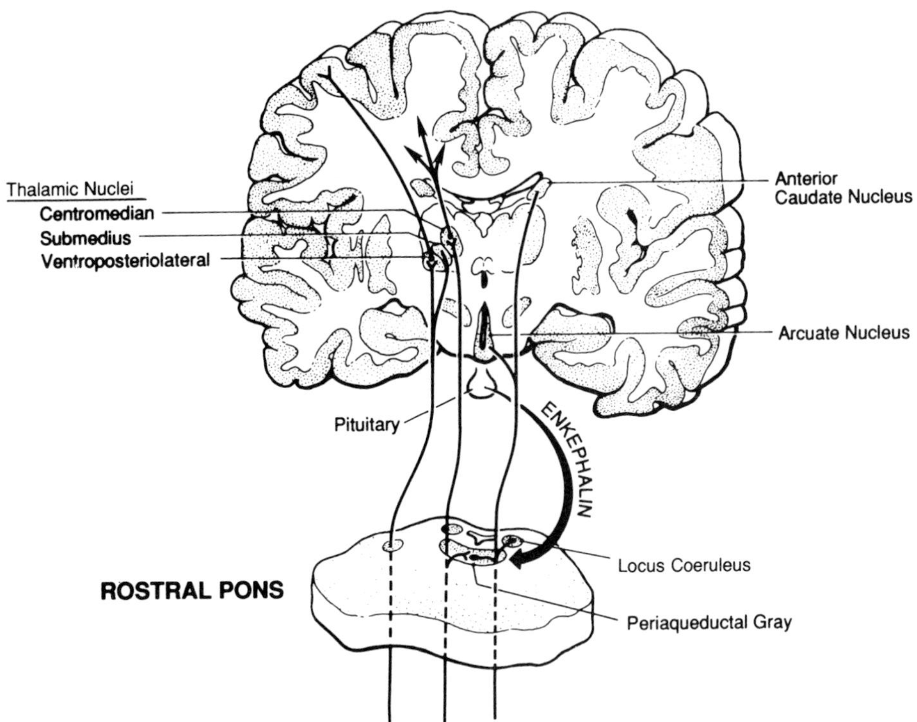

Figure 10–7. Rostral projections of nociceptive processing. Ascending stimuli (*left side of diagram*) travelling in the anterolateral funiculus, as well as impulses relayed from the medulla, pons, and midbrain, are projected to the thalamic nuclear complex. The centromedian, submedius, and ventroposteriolateral nuclei receive nociceptive information. The ventroposteriolateral nucleus projects discretely to the cortex. The centromedian nucleus projects more diffusely, particularly to the limbic region. The descending fibers (*right side of diagram*) inhibit the transmission of nociceptive information between primary afferents and the projection neurons in the dorsal horn. The periaqueductal gray is controlled by projections from the anterior caudate, midline limbic nuclei, and the arcuate nucleus of the hypothalamus. In addition to direct neural connection, endorphins synthesized in the pituitary are released into the cerebrospinal fluid and blood, where they can exert an inhibitory effect at multiple centers including the periaqueductal gray.

tems. Experimental evidence of this supraspinal influence includes inhibition of nociceptive reflexes by electrical stimulation or microinjections of opioid at brain stem sites, both of which are naloxone reversible. Various nuclei of the medulla oblongata and the pons project caudally to the spinal gray matter and the spinal nucleus of the trigeminal nerve. Serotonergic neurons in the nucleus raphe magnus, catecholaminergic neurons of the lateral reticular formation, and the locus coeruleus are all believed to play a role in descending modulation (Basbaum and Fields 1978; Beeson and Chaouch 1987; Fields and Basbaum 1984). Axons from these centers project to all levels of the spinal cord through the dorsolateral funiculus (Figure 10–6).

Stimulation of the medullary centers prevents the activation of second-order neurons in the dorsal horn or trigeminal gray matter by primary afferent fibers through this descending inhibition (Basbaum 1985; Basbaum and Fields 1978; Beeson and Chaouch 1987). The exact mechanism of this inhibition has not been characterized, but several models have been proposed (Basbaum 1985; Dubner 1985). In addition to these different modulating pathways that have been partially characterized (Figure 10–8), there are undoubtedly additional descending inhibitory influences that have yet to be evaluated. The depression of spinothalamic neurons by cortical and pyramidal stimulation is an example of such an uncharacterized pathway. Continued research in this area will help to unravel the complex reaction between pain stimulus and response and perhaps suggest additional therapeutic modalities that may be applied to the treatment of pain.

❑ NEUROPHARMACOLOGY

Pharmacology of Pain

Basic research on the processing of nociceptive information by the central nervous system has led to an improved understanding of pain and pain treatment. Figure 10–6 also summarizes the site of action of several of the chemical substances that have been identified with nociceptive processing. Using this simplified picture of the pain pathway, we can focus on the pharmacological interventions

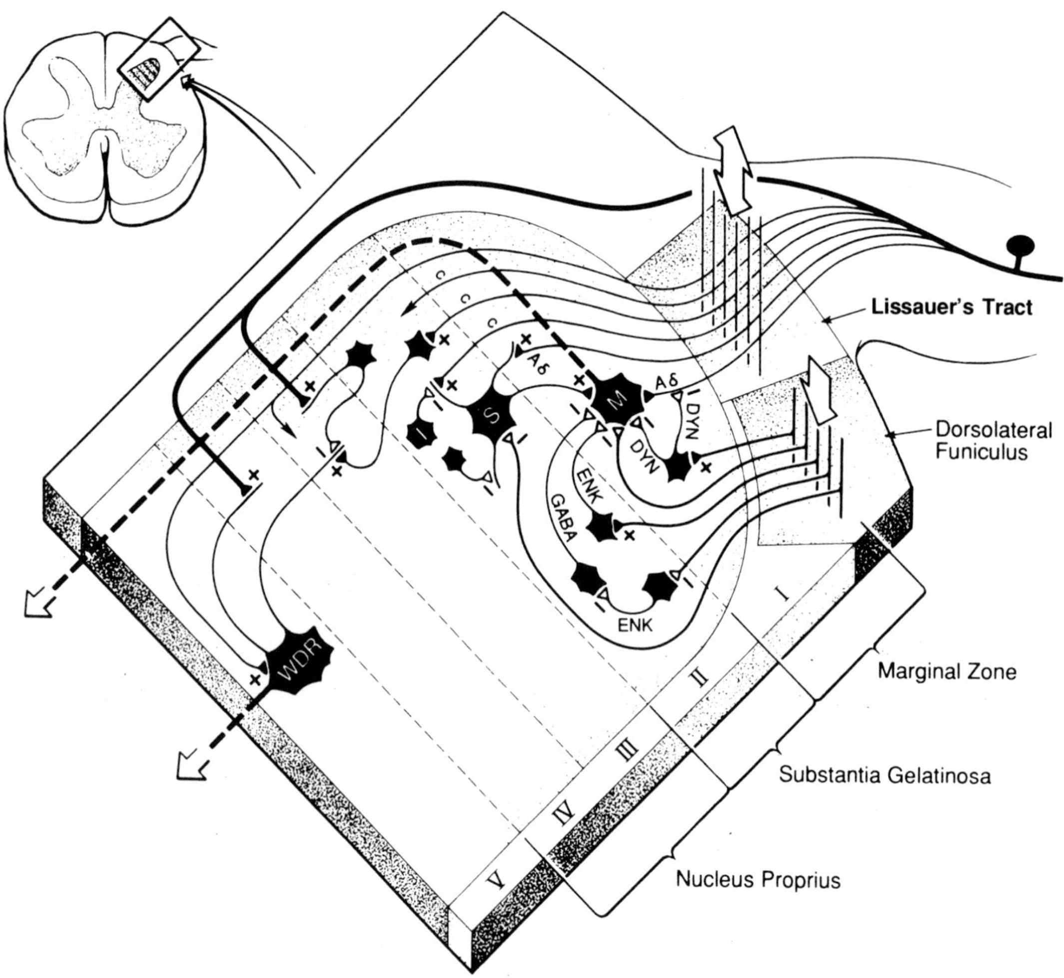

Figure 10–8. Dorsal horn processing. Large- and small-diameter primary neurons have their cell bodies in the dorsal root ganglia. These fibers segregate as they approach the spinal cord. Large-diameter afferents (*thick solid lines*) travel in the medial portion, whereas small-diameter afferents (*thin solid lines:* C and Aδ) segregate to the lateral portions of the entry zone. The spinal terminals of the small fibers enter the cord, where they may ascend or descend for several segments in the dorsolateral tract (Lissauer's tract) and subsequently terminate throughout the dorsal horn of the spinal cord. Aδ fiber afferents terminate primarily in lamina I (marginal zone), whereas C fiber afferents terminate in lamina II (substantia gelatinosa). In lamina I nociceptive fibers synapse on dendrites of the large marginal (M) neurons. Smaller neurons in lamina I may exert presynapse inhibition of the marginal neuron. Other nociceptive fibers (Aδ) synapse with stalked (S) neurons in lamina II. These S neurons stimulate M neurons in lamina I. The relay between primary afferent fibers and S neurons is also subject to modulation by inhibitory islet (I) neurons in lamina II. Central transmission is accomplished by M neurons directly, wide dynamic range neurons (WDRs) directly, or S neurons indirectly. M neurons are subject to inhibition by neurons in lamina II. Descending serotonergic neurons from the nucleus raphe magnus, which travel in the dorsolateral funiculus, are also shown. These neurons terminate throughout the spinal cord on interneurons (γ-aminobutyric acid [GABA] and enkephalins [ENK]) to provide inhibition of nociceptive transmission. DYN = dynorphin.

at different points in the pathway and determine a clinical effect on the relief of pain.

Peripheral Desensitization

A rough schematic drawing of the local circuitry involved in the detection of a noxious stimuli from the periphery is shown in Figure 10–9. As discussed previously, following trauma to peripheral site, an inflammatory reaction, including the activation of complement and coagulation-fibrinolytic pathways, will begin. Local release of histamine, serotonin, prostaglandins, and sP occurs. Subsequent changes in the local environment such as decreased tissue pH, changes in the microcirculation, and increase in efferent sympathetic activity all appear to increase the response of peripheral nociceptors.

Numerous drug therapies have been tried to interrupt these peripheral processes. Blockade of pain by aspirin-like drugs is one such peripheral action. Aspirin, indomethacin, ibuprofen, phenylbutazone, diclofenac, and ketorolac are all cyclooxygenase inhibitors. Cyclooxygenase is the enzyme that is responsible for the synthesis of prostaglandins, prostacyclins, and thromboxanes. All these endogenous substances have been proposed as mediators of the local pain response (Juan 1978). Clinical trials with topical capsaicin are also focused on peripheral action. This drug has been shown to deplete sP from cutaneous nerve endings (Gamse et al. 1980). Initially, the effect is a burning pain that is followed by insensitivity to subsequent painful stimuli.

The involvement of the sympathetic nervous system is also suspect. It is known that sympathetic fibers are present in large numbers near cutaneous nociceptors. Blockade of these sympathetic fibers can eliminate the pain of causalgia in some patients. The burning dysesthetic pain and hyperalgesia that are seen with this syndrome, which may be eliminated to sympathetic blockade, can be made to reappear with local application of norepinephrine, the sympathetic neurotransmitter.

Neural Blockade

In 1902 Cushing presented his theory that nerve block could prevent the pain and shock of amputation. Later, Crile (1910) proposed that disruption of the pain pathway might improve outcome from trauma. Indeed, a multitude of investigations have proven the beneficial effect of neural blockade with respect to neuroendocrine function following trauma and/or surgery (Kehlet 1988).

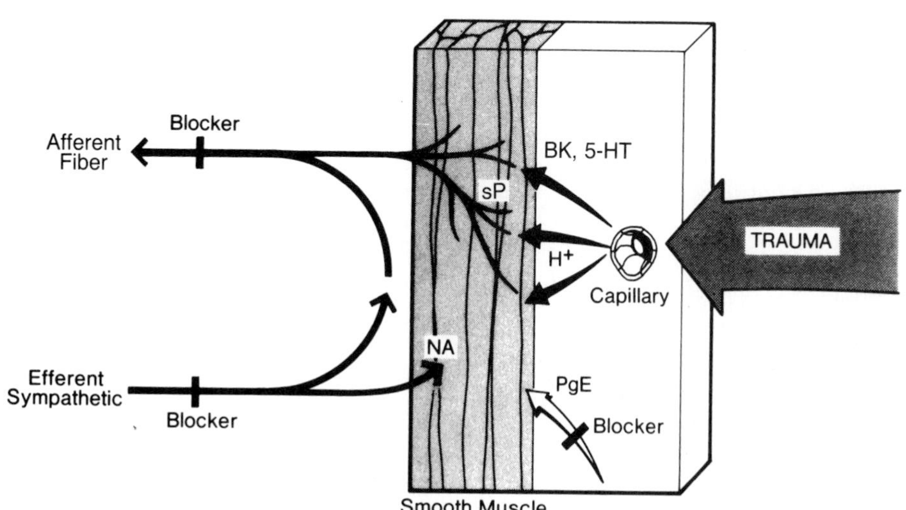

Figure 10–9. Local tissue factors and peripheral pain receptors. The physical stimuli of "trauma," the chemical environment (e.g., H^+), algesic substances (e.g., serotonin [5-hydroxytryptamine (5-HT)], and bradykinin [BK]), and the microcirculatory changes may all modify peripheral receptor activity. Efferent sympathetic activity may increase the sensitivity of receptors by means of noradrenaline (NA; norepinephrine) release. Substance P (sP) may be the peripheral pain transmitter. Points of potential blockade of nociception are shown as "Blocker"; other potential sites involve BK, 5-HT, NA, and sP. PgE = prostaglandin E. (Reprinted from Cousins MJ, Phillips GD [eds]: Acute Pain Management. London, Churchill Livingstone, 1986, p 742. Used with permission.)

Neural blockade can occur at any point along the pain pathway. The most common sites of neural block would be peripheral nerves, somatic plexuses, and dorsal roots. These blocks can be performed with relatively short-acting agents such as local anesthetics for acute pain, whereas long-acting (permanent) blockade with alcohol or phenol may be more appropriate for chronic pain. Surgical lesions at any of these points have also been suggested to provide long-lasting interruption of specific pain pathways. The disadvantage of permanent techniques is that they are neither specific for pain fibers nor reliable for protracted pain problems. The lack of anatomical separation of fibers carrying pain, motor, and other sensory information exposes the patient in whom neural blockade is employed to varying amounts of sympathetic, somatic, and perhaps motor dysfunction. Although these side effects may be well tolerated in certain acute pain situations where the patient is expected to improve rapidly, or in chronic cancer pain where the life expectancy of the patient is less than 12 months, the use of these techniques in chronic pain management situations is inappropriate.

Opioid Analgesia

In recent years researchers have identified multiple endogenous opioid chemicals that have analgesic effects (Yaksh 1988). Included among these are the enkephalins and β-endorphin. At least four different types of opioid receptors have also been located in the brain and spinal cord. Table 10–1 summarizes the pharmacodynamic effects obtained when each of these opioid receptors is stimulated. In 1973 Pert and Snyder demonstrated opioid receptors in the brain and brain stem. Afterward Yaksh and Rudy (1976) reported long-lasting analgesia following the introduction of intrathecal opioids. The discovery that spinally administered opioids produced dose-dependent, stereospecific, naloxone-reversible analgesia has led to development of an important clinical tool to combat pain.

TABLE 10–1. PHARMACODYNAMIC EFFECTS OBTAINED WHEN AN OPIOID AGONIST INTERACTS WITH THE VARIOUS TYPES OF OPIOID RECEPTORS

	Receptor subtype			
Effect	*Mu* (μ)	*Kappa* (κ)	*Sigma* (σ)	*Delta* (δ)
Pain relief	Yes	Yes, especially at spinal cord level	Yes	Yes
Sedation	Yes	Yes	—	—
Respiratory effects	Depression	Depression, but not as much as for μ (may reach plateau)	Stimulation	Depression
Affect	Euphoria	—	Dysphoria	—
Physical dependence	Marked	Less severe than with μ	—	Yes
Prototype agonist (other drugs with predominantly agonist activity)	Morphine (Meperidine) (Methadone) (Fentanyl) (Heroin) (Codeine) (Propoxyphene) (Buprenorphine)	Ketocyclazocine (Nalbuphine) (Dynorphin) (Butorphanol) (Nalorphine) (Pentazocine)	SKF 10,047	Enkephalins

Note. SKF = Smith Kline & French.
Source. Adapted from Gourlay et al. 1987b. Used with permission.

Brain receptors. Opium has been known for centuries to possess analgesic properties. Despite this being a well-recognized phenomenon, the location of the active sites for opium was not known. Microinjection techniques used in the 1960s have identified the periaqueductal gray of the midbrain and midline medullary nuclei to be the most sensitive sites. Through descending serotonergic and/or noradrenergic links with the spinal cord, morphine microinjections into these centers has been shown to inhibit spinal reflexes. This analgesic effect has also been shown to be similar to the effect achieved by systemically administered morphine. Further research has documented dose dependency, stereospecificity, naloxone reversibility, and well-defined structure activity relationships of these centers to other opiate agonists.

Spinal cord receptors. Equally interesting to the delineation of descending inhibition of nociception initiated by centrally administered opioids is the growing appreciation of opioid systems in spinal function. Opioids administered systemically will produce inhibition of nociceptive reflexes in spinal transected animals. Also, administration of opioids to the dorsal horn of the spinal cord will inhibit the discharge of nociceptive neurons. Multiple discrete populations of opioid receptors have been identified. Stimulation of μ (mu) and κ (kappa) systems present in the spinal cord depresses the response to noxious stimulation (Yaksh 1981).

Opiate systems appear to be active in the modulation of noxious impulses presented to the substantia gelatinosa via both direct action and indirect descending inhibition via serotonergic and noradrenergic systems (Yaksh 1988). In addition, other nonopioid systems appear to be functioning at this level to produce analgesic effects. Baclofen and clonidine also rely on both ascending and descending effects for antinociception (Sawynok and Labella 1981).

In summary, it appears that the substantia gelatinosa receives collaterals of nociceptive information and that information is subject to extensive modulation at the spinal level. Chemical mediators that have been shown to be associated with analgesia at this level include opioids, serotonin, norepinephrine, γ-aminobutyric acid (GABA), neurotensin, and acetylcholine. Some of the proposed endogenous and exogenous ligands for these neurotransmitter systems are shown in Table 10–2.

Electrical Stimulation

The prediction that large fiber activity could block certain noxious information at the level of the dorsal horn resulted in the introduction of transcutaneous electrical nerve stimulation (TENS). The clinical utility of TENS has yet to be established for individual pain syndromes. Dorsal column stimulation (DCS) excites descending inhibitory pathways with electricity to provide analgesia. The success of DCS has been mixed, but it may have a place in certain deafferentation pain syndromes.

The success of central morphine microinjection techniques to provide analgesia may have prompt-

TABLE 10–2. SPINAL NEUROTRANSMITTERS, RECEPTORS, AND LIGANDS

Neurotransmitter systems	*Proposed receptor*	*Endogenous ligand*	*Exogenous ligand*
Opioid	μ	β-Endorphin; Met/Leu-enkephalin	Morphine
	δ	Met/Leu-enkephalin	DADL
	κ	Dynorphin	U50488H
Adrenergic	α_1	Norepinephrine	Methoxamine
	α_2	Norepinephrine	Clonidine
	β	Epinephrine	Isoproterenol
Serotonergic	5-HT	Serotonin	Serotonin
GABAergic	A	GABA	Baclofen
	B	GABA	Muscimol
Neurotensin	—	Neurotensin	Neurotensin
Cholinergic	Muscarinic	Acetylcholine	Oxotremorine

Note. GABA = γ-aminobutyric acid; 5-HT = 5-hydroxytryptamine.
Source. Adapted from Yaksh 1988. Used with permission.

ed Reynolds (1969) to demonstrate similar results in animals using electrical stimulation of the periaqueductal gray. Hosobuchi has subsequently demonstrated naloxone-reversible analgesia in humans after implantation of brain stem electrodes (see Bonica and Ventafridda 1979). Each of these applications of electrical stimulation was predicted on the basis of improved understanding of the pain pathway. Electrical stimulation seems to have found a place in pain management by exciting intrinsic mechanisms used for the modulation of nociceptive information.

Nonsteroidal Anti-Inflammatory Drugs

The effect of nonsteroidal anti-inflammatory drugs (NSAIDs) to inhibit the synthesis of prostaglandins is currently thought to be the explanation of their pain-relieving properties. The prostaglandins, leukotrienes, and thromboxanes are oxygenated derivatives of arachidonic acid, an essential polyunsaturated fat. The term *eicosanoids* is often used to describe all of the products of arachidonic acid metabolism. This inhibition occurs by the inactivation of cyclooxygenase, which catalyzes the formation of cyclic endoperoxides from arachidonic acid. Anti-inflammatory steroids act at an earlier step in the arachidonic acid metabolism pathway (Raja et al. 1988). As discussed earlier, prostaglandins are formed in damaged tissue and appear to be involved in sensitizing the peripheral nociceptors to painful stimuli.

The indications for NSAIDs range from the treatment of aches and sprains and dysmenorrhea to long-term therapy for rheumatoid arthritis and osteoarthritis, as well as degenerative joint diseases (e.g., ankylosing spondylitis and gout). Their anti-inflammatory activities have also been shown to relieve pain in cancer patients with bony metastases. In contrast to the opioid drugs, there has not been a clear demonstration of a relationship between blood levels of NSAIDs and pain relief. The majority of NSAIDs can be classified into one of two groups based on their elimination half-lives (Table 10–3). The NSAIDs in the first group have half-lives between 2 and 4 hours. Acetaminophen is also included in this group, despite its lack of anti-inflammatory properties. The drugs in second group have longer half-lives, ranging from 6 to 60 hours. Patients with renal insufficiency are thought to be at risk for toxicity due to these agents because they are excreted through the kidney.

The use of NSAIDs alone has been supported through years of clinical practice. However, the different sites of action found with NSAIDs and opioids would also suggest additive or possibly even synergistic effects. Trials with a relatively new

TABLE 10–3. TERMINAL HALF-LIFE, RECOMMENDED DOSE, INFLUENCE OF FOOD ON ABSORPTION, AND INCIDENCE OF GASTRIC EROSION FROM NONSTEROIDAL ANTI-INFLAMMATORY DRUGS (NSAIDs)

Drug	*Terminal half-life (hours)*	*Oral dose and frequency (mg/hour)*	*Effect of food on absorption*[a]	*Incidence of gastric erosion (gastritis)*
Aspirin	0.2–0.3	600–900/4	1	High
Salicylate	2–3	600/4	1	Intermediate
Diflunisal	8–12	500/12	1	Low
Diclofenac	1.5–2	25–50/8	1	Low
Ibuprofen	2–3	200–400/8	1	Low
Naproxen	12–15	250–375/12	3	Low
Fenoprofen	2–3	400–600/6	2	Low
Indomethacin	6–8	50–75/8	1	Intermediate
Sulindac	6–8	100–200/12	2	Low
Piroxicam	30–60	20–30/24	1	Low
Flufenamic acid	8–10	500/6	1	—
Mefenamic acid	3–4	250/6	1	Intermediate
Ketoprofen	1–4	50/6	1	Low
Ketorolac[b]	5	10–30/6	?	?

[a]1 = decrease in rate of absorption; no change in oral bioavailability; 2 = decrease in rate of absorption and oral bioavailability; 3 = no change in rate of absorption and oral bioavailability.
[b]Not currently available for clinical use; doses based on review of scientific literature.
Source. Adapted from Gourlay et al. 1987b. Used with permission.

NSAID, ketorolac, indicate that this drug has strong analgesic properties and will significantly reduce opioid requirements. Ketorolac will likely find a place in the acute management of postoperative pain as it is available in a parenteral form.

Dosing of the individual agents is covered in Table 10–3. These doses have been derived from long-term therapy of rheumatologic disease and represent near maximal anti-inflammatory activity. Although these doses are considered safe for long-term therapy, careful monitoring of side effects is appropriate. Side effects of NSAIDs include gastric irritation, salt and fluid retention, platelet inhibition, and tinnitus. The gastric damage is caused by decreased prostaglandin levels, which cause less gastric mucus production, increased acid secretion, and decreased gastric mucosal blood supply. Acetaminophen does not share the potential for these prostaglandin-mediated side effects, but carries the potential for liver damage with excessive doses.

Antidepressants

The possible involvement of neurotransmitters in the transmission of pain is discussed above. Many of the antidepressant drugs act by blocking the uptake of noradrenaline and serotonin in the central nervous system. This effect may also occur in the medulla and increase the concentrations of these neurotransmitters at the synapses involved in descending inhibition of dorsal horn cells. Table 10–4 lists the names and properties of some of these antidepressants. Secondary amines are thought to be more effective blockers of norepinephrine, whereas the tertiary amines appear more effective in blocking serotonin reuptake.

Oral tricyclic antidepressants (TCAs) are well absorbed from the gastrointestinal tract. There is conflicting information regarding the existence of therapeutic ranges for antidepressants. All of the currently available pharmacokinetic information refers to the antidepressant activity of these drugs. The time taken for the perception of pain relief after the institution of these drugs is only 2–7 days, compared to the accepted time for antidepressant effect of 3–4 weeks. This observation suggests that different mechanisms may be involved in their analgesic effect and their antidepressant action.

Side effects from TCA use include autonomic, anticholinergic, and adrenergic effects. Dry mouth is the most common side effect and can be relieved by increased fluid intake and salivary stimulants such as sugarless candy. Blurring of vision is also common and usually interferes with reading. Orthostatic hypotension is also common. Patients should be warned to rise slowly and watch for dizziness. Constipation has also been described in association with these agents.

TABLE 10–4. TERMINAL HALF-LIFE, RECOMMENDED DAILY DOSES, AND OTHER PROPERTIES OF ANTIDEPRESSANT DRUGS

Drug	*Amine group*	*Terminal half-life (hours)*	*Inhibitor concentration*[a]		*Recommended daily dose (mg)*[b]
			NA	*5-HT*	
Amitriptyline	Tertiary	20–30	4.6	4.4	50–150
Nortriptyline	Secondary	18–36	0.9	17.0	50–150
Protriptyline	Secondary	50–90	—	—	10–50
Clomipramine	Tertiary	20–30	4.6	0.5	50–75
Imipramine	Tertiary	20–30	4.6	0.5	50–75
Desipramine	Secondary	12–24	0.2	35.0	75–150
Doxepin	Tertiary	10–25	6.5	20.0	75–150
Dothiepin	Tertiary	20–30	—	—	50–100
Mianserin	Tertiary	10–20	20.0	130.0	20–50
Nomifensine	Primary and tertiary	2–4	2.0	120.0	75–150
Zimelidine	Tertiary	5–10	630.0	14.0	200–300

[a]Inhibitor concentration (IC50) represents the antidepressant concentration (x 10^{-8} m) required to inhibit the uptake of either noradrenaline (NA) or serotonin (5-hydroxytryptamine [5-HT]) by 50% using rat midbrain synaptosomes.
[b]It is generally recommended that the antidepressant be administered as a single dose at night, unless significant side effects occur where a night and morning dose (divided dose) may be appropriate.
Source. Adapted from Gourlay et al. 1987b.

Analgesic Adjuvants

A multitude of agents have been purported to have analgesic qualities. The majority of these agents are thought to potentiate analgesia provided by opioid and nonopioid analgesics. Although the data in support of the use of such compounds may be anecdotal, a small number of these drugs do appear to have clinical utility in the management of cancer pain. Table 10–5 summarizes some of the currently available coanalgesics.

Corticosteroids are the first group of drugs to be considered as coanalgesics. These drugs have been used successfully for the management of neuropathic pain from direct neural compression and from pain due to increased intracranial pressure. Systemic steroids are thought to reduce perineural edema and lymphatic edema that may be contributing to pain by compressing individual nerves. This treatment appears to be especially helpful in cases of spinal cord compression. Treatment of such neural compression involves relatively high doses of dexamethasone (near 30 mg/day). Steroids are best employed on a trial basis. A single morning dose or twice daily dose of 2–4 mg/day of dexamethasone can be used over a 10- to 14-day period.

TABLE 10–5. COANALGESIC MEDICATIONS

Drugs, by classification	*Indications*	*Comments*
Antidepressant Amitriptyline Imipramine Mianserin Clomipramine Doxepin	Chronic pain, neuropathic pain associated with neuropathy and headache	Improves sleep, may improve appetite
Corticosteroid Dexamethasone Prednisolone Fludrocortisone	Neuropathic pain secondary to direct neural compression, pain secondary in increased intracranial pressure	May stimulate appetite, limit trial to 2 weeks and reassess efficacy
Anticonvulsant Carbamazepine Phenytoin Valproate Clonazepam	Neuropathic pain with paroxysmal character	Start slowly, increase gradually while observing for side effects
Membrane stabilizer Lidocaine 2-Chloroprocaine Tocainide Mexiletine	Neuropathic pain associated with peripheral neuropathy	Efficacy of oral preparations is not established
Phenothiazine Levomepromazine	Insomnia unresponsive to antidepressant or short-acting benzodiazepines	Increase dose slowly to achieve desired effect
Butyrophenone Haloperidol	Acute confusion, nausea, and vomiting	Prolonged use may be complicated by tardive dyskinesia
Antihistamine Hydroxyzine	Nausea, pruritus, and anxiety	Anticholinergic side effects
CNS stimulant Dextroamphetamine Cocaine Caffeine	Opioid-induced sedation, potentiation of NSAID, potentiation of opioid analgesia not proven in cancer	Should only be used as short-term therapeutic trial

Note. CNS = central nervous system; NSAID = nonsteroidal anti-inflammatory drug.

An additional benefit of corticosteroids is that they often stimulate appetite; this may aid in the nutritional support of patients with malignancy. The use of steroids is not without problems, however. Attention needs to be focused on the possible development of oral and vaginal candidiasis; in addition, this treatment may worsen peripheral edema.

Anticonvulsants are also often advocated as analgesic adjuvants. They suppress neuronal firing and have been successfully employed for treatment of neuropathic pain states, including trigeminal neuralgia and peripheral neuropathies. Anticonvulsant drugs probably exert their effects by blocking voltage-dependent sodium channels and thereby interfering with transduction and perhaps spontaneous depolarization seen in damaged neurons. Carbamazepine and phenytoin have been helpful in managing cancer pain with dysesthetic components. These drugs need to be started slowly and increased gradually, with particular attention being paid to the development of possible side effects. Common side effects can include dizziness, ataxia, drowsiness, blurred vision, and gastrointestinal irritation. In addition, carbamazepine has associated bone marrow toxicity, whereas sodium valproate is known to produce hepatic toxicity.

The use of lidocaine and 2-chloroprocaine in the treatment of certain peripheral neuropathies that have been refractory to other analgesic medications has led to the investigation of another group of drugs, which may be loosely classified as membrane stabilizers. In addition to intermittent intravenous infusion of these two local anesthetics, oral administration of the lidocaine congeners mexiletine and tocainide has been reported as useful in certain patients (Dejard et al. 1988; Lindstrom and Lindblom 1987). Typically, these patients are thought to have neuropathic components to their pain. In comparison with patients with episodic lancinating neuropathic pain who benefit from antiepileptics, those patients who benefit from membrane stabilizers may have a more constant pain.

Antipsychotics have long been purported to potentiate the analgesic effect of opioids. Most studies employing these drugs are uncontrolled, however, and the enthusiasm for their continued use is in contrast to available literature. The phenothiazines are the most commonly employed antipsychotics for analgesia. Dundee and colleagues (Dundee et al. 1963; Moore and Dundee 1961a, 1961b) published data regarding the analgesic potency of 14 different phenothiazines in an uncontrolled trial of experimental pain. The results of these studies suggested that the action of a few potentially analgesic phenothiazines was initially antianalgesic and after 2–3 hours only mildly analgesic (Atkison et al. 1985).

Review of phenothiazines in both experimental and clinical pain reveals that only levomepromazine (methotrimeprazine) has established analgesic properties. Levomepromazine appears to have analgesic potency about one-half that of morphine in patients with cancer pain (Beaver et al. 1966). Haloperidol is a butyrophenone antipsychotic that has found a useful position in the management of acute confusional states associated with terminal cancer. Haloperidol also has useful antiemetic properties, which can be helpful in the management of cancer pain. The appropriate utilization of antipsychotics in the management of chronic cancer pain has not been established. Care must be used in the long-term administration of these drugs because of the potential for developing tardive dyskinesia.

Benzodiazepines are often discussed as coanalgesics. These drugs do not have any demonstrated analgesic effect. Diazepam has been studied extensively with respect to analgesic activity, and it does not alter sensitivity to pain or potentiate the analgesic activity of opioids. These drugs do decrease affective responses to acute pain, however, and may produce extended relief in chronic pain due to musculoskeletal disorders, perhaps due to their muscle relaxant properties. Judicious use of benzodiazepines in cancer pain is appropriate for short-term relief of anxiety, but superior analgesic effects and night time sedation can be achieved by employing a TCA.

Hydroxyzine is an antihistaminic agent. It has proven analgesic properties at high doses. It does not consistently improve analgesia obtained with opioids, but it does potentiate the effect of opioids on the affective components of pain. It appears that hydroxyzine administered intramuscularly has analgesic properties similar to those of low doses of morphine (Beaver and Feise 1976). In addition, the sedative and antipruritic properties of this drug are useful in the setting of chronic cancer pain.

The final group of analgesic adjuvants to be considered are the stimulants. This group includes amphetamines, cocaine, and caffeine. Chronic cancer pain has been treated for nearly a century with combinations of opioid and stimulant in Brompton's cocktail. This mixture contains morphine, cocaine, and a phenothiazine. Despite years of clinical experience with such a mixture, no controlled studies have demonstrated superior analgesia with this combination compared with opioid alone. Potentiation of analgesia by sympathomimetics has been well described. Caffeine is known to increase the analgesic effects of aspirin and acetaminophen, and one study suggested that dextroamphetamine doubled the analgesic potency of morphine (Forrest et al. 1977). The long-term use of these stimulants in pain has not been systematically evaluated. The use of these drugs should probably be limited to a therapeutic trial period of several days to determine efficacy for individual patients.

Opioids

Opioids are extremely effective agents in the treatment of nociceptive components of acute pain. Many misconceptions surround the use of opioid drugs, which results in a marked tendency for inadequate doses and inappropriately long dosing intervals. Once a decision has been made to use opioid medications, it is both logical and essential to use an effective dosage regimen.

Although vast sums of money have been invested in the development of new opioids over the last decade, an increased understanding of the pharmacokinetics and pharmacodynamics involved in opioid administration has done more to improve the treatment of pain than any new drug. The introduction of concepts such as the minimum effective analgesic concentration (MEC) has helped health care providers conceptualize the association between blood opioid concentrations and analgesic effect. Equally important to effective pain treatment has been the realization that there may be as much as a five- to sixfold interpatient variability in the value of MEC for any one agent. Many factors, both physical and psychological, influence MEC. It is impossible to predict the value of MEC for any patient-opioid combination. It is therefore necessary that the dose for each individual be titrated to the desired effect. Although MEC and other pharmacokinetic variables cannot be used ahead of time to predict exact analgesic doses of opioids necessary to obtain analgesia, these concepts provide a good starting point. They also allow the prediction of the effect that certain disease states will have on opioid requirements.

In addition to planning effective analgesic therapy with opioids individualized to a particular patient, the use of opioids often involves management of side effects. The major side effects that limit the effectiveness of opioid therapy are nausea, vomiting, sedation, and respiratory depression. The incidence and severity of the side effects seen with the different μ agonists are probably similar at equianalgesic doses. Rather than restrict the dose of opioids to the point at which a patient is free from side effects but experiencing pain, one should consider administering other medications to treat these side effects.

Delivery Systems

The continued reports of inadequate pain relief, despite the vast numbers of newly developed opioids, point to the problems associated with opioid delivery rather than to any defect in the individual drugs, per se. There are many different delivery systems and dosing regimens that can provide good pain relief when used properly. The association between stable blood levels of opioids and continuous analgesia must be remembered when planning any systemic opioid therapy. The effective dose of opioid medication is the minimum dose that provides acceptable pain relief with a low incidence of side effects.

Oral opioids. The rapid clearance of the majority of opioids, combined with the extensive hepatic metabolism, has important implications for oral dosing. Drugs are absorbed from the gastrointestinal tract directly into the portal circulation, where they travel to the liver. Therefore, allowing oral dosing, a significant percentage of the dose is metabolized to inactive products before the opioids reach the systemic circulation (Mather and Gourlay 1984). This phenomenon is referred to as the hepatic *first-pass effect*. This effect and the poor bioavailability seen with certain opioids lead to perceptions that oral administration of opioids is ineffective.

Oral bioavailability ranges from zero for heroin to 80% for methadone. Morphine oral bioavailability ranges from 10% to 40%, leading to very wide fluctuations in oral dosing requirements between different patients. Similar variability is seen in meperidine (pethidine) and other opioids (Table 10–6). The high bioavailability of methadone and the long terminal half-life suggest that stable blood levels of the drug could be obtained from oral dosing.

Much attention has also been focused on the development of effective sustained-release preparations of morphine. Although the concept of sustained release is fairly simple, obtaining a pharmacological preparation that maintains a steady dose release without tendency toward dose dumping, which can lead to a bolus effect, has proven more difficult. Currently, sustained-release morphine products are available in many countries. The actual changes in pharmacokinetics of these sustained-release preparations with regard to food intake, activity, and posture have not been evaluated. As continued progress is made in this area, the availability of a reliable sustained-release preparation should be forthcoming.

In summary, satisfactory analgesia with oral dosing can be obtained if attention is focused on the pharmacokinetics of the particular opioid to be administered, the oral bioavailability of the drug, and titration of the drug to achieve adequate analgesia in each patient.

Sublingual administration. Ongoing interest in the improved pain management of patients with terminal malignancy has led to the investigation of sublingual administration. The sublingual route is particularly useful in patients who cannot tolerate oral medication because it causes nausea, vomiting, or dysphagia. This method of administration has theoretical advantages in that the oral cavity is well perfused, providing rapid onset of action; subsequent absorption results in systemic rather than portal drug delivery. The sublingual absorption of lipid-soluble drugs (methadone, fentanyl, and buprenorphine) from alkaline solution was shown to provide analgesic concentrations very quickly (Weinberg et al. 1988). The utility of this technique in comparison with other methods of administration still needs to be assessed.

Rectal administration. Rectal administration of opioids has been advocated for patients who cannot swallow or those who have a high incidence of nausea or vomiting with oral administration. Studies of rectal administration of meperidine have indicated a bioavailability similar to that seen following oral dosing: 50% (Ripamonti and Bruera 1991). Prolonged pain relief of 6–8 hours is observed following large doses (400 mg) of rectal meperidine, but a significant latency of 2–3 hours after administration can be seen. Rectal oxycodone has also been shown to have clinical utility providing pain relief for up to 8 hours.

Intramuscular administration. The most commonly used approach for managing postoperative pain is intramuscular administration of morphine or meperidine. The typical prescription would read: "Morphine 10 mg (or meperidine 100 mg) intramuscularly every 3–4 hours as needed for pain." This approach has been shown to provide inadequate analgesia for many reasons. The patient may not request medication despite experiencing severe pain. The nurse may not administer the medication. The dose may not be adequate for the patient's needs. Even controlling all of these potential problems, the variable blood levels seen after intramuscular dosing usually results in periods of pain, alternating with periods of toxicity (Austin et al. 1980).

Subcutaneous administration. Subcutaneous administration of opioids has been used for decades to provide analgesia. More recent attention has been focused on this technique with the availability of small infusion pumps for delivering continuous opioids to ambulatory patients. Recent applications include subcutaneous infusion for cancer pain and subcutaneous patient-controlled analgesia (PCA). Bruera et al. (1988b) recently presented data confirming the efficacy of subcutaneous infusion in treating patients with severe pain due to malignancy, both at home and in the hospital. The pharmacokinetic information available for subcutaneous administration of opioids is very limited. Continuous infusion of subcutaneous morphine has been demonstrated to provide equivalent analgesia and blood levels to intravenous infusion in postoperative patients (Waldeman et al. 1984). Other drugs have been delivered by this route, but no definitive information is available on blood levels achieved. Subcutaneous infusion appears to act clinically like a continuous infusion, but more carefully controlled trials need to be carried out to determine if this similarity is true for all opioids.

Intravenous administration. The use of intravenous opioids, by intermittent injection as well as continuous infusion, has been known for years to provide more rapid and effective analgesia. The clinical utility of this technique in the management of cancer pain was recently reviewed by the Sloan Kettering Group (Portenoy et al. 1986). The pharmacokinetic support for this clinical observation has been developed over the last several years. Intrave-

TABLE 10–6. DOSES, PHARMACOKINETIC PARAMETERS, MINIMUM EFFECTIVE CONCENTRATION, AND DURATION OF PAIN RELIEF FOR VARIOUS OPIOID DRUGS

			Pharmacokinetic parameters				
	Dose (mg)		*Terminal half-life*	*Bioavailability*	*MEC*	*Duration of pain relief*	
Opioid	*im/iv*	*po*	*(hours)*	*(%)*	*(ng/ml)*	*(hours)*	*Comments*
Codeine	130	250	2–3	50	—	3–4	Weak opiate, frequently combined with aspirin. Useful for pain with visceral and integumentary components.
Propoxyphene	240	500	8–24	40	—	4–6	Weak opioid. Unacceptable incidence of side effects.
Oxycodone	10	30	—	30–50	—	4–6	Suppository (30 mg) can provide pain relief for 8–10 hours.
Diamorphine	5	15	0.05	—	—	2–3	Very soluble, rapidly converted to 6-mono-acetyl morphine and morphine in vivo. No oral bioavailability.
Morphine	10	40	2–4	10–40	10–40	3–4	Standard opiate to which new opioids are compared. New sustained-release formulation available in some countries is of considerable benefit in chronic cancer pain.
Methadone	10	10–15	10–80	70–95	20–80	10–60	Duration of pain relief ranges from 10 to 60 hours both postoperatively and for cancer pain. Variable half-life. Requires initial care to establish dose for each patient to avoid accumulation. Otherwise of great value.
Hydromorphone	2	4–6	2–3	50–60	4	3–4	More potent but shorter acting than morphine.
Levorphanol	2	4	12–16	40–60	—	4–6	Good oral availability, but long half-life compared to analgesia may lead to accumulation.
Phenazocine	3	10–20	—	20–30	—	4–6	Similar to morphine, only more potent.
Oxymorphone	1	6	—	10–40	—	3–4	Similar to morphine, only more potent.

TABLE 10–6. (Continued)

			Pharmacokinetic parameters				
	Dose (mg)		Terminal half-life	Bioavailability	MEC	Duration of pain relief	
Opioid	*im/iv*	*po*	*(hours)*	*(%)*	*(ng/ml)*	*(hours)*	*Comments*
Meperidine	100	300	3–5	30–60	200–800	2–4	Not as effective in relieving anxiety as morphine. Suppositories (200–400 mg) have slow onset (2–3 hours) but can last for 6–8 hours. Normeperidine toxicity.
Dextromoramide	7.5	10	—	75	—	2–3	Methadone-like chemical structure. Short acting. Useful in covering exacerbation pain. Supposed as iv form.
Buprenorphine	0.3	0.2–1.2	2–3	30	—	6–8	Available in many countries as a sublingual tablet, which appears useful in treatment of cancer pain. Ceiling in analgesic effect at dose near 5 mg/day. Should not be used with a pure opioid agonist.
Butorphanol	2	—	2.5–3.5	—	—	3–6	Oral form unavailable in many countries. Value in treatment of chronic pain not established.
Nalbuphine	10	40	4–6	20	—	3–6	Oral form unavailable in many countries. Value in treatment of chronic pain not established.

Note. Data presented are estimates obtained from the literature. MEC = minimum effective analgesic concentration.
Source. Adapted from Gourlay et al. 1987b. Used with permission.

nous administration of opioid can maintain analgesia as long as the blood opioid concentration is kept above the MEC in a given patient. Knowledge of the systemic clearance of a drug will allow close approximation of the MEC value for a specific opioid to be delivered via continuous infusion. Using infusion alone, however, will require approximately four times the terminal half-life to achieve stable concentrations. The clinical utilization of continuous-infusion opioids is best simplified by providing a loading dose followed by a continuous infusion. The amount of the loading dose and the initial infusion can be predicted if the MEC, volume of distribution (Vd), and clearance (Cl) are known. The practical steps in calculating such an analgesic infusion are

1. Loading dose = Vd × MEC
2. Maintenance infusion = Cl × MEC

Providing the loading dose as an infusion over 10–15 minutes (followed by the maintenance rate) will allow good analgesia to be rapidly established with a minimum of toxicity. Subsequently, the maintenance infusion rate should be titrated to patient comfort.

Patient-controlled analgesia. The wide interpatient variability of the pharmacokinetic parameters discussed thus far is a primary reason that individual titration of opioid dosing is required to achieve adequate analgesia. Although the physician can do this by evaluating patients at a given time after the therapy has been initiated, the option of PCA is well suited to accommodate the differences between the theory and practice of pain relief. Using PCA, the physician decides the drug to be employed and the dose to be given. The patient can decide when a dose should be administered and the timing between doses.

Although there are several variants of PCA, the most commonly employed is a bolus demand form. With this type of PCA the physician prescribes the drug based on his or her personal preferences. The usual practice is to prescribe a bolus dose range that can be adjusted if inadequate analgesia or toxicity develops from a single demand. In addition, the minimum time between doses is also prescribed by the physician to avoid potential toxicity from repeated demands being provided before the peak effect of each bolus has been seen.

The majority of pharmacokinetic information that has been applied to PCA is inferred from single dose or continuous infusion of opioids. The applicability of this information to the multiple dose system of PCA has yet to be investigated. Despite this theoretical uncertainty, the clinical practice of PCA is successful. Several investigators have reported higher patient satisfaction and lower pain scores when this therapy is employed compared with other forms of parenteral opioid analgesia in acute pain management. Recently, the efficacy of short-term subcutaneous PCA was also demonstrated in cancer pain management (Bruera et al. 1988a).

Spinal administration. The use of spinal opioids for acute pain management dates back only into the last decade. As compared with all of the delivery systems discussed above, which use indirect delivery of the opioid to the receptor site via the systemic circulation, spinal delivery is a system in which the opioids are delivered directly to the receptors in the spinal cord via local mechanisms. The presence of opioid receptors in the dorsal horn of the spinal cord was suggested by Calvillo et al. (1974). The localization of high concentrations of opioid receptors in the substantia gelatinosa followed (Atweh and Kuhar 1977). Behavioral analgesia from intrathecal administration of morphine in rats was reported by Yaksh and Rudy in 1976. Large numbers of clinical reports of long-lasting analgesia obtained with spinal opioids followed, but these were also accompanied by frequent reports of side effects. These side effects included nausea, vomiting, sedation, pruritus, urinary retention, and respiratory depression. Fortunately, the identification of these side effects tempered the rampant application of this technique. Meanwhile, fundamental knowledge about the use of spinal opioids was obtained through extensive animal studies (Yaksh 1981; Yaksh and Noueihed 1985).

The term *spinal opioid* as applied in this section is used to describe intrathecal, epidural, and intracerebroventricular administration of opioids. In an effort to present some of the data concerning spinal opioids, the remainder of this section deals with the epidural opioids except where specifically stated.

The pharmacokinetics of epidurally administered morphine applied in the lumbar epidural space are still incompletely studied. It appears that after epidural injection of morphine, only low concentrations of lipid soluble, un-ionized drug will be present in the epidural space. Movement of the drug into the cerebrospinal fluid (CSF) by diffusion across the dura mater and transfer across the arachnoid granulation, as well as vascular uptake by spinal arteries and the epidural venous system, all regulate the distribution of epidural morphine (Figure 10–10). Because only small concentrations of the morphine present in the CSF will be un-ionized, the transfer across the spinal cord to the dorsal horn receptors will be slow. Morphine will also be available to move upward with the flow of CSF toward the brain. This explanation of epidural morphine distribution correlates well with the delayed onset of analgesia and the late respiratory depression seen.

Much of the concern about the utilization of spinal opioids has focused on the concern for respiratory depression. This can be early (associated with the peak blood levels following epidural administration) or late (perhaps due to the rostral migration of morphine into sensitive respiratory centers). Outcome studies (Rawal et al. 1987) generated from

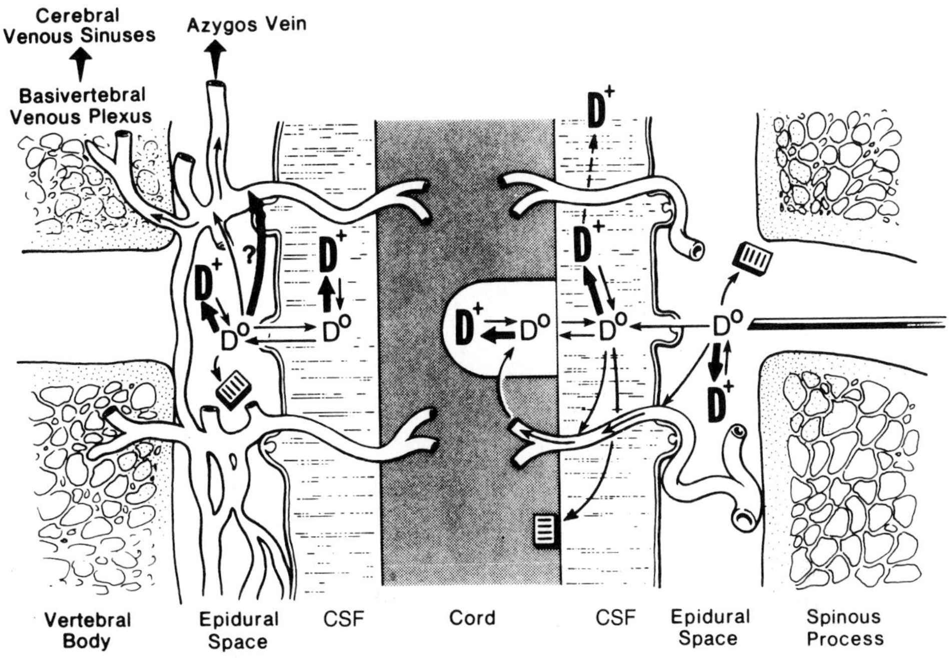

Figure 10–10. Pharmacokinetics model of an epidural injection of a hydrophilic opioid such as morphine. D° = un-ionized, lipophilic drug; D^+ = ionized, hydrophilic drug; CSF = cerebrospinal fluid. An epidural needle is shown delivering drug to the epidural space. The role of absorption by way of the radicular arteries remains speculative. The *shaded squares* represent nonspecific binding sites. (Reprinted from Cousins MJ, Bridenbaugh PO [eds]: Neural Blockade in Clinical Anesthesia and Management of Pain, 2nd Edition. Philadelphia, PA, JB Lippincott, 1988, p 987. Used with permission.)

large groups of patients in Sweden who received spinal opioids indicate that the incidence of severe delay respiratory depression after epidural morphine is approximately 1 in 1,000 patients. Although certain demographic characteristics of at-risk populations have been identified, the inability to predict the occurrence of delayed respiratory depression in healthy patients points out the need for increased surveillance of all patients who are receiving opioid analgesia.

The spinal administration of opioids is appropriate for pain in virtually any region of the body. Spinally administered morphine has been shown to migrate over the entire distance of the spinal cord, even when injected in the lumbar epidural space (Gourlay et al. 1985, 1987a). Pain relief from such spinal opioid systems has been shown for pain in cervical dermatomes and even in the trigeminal system.

Continued efforts to refine and evaluate spinal opioids should help to determine the appropriate utilization of this therapy. The high quality of analgesia and the tremendous reports of patient satisfaction seen following epidural morphine analgesia provide ample support for research in this field.

As mentioned above, multiple endogenous chemicals, which are thought to modulate nociceptive processing, have been identified in the region of the dorsal horn of the spinal cord. The clinical success of opioids to provide selective spinal analgesia has prompted the evaluation of other proposed analgesic agents. Intrathecal and epidural administration of clonidine has been shown to provide analgesia both in acute and chronic pain states. Clonidine is thought to mediate analgesia by blocking α_2- adrenergic transmission in the spinal cord. The activity of GABA in nociceptive processing at the dorsal horn has also promoted the evaluation of intrathecally administered baclofen. Although these and many other drugs have been demonstrated to be effective when administered spinally, the appropriate place for them in the treatment of pain is not known. These and other spinally active drugs may prove useful in patients who develop tolerance to spinal opioids. Alternatively, as more characterization of the neuropharmacology of the dorsal horn becomes available, these drugs may be applied to particular clinical situations in which spinal opioids have not been successful.

❑ ELECTRICAL STIMULATION

Transcutaneous Electrical Nerve Stimulation

The origin of transcutaneous electrical nerve stimulation (TENS) in Western medical society dates back to Roman times when use of electric fish was ascribed analgesic properties. Publication of the gate theory of pain by Melzack and Wall (1965) renewed interest in electrical stimulation to produce analgesia. The excitation of large fiber peripheral afferents by electrical stimulation at the periphery has been successful in treating nociceptive pain. TENS is a low-intensity stimulation, stimulating skin and muscle afferents in a specific segmental distribution. Numerous studies have documented the efficacy of TENS in certain pathologic pain states. In addition, TENS has been shown to decrease opioid requirements seen after surgery when used as an adjunct for postoperative analgesia.

Acupuncture

Classical acupuncture differs from modern concepts of acupuncture analgesia in that the techniques for the former evolved initially for the management of disease. Acupuncture analgesia uses stimulation of designated body sites by manual rotation of needles to produce a sensation known as *teh chi*. The classical acupuncture stimulation has been modernized more recently by the application of slow frequency (< 5 Hz) stimulation of the needles, which also produces powerful muscle contractions. Acupuncture produces a high-intensity stimulation that is believed to induce a chemical modulation of pain, which explains why the relief is not confined to a local segmental distribution.

Dorsal Column Stimulation

Many patients with deafferentation pain are candidates for dorsal column stimulation. This technique uses percutaneously positioned electrical leads that deliver a high-frequency current over the dorsal spinal cord in a effort to stimulate descending analgesic pathways. Effective electrical stimulation suggests that implantation of a self-contained battery-powered device may be efficacious in selected patients. There have been no prospective trials of this therapy in the management of neuropathic terminal cancer pain, but the responses achieved with other deafferentation pain syndromes point to possible efficacy in this difficult problem.

❑ NEURAL BLOCKADE

Patients who exhaust the analgesics or who develop toxicity problems from other medications may benefit from techniques of neurolytic blockade. The most common approach is to proceed from the least invasive to the more invasive techniques, as required for pain management. In one major study (Ventafridda et al. 1987) undertaken in a comprehensive cancer care center, only 20% of patients required treatment with neurolytic blocks or other neurodestructive techniques. The continued advancement of spinal opioid techniques, as well as the success of continuous subcutaneous opioid infusions, will likely continue to decrease the need for neurodestructive techniques. In cancer pain, local anesthetics may be used for diagnostic, prognostic, and therapeutic blocks.

Diagnostic blocks are used to localize the pain pathway and to pharmacologically differentiate the fiber type involved in mediating the pain. It is difficult to be certain that only a specific fiber type will be blocked by using differing concentrations of local anesthetics. Thus many pain clinicians prefer to block at sites where the fibers are anatomically separated (e.g., lumbar sympathetic block and individual somatic nerve blocks). The interpretation of diagnostic neural blockade is both difficult and crucial to the appropriate utilization of these techniques. This interpretation is discussed in detail by Boas and Cousins (1988).

Prognostic blocks should always be carried out at least twice before neurolytic or surgical ablation. This permits confirmation that the pain is relieved and also gives the patient an opportunity to decide if any side effects are acceptable.

Therapeutic blocks with local anesthetic cannot be expected to permanently relieve pain. However, pain may be due to muscle spasms, postoperative neuralgia, denervation phenomena, or neuroma formation. In some of these cases a series of long-acting local anesthetic blocks will produce long-lasting or permanent pain relief.

❑ NEURODESTRUCTIVE PROCEDURES

The continued progress in pain management with multidisciplinary therapies has decreased utilization of neurodestructive procedures. Despite the continued success of less invasive and nondestructive techniques, neurolytic blockade still provides valuable adjunctive treatment of nociceptive and neuropathic pain in terminal cancer (Cousins 1988). Often, a properly performed neurodestructive procedure can markedly decrease medication use and control the unwanted side effect associated with high doses of analgesics. Virtually all neurodestructive techniques should be confined to the treatment of nociceptive pain. The central and peripheral changes associated with neuropathic pain are not only never relieved by neurodestructive techniques, they are often aggravated by such procedures. Neurolytic blocks are mainly indicated for localized unilateral pain, except for pituitary ablation, which is suitable for diffuse areas of pain.

❑ HYPNOSIS

Central psychological approaches to pain control can also be effective and are underutilized. It has been known since the middle of the 1800s that hypnosis is effective in controlling even severe surgical pain (Esdaile 1846). Hypnosis and similar techniques work through two primary mechanisms: muscle relaxation and a combination of perceptual alteration and cognitive distraction. Pain is not infrequently accompanied by reactive muscle tension. Patients frequently splint the part of their body that hurts. Yet because muscle tension can by itself cause pain in normal tissue and because traction on a painful part of the body can produce more pain, techniques that induce greater physical relaxation can reduce pain in the periphery. Therefore, having patients enter a state of hypnosis so they can concentrate on an image that connotes physical relaxation such as floating or lightness often produces physical relaxation and reduces pain.

The second major component of hypnotic analgesia is perceptual alteration. Patients can be taught to imagine that the affected body part is numb. This is especially useful for extremely hypnotizable individuals who can, for example, relive an experience of dental anesthesia and reproduce the drug-induced sensations of numbness in their cheek, which they can then transfer to the painful part of their body. Temperature metaphors are often especially useful, which is not surprising given the fact that pain and temperature sensations are part of the same sensory system, as noted above. Thus imagining that an affected body part is cooler or warmer using an image of dipping it in ice water or heating it in the sun can often help patients transform pain signals. Some patients prefer to imagine that the pain is a substance with dimensions that can be moved or can flow out of the body as if it were a viscous liquid. Others like to imagine that they can step outside their body to, for example, visit another room in the house. Less hypnotizable individuals often do better with distraction techniques that help them focus on competing sensations in another part of the body.

Hypnotic techniques can easily be taught to patients for self-administration (Spiegel 1988). Pain patients can be taught to enter a state of self-hypnosis in a matter of seconds with some simple induction strategies such as looking up while slowly closing their eyes, taking a deep breath, and then letting the breath out, eyes relax, body float, and one hand float up in the air like a balloon. They are then instructed in the pain control exercise and taught to bring themselves out by reversing the induction procedure, again looking up, letting the eyes open, and letting the raised hand float back down. Patients can use this exercise every 1–2 hours initially and anytime they experience an attack of pain. They can evaluate their effectiveness in conducting the pain control exercise by rating on a scale from 0 to 10 the intensity of their pain before and after the self-hypnosis session. As with any pain treatment technique, hypnosis is more effective when employed early in the pain cycle, before the pain has become so overwhelming it impairs concentration. Patients should be encouraged to use this technique early and often because it is simple and effective (Spiegel and Bloom 1983b) and has no side effects (Spiegel 1986).

Although not all patients are sufficiently hypnotizable to benefit from these techniques, two out of three adults are at least somewhat hypnotizable (Spiegel and Spiegel 1987), and it has been estimated that hypnotic capacity is correlated at a .5 level with effectiveness in medical pain reduction (Hilgard and Hilgard 1975).

Hypnosis is especially effective in comforting children who are in pain. Several good studies have shown greater efficacy than placebo attention control (Hilgard and LeBaron 1982; Kellerman et al. 1983; Zeltzer and LeBaron 1982). This is likely due to the fact that children as a group are more hypnotizable than adults (Morgan and Hilgard 1973). Their imaginative capacities are so intense that separate relaxation exercises are not necessary. Children naturally relax when they mobilize their imagination during the sensory alteration component of hypnotic analgesia.

❑ SECONDARY GAIN

Secondary gain is a major problem with chronic pain. The term refers to the secondary reinforcements that accompany a primary loss involving physical function, ability to work, ability to engage in sexual activity, or other concomitants of injury and illness. A pain syndrome can set off a downward social spiral in which a patient loses the ordinary reinforcement that comes from contact with colleagues at work and the self-esteem that comes from being productive. Increasing depression can result in a loss of energy and an inability to interact rewardingly with others, leading to social withdrawal. Social contact becomes increasingly organized around pain complaints. Patients who seem to lose the ability to elicit enjoyable and rewarding social interactions increasingly coerce attention from health care providers, family, and friends over their disabilities, which contributes part of the secondary gain. Additional secondary gain may come in the form of being able to avoid unwanted responsibilities such as the pressures of work or unwelcome aspects of social interaction such as sexual activity.

Another major form of secondary gain is financial reinforcement. Disability systems frequently intensify this form of secondary gain by creating an adversarial system in which any evidence of the patient's ability to return to normal function endangers financial support, which in essence requires complete disability. Thus disability systems designed to provide a decent level of financial support for persons who have suffered physical and psychiatric illness have become rather rigid and wind up providing financial reinforcement for continued disability. In such an adversarial system, efforts at rehabilitation are used as evidence that there was never any serious disability in the first place. Furthermore, attaining disability status is often a protracted and unpleasant process. During a consolidation phase after an acute injury when patients might be able to return to some level of functioning despite continuing symptoms, they are instead engaged in a battle to prove the extent of their disability. Any improvement results in the reduction or elimination of the case for some disability payment.

Many patients are victims of this system. Others manipulate it, exaggerating their disability to obtain financial benefits, further reinforcing the system's adversarial nature. On the other hand, many more patients are accused of such exaggeration than actually commit it. This is in part because it is very difficult to communicate pain complaints in a rational and believable manner to others. Pain, after all, is not directly observable. It can only be interpreted through the report, both verbal and nonverbal, of the patient. In their own desire to control their pain, patients tend to either over- or undermodulate it. At times they seem perfectly composed and comfortable when in fact they are suffering; at other times they are histrionic and disruptive and apparently exaggerating the extent of their discomfort.

Secondary gain factors, both social and financial, substantially complicate treatment, and it is best to do everything possible to minimize them. Useful social strategies include the behavioral therapy principle of requesting health care personnel and family members to provide attention and positive reinforcement for non-pain-related behaviors (Fordyce et al. 1973) while diminishing reinforcement for pain-related interactions. Thus a nurse would be encouraged to walk up to a patient and say, "How nice to see you walking around," and engage him in other conversation when the patient does in fact walk, but to minimize social contact when responding to a demand for more pain medication.

Interactions with the legal system can be handled by advising the patient to discuss with his/her attorney ways to obtain the largest lump sum settlement possible as quickly as possible to avoid losing years in an emotionally and physically depleting struggle to prove how damaged they really are. Direct contact with attorneys after the patient's permission has been obtained is also a good way to reinforce the urgency of settling the complaint before the situation deteriorates further.

❑ CONCLUSIONS

As we continue to enrich the knowledge base on which we understand the causes, transmission, and processing of pain signals, we can make pain treatment more comprehensive, humane, and effective. There are multiple levels at which the pain problem can be approached, including removing the cause of the pain at the periphery, reducing muscle tension that exacerbates pain input, blocking pain transmission through competitive electrical stimulation, infusions into the central nervous system, and drugs that block pain transmission or perception. There are also important cognitive interventions that can help reduce patients' focus on pain and ameliorate their reaction to it.

In addition, there are interventions that can reduce the social reinforcement of pain perception and behavior. The old dichotomy between peripheral and central pain is being replaced by a more complex and comprehensive analysis that evaluates central and peripheral components of pain and designs interventions that take advantage of therapeutic opportunities at all levels of pain perception processing. This point of view is important because it underscores the fact that successful psychosocial intervention for reducing pain may occur via understandable neurological mechanisms and does not prove that the pain is largely functional. In the same way, successful pharmacological intervention does not prove that the pain is completely peripheral in origin. Most pain syndromes are a combination of physical and neuropsychiatric distress and dysfunction and require a combination of biological and psychosocial intervention to be optimally effective. The strain in pain lies mainly in the brain.

❑ REFERENCES

Ahles TA, Blanchard EB, Ruckdeschel JC: Multidimensional nature of cancer-related pain. Pain 17:277–288, 1983

Atkison JH, Kremer EF, Garfin SR: Current concepts review: psychopharmacologic agents in the treatment of pain. J Bone Joint Surg [Am] 67:337–339, 1985

Atweh SF, Kuhar MJ: Autoradiographic localization of opiate receptors in rat brain, I: spinal cord and lower medulla. Brain Res 124:53–67, 1977

Austin KL, Stapleton JV, Mather LE: Multiple intramuscular injections: a major source of variability in analgesic response to pethidine. Pain 8:4–19, 1980

Basbaum AI: Functional analysis of the cytochemistry of the spinal dorsal horn, in Advances in Pain Research and Therapy, Vol 9. Edited by Fields HL, Dubner R, Cervero F. New York, Raven, 1985, p 149

Basbaum AI, Fields HL: Endogenous pain control mechanisms: review and hypothesis. Ann Neurol 4:451–462, 1978

Beaver WT, Feise G: Comparison of the analgesic effects of morphine, hydroxyzine, and their combination in patients with postoperative pain, in Advances in Pain Research and Therapy, Vol 1. Edited by Bonica JJ, Albe-Fessard DG. New York, Raven, 1976, p 553

Beaver WT, Wallenstein SL, Houde RW, et al: A comparison of the analgesic effects of methotrimeprazine and morphine in patients with cancer. Clin Pharm Therapeut 7:436–446, 1966

Beecher HK: Relationship of significance of wound to pain experienced. JAMA 161:1609–1616, 1956

Beeson JM, Chaouch A: Peripheral and spinal mechanisms of nociception. Physiol Rev 67(1):67, 1987

Berkley KJ, Palmer R: Somatosensory cortical involvement in response to noxious stimulation in the cat. Exp Brain Res 20:363–374, 1974

Blumer D, Heilbronn M: Chronic pains as a variant of depressive disease: the pain prone disorder. J Nerv Ment Dis 170:381–406, 1982

Boas RA, Cousins MJ: Diagnostic neural blockade, in Neural Blockade in Clinical Anesthesia, 2nd Edition. Edited by Cousins MJ, Bridenbaugh PO. Philadelphia, PA, JB Lippincott, 1988, p 885

Bond MR: Personality studies in patients with pain secondary to organic disease. J Psychosom Res 17:257–263, 1973

Bond MR, Pearson IB: Psychological aspects of pain in women with advanced cancer of the cervix. J Psychosom Res 13:13–19, 1969

Bonica JJ: Evolution and current status of pain programs. Journal of Pain Symptom Management 5:368–374, 1990

Bonica JJ, Ventafridda V: Advances in Pain Research and Therapy: International Symposium on Pain of Advanced Cancer. New York, Raven, 1979

Brose WG, Cousins MJ: Gynecologic pain, in Gynecologic Oncology. Edited by Coppelson M, et al. Edinburgh, Churchill Livingstone (in press)

Bruera E, Brenneis C, Michaud M, et al: Patient controlled subcutaneous hydromorphone versus continuous subcutaneous infusion for the treatment of cancer pain. J Natl Cancer Inst 80(14):1152–1154, 1988a

Bruera E, Brenneis C, Michaud M, et al: Use of subcutaneous route for the administration of narcotics in patients with cancer pain. Cancer 62:407–411, 1988b

Calvillo O, Henry JL, Newman RS: Effects of morphine and naloxone on dorsal horn neurons in the cat. Can J Physiol Pharmacol 52:1207–1211, 1974

Cousins MJ: Chronic pain and neurolytic blockade, in Neural Blockade in Clinical Anesthesia and Management of Pain, 2nd Edition. Edited by Cousins MJ, Bridenbaugh PO. Philadelphia, PA, JB Lippincott, 1988, p 1053

Cousins MJ, Bridenbaugh PO (eds): Neural Blockade in Clinical Anesthesia and Management of Pain, 2nd Edition. Philadelphia, PA, JB Lippincott, 1988

Cousins MJ, Phillips GD (eds): Acute Pain Management. London, Churchill Livingstone, 1986

Crile GW: Phylogenetic association in relation to certain medical problems. Boston Medical and Surgical Journal 163:893, 1910

Cushing H: On the avoidance of shock in major amputations by cocainization of large nerve-trunks preliminary to their division. Ann Surg 36:321–345, 1902

Dejard A, Peterson P, Kestrup J: Mexiletine for the treatment of chronic painful diabetic neuropathy. Lancet 1:9–11, 1988

Derogatis LR, Morrow GR, Fetting J, et al: The prevalence of psychiatric disorders among cancer patients. JAMA 249:751–757, 1983

Dubner R: Specialization of nociceptive pathways: sensory discrimination, sensory modulation, and neural connectivity, in Advances in Pain Research and Therapy, Vol 9. Edited by Fields HL, Dubner R, Cervero F. New York, Raven, 1985, p 111

Dundee JW, Love WJ, Moore J: Alterations in response to somatic pain associated with anesthesia, XV: further studies with phenothiazine derivatives and similar drugs. Br J Anaesth 35:597–610, 1963

Dworkin SF, Von Koroff M, LeResche L: Multiple pains and psychiatric disturbance: an epidemiologic investigation. Arch Gen Psychiatry 47:239–244, 1990

Esdaile J: Hypnosis in Medicine and Surgery (1846), Reprinted. New York, Julian Press, 1957

Eysenck HJ, Eysenck BG: Manual of the Eysenck Personality Inventory. London, University of London Press, 1964

Fields HL: Pain. New York, McGraw-Hill, 1987

Fields HL, Basbaum AI: Endogenous pain control mechanisms, in Textbook of Pain. Edited by Wall PD, Melzack R. Edinburgh, Churchill-Livingstone, 1984, p 142

Fordyce WE, Fowler RS, Lehmann JR, et al: Operant conditioning in the treatment of chronic pain. Arch Phys Med Rehabil 54:399–408, 1973

Forrest WH, Brown BW, Brown CR, et al: Dextroamphetamine with morphine for the treatment of postoperative pain. N Engl J Med 296:712–715, 1977

Gamse R, Holzer P, Lembeck F: Decrease of substance P in primary afferent neurones and impairment of neurogenic plasma extravasation by capsaicin. Br J Pharmacol 68:207–213, 1980

Gourlay GK, Cherry DA, Cousins MJ: Cephalad migration of morphine in CSF following lumbar epidural administration in patients with cancer pain. Pain 23:317–326, 1985

Gourlay GK, Cherry DA, Plummer JL, et al: The influence of drug polarity on the absorption of opioid drugs into the CSF and subsequent cephalad migration following lumbar epidural administration: application to morphine and pethidine. Pain 31:297–305, 1987a

Gourlay GK, Cousins MJ, Cherry DA: Drug therapy, in Handbook of Chronic Pain Management. Edited by Burrows GD, Elton D, Stanley GV. Amsterdam, Elsevier Science, 1987b

Hagbarth KE, Kerr DIB: Central influences on spinal afferent conduction. J Neurophysiol 17:295, 1954

Hilgard ER, Hilgard JR: Hypnosis in the Relief of Pain. Los Altos, CA, William Kaufmann, 1975

Hilgard JR, LeBaron S: Relief of anxiety and pain in children and adolescents with cancer: quantitative measures and clinical observations. Int J Clin Exp Hypn 4:417–442, 1982

Juan H: Prostaglandins as modulators of pain. Journal of General Pharmacology 9:403, 1978

Katon W, Egan K, Miller D: Chronic pain: lifetime psychiatric diagnosis and family history. Am J Psychiatry 142:1156–1160, 1985

Kehlet H: Modification of responses to surgery by neural blockade: clinical implications, in Neural Blockade in Clinical Anesthesia and Management of Pain, 2nd Edition. Edited by Cousins MJ, Bridenbaugh PO. Philadelphia, PA, JB Lippincott 1988, p 145

Kellerman J, Zeltzer L, Ellenberg L, et al: Adolescents with cancer: hypnosis for the reduction of the acute pain and anxiety associated with medical procedures. J Adolesc Health Care 4:35–90, 1983

Kuhn CC, Bradnan WA: Pain as a substitute for fear of death. Psychosomatics 20:494–495, 1979

Lansky SB, List MA, Herrmann CA, et al: Absence of major depressive disorder in female cancer patients. J Clin Oncol 3:1553–1560, 1985

Levine JD, Coderre JJ, Basbaum AI: The peripheral nervous system and the inflammatory process, in Proceedings of the Fifth World Congress on Pain. Edited by Dubner R, Gebhart GF, Bond MR. Amsterdam, Elsevier Science, 1988, p 33

Lindstrom P, Lindblom U: The analgesic effect of tocainide in trigeminal neuralgia. Pain 28:45–50, 1987

Massie MJ, Holland JC: The cancer patient with pain: psychiatric complications and their management. Cancer Pain 71:243–258, 1987

Mather LE, Gourlay GK: The biotransformation of opioids, in Opioid Agonist/Antagonist Drugs in Clinical Practice. Edited by Nimmo WS, Smith G. Amsterdam, Excerpta Medica, 1984

Melzack R: Recent concepts of pain. J Med 13:147–160, 1982

Melzack R, Wall PD: Pain mechanisms: a new theory. Science 150:971–979, 1965

Moore J, Dundee JW: Alterations in response to somatic pain associated with anesthesia, V: the effect of promethazine. Br J Anaesth 33:3–8, 1961a

Moore J, Dundee JW: Alterations in response to somatic pain associated with anesthesia, VII: the effects of nine phenothiazine derivatives. Br J Anaesth 33:422–431, 1961b

Morgan AH, Hilgard ER: Age differences in susceptibility to hypnosis. Int J Clin Exp Hypn 21:78–85, 1973

Müller J: Von den Ergentumlichkeiten der ein zelnen Nerve, in Handbuch der Physiologie de Menschen. Edited by Kobling L. Coblenz, Holscher, 1844

Pert CB, Snyder SH: Opiate receptors: demonstration in nervous tissue. Science 179:1011–1014, 1973

Peteet J, Tay V, Cohen G, et al: Pain characteristics and treatment in an outpatient cancer population. Cancer 57:1259–1265, 1986

Pilowski I, Chapman CR, Bonica JJ: Pain, depression and illness behavior in a pain clinic population. Pain 4:183–192, 1977

Portenoy RK, Moulin DE, Rodgers A, et al: IV infusion of opioids for cancer pain: clinical review and guidelines for use. Cancer Treat Rev 70:575, 1986

Posner MI, Petersen SE: The attention system of the human brain. Annual Review of Neuroscience 13:125–142, 1990

Raja SN, Meyer RA, Campbell JN: Peripheral mechanisms of somatic pain. Anesthesiology 68:571–590, 1988

Rawal N, Arner S, Gustaffson LL, et al: Present state of extradural and intrathecal opioid analgesia in Sweden: a nationwide follow-up survey. Br J Anesth 59:791–799, 1987

Reich J, Tupin JP, Abramowitz SI: Psychiatric diagnosis of chronic pain patients. Am J Psychiatry 140:1495–1498, 1983

Reynolds DV: Surgery in the rat during electrical analgesia induced by focal brain stimulation. Science 164:444–445, 1969

Rexed B: Cytoarchitectonic organization of the spinal cord in the cat. J Comp Neurol 96:415–495, 1952

Ripamonti C, Bruera E: Rectal, buccal and sublingual narcotics for the management of cancer pain. J Palliat Care 7:30–35, 1991

Sawynok J, Labella L: GABA and baclofen potentiate the K^+-evoked release of methionine-enkephalin from rat striatal slices. Eur J Pharmacol 70(2):103–110, 1981

Spiegel D: Oncological and pain syndromes, in Psychiatry Update: American Psychiatric Association Annual Review, Vol 5. Edited by Frances AJ, Hales RE. Washington, DC, American Psychiatric Press, 1986, pp 561–579

Spiegel D: Hypnosis, in The American Psychiatric Press Textbook of Psychiatry. Edited by Tablbott JA, Hales RE, Yudofsy SC. Washington, DC, American Psychiatric Press, 1988, pp 907–928

Spiegel D, Bloom JR: Pain in metastatic breast cancer. Cancer 52:341–345, 1983a

Spiegel D, Bloom JR: Group therapy and hypnosis reduce metastatic breast carcinoma pain. Psychosom Med 45: 333–339, 1983b

Spiegel D, Sands S: Pain management in the cancer patient. Journal of Psychosocial Oncology 6:205–216, 1988

Spiegel D, Hunt T, Dondershine H: Dissociation and hypnotizability in post traumatic stress disorder. Am J Psychiatry 145:301–355, 1988

Spiegel H, Spiegel D: Trance and Treatment: Clinical Uses of Hypnosis. Washington, DC, American Psychiatric Press, 1987

Ventafridda V, Tamburini M, Carceni A, et al: A validation study of the WHO method for cancer relief. Cancer 59:850–856, 1987

Waldeman C, Eason J, Rambohui E, et al: Serum morphine levels: a comparison between continuous subcutaneous and intravenous infusions in post-operative patients. Cancer Treat Rev 71(10):953, 1984

Wall PD: An eye on the needle. New Scientist July:129–131, 1972

Weinberg DS, Inturrisi CE, Reidenberg B, et al: Sublingual absorption of selected opioid analgesics. Clin Pharmacol Ther 44:335–342, 1988

Willis WD: Thalamocortical mechanisms of pain, in Advances in Pain Research and Therapy, Vol 9. Edited by Fields, Dubner R, Cervero F. New York, Raven, 1985

Woodforde JM, Fielding JR: Pain and cancer. J Psychosom Res 14:365–370, 1970

Yaksh TL: Spinal opiates analgesia: characteristics and principles of action. Pain 11:293, 1981

Yaksh TL: Neurologic mechanisms of pain, in Neural Blockade in Clinical Anesthesia and Management of Pain, 2nd Edition. Edited by Cousins MJ, Bridenbaugh PO. Philadelphia, PA, JB Lippincott, 1988, p 79

Yaksh TL, Noueihed R: The physiology and pharmacology of spinal opiates. Annu Rev Pharmacol Toxicol 25:433–462, 1985

Yaksh TL, Rudy TA: Narcotic analgesia produced by a direct action on the spinal cord. Science 192:1357–1358, 1976

Zeltzer L, LeBaron S: Hypnosis and nonhypnotic techniques for reduction of pain and anxiety during painful procedures in children and adolescents with cancer. J Pediatr 101:1032–1035, 1982

Chapter

11

Neuropsychiatric Aspects of Attention and Consciousness: Stupor and Coma

John Cutting, M.D.

ATTENTION IS A MULTIFACETED mental function, but, in general, it denotes the capacity of an individual to focus the mind on some aspect of the environment or the contents of the mind itself. The nature of attention can be illustrated through the situation of someone in front of a television set. This person can select a channel, stay with this channel and take in the scope of its program, or switch to another channel. Attention encompasses these three possibilities.

Indeed, these possibilities correspond to the four components of attention identified by Posner and Boies (1971) and Zubin (1975): 1) selectivity (the ability to select one source of information rather than another); 2) vigilance or concentration (the capacity to sustain interest over time in one direction alone); 3) the fact that attention is not limitless in scope (it can only cope with a finite span of information; Miller's rule [1956] for auditory-verbal items—"the magical number seven, plus or minus two"—illustrates this well); and 4) the ability to be ready to heed new information when its importance outweighs that in the current channel (this is connoted by the term *alertness,* but its exact nature is better conveyed by the term *ability to disattend*). In addition to these four components is the fact that attention is distributed over space, as well as over time, and with respect to all modalities of sensation. Finally, none of these components can function unless there is an underlying level of arousal.

Brain Regions Subserving Attention

Each of the components of attention can be affected, alone or in combination, by different neurological and psychiatric conditions (Table 11–1). This information throws considerable light on the contribution to attention made by different brain regions.

The selectivity component is primarily a function of the left hemisphere: predominantly left parietal, with temporal, frontal, and striatal-limbic contributions. Dimond and Beaumont (1973) first demonstrated this neatly in a vigilance task in control subjects, presented to each hemisphere separately by means of carefully arranged mirrors. In the first quarter of an 80-minute stretch the left hemisphere's detection rate for randomly appearing signals was better than that of the right hemisphere. However, the left hemisphere's performance fell off rapidly after this, whereas that of the right hemisphere remained constant throughout the entire period. The investigators suggested that the right hemisphere excelled at providing a "skeleton service," whereas the left was superior if required to focus attention in short bursts. Kinsbourne (1974) and Heilman and Satz (1983) came to the same conclusion.

The capacity to sustain attention, on the other hand, is primarily a function of the right parietal lobe and its neighboring connections. Dimond's and Beaumont's experiment (1973) demonstrated this, and subsequent investigators (Warm et al. 1980; Wilkins et al. 1987) confirmed it.

Warrington et al. (1971) concluded that the span of attention is probably determined by the efficiency of left-hemisphere activity, certainly within the left parietal lobe in the case of auditory-verbal span. In their study, the investigators reported several patients with focal damage to the left parietal zone who had an auditory span of less than three items.

The frontal lobes are generally credited with allowing the mind to be versatile, hence, in the sphere of attention, rendering it capable of disattending from a stimulus if necessary. Certainly, one of the most characteristic symptoms of a frontal lobe lesion is perseveration (Stuss and Benson 1987).

Limbic contributions to attention include, in particular, the cingulate gyrus (Watson et al. 1973). Subcortical influences emanate chiefly from the reticular formation in the upper brain stem (Watson et al. 1974).

Some of the interactions between these various regions are illustrated by Mesulam's model (1981) of the mechanisms by which attention is directed toward the outside world. He proposed that four systems participate in a network: the right parietal cortex provides a spatial map of the world; the frontal lobes contain a representation of oculomotor programs for exploring this world; the cingulate cortex regulates the spatial distribution of motives and drives; and the reticular formation is responsible for the overall level of arousal.

Range of Attention Disorders

The range of attention disorders includes poor concentration, distractibility, reduced attention span, widened attention span, neglect, extinction, and perseveration (Table 11–2).

Poor concentration. Poor concentration denotes an impaired ability to sustain attention over time. It is almost universal in delirium and dementia and is common in depressive psychosis and schizophrenia. Poor concentration is also a characteristic feature of right parietal damage.

TABLE 11–1. EFFECTS OF NEUROLOGICAL AND PSYCHIATRIC CONDITIONS ON COMPONENTS OF ATTENTION

Neurological or psychiatric condition	*Component(s) of attention most affected*
Delirium	Sustained attention, span, and selectivity
Dementia	Sustained attention, span, selectivity, and ability to disattend
Frontal lobe lesion	Ability to disattend
Left parietal lesion	Span and selectivity
Right parietal lesion	Sustained attention and spatial distribution of attention
Schizophrenia	Sustained attention
Depressive psychosis	Span and selectivity
Mania	Selectivity
Cingulate lesion	Spatial distribution of attention
Midbrain lesion	Arousal

TABLE 11–2. RANGE OF ATTENTION DISORDERS

Poor concentration	
Distractibility	
Reduced attention span	
Widened attention span	
Neglect	
Visual:	Unilateral visuospatial agnosia
	Balint's syndrome
Somatic:	Hemiasomatognosia
	Anosognosia for hemiplegia
Tactile:	Alloesthesia
	Exosomesthesia
Auditory	
Olfactory	
Extinction	
Perseveration	

Distractibility. Distractibility mainly derives from a lability of the selectivity component, but an increased tendency to disattend and inadequately sustained attention probably play a part. It is a characteristic feature of mania (Andreasen 1979; Kraepelin 1921) and is common in delirium (Lipowski 1980).

Altered attention span. Reduced attention span is common in delirium (Cutting 1980; Lipowski 1980), dementia (McGhie 1969), and depressive psychosis (Strömgren 1977), as well as in the left parietal lesions mentioned above. Widened attention span is not as well documented, but has been reported in acute schizophrenia (Cegalis et al. 1977) and during intoxication with hallucinogenic drugs (Lishman 1987).

Neglect and extinction. There are several neuropsychological terms and neuropsychiatric conditions that have as their basis a selective failure to attend to one part of space, somatic or environmental. Numerous terms have been used for what are only a few discrete disorders. The most common disorder is visual neglect for a half-field, almost always the left, and the most widely used term for this is *unilateral visuospatial agnosia. Balint's syndrome* (Balint 1909; Hecaen and Ajuriaguerra 1954) is a bilateral form of visual neglect, but only in the peripheral field and only when a subject actively searches for something: an object may be "seen" by chance as the eyes wander at random over the field. For somatic neglect, which is always unilateral, the preferred term is *hemiasomatognosia,* of which anosognosia is a special case, if there is a hemiplegia. In the auditory, olfactory, and tactile modalities, the term *neglect* is retained. *Alloesthesia* is a variety of tactile neglect where a touch on one side is "felt" on the other side, as is *exosomesthesia,* in which a touch is felt outside of the body entirely. *Extinction* refers to a situation in which one of two simultaneous stimuli, one on each side of the body, is ignored.

There is a vast literature on the subject of neglect, much of it confusing or patently wrong, because until recently few neurologists or neuropsychologists fully appreciated the single most important fact about neglect: the area of space that is ignored is almost always on the left, and the site of the brain lesion is almost always on the right. Weintraub and Mesulam (1987), Kosslyn (1987), and Gainotti et al. (1989) provide the best current accounts.

Perseveration. Perseveration is a tendency to persist in some activity (e.g., speech, action, ideation, and perceptual frame) when it is no longer appropriate to do so. Inability to disengage attention is only part of this disorder. Some forms of perseveration may be very complex, as illustrated by the so-called environmental dependency syndrome (Lhermitte 1986).

❑ THE NATURE OF CONSCIOUSNESS

The nature of consciousness has been a subject of continuing speculation from the era of ancient Greek philosophy up to the present day. Indeed, it is easier to say what consciousness is not, than what it is. It is certainly not a system for analyzing information currently available to us in the real world; that is the domain of perception. Nor is it a system for representing information pertaining to experiences that we have had in the past; language and memory cover that. It is rather the product of what these systems, particularly perception and memory, present to us for our inspection.

Pribram (1976) regarded consciousness as a holographic construction of the world by the brain. I would agree with this, with the proviso that its constructions can be internal images of events or objects experienced in the past (e.g., the dog I saw the day before yesterday) as equally well as events or objects that are unfolding or appearing in the present. To use an earlier analogy, consciousness is like a television screen on which events flash up. But, to continue the analogy, one should not assume that the television set determines what appears on the screen. What we see is controlled at a distance by the studio team. Similarly, what is presented in consciousness is the product of a number of systems including perception, attention, memory, and even will.

Brain Regions Subserving Consciousness

There are two regions of the brain that have a known role in maintaining consciousness, as evidenced by the fact that damage to either of these results in an altered level of consciousness or else unconsciousness. One is the brain stem; the other is the posterior part of the left cerebral cortex.

The critical area of the brain stem is the paramedian reticular formation, the ascending limb of which extends into the thalamus and hypothalamus and is known as the *reticular activating system* (Moruzzi and Magoun 1949). This system of neurons "serves as a converging point for signals from the external and internal environments" (Jouvet 1969, p. 64), and determines the arousal level of the cortex. Animals in which this system is experimentally destroyed remain immobile and comatose; powerful stimuli fail to arouse them. In humans, the lower down the brain stem the lesion is, the more likely it is that complete loss of consciousness will occur. On the other hand, lesions higher up, particularly if they involve the thalamus and hypothalamus, tend to result in disordered consciousness rather than complete loss of consciousness. These disorders include the varieties of stupor and disturbances of sleep.

Evidence for the involvement of the posterior part of the left cerebral cortex in consciousness is abundant. Alford (1933) observed that whereas 27 of 55 patients with an acute right hemiplegia had clouding of consciousness, none of 33 with an acute left hemiplegia did. Serafetinides et al. (1965) injected Amytal Sodium into the left and then the right carotid arteries of 18 subjects as part of a preoperative assessment of cerebral dominance in patients with temporal lobe epilepsy. Among the 8 right-handed subjects, 7 lost consciousness only when the left carotid artery was injected, and 1 lost consciousness only when the right was injected. Among the 7 left-handed subjects with unilateral dominance for speech (3 in the right hemisphere, 4 in the left), consciousness was lost in 5 only when the injection was on the speech-dominant side, in 1 only when the injection was on the speech-nondominant side, and in 1 with injection to either side. All 3 subjects with bilateral representation of speech lost consciousness when either hemisphere was injected.

Albert et al. (1976) noted that 57% of 23 patients with an acute cerebrovascular accident (CVA) affecting the left hemisphere had a disturbance of consciousness, whereas only 25% of 24 patients with a CVA affecting the right hemisphere did so. Devinsky et al. (1988) found that 4 of 7 patients with a left-sided infarct in the region of the posterior cerebral territory developed a confusional state, whereas none of 7 with an infarct in the comparable region on the right did so. They consulted the literature on the matter and discovered that of 15 extant cases of confusion following posterior cerebral artery infarction, 14 had a left-sided lesion.

The contribution of each of these two brain regions to the maintenance of consciousness is almost certainly very different in quality. The brain stem contains the reticular activating system and can be regarded as the powerhouse of the brain, creating the conditions for the efficient working of the rest of the brain. The posterior part of the left cerebral cortex is credited by Farah (1984) and Kosslyn (1987) with the ability to manufacture multipart images of objects. Damage in this region, if it does not lead to unconsciousness, may give rise to selective imagery loss for objects and colors and to cessation of dreaming. Therefore (returning to the analogy of the television set), put crudely, brain stem damage is equivalent to pulling the plug of the set, whereas left posterior cortical damage is equivalent to there being a defective tube. In the former case the power is lost, in the latter the image-generating mechanism is defunct.

Range of Disorders of Consciousness

A suggested classification of disorders of consciousness is shown in Table 11–3. The terminology in the literature is confusing because some varieties are synonymous with the main three disorders: delirium, stupor, and coma. Others are subclasses or integral phenomena of these three. Still others (which I call the "apparent disorders of consciousness") are not intrinsic disorders of consciousness at all, although superficially they appear to be so.

TABLE 11–3. SUGGESTED CLASSIFICATION OF DISORDERS OF CONSCIOUSNESS

Main disorders	
Delirium	
Synonyms:	Confusional state, toxic confusional state, and acute organic reaction
Integral phenomena:	Confusion and clouding of consciousness
Varieties:	Amentia, twilight state, hallucinosis, and subacute delirium
Stupor	
Synonym:	Parasomnia
Integral phenomenon:	Coma vigil
Varieties:	Akinetic mutism, apallic syndrome, catatonic stupor, depressive stupor, manic stupor,[a] and hysterical stupor[a]
Coma	
Synonym:	Unconsciousness
Other intrinsic disorders	
Perplexity	
Dissociative states:	Hysterical fugue, multiple personality, and hysterical twilight state[a]
Ganser syndrome	
Apparent disorders	
"Dreamy states"	
Derealization	
Depersonalization	
Anosognosia	

[a]Doubtful entity.

Apparent Disorders of Consciousness

Dreamy states. "Dreamy states" were first described by Jackson (1889) as an accompaniment of some forms of epilepsy. From the examples he gave, it is clear that these states are an amalgam of several separate phenomena, and the term is rarely used now. In some instances it is déjà vu that dominates the picture:

> Case 3 . . . the first stage is a dreamy state or reminiscence, in which everything around her seems familiar or to have happened before. (Jackson 1889, p. 197)

In others, hallucinations predominate:

> Case 2 . . . the next thing was his "dreamy state." He seemed to actually see large buildings which he had once seen; it might be that he seemed near a church, "close to its wall." In the last attack he "saw" certain alms-houses, "all in a moment saw that building and could actually see the clock." (Jackson 1889, p. 195)

In still others, certain thoughts are experienced in a pathological fashion, a phenomenon that Penfield and Erickson (1941) referred to as "forced thinking":

> Case 1 . . . . He said that he began to think of things years gone by. He thinks of things he has, might, or will do. (Jackson 1889, p. 188)

Some subjects do describe the experience as "like a dream," but Jackson's claim (1889) that the dreamy state reflected "over-consciousness" is difficult to accept. The most one can say is that dreamy states represent what several writers on the subject of disorders of consciousness have recently referred to as "disorders of the content of consciousness" (Frederiks 1969; Saper and Plum 1985). In other words, the original cause of dreamy states lies external to the apparatus of consciousness itself—in memory, perception, or thinking.

Derealization. Derealization has been regarded as a disorder of consciousness (Janet 1903). However, in my view, it is better considered as a disorder of perception. The world certainly looks different from how it did before—stranger, maybe more two-dimensional—and a subject is often acutely conscious of this and distressed by it, but there is no intrinsic disorder of consciousness. It is just that a different worldview has been transmitted from the faulty perceptual system to a normally functioning consciousness channel, which then faithfully projects what it receives.

Depersonalization. The same argument applies to depersonalization, but in this case it is a subject's body- and self-image that are distorted, the raw data that consciousness again efficiently receives and generates for the subject's inspection.

Anosognosia. The case of anosognosia—denial of hemiplegia (nearly always a left hemiplegia in conjunction with a right-hemisphere lesion)—is slightly different. A plausible argument has been put forward for why anosognosia should be regarded as a "sectional disorder of consciousness" (Purdon Martin 1949). The self, or at least the self's spokesperson, is genuinely unaware of the existence of its paralyzed limb, ignores it, and confabulates when asked searching questions about its disability. It is true to say, therefore, that the existence of the limb and its paralyzed state have been blotted out of consciousness. But this is not caused by the consciousness-generating system itself. It is simply being denied a class of information about the body, which is caused by a breakdown in a system in the right hemisphere that distributes attention over the left side of the body. The problem is thus again extrinsic to the consciousness-generating system itself.

Intrinsic Disorders of Consciousness (Excluding Delirium, Stupor, and Coma)

Perplexity. The phenomenon of perplexity is a troublesome one with respect to its exact phenomenological status. A minority of acutely psychotic schizophrenic patients, a substantial minority of severely psychotic depressive patients, and the majority of patients with an atypical functional psychosis such as cycloid psychosis (Cutting et al. 1978) have a perplexed facial appearance and will admit to feeling puzzled about the world and themselves. Many will actually use the word "confused" to describe their mental state. To all intents and purposes their mental state cannot be distinguished from that of a delirious subject with known cerebral dysfunction. According to Storring (1939), one of the few psychiatrists to have written on the subject, the reason for the perplexity is different in each of the functional psychoses mentioned. Storring takes the view that perplexity (*Ratlosigkeit*, in German) is

> the oppressive awareness of one's inability to cope with a given internal or external situation, this awareness being experienced as something that cannot be explained, something that has to do with one's own self. (p. 79)

This may be a good account of the perplexity that accompanies the delusional mood in the early stage of schizophrenia, but in psychotic depression and cycloid psychosis (which most authorities believe to be an atypical affective psychosis), I believe there is often a true disturbance of consciousness. Because of the traditional distinction between organic and functional psychoses, psychiatrists have been unwilling to accept the existence of a delirious-like picture in affective psychosis and have sought to maintain the traditional nosological distinction by calling the same phenomenon *perplexity* if it occurs in a "functional" setting and *clouding of consciousness* if in an undeniably "organic" setting.

Dissociative states. The so-called dissociative states, such as hysterical fugue, multiple personality, and hysterical twilight state, also pose phenomenological and nosological problems with respect to more clear-cut disorders of consciousness. (Hysterical stupor is considered in the section on stupor.) Most writers on the subject (e.g., Abse 1982) regard these as examples of "distinctive alterations in consciousness." But there is a case (as with Jackson's dreamy states [1889], derealization, and so on) for regarding them as merely disorders of the content of consciousness.

Hysterical fugue and multiple personality have a common basis in the fact that certain autobiographical information is temporarily unavailable to the conscious self and that this state of affairs occurs in the absence of any identifiable brain damage that might account for this. Taylor and Kopelman (1984) suggested that some cases of hysterical amnesia, particularly the relatively common form in murderers for the period around the murder, might be adequately explained by assuming that the emotional arousal induced by the event could have impaired registration of information. But this cannot explain fugues lasting weeks, such as the case of the Reverend Ansel Bourne (James 1891), whose "lost weeks" were subsequently regained under hypnosis. Here, information about daily events was being registered and assimilated and was determining behavior, and it was the previous record of autobiographical experience that was unavailable to consciousness. Also, in the condition of multiple personality, a subject is capable of shifting between two or more integrated personalities, at least one of which is not based on a true autobiographical record at all.

In my view, hysteria is one of the most mysterious of all psychiatric disorders. In hysteria and multiple personality there are two explanations:

1. The consciousness-generating system efficiently, albeit naively, carries out the will of some other pathological process in the brain, temporarily blocking out vast tracts of autobiographical experience and substituting false bits.
2. The consciousness-generating system itself is so fragile that it is at the mercy of other systems in the brain, which try to foist on to it inaccurate information.

Unlike the previous dissociative disorders, which, although uncommon, do exist (I have seen three of each in 17 years of psychiatric practice), a hysterical twilight state is a doubtful entity. It is mentioned in most of the major textbooks of psychiatry written earlier this century (Bleuler 1916; Lange 1934), but to my knowledge no indisputable case has been reported in the literature of the latter half of the century. Bleuler's case (1916), however, is quite convincing. The case involved a bookkeeper, whose fiancé died in a mental hospital of general paralysis of the insane just before their wedding. She devoted herself to nursing a sick brother and a sick child, but, while taking a holiday from these cares in Germany, she began behaving peculiarly, digging up graves in a cemetery. On admission to the hospital she had regular episodes in which she imagined herself in the cemetery and heard and saw dead people. In between these episodes she was completely well, and at such times claimed to know nothing of the "twilight states." However, when she was in a twilight state she could recall events of a previous twilight state. Hypnosis could abort an episode.

Ganser syndrome. In 1898 Ganser described what he thought was a "peculiar" variety of the hysterical twilight state, a condition that soon after was named the *Ganser syndrome*. There is considerable dispute not only as to the nature of this syndrome but even as to its essential features (Whitlock 1982). The central feature is the phenomenon of approximate answers (or *Vorbeireden*) to questions about things that even the dullest person should know (e.g., the question "How many legs has an elephant?" is answered "Five"). In addition, the complete syndrome is said to require the existence of hysterical symptoms, hallucinations, and clouding of consciousness. In my opinion (Cutting 1990), the syndrome is a manifestation of either psychotic depression or left-hemisphere damage and has nothing to do with hysteria at all. The clouding of consciousness that may occur is genuine and is the result of intrinsic dysfunction of the consciousness-generating apparatus in the left hemisphere, disrupted either as a direct consequence of left-hemisphere damage or in the course of the transient left-hemisphere dysfunction that many authorities claim underlies psychotic depression (Finset 1988; Starkstein and Robinson 1989).

❑ STUPOR

Definition and Nosology

Stupor is generally held to comprise the following triad: loss of speech (mutism), markedly reduced movement (usually referred to as *akinesis* but more correctly as *hypokinesis*), and reduced level of consciousness.

The loss of speech is absolute or virtually so. The reduction in voluntary movement, however, is not complete. In one variety at least—akinetic mutism—the eyes are open and "regard the observer steadily or follow the movement of objects" (Cairns et al. 1941, p. 273). The level of consciousness differs between the varieties that have been described but is somewhere along a spectrum ranging from just short of normal wakefulness or sleep at one end to just short of complete unconsciousness (coma) at the other.

From a psychopathological point of view, there are no more than four definite varieties (Table 11–3)—if one excludes hysterical stupor, which is extremely rare (if not extinct) these days, and manic stupor, which is a dubious entity (see below). Moreover, two of these varieties—catatonic stupor and depressive stupor—cannot easily be distinguished by mere observation of the patient during the stuporous state; a differential diagnosis can only be made on the basis of the patient's past psychiatric history or, when he or she is recovered, by subsequent mental state examination. Nevertheless, there are good reasons for supposing that the reasons for the stupor (i.e., the essential psychological dysfunction) are different in each case. The term *apallic syndrome* is not used much by English-speaking psychiatrists and neurologists. It was coined by Kretschmer in 1940, who described it as follows:

> The patient is prostrate, awake, with his eyes open. He either stares straight ahead or his eyes travel back and forth without understanding or being able to focus on anything. Attempts to attract his attention are unsuccessful or only slightly successful. Talking to the patient, touching him or showing him objects does not result in any sensible response. (p. 577)

Compare this description with that of *akinetic mutism,* a term introduced by Cairns et al. in 1941:

> The patient sleeps more than normally, but he is easily roused. In the fully developed state he makes no sound and lies inert, except that his eyes regard the observer steadily, or follow the movement of objects, and they may be diverted by sound . . . . Oft-repeated commands may be carried out in a feeble, slow, and incomplete manner. (p. 273)

The term *coma vigil* appears most commonly in the French literature, where it probably covers both the apallic syndrome and akinetic mutism, but Peters and Gerstenbrand (1977) suggested that it be used as a phenomenological description for the particular disturbance of consciousness that is seen in the apallic syndrome. The term *parasomnia* was introduced by Jefferson (1944), who defined it as a "state in which there is no response to stimuli, verbal or mechanical, except those of a reflex nature" (p. 1). Defined in this way, it would appear to be no more than a description of a severe stupor.

Clinical Picture

In practice, the fine shades of psychopathological difference between functional psychotic stupor (depressive or catatonic stupor) and organic stupor (apallic syndrome and akinetic mutism) are not easy to identify. But because this bipartite distinction is the most crucial for the purposes of management, it is worth examining claims made in the literature as to useful clues to differential diagnosis.

One general rule is that depressive and catatonic stupor are milder in degree, in that the disturbances of consciousness and movement are less than those that occur in the organic varieties. Raskin and Frank (1974), for example, claimed that the stupor in their single patient, which was attributed to herpes encephalitis, differed from the stupor of a depressive or schizophrenic patient in five ways: 1) the patient's eyelids tended to drift back to the closed position after they had opened in response to strong stimulation, 2) there were roving eye movements, 3) the respiration rate was irregular, 4) associated seizures or adoption of a decorticate body posture could occur, and 5) an abreaction with Amytal Sodium made the patient confused, not lucid. Unfortunately, not all these purported discriminating features are reliable. There are several case reports in the literature in which patients were confidently regarded for months as functional instead of organic, or vice versa, until subsequent events proved the clinicians wrong (Cooper and Schapira 1973; Hoenig and Toakley 1959). The most well-established clinical differences between the various types of stupor are summarized in Table 11–4 (Akhtar and Buckman 1977; Johnson 1984; Peters and Gerstenbrand 1977; Raskin and Frank 1974).

Hysterical stupor, like hysterical twilight states, was regularly mentioned in textbooks of psychiatry in the first half of the century. It must be exceedingly rare now, because there was no pure case of this among 100 instances of various kinds of stupor in the series reported by Joyston-Bechal (1966) nor among 27 cases of stupor in the series reported by Smith (1959). There was one case, about which no details were given, among 25 stuporous patients in a series reported by Johnson (1984). Neustatter's case report (1942) is the last descriptive account I could find: a soldier, who deserted soon after conscription.

Manic stupor is another variety that is passed on from textbook to textbook without question of its validity. There were no instances of it in any of the three comprehensive studies mentioned above, and its provenance is Kraepelin's account in 1921, which, on careful reading, actually refers to cases of *mixed* affective psychosis.

Course of Stupor

The course of a stupor depends largely on the variety and cause involved and on what treatment is given. Joyston-Bechal's series (1966) of 100 cases, only 23 of whom definitely had organic stupor, provides the best information on this issue. One-third of these patients remitted spontaneously, one-half recovered following electroconvulsive therapy (ECT), and 8 died (6 of the organic cases and 2 of the schizophrenic cases). In 43 of the patients the duration of illness was less than 1 week, in another 43 patients it was between 1 and 4 weeks, in 16 it was between 1 and 6 months, and in 4 (all organic) it was more than 6 months. In 18% of all the cases, the patient, when recovered, could remember much of what had gone on during the stuporous state. Hoch (1915) described what he referred to as *benign*

TABLE 11–4. PURPORTED CLINICAL DIFFERENCES BETWEEN MAIN VARIETIES OF STUPOR

Depressive	Diurnal variation (better in evening) Depressive facial appearance Occasional muttered reply to questions on nonemotive topics Increased lucidity with depressive themes during Amytal Sodium abreaction
Catatonic	Negativism and waxy flexibility Bizarre body posture Movement of eyes and laughter or grimacing to presumed intrapsychic events Sudden outbursts of explosive activity Increased talkativeness with illogical themes during Amytal Sodium abreaction
Apallic syndrome	Abnormal electroencephalogram (EEG) (slow waves) Lack of coordination of eye movements No emotional reactions Primitive reflexes (e.g., snout reflex) No response to stimulation Upper limbs flexed and lower limbs extended Bilateral pyramidal signs
Akinetic mutism	Abnormal EEG (slow waves) Eyes coordinated Some response to stimulation Bilateral pyramidal signs

stupor, the condition of patients whom he believed had an atypical depressive illness with a good prognosis. However, when 20 years later a student of his (Rachlin 1935) traced these patients, most had pursued a rather unfavorable course, with either subsequent episodes of stupor, or other schizophrenic symptoms.

Cause of Stupor

General mechanism. The general mechanism whereby stupor comes about is almost certainly different according to the variety involved. Within the functional varieties, Bleuler's suggestion (1916) is to my mind insightful and probably correct. He suggested that the outward similarity of the stupor in schizophrenia and depressive psychosis concealed the fact that it was the end product of two entirely separate psychological mechanisms. In the former case there was what he called blocking (*Sperrung*) and in the latter inhibition or retardation (*Hemmung*). In other words (see Cutting 1990), the schizophrenic individual's problem is that the consciousness, speech, and movement systems are inherently intact, but the will to use them has been lost. In a depressive psychosis these three systems are themselves failing in efficiency and cannot execute the will of the remaining viable parts of the mind.

The situation with regard to the organic varieties is yet different from either of these proposed mechanisms. The main, and only clear, fact to emerge from clinical-pathological correlations of subcortical disorders of consciousness (Cairns 1952) is that the lower down the brain stem the lesion is, the more likely it is that complete unconsciousness will result and the more quickly this will be fatal. Therefore, lesions of the pons and medulla lead to unconsciousness and rapid death. Lesions of the upper brain stem (the midbrain) are more likely to produce the apallic syndrome or akinetic mutism. It is not at all clear from the literature whether different mechanisms or different locations of brain damage are responsible for the likelihood that the apallic syndrome or akinetic mutism will occur.

There is a suggestion from the original case report of Cairns et al. (1941), from the collection of cases by Cairns (1952), and from accounts of the apallic syndrome by Peters and Gerstenbrand (1977) and Avenarius and Gerstenbrand (1977) that akinetic mutism is more likely if a focal lesion is disrupting "the hypothalamic-thalamic pathways alongside the third ventricle" (Cairns et al. 1941, p. 286) (i.e., the diencephalon), whereas the apallic syndrome is more likely a consequence of diffuse damage to the midbrain itself. This would certainly fit with the clinical differences between the two, which, in summary, is that akinetic mutism is associated with less overall mental disturbance, suggesting a lesion higher up the brain stem.

Specific causes. Akinetic mutism was first described in a girl who had an epidermoid cyst of the third ventricle (Cairns et al. 1941). Cairns (1952) then observed a very similar picture in patients with pineal or thalamic tumors and stricture of the aqueduct of Sylvius causing an obstructive hydrocephalus. The apallic syndrome has been reported following head injury (Lehmann 1977); metabolic disorders, such as liver or renal failure (Gerstenbrand et al. 1977); and drug intoxication, particularly with lithium (Kanowski 1977). Among cases of organic stupor, without psychopathological division into akinetic mutism and apallic syndrome, the commonest causes are tumor, encephalitis, and dementia (Table 11–5).

Management

It is imperative to establish as soon as possible whether the cause of a stupor is organic or functional. In the case of organic stupor, it may be possible to eliminate the cause (e.g., by surgery or restoration of normal metabolic state). In the case of functional stupor, the most common, by far, is depressive stupor, and this usually responds promptly and completely to ECT, sometimes after only one application (Barnes et al. 1986).

A full clinical history from an informant should be taken, with special emphasis on eliciting any previous history of an affective disorder. Physical examination, biochemical screening, and radiological investigation should then be carried out. A good illustration of the problems in management is given by the following personal case example.

Case example

A 24-year-old man had been admitted to his local psychiatric hospital on the outskirts of London 3 months before I was asked to see him. He was stuporous on admission, and it was established that he had had a previous manic illness 2 years before. ECT was commenced, but after two applications he appeared to be worse. The psychiatrist panicked, fearing the patient might have an organic cause for the stupor, and referred him to the regional neurological center in the center of London. Here he remained for 10 weeks undergoing a series of radiological and biochemical investigations, without treatment, and with no change in his stuporous state.

I was asked to see him and decided to carry out an Amytal Sodium abreaction. (By this time the patient had developed contractures.) During the abreaction he talked for the first time for 3 months, saying, in a rather muddled way, that he believed he was on the floor of the ocean, being eaten by fishes. I decided that the previous psychiatric history of affective disorder, a strong family history of depression that I uncovered, and the morbid statements under abreaction all pointed to a diagnosis of depressive stupor. I arranged for a further course of ECT, and after the first application he recovered completely.

TABLE 11–5. CAUSES OF STUPOR IN FOUR SERIES OF PATIENTS WITH MIXED ORGANIC AND FUNCTIONAL VARIETIES (BY PERCENTAGE OF POPULATION)

	Causes[a]					
Study	*Depressive*	*Schizophrenic*	*Organic*	*"Mixed neurotic" (depressive features)*	*Hysterical*	*Uncertain*
Smith 1959 (n = 27)	44	33	8	15	0	0
Joyston-Bechal 1966 (n = 100)	25	31	20	10	0	14
Johnson 1984 (n = 25)	40	16	40	0	4	0
Barnes et al. 1986 (n = 25 catatonic patients; "most stuporous")	36	4	20	0	0	40

[a]Of the 36 organic cases in the four studies the breakdown was as follows: dementia, 7 patients; encephalitis, 5; cerebral malignancy, 5; confusional state—cause not specified, 5; neurosyphilis, 3; epilepsy, 2; lithium intoxication, 1; cerebral cyst, 1; neuroleptic intoxication, 1; traumatic encephalopathy in boxer, 1; pontine infarct, 1; epiloia, 1; multiple sclerosis, 1; tuberculous meningitis, 1; cerebellar hemangioblastoma, 1.

TABLE 11–6. TYPICAL SIGNS OF THE FIVE CATEGORIES OF CAUSES OF COMA

	Signs					
Causes	*Pupils*	*Eye movements*	*Respiration*	*Limbs*	*Progression of coma*	*Face*
Focal left cortical lesion	Normal	Conjugate deviation of eyes to side of lesion	Normal	Asymmetrical tone and reflexes	Maximum at onset unless enlarging space-occupying lesion	Unilateral facial weakness
Brain stem activity damage						
Uncal herniation	One dilated	Failing elevation, depression and adduction of one eye	Progression from normal to hyperventilation	Progression from normal through decorticate[a] to flaccid	Progression	Not helpful
Central herniation	Both become gradually fixed and dilated	Early loss of conjugate upward movement	Progression from normal to hyperventilation	Progression from normal through decorticate to flaccid	Progression	Not helpful
Infratentorial lesion	Both fixed or pin-point	Dysconjugate movement	Hyperventilation or apneic breathing	Bilateral pyramidal signs	Maximum at onset	Bilateral facial weakness possibly
Generalized cerebral dysfunction	Normal	Normal	Regular or Cheyne-Stokes	Symmetrical reflexes and hypotonia	Progression	Not helpful

[a]Decorticate posture = flexion of joints in upper limbs and extension of those in lower limbs.

❑ COMA

Definition and Nosology

Coma denotes unconsciousness. There are degrees of coma, but no varieties.

Clinical Features and Course

When establishing the diagnosis and planning the management of a comatose patient, the two important aspects of the clinical state are 1) a record of the progression of coma and 2) the pattern of associated abnormalities of pupil size, respiration, and movement response to stimulation. The progression of the coma is best established by ensuring that the nursing staff regularly record the items in the Glasgow Coma Scale (Teasdale and Jennett 1974) (see also Chapter 16, Table 16–3). This allows a differentiation between the main categories of causes of coma.

Causes of Coma

General mechanism. Three general situations can lead to coma: 1) there may be a focal lesion in the left cerebral hemisphere that damages the cortical mechanism projecting the contents of consciousness; 2) there may be damage to the brain stem activity that activates consciousness, and this may occur through three main ways: a) uncal herniation (herniation of the inferomedial part of the temporal lobe over the free edge of the tentorial membrane, by pressure from a unilateral supratentorial mass); b) central herniation (midline downward displacement at the tentorial opening, usually from generalized raised intracranial pressure); and c) intratentorial lesions themselves; and 3) generalized cerebral dysfunction may affect the activity of cortex and brain stem alike. The patterns of coma and associated abnormalities in each of these situations are shown in Table 11–6.

Specific causes. The most common cause of an intrinsic disturbance in the cortical consciousness-generating system is an acute CVA in the territories of the left-middle and posterior cerebral arteries. Uncal herniation is a consequence of a rapidly enlarging supratentorial space-occupying lesion, such as a neoplasm, subdural hematoma, or intracerebral hematoma. Central herniation results from raised intracranial pressure from cerebral edema as well as space-occupying lesions. Infratentorial lesions themselves include brain stem infarction and subtentorial tumors. Generalized cerebral dysfunction leading to coma results from the same set of causes that produces delirium (see Chapter 12).

Management

After emergency treatment to ensure an airway and provide effective respiratory support, the management of coma consists of trying to establish which of the general categories of causes listed in Table 11–6 exists. This should be followed by a neurosurgical opinion as to whether uncal or central herniation is suspected and attempts to identify the precise cause of focal or generalized cerebral dysfunction if herniation is not present.

❑ REFERENCES

Abse W: Multiple personality, in Hysteria. Edited by Roy A. Chichester, England, John Wiley, 1982, pp 165–184

Akhtar S, Buckman J: The differential diagnosis of mutism: a review and a report of three unusual cases. Diseases of the Nervous System 38:558–563, 1977

Albert ML, Silverberg R, Reches A, et al: Cerebral dominance for consciousness. Arch Neurol 33:453–454, 1976

Alford LB: Localization of consciousness and emotion. Am J Psychiatry 89:789–799, 1933

Andreasen NC: Thought, language and communication disorders. Arch Gen Psychiatry 36:1315–1330, 1979

Avenarius HJ, Gerstenbrand F: The transition stage from midbrain syndrome to traumatic apallic syndrome, in The Apallic Syndrome. Edited by Dalle Ore G, Gerstenbrand F, Lücking CH, et al. Berlin, Springer, 1977, pp 22–25

Balint R: Die Seelenlahmung des "Schauens." Monatsschrift für Psychiatrie und Neurologie 1:51–81, 1909

Barnes MP, Saunders M, Walls TJ, et al: The syndrome of Karl Ludwig Kahlbaum. J Neurol Neurosurg Psychiatry 49:991–996, 1986

Bleuler E: Textbook of Psychiatry, 4th Edition (1916). Translated by Brili AA. New York, Dover, 1951

Cairns H: Disturbances of consciousness with lesions of the brain-stem and diencephalon. Brain 75:109–146, 1952

Cairns H, Oldfield RC, Pennybacker JB, et al: Akinetic autism with an epidermoid cyst of the 3rd ventricle. Brain 64:273–290, 1941

Cegalis JA, Leen D, Solomon EJ: Attention in schizophrenia: an analysis of selectivity in functional visual field. J Abnorm Psychol 86:470–482, 1977

Cooper AF, Schapira K: Case report: depression, catatonic stupor, and EEG changes in hyperparathyroidism. Psychol Med 3:509–515, 1973

Cutting J: Physical illness and psychosis. Br J Psychiatry 136:109–119, 1980
Cutting J: The Right Cerebral Hemisphere and Psychiatric Disorders. Oxford, England, Oxford University Press, 1990
Cutting J, Clare AW, Mann AH: Cycloid psychosis: an investigation of the diagnostic concept. Psychol Med 8:637–648, 1978
Devinsky O, Bear D, Volpe BT: Confusional states following posterior cerebral artery infarction. Arch Neurol 45:160–163, 1988
Dimond SJ, Beaumont JG: Differences in the vigilance performance of the right and left hemispheres. Cortex 9:259–265, 1973
Farah MJ: The neurological basis of mental imagery: a componential analysis. Cognition 18:245–272, 1984
Finset A: Depressed mood and reduced emotionality after right hemisphere brain damage, in Cerebral Hemisphere Function in Depression. Edited by Kinsbourne M. Washington, DC, American Psychiatric Press, 1988, pp 49–64
Frederiks JAM: Consciousness, in Handbook of Clinical Neurology, Vol 3. Edited by Vinken PJ, Bruyn GW. Amsterdam, North-Holland, 1969, pp 48–61
Gainotti G, D'Erme P, De Bonis C: Components of visual attention disrupted in unilateral neglect, in Neuropsychology of Visual Perception. Edited by Brown JW. Hillsdale, NJ, Lawrence Erlbaum, 1989, pp 123–144
Ganser SJM: Ueber einen eigenartigen hysterischen Dammerzustand (1898), translated in British Journal of Criminology 5:120–126, 1965
Gerstenbrand F, Avenarius HJ, Preissler HP: The apallic syndrome in metabolic disorders of the brain, in The Apallic Syndrome. Edited by Dalle Ore G, Gerstenbrand F, Lücking CH, et al. Berlin, Springer, 1977, pp 29–36
Hecaen H, Ajuriaguerra J: Balint's syndrome. Brain 77: 373–400, 1954
Heilman KM, Satz P: Neuropsychology of Human Emotion. London, Guilford, 1983
Hoch A: A study of the benign psychoses. Johns Hopkins Hospital Bulletin 26:165–169, 1915
Hoenig J, Toakley JG: The diagnosis of stupor. Psychiatria et Neurologia Basel 137:128–144, 1959
Jackson JH: On a particular variety of epilepsy ("intellectual aura"), one case with symptoms of organic brain disease. Brain 11:179–207, 1889
James W: The Principles of Psychology, Vol 1. London, MacMillan, 1891, pp 391–393
Janet P: Les Obsessions et la Psychasthénie. Paris, Alcan, 1903
Jefferson G: The nature of concussion. Br Med J 1:1–5, 1944
Johnson J: Stupor and akinetic mutism, in Contemporary Neurology. Edited by Harrison MJG. London, Butterworths, 1984, pp 96–102
Jouvet M: Coma and other disturbances of consciousness, in Handbook of Clinical Neurology. Edited by Vinken PJ, Bruyn GW. Amsterdam, North-Holland, 1969, pp 62–79
Joyston-Bechal MP: The clinical features and outcome of stupor. Br J Psychiatry 112:967–981, 1966
Kanowski S: Apallic syndrome due to pharmacotoxic effects, in The Appallic Syndrome. Edited by Dalle Ore G, Gerstenbrand F, Lücking CH, et al. Berlin, Springer, 1977, pp 46–49
Kinsbourne M: Mechanisms of hemispheric interaction in man, in Hemisphere Disconnection and Cerebral Function. Edited by Kinsbourne M, Smith WL. Springfield, IL, Charles C Thomas, 1974, pp 260–285
Kosslyn SM: Seeing and imagining in the cerebral hemispheres. Psychol Rev 94:148–175, 1987
Kraepelin E: Manic-Depressive Insanity and Paranoia. Edinburgh, Livingstone, 1921
Kretschmer E: Das apailische Syndrom. Zeitschrift für Neurologie und Psychiatrie 169:576–579, 1940
Lange J: Spezielle gerichtliche Psychopathologie, in Handbuch der gerichtlichen Psychiatrie. Edited by Hoche A. Berlin, Springer, 1934, p 547
Lehmann HJ: Apallic syndrome in diseases of the cerebral white matter, in The Apallic Syndrome. Edited by Dalle Ore G, Gerstenbrand F, Lücking CH, et al. Berlin, Springer, 1977, pp 57–58
Lhermitte F: Human autonomy and the frontal lobes, part II: patient behavior in complex and social situations: the "environmental dependency syndrome." Ann Neurol 19:335–343, 1986
Lipowski ZJ: Delirium: Acute Brain Failure in Man. Springfield, IL, Charles C Thomas, 1980
Lishman WA: Organic Psychiatry, 2nd Edition. Oxford, England, Blackwell, 1987
McGhie A: Pathology of Attention. Harmondsworth, England, Penguin, 1969
Mesulam M-M: A cortical network for directed attention and unilateral neglect. Ann Neurol 10:309–325, 1981
Miller GA: The magical number seven, plus or minus two: some limits on our capacity for processing information. Psychol Rev 63:81–97, 1956
Moruzzi G, Magoun HW: Brain-stem reticular formation and activation of the EEG. Electroencephalogr Clin Neurophysiol 1:455–460, 1949
Neustatter WL: A case of hysterical stupor recovering after cardiazol treatment. Journal of Mental Science 88: 440–443, 1942
Penfield W, Erickson TC: Epilepsy and Cerebral Localization. Springfield, IL, Charles C Thomas, 1941
Peters UH, Gerstenbrand F: Clinical picture and problems in terminology, in The Apallic Syndrome. Edited by Dalle Ore G, Gerstenbrand F, Lücking CH, et al. Berlin, Springer, 1977, pp 8–13
Posner MI, Boies SJ: Components of attention. Psychol Rev 78:391–408, 1971
Pribram KH: Problems concerning the structure of consciousness, in Consciousness and the Brain. Edited by Globus GG, Maxwell G, Savodnik I. New York, Plenum, 1976, pp 297–313
Purdon Martin J: Consciousness and its disturbances. Lancet 1:48–53, 1949
Rachlin HL: A follow-up study of Hoch's benign stupor cases. Am J Psychiatry 92:531–558, 1935
Raskin DE, Frank SW: Herpes encephalitis with catatonic stupor. Arch Gen Psychiatry 31:544–546, 1974
Saper CB, Plum F: Disorders of consciousness, in Handbook of Clinical Neurology, Vol 45. Edited by Frederiks JAM. Amsterdam, Elsevier, 1985, pp 107–128

Serafetinides EA, Hoare RD, Driver MV: Intracarotid sodium amylobarbitone and cerebral dominance for speech and consciousness. Brain 88:107–130, 1965

Smith S: An investigation and survey of 27 cases of akinesis with mutism (stupor). Journal of Mental Science 105:1088–1094, 1959

Starkstein SE, Robinson RG: Affective disorders and cerebral vascular disease. Br J Psychiatry 154:170–182, 1989

Storring GE: Wesen und Bedeutung des Symptoms der Ratlosigkeit bei Psychischen Erkrankungen (1939), translated in The Clinical Roots of the Schizophrenia Concept. Edited by Cutting J, Shepherd M. Cambridge, England, Cambridge University Press, 1986, pp 79–82

Strömgren LS: The influence of depression on memory. Acta Psychiatr Scand 56:109–128, 1977

Stuss DT, Benson DF: The frontal lobes and control of cognition and memory, in The Frontal Lobes Revisited. Edited by Perecman E. New York, IRBN Press, 1987, pp 141–158

Taylor PJ, Kopelman MD: Amnesia for criminal offences. Psychol Med 14:581–588, 1984

Teasdale G, Jennett B: Assessment of coma and impaired consciousness: a practical scale. Lancet 2:81–84, 1974

Warm JS, Richter DO, Sprague RL, et al: Listening with a dual brain: hemisphere asymmetry in sustained attention. Bulletin of the Psychodynamic Society 15:229–232, 1980

Warrington EK, Logue V, Pratt RTC: The anatomical localisation of selective impairment of auditory verbal short-term memory. Neuropsychologia 9:377–387, 1971

Watson RT, Heilman KM, Cauthen JC, et al: Neglect after cingulectomy. Neurology 23:1003–1007, 1973

Watson RT, Heilman KM, Miller BD, et al: Neglect after mesencephalic reticular formation lesions. Neurology 24:294–298, 1974

Weintraub S, Mesulam M-M: Right cerebral dominance in spatial attention. Arch Neurol 44:621–625, 1987

Whitlock FA: The Ganser syndrome and hysterical pseudo-dementia, in Hysteria. Edited by Roy A. Chichester, England, John Wiley, 1982, pp 185–209

Wilkins AJ, Shallice T, McCarthy R: Frontal lesions and sustained attention. Neuropsychologia 25:359–369, 1987

Zubin J: Problem of attention in schizophrenia, in Experimental Approaches to Psychopathology. Edited by Kietzman ML, Sutton S, Zubin J. New York, Academic, 1975, pp 139–166

Chapter

12

Delirium

Michael G. Wise, M.D.
George T. Brandt, M.D.

DELIRIUM MAY WELL BE the most common psychiatric syndrome found in a general medical hospital. Its mortality and morbidity may surpass all other psychiatric diagnoses. Only dementia, when followed for several years, has a higher mortality rate (Roth 1955; Varsamis et al. 1972). In addition, patients with dementia or other brain damage have a lower threshold for developing a delirium and do so with greater frequency (Epstein and Simon 1967; Hodkinson 1973; Lipowski 1990). Although commonly seen by consultation psychiatrists and other physicians, delirium remains an ignored, underresearched phenomenon. Lipowski's comment in 1978, "Organic brain syndromes are the most neglected areas of psychiatry in this country. Little is known about their epidemiology, their classification is inadequate, and their terminology is a prime example of semantic bedlam" (p. 309), continues to be true today.

Figure 12–1 presents a conceptual overview of delirium. Note the wide variety of different physiological insults that can produce the symptom cluster of the delirium syndrome. This multifactorial etiology accounts both for the high incidence of the syndrome and for the evolution of so many "equivalent" diagnostic terms. Delirium can manifest clinically as a hypoactive state (decreased arousal), hyperactive state (increased arousal), or as a mixed state with fluctuations between hypoactive and hyperactive forms. Accurate diagnosis, of course, precedes treatment. However, if the clinician cannot find a specific reason or reasons for a delirium, there are nonspecific treatments that can decrease symptoms, decrease morbidity, and possibly decrease mortality. The prognosis for delirium, without proper diagnosis and treatment, is bleak.

❑ DEFINITION

Defining *delirium* is not an easy task because many terms have been used to describe this clinical syndrome (Table 12–1). These terms are sometimes used synonymously and at other times are used as though they describe different clinical syndromes. For example, Peura and Johnson (1985), who described the side effects of intravenous cimetidine in patients who had gastroduodenal mucosal lesions, stated that one patient developed delirium, one patient had hallucinations, and a third patient had mental confusion. These three patients did not have different disorders. All three had a delirium. It

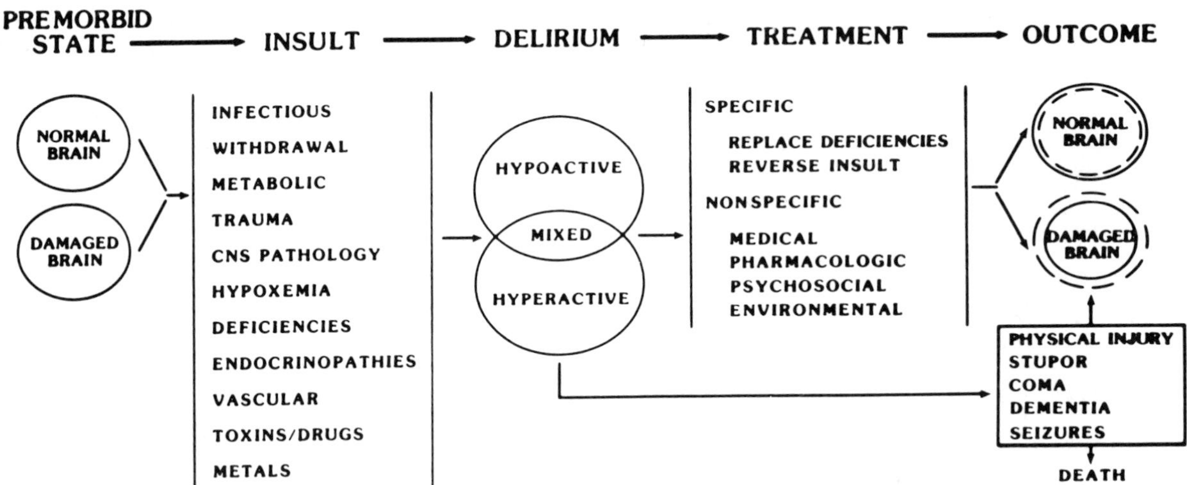

Figure 12–1. Conceptual overview of delirium.

would sometimes appear that confusion describes both delirium and its literature.

The diagnostic criteria for delirium found in DSM-III-R (American Psychiatric Association 1987) are outlined in Table 12–2. Both DSM-III (American Psychiatric Association 1980) and DSM-III-R criteria evolved from a committee effort but underrepresent the wide array of neuropsychiatric abnormalities found in the delirious patient. In the section of this chapter on clinical features we attempt to amplify and expand these criteria. DSM-III-R does unite a broad spectrum of clinical states (i.e., hypoactive, hyperactive, and mixed confusional states) under the diagnostic umbrella of delirium. This approach is not accepted by many of our medical colleagues, particularly neurologists. Adams and Victor (1989), for example, suggested that the diagnosis of delirium should be reserved for a subgroup of confused patients with agitation, autonomic instability, and hallucinations. Delirium tremens (DTs) was the conceptual model they used. Patients who become acutely confused, incoherent, and disoriented, but without autonomic instability and hallucinations, would be said to have "acute confusional states," not delirium. These classification disparities are rooted in the history and evolution of the concept of delirium and have been discussed by Lipowski (1980b, 1990) and Berrios (1981).

Pending further research, the unified approach of DSM-III-R, which labels both hyperactive and

TABLE 12–1. TERMS USED TO DENOTE DELIRIUM

Acute brain failure	Exogenous psychosis
Acute brain syndrome	Infective-exhaustive psychosis
Acute brain syndrome with psychosis	Intensive care unit (ICU) psychosis
Acute confusional state	Metabolic encephalopathy
Acute dementia	Oneiric state
Acute organic psychosis	Organic brain syndrome
Acute organic reaction	Reversible cerebral dysfunction
Acute organic syndrome	Reversible cognitive dysfunction
Acute reversible psychosis	Reversible dementia
Acute secondary psychosis	Reversible toxic psychosis
Cerebral insufficiency	Toxic confusion state
Confusional state	Toxic encephalopathy
Dysergastic reaction	

TABLE 12–2. DSM-III-R DIAGNOSTIC CRITERIA FOR DELIRIUM

A. Reduced ability to maintain attention to external stimuli (e.g., questions must be repeated because attention wanders) and to appropriately shift attention to new external stimuli (e.g., perseverates answer to a previous question).

B. Disorganized thinking, as indicated by rambling, irrelevant, or incoherent speech.

C. At least two of the following:

(1) reduced level of consciousness, e.g., difficulty keeping awake during examination
(2) perceptual disturbances: misinterpretations, illusions, or hallucinations
(3) disturbance of sleep-wake cycle with insomnia or daytime sleepiness
(4) increased or decreased psychomotor activity
(5) disorientation to time, place, or person
(6) memory impairment, e.g., inability to learn new material, such as the names of several unrelated objects after five minutes, or to remember past events, such as history of current episode of illness

D. Clinical features develop over a short period of time (usually hours to days) and tend to fluctuate over the course of a day.

E. Either (1) or (2):

(1) evidence from the history, physical examination, or laboratory tests of a specific organic factor (or factors) judged to be etiologically related to the disturbance
(2) in the absence of such evidence, an etiologic organic factor can be presumed if the disturbance cannot be accounted for by any nonorganic mental disorder, e.g., manic episode accounting for agitation and sleep disturbance

Source. Reprinted from American Psychiatric Association: Diagnostic and Statistical Manual of Mental Disorders, 3rd Edition, Revised. Washington, DC, American Psychiatric Association, 1987, p 103. Used with permission.

hypoactive forms as delirium, seems appropriate. This concept was supported by Engel and Romano (1959), who hypothesized that delirium represents a metabolic derangement. Several other aspects of the syndrome must be incorporated into a definition. Delirium usually has a sudden onset, a brief duration, and is reversible. Therefore, delirium is herein defined as *a transient, essentially reversible dysfunction in cerebral metabolism that has an acute or subacute onset and is manifest clinically by a wide array of neuropsychiatric abnormalities.*

❑ EPIDEMIOLOGY

A discussion of the epidemiology of delirium implies the existence of a reasonable body of scientific study into the factors that influence its frequency and distribution. However, systematic research on the epidemiology of delirium is, for the most part, lacking. In addition, terms such as *incidence,* which considers the number of new cases over a span of time and population at risk, as well as *prevalence,* which considers identified cases in a population, are inconsistently used in the literature.

Incidence and Prevalence

The frequency of delirium varies depending on the type of insult and the predisposition of the individual involved. Engel (1967) estimated that 10%–15% of patients on acute medical and surgical wards were delirious. Lipowski (1990) agreed with this estimate but noted that the increasing age of the population may make the estimate low.

Anthony et al. (1982) used the Mini-Mental State Exam (MMSE; Folstein et al. 1975) and tested consecutively admitted patients to a general medical ward of the Johns Hopkins Hospital. They found a point prevalence for delirium of 24% and also found that 34% of patients had some cognitive impairment on the day of admission. Cameron et al. (1987), using DSM-III diagnostic criteria, found 13.5% of 133 consecutive patients admitted to a medical ward were delirious and that an additional 3.3% became delirious during hospitalization.

Predisposing Factors

Six groups of patients have a high risk of developing a delirium: 1) elderly patients, 2) postcardiotomy patients, 3) burn patients, 4) patients with preexisting brain damage (e.g., dementia and strokes), 5) patients with drug dependency who are experiencing withdrawal, and 6) patients with acquired immunodeficiency syndrome (AIDS) (Table 12–3). Advancing age increases the risk, with persons aged 60 or over usually cited as the highest risk group (Lipowski 1980a, 1990). If children are excluded, the incidence of delirium increases with the age of the patient population studied. While studying the natural history of mental disorders in older people, Sir Martin Roth (1955) reported acute confusional states among psychiatric patients in 7.5% of patients aged 60–69, 9% in patients aged 70–79, and 12% in patients over age 80. Bedford (1959) reported that 80% of the 5,000 patients aged 65 years or over admitted to the Oxford Geriatric Unit during an 8-year period had confusional states. Inouye et al. (1989) and Francis et al. (1988) reported that 23% and 25.3%, respectively, of patients over the age of 70 were delirious during hospitalization.

Postcardiotomy delirium has been the focus of more neuropsychiatric research than any other aspect of delirium (Smith and Dimsdale 1989). Dubin et al. (1979) wrote a thorough review of postcardiotomy delirium in which they reported that the frequency across studies varied from 13% to 67%. In more recent studies, Calabrese et al. (1987) and Nussmeier et al. (1986) reported a lower frequency of delirium. Nussmeier noted that 8.6% of patients who received narcotic anesthesia and 5.6% who received barbiturate coma developed delirium. Several factors, in addition to increased age and preexisting brain damage, may increase the risk of postcardiotomy delirium. These include time on bypass (Heller et al. 1970; Kornfeld et al. 1974), severity of postoperative illness (Kornfeld et al. 1974), serum levels of anticholinergic drugs (Tune et al. 1981), increased levels of central nervous system (CNS) adenylate kinase and subclinical brain injury (Aberg et al. 1982, 1984), decreased cardiac output (Blachly and Kloster 1966), complexity of the surgical procedure (Dubin et al. 1979), complement activation (Chenoweth et al. 1981), embolism (Nussmeier et al. 1986), and nutritional status as measured by albumin levels (M. G. Wise, N. H. Cassem, K. Gray, 1980–1981, unpublished observations). Preoperative psychiatric interviews may reduce postoperative psychosis by 50% (Kornfeld et al. 1974; Layne and Yudofsky 1971). In a factor analysis of 28 risk factors from 44 studies, Smith and Dimsdale (1989) found that only preoperative psychiatric intervention correlated with the occurrence of postcardiotomy delirium. The correlation was negative.

According to Andreasen (1974), about 30% of adult burn patients have symptoms of delirium and the "frequency increases with both the age of the patient and the severity of the burn" (Andreasen et al. 1972, p. 68). Blank and Perry (1984) described an 18% incidence of delirium in burn patients. Antoon et al. (1972) reported a 14% incidence of burn encephalopathy in children, but they defined burn encephalopathy, as "neurologic disturbances ranging from hallucination, personality changes, and delirium to seizures and coma" (p. 609), so the actual frequency of delirium in this study was much lower.

The presence of preexisting brain damage, whether preoperative CNS neurological abnormalities (Branthwaite 1972; Kornfeld et al. 1974; Layne and Yudofsky 1971) or dementia (Epstein and Simon 1967; Hodkinson 1973; Purdie et al. 1981), lowers the patient's threshold for developing a delirium. Koponen et al. (1989a) found that 81% of delirious patients in their study had dementia. Rapid drug withdrawal in a patient with drug dependence, particularly rapid withdrawal from alcohol and benzodiazepines, is without question a risk factor for developing delirium. Perry (1990) reported a 90% frequency of organic mental disorders in patients with far-advanced AIDS. In another study (Fernandez et al. 1989), delirium was found to be the most frequent neuropsychiatric complication of AIDS.

In an earlier review (Wise 1987), children were listed as predisposed to delirium. However, there still exists only one study of delirium in children and adolescents (Prugh et al. 1980). Kornfeld et al.'s sample of 119 unselected open-heart surgery patients included 20 children who had surgical proce-

TABLE 12–3. PATIENTS WITH HIGH RISK FOR DEVELOPING DELIRIUM

Elderly patients
Postcardiotomy patients
Burn patients
Patients with brain damage
Patients in drug withdrawal
Acquired immunodeficiency syndrome (AIDS) patients

dures for repair of congenital lesions (Kornfeld et al. 1965). None of the children developed delirium, but 30% of the adults operated on for congenital repairs did. Based on lack of data, childhood was removed in this review as a risk factor for developing delirium.

Additional factors, such as sleep deprivation and perceptual (sensory) deprivation, are believed to facilitate the development of a delirium. After a thorough review of the literature on the relationship between sleep and delirium Lipowski (1990) stated, "In summary, experimental and clinical studies indicate a relationship between sleep disturbance and delirium but fail to clarify its exact nature" (p. 123). Without question, sleep-wake abnormalities are frequently an integral part of the symptomatology found in delirium. How critical sleep deprivation is to the development of the delirium remains an unanswered question. Harrell and Othmer (1987) found that sleep disturbance developed after patients' scores on the MMSE decreased (i.e., after the delirium developed) and not before. Both sensory deprivation and sensory overload are believed to be facilitating factors in delirium (Lipowski 1980a, 1990). The crucial issue may not be the quantity of stimuli but rather the quality. It is known, for example, that the electroencephalogram (EEG) of a subject exposed to monotonous stimuli shows more slowing than the EEG of a sensory-deprived subject (Zubek and Welch 1963). Patients in an intensive care unit (ICU) do not lack stimulation; rather, they lack the kinds of stimuli that orient them to time and environment. In his most recent book, Lipowski (1990) stated that, "there is no evidence that sensory deprivation alone can cause delirium" (p. 128).

The predisposition associated with personality and psychological variables has been investigated as well. In their review of the postoperative literature, Dubin et al. (1979) indicated that no specific personality profile correlated with delirium. Lipowski (1980a) agreed, reporting that "it may be stated that so far not a single psychological variable has been conclusively shown to predispose one to delirium" (p. 115).

❑ CLINICAL FEATURES OF DELIRIUM

Prodrome

The patient will often manifest symptoms such as restlessness, anxiety, irritability, or sleep disruption before the onset of a delirium. Review of the delirious patient's hospital medical chart, particularly the nursing notes, will often reveal these prodromal features.

Fluctuating Course

The clinical features of delirium are protean (Table 12–4) and, to complicate the picture further, vary rapidly over time. This variability and fluctuation of clinical findings are not only characteristic of delirium but can lead to diagnostic confusion. Thus the surgery team that sees Mr. Jones on early morning rounds may find him friendly, sleepy, and noncomplaining, but the psychiatric consultant later

TABLE 12–4. CLINICAL FEATURES OF DELIRIUM

- Prodrome (restlessness, anxiety sleep disturbance, and irritability)
- Rapidly fluctuating course
- Attention decreased (easily distractible)
- Altered arousal and psychomotor abnormality
- Disturbance of sleep-wake cycle
- Impaired memory (cannot register new information)
- Disorganized thinking and speech
- Disorientation (time, place, and person [very rare])
- Altered perceptions (misperceptions, illusions, delusions [poorly formed], and hallucinations
- Neurological abnormalities
  - Dysgraphia
  - Constructional apraxia
  - Dysnomic aphasia
  - Motor abnormalities (tremor, asterixis, myoclonus, and reflex and tone changes)
  - Electroencephalogram (EEG) abnormalities (almost always global slowing)
- Other features (sadness, anger, euphoria, or other affects)

that day may find Mr. Jones grossly confused, paranoid, agitated, uncooperative, and visually hallucinating. To convince the surgeon(s) that Mr. Jones has a severe delirium that requires immediate evaluation and treatment is often a difficult and frustrating task. The appearance of lucid intervals in the clinical course of a patient is an important observation and is diagnostic of a delirium.

What Wells and Duncan (1980) suggested—that the symptom complex of delirium is manifest by a "marked variability from patient to patient and from time to time in the same patient" (p. 46)—is certainly true. There is a subgroup of patients who manifest what has been called "reversible dementia" (Cummings et al. 1980; Task Force Sponsored by the National Institute on Aging 1980). These patients lack the dramatic fluctuations that are so typical of delirium and, as a result, are often misdiagnosed as having dementia.

Attentional Deficits

The patient with a delirium has difficulty sustaining attention. Such a patient is easily distracted by incidental activities in the environment. If a clinician was interviewing a delirious patient in the hospital and a housekeeping person walked by, the patient would most likely attend to the distraction. When the patient then looked back, the patient might say, "Did you ask me a question?" The patient's inability to sustain attention undoubtedly plays a key role in memory and orientation difficulties.

Arousal Disturbance and Psychomotor Abnormalities

In delirium, the reticular activating system of the brain stem may be hypoactive, in which case the patient would appear apathetic, somnolent, and quietly confused. In other patients, the brain stem's activating system may be hyperactive, in which case the patient is agitated and hypervigilant, exhibiting psychomotor hyperactivity. Some patients have a mixed picture, with swings back and forth between hypoactive and hyperactive states. According to Lipowski (1990), "the frequency of the respective variants in clinical practice is unknown" (p. 65). The patient with a retarded (hypoactive) type delirium is less apt to be diagnosed as delirious and is often labeled as depressed, uncooperative, or character disordered. The diagnosis of clinical depression in an apathetic, quietly confused patient can lead to inappropriate treatment with antidepressants. This misdiagnosis increases morbidity and mortality, from failure to diagnose and treat underlying causes for the delirium, and adds the anticholinergic burden from antidepressants to the already malfunctioning brain.

Sleep-Wake Disturbance

Sleep-wake disturbance is not only symptomatic of a delirium, it exacerbates the confusion via sleep deprivation. The sleep-wake cycle of the delirious patient is often reversed. The patient may be somnolent during the day and active during the night when the nursing staff is sparse. Restoration of the normal diurnal sleep cycle is an important part of treatment.

Impaired Memory

The ability of a delirious patient to register events into memory is severely impaired. Whether because of attentional deficits, perceptual disturbances, or malfunction of the hippocampus, the patient will fail tests of immediate and recent memory. After recovery from a delirium, some patients will be amnestic for the entire episode; others will have islands of memory for events during the episode. Whether these islands of memory correspond to the previously described lucid intervals is unknown.

Disorganized Thinking and Impaired Speech

The delirious patient's thought patterns are disorganized and reasoning is defective. Ask a presumptively delirious patient to explain the following story: "I have a friend by the name of Frank Jones whose feet are so large he has to put on his pants by pulling them over his head. Can Mr. Jones do that?" Typical responses from a delirious patient, usually with a smile and a laugh, are, "Sure, as long as he unzips his fly" or "I guess so, if he does one leg at a time." The delirious patient does not understand the problem at hand and is unable to reason normally. Using DSM-III-R terminology, the patient's consciousness is *clouded*. In addition, as the severity of the delirium increases, spontaneous speech becomes "incoherent, rambling, and shifts from topic to topic" (Cummings 1985, p. 68).

Disorientation

The patient with a delirium, except for lucid intervals, is usually disoriented to time, often disoriented to place, but very rarely, if ever, disoriented to person. It is not unusual for a delirious patient to feel that he or she is in a familiar place (e.g., "a room in the attic of my house") while also nodding agreement that he or she is being monitored in a surgical ICU. The extent of the patient's disorientation will fluctuate with the severity of the delirium.

Altered Perceptions

The delirious patient will often experience misperceptions that involve illusions, delusions, and hallucinations. Virtually all patients with a delirium will have misperceptions. The patient will often weave these misperceptions into a loosely knit delusional, often paranoid system. The patient may, for example, overhear the nurses say, "We're going to move him out" (i.e., move the patient to another room). The patient may then hear a postoperative patient moaning and hear a bedpan fall on the floor (i.e., "A shot?!"). The patient may then put these events together and suspect that he is about to be transferred to a torture chamber and killed.

Visual hallucinations are common and can involve simple visual distortions or complex scenes. During a delirium, visual hallucinations occur more frequently than auditory hallucinations. Tactile hallucinations are the least frequent. In our experience, most auditory and tactile phenomena that are labelled as hallucinations are, in fact, illusions. For example, intravenous tubing may brush against the skin and be perceived as a snake crawling on the arm.

Neurological Abnormalities

There are a number of neurological abnormalities that are found in delirium. Testing for these signs at the bedside not only strengthens the clinician's suspicion of the diagnosis but, when added to the chart, helps other physicians recognize the presence of a confusional state. One easy bedside test is to draw a large circle on an unlined blank sheet of paper and ask the patient to draw a clock face with the hands showing 10 minutes before 11 o'clock (Figure 12–2). This and other constructional tasks are very sensitive indicators for the degree of confusion present. Ask the patient to name objects (testing for dysnomia) and to write a sentence (testing for dysgraphia). Dysgraphia is one of the most sensitive indicators of a delirium. In Chedru's and Geschwind's study (1972), 33 of 34 acutely confused patients had impaired writing. Writing shows motor impairment (from tremor to illegible scribble), spatial impairment (letter malalignment and line disorientation), misspelling, and linguistic errors. Patten and Lemarre (1989) examined 250 psychiatric patients and noted that dysgraphia is not specific to delirium and can occur with dementia and acute psychiatric disorders. However, dysgraphia in delirious patients tended to be more severe.

Delirious patients may not have motor system abnormalities, although many patients manifest tremor, myoclonus, asterixis, or reflex and muscle tone changes. The tremor associated with delirium, particularly toxic-metabolic delirium, is absent at rest but apparent during movement. Myoclonus and asterixis (so-called liver flap) occur in many toxic and metabolic conditions. Symmetric reflex and muscle tone changes can also occur.

Other Features

Emotional disturbances are common among delirious patients. The intensity of patients' emotional response to mental confusion may fluctuate relatively rapidly and may also change in character with the passage of time (i.e., from fear with associated hyperarousal to apathy with hypoarousal). Thus delirious patients are often described as emotionally labile.

The emotional responses seen in delirious patients include anxiety, panic, fear, anger, rage, sadness, apathy, and (rarely, except in steroid-induced delirium) euphoria. Medical caregivers may identify the emotional or behavioral disturbance of the critically ill patient without recognizing the underlying confusional state. Lipowski (1967, 1980a) noted that the determinants of the individual's response to delirium are personality structure, the nature of the underlying illness, the contents of thoughts and hallucinations, and the characteristics of the environment.

❑ PATHOPHYSIOLOGY AND EEG ABNORMALITIES

Although delirium is a common clinical entity, remarkably little of its pathophysiology has been studied. Significant information has been provided by early EEG investigators. From 1944 to 1947, Engel, Romano, and others (Engel et al. 1947; Romano and Engel 1944) wrote a series of classic papers that correlated the severity of delirium (i.e., cognitive dysfunction) with EEG findings (Figure

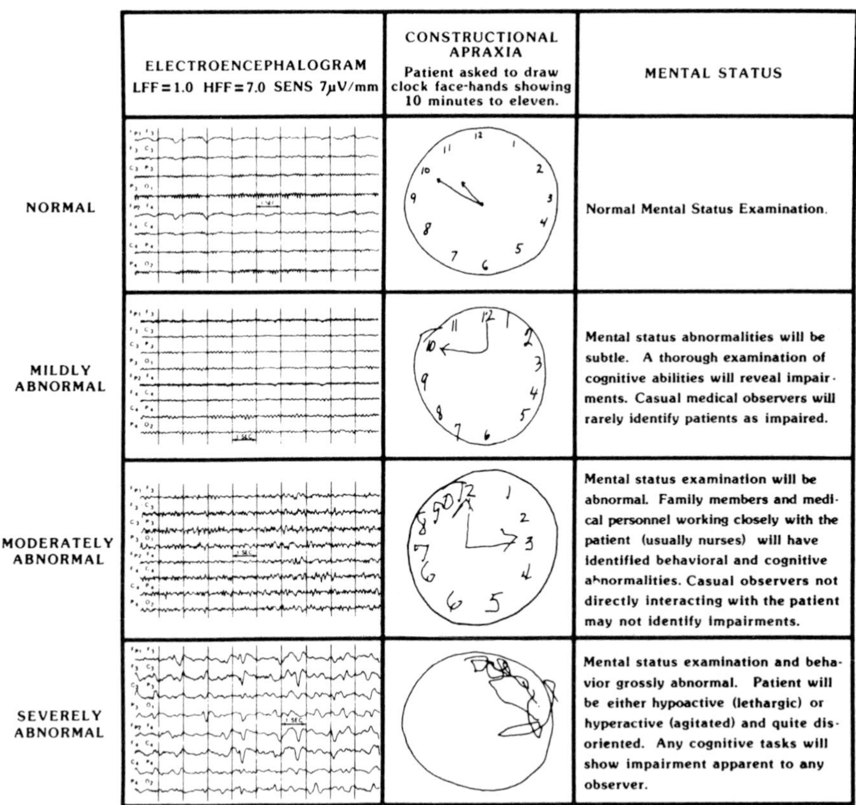

Figure 12–2. Comparison of electroencephalogram, constructional apraxia, and mental status.

12–2). Their clinical research established that 1) a correlation existed between the electrical abnormality and disturbance of consciousness, which they termed "the primary psychological symptom of delirium"; 2) EEG changes were reversible to the extent that the clinical delirium was reversible; 3) the character of the EEG change appeared to be independent of the specific underlying disease process; 4) the character of the EEG changes was determined by the intensity, duration, and reversibility of the noxious factors as modified by the essential premorbid integrity of the CNS; and 5) clinical interventions (e.g., administration of oxygen in congestive heart failure and pulmonary insufficiency) improved (normalized) the EEG and improved the mental status. Spectral EEG analyses, which measure the quality of alpha, beta, theta, and delta background activity, have further supported Engel's and Romano's proposed correlation between EEG slowing and cognitive deterioration (Koponen et al. 1989b).

Engel's and Romano's classic article (1959)—"Delirium, a Syndrome of Cerebral Insufficiency"—proposed that the basic etiology of all delirium was a derangement in functional metabolism that was manifest at the clinical level by characteristic disturbances in cognitive functions and at the physiological level by characteristic slowing of the EEG. Pro and Wells (1977) reported that EEG changes virtually always accompany delirium. The EEG changes found in delirium are not always slowing and the pattern can be low-voltage fast activity, as in DTs (Kennard et al. 1945). Low-voltage fast activity, is usually found in hyperactive, agitated patients with heightened arousal (Pro and Wells 1977). EEG slowing is found in lethargic, anergic, abulic patients. The EEG slowing illustrated in Figure 12–2 is typical for deliriums caused by toxic-metabolic etiologies.

An individual's EEG can have significant slowing but still be read as normal if, for example, his or her normal background activity is 12 cycles/second and during a metabolic encephalopathy the background slows to 8 cycles/second. Significant slowing has occurred, although the reported rate (8 cycles/second) still falls within the "normal" range, and the EEG could be read as normal. Documentation of the encephalopathy might only occur if the patient has a previous EEG on record or if a second EEG is obtained once the patient is again cognitively normal. EEG abnormalities can also occur before, and also linger after, the clinical manifestations of a delirium (Andreasen et al. 1977).

Since Engel's and Romano's 1959 hypothesis that delirium represents a metabolic derangement, little additional research information has been forthcoming. When Lipowski (1980a) reviewed the studies on cerebral metabolism, cerebral blood flow, and delirium, he suggested that studies of regional cerebral blood flow (rCBF) in delirium have only begun. This is still an accurate assessment. Two textbooks, *Cerebral Blood Flow and Metabolism Measurement* (Hartmann and Hayer 1985) and *Positron Emission Tomography* (Reivich and Abass 1985) contain information on psychiatric disorders, but neither sheds any further light on the pathophysiology of delirium. Lipowski (1990) stated, "Unfortunately, this superior research technique [positron-emission tomography] has not yet been used to study delirium and to elucidate its pathophysiology" (p 146). Koponen (1989d, 1989e) reported a correlation between a decrease in MMSE scores and a decrease in somatostatin and β-endorphin-like immunoreactivity in the cerebrospinal fluid (CSF).

Some neurologists (Adams and Victor 1989; Mesulam 1985; Mori and Yamadori 1987) divide the DSM-III-R concept of delirium into two different types, an acute confusional state (ACS) and an acute agitated delirium (AAD). Mori and Yamadori (1987) studied 41 consecutive patients with infarction in the territory of the right middle artery. They concluded that ACS reflects a disturbance of attention secondary to damage of the frontostriatal region and that AAD is a disturbance of emotion and affect secondary to injury of the middle temporal gyrus. Koponen (1989c) noted that delirium was more common with vascular lesions of the high-order association areas of the prefrontal and posterior parietal regions.

❑ DIFFERENTIAL DIAGNOSIS FOR DELIRIUM

The differential diagnosis of delirium is so extensive that there may be a tendency to avoid the search for etiologies. It is also important to realize that confusional states, particularly in the elderly, may have multiple causes. For example, an elderly patient with delirium may be found to have a low-hematocrit, multiorgan system disease (e.g., pulmonary insufficiency, cardiac failure, or dementia) and to be taking multiple medications. Each potential contributor to the delirium needs to be pursued and reversed independently.

Nonspecific terms such as *ICU psychosis* are sometimes used as an explanation for delirium, when, in fact, these nonspecific terms simply mask ignorance. Koponen (1989a) found clear organic etiologies in 87% of delirious patients and also found that patients who became confused because of psychological and environmental events were severely demented. The task for the clinician is to organize the wide array of potential causes of delirium into a usable diagnostic system. The following mnemonics are an attempt to present a systematic approach to the differential diagnosis of delirium.

Emergent Items (WHHHHIMP)

A two-tiered differential diagnostic system is very helpful when consulting on a delirious patient. The first level of this diagnostic system is demonstrated in Table 12–5 and is represented by the mnemonic *WHHHHIMP*. Diagnoses using this mnemonic must be made early in the course of a delirium because failure to do so may result in irreversible damage to the patient. WHHHHIMP can help the clinician recall these critical items. Table 12–5 also contains many of the clinical questions that must be asked by the clinician to determine the etiology.

W—Wernicke's encephalopathy or Withdrawal. A patient with Wernicke's encephalopathy will have a triad of findings consisting of confusion, ataxia, and ophthalmoplegia (usually lateral gaze paralysis). If Wernicke's encephalopathy is not promptly treated with parenteral thiamine, the patient will be left with a permanent Korsakoff's psychosis (called *organic amnestic syndrome* in DSM-III-R).

A precise history of alcohol intake is critical for the diagnosis of alcohol withdrawal or DTs. Other findings that increase the suspicion of alcohol withdrawal or DTs are a history of alcohol-related arrests, alcoholic blackouts, medical complications associated with alcohol abuse, liver function abnormalities, and elevated red cell mean corpuscular volume (MCV). Hyperreflexia and increased sym-

TABLE 12–5. DIFFERENTIAL DIAGNOSIS FOR DELIRIUM: EMERGENT ITEMS (WHHHHIMP)

Diagnoses	*Clinical questions*
Wernicke's encephalopathy or **W**ithdrawal	Ataxia? Ophthalmoplegia? Alcohol or drug history? Increased mean corpuscular volume (MCV)? Increased sympathetic activity (e.g., increased pulse, increased blood pressure (BP), or sweating)? Hyperreflexia?
Hypertensive encephalopathy	Increased BP? Papilledema?
Hypoglycemia	History of insulin-dependent diabetes mellitus? Decreased glucose?
Hypoperfusion of central nervous system	Decreased BP? Decreased cardiac output (e.g., myocardial infarct, arrhythmia, cardiac failure)? Decreased hematocrit?
Hypoxemia	Arterial blood gases (decreased PO_2)? History of pulmonary disease?
Intracranial bleeding or **I**nfection	History of unconsciousness? Focal neurological signs?
Meningitis or encephalitis	Meningeal signs: Increased white blood count? Increased temperature? Viral prodrome?
Poisons or medications	Should toxic screen be ordered? Signs of toxicity (e.g., pupillary abnormality, nystagmus, or ataxia)? Is the patient on a drug that can cause delirium?

pathetic tone (e.g., tachycardia, tremor, sweating, and hyperarousal) at the time of examination should lead the clinician to suspect a hyperadrenergic withdrawal state.

HHHH—Hypoxemia, Hypertensive encephalopathy, Hypoglycemia, or Hypoperfusion. A check of the arterial blood gases, and current and past vital signs, should quickly establish whether hypoxemia or hypertensive encephalopathy is present. The patient with hypoglycemic-induced delirium almost always has a history of insulin-dependent diabetes mellitus. Hypoglycemic delirium is also a hyperadrenergic delirium. There are a number of clinical phenomena that can singularly, or additively, decrease brain perfusion. These phenomena cause "relative" hypotension (relative to usual perfusion pressures), such as decreased cardiac output from a myocardial infarction, cardiac failure or arrhythmias, and anemia.

I—Intracranial bleeding or Infection. If the patient has had a brief period of unconsciousness, with or without headache, and is now delirious, or if the patient had or now has focal neurological signs, an intracranial bleed or infection must be suspected. In such cases, immediate neurological or neurosurgical evaluation is necessary. Also, the clinician must look for signs of an infectious process, such as fever or an elevated white blood cell count.

M—Meningitis or encephalitis. These are typically acute febrile illnesses (check vital signs for fever) and usually have either nonspecific localizing neurological signs (e.g., meningismus with stiff neck) or more focal neurological signs.

P—Poisons or medications. When a delirious patient is encountered in the emergency room, the clinician must consider a toxic organic reaction and order a toxic screen. Other considerations such as pesticide or solvent poisoning are less likely but should be considered. Among hospital and emergency room patients, a very common cause of delirium is prescribed medications (Table 12–6). The importance of taking a thorough medication history cannot be overemphasized. For hospitalized patients who become delirious, the examiner must thoroughly review the patient's medication records. The doctor's order sheets can be misleading because drugs may have been ordered but not given. Correlation of behavior with medication administration or discontinuation can be very helpful in sorting through a difficult case.

Critical Items (I WATCH DEATH)

Space limitations in this text preclude a complete discussion of each category contained within the *I WATCH DEATH* mnemonic. Table 12–7 lists many of the insults that can cause delirium. Because the list is lengthy, it may be helpful for the clinician to carry a card containing the entire differential diagnosis of delirium.

The use of I WATCH DEATH may sound melodramatic. This is not the case. The appearance of a delirium, which is equivalent to acute brain failure, should marshal the same medical forces as failure of any other vital organ. The morbidity and mortality that result from an untreated or undertreated delirium are substantial and should not be ignored.

❑ COURSE (PROGNOSIS)

The clinical course of a delirious patient is variable. The possibilities are 1) full recovery, 2) progression

TABLE 12–6. DRUGS THAT CAN CAUSE DELIRIUM

Antibiotic	**Anti-inflammatory**	**Drug withdrawal**
Acyclovir (antiviral)	Adrenocorticotropic hormone	Alcohol
Amphotericin B (antifungal)	Corticosteroids	Barbiturates
Cephalexin (Keflex)	Ibuprofen (Motrin and Advil)	Benzodiazepines
Chloroquine (antimalarial)	Indomethacin (Indocin)	**Sedative-hypnotic**
Anticholinergic	Naproxen (Naprosyn)	Barbiturates (Miltown and Equanil)
Antihistamines	Phenylbutazone (Butazolidin)	Benzodiazepines
Chlorpheniramine	**Antineoplastic**	Glutethimide (Doriden)
(Ornade and Teldrin)	5-Fluorouracil	**Sympathomimetic**
Antiparkinson drugs	**Antiparkinson**	Amphetamines
Benztropine (Cogentin)	Amantadine (Symmetrel)	Phenylephrine
Biperiden (Akineton)	Carbidopa (Sinemet)	Phenylpropanolamine
Antispasmodics	Levodopa (Larodopa)	Cimetidine (Tagamet)
Atropine/homatropine	**Antituberculous**	Disulfiram (Antabuse)
Belladonna alkaloids	Isoniazid	Lithium
Diphenhydramine (Benadryl)	Rifampin	Metrizamide (Amipaque)
Phenothiazines (especially	**Analgesic**	Metronidazole (Flagyl)
thioridazine)	Opiates	Podophyllin by absorption
Promethazine (Phenergan)	Salicylates	Propylthiouracil
Scopolamine	Synthetic narcotics	Quinacrine
Tricyclic antidepressants	**Cardiac**	Theophylline
(especially amitriptyline)	β-Blockers	Timolol ophthalmic
Trihexyphenidyl (Artane)	Propranolol (Inderal)	**Over-the-counter**
Anticonvulsant	Clonidine (Catapres)	Compoz
Phenobarbital	Digitalis (Digoxin and Lanoxin)	Excedrin P.M.
Phenytoin (Dilantin)	Disopyramide (Norpace)	Sleep-Eze
Sodium valproate (Depakene)	Lidocaine (Xylocaine)	Sominex
	Mexiletine	**Miscellaneous**
	Methyldopa (Aldomet)	Aminophylline
	Quinidine (Quinidine,	Bromides
	Quinaglute, and Duraquine)	Chlorpropamide (Diabinese)
	Procainamide (Pronestyl)	

TABLE 12–7. DIFFERENTIAL DIAGNOSIS FOR DELIRIUM: CRITICAL ITEMS (I WATCH DEATH)

Infectious	Encephalitis, meningitis, and syphilis
Withdrawal	Alcohol, barbiturates, sedative-hypnotics
Acute metabolic	Acidosis, alkalosis, electrolyte disturbance, hepatic failure, and renal failure
Trauma	Heat stroke, postoperative, and severe burns
CNS pathology	Abscesses, hemorrhage, normal pressure hydrocephalus, seizures, stroke, tumors, and vasculitis
Hypoxia	Anemia, carbon monoxide poisoning, hypotension, and pulmonary or cardiac failure
Deficiencies	Vitamin B_{12}, niacin, and thiamine and hypovitaminosis
Endocrinopathies	Hyper- or hypoadrenocorticism and hyper- or hypoglycemia
Acute vascular	Hypertensive encephalopathy and shock
Toxins or drugs	Medications (see Table 12–6), pesticides, and solvents
Heavy metals	Lead, manganese, and mercury

to stupor and/or coma, 3) seizures, 4) chronic brain syndromes, 5) death, or 6) *1* through *4* above with associated morbidity (e.g., fracture or subdural hematomas from falls). The majority of patients who experience delirium probably have a full recovery (Lipowski 1990), although the actual probability of this outcome is unknown. Some patients will progress to stupor and/or coma and either recover, with or without chronic brain damage, or become chronically vegetative or die. Seizures can accompany delirium but are more likely to occur with drug withdrawal, particularly alcohol, and burn encephalopathy (Antoon et al. 1972). Finally, some patients will not completely recover and will have residual brain injury. The chronic brain syndrome may be global or focal (e.g., amnestic syndrome or organic personality disorder).

Morbidity

Although there are no direct studies of morbidity in delirium, research does indicate that hospitalization is prolonged (Kay et al. 1956). In one study (Titchener et al. 1956), 38.9% of acute brain syndromes became chronic brain syndromes. In another study (Tufo et al. 1970), 15% of postcardiotomy delirious patients had persistent neurological signs at discharge. Fernandez et al. (1989) found that only 37% of AIDS patients who became delirious had a complete recovery of cognitive function.

Patients who undergo orthopedic surgery are a fertile ground for research in delirium. Rogers et al. (1989) reported that patients who were cognitively normal when tested preoperatively showed no improvement in level of physical function at 6 months postoperatively if they developed delirium. In other words, patients who became delirious gained no functional benefit from the surgery (Berggren et al. 1987). Gustafson et al. (1988), found that delirium seemed to be the best predictor of outcome in patients who presented with femoral neck fractures. They reported that 37 of 111 patients were delirious preoperatively and another 31 became delirious postoperatively. The delirious patients had longer hospital stays than the patients who were not delirious (21.7 days vs. 13.5 days) and were more likely to require walking aids, be bedridden, die, or require rehabilitation. The delirious group spent four times as long in recuperation before discharge.

Any clinician who performs hospital consultations has seen patients, as Moore (1977) described, who "became agitated, struck a nurse, and pulled out his nasogastric tube" (p. 1431). Delirious patients pull out intravenous lines, nasogastric tubes, arterial lines, nasopharyngeal tubes, and intra-aortic balloon pumps. Inouye et al. (1989) reported that the risk of complications such as decubiti and aspiration pneumonia was more that six times greater for the delirious elderly patient compared with elderly patients who were not delirious. Levkoff et al. (1986) projected a $1–$2 billion savings if the hospital stay of each delirious patient could be reduced by 1 day.

Mortality

Most psychiatrists, and physicians in general, underestimate the mortality associated with delirium. Of 77 patients who received a DSM-III diagnosis of delirium from a consultation psychiatrist, 19 (25%) died within 6 months (Trzepacz et al. 1985). Three months after diagnosis, the mortality rate for delirium is 14 times greater (Weddington 1982) than the mortality rate for affective disorders. A patient diagnosed with delirium during a hospital admission has a 5.5 times greater hospital mortality rate than a patient diagnosed with dementia (Rabins and Folstein 1982). Furthermore, the elderly patient who develops a delirium in the hospital has a 22% (Rabins and Folstein 1982) to 76% (Flint and Richards 1956) chance of dying during that hospitalization. Patients who survive hospitalization have a very high death rate during the months immediately after discharge. Patients with a diagnosis of delirium followed for several months showed a mortality rate equal to that of dementia patients followed for several years (Roth 1955; Varsamis et al. 1972). Cameron et al. (1987) reported that 13 of 20 (65%) delirious patients died during hospitalization.

❑ MAKING THE DIAGNOSIS OF DELIRIUM

Regardless of the suspected diagnosis, the neuropsychiatric evaluation of a patient follows a particular generic process. A specific diagnosis, such as delirium, follows from an appreciation of the clinical features of the syndrome (Table 12–4) and a thorough evaluation of the patient's mental and physical status (Table 12–8). In addition to the usual mental status examination, the examiner should, at a minimum, test for construction praxis (Figure 12–2), writing ability, and the ability to name objects. If a delirium is present, every effort should be made to identify the specific etiology (etiologies). Francis et al. (1990) noted that 56% of delirious patients had a single definite or probable etiology and the remaining 44% had an average of 2.8 etiologies per patient. When no apparent etiology exists at the time of consultation, the etiology will often declare itself within a few days.

The gold standard for diagnosis is the clinical evaluation, and the most useful diagnostic laboratory measure is the EEG. Several paper-and-pencil tests exist to aid the clinician in diagnosis, although it is not clear that these bedside cognitive screening tools improve diagnostic accuracy (Nelson et al. 1986). Folstein et al.'s Mini-Mental State Exam (1975) (Appendix 12–1) provides a screening tool for organicity and is also used to follow the patient's clinical course serially. A score on the MMSE of 20 or less out of 30 indicates cognitive impairment in a patient who has at least an 8th grade education and a good understanding of English. The major problem with the MMSE is its lack of sensitivity (i.e., high rate of false negatives). For example, several patients in a recent study (M. G. Wise, N. Boutros, D. Pearson, et al., February–June 1989, unpublished observations), who had slowed background activity on EEG at the time of evaluation, scored in the mid to upper 20s on the MMSE. The Delirium Rating Scale (DRS; Trzepacz et al. 1988) and the Confusion Assessment Method (CAM; Inouye et al. 1990) are two recently developed tests. Both tests basically translate DSM-III-R diagnostic criteria for delirium into an assessment instrument. Some training is required for optimal use of the CAM.

The laboratory evaluation of a delirious patient can be conceptualized as having two levels. The basic laboratory battery will be ordered in virtually every patient with a diagnosis of delirium. Other tests are available to the clinician. When information concerning the patient's mental and physical status is combined with the basic laboratory battery, the specific etiology (etiologies) is often apparent. If not, the clinician should review the case and consider ordering further diagnostic studies.

❑ TREATMENT

After thoroughly evaluating the patient, the consulting psychiatrist is often faced with one the following situations: 1) a specific etiology or several etiologies have been identified, and the patient's inappropriate behavior endangers medical care and requires treatment; or 2) no specific etiology has been identified, and the patient's inappropriate behavior endangers medical care and requires treatment. When faced with managing a patient in one of these situations, it is helpful to divide the treatment of delirium into specific and nonspecific treatments.

Etiologies Known

Because many causes of delirium have specific treatments, the clinician must systematically attempt to establish a diagnosis. The goal of diagnosis is to

TABLE 12–8. NEUROPSYCHIATRIC EVALUATION OF THE PATIENT

Mental status
Interview (assess level of consciousness, psychomotor activity, appearance, affect, mood, intellect, and thought processes)
Performing tests (memory, concentration, reasoning, motor and constructional apraxia, dysgraphia, and dysnomia)
Physical status
Brief neurological exam (reflexes, limb strength, Babinski reflex, cranial nerves, meningeal signs, and gait)
Review past and present vital signs (pulse, temperature, blood pressure, and respiration rate)
Review chart (labs, abnormal behavior noted and if so when it began, medical diagnoses, VDRL, or FTA-ABS+?)
Review medication records (correlate abnormal behavior with starting or stopping medications)
Laboratory examination—basic
Blood chemistries (electrolytes, glucose, calcium, albumin, blood urea nitrogen, ammonia [NH_4^+], and liver functions)
Blood count (hematocrit, white count and differential, mean corpuscular volume, sedimentation rate)
Drug levels (need toxic screen? medication blood levels?)
Arterial blood gases
Urinalysis
Electrocardiogram
Chest X ray
Laboratory—based on clinical judgment
Electroencephalogram (seizures? focal lesion? and confirm delirium)
Computed tomography (normal pressure hydrocephalus, stroke, and space occupying lesion)
Additional blood chemistries (heavy metals, thiamine and folate levels, thyroid battery, LE prep, antinuclear antibodies, and urinary porphobilinogen)
Lumbar puncture (if indication of infection or intracranial bleed)

Note. FTA-ABS = fluorescent treponemal antibody absorption; VDRL = Venereal Disease Research Laboratory; LE prep = lupus erythematosus prep.

discover reversible causes for delirium. For example, a delirious patient found to have a blood pressure of 260/150 and papilledema must immediately receive antihypertensive medications. The alcoholic patient having withdrawal symptoms must receive appropriate pharmacological intervention with drugs such as thiamine and oxazepam. Without an organized approach to diagnosis, one might attempt to treat the agitation and hallucinations of the patient having DTs with chlorpromazine. This would increase the likelihood of withdrawal seizures.

Etiologies Unknown

There are nonspecific treatments that will help the patient medically and psychologically through the ordeal of a delirium. These treatments are particularly applicable for the patient who is delirious and the exact etiology is unknown. These interventions are divided into medical, pharmacological, psychosocial, and environmental categories.

Medical. In addition to ordering the laboratory tests essential to identify the cause of a delirium, one of the important roles of the neuropsychiatrist is to raise the level of awareness of the medical and nursing staff concerning the morbidity and mortality associated with a delirium. The patient should be placed in a room near the nursing station. Obtaining frequent vital signs is essential. Increased observation of the patient ensures closer monitoring for medical deterioration and for dangerous behaviors, such as trying to crawl over bed rails or pulling out intravenous lines. Fluid input and output must be monitored, and good oxygenation must be ensured. All nonessential medications should be discontinued.

It is important to remember that the brain is a very sensitive forecaster of medical perils ahead. When an etiology for the confusional state has not been identified, daily laboratory examinations (e.g., blood count, blood chemistries, and urinalysis) and physical examinations are essential.

Pharmacological. There is no consensus in the literature on the pharmacological treatment of delirium when the etiology is unknown. To our knowledge, there have been no double-blind trials using drug(s) to treat delirium. Therefore, we must rely on clinical experience, known properties of drugs (particularly side effects), and anecdotal reports of various treatments. The scenario for pharmacological intervention often involves consultation on an agitated, combative, hallucinating, paranoid, medically ill patient whose behavior is a threat to continuing medical treatment.

A drug used to control agitated psychotic behavior in an ICU should calm the patient, without obtunding consciousness, and stop hallucinations and paranoid ideation. A drug should not suppress respiratory drive, cause hypotension, or be deliriogenic (e.g., anticholinergic). The drug should also be available in a parenteral form. Review of the literature and clinical experience indicate that haloperidol comes closest to meeting these criteria and is the drug of choice when treating an agitated delirium with an unknown etiology (Lipowski 1980b, 1990). Haloperidol is a potent antipsychotic with virtually no anticholinergic or hypotensive properties, and it can be given parenterally. In fact, intravenous haloperidol has been used in very high doses for many years in seriously ill patients without harmful side effects (Fernandez et al. 1988; Sos and Cassem 1980; Tesar et al. 1985).

Severe refractory agitation has also been controlled with a continuous intravenous infusion of haloperidol (Fernandez et al. 1988). (**Note:** Haloperidol is not approved by the Food and Drug Administration for intravenous use.) Although extrapyramidal side effects are more likely with the higher-potency antipsychotic drugs, the actual occurrence rate of these side effects in medically ill patients, particularly when using intravenous administration, is strikingly low. When extrapyramidal symptoms of oral versus intravenous haloperidol were measured in a blind fashion, intravenous administration of haloperidol was associated with less severe extrapyramidal symptoms (Menza et al. 1987).

Other antipsychotic medications that have been found useful are thiothixene (Navane) and droperidol (Inapsine). Droperidol is used by anesthesiologists as a preanesthetic agent and by other physicians for the control of nausea and vomiting. It is, like haloperidol, a butyrophenone and has comparable antipsychotic potency. Droperidol is approved for intravenous use but is more sedating than haloperidol and has a slight risk of hypotension. In a double-blind study (Resnick and Burton 1984) that compared intramuscular haloperidol to droperidol in actively agitated patients, droperidol appeared to give more rapid relief. Antipsychotic medications that are less potent, such as chlorpromazine and thioridazine, are more likely to cause hypotension and anticholinergic effects.

Regardless of the route of administration, the usual initial dosage of haloperidol in the agitated younger patient is 2 mg for mild agitation, 5 mg for moderate agitation, and 10 mg for severe agitation. The initial dosage for the elderly patient is 0.5 mg for mild agitation, 1 mg for moderate agitation, and 2 mg for severe agitation. The dose is repeated every 30 minutes until the patient is sedated or calm.[1] After the confusion has cleared, the medications are continued for 3–5 days. Abrupt discontinuation of medication immediately after improvement (within 24 hours) may be followed by recurrence of the delirium. A more rational approach is to taper the medication over a 3- to 5-day period, administering the largest dose of the medication before bedtime to help normalize the sleep-wake cycle.

The use of benzodiazepines in delirium has its proponents. Benzodiazepines are the drugs of choice in DTs. However, the sedation that accompanies benzodiazepines may further impair the delirious patient's sensorium. In addition, some patients may be further disinhibited when given benzodiazepines. Therefore, except in cases of drug-withdrawal states, benzodiazepines are not recommended as a sole agent in the treatment of the delirious patient. Benzodiazepines have been used with success as adjuncts to high-potency neuroleptics like haloperidol (Adams 1984; Garza-Trevino et al. 1989). Small doses of intravenous lorazepam, particularly in patients who have not responded to high doses of haloperidol alone, have been found useful.

Psychosocial. The psychological support of a patient both during and after a delirium is important.

[1]Neuroleptic prescribing practices remain controversial. Issues of rapid neuroleptization, speculation regarding the presence of a therapeutic window, and appropriate dosage levels continue to be debated. The clinical issue, however, must be the individual patient's situation and response to medications. Delirium is defined by its variability; thus one consultation assessment will evoke management and medical recommendations that are time limited in efficacy. Only constant follow-up of the delirious patient will suffice, regardless of what eventually prevails about the pharmacology of specific neuroleptics.

Having a calm family member remain with the paranoid, agitated patient is reassuring to the patient and can stop mishaps (e.g., pulling out arterial lines or falling out of bed). In lieu of a family member, close supervision by reassuring nursing staff is crucial.

After the delirium has resolved, helping the patient understand the bizarre experience can be therapeutic (MacKenzie and Popkin 1980). An explanation to the family about delirium can reduce anxiety and calm fears. Many patients, if they remember the delirious period, will be reluctant to discuss their experiences. Patients may be encouraged to talk if the physician makes a statement such as, "Many patients get confused after . . . [e.g., surgery]. Some patients experience frightening visions, some hear strange conversations or noises, and others believe that people they trust are trying to harm them. These experiences, if you had any of them, might cause you to worry." Simple explanation is usually all that is required to reduce this type of morbidity.

Environmental. Environmental interventions are sometimes helpful but should not be considered as the primary treatment. Both nurses and family members can frequently reorient the patient to date and surroundings. Placing a clock, calendar, and familiar objects in the room may be helpful. Adequate light in the room during the night will usually decrease frightening illusions. Despite recommendations to the contrary, a private room for the delirious patient is appropriate only if adequate supervision can be assured. A room with a window may be helpful to orient the patient to normal diurnal cues (Wilson 1972). If the patient normally wears eyeglasses or a hearing aid, improving the quality of sensory input by returning these devices may help the patient better understand the surroundings.

A common error occurring on medical and surgical wards is to place delirious patients in the same room. This makes reorientation of these patients impossible and often leads to confirmation, based on conversations with a paranoid roommate, that strange things are indeed happening in the hospital.

❑ FUTURE DIRECTIONS

The need for future research into delirium is clear, given its high morbidity, mortality, and cost. Basic questions still need to be answered. Does delirium represent the final common pathway in brain dysfunction? Are hyperactive and hypoactive forms of delirium truly different entities, or is delirium similar to bipolar disorder in its dichotomous clinical presentations? What are the predisposing physiological, personality, emotional, genetic, and environmental factors in the development of a delirium? The resurgence of interest in the neurosciences, neuropsychiatry, and geriatric psychiatry may provide the impetus that is needed to perform this crucial research. Unfortunately, lack of research funds to study delirium and lack of psychiatrists or neurologists who are interested in delirium research bodes poorly for the future.

❑ REFERENCES

Aberg T, Ronquist G, Tyden H, et al: Release of adenylate kinase into cerebrospinal fluid during open-heart surgery and its relation to postoperative intellectual function. Lancet 1:1139–1141, 1982

Aberg T, Ronquist G, Tyden H, et al: Adverse effects on the brain in cardiac operations as assessed by biochemical, psychometric, and radiologic methods. J Thorac Cardiovasc Surg 87:99–105, 1984

Adams F: Neuropsychiatric evaluation and treatment of delirium in the critically ill cancer patient. Cancer Bulletin 36:156–160, 1984

Adams RD, Victor M: Principles of Neurology. New York, McGraw-Hill, 1989

American Psychiatric Association: Diagnostic and Statistical Manual of Mental Disorders, 3rd Edition. Washington, DC, American Psychiatric Association, 1980

American Psychiatric Association: Diagnostic and Statistical Manual of Mental Disorders, 3rd Edition, Revised. Washington, DC, American Psychiatric Association, 1987

Andreasen NJC: Neuropsychiatric complications in burn patients. Int J Psychiatry Med 5:161–171, 1974

Andreasen NJC, Noyes R, Hartford C, et al: Management of emotional reactions in seriously burned adults. N Engl J Med 286:65–69, 1972

Andreasen NJC, Hartford CE, Knott JR, et al: EEG changes associated with burn delirium. Diseases of the Nervous System 38:27–31, 1977

Anthony JC, LeResche L, Niaz U, et al: Limits of the Mini-Mental State as a screening test for dementia and delirium among hospital patients. Psychol Med 12:397–408, 1982

Antoon AY, Volpe JJ, Crawford JD: Burn encephalopathy in children. Pediatrics 50:609–616, 1972

Bedford PD: General medical aspects of confusional states in elderly people. Br Med J 2:185–188, 1959

Berggren D, Gustafson Y, Eriksson B, et al: Postoperative confusion after anesthesia in elderly patients with femoral neck fractures. Anesth Analg 66:497–504, 1987

Berrios GE: Delirium and confusion in the 19th century: a conceptual history. Br J Psychiatry 139:439–449, 1981

Blachly PH, Kloster FE: Relation of cardiac output to postcardiotomy delirium. J Thorac Cardiovasc Surg 52: 423–427, 1966

Blank K, Perry S: Relationship of psychological processes during delirium to outcome. Am J Psychiatry 141:843–847, 1984

Branthwaite MA: Neurological damage related to open-heart surgery: a clinical survey. Thorax 27:748–753, 1972

Calabrese J, Skwerer R, Gulledge A, et al: Incidence of postoperative delirium following myocardial revascularization. Cleve Clin J Med 54:29–32, 1987

Cameron D, Thomas R, Mulvihill M, et al: Delirium: a test of the Diagnostic and Statistical Manual III criteria on medical inpatients. J Am Geriatr Soc 35:1007–1010, 1987

Chedru F, Geschwind N: Writing disturbances in acute confusional states. Neuropsychologia 10:343–353, 1972

Chenoweth DE, Cooper SW, Hugli TE, et al: Complement activation during cardiopulmonary bypass. N Engl J Med 304:497–502, 1981

Cummings J, Benson DF, LoVerme S: Reversible dementia. JAMA 243:2434–2439, 1980

Cummings JL: Acute confusional states, in Clinical Neuropsychiatry. Edited by Cummings JL. New York, Grune & Stratton, 1985, pp 68–74

Dubin WR, Field NL, Gastfriend DR: Postcardiotomy delirium: a critical review. J Thorac Cardiovasc Surg 77: 586–594, 1979

Engel GL: Delirium, in Comprehensive Textbook of Psychiatry. Edited by Friedman AM, Kaplan HS. Baltimore, MD, Williams & Wilkins, 1967

Engel GL, Romano J: Delirium, a syndrome of cerebral insufficiency. Journal of Chronic Disease 9:260–277, 1959

Engel GL, Romano J, Ferris EB: Effect of quinacrine (Atabrine) on the central nervous system. Archives of Neurology and Psychiatry 58:337–350, 1947

Epstein LJ, Simon A: Organic brain syndrome in the elderly. Geriatrics 22:145–150, 1967

Fernandez F, Holmes V, Adams F, et al: Treatment of severe, refractory agitation with a haloperidol drip. J Clin Psychiatry 49:239–241, 1988

Fernandez F, Levy J, Mansell P: Management of delirium in terminally ill AIDS patients. Int J Psychiatry Med 19(2):165–172, 1989

Flint FJ, Richards SM: Organic basis of confusional states in the elderly. Br Med J 2:1537–1539, 1956

Folstein MF, Folstein SE, McHugh PR: Mini-Mental State: a practical method for grading the cognitive state of patients for the clinician. J Psychiatr Res 12:189–198, 1975

Francis J, Strong S, Martin D, et al: Delirium in elderly general medical patients: common but often unrecognized. Clin Res 36(3):711A, 1988

Francis J, Martin D, Kapoor W: A prospective study of delirium in hospitalized elderly. JAMA 263:1097–1101, 1990

Garza-Trevino E, Hollister L, Overall J, et al: Efficacy of combinations of intramuscular antipsychotics and sedative-hypnotics for control of psychotic agitation. Am J Psychiatry 146:1598–1601, 1989

Gustafson Y, Berggren D, Brannstrom B, et al: Acute confusional states in elderly patients treated for femoral neck fracture. J Am Geriatr Soc 36:525–530, 1988

Harrell R, Othmer E: Postcardiotomy confusion and sleep loss. J Clin Psychiatry 48:445–446, 1987

Hartmann A, Hayer S: Cerebral Blood Flow and Metabolism Measurement. New York, Springer-Verlag, 1985

Heller SS, Frank KA, Malm JR, et al: Psychiatric complications of open-heart surgery. N Engl J Med 283:1015–1020, 1970

Hodkinson HM: Mental impairment in the elderly. J R Coll Physicians Lond 7:305–317, 1973

Inouye S, Horwitz R, Tinetti M, et al: Acute confusional states in the hospitalized elderly: incidence, factors, and complications. Clin Res 37(2):524A, 1989

Inouye S, van Dyck C, Alessi C, et al: Clarifying confusion: the Confusion Assessment Method. Ann Intern Med 113:941–948, 1990

Kay DWK, Norris V, Post F: Prognosis in psychiatric disorders of the elderly. Journal of Mental Science 102: 129–140, 1956

Kennard MA, Bueding E, Wortis WB: Some biochemical and electroencephalographic changes in delirium tremens. Quarterly Journal of Studies on Alcohol 6:4–14, 1945

Koponen H, Stenback U, Mattila E, et al: Delirium among elderly persons admitted to a psychiatric hospital: clinical course during the acute stage and one-year follow-up. Acta Psychiatr Scand 79:579–585, 1989a

Koponen H, Partanen J, Paakkonen A, et al: EEG spectral analysis in delirium. J Neurol Neurosurg Psychiatry 52:980–985, 1989b

Koponen H, Hurri L, Stenback U, et al: Computed tomography findings in delirium. J Nerv Ment Dis 177:226–231, 1989c

Koponen H, Stenback U, Mattila E, et al: CSF beta-endorphin-like immunoreactivity in delirium. Biol Psychiatry 25:938–944, 1989d

Koponen H, Stenback U, Mattila E, et al: Cerebrospinal fluid somatostatin in delirium. Psychol Med 19:605–609, 1989e

Kornfeld DS, Zimberg S, Malm JR: Psychiatric complications of open-heart surgery. N Engl J Med 273:287–292, 1965

Kornfeld DS, Heller SS, Frank KA, et al: Personality and psychological factors in postcardiotomy delirium. Arch Gen Psychiatry 31:249–253, 1974

Layne OL, Yudofsky SC: Postoperative psychosis in cardiotomy patients: the role of organic and psychiatric factors. N Engl J Med 284:518–520, 1971

Levkoff SE, Besdine RW, Wetle T: Acute confusional states (delirium) in the hospitalized elderly. Ann Rev Gerontol Geriatr 6:1–26, 1986

Lipowski ZJ: Delirium, clouding of consciousness and confusion. J Nerv Ment Dis 145:227–255, 1967

Lipowski ZJ: Organic brain syndromes: a reformulation. Compr Psychiatry 19:309–322, 1978

Lipowski ZJ: Delirium: Acute Brain Failure in Man. Springfield, IL, Charles C Thomas, 1980a

Lipowski ZJ: Delirium updated. Compr Psychiatry 21: 190–196, 1980b

Lipowski ZJ: Delirium: Acute Confusional States. New York, Oxford University Press, 1990

MacKenzie TB, Popkin MK: Stress response syndrome occurring after delirium. Am J Psychiatry 137:1433–1435, 1980

Menza M, Murray G, Holmes V, et al: Decreased extrapyramidal symptoms with intravenous haloperidol. J Clin Psychiatry 48:278–280, 1987

Mesulam M-M: Attention, confusional states, and neglect, in Principles of Behavioral Neurology. Edited by Mesulam M-M. Philadelphia, PA, FA Davis, 1985, pp 125–168

Moore DP: Rapid treatment of delirium in critically ill patients. Am J Psychiatry 134:1431–1432, 1977

Mori E, Yamadori A: Acute confusional state and acute agitated delirium. Arch Neurol 44:1139–1143, 1987

Nelson A, Fogel B, Faust D, et al: Bedside cognitive screening instruments: a critical assessment. J Nerv Ment Dis 174:73–83, 1986

Nussmeier N, Arlund C, Slogoff S: Neuropsychiatric complications after cardiopulmonary bypass: cerebral protection by a barbiturate. Anesthesiology 64(2):165–170, 1986

Patten S, Lamarre C: Dysgraphia (letter). Can J Psychiatry 34:746, 1989

Perry S: Organic mental disorders caused by HIV: update on early diagnosis and treatment. Am J Psychiatry 147: 696–710, 1990

Peura DA, Johnson LF: Cimetidine for prevention and treatment of gastroduodenal mucosal lesions in patients in an intensive care unit. Ann Intern Med 103: 173–177, 1985

Pro JD, Wells CE: The use of the electroencephalogram in the diagnosis of delirium. Diseases of the Nervous System 38:804–808, 1977

Prugh DG, Wagonfeld S, Metcalf D, et al: A clinical study of delirium in children and adolescents. Psychosom Med 42 (suppl):177–197, 1980

Purdie F, Honigman B, Rosen P: Acute organic brain syndrome: a review of 100 cases. Ann Emerg Med 10:455–461, 1981

Rabins PV, Folstein MF: Delirium and dementia: diagnostic criteria and fatality rates. Br J Psychiatry 140:149–153, 1982

Reivich M, Abass A: Positron Emission Tomography. New York, Alan R Liss, 1985

Resnick M, Burton B: Droperidol vs. haloperidol in the initial management of acutely agitated patients. J Clin Psychiatry 45:298–299, 1984

Rogers M, Liang M, Daltroy L: Delirium after elective orthopedic surgery: risk factors and natural history. Int J Psychiatry Med 19:109–121, 1989

Romano J, Engel GL: Delirium, I: electroencephalographic data. Archives of Neurology and Psychiatry 51:356–377, 1944

Roth M: The natural history of mental disorder in old age. Journal of Mental Science 101:281–301, 1955

Smith L, Dimsdale J: Postcardiotomy delirium: conclusions after 25 years? Am J Psychiatry 146:452–458, 1989

Sos J, Cassem NH: Managing postoperative agitation. Drug Therapy 10(3):103–106, 1980

Task Force Sponsored by the National Institute on Aging: Senility reconsidered. JAMA 244:259–263, 1980

Tesar GE, Murray GB, Cassem NH: Use of high-dose intravenous haloperidol in the treatment of agitated cardiac patients. J Clin Psychopharmacol 5:344–347, 1985

Titchener JL, Swerling I, Gottschalk L, et al: Psychosis in surgical patients. Surg Gynecol Obstet 102:59–65, 1956

Trzepacz P, Teague G, Lipowski Z: Delirium and other organic mental disorders in a general hospital. Gen Hosp Psychiatry 7:101–106, 1985

Trzepacz P, Baker R, Greenhouse J: A symptom rating scale for delirium. Psychiatry Res 23:89–97, 1988

Tufo HM, Ostfeld AM, Shekelle R: Central nervous system dysfunction following open-heart surgery. JAMA 212: 1333–1340, 1970

Tune LE, Dainlouh NF, Holland A, et al: Association of postoperative delirium with raised serum levels of anticholinergic drugs. Lancet 2:651–653, 1981

Varsamis J, Zuchowski T, Maini KK: Survival rates and causes of death in geriatric psychiatric patients: a six-year follow-up study. Canadian Psychiatric Association Journal 17:17–21, 1972

Weddington WW: The mortality of delirium: an underappreciated problem? Psychosomatics 23:1232–1235, 1982

Wells CE, Duncan GW: Neurology for Psychiatrists. Philadelphia, PA, FA Davis, 1980

Wilson LM: Intensive care delirium. Arch Intern Med 130: 225–226, 1972

Wise MG: Delirium, in The American Psychiatric Press Textbook of Neuropsychiatry. Edited by Hales RE, Yudofsky SC, Washington DC, American Psychiatric Press, 1987, pp 89–1O5

Zubek JP, Welch G: Electroencephalographic changes after prolonged sensory and perceptual deprivation. Science 139:1209–1210, 1963

❑ APPENDIX 12–1

MINI-MENTAL STATE EXAM AND INSTRUCTIONS

Patient ____________________

Examiner ____________________

Date ____________________

Mini-Mental State Exam

Maximum score	Score	
		Orientation
5	( )	What is the (year) (season) (date) (day) (month)?
5	( )	Where are we: (state) (county) (town) (hospital) (floor)?
		Registration
3	( )	Name 3 objects: 1 second to say each. Then ask the patient all 3 after you have said them. Give 1 point for each correct answer. Then repeat them until he learns all 3. Count trials and record. Trials ____________________
		Attention and Calculation
5	( )	Serial 7s. 1 point for each correct. Stop after 5 answers. Alternatively spell "world" backwards.
		Recall
3	( )	Ask for the 3 objects repeated above. Give 1 point for each correct.
		Language
9	( )	Name a pencil, and watch (2 points) Repeat the following "No ifs, ands, or buts." (1 point) Follow a 3-stage command: "Take a paper in your right hand, fold it in half, and put it on the floor" (3 points) Read and obey the following: **Close your eyes** (1 point) Write a sentence (1 point) Copy design (1 point) Total score ASSESS level of consciousness along a continuum

Alert	Drowsy	Stupor	Coma

APPENDIX 12–1 (Continued)

INSTRUCTIONS FOR ADMINISTRATION OF MINI-MENTAL STATE EXAM

Orientation

1. Ask for the date. Then ask specifically for parts omitted, e.g., "Can you also tell me what season it is?" One point for each correct.
2. Ask in turn "Can you tell me the name of this hospital?" (town, county, etc.). One point for each correct.

Registration

Ask the patient if you may test his memory. Then say the names of 3 unrelated objects, clearly and slowly, about one second for each. After you have said all 3, ask him to repeat them. This first repetition determines his score (0–3) but keep saying them until he can repeat all 3, up to 6 trials. If he does not eventually learn all 3, recall cannot be meaningfully tested.

Attention and Calculation

Ask the patient to begin with 100 and count backwards by 7. Stop after 5 subtractions (93, 86, 79, 72, 65). Score the total number of correct answers.

If the patient cannot or will not perform this task, ask him to spell the word "world" backwards. The score is the number of letters in correct order, e.g., dlrow = 5, dlorw = 3.

Recall

Ask the patient if he can recall the 3 words you previously asked him to remember. Score 0–3.

Language

Naming: Show the patient a wrist watch and ask him what it is. Repeat for pencil. Score 0–2.

Repetition: Ask the patient to repeat the sentence after you. Allow only one trial. Score 0 or 1.

3-Stage command: Give the patient a piece of plain blank paper and repeat the command. Score 1 point for each part correctly executed.

Reading: On a blank piece of paper print the sentence "Close your eyes", in letters large enough for the patient to see clearly. Ask him to read it and do what it says. Score 1 point only if he actually closes his eyes.

Writing: Give the patient a blank piece of paper and ask him to write a sentence for you. Do not dictate a sentence; it is to be written spontaneously. It must contain a subject and verb and be sensible. Correct grammar and punctuation are not necessary.

Copying: On a clean piece of paper, draw intersecting pentagons, each side about 1 in., and ask him to copy it exactly as it is. All 10 angles must be present and 2 must intersect to score 1 point. Tremor and rotation are ignored.

Estimate the patient's level of sensorium along a continuum, from alert on the left to coma on the right.

Source. Reprinted from Folstein MF, Folstein SE, McHugh PR: Mini-Mental State: a practical method for grading the cognitive state of patients for the clinician. J Psychiatr Res 12:189–198, 1975.

Chapter

13

Neuropsychiatric Aspects of Aphasia and Related Language Impairments

D. Frank Benson, M.D.

ALTHOUGH NOT THE MOST common neuropsychiatric problem, aphasia is such a dramatic and devastating disorder that it ranks among the most thoroughly investigated of human behavioral alterations. By definition, aphasia is *the loss or impairment of language caused by brain damage. Language,* the key word in the definition, pertains to the ability to handle (decode, encode, and interpret) the symbols used within a cultural group for the communication of information, feelings, and thoughts. Inherent in the definition is that aphasia is acquired; language function must have been present and then impaired by brain disorder. In most instances focal structural damage is the source of the impairment.

It has been estimated that between 300,000 and 400,000 individuals sustain a cerebrovascular accident (CVA) annually, that about 40% of CVAs produce some degree of aphasia, and that about half of these individuals sustain permanent language disability. Two other common problems—intracranial neoplasm and traumatic brain injury—also produce language disturbance. More than 100,000 Americans acquire aphasia each year, and, because the underlying disorders are often stable, their numbers accumulate over the years. Aphasia represents a numerically prominent and behaviorally significant cause of chronic medical disability.

Aphasia has obvious psychiatric consequences, both immediate and for long-term management. The problems of the aphasic patient encompass the entire spectrum of neuropsychiatry, from the circumscribed effects of focal brain destruction on linguistic processing through emotional and motivational problems based on disordered subcortical networks to the personal predicaments produced by the considerable change in life-style. In addition, aphasia produces serious problems for the caregiver, family members, friends, business associates, and social acquaintances. Appreciation of the problem at only one level is manifestly inadequate.

Although aphasia has been studied for over a century and sizable, formal subspecialties have arisen to study the anatomical-language correlations and to treat the language disorder, relatively little attention has been paid to the psychiatric complications. Little more than sympathy and superficial support have been available for most aphasic patients and their families, and yet the neuropsychiatric complications are often crucial to the well-being and ultimate outcome of the aphasic condition.

❑ BACKGROUND

History

Although the formal history of aphasia is relatively short, it evolved from several millennia of speculation about language and thought. The study of acquired language impairment has proved to be a fruitful means of bridging these entities. Individual cases of aphasia were described in antiquity and additional cases recorded through the centuries (Benton and Joynt 1960), but all current approaches to aphasia stem from 1861 when Broca presented the first clinical-anatomical correlation of aphasia. Broca's methodology was successful, a powerful technique for the study of mental functions. Since 1861 a vast literature has been accumulated, multiple observations have been collected, and numerous theories of language function have evolved. Many reviews of this fascinating early history are available (Benson 1979; Brain 1961; Freud 1891; Head 1926; Hécaen and Albert 1978; Kertesz 1979; Lecours and Lhermitte 1983; Weisenburg and McBride 1935). For this chapter the historical base will be severely abridged and presented as four separate but interrelated epochs.

With Broca's original description (1861) of a patient who had lost the ability to speak and demonstration that a focal brain injury involved the frontal region, a novel technique—the correlation of clinical behavior with a focal brain defect—became available. Broca's observations were rapidly replicated and, in some instances, refuted. A body of clinical and anatomical data developed. Important observations, particularly the dominance of the human left hemisphere for language function (Broca 1865), were established, and after Wernicke (1874) an anterior-posterior dichotomy of language function was solidly demonstrated. Many investigators (Bastian 1898; Henschen 1922; Kleist 1934; Lichtheim 1885) presented classifications of brain-language correlations, often based on individual case observations. With limited exception, all language functions were localized to the cerebral cortex and were diagrammed in a phrenological, mosaic manner (Figure 13–1). The various classifications did not agree in nomenclature and, not infrequently, were based on individual case studies that could not be replicated.

The second epoch was a reaction against the mechanical dictum that a focal brain lesion produces a specific clinical finding. Early investigators (Freud 1891; Jackson 1864) raised arguments against strict localization, but it was Marie (1906), stating that Broca's original patient was not aphasic and presenting a holistic theory of language function, who prevailed. For half a century Marie's thesis of a single aphasia was championed by many investigators including Head (1926), Pick (1931), Weisenburg and McBride (1935), Wepman (1951), Bay (1964a), Schuell et al. (1964), and Critchley (1970). The holistic approach reached its acme in the 1960s when Bay (1964a), Schuell et al. (1964), Wepman (1961), and Brown (1968), among others, championed brain-language theories featuring a central language area, vaguely localized to the thalamus. Aphasia was the product of a disordered central language area with clinical variation based on damage to surrounding areas carrying out basic functions (e.g., auditory, visual, and motor) (Figure 13–2). Language was considered a single, unitary, nondivisible function.

The third major epoch in the history of aphasia came in the 1960s and was strongly influenced by Geschwind's rediscovery and powerful demonstration (1965) that separation (disconnection) of cortical areas could produce distinctive language impairments. Material from the 19th-century continental aphasia classifications was reinstituted and then correlated with improved clinical and laboratory studies. The 19th-century localizationist approach was reborn (Figure 13–3) and continues (Alexander and Benson 1991; Kirshner 1986).

A fourth epoch stemmed from and accompanied the third but has produced a far broader and more divergent approach to aphasia. Concomitant

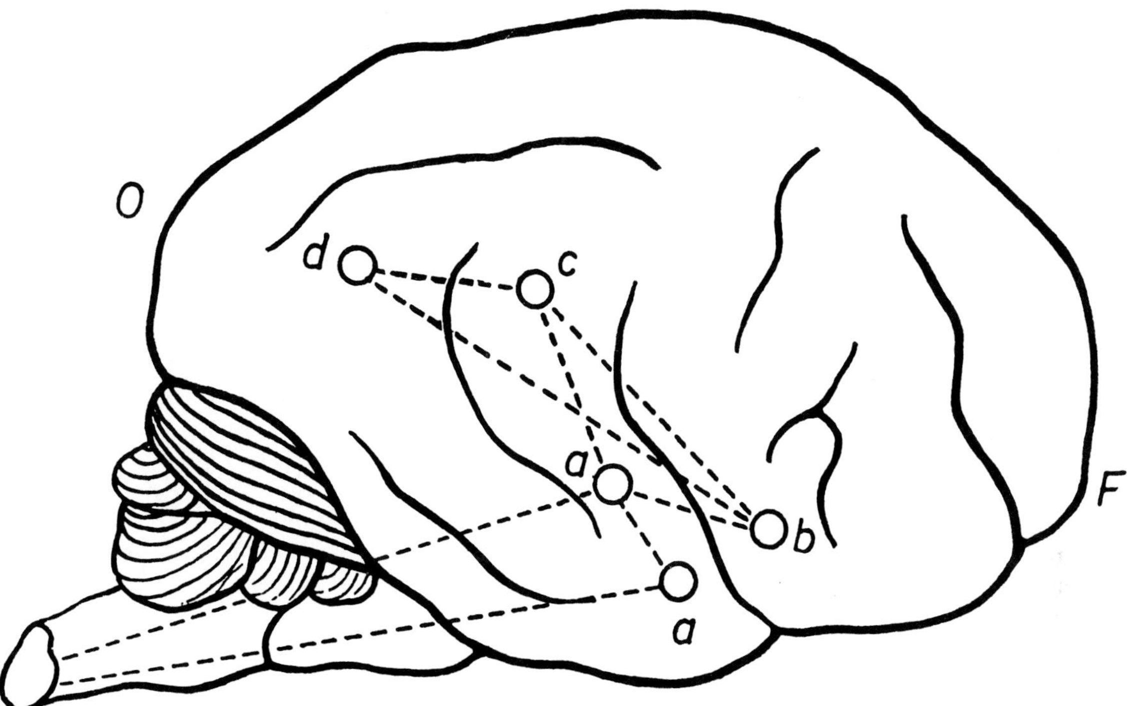

Figure 13–1. Wernicke's diagram of language centers and pathways; a = auditory centers; b = motor speech centers; c and d are central language processing areas; F = frontal; O = occipital.

with renewed interest in the localizationist approach, the field of neuropsychology expanded, major advances occurred in linguistics (neurolinguistics and psycholinguistics), computer-based artificial intelligence studies were started, and cognitive science was born. Assessment and delineation of language disorders were greatly enhanced. During these same years, the ability to image the brain of a living individual was born and developed. Radioisotope brain scans gave way to X-ray computerized tomographs, magnetic resonance images, and isotope computed tomographs to provide greatly improved anatomical correlates for the new language observations. Greater or lesser degrees of the localizationist approach to language were incorporated in these studies to greatly enrich both approaches. Although some (e.g., linguistics and artificial intelligence) have become increasingly theoretical, each adds observations and factual data to the growing body of information concerning language functions in the brain. The study of aphasia has been and remains a rich source of information of pertinence to human behavior.

Terminology and Classification

> Aphasiology . . . became precociously addicted to the game of linguistic ambiguities. More than any other medical discipline, with the possible exception of psychiatry, aphasia generated and tolerated (apparent) terminological confusions in its own vocabulary and, particularly, in its classification. (Lecours et al. 1983b, p. 243)

The study of aphasia has been plagued by terms invented to describe variations in language disorder and classifications invented to contain the described entities. Head (1926) described the situation as "chaos," then compounded the problem with a totally different classification using elementary linguistic terminology. In the second epoch, the classification problem was solved by simply declaring that all aphasia represented a single, holistic entity, but this approach proved inadequate. Subdivisions based on severity (Schuell et al. 1964), developmental regression (Wepman and Jones 1961), the effects of neighborhood findings (Brown 1968), and others were created. These steps not only increased the

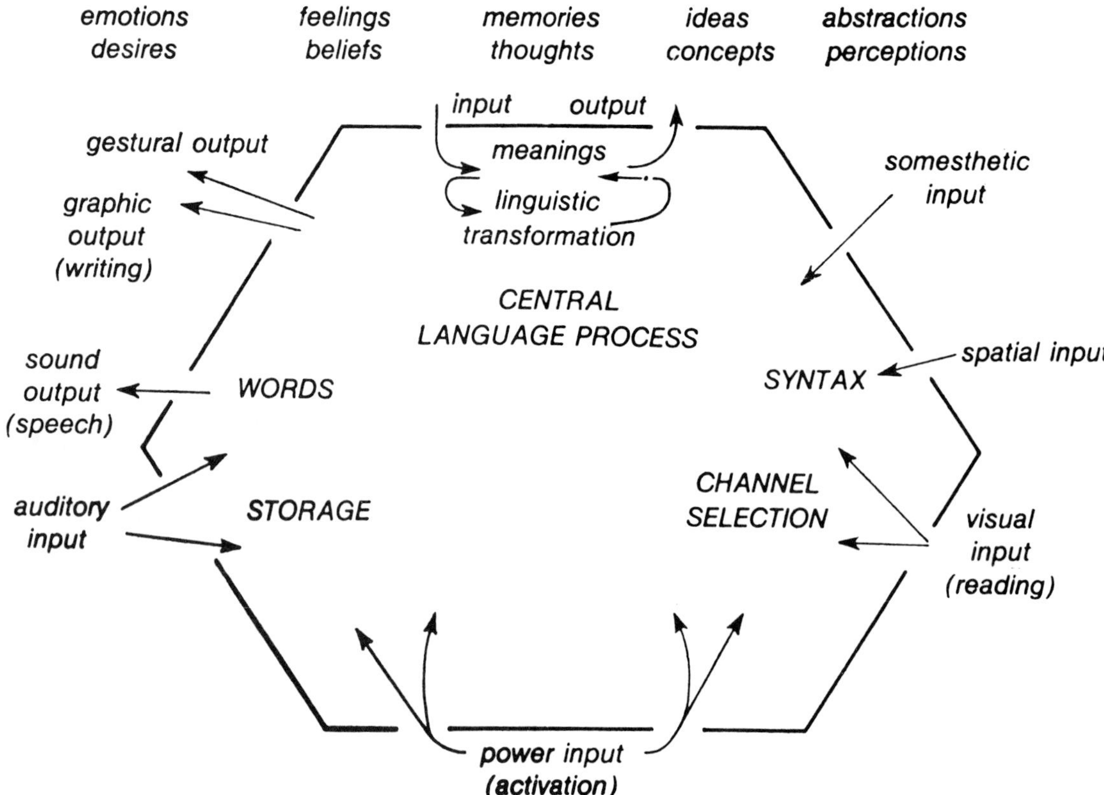

Figure 13–2. Hypothetical model of cerebral mechanisms of speech—attributed to J. R. Brown. (Reprinted from Maruszewski M: Language, Communication and the Brain. The Hague, Mouton, 1975. Used with permission.)

terminological-classification confusion but also limited interest in the study of aphasia for many decades. Although it was obvious that a finite, indeed a limited, number of clinical variations were being described (Howes 1964), dozens of aphasia classifications tended to produce a cacophony of terminology (Benson 1979; Kertesz 1979).

One accomplishment of the third epoch was reintroduction, augmentation, and clarification of the 19th-century classification efforts (Benson and Geschwind 1971). Primarily the work of the Boston Aphasia Group, the establishment of a practical classification with consistent terms based on clinical and anatomical correlates provided a stable structure for later investigations. Although imperfect, the syndrome classification outlined by the Boston group remains the core of both clinical and academic studies of aphasia. Table 13–1 presents an abridged version of this classification with the major language abnormalities, basic neurological dysfunctions, and characteristic anatomical findings associated with each syndrome. Only a bare listing of the basic language and neurological findings of the more common syndromes can be presented in this chapter. Detailed descriptions are available in some neurological textbooks and in a number of texts dedicated to aphasiology and behavioral neurology (Benson 1979; Heilman and Valenstein 1979; Kertesz 1979; Kirshner 1986; Lecours et al. 1983a; Mesulam 1985).

It must be emphasized that the entities outlined in Table 13–1 and discussed here are syndromes, not disease entities. A *syndrome*, by definition, is a collection of clinical findings that, when occurring together, suggest a specific disorder to a physician. Paraphrasing that definition, a *syndrome* is a fantasy devised by the clinician seeking order in the plethora of clinical findings presented by a patient. A syndrome is not a real entity; it is not fixed and does not have constant constituents. All aphasic patients vary in symptom presentation, and yet, for most of them, one syndrome better describes the clinical status than do the others. The syndromes of aphasia

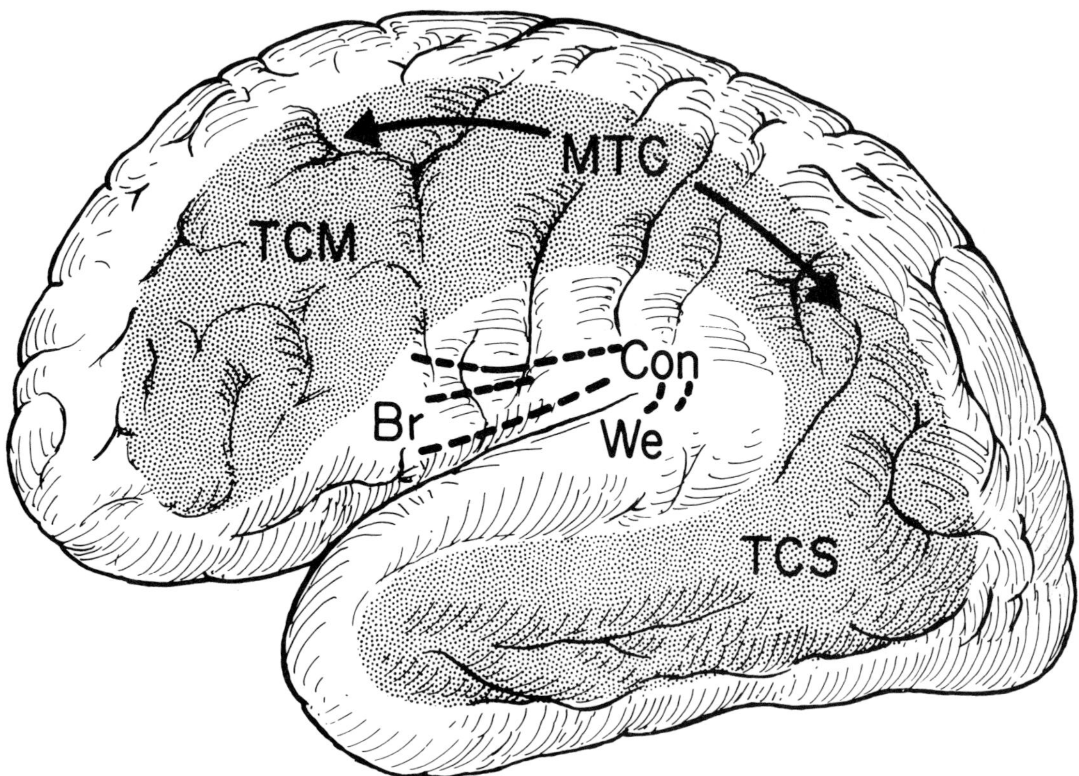

Figure 13–3. Outline of left lateral hemisphere outlining central (*clear*, perisylvian) and outer, border zone language areas (*stippled*). The letters indicate most common situation of structural pathology in the syndromes of aphasia. Br = Broca's area; We = Wernicke's area; Con = supramarginal gyrus–conduction aphasia; TCM, TCS, and MTC demarcate areas most involved in cases of transcortical motor, transcortical sensory, and mixed transcortical aphasias, respectively. (Reprinted from Benson DF, Geschwind N: The aphasias and related disturbances, in Clinical Neurology, Vol 1. Edited by Baker AB, Joynt R. Philadelphia, PA, Harper & Row, 1985, Chapter 10, pp 1–34. Used with permission.)

were invented by the 19th-century investigators on the basis of postmortem correlations. Contemporary neurologists, matching advanced localization techniques with clinical observations, have both supported and corrected the early observations linking brain damage locus to specific language syndromes (Alexander and Benson 1991; Benson and Geschwind 1971; Kertesz 1979). The original syndrome classification of aphasia was upheld and strengthened by the introduction of new brain-imaging techniques. It remains the gold standard for aphasia deliberations.

Syndromes of Aphasia

Broca's aphasia. The best known syndrome of language impairment—Broca's aphasia—is an acquired disorder with strikingly nonfluent verbal output (sparse, effortful, dysarthric, dysprosodic, short-phrase length, and agrammatic) with relatively preserved comprehension (relational words may be poorly understood), distinct disturbance in repetition and naming, usually a disturbance in reading (again, it is the relational and syntactic words that are not understood), and striking disturbance in writing. Most patients with Broca's aphasia have a right-sided weakness, varying from mild paresis to total hemiplegia, and some have mild sensory loss. The pathology involves the dominant hemisphere frontal opercular area. If the lesion is superficial and involves only cortex, the prognosis for improvement is good. If, however, the lesion extends sufficiently deep to involve the basal ganglia and internal capsule, the language defect tends to be permanent.

TABLE 13–1. APHASIA SYNDROMES

	Major language characteristics						*Major neurological characteristics*			
Syndrome	*Spontaneous speech*	*Repetition*	*Comprehension*	*Naming*	*Reading*	*Writing*	*Motor*	*Sensory*	*Visual field*	*Site of pathology (dominant hemisphere)*
Broca	NF	0	+	±	0	0	0	±	++	Posterior inferior frontal lobe
Wernicke	F, P	0	0	0	0	0	++	±	±	Posterior superior temporal lobe
Conduction	F, P	0	++	±	+	±	+	±	+	Deep to supramarginal gyrus
Global	NF	0	0	0	0	0	0	0	0	Combinations of above three
Transcortical motor	NF	+	++	±	+	0	0	+	++	Frontal, anterior, or superior to Broca's area
Transcortical sensory	F	+	0	0	0	0	+	0	0	Parietal-temporal junction
Transcortical mixed	NF	+	0	0	0	0	0	0	0	Combination of above two
Anomic	F	+	+	0	±	±	±	±	±	Multiple sites
Subcortical	F, P, or NF, P	+	±	±	±	±	±	±	±	Putamen and thalamus

Note. NF = nonfluent; F = fluent; P = paraphasic; ++ = normal; + = relatively normal; ± = variable; 0 = abnormal.
Source. Reprinted from Benson DF: Aphasia managment: the neurologist's role, in Seminars in Speech, Language and Hearing, Vol 2. Edited by Wertz RT. New York, Thieme-Stratton, 1981, pp 237–247. Used with permission.

Wernicke's aphasia. Named for the person who first described it, Wernicke's aphasia features a fluent verbal output with normal word count and phrase length; no effort, articulatory problems, or prosodic difficulties; but difficulty in word finding and frequent paraphasic substitutions. The most striking abnormality of Wernicke's aphasia is a disturbance of comprehension, which may range from a total inability to understand spoken language (word deafness) to a partial difficulty in understanding. The ability to repeat reflects the limitations of comprehension. Often there are no basic neurological defects, but a superior quadrantopia may be present. Pathology involves the posterior superior temporal lobe of the dominant hemisphere (the auditory association cortex) and, in some cases, the primary auditory sensory area.

Conduction aphasia. Conduction aphasia, a relatively common disorder, features a fluent verbal output and good ability to comprehend, but severe disturbance in repetition. Paraphasias are common, particularly substitutions of phonemes. Naming tends to be limited by paraphasic intrusions. Reading aloud is severely disturbed, but reading comprehension may be fully normal. Writing is often abnormal. Most cases of conduction aphasia have pathology involving anterior inferior parietal lobe (supramarginal gyrus) (Damasio and Damasio 1980), but exceptions are recognized (Mendez and Benson 1985). Paresis and visual field defects are variable, but cortical sensory loss is frequently present.

Global aphasia. A severe language impairment in which all modalities—verbal output, comprehension, repetition, naming, reading, and writing—are seriously impaired is known as *global* or *total aphasia*. Most often this is caused by a total middle cerebral artery occlusion, although exceptions are noted, including some in which there is global aphasia with no hemiparesis or other basic neurological disturbance.

Transcortical aphasias. The major factor underlying the transcortical aphasias is preservation of the ability to repeat spoken language in the face of distinct language impairment. *Transcortical motor aphasia* is an anterior aphasia, resembling Broca's aphasia except for a normal or near-normal ability to repeat. Pathology is most frequently seen in the supplementary motor area of the dominant hemisphere or in the frontal tissues between that region and the dominant hemisphere opercular area. *Transcortical sensory aphasia* features significant comprehension disorder, a fluent paraphasic verbal output, and good ability to repeat. The normal repetition demonstrates that heard language is processed but cannot be interpreted. The most common site of pathology in transcortical sensory aphasia is in the dominant parietal region (angular gyrus). *Mixed transcortical aphasia,* also known as *isolation of the speech area,* features a combination of the motor and sensory forms: the patient has a global aphasia except for preservation of the ability to repeat. Pathology in the mixed transcortical syndrome involves the vascular border zone area in both the frontal and parietal lobes.

Anomic aphasia. A common residual following improvement from other types of aphasia has been called anomic aphasia. In this syndrome the primary problem concerns difficulty with word finding causing multiple pauses, a tendency to circumlocution, and a somewhat stumbling verbal output. The verbal output is fluent with repetition and comprehension relatively intact, but naming to confrontation is significantly disturbed. Many individuals with anomic aphasia also have reading and writing disturbance (alexia and agraphia). There is no specific location for pathology, although pathology often involves the dominant hemisphere angular gyrus. In this situation, anomic aphasia can be considered a lesser degree of transcortical sensory aphasia.

Subcortical aphasia. With the advent of brain imaging, particularly computed tomography (CT) scans, it became apparent that subcortical lesions (hemorrhage or infarction) could produce an acute aphasic syndrome, but the symptomatology varied considerably depending on the subcortical anatomical structures involved. Most subcortical aphasias are initiated by a period of mutism followed by a period of abnormal motor speech (hypophonia and articulatory problems), with either fluent or nonfluent output with many paraphasias. In contrast, repetition is near normal (without paraphasia), although comprehension, naming, reading, and writing may or may not show abnormality. If the lesion is entirely subcortical, a tendency for recovery is strong; many individuals recover totally from the aphasia but are left with residual speech impairments. If there is concomitant cortical involvement, aphasia may persist.

In addition to the classic aphasias (almost always based on left-hemisphere damage), several disturbances affecting communication can result from right-hemisphere damage. Two of these produce psychiatrically significant symptomatology.

Amelodia (also called affective motor aprosodia) is a disturbance characterized by a flat, monotonous verbal output; inability to produce a melody when singing; decreased facial grimacing; and sparse use of gestures. The result is an emotionless response, easily misinterpreted as depression. Originally described as a right-hemisphere language dysfunction (Ross and Mesulam 1979) and later considered a defect in prosody (Ross 1981), the disorder is most clearly defined by the loss of melody (amelodia) in verbal output and singing. Numerous cases have been reported including some associated with significant depression (Ross and Rush 1981). Pathology invariably involves the right frontal opercular area or its connections, the right-hemisphere equivalent of Broca's area. Inasmuch as the causative lesion (usually a CVA) may be small and otherwise silent, the apparently depressed subject with inability to produce melody deserves special consideration. CT or magnetic resonance imaging will usually confirm presence of the lesion and direct the physician toward appropriate therapy.

Verbal dysdecorum, a newly described phenomenon (Alexander et al. 1989), features decreased ability to monitor and control the contents of verbal output. Individuals with verbal dysdecorum speak too freely, discuss improper topics, make snide or cruel (but often true) remarks about themselves and others, argue, and are otherwise disagreeable without realizing the social consequences of their conversations. There is a tendency for these patients to confabulate. Often these patients' presenting complaint is an inability to maintain friendships; even a short exposure to such an individual identifies the problem. Verbal dysdecorum may or may not be associated with physical impropriety. Current evidence suggests a right-hemisphere frontal, probably lateral convexity, site of pathology (Alexander et al. 1989). Although language itself is not defective in verbal dysdecorum, the serious psychological problems caused by poorly monitored output have an organic source. Demonstration of the pathology and correction of any problem likely to produce further brain damage should be part of psychiatric therapy; remediation of the defect is difficult.

❑ NEUROPSYCHIATRIC ASPECTS OF APHASIA

The sudden loss of the ability to use language for communication has obvious consequences and has been the subject of a range of psychological investigations and interpretations. Early aphasia treatment (Wepman 1951) focused on psychogenic support (sympathy and understanding), an approach that remains valuable. Relatively little attention, however, has been given to psychiatric care for the aphasic patient, in part based on the communication disability. Aphasia is obviously "organic," not psychogenic, and the language disorder interferes with verbal communication. Both factors excluded aphasic patients from the "talk therapy" approach of mid-20th-century psychiatry, and aphasia has been largely ignored by psychiatrists. Psychological considerations, however, often prove crucial to the outcome of aphasia rehabilitation and are almost invariably significant in long-term care. Some of the problems are general and can be termed *psychosocial*; some are directly related to the type of aphasia (neurobehavioral).

Psychosocial Aspects

Altered life-style. An important but easily overlooked factor that affects most individuals with acquired aphasia stems from the sudden, unexpected, and truly calamitous alteration of life-style produced by the language disorder. Any impairment of language function is disturbing, but in many aphasic patients the magnitude of language loss, particularly in the early stages, is overwhelming. Language is such a basic human function that, in shock value, its acute loss ranks with sudden blindness, quadriplegia, or the diagnosis of an incurable disease. Along with the sudden loss of this critical function, many of the stabilizing factors of personal existence are lost. Employment status, social and family position, recreational opportunities, and physical and sexual status are all threatened. The sudden onset of aphasia is catastrophic, and the acute change in life-style caused by the disorder produces massive psychosocial problems.

Threatened economic status. Of real concern for many aphasic individuals is a serious alteration of economic status. Aphasia often occurs at an age when a person's earning capacity is near its prime;

most are comparatively independent and self-sufficient when the disorder occurs. Suddenly, this desirable status disappears, and even though medical and disability insurance, family savings, and other sources of income may be available, a growing awareness that economic independence is permanently lost can be a crushing blow. Real problems of financial solvency loom for many. Financial problems become a matter of deep concern and may produce, by themselves, a serious psychological threat.

Social position. Another matter of concern for the aphasic individual concerns altered position in society. Most aphasic individuals have established fixed, relatively secure patterns in both employment and social activities by the time they become aphasic. Well-established relationships with co-workers, employees, neighbors, social and recreational associates, and many others in their social community have been developed. This status changes abruptly with the onset of aphasia. The changes in social status do not occur immediately, and realization of the degree of change may not be recognized for some time after onset. Eventually, however, the real change in social position produced by the disorder represents an important psychosocial vexation for the aphasic individual.

Family position. In a similar manner, aphasia produces an alteration of family status. Most individuals who become aphasic have developed a stable role in a family setting, either as the true leader or as a major contributor to family activities. If the language disturbance is relatively mild, the aphasic individual may retain or eventually regain previous status within the family, but when the language disturbance is more severe, the spouse or some other family member must assume much of the leadership, decision-making role. Aphasia can place an individual in a passive, childlike position within the family. He or she may need help from the family to carry out everyday activities, and most family decisions are made by the spouse. Not infrequently, the reaction to this downgrading of family status is violent, with negative, hostile, paranoid, and downright cruel behavior directed toward close family members. Realization by the patient that his or her position within the family is altered is often delayed after the onset of aphasia, and, if family members intelligently and carefully manage the situation, adverse reactions may be minimized.

Unfortunately, many (perhaps most) families are incapable of gracefully carrying out this alteration. The spouse often feels and expresses anger and hostility because of decreased income, altered social position, and the many added responsibilities. Instead of providing support for the aphasic patient, family members may become additional vexations for the patient's psychological affliction. Alteration (in most cases deterioration) of family position affects most aphasic individuals and represents a significant behavioral factor.

Physical status. Some (not all) aphasic individuals suffer significant alterations in physical capability. A previously active, self-caring individual may become hemiparetic, must learn to stand and to walk again, and can never again hope to participate freely in physical activities such as athletics, dancing, hiking, or even just walking. Serious but less obvious functional changes are common and just as disabling. Balance insecurity, visual field defect, unilateral attention disorder, paresthesias, vague or not-so-vague pain, epileptic seizures, the need for major medical or surgical treatments, and many other physical problems plague the aphasic patient. Physical disability routinely demands a considerably more confined life-style than previously enjoyed. The onus of physical impairment, the threat of additional impairment, and the demonstration of one's mortal status hang heavily. Physical disability produces a significant psychological distress that affects self-esteem.

Recreational status. Physical disability, communication problems, concern for underlying disease processes, and similar problems force most newly aphasic individuals to change their established recreational patterns. Demanding physical activities (e.g., hunting, hiking, swimming, tennis, golf, and bowling) may be precluded by physical problems; less demanding activities (e.g., card games, reading, and going to parties) may not be possible or enjoyable because of communication disability. For a normally active adult, the physical limitations of the postaphasic state produce aggravating adjustment problems.

Sexual status. Not to be overlooked among the psychological problems of the aphasic individual is the real or imagined loss of sexual capability. Aphasia-producing pathology does not, by itself, affect sexual competency in most individuals. Nonetheless, a major degree of paralysis, an inability to communicate accurately, and an underlying uncertainty of residual sexual competency hinder healthy sexual relationships. Many aphasic individuals silently suspect that they will never regain sexual prowess, a belief frequently shared by the spouse. In most instances the acquired lack of sexuality is physiologically unfounded, but if both partners believe the situation is real, normal sexual responses are discouraged. Not infrequently, the spouse refuses to partake in sexual activities based on fear of causing additional brain damage. Sexual maladjustment may be a significant problem and is often hidden from and almost routinely overlooked by physicians and therapists.

Neurobehavioral Aspects

Concomitant with the alterations in psychosocial status, the brain of an aphasic patient has undergone structural damage, and the subsequent alteration of function can produce significant neuropsychiatric findings. For convenience, brain-damage findings are discussed here in two segments: one describing a more general disability present in the early postonset stages and the other outlining anatomically based psychiatric syndromes appearing later.

Early neurobehavioral alterations. If the brain insult is sufficiently large the patient with aphasia is often lethargic and/or confused in the early stage. Appropriate medical care can correct life-threatening situations within hours or days, but a considerably more prolonged period ensues in which the aphasic patient fails to fully realize the alterations that have occurred. A combination of decreased mental functioning (clouding of consciousness) and disturbed language decoding capability (comprehension defect) is present.

Over a period of days to weeks, the clouding of consciousness will clear, leaving an alert patient who remains unaware of the full extent of the problem. Although responsive, the patient does not grasp the meaning of the language defect (or of paralysis, if present) and fails to show appropriate concern. Although not truly denying disability, many aphasic patients in this stage are unable (rather than unwilling) to monitor their own defects and to see the problem in appropriate perspective. The early unawareness-unconcern stage protects the patient and makes the initial period somewhat easier for family and friends. At this stage, however, the patient cannot participate rationally in plans for the future because of decreased reality appreciation. In some patients with aphasia, particularly those with large posterior dominant-hemisphere lesions, disturbed language comprehension is long lasting, but for most the realization problem disappears, sometimes rather acutely, and can lead directly into a reactive depression.

Because of the many losses incurred, it would appear appropriate for an aphasic patient to enter a period of bereavement, a grief reaction. Losses involving most life activities depress self-image. Feelings of self-deprecation and worthlessness may lead to a severe dysphoria. As a rule, however, such feelings do not develop immediately with the onset of acquired language impairment. In many such patients these feelings build over a variable period after onset of aphasia, and the interval may be extended, measured in weeks or even months.

It could be expected that most aphasic patients would, at some stage, experience a period of reactive depression, but the problem is far from universal. In fact, the observer would anticipate that the problems of disordered self-image should be considerably greater than is apparent in many aphasic patients. In many cases the discrepancy (an apparent lack of personal concern) reflects a degree of mental deterioration caused by brain injury, a disturbance of self-awareness. The absence of depressive reaction cannot be automatically accepted as a product of intrinsic ego strength. Reactive depression never becomes serious for many aphasic patients, but some do develop a characteristic depression featuring intense feelings of personal worthlessness and hopelessness.

The reaction typically starts with feelings of futility that lead to an unwillingness to participate in self-care or rehabilitation activities. During the episode the aphasic patient may sink deeply within himself or herself; stop eating; refuse social interaction with therapists, with other patients, or even with family members; and manifest a strong but passive noncooperation. Withdrawal and negativism are the key features. In some instances the negative reaction may become intense, a catastrophic reaction (Goldstein 1948). The aphasic patient may cry and moan for hours, the reaction vigorously accentuated by any effort to divert attention or provide emotional support. The patient may forcefully avoid attention, refuse to eat or take medications, and actively fight off therapists, attendants, and family. The reaction may be sufficient to produce exhaustion and actually represent a threat to the patient's health.

Catastrophic reactions are rare, however, and need not occur. Awareness of the onset of a reactive depression in an aphasic patient should immediately be followed by strong, radical support measures. Challenging therapies (e.g., language, occupational, and physical) should be halted and replaced by activities that the patient can perform successfully. Praise for success can be given, but, more important, the patient should not be allowed to fail, particularly at tasks that would be considered simple and mundane in normal life. The real treatment of a catastrophic reaction is prophylactic: recognition of the aphasic patient's increasing awareness of the deficits and avoidance of damaging failures.

Critical to treatment of reactive depression are early recognition and prompt response. Hospital personnel and family members who deal with the patient should be alerted to the possibility, and, at the first sign of negativism, withdrawal, sleep problems, poor appetite, and so on, countermeasures should be taken. Reactive depression is a healthy psychic phenomenon and, within limits, should be allowed to run its course. It is a painful time, however, for both the patient and those about him or her and demands attention. Extra amounts of sympathy and personal attention (old-fashioned tender, loving care) are often the best treatment and are rewarded with a rapid recovery.

If the patient is in language therapy, this effort should be continued, but emphasis should be directed toward positive language competency, allowing few failures and many successes rewarded with approval by the therapist. Similar approaches are also correct for physical and occupational therapy. Eating and sleeping patterns may need to be altered and medical supports offered (e.g., bedtime hypnotic medication), but reactive depression is best controlled by intelligent manipulation as it is self-limited with a basically favorable long-term prognosis. In most instances, the reaction runs its course in a few to 10 days. Antidepressant medications are rarely necessary because, in most instances, the depression disappears before the medications become effective. Antidepressants act mainly to reassure concerned family, physicians, and nursing staff that everything possible is being done, and the known side effects of these powerful drugs necessitate caution.

Despite its morbid appearance, reactive depression is a healthy sign in the aphasic patient because it indicates sufficient recovery of intellectual competency for the patient to recognize the severity of the problem and the need to alter life-style. With this more realistic status, rehabilitation measures can become more problem oriented, and the potential for success increases considerably.

Long-term neurobehavioral complications. Two distinct and powerful behavioral reactions seen in aphasic patients have been correlated with the anatomical locus of pathology. One accompanies nonfluent (anterior) aphasia; the other appears in cases of fluent (posterior) aphasia (Benson 1973).

The behavioral reaction of patients with *anterior aphasia behavioral reaction* is definitive with time. With time, most nonfluent aphasic individuals become aware, at least to a considerable degree, of their new problems. They know exactly what they wish to say, but their output is restricted and barely intelligible. Inability to explain their wishes or thoughts is an intensely frustrating situation, and many patients with nonfluent aphasia experience both frustration and depression, problems that tend to aggravate each other. A catastrophic reaction may develop, but most depression with anterior aphasia is not this dramatic. It can, however, extend well beyond a time-limited reactive depression and represent a serious problem, both in its own right and as an impediment to rehabilitation. Suicide intentions may be suggested by aphasic patients and must be accepted as real possibilities.

Just as in reactive depression, recognition and appropriate alteration of management can help combat the depression of anterior aphasia. Nursing personnel and family members must be alerted to the potential of suicide and should offer increased attempts at meaningful interrelationships. Careful monitoring is needed, and suicide precautions may become necessary. Institution of appropriate antidepressant medication may be of value. The depression of nonfluent aphasia deserves the comprehensive management given to stroke patients with left frontal pathology (Robinson and Chait 1985) with the caveat that physical treatments (e.g., drugs and electroconvulsive therapy) be prescribed judiciously in a patient with brain damage and that the language therapist's position as a psychotherapist be recognized and used intelligently.

Depression is considerably more common in anterior than in posterior aphasia (Robinson and Benson 1981); several suggestions have been made to explain this observation. The first centers on the psychodynamic significance of the patient's ability to recognize the disability, the frustration of not being able to express thoughts and desires, and the realization that this frustrating status may continue indefinitely. Robinson and Szetela (1981) demonstrated a strong correlation between the anatomical locus of brain damage and the degree of depression in stroke patients; the more anterior a left cerebral infarct extends, the more likely the patient is to suffer significant depression. Robinson et al. (1975) suggested neurotransmitter asymmetry (stroke damage to dopamine and/or norepinephrine channels) as the cause of the depression. Whether explained neurochemically or psychodynamically, the increased frequency of depression in left anterior stroke patients is a reality of consequence in the care of aphasic patients.

The psychiatric problems of patients with *posterior aphasia* (fluent aphasia) are dramatically different. Most patients with posterior aphasia have difficulty comprehending spoken language and are frequently unaware of the deficit, producing an unconcern that is pathological. Fluent aphasic patients, unable to monitor their own verbal output, often fail to realize that they are producing an incomprehensible jargon. In fact, when tape recordings have been made of the jargon and replayed immediately, many patients with posterior aphasia deny that it is their output. The combination of unawareness and unconcern in posterior aphasia stands in sharp contrast to the frustrated, depressed condition in anterior aphasia.

Unaware of their own comprehension disturbance, individuals with posterior aphasia tend to blame their communication difficulties on others. They suggest that the person they are talking to is not speaking clearly or is not paying sufficient attention; some come to believe that persons they observe talking together must be using a special code because their conversation cannot be understood. Placing blame outside the self is a classic paranoid reaction and is similar, if not identical, to the well-recognized paranoia of acquired deafness. In addition, some posterior aphasia patients display impulsive behavior; the combination of unawareness, paranoia, and impulsiveness makes them potentially dangerous, both to themselves and to others. Physical attacks against medical personnel, family members, other patients, or themselves can occur. Almost all aphasic patients who need custodial management because of dangerous behavior have a posterior, fluent aphasia (Benson and Geschwind 1971).

The cause of the characteristic behavior pattern of posterior aphasia also remains conjectural. Impulsive paranoid behavior is particularly common when the left temporal lobe is involved. It is almost universally present in pure word deafness, is less common but still occurs when damage is limited to the posterior temporal lobe (Wernicke's aphasia), is much less common in transcortical sensory aphasia, and is virtually unknown in anterior aphasia. A psychodynamic interpretation would stress that the unawareness of disability accounts for the tendency to place blame for the problem on others. A more neurological interpretation would note the consistent involvement of left temporal tissues, suggesting that damage in this particular anatomical locus decreases behavioral control, complicating the language comprehension problem. The interpretations are not necessarily exclusive.

In addition to the site-based emotional complications, brain damage alters psychiatric reactivity in another manner. Loss of cerebral tissue and connections alters (usually decreases) mental control; the damaged brain is less competent to monitor, manage, and control cerebral operations. Aphasia is not just a disorder of language; it is one manifestation of a structurally damaged mental apparatus. The aphasic patient is changed, just as nonaphasic brain-damaged patients are changed, and in many instances the personality and/or mental competence present before brain injury are not recovered.

Suicide. A potential psychiatric complication of aphasia is suicide. Although relatively rare, some aphasic patients do commit suicide, and the possibility must be considered seriously. The depression, frustration, and catastrophic reaction of the patient with anterior aphasia suggest a strong potential for suicide, but, although individuals with anterior aphasia may threaten, suicide is rarely reported in this group. It occurs more often among patients with posterior aphasia, particularly when they are both paranoid and impulsive. With the patient's increasing awareness of the disability, its permanence, and the profound alterations in his or her life-style that are imposed, the possibility of premeditated self-destruction by a posterior aphasic patient must be considered.

Treatment of potential suicide in patients with posterior aphasia is extremely difficult. Their aphasia makes free communication impossible and precludes most traditional person-to-person psychotherapy measures. Standard suicide precautions should be put into effect with removal of potential self-destructive devices, careful monitoring of activities, and, if deemed necessary, transfer to a more secure situation (i.e., locked ward or seclusion room). Extra efforts should be made to establish and/or maintain interpersonal relationships and minimize frustration. However, even when suicide potential is recognized and appropriate measures are taken, a well-planned, life-ending act may occur. Management of the potentially suicidal aphasic patient is a tremendous burden, one that must be shared by the nursing staff, rehabilitation team, physicians, and family members.

Legal Aspects

The psychiatrist may be asked to give expert opinion concerning the mental competency of an individual with aphasia. Even decisions as to whether there is sufficient intelligence to warrant investment in a long-term rehabilitation program may prove difficult; determination of legal competency can be almost impossible. These two aspects deserve discussion.

Intelligence in aphasia. Whether an aphasic patient retains sufficient intelligence for personal decision making has produced considerable disagreement. Following Bastian (1898), who dogmatically stated, "We think in words," many experts emphasize the symbolic nature of language and declare that defective use of language symbols produces defective thinking. This view was strongly stressed by Gestalt psychology; both Goldstein (1948) and Bay (1964b) accepted aphasia as proof that thinking was abnormal, either regressed or concrete. Most aphasic subjects perform poorly on standard tests of intellectual competency, some in both verbal and nonverbal portions, but many retain considerable nonverbal capability. Standard IQ tests unfairly penalize the aphasic individual and exaggerate any intellectual disorder that may be present. Numerous studies to determine intelligence in aphasia have been attempted (Basso et al. 1981; Lebrun 1974; Tissot et al. 1963; Zangwill 1964) but, at best, provide nebulous results. Most such studies treat aphasia as a single, unitary disturbance, failing to note that intellectual dysfunction varies considerably with the neuroanatomical locus of damage (the syndromes of aphasia). It has been suggested that posterior language area pathology is more likely to interfere with intellectual competency than is anterior damage (Benson 1979), but this observation has yet to be systematically documented.

One major problem, crucial to the discussion of intelligence in aphasia, stems from inadequate definitions of intelligence. Hamsher (1981) reiterated a broadly held notion: "[I]n civilized cultures the concept of intelligence has appeared self-evident" (p. 334); attempts at more precise definition invariably fuel controversy. As a concept, intelligence can be dated to the discourses of Plato, Aristotle, and other early philosophers; the term was coined by Cicero (Burt 1955). Some scholars suggest that intelligence equals stored knowledge, whereas others emphasize performance capability. The problem has been compounded by the use of intelligence testing; many contemporary investigators define intelligence as a complex trait that is measured by intelligence tests (Wechsler 1971). Most aphasic patients are severely penalized by the verbal nature of intelligence tests, and, if the tests themselves are used to define the concept, intelligence must be defective in aphasia. On the other hand, if intelligence is equated with thought processing or other performance capabilities, aphasic patients may perform in the normal range. In real life the examiner must base a decision concerning the intelligence of an aphasic patient on observations; test results alone are not competent.

One approach to neuropsychological test administration and interpretation, the process method (Kaplan 1990), stresses observation of procedures used by the subject to solve test problems. The method holds promise for interpreting an aphasic patient's capabilities but, to date, is neither fully developed nor widely practiced. Important information such as the retention of social graces; counting; making change; exhibiting appropriate concern about family, business, and personal activities; finding the way about; socializing; and showing self-concern may provide valuable indications of residual intelligence in the individual with aphasia. It has been suggested that "most aphasics comprehend more than they can indicate and think more clearly than their expressive capability demonstrates" (Benson 1979, p. 180). Demonstration of the degree of intellectual competency almost invariably proves difficult.

Legal competency. Determination of whether an aphasic patient is sufficiently sound mentally to sign checks or business papers, to dispense money, to manage property or other holdings, to make a will or other testamentary documents, and so on often hinges on informed medical opinion. This demands correlated judgment of both the aphasic disability and the legal problem. Many aphasic patients can manage their own affairs whereas others are obviously unable to make decisions and deserve the protection of a conservator or a guardian, a status that demands medical opinion. Most troublesome is an intermediate group, those seriously disabled patients who, with appropriate aid, are capable of making decisions. These patients can easily lead a practitioner into legal controversy.

If a legal act (e.g., signing a will or entering into a contract) is to be performed by an aphasic patient, a physician should evaluate and carefully record the patient's ability to comprehend both spoken and written language and to express personal decisions. Then with the aid of an attorney, the document in question should be reviewed with the patient, bit by bit, until both the physician and attorney are satisfied that the patient understands the basic meaning. Such a procedure may require several sessions and, for practical reasons, the document should be kept short, simple, and as free of legal jargon as possible. It is often advisable to have the entire process videotaped to provide adequate documentation of both the process used and the patient's response to the information offered.

An even more difficult problem arises when a physician is asked to provide retrospective testimony about an aphasic patient's legal competency, the question of whether the patient did or did not understand a legal document consummated after onset of aphasia. A physician's testimony can relate only to observations of the patient's mental and language capabilities recorded at or near the time of the signing of the document. Although the physician's testimony may entail description of the patient's ability to understand spoken and written language and the ability to express ideas, it may not be possible to present a firm opinion of mental competency. A final decision will ultimately depend on whether the document reflected the patient's wishes at the time of signing; this is a legal decision based on testimony from individuals dealing with the patient at the time. It is not a medical matter.

In regard to both legal and personal decisions, aphasic patients should be given the benefit of a great deal of extra effort to allow maintenance of as much control of their own affairs as is reasonable.

❑ TREATMENT

In the past several decades neurological rehabilitation has become standardized and disciplined. Many different treatment modalities are available, and the program selected will reflect both the patient's disabilities and the available treatment resources. Some aphasic patients need considerable physical therapy, gait training, and/or mechanical aids such as crutches and leg braces; most need occupational therapy, particularly instruction and training in daily living activities. Language therapy is now presented to most (but not all) aphasic patients. These rehabilitation efforts are overlapping; all stress rote practice, repetitive attempts at an action until successful. Although tiring, demanding, and frustrating, these activities do influence behavior and can be used as positive features when an aphasic patient needs psychiatric care.

Not infrequently, patients with aphasia are being treated with medications. Drugs for heart failure, arrhythmia, and hypertension are common. Some are treated with anticoagulants, and many take aspirin as antiembolus therapy. Some have more esoteric problems such as liver or renal failure, collagen disorder, arteritis, brain tumor, and pulmonary insufficiency; all are likely to be treated with potent medications. The neuropsychiatrist asked to evaluate and treat a patient with aphasia must be aware of the medications and the potential complications of these or additional pharmaceuticals.

Two approaches to the treatment of neuropsychiatric complications in the aphasic patient are in use: pharmacological management and traditional psychotherapy. Both may be used successfully, but precautions are needed.

Pharmaceutical Approach

The entire panoply of pharmaceuticals currently used by psychiatrists may find use in the treatment of aphasia. Antidepressant medications are often considered and used, particularly in patients with left anterior lesions. The risk of adrenergic or anticholinergic side effects with antidepressants demands concern, and pharmaceuticals with fewer of these side effects (e.g., nortriptyline and desipramine) may be preferable, based on the individual situation.

Tranquilizers may be helpful in management of an aphasic patient. Benzodiazepines may help control anxiety and/or hyperactivity, but their addicting qualities and potential suppression of learning ability (amnesia) demand caution; they are not frequently used in aphasic patients. Psychotropic medications (e.g., phenothiazines and butyrophenones) are useful in selected aphasic patients, particularly those with posterior aphasia who have impulsive, paranoid behavior. Pure word-deaf and Wernicke's aphasia patients treated with these medications appear to have less agitation and are more compliant with rehabilitation measures. Dosage should be kept low to avoid interference with residual mental functions.

A third class of drugs, stimulants, are infrequently used but may be appropriate in selected cases. When brain damage causes apathy, lethargy, and decreased drive, judicious use of a stimulant such as methylphenidate may be beneficial. Fluoxetine, a relatively new antidepressant with mild stimulant side effects, may be appropriate for some aphasic patients. Again, the potential complications of these drugs on damaged brain or systemic disorder must be recognized, and their actions must be monitored carefully.

Crucial to the pharmaceutical treatment of psychiatric complications of aphasia is the possibility of adverse reactions to the medication or cross-reaction with other medications the patient is taking. Before ordering medications, the neuropsychiatrist must be aware of all other medications taken by the patient and of possible cross-complications. In general, drugs should be recognized as adjuncts to more formal rehabilitation measures, not as primary treatment modalities. With these caveats in mind, judicious use of pharmaceutical products can often be rewarding in treatment of psychiatric complications of aphasia.

Psychotherapy Approach

Despite the language disturbance, many forms of psychotherapy can be used for aphasic patients, not the least of which is the support provided by family members, nursing staff, therapists, physicians, and others in contact with the patient. Although they rarely express appreciation for such encouragement, many aphasic patients are dependent on a great deal of personal consideration.

Group psychotherapy can be attempted but is difficult because of the individual differences in language disorder. Most aphasia groups are made up of individuals with similar language disorders and stress practice of language skills. If properly managed, however, such a group also provides considerable psychic assurance. The individual bereft of language often considers the disturbance unique (most patients and their families have never heard of aphasia before the onset). Inclusion with other individuals with a similar disturbance can be helpful. First, it tends to decrease their feeling of isolation; second, seeing the improving status of members of the group offers hope; and finally, seeing one's own status becoming better in comparison with others provides additional encouragement. In a properly managed aphasic group these factors can be manipulated and used as positive treatment measures.

The use of family members for psychotherapy in aphasia deserves attention. Two aspects are obvious. First, an intelligent, well-motivated spouse or child can provide support and encouragement. Unfortunately, the opposite (disturbed family members) can be a problem. Not infrequently the spouse or children are sufficiently upset by the altered circumstances caused by the patient's aphasia that they represent a serious negative influence. Family counseling, distancing of certain family members from the patient, and/or suggestion for their own psychiatric care may be needed. Management of the family, although difficult, often represents a crucial factor in successful management of an aphasic patient's neuropsychiatric problems.

Finally, attention should be given to the position of the language therapist in psychotherapy for the aphasic patient. The aphasic patient gets considerable emotional support by working with a person who understands aphasia and is dedicated to the improvement of the patient's language deficit. There is almost always a positive transference between the patient with aphasia and the therapist, a phenomenon that can be used therapeutically. Most language therapists are neither trained nor experienced in psychiatric management; they need both coaching and encouragement to maintain treatment of a psychiatrically disturbed aphasic patient. In fact, many language therapists attempt to "dump" a disturbed patient into the psychiatrist's lap, correctly claiming that the patient's psychiatric problems obviate good language rehabilitation. It should be recognized, however, that the professional best capable of dealing with the aphasic patient is one trained in language disorders. Whenever possible, the bulk of psychotherapy provided to an aphasic patient should be performed by the language therapist.

❑ SUMMARY

The aphasic patient often suffers significant psychiatric complications, based on both damage to the brain and altered personal status. The complications hamper rehabilitation and may produce significant behavioral problems. Formulation of a rational treatment demands understanding of both the neurological and the psychological aspects, the realm of the neuropsychiatrist.

❑ REFERENCES

Alexander MP, Benson DF: The aphasias and related disturbances, in Clinical Neurology, Vol 1. Edited by Joynt R. Philadelphia, PA, JB Lippincott, 1991, Chapter 10, pp 1–58

Alexander MP, Benson DF, Stuss DT: Frontal lobes and language. Brain Lang 37:643–691, 1989

Basso A, Capitani E, Luzzatti C, et al: Intelligence and left hemisphere disease: role of aphasia, apraxia and size of lesion. Brain 104:721–734, 1981

Bastian HC: Aphasia and Other Speech Defects. London, HK Lewis, 1898

Bay E: Principles of classification and their influence on our concepts of aphasia, in Disorders of Language. Edited by De Reuck AV, O'Connor M. Boston, MA, Little, Brown, 1964a, pp 122–139

Bay E: Aphasia and intelligence. International Journal of Neurology 4:252–264, 1964b

Benson DF: Psychiatric aspects of aphasia. Br J Psychiatry 123:555–566, 1973

Benson DF: Aphasia, Alexia, and Agraphia. New York, Churchill Livingstone, 1979

Benson DF: Aphasia managment: the neurologist's role, in Seminars in Speech, Language and Hearing, Vol 2. Edited by Wertz RT. New York, Thieme-Stratton, 1981, pp 237–247

Benson DF, Geschwind N: The aphasias and related disturbances, in Clinical Neurology. Edited by Baker AB, Baker LH. New York, Harper & Row, 1971, Chapter 8, pp 1–33

Benson DF, Geschwind N: The aphasias and related disturbances, in Clinical Neurology, Vol 1. Edited by Baker AB, Joynt R. Philadelphia, PA, Harper & Row, 1985, Chapter 10, pp 1–34

Benton AL, Joynt RJ: Early descriptions of aphasia. Arch Neurol 3:205–222, 1960

Brain R: Speech Disorders—Aphasia, Apraxia and Agnosia. London, Butterworths, 1961

Broca P: Remarques sur le siège de la faculté du langage articulé, suivies d'une observation d'aphemie. Bulletin-Societé Anatomique de Paris 2:330–357, 1861

Broca P: Sur la faculté du langage articulé. Bulletin Societé Anthropologie 6:337–393, 1865

Brown JR: A model for central and peripheral behavior in aphasia. Paper delivered at the annual meeting of the Academy of Aphasia, Rochester, MN, 1968

Burt C: The evidence for the concept of intelligence. Br J Educ Psychol 25:158–177, 1955

Critchley M: Aphasiology. London, Edward Arnold, 1970, pp 159–173

Damasio H, Damasio A: The anatomical basis of conduction aphasia. Brain 103:337–350, 1980

Freud S: On Aphasia (1891). Translated by Stengel E. New York, International Universities Press, 1953

Geschwind N: Disconnexion syndromes in animals and man. Brain 88:237–294, 585–644, 1965

Goldstein K: Language and Language Disturbances: Aphasic Symptom Complexes and Their Significance for Medicine and Theory of Language. New York, Grune & Stratton, 1948

Hamsher K: Intelligence and aphasia, in Acquired Aphasia. Edited by Sarno MT. New York, Academic, 1981, pp 327–359

Head H: Aphasia and Kindred Disorders of Speech, Vols I and II (1926). New York, Hafner, 1963

Hécaen H, Albert ML: Human Neuropsychology. New York, Wiley, 1978

Heilman KM, Valenstein E (eds): Clinical Neuropsychology. New York, Oxford University Press, 1979

Henschen SE: Klinische und Anatomische Beitrage zur Pathologie der Gehirns. Stockholm, Almqvist and Wiksell, 1922

Howes D: Application of the word frequency concept to aphasia, in Disorders of Language. Edited by De Reuck AV, O'Connor M. Boston, MA, Little, Brown, 1964, pp 47–78

Jackson JH: Clinical remarks on cases of defects of expression (by words, writing, signs, etc.) in diseases of the nervous system. Lancet 1:604–605, 1864

Kaplan E: The process approach to neuropsychological assessment of psychiatric patients. Journal of Neuropsychiatry and Clinical Neurosciences 2:72–87, 1990

Kertesz A: Aphasia and Associated Disorders. New York, Grune & Stratton, 1979

Kirshner HS: Behavioral Neurology: A Practical Approach. New York, Churchill Livingstone, 1986

Kleist K: Gehirnpathologie. Leipzig, Barth, 1934

Lebrun Y: Intelligence and Aphasia. Amsterdam, Swets and Zeitlinger, 1974

Lecours AR, Lhermitte F: Historical review, in Aphasiology. Edited by Lecours AR, Lhermitte F, Bryans B. London, Bailliere-Tindall, 1983, pp 11–29

Lecours AR, Lhermitte F, Bryans B (eds): Aphasiology. London, Bailliere-Tindall, 1983a

Lecours AR, Poncet M, Ponzio J, et al: Classification of the aphasias, in Aphasiology. Edited by Lecours AR, Lhermitte F, Bryans B. London, Bailliere-Tindall, 1983b, pp 243–268

Lichtheim L: On aphasia. Brain 7:434–484, 1885

Marie P: Revision de la question de l'aphasie. Semaine Médicale 26:241–247, 493–500, 565–571, 1906

Maruszewski M: Language, Communication and the Brain. The Hague, Mouton, 1975

Mendez MF, Benson DF: Atypical conduction aphasia: a disconnection syndrome. Arch Neurol 42:886–891, 1985

Mesulam M-M: Principles of Behavioral Neurology. Philadelphia, PA, FA Davis, 1985

Pick A: Aphasia (1931). Springfield, IL, Charles C Thomas, 1973

Robinson RG, Benson DF: Depression in aphasic patients: frequency, severity, and clinical-pathological correlations. Brain Lang 14:282–291, 1981

Robinson RG, Chait RM: Emotional correlates of structural brain injury with particular emphasis on post-stroke mood disorders. CRC Critical Review of Clinical Neurobiology 4:285–318, 1985

Robinson R, Szetela B: Mood change following left hemisphere brain injury. Ann Neurol 9:447–453, 1981

Robinson RG, Shoemaker WJ, Schlumpf M, et al: Effect of experimental cerebral infarction in rat brain: effect on catecholamines and behavior. Nature 255:332–334, 1975

Ross ED: The aprosodias: functional-anatomic organization of the affective components of language in the right hemisphere. Arch Neurol 38:561–569, 1981

Ross ED, Mesulam M-M: Dominant language functions of the right hemisphere? Prosody and emotional gesturing. Arch Neurol 36:144–148, 1979

Ross ED, Rush J: Diagnosis and neuroanatomical correlates of depression in brain-damaged patients. Arch Gen Psychiatry 38:1344–1354, 1981

Schuell H, Jenkins JJ, Jiminez-Pabon E: Aphasia in Adults: Diagnosis, Prognosis and Treatment. New York, Harper & Row, 1964

Tissot R, Lhermitte F, Ducarne B: Etat intellectuel des aphasiques. Encéphale 52:285–320, 1963

Wechsler D: Intelligence: definitions, theory and the IQ, in Intelligence: Genetic and Environmental Influences. Edited by Cancro R. New York, Grune & Stratton, 1971, pp 50–55

Weisenburg TS, McBride KL: Aphasia (1935). New York, Hafner, 1964

Wepman JM: Recovery From Aphasia. New York, Ronald, 1951

Wepman J, Jones L: Dimensions of language performance in aphasia. J Speech Hear Res 4:220–232, 1961

Wernicke C: Das Aphasiche Symptomenkomplex. Breslau, Cohn and Weigart, 1874

Zangwill OL: Intelligence in aphasia, in Disorders of Language. Edited by De Reuck AV, O'Connor M. Boston, Little, Brown, 1964, pp 261–274

Chapter

14

Practical Pathophysiology in Neuropsychiatry: A Clinical Approach to Depression and Impulsive Behavior in Neurological Patients

Barry S. Fogel, M.D.
Andrea B. Stone, M.D.

DEPRESSION AND IMPULSIVE BEHAVIOR are two of the most common clinical problems encountered by neuropsychiatrists. The linkage of these symptoms to dysfunction in specific brain areas has been a main objective of neuropsychiatric research on major neurological diseases. The twin goals of this research effort have been functional localization and establishing that the behavioral symptoms of neurological diseases are not merely general emotional reactions to discomfort or disability (Fogel 1990a, 1990b). Many of the disease-specific chapters of this textbook illustrate the success of this general research line. However, the clinician encountering a specific patient with brain disease and depression, or brain disease and impulsive behavior, must develop a unique working formulation of the mechanism of symptom production in that patient's case. Such formulations are necessary for the development of an effective therapeutic plan. They must go well beyond general statements about the association of the patient's symptoms with regional brain injury. In this chapter we set forth some basic principles for approaching depression and impulsive behavior in patients with known neurological disease. We do not discuss the differential diagnosis of systemic and neurological diseases that may present with these neuropsychiatric syndromes. Instead, we address the problems of the clinician confronted with a specific patient with depression or impulsive behavior, providing guidelines for analyzing mechanisms of symptom production and setting priorities for therapeutic intervention.

❑ REASONS TO DISCUSS DEPRESSION AND IMPULSIVE BEHAVIOR TOGETHER

In this chapter we discuss depression and impulsive behavior together, not only because they are both common consequences of neurological disease, but also because they are linked in many patients and may share common pathophysiological mechanisms. Thus any patient with recurrent impulsive behavior deserves an assessment for depression, taking into account the special considerations described below.

Depression is a risk factor for self-injurious acts, such as suicide attempts, but it also may increase the risk of violence or impulsive acts directed at others. For example, the manifestations of personality disorders of the dramatic (acting-out) cluster are aggravated by concurrent major depression (Akiskal 1981). In many patients, major depression is associated with diminished frontal lobe metabolism; impaired judgment and impulse control may be a consequence. Depressive agitation increases arousal and, consequently, the risk of impulsive action. Low serotonin levels—frequent accompaniments of depressive states—have been directly associated with suicide, with agitation, and with impulsive or violent acts (Lidberg et al. 1985; Roy et al. 1986; Traskman-Bendz et al. 1986).

Depression may be associated with diminished frontal lobe function and metabolism, which may in turn disinhibit impulsive behavior, or impair the generation of socially appropriate alternative responses. Finally, the neuropsychiatric approaches to depression and impulsive behavior must address a shared set of neuropsychiatric concerns. These include the effects of right-hemisphere damage on the accurate reception and expression of emotional communication, as well as the need to scrupulously check for drug interactions between psychotropic drugs and the nonpsychotropic medications that neurological patients are very likely to be receiving. Although the latter topic is beyond the scope of this chapter, several recent reviews have addressed various aspects of drug interaction problems in neuropsychiatry (Fogel 1988; Stoudemire et al. 1990, 1991a, 1991b).

❑ DEPRESSION

Depression in its various forms is probably the most common psychiatric complication of neurological disease. Because depression is a common reaction to disability and to discomfort, it is therefore common in all clinical populations. Additionally, a range of anatomical, physiological, and biochemical changes associated with specific neurological diseases produces depression by a direct influence on the physiological mechanisms that underlie mood and affect. Several lines of evidence have been brought forth to demonstrate these specific linkages in particular neurological populations, including the following:

1. Studies showing that the prevalence of depression in patients with a particular neurological disease is greater than that seen in a matched comparison population equally disabled by nonneurological disease
2. Studies showing that the prevalence or severity of depression in the disease is poorly correlated with the severity of physical disability or length of illness
3. Studies showing that depression is correlated to a specific anatomical, biochemical, or physiological change intrinsic to the disease
4. Studies showing that clinical features of the depression differ significantly from those encountered in equally ill patients with primary depression
5. Studies showing alleviation of the depression with therapies directed at the neurological disease that are not thought to have antidepressant effects in patients with primary depression

Common to all these approaches, except possibly the last, is that they are based on studying *populations* of patients rather than *individuals*. The clinician's task when confronted with a particular depressed patient is to formulate a working hypothesis of etiology for that individual that will be helpful in planning therapy. The next section of this chapter begins with a general model for depression in neurological disease. It also offers 13 general principles for approaching depression in the patient with neurological disease and illustrates them with commonly occurring examples from the practice of clinical neuropsychiatry. These principles are summarized in Table 14–1. As indicated, the principles also are applicable in evaluating patients with impulsive or self-injurious behavior because these behaviors may be driven by dysphoric mood.

A General Model of Depression in the Neurological Patient

A general model of mood and its expression in neurological patients is shown in Figure 14–1. Applied to depression, it represents in schematic form the idea that although depressive mood arises from the limbic system, itself under the influence of brain stem monoamine inputs, the full expression of a depressive *syndrome* involves the hypothalamus (vegetative and autonomic signs), the left parietotemporal cortex (depressive cognitions and their verbal expression), the right parietotemporal cortex (nonverbal expression of mood), and the frontal lobes (via articulation of action, maintenance of mental set, responsiveness to environmental contingencies, inhibition of socially proscribed behavior, and direct inputs to the limbic system).

The model also notes that the limbic system has extensive reciprocal connections with the frontal lobes, the basal ganglia, and the limbic thalamus. By these routes, factors such as pain and immobility may directly influence the development of a mood state in the limbic system.

Brain damage, particularly to brain areas and circuits referred to in the model, increases the likelihood that the symptoms and signs of a depressed mood will not resemble the syndromes typical of primary depression in neurologically intact patients. The concept of reciprocal connections, indicated by the arrows throughout the diagram, implies that cortical damage may lead to altered function not only of the limbic system, but also of the brain stem. Thus cortical damage may simultaneously alter mood and modify its symptomatic expression.

Principles of the Clinical Approach to Depression in the Neurological Patient

With this model in mind, the literature on mood disorder in neurological patients was analyzed to yield 13 principles to guide the clinician in approaching depressed patients with known or suspected neurological disease and neurological pa-

TABLE 14–1. PRINCIPLES FOR EVALUATING DEPRESSION IN THE NEUROLOGICAL PATIENT

1. Perform a functional assessment and thorough symptom review to identify remediable discomforts and disabilities.
2. Check the medication list for potentially psychotoxic agents and substitute less psychotoxic agents whenever possible.
3. Identify and treat underlying systemic diseases.
4. Consider seizures, increased intracranial pressure, and hydrocephalus.
5. Identify and treat endocrinopathies.
6. Consider secondary brainstem consequences of cortical injury.
7. Allow for modification of the expression of mood by aphasia, frontal lobe disorder, or right frontotemporal damage.
8. Differentiate neurologically based apathy, bradykinesia, and anhedonia from true depression.
9. Consider variations in neuroanatomical involvement by the underlying neurological disease.
10. Allow for aggravating effects of depression when interpreting cognitive and functional deficits.
11. Evaluate the possibility of episodic or paroxysmal mood changes, using direct observation and collateral history; consider mechanisms including partial seizures, subictal phenomena, migraine, and dissociation.
12. Attend to social and developmental issues.
13. Identify and treat persistent preexisting psychiatric disorders, especially substance abuse in head injury patients.

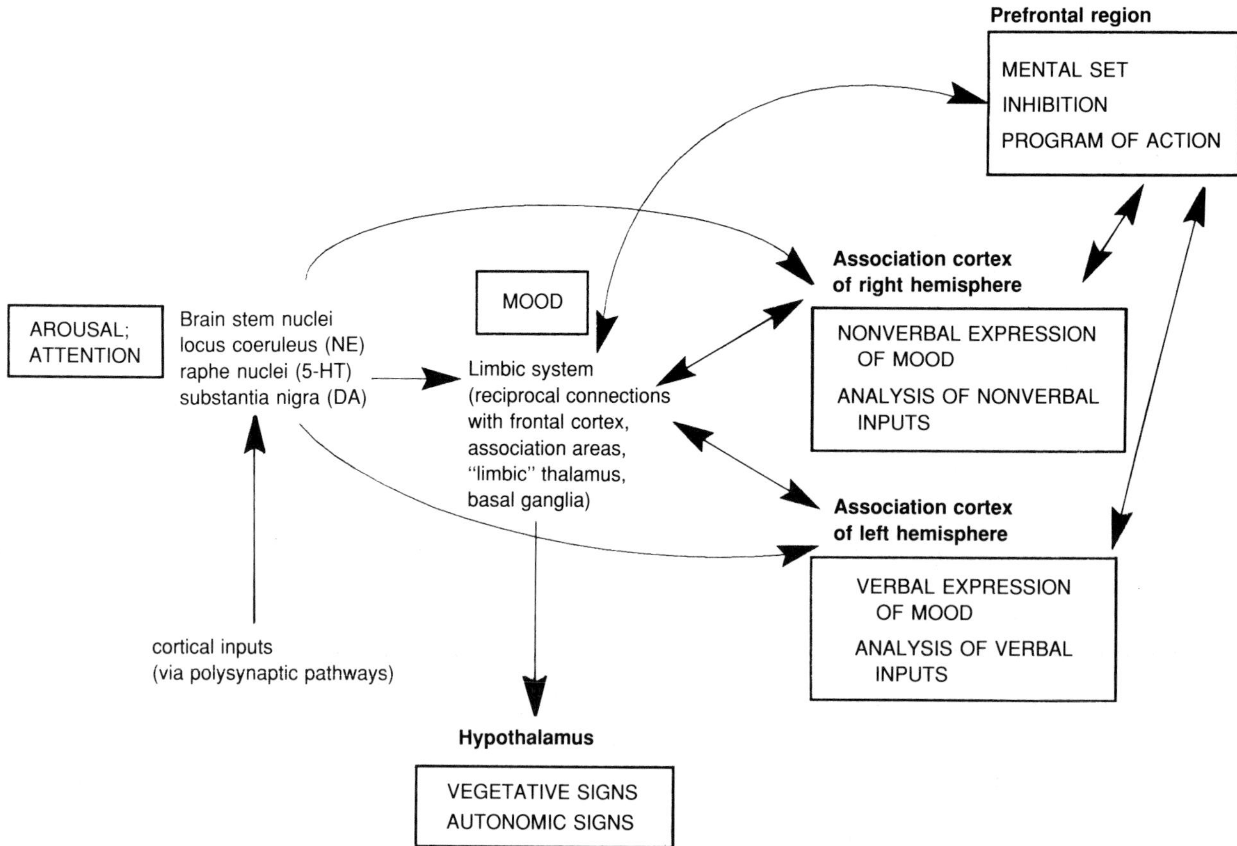

Figure 14–1. Mood and its expression. NE = norepinephrine; 5-HT = 5-hydroxytryptamine (serotonin); DA = dopamine.

tients with known or suspected depression. These principles stress the identification of opportunities for therapeutic intervention and consider the patient's medical and neurological regimen as subject to modification if necessary to improve mood and behavior.

1. **Even when depression is a direct consequence of brain damage, disability and discomfort may aggravate the patient's dysphoria.** Therefore, the depressed patient with neurological disease requires a thorough functional assessment and review of systems to identify remediable disabilities and discomforts. Several clinical examples can be offered. In Parkinson's disease, decreased mobility of the upper extremities may lead to bursitis or frozen shoulder or contractures—conditions that may be both painful and disabling (Kase and O'Riordan 1987). The treatment of these conditions with anti-inflammatory drugs and physical therapy may indirectly alleviate some of the patient's depressive symptoms. In multiple sclerosis, patients may have troublesome paroxysmal symptoms, such as intermittent paresthesias and dysesthesias, that are uncomfortable in themselves and continual reminders to the patient of the illness. Some of these symptoms are exquisitely responsive to anticonvulsant medications (Matthews 1985). Abolition of the paroxysmal symptoms may be associated with the lifting of mood.

   For each of the major neurological diseases, there are associated discomforts and disabilities that are particularly frequent. Parkinson's disease is associated with orthopedic problems, constipation, and sleep disturbance (Nausieda 1987). Hemiparetic stroke is associated with impaired gait and associated musculoskeletal discomfort. Early Alzheimer's disease may combine with primary urologic disease to produce incontinence, which (by producing discomfort and embarrassment) aggravates the patient's dysphoria (Ouslander 1990). For each of these situations, specific and effective treatments may exist (Ouslander 1990). The patient's depression, however, and a general atmosphere of pessimism concerning the disease, may interfere with these functional problems being identified and addressed. It may fall to the neuropsychiatrist to identify and respond to these issues.

2. **Drugs used to treat the neurological disease, or associated medical conditions, may cause or aggravate depression.** Therefore, the drug list must be examined carefully for potentially psychotoxic agents that can be either eliminated or substituted. Some psychotoxic drug situations are so common in neuropsychiatric practice that they deserve specific mention. These include

   a. The use of barbiturates or phenytoin to control seizures associated with neurological disease. Carbamazepine and valproate are less likely to cause depression (Mattson 1989).
   b. The use of centrally acting antihypertensive drugs, such as methyldopa or propranolol, to manage hypertension in stroke patients. These drugs, particularly methyldopa, may cause or aggravate depression. Acceptable substitutes, such as angiotensin-converting enzyme (ACE) inhibitors and calcium channel blockers, are less psychotoxic (Pasqualy and Veith 1989; Pottash et al. 1981).
   c. The use of antiarrhythmic agents, such as quinidine and procainamide, to treat cardiac arrhythmia associated with embolic stroke. These agents are known to be psychotoxic. Therapeutic alternatives often exist that are better tolerated with respect to mental and behavioral side effects (Caird and Scott 1986).
   d. The use of corticosteroids such as prednisone in multiple sclerosis, lupus, and other inflammatory diseases (Lewis and Smith 1983). Alternative anti-inflammatory or immunosuppressant treatments sometimes can be substituted in patients who are unable to tolerate the mental side effects of steroids.
   e. The use of cimetidine to treat or prevent peptic symptoms, occurring due to the stress of acute illness, or to mitigate the gastrointestinal side effects of anti-inflammatory drugs or corticosteroids. Cimetidine can cause or aggravate depression (Pasqualy and Veith 1989). Other agents that have few or no psychiatric side effects, such as sucralfate, often can be substituted successfully.

   These issues are summarized in Table 14–2.

3. **The neurological disorder may be due to an underlying systemic disease that causes or aggravates depression in itself.** This underlying disease must be identified and optimally treated. Systemic lupus erythematosus, which may present with a stroke or seizure in a young person, offers a classic example (Giang, in press). In general, strokes occurring in young people, or the new onset of seizures in later life, are due to other medical conditions (Hachinski and Norris 1985; Schold et al. 1977).
4. **The primary neurological disorder may have neurological complications that contribute to the depression and require independent treatment.** Patients with a variety of focal lesions may develop partial seizures, which in turn may cause depressive symptoms (Engel 1989). The development of new depressive symptoms, particularly of an episodic or fluctuating character, in a patient with an established focal lesion should always raise the consideration of focal seizure activity.

   Patients with tumors may develop not only seizures, but also increased intracranial pressure, which may present initially with a change in mood. Patients with a history of head trauma, central nervous system infection, or brain hemorrhage are vulnerable to the subsequent development of hydrocephalus, which may also present initially with mood changes (Benson 1985; Price and Tucker 1977). As with seizures, hydrocephalus may develop relatively late after the acquisition of an apparently stable lesion.
5. **Several neurological diseases, or their treatments, have endocrine complications or concomitants that may contribute to alterations in mood.** Remediation of the endocrine problem may improve the patient's well-being and function.

   Patients receiving anticonvulsant drugs, such as carbamazepine and phenytoin, may show pharmacological suppression of thyroid function. The problem is particularly complex because these drugs suppress the secretion of

TABLE 14–2. COMMON SITUATIONS FOR DRUG-INDUCED AGGRAVATION OF DEPRESSION IN NEUROLOGICAL DISEASE

Neurological disease	*Drug and indication*	*Possible alternatives*
Epilepsy	Barbiturates, benzodiazepines, or phenytoin as anticonvulsants	Carbamazepine Valproate
Stroke or multi-infarct dementia	Methyldopa, reserpine, or propranolol for hypertension	Angiotensin-converting enzyme (ACE) inhibitors Calcium channel blockers
Embolic stroke or multi-infarct dementia	Quinidine or procainamide for cardiac arrhythmias	Disopyramide Verapamil, β-Blockers
Lupus or multiple sclerosis	Corticosteroids as immunosuppressants	Other immunosuppressants (e.g., methotrexate and cyclophosphamide)
Head trauma, stroke, or other acute severe brain disease	Cimetidine to treat or prevent stress ulcers	Sucralfate Antacids

thyrotropin (TSH) by the pituitary. It may be impossible to tell whether a low-normal thyroid level is clinically significant because the usual sign of elevated TSH may be blocked. When the patient's symptoms suggest hypothyroidism, an empiric trial of thyroid hormone may be necessary (Hein and Jackson 1990).

Complex partial epilepsy is frequently associated with abnormalities in the reproductive endocrine system, which in turn may be associated with mood symptoms. Among women, there is an increased prevalence of polycystic ovary syndrome; among men, testosterone may be low (Barragry et al. 1978; Herzog 1989; Herzog et al. 1986; Toone et al. 1983). The specific pharmacological treatment of these disorders may improve patients' mood.

Both stroke and Parkinson's disease, two neurological disorders highly associated with depression, are also associated with a high prevalence of nonsuppression on the dexamethasone suppression test (Finkelstein et al. 1982; Pfeiffer et al. 1987). This raises the possibility that the elevated cortisol itself seen in these patients may contribute to their depressed mood, because depression is the most common psychiatric correlate of primary Cushing's disease (Gottlieb and Greenspan 1989).

6. **Focal cortical lesions may have remote effects on the function of subcortical and brain stem nuclei, leading to more general and bilateral biochemical changes.** This has been demonstrated most convincingly in Robinson's animal model of poststroke depression (Robinson 1979). Function of the noradrenergic locus coeruleus is altered in response to unilateral hemisphere damage, leading to decreased norepinephrine contralaterally. Eventually, pharmacological interventions may be aimed at reversing the abnormalities and biochemical systems known to be altered by the remote effects of cortical damage. Positron-emission tomography (PET) and single photon emission computed tomography (SPECT) offer the prospects of identifying these mechanisms noninvasively.
7. **Focal hemispheric lesions may alter the expression of mood, leading to an underdiagnosis of significant and treatable depression.** The three major situations in which this occurs are frontal lobe lesions, right frontotemporal lesions, and lesions causing aphasia.

Frontal lobe lesions may lead to a shallowness of affective expression, so that a patient with intense depressive feelings may seem superficially unconcerned or even facetious (Stuss and Benson 1986). Direct questioning, however, may identify the core elements of a major depressive syndrome. In the presence of frontal lobe damage, the apparent incongruity of the patient's affect with his or her verbally expressed mood should not negate the significance of the verbally reported mood state. Also, the lack of spontaneity in many patients with frontal damage requires that depressive symptomatology be sought by direct questions; the clinician cannot rely on the patient to volunteer the information or to offer consistent facial expressions of depressed affect.

Patients with right frontotemporal lesions may be unable to express emotion by means of prosody or other paralinguistic dimensions of speech (Ross 1985). As with patients with frontal lesions, patients with right frontotemporal lesions may yield significant depressive ideation on direct questioning, even though their spontaneous speech does not suggest a low mood. They may also show severe vegetative signs and behavioral signs of depression while verbally denying depressed mood (Ross and Rush 1981). Lesions in the right hemisphere are differentially associated with denial of deficit. Bear (1983) described the fundamental deficit of many patients with right-hemisphere damage as a "failure in emotional surveillance." This may on occasion produce strange inconsistencies in the clinical interview. Patients may, for example, answer no to "Are you depressed?" while pouring forth negative feelings when asked if they have considered suicide. Accuracy of assessment of these patients is best promoted by the most comprehensive questioning.

Patients with aphasia may be unable to express the cognitive elements of a major depressive syndrome, even though mood, behavior, and vegetative signs may be compatible with a clinical depression (Ross and Rush 1981). In these patients, in whom the right hemisphere usually is intact, the facial expression of affect may be a reliable clue to the patient's mood. Patients with nonfluent aphasia but with intact comprehension can be questioned about their mood with yes-or-no questions because most are able to respond to such questions with some kind of signal. Patients with impaired comprehension often can be questioned about mood by using a nonverbal form of the Visual Analog Mood Scale (Stern and Bachman 1991). This scale, shown in Figure 14–2, consists of a vertical line with a smiling (happy) face at the top and a frowning (sad) face at the bottom. The patient is instructed to mark on the line the place best describing their current mood.

8. **Apathy, bradykinesia, and anhedonia may occur as consequences of brain lesions in the absence of depression.** These conditions are most often seen in individuals with right-hemisphere disease (Bear 1983), with frontal lobe damage (Stuss and Benson 1984), or with disordered dopaminergic transmission (as may occur in Parkinson's disease and other basal ganglia disorders) or with administration of drugs that deplete dopamine or block dopamine receptors (Marin 1990). When these symptoms and signs occur in the absence of depressed mood, they may be more likely to respond to dopamine agonist therapy than to generic antidepressant therapy. The distinction can be made by questioning patients carefully about the cognitive features of depression and by demonstrating motor signs, such as rigidity. Of course, patients with frontal lobe disease and basal ganglia disorders are at risk for developing depres-

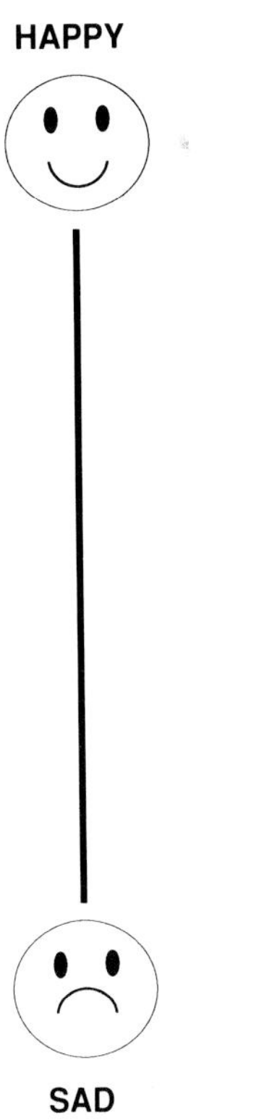

Figure 14–2. Visual Analog Mood Scale.

sion and often require concomitant therapy with antidepressants.

9. **Depression may be related to the regional emphasis of diffuse diseases or to the specific involvement of anatomical structures inconstantly affected by a particular disease.** For example, in Alzheimer's disease, depression occurs more frequently among patients in whom greater frontal involvement is demonstrable by PET scan or in whom greater pathological involvement of the substantia nigra and locus coeruleus is seen at postmortem (Zubenko and Moossy 1988). Similarly, in Parkinson's disease, greater involvement of the serotonergic raphe nuclei, as demonstrated by decreased cerebrospinal fluid 5-hydroxyindoleacetic acid (5-HIAA), is associated with depression (Mayeux et al. 1987).
10. **Depression may aggravate cognitive and functional deficits of fixed brain lesions, possibly leading to erroneous conclusions about their extent or severity.** Not only can generalized cognitive impairment be aggravated by depression, the cognitive manifestations of focal or lateralized disease may also be intensified by depression (Fogel and Sparadeo 1985). Localization of neuropsychological dysfunction in the depressed patient by neuropsychological testing or bedside cognitive examination may thus be unreliable. From the standpoint of diagnostic formulation, there is a risk of attribution of a patient's depressed mood to profound cognitive disability that actually is due largely to the depression itself.

    Recent evidence that major depression is associated with alterations in regional brain metabolism (Holcomb et al. 1989) suggests a possible mechanism for aggravation of cognitive and functional disturbances by depression. It further suggests that functional imaging (e.g., fluorodeoxyglucose PET scans) of specific brain lesions may be affected by depression just as much as neuropsychological investigation of those lesions (Fogel and Eslinger 1991).
11. **Disturbances of mood in neurological patients may be episodic, rather than continuous.** Thus a single evaluation showing a normal mood may not be conclusive, and an accurate history is crucial. For many individuals with brain damage, this requires extensive history from observers and other collateral sources. Several mechanisms, each with treatment implications, should be considered when patients have episodic but clinically significant depression in the context of neurological disease. These include focal seizures, subictal phenomena, migrainous phenomena, and dissociative states.

    a. *Focal seizures* are a frequent concomitant of focal brain injury from a number of causes. Focal seizures in individuals with brain damage may present as sudden mood changes (Engel 1989; Robertson and Trimble 1983). If the patient is impaired in cognition or communication, he or she may be unable to describe the mood shift that is evidenced by a change in behavior or affect. Changes occurring within seconds, and having a stereotypic quality and time course, are a clue that an ictal mechanism may be involved. The appropriate clinical response is electroencephalographic (EEG) investigation, and possibly an empiric anticonvulsant trial.
    b. *Subictal phenomena*, as described by Himmelhoch, Blumer, and others (Blumer et al. 1988; Himmelhoch 1984), are paroxysmal shifts in mental state that are not sufficiently stereotypic to warrant a diagnosis of epilepsy but have features suggestive of epileptic seizures and a definite anticonvulsant response. For example, patients with such phenomena might have episodic shifts into depressed mood that lack the rapid onset and stereotypic course that is typical of epileptic seizures. EEG changes may be absent, or nonspecific, such as temporal lobe sharp activity. The psychiatric diagnoses carried by such patients include atypical depression, atypical psychosis, and panic disorder. Most reported cases have been in patients without known gross neurological disease, but patients with focal brain lesions, such as those from past head trauma, would be expected to be at higher risk if the condition really were a variant of focal epilepsy. However, the validity of the subictal concept is controversial because seizure activity is inferred rather than definitively recorded, and the direct psychotropic effects of anticonvulsants are powerful, confounding the interpretation of treatment response. In any case, the use of mood-stabilizing anticonvulsants such as carbamazepine and valproate is becoming

widespread for atypical and refractory mood disorders (Amsterdam 1990; McElroy and Pope 1988), without resolution of the issue of whether the disorder is related to epilepsy, either for the patient in particular or for such patients in general.

c. *Migraine*, a common disorder, is overrepresented among neurological patients. Not only do migraine patients consult neurologists for their headaches, but migraine is associated with several other neurological conditions, such as epilepsy and stroke. Moreover, brain injury patients may have migraine-type headaches as a posttraumatic sequel. Migraine with aura is characterized by the combination of headache and neurological symptoms that slowly develop and spread over a period of minutes. Often, the prodrome, aura, and headache itself are associated with shifts in mood, with depression and irritability being common accompaniments (Harvey and Hay 1984; Welch 1987). Specific antimigraine therapy is helpful for the mood shifts as well as the headaches. Notably, some of the most effective antimigraine drugs are antidepressants (e.g., amitriptyline and phenelzine [Merikangas 1991]).

d. *Dissociative phenomena* may cause changes in mood and behavior, and some forms of brain disease may be connected with an increased risk of dissociative phenomena. Complex partial epilepsy may be associated with an increased risk of dissociation (Engel 1989). The greater tolerance of inconsistency by patients with frontal lobe damage may be a risk factor for dissociation in such patients. Clues to dissociation include absolute amnesia, the occurrence of socially unacceptable behavior during the episode, a duration of hours, and precipitation of the episode by a specific psychological stressor. Treatment may emphasize psychotherapy, but in specific cases anticonvulsant and antipsychotic medications may be useful adjuncts (Ford 1989; Linn 1989; Wilbur and Kluft 1989).

12. **Social and developmental issues are important determinants of depression in patients with brain injury.** Consideration of the patient's developmental history and social situation is crucial to formulating a particular case of depression, and appropriate psychotherapeutic and social intervention may be a necessary condition for a good therapeutic outcome (Taylor 1982). A number of generic themes recur among neuropsychiatric patients: familial overprotectiveness, self-blame or familial blame for involuntary symptoms, linkage of self-esteem to a particular competence that is impaired by the neurological lesion, conflicts over dependency, and interference with an age-specific developmental task due to the brain disease.

    From a practical point of view, brief focal psychotherapy is often an effective adjunct to the medical and pharmacological interventions alluded to above. It is often helpful for the neuropsychiatrist to define one or two focal points for psychotherapeutic and social intervention, so that psychotherapy can go beyond the generic provision of support and concern.

13. **A psychiatric disorder, responsible for the acquisition of the neurological lesion, may persist and be relevant to the present symptoms.** The most frequent example is the association of alcohol and drug abuse with head injury. When approaching depression in a patient with a recent head injury, it is relevant to know whether the injury was acquired when the patient was under the influence of alcohol or cocaine. In addition to substance abuse diagnoses, premorbid problems such as attention-deficit hyperactivity disorder (ADHD) and antisocial personality may also predispose both to head trauma and to mood disorder (Akiskal et al. 1983; Popper 1988; Widiger and Frances 1988).

❑ IMPULSIVE BEHAVIOR

Impulsive behavior, particularly violence, but also impulsive sexual behavior or eating behavior, is a central concern of neuropsychiatrists because of its dramatic quality and its potential for harm. Since the 1950s, a frequent "psychiatric" response to impulsive and violent behavior has been neuroleptic therapy, an approach that is neither universally helpful nor particularly safe, particularly for patients with brain injury. A major theme in clinical neuropsychiatric research has been the demonstration that various nonneuroleptic treatments might alleviate violent and impulsive behavior in patients with brain damage. Anticonvulsant drugs, particularly carbamazepine, and β-adrenergic blocking drugs (Ratey et al. 1983; Yudofsky et al. 1984), have a well-established record in this area; for many years neuropsychiatrists were distinguishable from general psychiatrists by their comfort in using these agents as alternatives to neuroleptics. As with depression, a line of neuropsychiatric studies has aimed at linking impulsive or aggressive behavior with damage to specific brain areas, particularly in the frontotemporal region. With a few exceptions, such as the human Klüver-Bucy syndrome from bilateral anterior temporal damage, associations between specific regional brain damage and impulsive behavior have been imprecise, and the matching of patients and therapies for impulsive behavior has relied extensively on clinical intuition and sequential drug trials. This creates a therapeutic dilemma for the neuropsychiatric clinician, particularly when promising new agents for treating impulsive behavior are continually being reported, usually in open, uncontrolled trials.

In this section we offer a general model for understanding impulsive behavior in neurological patients that may be of some help in organizing a therapeutic strategy for the individual patient with impulsive behavior and known brain damage or dysfunction. The model is similar to that described by Bear (1989), but is framed in language that is more clinical than neuroanatomical.

Application of the model will assume that the general clinical considerations discussed above for depression have also been considered and applied. The model emphasizes the multifactorial etiology of impulsive behavior. The attribution of purposeful violence, in particular, to a sole neurological cause, such as epilepsy, is usually unsound (Delgado-Escueta et al. 1981). An example of an appropriately multifactorial analysis was the study by Lewis et al. (1983) of homicidally aggressive young children. Comparing homicidally aggressive children with psychiatric inpatient control subjects, they found that fathers' violence toward mothers, seizures, suicidal behavior, and psychiatric hospitalization of the mother were associated with homicidal aggression. Family violence and disrupted relationships can be seen as providing a motive and context for violence, whereas seizures might have affected arousal or mood or might be a marker for gross brain injury affecting inhibitory mechanisms.

A General Model for Impulsive Behavior in Neurological Patients

A general model for impulsive behavior in neurological patients is shown in Figure 14–3. It represents in schematic form the idea that a particular impulsive action requires arousal, a motive, and a plan, however rudimentary; to be acted on, the plan must escape from inhibition. Both the formulation of a plan and the activation of inhibitory mechanisms depend on the perception of situational context, mediated by the dorsolateral frontal lobes. The development of the motive for impulsive action de-

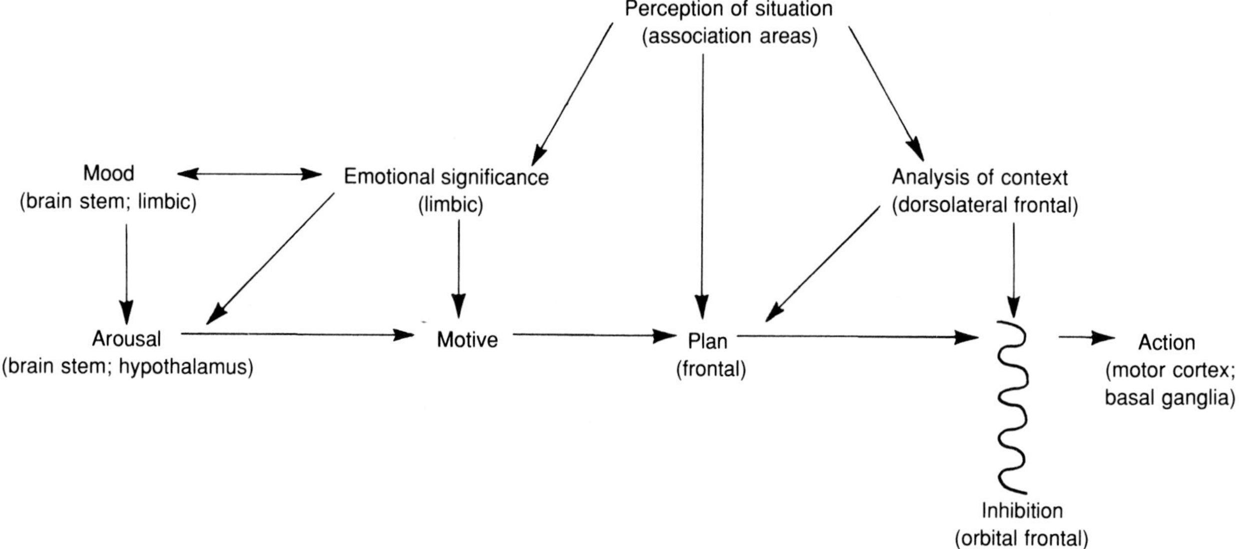

Figure 14–3. A model of impulsive behavior.

pends on the individual's perception of the emotional significance of the situation, which in turn is related to the individual's mood. Both the mood and the perceived emotional context may lead to an alteration in the individual's level of arousal.

Brain lesions predispose patients to impulsive action by affecting one or more of the functions described; neuropsychiatric therapies likewise work by altering one or more specific mechanisms. The failure of an attempted therapy may relate to its targeting the wrong mechanism or its having unwanted effects on other mechanisms. A classic example is when a neuroleptic drug causes akathisia. The increase in arousal due to the akathisia may outweigh benefits of the neuroleptic in improving a paranoid perception of the present situation.

Therapeutic intervention may be aimed at specifically reversing a causative mechanism such as correcting a manic mood or delusional perception. It may have the more general aim of reducing arousal and thereby diminishing the likelihood of any impulsive behavior. In the remainder of this section we discuss how each aspect of the impulsive behavior may be affected by specific brain dysfunction and how particular therapies for impulsive behavior may be linked to specific mechanisms.

First of all, anxiety, tension, or fear due to neuropsychiatric disorders may increase arousal, leading to impulsive action. A wide range of neuropsychiatric disorders have been linked to increased anxiety, and some of them have been specifically linked to impulsive and unplanned violence or self-injury. Partial seizures with ictal fear, or with postictal agitation, may be associated with unplanned violence. Furthermore, behaviorally relevant anxiety may also occur interictally in patients with epilepsy (Fedio 1986). Delirium, during its agitated phases, is associated with increased arousal; focal vascular lesions particularly likely to cause delirium are strokes in the right parietal region and the basal occipital regions (Lipowski 1990). Increased arousal, particularly in the form of irritability, may accompany migrainous phenomena (Welch 1987). A range of drugs frequently encountered in neurological patients may raise arousal levels, even in the absence of delirium. Common examples are antidepressants, dopamine agonists, stimulants, and xanthines such as theophylline.

Weissman et al.'s recent work (1989) associating panic disorder with an increased risk of suicide attempts may be explained by increased impulsivity secondary to the increased arousal caused by anxiety. However, as suggested by Fogel (1990a), panic disorder may be an insufficient condition to explain suicidal behavior without additional psychopathology. Other psychiatric syndromes that cause increased arousal include mania or hypomania. They may be secondary to neurological disease; right-hemisphere lesions are the most common neurological causes of secondary mania (Cummings and Mendez 1984; Robinson et al. 1988; Starkstein et al. 1987).

Arousal can be reduced by a variety of agents including antianxiety drugs, neuroleptics, and β-blockers, and also by correcting the primary causes of increased arousal discussed above. For example, Ratey et al. (1987) attributed their success with β-blockers in treating aggressive behaviors in autistic patients to the reduction of a hyperaroused state.

Second, patients' perceptions of their current environment, including contingencies that might lead to impulsive action, depend on the intactness of primary sensory cortex and association areas. Patients who misperceive their environment may perceive threats when none are there, leading to inappropriate impulsive behavior as a defense against the perceived threat. One of the best established examples is the paranoia that often accompanies Wernicke's aphasia (Benson 1979). Some patients with visual agnosia, or with geographic disorientation due to right-hemisphere lesions, may become frightened by their misperceptions, leading to an increased state of arousal and vulnerability to impulsive action. Assessment of sensory function therefore becomes relevant in evaluating impulsive behavior. This should include both primary sensory function as well as sensory gnosis and language function.

Third, the emotional significance of a perceived situation is relevant both to the level of arousal and to the development of a motive for an impulsive act. Perceptions of emotional significance in neuropsychiatric patients may be colored by altered mood, disordered thinking, or the "hyperconnection" of temporolimbic epilepsy. The despair and irritability of a major depression, or the euphoria and grandiosity of mania, clearly can alter the emotional significance of a situation and lead to the development of a motive for impulsive action. (The wide range of neurological lesions associated with the development of secondary depression or mania is discussed in Chapter 9.) When these conditions exist, treatment of impulsive behavior is best directed initially toward normalization of mood.

Delusional or paranoid thinking (see Chapter 9 for its multiple neurological causes) leads to impulsive behavior by the misperception of benign events as threatening. Neuroleptic therapy is most appropriate and specific for altering these paranoid and delusional perceptions.

Patients with temporolimbic epilepsy may show hyperemotionality, thought by Bear (1979) to be due to a "hyperconnection" of limbic areas with association areas brought about by the continual abnormal electrical activity of the seizure focus. The excessively deep feeling of patients with this condition may lead them to act impulsively on abnormally intensified emotions. This may explain the striking increase in suicidal behavior among depressed epileptic patients compared with patients with uncomplicated depression (Mendez et al. 1986). Excessive self-righteous anger or self-punitive guilt have also been described (Blumer and Benson 1982). Anticonvulsant therapy, particularly with carbamazepine, may alleviate some of the overly intense emotion, although the syndrome of hyperconnection may persist even when seizures are controlled. Dramatic changes in impulsive behavior, related to changes in emotional function, have been observed after surgical therapy of temporal lobe epilepsy (Rausch and Crandall 1982; Taylor 1972).

Fourth, because action requires a plan, neurologically based impairment in planning may lead to simpler and less appropriate actions. The development of motor plans is linked with the basal ganglia and frontal lobes. In particular, damage to the frontal lobes impairs the ability to develop complex plans (Mesulam 1986; Stuss and Benson 1986). Thus the patient with frontal lobe damage or dysfunction may respond to an arousing situation with a relatively simple, and sometimes inappropriate, action.

Finally, appropriate inhibition of action depends both on appreciation of contingencies and on the ability to control impulses in response to them. The dorsolateral frontal region is associated with the perception of contextual cues to appropriate behavior, whereas the orbital frontal region is thought to be necessary to make actions conform to the perceived cues (Fogel and Eslinger 1991). Thus the patient with severe dorsolateral frontal damage may not perceive the significance of the police officer standing by his elbow, whereas the patient with more isolated orbital frontal damage may be aware that this calls for restraint but may be unable to control himself. The relevance of focal frontal lesions to violence is supported by recent work by Heinrichs (1989), who studied neurological, psychiatric, and demographic predictors of violent incidents in a provincial psychiatric hospital. The presence of a focal frontal lesion was the best single predictor of violent incidents, accounting for 11% of the variance.

Anatomical localization of frontal lobe damage and neuropsychological investigation of abstract reasoning and impulse control capabilities may be useful in determining the specific reason why an individual with frontal damage or dysfunction has difficulty inhibiting inappropriate behavior. However, anatomical localization based on cognitive and behavioral signs alone is at best tentative. Deficits in appreciation of context or in impulse control suggesting frontal lobe dysfunction may be due to changes in subcortical input to the frontal lobe, including dopaminergic, noradrenergic, and serotonergic inputs from the brain stem. Furthermore, diseases of the basal ganglia may produce "frontal" signs, because output from the prefrontal cortex goes to the basal ganglia, which in turn feed back to the frontal lobes via the thalamus (Goldman-Rakic 1987).

A specific example of disinhibition probably due to subcortical influences on the frontal lobe is ADHD. In this condition, aggressive behavior is ameliorated by administration of methylphenidate, a dopamine agonist. Detailed study of behavioral effects of methylphenidate in a group of boys with ADHD showed that the drug decreased rule breaking but did not increase positive prosocial behavior (Hinshaw et al. 1989). This suggests a relatively specific therapeutic action on a deficient inhibitory system.

The distinction between orbital frontal and dorsolateral frontal mechanisms may have therapeutic implications. The patient with impaired perception of cues might benefit from a strengthening of environmental cues or repeated practice to overlearn the response to particular inhibitory cues. By contrast, the individual with severe orbital frontal damage, who simply cannot inhibit impulses even when context is clear to him or her, may do better with treatments directed at reducing arousal.

Applications of the Model

The model described above can be used to hypothesize specific mechanisms in formulating a case of impulsive behavior and to select a plan and sequence of drug trials. If assessment reveals that paranoid ideation is the primary stimulus for a patient's impulsive behavior, neuroleptic therapy should be tried first. If excess arousal appears to be the major problem, treatment should begin with eliminating stimulants, such as caffeine, and using agents such as benzodiazepines, β-blockers, or buspirone. If agitated or irritable affect associated with depression is a major feature, an antidepressant should be tried first. If diminished self-monitoring and self-control due to poor frontal performance are the primary issues, stimulants or dopamine agonists should be considered to enhance residual frontal lobe function. If impaired appraisal of environmental contingencies is a conspicuous feature, a cognitive behavioral approach, potentially using external clues, should be attempted. For patients in whom multiple mechanisms are likely, combined pharmacotherapy or combined medical-behavioral intervention is prescribed, according to the mechanisms thought to be involved.

In future research on drug therapies for impulsive behavior in patients with brain damage, patients should be characterized as precisely as possible regarding lesion localization, neuropsychological features, and the precise details of their mental status and the circumstances in which they act impulsively. This would allow application of the lessons of case series to the kind of analyses illustrated here.

The general model offered here for impulsive behavior may also be helpful in understanding why therapies attempted for impulsive behavior may not work or may actually make the behavior worse:

1. Behavioral treatments based on negative reinforcement of impulsive behavior may fail if the patient's basic inhibitory mechanisms are inadequate, for example, because of severe orbital frontal damage. In this situation, an increase in arousal due to punishment actually could aggravate the behavior.
2. Neuroleptic therapy, appropriately prescribed because of paranoid perceptions, may actually aggravate impulsive behavior if it increases arousal by causing akathisia, if it causes depression, or if its inhibitory effect on frontal lobe function leads to a worsening of reasoning and judgment.
3. β-Blockers, given to improve impulsive behavior by reducing arousal, may aggravate the behavior if they cause depression, or, as may occur rarely, if they cause hallucinations or other abnormal perceptions.
4. Benzodiazepines, given to reduce arousal or possibly to treat a hypomanic state, may aggravate impulsive behavior by impairing the inhibitory mechanisms of the frontal lobes. Barbiturates may have similar effects.
5. Stimulants or dopamine agonists, given to improve frontal lobe function and enhance inhibition (as in stimulant treatment of ADHD) may aggravate impulsive behavior if they excessively increase arousal, induce a manic mood, or lead to the development of paranoid ideation.
6. Antidepressants, given to improve impulsive behavior by correcting depressed mood and perhaps indirectly by improving frontal lobe function (which is diminished in severe depression), may at times induce a hyperaroused state with an increase in impulsive behavior. This issue has recently been raised in connection with suicidal or violent behavior in patients initiating therapy with fluoxetine, but hyperarousal can be seen with any of the antidepressants (Teicher et al. 1990). It is perhaps less common with the more sedating agents, such as trazodone and amitriptyline.

Application of the model to violence associated with substance abuse. Alcohol (Roy and Linnoila 1986; Skog 1986; Virkkunen 1974) and other drugs of abuse, including phencyclidine, cocaine, and anabolic steroids (Pope and Katz 1990), have been linked to violent behavior. Drug-related violence can be understood in relation to the general model, and the model assists differentiation of cases requiring different treatments. For example, cocaine may induce a paranoid psychosis, mania, or hyperarousal without thought disorder, or there may be frontal dysfunction from subcortical brain damage from cocaine-associated vasculopathy. Similarly, acute alcohol intoxication can produce disinhibition similar to that seen with frontal lobe damage, and chronic use may lead to a mood disorder or paranoid state. Withdrawal is associated with marked hyperarousal. Violence related to anabolic steroid use was linked in three cases to a drug-induced manic episode (Pope and Katz 1990), which presumably increased arousal and altered the patients' judgment of their situation. As with impulsive behavior in general, therapy should be aimed at the specific underlying dysfunction that leads to the common outcome of violence.

❑ CONCLUSIONS

The assessment and management of depression and impulsive behavior are daily tasks for the practicing neuropsychiatrist. At present, we are far from a comprehensive pathophysiology of either of these problems. The clinician's dilemma is that controlled trials and case series must necessarily simplify the complexities actually encountered in approaching patients with these syndromes. Nonetheless, practical guidelines can be offered to inform therapeutic choices. Basing clinical decisions on hypotheses, even if they are ultimately proved wrong, makes therapy a more systematic and rational process and helps the clinician learn from experience. This chapter is intended as an invitation to the reader to pursue "practical pathophysiology" with neuropsychiatric patients.

❑ REFERENCES

Akiskal HS: Subaffective disorders: dysthymic, cyclothymic and bipolar, II: disorders in the "borderline" realm. Psychiatr Clin North Am 4:26–46, 1981

Akiskal HS, Hirschfeld FMA, Yerevanian BI: The relationship of personality to affective disorders: a critical review. Arch Gen Psychiatry 40:801–810, 1983

Amsterdam JD: Pharmacotherapy of refractory depression. Symposium presented at the 143rd annual meeting of the American Psychiatric Association, New York, May 1990

Barragry JM, Makin HLJ, Trafford DJH, et al: Effect of anticonvulsants on plasma testosterone and sex hormone binding globulin levels. J Neurol Neurosurg Psychiatry 41:913–941, 1978

Bear DM: The temporal lobes: an approach to the study of organic behavioral changes, in Handbook of Behavioral Neurobiology-Neuropsychology. Edited by Gazzaniga M. New York, Plenum, 1979

Bear DM: Hemispheric specialization and the neurology of emotion. Arch Neurol 40:195–202, 1983

Bear DM: Hierarchical neural regulation of aggression: some predictable patterns of violence, in Current Approaches to the Prediction of Violence. Edited by Brizer DA, Crowner M. Washington, DC, American Psychiatric Press, 1989, pp 85–99

Benson DF: Aphasia, Alexia, and Agraphia. New York, Churchill Livingstone, 1979

Benson DF: Hydrocephalic dementia, in Handbook of Clinical Neurology, Vol 2(46): Neurobehavioral Disorders. Edited by Frederiks JAM. Amsterdam, Elsevier, 1985, pp 323–333

Blumer D, Benson DF: Psychiatric manifestations of epilepsy, in Psychiatric Aspects of Neurologic Disease, Vol II. Edited by Benson DF, Blumer D. New York, Grune & Stratton, 1982, pp 25–48

Blumer D, Heilbronn M, Himmelhoch J: Indications for carbamazepine in mental illness: atypical psychiatric disorder or temporal lobe syndrome? Compr Psychiatry 29:108–122, 1988

Caird FI, Scott PJW: Drug-Induced Diseases in the Elderly. Amsterdam, Elsevier, 1986, pp 71–82

Cummings JL, Mendez MF: Secondary mania with focal cerebrovascular lesions. Am J Psychiatry 141:1084–1087, 1984

Delgado-Escueta AV, Mattson RH, King L, et al: The nature of aggression during epileptic seizures. N Engl J Med 305:711–716, 1981

Engel J: Seizures and Epilepsy. Philadelphia, PA, FA Davis, 1989

Fedio P: Behavioral characteristics of patients with temporal lobe epilepsy. Psychiatr Clin North Am 9:267–281, 1986

Finkelstein S, Benowitz L, Baldessarini RJ, et al: Mood, vegetative disturbance, and dexamethasone suppression test after stroke. Ann Neurol 12:463–468, 1982

Fogel BS: Combining anticonvulsants with conventional psychopharmacologic agents, in Anticonvulsants in Psychiatry. Edited by McElroy SL, Pope HG. Clifton, NJ, Oxford Health Care, 1988, pp 77–94

Fogel BS: Panic attacks and the risk of suicide attempts (letter). N Engl J Med 322:1320–1321, 1990a

Fogel BS: Localization in neuropsychiatry (editorial). Journal of Neuropsychiatry and Clinical Neuroscience 2: 361–362, 1990b

Fogel BS, Eslinger PJ: Diagnosis and management of patients with frontal lobe syndromes, in Medical Psychiatric Practice, Vol I. Edited by Stoudemire A, Fogel BS. Washington, DC, American Psychiatric Press, 1991, pp 349–392

Fogel BS, Sparadeo F: Focal cognitive deficits accentuated by depression: a case study. J Nerv Ment Dis 173:120–124, 1985

Ford CV: Psychogenic fugue, in Treatments of Psychiatric Disorders: A Task Force Report of the American Psychiatric Association. Washington, DC, American Psychiatric Association, 1989, pp 2190–2196

Giang DL: Depression in systemic lupus erythematosus. Journal of Neuropsychiatry, Neuropsychology and Behavioral Neurology (in press)

Goldman-Rakic PS: Circuitry of the frontal association cortex and its relevance to dementia. Archives of Gerontology and Geriatrics 6:299–309, 1987

Gottlieb GL, Greenspan D: Depression and endocrine disorders, in Depression and Coexisting Disease. Edited by Robinson RG, Rabins PV. New York, Igaku-Shoin, 1989, pp 83–102

Hachinski V, Norris JW: The Acute Stroke. Philadelphia, PA, FA Davis, 1985, pp 141–164

Harvey PG, Hay KM: Mood and migraine: a preliminary prospective study. Headache 24:225–228, 1984

Hein MD, Jackson IMD: Thyroid function in psychiatric illness. Gen Hosp Psychiatry 12:232–244, 1990

Heinrichs RW: Frontal cerebral lesions and violent incidents in chronic neuropsychiatric patients. Biol Psychiatry 25:174–178, 1989

Herzog AG: A hypothesis to integrate partial seizures of temporal lobe origin and reproductive endocrine disorders. Epilepsy Res 3:151–159, 1989

Herzog AG, Siebel MM, Schomer DL, et al: Reproductive endocrine disorders in men with partial seizures of temporal lobe origin. Arch Neurol 43:347–350, 1986

Himmelhoch JM: Major mood disorders related to epileptic changes, in Psychiatric Aspects of Epilepsy. Edited by Blumer D. Washington, DC, American Psychiatric Press, 1984, pp 271–294

Hinshaw SP, Henker B, Whalen CK, et al: Aggressive, prosocial, and nonsocial behavior in hyperactive boys: dose effects of methylphenidate in naturalistic settings. J Consult Clin Psychol 57:636–643, 1989

Holcomb HH, Links J, Smith C, et al: Positron emission tomography: measuring the metabolic and neurochemical characteristics of the living human nervous system, in Brain Imaging: Applications in Psychiatry. Edited by Andreasen NC. Washington, DC, American Psychiatric Press, 1989, pp 235–370

Kase SE, O'Riordan CA: Rehabilitation approach, in Handbook of Parkinson's Disease. Edited by Koller WC. New York, Marcel Dekker, 1987, pp 455–464

Lewis DA, Smith RE: Steroid induced psychiatric syndrome. J Affective Disord 5:319–332, 1983

Lewis DO, Shanok SS, Grant M, et al: Homicidally aggressive young children: neuropsychiatric and experiential correlates. Am J Psychiatry 140:148–153, 1983

Lidberg L, Tuck JR, Asberg M, et al: Homicide, suicide and CSF 5-HIAA. Acta Psychiatr Scand 71:230–236, 1985

Linn L: Psychogenic amnesia, in Treatments of Psychiatric Disorders: A Task Force Report of the American Psychiatric Association. Washington, DC, American Psychiatric Association, 1989, pp 2186–2190

Lipowski ZJ: Delirium: Acute Confusional States. New York, Oxford University Press, 1990, pp 375–398

McElroy SL, Pope HG (eds): Use of Anticonvulsants in Psychiatry: Recent Advances. Clifton, NJ, Oxford Health Care, 1988

Marin RS: Differential diagnosis and classification of apathy. Am J Psychiatry 147:22–30, 1990

Matthews WB: Symptoms and signs, in McAlpine's Multiple Sclerosis. Edited by Matthews WB. Edinburgh, Churchill Livingstone, 1985, pp 96–118

Mattson RH: Selection of antiepileptic drug therapy, in Antiepileptic Drugs, 3rd Edition. Edited by Levy RH, Dreifuss FE, Mattson RH, et al. New York, Raven, 1989, pp 103–116

Mayeux R, Stern Y, Williams JBW, et al: Depression and Parkinson's disease, in Advances in Neurology, Vol 45: Parkinson's Disease. Edited by Yahr MD, Bergmann KJ. New York, Raven, 1987, pp 451–455

Mendez MF, Cummings JL, Benson DF: Depression in epilepsy. Arch Neurol 43:766–770, 1986

Merikangas JR: Headache syndromes, in Medical Psychiatric Practice, Vol 1. Edited by Stoudemire A, Fogel BS. Washington, DC, American Psychiatric Press, 1991, pp 393–424

Mesulam M-M: Frontal cortex and behavior (editorial). Ann Neurol 19:320–325, 1986

Nausieda PA: Sleep disorders, in Handbook of Parkinson's Disease. Edited by Koller WC. New York, Marcel Dekker, 1987, pp 371–380

Ouslander JG: Incontinence, in Alzheimer's Disease: Treatment and Long-Term Management. Edited by Cummings JL, Miller BL. New York, Marcel Dekker, 1990, pp 177–206

Pasqualy M, Veith RC: Depression as an adverse drug reaction, in Depression and Coexisting Disease. Edited by Robinson RG, Rabins PV. New York, Igaku-Shoin, 1989, pp 132–151

Pfeiffer RF, Hsieh HH, Diercks MJ, et al: Dexamethasone suppression test in Parkinson's disease, in Advances in Neurology, Vol 45: Parkinson's Disease. Edited by Yahr MD, Bergmann KJ. New York, Raven, 1987, pp 439–442

Pope HG, Katz DL: Homicide and near-homicide by anabolic steroid users. J Clin Psychiatry 51:28–31, 1990

Popper CW: Disorders usually first evident in infancy, childhood, or adolescence, in American Psychiatric Press Textbook of Psychiatry. Edited by Talbott JA, Hales RE, Yudofsky SC. Washington, DC, American Psychiatric Press, 1988, pp 649–735

Pottash ALC, Black HR, Gold MS: Psychiatric complications of antihypertensive medications. J Nerv Ment Dis 169:430–438, 1981

Price TR, Tucker GJ: Psychiatric and behavioral manifestations of normal pressure hydrocephalus. J Nerv Ment Dis 154:51–55, 1977

Ratey JJ, Morrill R, Oxenkrug G: Use of propranolol for provoked and unprovoked episodes of rage. Am J Psychiatry 140:1356–1357, 1983

Ratey JJ, Mikkelsen E, Sorgi P, et al: Autism: the treatment of aggressive behaviors. J Clin Psychopharmacol 7:35–41, 1987

Rausch R, Crandall PH: Psychological status related to surgical control of temporal lobe seizures. Epilepsia 23:191–202, 1982

Robertson MM, Trimble MR: Depressive illness in patients with epilepsy: a review. Epilepsia 24 (suppl 2):S109–S116, 1983

Robinson RG: Differential behavioral and biochemical effects of right and left hemispheric cerebral infarction in the rat. Biol Psychiatry 12:669–680, 1979

Robinson RG, Boston JD, Starkstein SE, et al: Comparison of mania and depression after brain injury: causal factors. Am J Psychiatry 145:172–178, 1988

Ross ED: Modulation of affect and nonverbal communication by the right hemisphere, in Principles of Behavioral Neurology. Edited by Mesulam M-M. Philadelphia, PA, FA Davis, 1985, pp 239–257

Ross ED, Rush AJ: Diagnosis and neuroanatomical correlates of depression in brain-damaged patients: implications for a neurology of depression. Arch Gen Psychiatry 38:1344, 1981

Roy A, Linnoila M: Alcoholism and suicide. Suicide Life Threat Behav 16:244–273, 1986

Roy A, Virkkunen M, Guthrie S, et al: Indices of serotonin and glucose metabolism in violent offenders, arsonists, and alcoholics. Ann N Y Acad Sci 487:202–220, 1986

Schold C, Yarnell PR, Earnest MP: Origins of seizures in elderly patients. JAMA 238:1177–1178, 1977

Skog O-J: Trends in alcohol consumption and violent deaths. Br J Addict 81:365–379, 1986

Starkstein SE, Pearlson GD, Boston J, et al: Mania after

brain injury: a controlled study of causative factors. Arch Neurol 44:1069–1073, 1987
Stern RA, Bachman DL: Depressive symptoms following stroke. Am J Psychiatry 148:351–356, 1991
Stoudemire A, Moran MG, Fogel BS: Psychotropic drug use in the medically ill: part I. Psychosomatics 31:377–391, 1990
Stoudemire A, Moran MG, Fogel BS: Psychotropic drug use in the medically ill: part II. Psychosomatics 32:34–46, 1991a
Stoudemire A, Fogel BS, Gulley LR: Psychopharmacology in the medically ill: an update, in Medical Psychiatric Practice, Vol 1. Edited by Stoudemire A, Fogel BS. Washington, DC, American Psychiatric Press, 1991b, pp 29–97
Stuss DT, Benson DF: Neuropsychological studies of the frontal lobes. Psychol Bull 95:3–28, 1984
Stuss DT, Benson DF: The Frontal Lobes. New York, Raven, 1986
Taylor DC: Mental state and temporal lobe epilepsy: a correlative account of 100 patients treated surgically. Epilepsia 13:727–765, 1972
Taylor DC: The components of sickness: disease, illness and predicaments, in One Child. Edited by Apley J, Ounsted C. London, Heinemann, 1982, pp 1–13
Teicher MH, Glod C, Cole JO: Emergence of intense suicidal preoccupation during fluoxetine treatment. Am J Psychiatry 147:207–210, 1990
Toone BK, Wheeler M, Nanjee M, et al: Sex hormones, sexual activity and plasma anticonvulsant levels in male epileptics. J Neurol Neurosurg Psychiatry 46:824–826, 1983
Traskman-Bendz L, Asberg M, Schalling D: Serotonergic function and suicidal behavior in personality disorders. Ann N Y Acad Sci 487:168–174, 1986
Virkkunen M: Alcohol as a factor precipitating aggression and conflict behaviour leading to homicide. Br J Addict 69:149–154, 1974
Weissman MM, Klerman GL, Markowitz JS, et al: Suicidal ideation and suicide attempts in panic disorder and attacks. N Engl J Med 321:1209–1214, 1989
Welch KMA: Migraine: a biobehavioral disorder. Arch Neurol 44:323–327, 1987
Widiger TA, Frances AJ: Personality disorders, in The American Psychiatric Press Textbook of Psychiatry. Edited by Talbott JA, Hales RE, Yudofsky SC. Washington, DC, American Psychiatric Press, 1988, pp 621–648
Wilbur CB, Kluft RP: Multiple personality disorder, in Treatments of Psychiatric Disorders: A Task Force Report of the American Psychiatric Association. Washington, DC, American Psychiatric Association, 1989, pp 2197–2216
Yudofsky SC, Stevens L, Silver J, et al: Propranolol in the treatment of rage and violent behavior associated with Korsakoff's psychosis. Am J Psychiatry 141:114–115, 1984
Zubenko GS, Moossy J: Major depression in primary dementia. Arch Neurol 45:1182–1186, 1988

Chapter

15

Neuropsychiatric Aspects of Memory and Amnesia

Arthur P. Shimamura, Ph.D.
Felicia B. Gershberg, Sc.B.

COMPLAINTS ABOUT MEMORY are prominent symptoms among psychiatric and neurological patients (Strubb and Black 1977). This symptomatology is not surprising, because memory influences nearly all aspects of daily living, and thus any disturbance of mood or thought will likely affect the ability to learn and remember. The ubiquity of memory in daily activities is one reason why an understanding of the neural systems that mediate memory is so important for neuropsychiatry. Moreover, it is vital to understand how these neural systems are affected by pharmacological treatments or other psychiatric treatments, such as electroconvulsive therapy (ECT).

Advances in our understanding of brain organization and memory have come from many diverse fields, including neuroanatomy, physiology, behavioral neurology, biological psychiatry, neuropsychology, and cognitive science. In this chapter we review some of these recent advances. In the first section we review neurobehavioral findings concerning the "amnestic syndrome" and describe how these findings contribute to our understanding of normal memory functions. In the second section we highlight advances in neuroanatomical, physiological, and biochemical approaches and describe biological mechanisms that mediate memory functions. Finally, in the third section we address related issues such as the role of the frontal lobes in memory, the effects of depression on memory, and the notion of psychogenic or functional amnesia.

This work was supported by a Biomedical Research Support Grant (No. 89-6-82), a National Institute on Aging Grant (AG-09055), and a National Science Foundation Predoctoral Fellowship (to F. B. Gershberg).

❑ THE AMNESTIC SYNDROME

Memory and the Hippocampus

Across a lifetime, we retain and recollect a plethora of memories, many of which have been held for more than several decades. How does the brain accomplish such extraordinary feats of learning and remembering? An important clue to this process was discovered serendipitously with the investigation of patient H. M., who in 1953 underwent surgery for relief of severe epilepsy (Scoville and Milner 1957). The surgery involved bilateral excision of the medial temporal region, which reportedly included removal of the uncus (including the amygdala), anterior two-thirds of the hippocampus, and hippocampal gyrus (Figure 15–1).

After surgery, H. M. exhibited a profound *anterograde amnesia* (i.e., he was unable to remember events and information encountered since his operation) (Corkin 1984; Milner 1959; Milner et al. 1968). Despite this severe impairment in new learning ability, there was no detectable impairment in intellectual or language abilities. There was some *retrograde amnesia,* which refers to impairment of memory for events that occurred before the onset of amnesia. For example, H. M. could not recognize previously familiar members of the medical staff nor could he remember the layout of the hospital ward, which was also familiar to him before surgery. Furthermore, he could not recall the death of a favorite uncle who had died 3 years previously. H. M. is still alive, and more recent evidence suggests that he has some retrograde amnesia for even more remote events (Corkin 1984). Nevertheless, H. M.'s retrograde amnesia is not severe, as indicated by the fact that he performed as well as control subjects on a test of memory for faces of celebrities who became famous before 1950 (Marslen-Wilson and Teuber 1975). He was also able to recall well-formed autobiographical episodes from his adolescence (Corkin 1984).

The central feature of H. M.'s memory disorder is new learning impairment, which affects information received from all sensory modalities and includes impairment of both verbal and nonverbal memory. For example, H. M. exhibits severe impairment on tests of word and picture recall, paired-associate learning, and recognition memory. His impairment also includes the inability to learn new vocabulary words that have been added to the dictionary since his surgery. In conjunction with these findings from psychometric tests, clinical observations of H. M. indicate that memory for ongoing events is severely impaired. For example, 30 minutes after eating lunch, H. M. could not recall what he had eaten or whether he had even had lunch. H. M. is aware of his disorder and has reflected on his impairment as always "waking from a dream." In other words, he seems to lack continuity in the memory of events across time, even when the events are separated by only a few minutes.

Despite the severity of his amnesia, H. M. can think and act normally, as indicated by his pre-

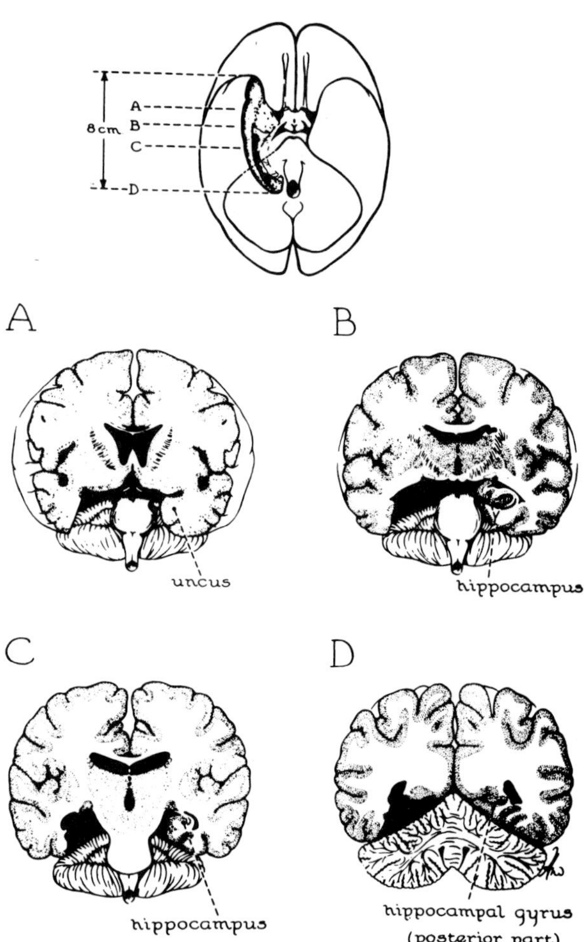

Figure 15–1. Diagram of the extent of tissue removal in the bilateral medial temporal lobe surgery of patient H. M. Surgery included removal of anterior two-thirds of the hippocampus, uncus (including the amygdala), and hippocampal gyrus. Lesioned area is indicated by the darkened region in the area of the left medial temporal lobe of each orbital view, although actual lesion was bilateral. (Reprinted from Milner B: The memory defect in bilateral hippocampal lesions. Psychiatric Research Reports 11:43–52, 1959. Used with permission.)

served I.Q. Indeed, even some memory functions are spared, such as *immediate memory*, which is exemplified by intact performance on tests of digit span. Nevertheless, as soon as information is out of conscious experience, it is forgotten. The analysis of H. M.'s amnesia stands as a milestone in our progress to understanding memory in the brain. He has provided the crucial evidence for the specific role of the medial temporal region in the process of memory formation and storage. Indeed, the analysis of H. M. by Milner and colleagues has provided the impetus for thousands of animal studies on the role of the hippocampus in learning and memory.

Other neurological disorders can produce an amnestic syndrome similar to that seen in patient H. M. The DSM-III-R diagnostic criteria (American Psychiatric Association 1987) for this syndrome are shown in Table 15–1. The diagnostic criteria define anterograde amnesia as impairment of "short-term" memory and retrograde amnesia as impairment of "long-term" memory. (These terms are avoided here so as not to confuse readers familiar with the way in which psychologists and neuroscientists use the terms "short-term memory," which refers to memory that lasts for seconds, and "long-term memory," which refers to memory that lasts beyond the span of short-term or immediate memory.) Tumors, head injuries, or vascular disorders that impinge on the medial temporal region can produce an amnestic syndrome. Also, a persistent and selective amnesia can occur following viral encephalitis, ischemia, or hypoxia (Cermak 1976; Damasio et al. 1985; Whitty et al. 1977; Zola-Morgan et al. 1986). In these cases, anterograde amnesia is typically the outstanding cognitive impairment, but retrograde amnesia can also occur (Squire and Shimamura 1986). General intellectual abilities and immediate memory (i.e., digit span) are often intact. Although the medial temporal region is typically affected in these disorders, damage to other brain regions can also occur.

One case of amnesia (patient R. B.) provided additional clues about the role of the hippocampus in memory (Zola-Morgan et al. 1986). Patient R. B. became amnesic in 1978, when he experienced an ischemic episode that occurred during open-heart surgery. During the 4 years after this episode, R. B. was given extensive neuropsychological assessment. He exhibited the hallmark features of medial temporal amnesia: severe anterograde amnesia, little if any retrograde amnesia, and preserved intellectual abilities. In 1983, R. B. suffered a fatal cardiac arrest, and, with the encouragement of his family, a comprehensive histological examination of his brain was performed. This examination revealed a circumscribed, bilateral lesion restricted to the CA_1 subfield of the hippocampus. R. B. represents the first extensively studied case of amnesia that occurred as a result of a lesion restricted to the hippocampus. Along with patient H. M., patient R. B. demonstrates the crucial role of the hippocampus in memory. It is important to note that although R. B.'s amnesia was clinically significant, it was not as severe as that of H. M. This difference is probably due to the fact that H. M.'s lesion extended beyond the hippocampus and included bilateral removal of parahippocampal gyrus and amygdala. Thus it is likely that the extent of the damage within the medial temporal region can determine the severity of amnesia.

TABLE 15–1. DSM-III-R DIAGNOSTIC CRITERIA FOR AMNESTIC SYNDROME

A. Demonstrable evidence of impairment in both short- and long-term memory; with regard to long-term memory, very remote events are remembered better than more recent events. Impairment in short-term memory (inability to learn new information) may be indicated by inability to remember three objects after five minutes. Long-term memory impairment (inability to remember information that was known in the past) may be indicated by inability to remember past personal information (e.g., what happened yesterday, birthplace, occupation) or facts of common knowledge (e.g., past Presidents, well-known dates).

B. Not occurring exclusively during the course of delirium, and does not meet the criteria for dementia (i.e., no impairment in abstract thinking or judgment, no other disturbances of higher cortical function, and no personality change).

C. There is evidence from the history, physical examination, or laboratory tests of a specific organic factor (or factors) judged to be etiologically related to the disturbance.

Source. Reprinted from American Psychiatric Association: Diagnostic and Statistical Manual of Mental Disorders, 3rd Edition, Revised. Washington, DC, American Psychiatric Association, 1987, p 109. Used with permission.

Advances in in vivo neuroimaging techniques, such as magnetic resonance imaging (MRI) and positron-emission tomography (PET), have allowed more detailed analysis of the brain areas that are damaged in neurological patients (Andreasen 1988; Damasio and Damasio 1989). For example, a new technique has been developed for high-resolution MRI imaging of the hippocampus (Press et al. 1989). This technique involves positioning the head so the image plane is perpendicular to the long axis of the hippocampal formation. As a result, a clear cross-sectional image of the hippocampal formation can be obtained. This technique has already provided remarkable data concerning the extent of hippocampal damage in patients with amnesia (Press et al. 1989). For example, quantitative analyses of MRI scans using this new technique have revealed that, compared with control subjects, patients with amnesia exhibit an average loss of 49% of tissue in the area of the hippocampal formation. Despite this tissue loss, the average area of the temporal lobe in these patients was nearly identical to that of the control subjects. These data confirm and extend the findings from patients H. M. and R. B. and offer a new approach to the analysis of amnestic disorders.

Diencephalic Amnesia

Damage to the diencephalic midline can also produce an amnestic disorder that is often indistinguishable from the behavioral consequences of medial temporal damage. Patients with thalamic infarction in the area surrounding the paramedian arteries often exhibit an amnestic syndrome (Graff-Radford et al. 1990; Von Cramon et al. 1985). Also, a noted patient with amnesia (patient N. A.), who sustained left-thalamic damage after a penetrating head injury with a miniature fencing foil, exhibited a severe amnesia for verbal information (Kaushall et al. 1981). The two structures within the diencephalon that have been implicated as critical for memory processes are the mediodorsal nucleus of the thalamus and the mammillary bodies of the hypothalamus.

The best-studied cases of amnesia due to diencephalic damage are those of patients with Korsakoff's syndrome. Korsakoff's syndrome can develop after nutritional deficiency resulting from many years of chronic alcohol abuse (Butters and Cermak 1980; Victor et al. 1989). Neuropathological studies have indicated bilateral lesions along the walls of the third and fourth ventricles, typically involving the dorsomedial thalamic nuclei and mammillary bodies (Mair et al. 1979; Mayes et al. 1988; Victor et al. 1989). In addition, cortical atrophy and cerebellar damage are often observed. A study (Shimamura et al. 1988) using quantitative analyses of computed tomography (CT) data from patients with Korsakoff's syndrome corroborated these neuropathological findings by identifying increased fluid volume and low density values in the medial thalamic region and the frontal and temporal lobes.

Patients with Korsakoff's syndrome exhibit severe anterograde amnesia in the presence of relatively preserved intellectual abilities. Extensive retrograde amnesia can occur and encompass memory loss that can span several decades (Albert et al. 1979). The extent and severity of retrograde amnesia, however, is variable among these patients, with some showing extensive retrograde amnesia and others showing little (Squire et al. 1989a). One factor that complicates the characterization of the memory impairment in Korsakoff's syndrome is generalized cortical atrophy, which is presumed to be a consequence of chronic alcohol abuse. Indeed, some memory functions, such as memory for temporal order, immediate memory, and stimulus encoding, are impaired in patients with Korsakoff's syndrome but not in other patients with amnesia (Huppert and Piercy 1976; Meudell et al. 1985; Shimamura et al., in press; Squire 1982). Moreover, patients with Korsakoff's syndrome are often emotionally flat, apathetic, and lacking insight about their deficit (Butters and Cermak 1980; Squire and Zouzounis 1988; Talland 1965). These additional cognitive and personality disorders may occur as a result of extensive cortical damage and, in particular, damage to the frontal lobes.

Transient Amnesias

Not all amnestic syndromes are permanent. Traumatic head injury, for example, can cause a transient and selective memory impairment (Barbizet 1970; Whitty and Zangwill 1977). After the initial stages of unconsciousness or confusion, both anterograde and retrograde amnesias occur, and the severity of anterograde amnesia is often correlated with the temporal extent of retrograde amnesia (Russell and Nathan 1946). Retrograde amnesia tends to follow *Ribot's Law* (Ribot 1881), which states that memory for the recent past is affected more severely than memory for the distant past. Amnesia following head trauma can last for minutes, days, or even weeks. In mild trauma cases, new learning ability recovers to premorbid levels. In more severe cases, both amnesia and other cognitive impairment can be long lasting and sometimes permanent (Whitty and Zangwill 1977).

Figure 15–2 illustrates a time course of posttraumatic, transient amnesia in a case reported by Barbizet (1970). During the first examination, which occurred 5 months after trauma, the patient exhibited rather extensive anterograde and retrograde amnesia. The second examination revealed some recovery of new learning ability with shrinking of the temporal extent of retrograde amnesia. The third examination revealed almost complete recovery from anterograde and retrograde amnesia. However, there was a permanent residual loss of memories for the events that occurred just before the traumatic event and throughout the period of severe anterograde amnesia. This gap in memory—often described as a *memory lacuna*—occurs because memory formation or storage was dysfunctional during that time period.

Another form of memory impairment is *transient global amnesia* (TGA), which closely resembles the permanent amnestic syndrome seen in patients with medial temporal or diencephalic amnesia (Fisher and Adams 1964; Kritchevsky et al. 1988; Whitty et al. 1977). The onset of anterograde and retrograde amnesias is sudden, and the amnesia typically lasts for several hours. Patients can appear neurologically intact when examined on the day after a TGA attack (Kritchevsky et al. 1988). Both epileptic seizures and transient cerebrovascular disorder have been considered as causes of TGA, but vascular etiology is widely favored (Fisher and Adams 1964; Whitty et al. 1977).

Amnesia can also occur after ECT. After a postictal confusional period of 30–60 minutes, amnesia is present as a relatively circumscribed disorder (Squire 1977; Williams 1977). ECT causes both an-

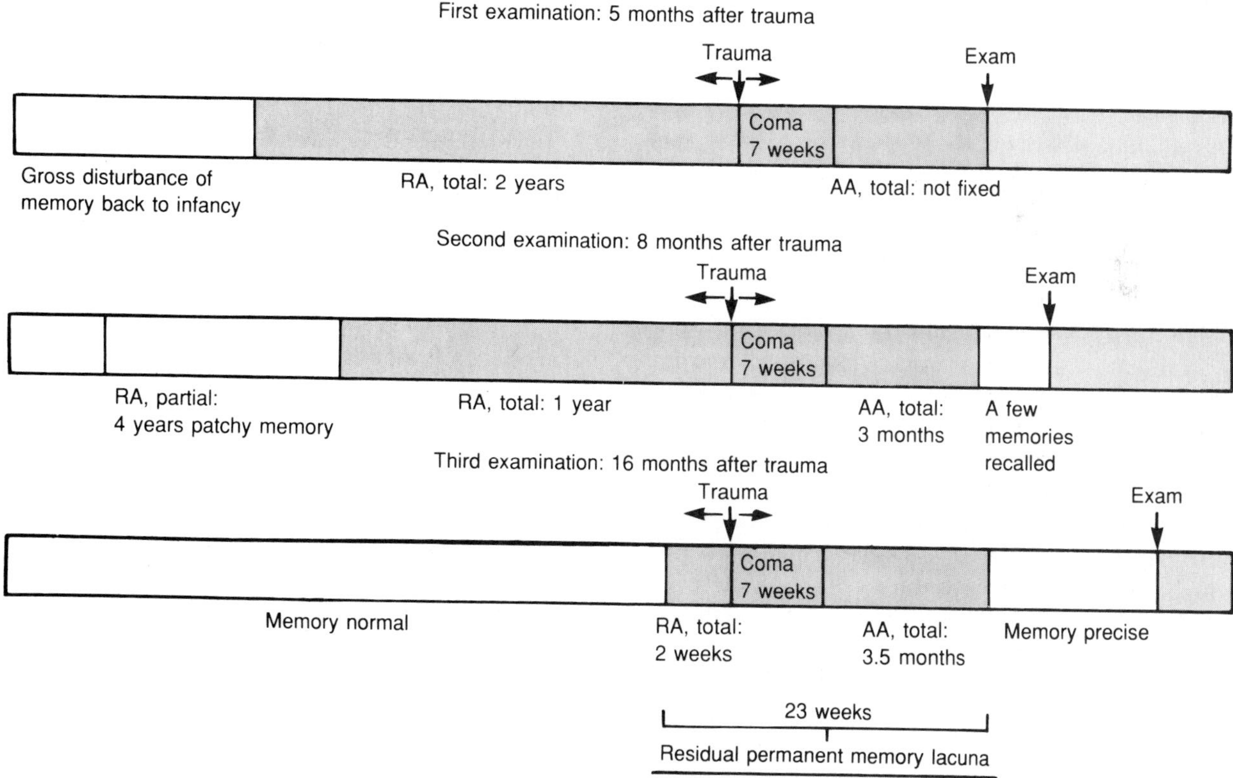

Figure 15–2. Description of posttraumatic amnesia during three examinations of a case reported by Barbizet (1970). Note the shrinking of retrograde amnesia (RA), diminution of anterograde amnesia (AA), and residual permanent memory lacuna. (Reprinted from Barbizet J: Human Memory and Its Pathology. New York, WH Freeman, 1970. Copyright 1970 by W. H. Freeman and Company. Used with permission.)

terograde and retrograde amnesias. Anterograde amnesia can be quite severe, particularly in patients who receive bilateral ECT. Retrograde amnesia is often temporally graded, affecting memory for recent events more than memory for very remote events. By several months after ECT treatment, there is extensive recovery of new learning capacity (Squire and Chace 1975). In fact, performance on memory tests given 6–9 months after ECT is similar to pre-ECT performance. Retrograde amnesia also resolves considerably when testing occurs 6–9 months after ECT. Despite good recovery of memory functions, however, patients prescribed ECT often complain that their memory is not as good as it used to be (Squire and Chace 1975). These complaints may be mediated by 1) the permanent absence of memory for events during the amnesic lacuna, 2) misattributions of instances of normal forgetting to the ECT treatment, or 3) subtle, persisting memory problems that are too mild to detect on psychometric tests. Although the biological factors that cause the transient amnesic disorder after ECT are not well understood, it is known that the hippocampus has one of the lowest seizure thresholds of all brain structures (Inglis 1970). Thus hippocampal functioning may be disproportionately compromised after ECT.

Preserved Memory Functions in Amnesia

One of the most striking findings of the past decade is evidence of preserved memory functions in patients with amnesia (Schacter 1987; Shimamura 1986; Squire 1987). Specifically, amnesic patients can perform in an entirely normal fashion on certain "implicit" or "nondeclarative" memory tests, such as tests of skill learning, classical conditioning, and priming. For example, H. M. showed considerable retention of perceptual-motor skill on a mirror-drawing task in which he was required to trace the outline of a star while viewing the star in a mirror (Milner 1962). Corkin (1968) also found good perceptual skill learning by H. M. on a pursuit-rotor task in which a stylus must be kept on a rotating target. Preserved skill learning has been observed in other cases of amnesia as well (Parkin 1982). Brooks and Baddeley (1976) found normal pursuit-rotor skill learning and 1-week retention in three patients with Korsakoff's syndrome and two patients with amnesia due to encephalitis. Also, in a jigsaw puzzle assembly task, these amnesic patients exhibited faster completion times across six trials and good retention when the same puzzle was given 1 week later.

Cohen and Squire (1980) observed preserved skill learning by amnesic patients doing a mirror-reading task. In this task, subjects were asked to read mirror-reversed words. Patients with Korsakoff's syndrome, patients prescribed ECT, and patient N. A. improved their reading speed of mirror-reversed words across training sessions to the same extent as control subjects (Figure 15–3). Moreover, amnesic patients exhibited normal retention of the mirror-reading skill even when they were tested 1 month after learning. Despite preserved skill learning, recognition memory for the words used in the task was severely impaired in amnesic patients. Moreover, the patients often did not recognize the testing apparatus nor did they have conscious recollection of having engaged in the task before. Performance by amnesic patients in these tasks indicates that skill learning can be preserved even when the patient has little or no recollection of having acquired the skill. These findings suggest that patients with amnesia can exhibit a certain form of knowledge ("knowing how") in the absence of explicit or conscious knowledge ("knowing that").

There are several other forms of preserved memory function in amnesia. One form is illustrated by an early anecdote of "unconscious" memory that was reported by Claparede (1911). During an interview with an amnesic patient, Claparede hid a pin between his fingers and surreptitiously pricked the patient on the hand. At a later time during the interview, he once again reached for the patient's hand, but the patient quickly withdrew her hand. The patient did not acknowledge the previous incident, and, when asked why she withdrew her hand, she simply stated, ". . . sometimes pins are hidden in people's hands." This anecdote is an example of stimulus-response learning without awareness.

Another form of such learning was demonstrated by Weiskrantz and Warrington (1979), who assessed classical conditioning of the blink response in two amnesic patients. These patients retained the conditioned response for as long as 24 hours, even though they did not recognize the test apparatus. A memory phenomenon known as *priming* is also preserved in amnesia (Schacter 1987; Shimamura 1986). Priming is a facilitation or bias in performance as a result of recently encountered information. The seminal evidence for preservation of priming in amnesia came from Warrington and Weiskrantz (1968, 1970). Amnesic patients were asked to identify

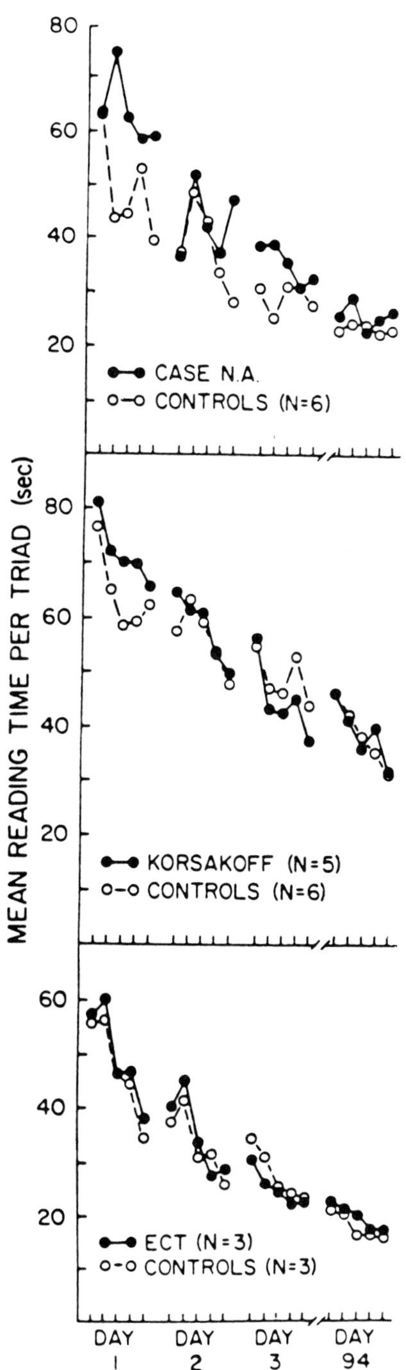

Figure 15–3. Acquisition of a mirror-reading skill during three daily sessions and retention of the skill 3 months later. The skill in reading nonrepeated mirror-reversed words was acquired at a normal rate by patient N. A., patients with Korsakoff's syndrome, and patients prescribed electroconvulsive therapy (ECT). (Reprinted from Cohen NJ, Squire LR: Preserved learning and retention of pattern analyzing skill in amnesia: association of knowing how and knowing that. Science 210:207–209, 1980. Copyright 1980 by the AAAS. Used with permission.)

words or pictures that were presented in a degraded form. If the subjects could not identify a stimulus, a succession of less degraded versions of the stimulus were shown until identification was successful. When amnesic patients were asked to identify the same degraded words or pictures at a later time, their performance was facilitated by the previous experience; that is, they were able to identify the stimuli more quickly. This priming effect occurred despite failure to discriminate previously presented stimuli from new ones in a recognition memory test.

Graf et al. (1984) used a word-completion task to study priming effects. In this task, words were presented (e.g., *motel*) to the subject and later cued by three-letter word stems (e.g., *mot*). Subjects were asked to say the first word that came to mind for each word stem. In both amnesic patients and control subjects, the tendency to use previously presented words in the word completion test was increased by 100%–200% over baseline levels. In this test, words appeared to "pop" into mind, and amnesic patients exhibited this effect to the same level as control subjects. However, when subjects were asked to use the same word stems as aids to recollect words from the study session, the control subjects exhibited better performance than amnesic patients.

A variety of priming paradigms have since been used to demonstrate preserved priming in amnesia. For example, Shimamura and Squire (1984) presented words (e.g., *baby*) and later asked subjects to "free associate" to related words (e.g., *child*). Amnesic patients exhibited a normal bias to use recently presented words in this word-association task (Figure 15–4). This finding suggests that semantic associations can also be used to prime information in memory. This priming effect, as well as others, are short lasting, and decline to baseline levels after a 2-hour delay. Although patients with circumscribed diencephalic or medial temporal lesions exhibit normal priming effects, patients with the clinical diagnosis of Alzheimer's disease do not. For example, impaired word completion and word association priming have been observed in patients with probable Alzheimer's disease (Salmon et al. 1988; Shimamura et al. 1987). These findings suggest that priming effects may depend critically on neocortical areas that are damaged in Alzheimer's disease.

Demonstrations of preserved memory functions in amnesic patients suggest that some memory processes can be dissociated from the brain regions that are damaged in amnesia. Various taxonomies have been used to distinguish the memory forms that are

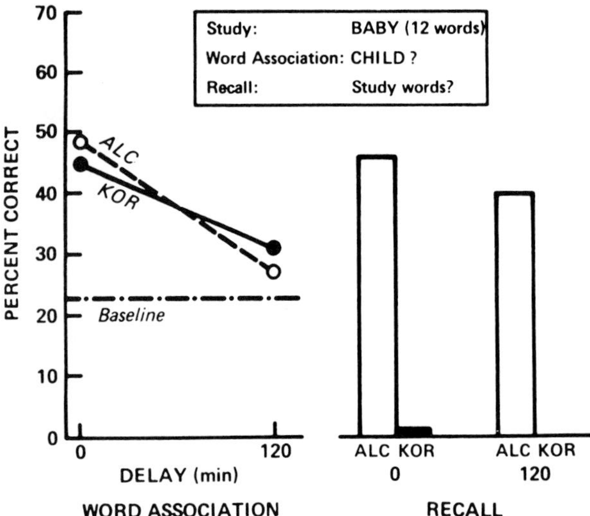

Figure 15–4. Patients with Korsakoff's syndrome (KOR) exhibited intact semantic priming as measured by a word-association test (*left panel*). After a 120-minute delay, performance dropped to baseline levels for both patients with KOR and alcoholic control subjects (ALC). Patients with KOR exhibited severely impaired free recall performance at both immediate and 120-minute delay conditions (*right panel*). (Reprinted from Shimamura AP, Squire LR: Paired-associate learning and priming effects in amnesia: a neuropsychological study. J Exp Psychol [Gen] 113:556–570, 1984. Copyright 1984 by the American Psychological Association. Used with permission.)

impaired in amnesia from those that are preserved (Squire 1987). For example, many distinguish *conscious* recollection from *unconscious* or *automatic memory*. Squire and colleagues (Cohen and Squire 1980; Squire 1987; Squire and Zola-Morgan 1988) suggested that amnesia impairs declarative memory and spares procedural or nondeclarative memory. Others have used related terms such as *explicit* and *implicit memory* (Graf and Schacter 1985; Schacter 1987) or *memory* and *habit* (Mishkin et al. 1984). Such descriptions provide a framework for theoretical views about the organization of memory in the brain.

❑ NEURAL MECHANISMS OF MEMORY

Memory at the Neural Systems Level

One important feature of declarative memory is the ability to report explicitly knowledge about facts and events of previous experiences (e.g., "I ate a chocolate doughnut for breakfast this morning at the cafeteria"). Such memories involve the formation, association, and organization of various pieces of information, including information about what occurred, when it occurred, and where it occurred. Thus to establish, maintain, and ultimately recollect such (declarative) memories, it is critical to have an efficient neural mechanism by which new pieces of information can be associated with each other and with previously stored information.

During the 1950s and 1960s, animal models of human amnesia proliferated. It was hoped that the models would allow a more detailed analysis of the neural systems that mediate memory processes. However, the field was scattered with inconsistent findings, and it was often suggested that animal models were inadequate and unsuccessful. This problem occurred because researchers were not aware that amnesia affects only a certain form of memory (i.e., declarative memory). Now it is understood that some memory functions are actually spared in animals models of amnesia, just as they are spared in human patients. For example, monkeys with medial temporal lesions exhibit severe impairment on a delayed, non-matching-to-sample test in which the animal must remember which of two toy objects was recently rewarded. Nevertheless, these lesioned monkeys perform normally on certain tests of skill learning (Squire and Zola-Morgan 1988). Recent studies using animal models (Mishkin 1982; Squire and Zola-Morgan 1988) have proven their usefulness by providing substantial information about the neural systems that contribute to memory.

One particular area that has received extensive analysis is the hippocampal formation, which includes the entorhinal cortex, dentate gyrus, subicular complex, and hippocampus proper (Figure 15–5). These structures form the *trisynaptic circuit* (Squire et al. 1989b; Swanson et al. 1982). In this circuit, the axons of entorhinal neurons form a fiber bundle known as the *perforant path,* which projects to the dentate gyrus granule cells where it forms its first set of synapses. The granule cells give rise to the mossy fibers, which synapse onto neurons in the CA_3 field of the hippocampus. The CA_3 neurons give rise to the Schaffer collaterals, which project to pyramidal cells of the CA_1 field. The CA_1 cells complete the circuit with projections to the subiculum and entorhinal cortex. The subiculum gives rise to the projections that exit through the fornix to diencephalic structures such as the mammillary bodies

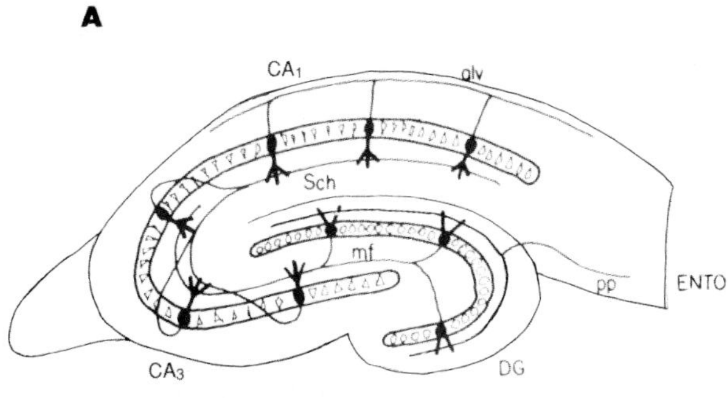

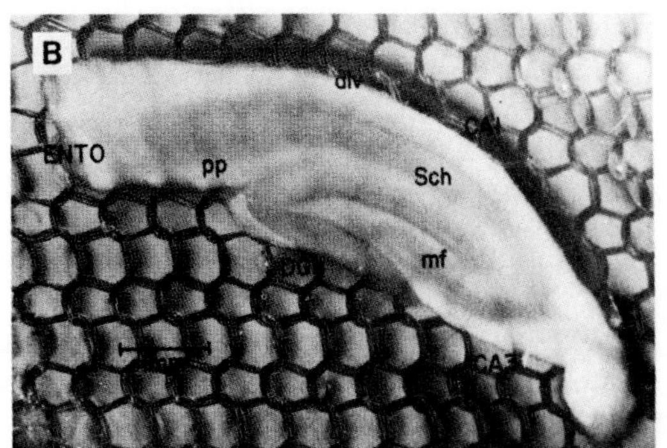

Figure 15–5. *Panel A*: Schematic diagram of the trisynaptic circuit in the hippocampus (ENTO = entorhinal cortex; pp = perforant path; DG = dentate gyrus; mf = mossy fibers; Sch = Schaffer collaterals; Alv = alveus). *Panel B*: Photograph of a hippocampal tissue slice preparation. (Reprinted from Teyler TJ: Memory: electrophysiological analogs, in Learning and Memory: A Biological View. Edited by Martinez JL Jr, Kesner RP. New York, Academic, 1984, pp 237–265. Used with permission.)

and the anterior thalamic nuclei. The complete neural circuitry of the hippocampal formation is exceedingly complex (Witter et al. 1989); however, this basic neural architecture (i.e., the trisynaptic circuit) is typical of hippocampal circuitry along its rostral-caudal extent.

What is the functional role of hippocampal circuitry? As illustrated in Figure 15–6, many areas of neocortex, such as the cingulate cortex, superior temporal gyrus, orbitofrontal cortex, and insula, project directly to the entorhinal cortex. In addition, the entorhinal cortex receives projections from adjacent cortical areas, such as the perirhinal cortex (areas 35 and 36) and the parahippocampal gyrus (areas TF/TH), which are located rostral and caudal to the entorhinal cortex, respectively. These adjacent areas themselves receive projections from many neocortical regions (as shown in the upper half of Figure 15–6). All of these projections to the entorhinal cortex have reciprocal projections back to neocortical regions. The neocortical regions that project to the entorhinal cortex have been classified as "polysensory associational cortices," which indicates that the entorhinal cortex receives highly processed, multimodal information (Squire et al. 1989b).

A functional model of the neural system within the medial temporal region has been developed from these anatomical findings. The entorhinal cortex receives a vast amount of information from var-

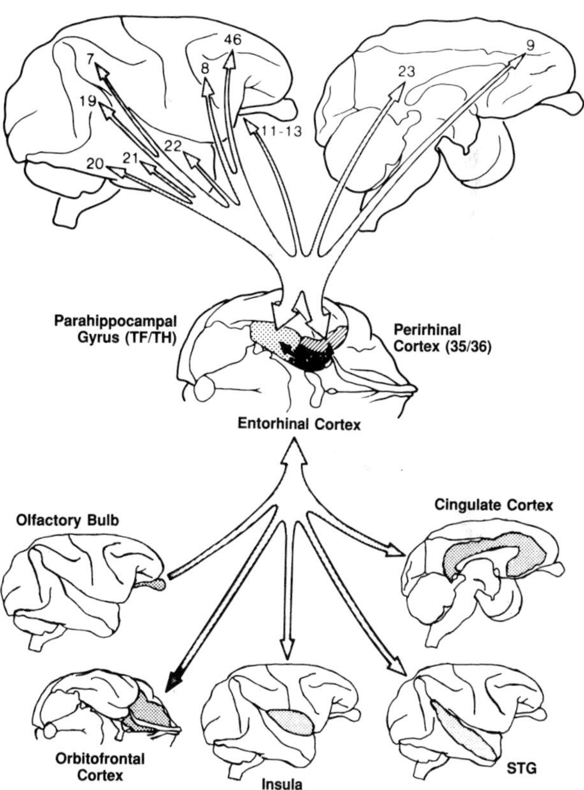

Figure 15–6. Diagram of the cortical areas that project to the entorhinal cortex either directly as shown by the projections below (e.g., orbitofrontal cortex and cingulate cortex) or indirectly by way of the parahippocampal gyrus or perirhinal cortex (e.g., Brodmann areas shown above). The entorhinal cortex projects to the hippocampus and also sends reciprocal projections back to cortical areas. STG = superior temporal gyrus. (Reprinted from Squire LR, Shimamura AP, Amaral DG: Memory and the hippocampus, in Neural Models of Plasticity: Experimental and Theoretical Approaches. Edited by Byrne JH, Berry WO. New York, Academic, 1989, pp 208–239. Used with permission.)

ious polysensory areas in neocortex, either directly or by way of the perirhinal cortex and parahippocampal gyrus. Neural activity courses through the trisynaptic circuit, enabling a process that acts to conjoin or index the information from various inputs. The product of this process influences or modulates activity in polysensory neocortical regions. In other words, the medial temporal region—particularly the hippocampus—is privy to extensive cortical activity from a variety of areas, and one possibility is that the hippocampus acts to associate or index cortical activity that otherwise would not occur because of the geographical disparity of the cortical sites (Rolls 1989; Squire et al. 1989b; Teyler and DiScenna 1986). In the following sections we further delineate findings concerning the functional role of hippocampal circuitry.

Memory at the Synaptic Level

Knowledge about memory at the synaptic level has benefited from physiological analyses of hippocampal tissue slice preparations. Hippocampal slice preparations are made by cutting thin slices (350–500 μm) perpendicular to the long axis of the hippocampus (Figure 15–5). With this slice preparation, electrophysiological stimulations and recordings can be performed selectively on each component of the trisynaptic circuit. For example, excitatory postsynaptic potentials (EPSPs) can be reliably recorded after electrical stimulation of the perforant path in hippocampal slice preparations. Such recordings can be made for as long as the tissue survives, which can be for several hours or even days.

Studies of hippocampal physiology have demonstrated that neural transmission along the trisynaptic circuit is excitatory (Swanson et al. 1982). Many of the pyramidal cell connections are mediated by excitatory amino acids, such as glutamic acid and aspartic acid. In addition, inhibitory interneurons in the hippocampus synapse on hippocampal pyramidal cells and thus may act to modulate excitatory activity in the trisynaptic circuit. Many of these interneurons, such as basket cells, modulate excitatory transmission with the neurotransmitter γ-aminobutyric acid (GABA).

An important discovery regarding the nature of hippocampal function has been the finding of *long-term potentiation* (LTP), a phenomenon in which long-lasting changes in synaptic efficacy are induced by brief, high-frequency stimulation (Lynch 1986; Teyler 1984). LTP is characterized by lowered firing thresholds and can be induced at every component of the trisynaptic circuit. Because LTP involves long-lasting synaptic changes, it has been useful as a model of memory formation at the synaptic level. Numerous studies of the nature of LTP have demonstrated several important properties of hippocampal physiology—and perhaps of the process by which declarative memory is formed (Lynch 1986). First, LTP can be induced quickly and can last for as long as the cell survives. Second, LTP is cumulative such that successive episodes of high-frequency stimulation increase the degree of synaptic efficacy.

A third property of LTP is cooperativity; that is, more effective potentiation occurs when stimulation is delivered to a group of axons that terminate at overlapping synaptic fields than when stimulation is restricted to a small number of axons (Lynch 1986; McNaughton and Morris 1987). This property suggests that excitation from different axons that terminate on the same synaptic area can cooperate to facilitate LTP. Finally, LTP is selective (i.e., it does not induce a general increase in the efficacy of all synapses on the postsynaptic membrane). Thus there is regional localization of LTP induction.

In summary, LTP provides a useful model for the physiology of hippocampal function and thus may be associated with the kinds of plastic changes that occur naturally in the formation of long-lasting memories. The properties of LTP—namely the fact that it is long-lasting, forms quickly, acts cooperatively, and has regional selectivity—are all features that would be advantageous for the formation of memory.

Memory at the Biochemical Level

At the biochemical level, many neural and intracellular processes must contribute to the formation, maintenance, and retrieval of memory. Indeed, it is most likely that many biochemical processes influence memory either directly or indirectly, via modulation of general activational or metabolic processes that occur throughout the brain (Dunn 1986; Martinez 1986). These direct and indirect effects include modulation of neurotransmitters, such as acetylcholine, norepinephrine, and serotonin, and modulation of intracellular processes, such as protein synthesis, enzymatic reactions, and cell metabolism (Kandel and Schwartz 1982; Lynch 1986). Even peripheral effects, such as hormonal influences, can affect memory functions rather dramatically (McGaugh 1990).

One important issue of memory at the biochemical level concerns mechanisms by which physiological activity leads to structural changes. One prominent candidate for an intracellular mechanism of long-term plasticity is protein phosphorylation (Dunn 1986; Kandel and Schwartz 1982; Schwartz and Greenberg 1989). Protein phosphorylation involves a cascade of processes that begins with the binding of neurotransmitters onto receptors. The binding of neurotransmitters onto receptors activates adenylate cyclase, which produces cyclic adenosine monophosphate (cAMP). The cAMP activates a protein kinase that phosphorylates proteins. The mechanism of protein phosphorylation is quite specific, depending on the cAMP-dependent protein kinase that is activated. For example, Kandel and Schwartz (1982) suggested that synaptic efficacy in the invertebrate *Aplysia californica* is induced by a specific form of protein phosphorylation that restricts potassium ion channels and thereby lowers the firing threshold of the neuron. This and other related mechanisms could lead to cellular or structural modifications that are long lasting (Dunn 1986; Schwartz and Greenberg 1989).

Another biochemical mechanism of cellular plasticity was proposed by Lynch (1986), who offered an elegant model of the way in which LTP increases synaptic efficacy. It was proposed that LTP involves a calcium-mediated process that produces structural changes in the cell membrane of the postsynaptic neuron. The model is supported by the finding that LTP increases the number of postsynaptic synapses and also produces changes in the shape of dendritic spines. The importance of calcium was suggested because injection of a calcium chelator was effective in greatly reducing the likelihood of LTP. It is presumed that calcium ions activate a proteolytic enzyme (calpain) within the postsynaptic neuron, which acts to break down the postsynaptic membrane, expose previously concealed or inactive glutamate receptors, and thus increase synaptic efficacy. The model is also supported by the finding that leupeptin, an inhibitor of calpain, prevents the morphological changes that occur in the postsynaptic membrane. Interestingly, when leupeptin was injected by intraventricular cannulas into living rats, memory on a maze learning task was significantly impaired (Lynch 1986).

The model proposed by Lynch (1986) has recently received further support from research on the biochemistry of glutamate receptors. One type of receptor channel is called the *N*-methyl-D-aspartate (NMDA) receptor, because of its affinity for binding with NMDA. Other related glutamate receptors are the so-called quisqualate and kainate receptors (Foster and Fagg 1984). All of these receptor types can be found in the hippocampus, but the NMDA receptors have unique properties that may contribute to the formation of long-term memory. NMDA receptors are most highly concentrated in the hippocampus—especially in the CA_1 field—although they are also found in moderate proportions throughout the brain, including the neocortex, corpus striatum, thalamus, hypothalamus, and cerebellum (Olverman et al. 1984).

Several findings have suggested a relationship between NMDA receptors and memory (Jahr and Stevens 1987). First, the formation of LTP is blocked by an antagonist of NMDA, 2-amino-5-phosphonovalerate (APV), though APV does not interfere with normal synaptic transmission (Harris et al. 1984). Second, rats that were given infusions of APV in sufficient doses to block LTP performed poorly on a spatial memory task (Morris et al. 1986). Third, the action of glutamate on NMDA receptors may be responsible for its excitotoxic effects on hippocampal cells during episodes of anoxia or ischemia (Meldrum 1985). Experimental prophylactic methods have been proposed that involve the injection of glutamate antagonists to protect against neuronal death following an anoxic or ischemic event. These methods may prove extremely useful in the prevention of amnesia following anoxia or ischemia.

Finally, the biomechanics of NMDA receptors provides a method by which associational synaptic connections can be strengthened as a result of experience. Specifically, synaptic transmission during normal EPSPs is mediated by the quisqualate and kainate receptors but not by the NMDA receptors because NMDA receptors are normally blocked by extracellular magnesium ions. However, this magnesium ion block of NMDA receptors is voltage dependent such that depolarization of the postsynaptic cell prior to an EPSP will open the NMDA channels and allow an influx of cations, such as calcium ions. By this process, further depolarization occurs, as well as the initiation of calcium-dependent mechanisms, such as those proposed by Lynch (1986). Thus there is a critical relationship between NMDA biomechanics and LTP induction in that high-frequency stimulation induces both activation of NMDA receptor channels and LTP.

The identification of a voltage-dependent mechanism that unblocks NMDA channels and increases the influx of calcium ions into the postsynaptic cell provides the necessary link between physiological activity and structural changes. NMDA receptors act as a gating mechanism that increases synaptic efficacy as a function of cotemporal activity. This process may be the essential mechanism by which the hippocampus makes associative connections. Because the hippocampus has a greater concentration of NMDA receptors than any other brain region, it may be critical for the formation and storage of conjunctions between two distinct but coactive inputs. As previously mentioned, the hippocampus receives inputs from many polysensory neocortical areas. Thus the mechanisms responsible for NMDA receptor activity and LTP appear to be excellent candidates for the processes by which new pieces of information can be conjoined and associated with previously stored information. This convergence of evidence from neural systems analyses, LTP physiology, and the biophysics of NMDA receptors has led to a remarkable understanding of memory functions in the brain.

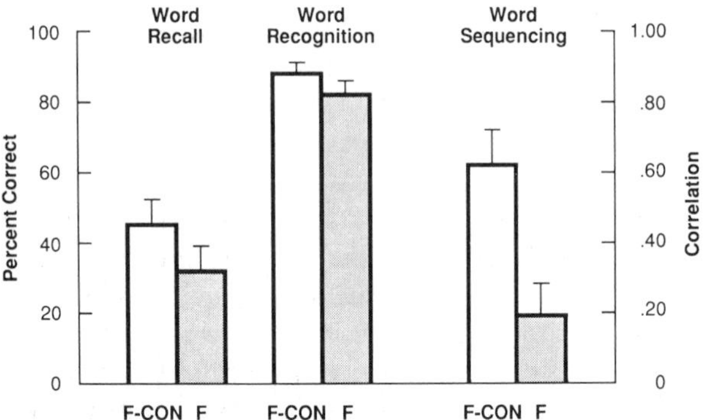

Figure 15–7. After the presentation of 15 words, subjects were asked to recall and recognize the words on the list or, on a different occasion, to reconstruct the order in which the words were presented. Word sequencing performance was based on the correlation of the judged order of the words with the actual list order. F = patients with frontal lobe lesions; F-CON = control subjects for patients with frontal lobe lesions. (Reprinted from Shimamura AP, Janowsky JS, Squire LR: Memory for the temporal order of events in patients with frontal lobe lesions and amnesic patients. Neuropsychologia 28:803–813, 1990. Used with permission.)

❑ RELATED NEUROPSYCHIATRIC ISSUES

The Role of the Frontal Lobes in Memory Disorders

Frontal lobe damage in human patients can cause changes in personality, language, planning, categorizing, attention, perseveration, verbal fluency, and inferential problem solving (Fuster 1989; Milner et al. 1985; Shimamura et al., in press). Despite these cognitive and personality changes, patients with circumscribed frontal lobe lesions can perform quite well on many standard tests of new learning ability (e.g., tests of paired-associate learning and recognition memory). Detailed studies of memory functions in patients with frontal lobe lesions, however, have demonstrated impairment on certain tests of memory, particularly those that require organizational or retrieval strategies. Some have described this form of memory impairment as a specific problem in spatial-temporal encoding, whereas others have characterized the disorder as an impairment in working memory (Baddeley 1986; Milner et al. 1985; Shimamura et al., in press).

To illustrate the effect of frontal lobe lesions on memory, Figure 15–7 displays data from a study of memory for the temporal order of events (Shimamura et al. 1990; see also, Milner et al. 1985). Patients with frontal lobe lesions and control subjects were shown 15 words, one at a time, and asked to remember the order in which the words were presented. After presentation, subjects were given the words arranged randomly on a table and asked to reassemble the cards in the original presentation order. Subjects were also given standard word recall and recognition tests with a second word list. Patients with frontal lobe lesions exhibited impairment on the test of temporal order memory, despite normal performance on tests of word recall and recognition. Another aspect of impaired temporal memory is the phenomenon of source amnesia. Patients with frontal lobe lesions performed well on tests of facts that were presented in a previous experimental session (e.g., Angel Falls is located in Venezuela), but they forget when and where the facts were learned (Janowsky et al. 1989a; Shimamura and Squire 1987). When source amnesia occurs, patients will often attribute the fact to an extraneous source such as a recent television show or magazine article. This finding suggests that the frontal lobes may be involved in connecting factual information with episodic or spatial-temporal information.

Other forms of memory impairment occur in patients with frontal lobe lesions, suggesting that the disorder extends beyond the domain of spatial-temporal memory. For example, patients with frontal lobe lesions exhibit impaired metamemory (i.e., they lack knowledge about their own memory capabilities and knowledge about strategies that can aid memory [Shimamura et al., in press]). In one study (Janowsky et al. 1989b), patients with frontal lobe lesions were unable to judge how well they would perform on a recognition test of factual information. This deficit is similar to the finding of poor cognitive estimation in patients with frontal lobe lesions (Shallice and Evans 1978). Specifically, patients were unable to make accurate inferential estimations (e.g., About how long is the average men's necktie?). Deficits in metamemory and cognitive estimation suggest that the frontal lobes may be involved in the ability to organize and retrieve information. This disorder can be contrasted with the impairment of new learning ability seen in patients with medial temporal or diencephalic damage.

Studies of patients with Korsakoff's syndrome have provided further evidence for the contribution of frontal lobe dysfunction to memory disorders. In addition to diencephalic damage, which presumably causes their new learning impairment, patients with Korsakoff's syndrome have frontal lobe atrophy, as indicated by quantitative analyses of CT scans (Shimamura et al. 1988). As one might predict, patients with Korsakoff's syndrome exhibit the cognitive and memory disorders associated with frontal lobe dysfunction in addition to their general amnestic disorder. For example, these patients have deficits in planning, attention, organization, temporal order memory, inferential reasoning, and metamemory (Butters and Cermak 1980; Shimamura 1989). Amnesic patients with discrete diencephalic lesions (i.e., without observable frontal damage) and patients with medial temporal lesions do not exhibit the cognitive and memory impairments associated with frontal lobe damage. Because the role of the frontal lobes in memory functions has not been analyzed extensively, it is as yet unclear exactly how to characterize frontal lobe function. Indeed, the prefrontal cortex in humans comprises more than 29% of the cortical mantle, and thus it is likely that different areas within the frontal lobes contribute to behavior in different ways.

Memory and Depression

Patients with affective disorders often exhibit memory impairment. For example, patients with depression perform poorly on tests of free recall, paired-associate learning, and recognition memory (Johnson and Magaro 1987; McAllister 1981). Depressed patients also describe their memory abilities as impaired relative to their abilities before the onset of depression (Squire et al. 1979). These deficits, however, are different from those observed in amnesic disorders. In amnesia, the ability to store new long-term memories is disrupted. In contrast, depression appears to cause a deficit in the initial processing of new information. Thus depressed patients encode less information initially but retain that which has been learned (Steif et al. 1986), whereas amnesic patients process information in a normal manner but fail to retain that information beyond the span of immediate memory.

How does depression disrupt learning processes? One hypothesis suggests that the ability to expend or sustain cognitive effort is reduced in depressed patients (Hasher and Zacks 1979). This decrease in effort results in a diminished use of learning strategies such as rehearsal and organization and thus leads to less effective acquisition of new information. On tests of recognition memory and free recall of word lists, clinically depressed patients, as well as non-clinically-depressed individuals who rate themselves high on a depression scale, exhibit deficient use of rehearsal and organizational strategies during learning (Hasher and Zacks 1979; Weingartner et al. 1981).

The effort hypothesis predicts that depressed patients will show a general impairment for any task that requires sustained effort. This prediction has been tested by examining depressed patients' performance on effortful, nonmemory tasks and on automatic (i.e., noneffortful) tasks that do rely on memory. For example, depressed patients showed marked impairment on a motor task that involved sustained effort (Cohen et al. 1982). On the other hand, individuals with high self-rated depression exhibited normal performance on an "automatic" memory task, such as estimating the number of times that a stimulus was presented (Hasher and Zacks 1979).

Depression can affect memory retrieval as well as learning, and in many instances individuals exhibit "state-dependent" retrieval. For example, a memory may be most easily retrieved during a mood state that is congruent with the emotional value of the memory. Indeed, depressed patients have been found to exhibit "negative selectivity": they retrieve unpleasant memories more readily than pleasant ones, recall more negative than positive words in a list learning task, and erroneously report having received more negative reinforcement than was actually delivered (for a review, see Johnson and Magaro 1987). Another example of state-dependent retrieval is the finding that memories are most easily retrieved when they are congruent with the mood state that was present when the memory was established. In one study (Weingartner et al. 1977), bipolar patients were asked to generate word associates during episodes of depression, mania, and normal affect. State-dependent retrieval was exhibited when recall of these word associates was assessed during subsequent episodes of depression, mania, and normal affect. For example, when tested during an episode of depression, recall was best for associates generated during a previous episode of depression.

In some instances, depression can cause profound deficits in memory and cognition that are nearly indistinguishable from the early stages of dementia. The possibility that a treatable psychiatric disorder could be mistaken for an untreatable dementia is of particular concern to clinicians. Kiloh (1961), who first described the phenomenon of pseudodementia, noted that in the elderly "the most common condition in which the erroneous diagnosis of dementia is made, is in endogenous depression" (p. 339). Wells (1979) suggested criteria for differentiating depression from dementia, including the rate of cognitive decline, which is often more rapid in depression than in dementia, and the pattern of test performance, which is more inconsistent in depression than in dementia. In addition, a diagnosis of dementia might be indicated if cognitive symptoms progressively worsen. The cognitive deficits associated with depression are generally transient, resolving on successful treatment of the affective disorder.

Psychogenic Amnesia

Psychogenic or functional amnesia is a rare psychiatric disorder that involves pathological memory loss of one's own identity or autobiography (Pratt 1977; Schacter and Kihlstrom 1989). The DSM-III-R diagnostic criteria for psychogenic amnesia are shown in Table 15–2. Typically, patients cannot recall their own name, address, or occupation. Psychogenic amnesia usually occurs after psychological trauma and lasts for days or weeks (Abeles and Schilder 1935) or sometimes even years (Pratt 1977). Typically, the patient is first observed in a fugue state—wandering aimlessly and acting confused and incoherent. After the fugue state, psychogenic amnesia occurs without apparent loss of other cognitive abilities, although in many cases the patient appears agitated and nervous and sometimes borders on hysteria. Retrograde amnesia may encompass virtually all personal memories or many personal memories with some pockets of preservation. In some patients, the amnesia involves a circumscribed traumatic episode or time period. Psychogenic amnesia can clear spontaneously, but it often clears as a result of an experience that is related to the traumatic event that induced the amnesia. This psychiatric disturbance is one of the more intriguing and dramatic forms of mental illness. Indeed, it has been characterized in numerous movies and television episodes, including such popular films as *Spellbound* and *Desperately Seeking Susan.*

Many case studies of psychogenic amnesia have been described. One of the more extensive reports was made by Abeles and Schilder (1935), who described 63 patients seen at the Bellevue Hospital in New York over a 4-year period. More recent cases exhibit the same pattern of disturbance as observed by Abeles and Schilder (1935) and have been re-

TABLE 15–2. DSM-III-R DIAGNOSTIC CRITERIA FOR PSYCHOGENIC AMNESIA

A. The predominant disturbance is an episode of sudden inability to recall important personal information that is too extensive to be explained by ordinary forgetfulness.

B. This disturbance is not due to multiple personality disorder or to an organic mental disorder (e.g., blackouts during alcohol intoxication).

Source. Reprinted from American Psychiatric Association: Diagnostic and Statistical Manual of Mental Disorders, 3rd Edition, Revised. Washington, DC, American Psychiatric Association, 1987, p 275. Used with permission.

viewed by Pratt (1977) and Schacter and Kihlstrom (1989). Psychogenic amnesia cannot be attributed to any known organic causes, although mild head trauma (e.g., head injury) is sometimes associated with the event that precipitated amnesia. In virtually all cases, the amnesia is preceded by some emotional or traumatic experience (e.g., death of a loved one, rape, and attempted suicide).

An example of the disorder and its pattern of recovery is the case of patient P. N. (Schacter et al. 1982). P. N., a 21-year-old man, approached a policeman on a street and complained of excruciating back pains. On entry into a hospital, P. N. could not remember his name, address, or almost any other information about himself or his past. In the following excerpt, Schacter et al. (1982) describe the events that led to P.N.'s recovery:

> The patient's picture was published in a newspaper; a cousin saw it and came to the hospital the next day. She identified the patient but he did not recognize her. The cousin reported that P. N.'s grandfather had died the previous week and that P. N. had been closer to his grandfather than to any other person. However, P. N. did not recall going to the funeral, and could not remember anything about his grandfather.... P. N.'s amnesia cleared on the next evening while he watched an elaborate cremation and funeral sequence in the concluding episode of the television series *Shogun*. P. N. reported that as he watched the funeral scene, an image of his grandfather gradually appeared in his mind. (p. 524)

The behavioral pattern of psychogenic amnesia is often easily discernible from amnesias with known organic etiologies, such as in patients with medial temporal or diencephalic damage. In psychogenic amnesia, memory loss is primarily for premorbid events and is often specific to personal memories rather than to memories for public events (Abeles and Schilder 1935; Schacter et al. 1982). Often the patient adapts to the disorder by relearning personal information after the onset of amnesia. Thus unlike cases of organic amnesia, patients with psychogenic amnesia exhibit good new learning ability. Conversely, patients with organic amnesia typically will recall their name, previous occupation, and other well-established personal memories, despite severe loss of new learning ability.

Perhaps the most difficult issue concerning psychogenic amnesia is determining whether the patient is truly amnesic or simply malingering. Cases of feigned amnesia have been reported (Baker 1901; Lennox 1943; Price and Terhune 1919), and the predominant motivation for this behavior is to avoid obligation or punishment (e.g., military duty or criminal prosecution). Some criteria for distinguishing true and feigned amnesia have been proposed. For example, true psychogenic amnesia is thought to include confused and/or hysterical behavior, whereas feigned amnesia may occur without affective disorders. Yet it is virtually impossible to determine with confidence whether a patient is amnesic or malingering. Indeed, the only sure way of identifying feigned amnesia is by a confession by the perpetrator. The following excerpt from Lennox (1943), describing a case of feigned amnesia reported by Baker (1901), illustrates a clever manner of exposing the farce:

> In the case mentioned by Baker (1901), the man had a grudge against his neighbor, he selected a weapon, went to the neighbor's house, asked for him and on his appearance, struck him a fatal blow. He said he recollected nothing from the day before the crime until several days afterwards and the defense of post-epileptic automatism was made. However, in an unguarded moment he revealed the identity of the policeman who arrested him and his occupation at the time of the arrest which he stated took place two hours afterwards. "After what?" asked the examiner. The prisoner looked chagrined, would answer no further questions, and was convicted. (p. 741)

One final issue is the relationship between psychogenic amnesia and the amnesia that can occur between personalities in multiple personality disorder (Pratt 1977; Putnam et al. 1986; Schacter and Kihlstrom 1989). There are several parallels between the two psychiatric disorders, including the presumed etiology of psychological or emotional trauma, the association of neurotic or hysterical behavior, and the failure to retrieve personal memories. One interesting feature of amnesia in multiple personality disorder is the asymmetry of the amnesia; that is, some personalities are amnesic for certain personal memories, whereas other personalities have complete access to personal memories. Another feature is the finding of implicit or unconscious knowledge of personal memories, despite failure to access the knowledge explicitly or consciously. For example, a patient exhibited an unconscious affective response to known people or places, despite claiming no explicit recollection of the people or places (Schacter and Kihlstrom 1989). An analysis of amnesia associated with multiple personality disorder may provide a better understanding of psychogenic amnesia because multiple personality disorder has been found to be more frequent than previously thought (Schacter and Kihlstrom 1989).

❑ CONCLUSIONS

The study of memory and amnesia is one of the most productive areas in neuropsychiatric research. Progress has occurred as a result of extensive interdisciplinary research—drawing on neuroanatomy, neurophysiology, psychiatry, neurology, psychology, and cognitive science. Based on this progress, investigations concerning memory assessment and rehabilitation have been conducted, but further studies in these clinical areas are needed (Glisky et al. 1986; Wilson 1987). In addition to providing clinical benefits, the research reviewed in this chapter has been of paramount importance in the elucidation of the neural organization of normal memory functions. Further developments in clinical and basic research are certainly forthcoming with the advent of better neuroanatomical and physiological techniques as well as more precise analyses of behavior.

❑ REFERENCES

Abeles M, Schilder P: Psychogenic loss of personal identity. Archives of Neurology and Psychiatry 34:587–604, 1935

Albert MS, Butters N, Levin J: Temporal gradients in the retrograde amnesia of patients with alcoholic Korsakoff's disease. Arch Neurol 36:211–216, 1979

American Psychiatric Association: Diagnostic and Statistical Manual of Mental Disorders, 3rd Edition, Revised. Washington, DC, American Psychiatric Association, 1987

Andreasen NC: Brain imaging: applications in psychiatry. Science 239:1381–1388, 1988

Baddeley A: Working Memory. Oxford, England, Oxford University Press, 1986

Baker JJ: Epilepsy and crime. Journal of Mental Science 47:260–277, 1901

Barbizet J: Human Memory and Its Pathology. New York, WH Freeman, 1970

Brooks DN, Baddeley AD: What can amnesic patients learn? Neuropsychologia 14:111–122, 1976

Butters N, Cermak LS: Alcoholic Korsakoff's Syndrome: An Information Processing Approach. New York, Academic, 1980

Cermak LS: The encoding capacity of a patient with amnesia due to encephalitis. Neuropsychologia 14:311–326, 1976

Claparede E: Reconnaissance et moiite. Archives de Psychologie 11:79–90, 1911 (Recognitive and "me-ness," translation in Organization and Pathology of Thought. Edited by Rapaport D. New York, Columbia University Press, 1951)

Cohen NJ, Squire LR: Preserved learning and retention of pattern analyzing skill in amnesia: association of knowing how and knowing that. Science 210:207–209, 1980

Cohen RM, Weingartner H, Smallberg SA, et al: Effort and cognition in depression. Arch Gen Psychiatry 39:593–597, 1982

Corkin S: Acquisition of motor skill after bilateral medial temporal lobe excision. Neuropsychologia 6:225–265, 1968

Corkin S: Lasting consequences of bilateral medial temporal lobectomy: clinical course and experimental findings in H. M. Semin Neurol 4:249–259, 1984

Damasio H, Damasio AR: Lesion Analysis in Neuropsychology. New York, Oxford University Press, 1989

Damasio AR, Eslinger PJ, Damasio H, et al: Multimodal amnesic syndrome following bilateral temporal and basal forebrain damage. Arch Neurol 42:252–259, 1985

Dunn AJ: Biochemical correlates of learning and memory, in Learning and Memory. Edited by Martinez JL, Kesner RP. San Diego, CA, Academic, 1986, pp 165–201

Fisher CM, Adams RD: Transient global amnesia. Acta Neurol Scand 39:605–608, 1964

Foster AC, Fagg GE: Acidic amino acid binding sites in mammalian neuronal membranes: their characteristics and relationship to synaptic receptors. Brain Research Review 7:103–164, 1984

Fuster JM: The Prefrontal Cortex, 2nd Edition. New York, Raven, 1989

Glisky EL, Schacter DL, Tulving E: Learning and retention of computer-related vocabulary in memory-impaired patients: method of vanishing cues. J Clin Exp Neuropsychol 8:292–312, 1986

Graf P, Schacter DL: Implicit and explicit memory for new associations in normal and amnestic subjects. J Exp Psychol [Learn Mem Cogn] 11:501–518, 1985

Graf P, Squire LR, Mandler G: The information that amnesic patients do not forget. J Exp Psychol [Learn Mem Cogn] 10:164–178, 1984

Graff-Radford NR, Tranel D, VanHoesen GW, et al: Diencephalic amnesia. Brain 113:1–25, 1990

Harris EW, Ganong AH, Cotman CW: Long-term potentiation in the hippocampus involves activation of *N*-methyl-D-aspartate receptors. Brain Res 323:132–137, 1984

Hasher L, Zacks RT: Automatic and effortful processes in memory. J Exp Psych [Gen] 108:356–388, 1979

Huppert FA, Piercy M: Recognition memory in amnesic patients: effect of temporal context and familiarity of material. Cortex 12:3–20, 1976

Inglis J: Shock, surgery, and cerebral symmetry. Br J Psychiatry 117:143–148, 1970

Jahr CE, Stevens CF: Glutamate activates multiple single channel conductances in hippocampal neurons. Nature 325:522–525, 1987

Janowsky JS, Shimamura AP, Kritchevsky M, et al: Cognitive impairment following frontal lobe damage and its relevance to human amnesia. Behav Neurosci 103: 548–560, 1989a

Janowsky JS, Shimamura A, Squire LR: Memory and metamemory: comparisons between patients with frontal lobe lesions and amnesic patients. Psychobiology 17:3–11, 1989b

Johnson MH, Magaro PA: Effects of mood and severity on memory processes in depression and mania. Psychol Bull 101:28–40, 1987

Kandel ER, Schwartz JH: Molecular biology of learning: modification of transmitter release. Science 218:433–442, 1982

Kaushall PI, Zetin M, Squire LR: A psychosocial study of chronic circumscribed amnesia. J Nerv Ment Dis 169: 383–389, 1981

Kiloh LG: Pseudo-dementia. Acta Psychiatr Scand 37:336–351, 1961

Kritchevsky M, Squire LR, Zouzounis JA : Transient global amnesia: characterization of anterograde and retrograde amnesia. Neurology 38:213–219, 1988

Lennox WG: Amnesia, real and feigned. Am J Psychiatry 732–743, 1943

Lynch G: Synapses, Circuits, and the Beginnings of Memory. Cambridge, MA, MIT Press, 1986

McAllister TW: Cognitive functioning in the affective disorders. Compr Psychiatry 22:572–586, 1981

McGaugh JL: Significance and remembrance: the role of neuromodulatory systems. Psychological Science 1:15–25, 1990

McNaughton B, Morris RGM: Hippocampal synaptic enhancement and information storage within a distributed memory system. Trends Neurosci 10:408–415, 1987

Mair WGP, Warrington EK, Weiskrantz L: Memory disorder in Korsakoff's psychosis: a neuropathological and neuropsychological investigation of two cases. Brain 102:749–783, 1979

Marslen-Wilson WD, Teuber H: Memory for remote events in anterograde amnesia: recognition of public figures from news photographs. Neuropsychologia 13: 353–364, 1975

Martinez JL: Memory: drugs and hormones, in Learning and Memory. Edited by Martinez JL, Kesner RP. San Diego, CA, Academic, 1986, pp 127–163

Mayes AR, Meudell PR, Mann D, et al: Location of lesions in Korsakoff's syndrome: neuropsychological and neuropathological data on two patients. Cortex 24:367–388, 1988

Meudell PR, Mayes AR, Ostergaard A, et al: Recency and frequency judgements in alcoholic amnesics and normal people with poor memory. Cortex 21:487–511, 1985

Meldrum B: Excitatory amino acids and anoxic/ischaemic brain damage. Trends Neurosci 8:47–48, 1985

Milner B: The memory defect in bilateral hippocampal lesions. Psychiatric Research Reports 11:43–52, 1959

Milner B: Les troubles de la memoire accompagnant des lesions hippocampiques bilaterales (Memory impairment accompanying bilateral hippocampal lesions), in Physiologie de l'Hippocampe. Paris, Centre Nationale de la Recherche Scientifique, 1962, pp 257–272

Milner B, Corkin S, Teuber H: Further analysis of the hippocampal amnesic syndrome: 14-year follow-up study of H.M. Neuropsychologia 6:215–234, 1968

Milner B, Petrides M, Smith ML: Frontal lobes and the temporal organization of memory. Human Neurobiology 4:137–142, 1985

Mishkin M: A memory system in the monkey, in The Neuropsychology of Cognitive Function. Edited by Broadbent DE, Weiskrantz L. London, The Royal Society, 1982, pp 85–95

Mishkin M, Malamut B, Bachevalier J: Memories and habits: two neural systems, in The Neurobiology of Learning and Memory. Edited by McGaugh JL, Lynch G, Weinberger N. New York, Guilford, 1984, pp 65–77

Morris RGM, Anderson E, Lynch GS, et al: Selective impairment of learning and blockade of long-term potentiation by an N-methyl-D-aspartate receptor antagonist, AP5. Nature 319:774–776, 1986

Olverman HJ, Jones AW, Watkins JC: L-Glutamate has higher affinity than other amino acids for [3H]-D-AP5 binding sites in rat brain membranes. Nature 307:460–462, 1984

Parkin AJ: Residual learning capability in organic amnesia. Cortex 18:417–440, 1982

Pratt TRC: Psychogenic loss of memory, in Amnesia. Edited by Whitty CWM, Zangwill OL. London, Butterworths, 1977, pp 224–232

Press, GA, Amaral DG, Squire LR: Hippocampal abnormalities in amnesic patients revealed by high-resolution magnetic resonance imaging. Nature 341:54–57, 1989

Price GE, Terhune WB: Feigned amnesia as a defense reaction. JAMA 72:565–567, 1919

Putnam FW, Guroff JJ, Silberman EK, et al: The clinical phenomenology of multiple personality disorder: 100 recent cases. J Clin Psychiatry 47:285–293, 1986

Ribot T: Les Maladies de la Memoire. Paris, Germer Baillere, 1881 (translation: Diseases of Memory. New York, Appleton-Century-Crofts, 1882)

Rolls ET: Functions of neuronal networks in the hippocampus and neocortex in memory, in Neural Models of Plasticity. Edited by Byrne J, Berry W. New York, Academic, 1989

Russell WR, Nathan PW: Traumatic amnesia. Brain 69: 280–300, 1946

Salmon DP, Shimamura AP, Butters N, et al: Lexical and semantic priming deficits in patients with Alzheimer's disease. J Clin Exp Neuropsychol 10:477–494, 1988

Schacter DL: Implicit memory: history and current status. J Exp Psychol [Learn Mem Cogn] 13:501–518, 1987

Schacter DL, Kihlstrom JF: Functional amnesia, in Handbook of Neuropsychology, Vol 3. Edited by Boller F, Grafman J. New York, Elsevier, 1989, pp 209–231

Schacter DL, Wang PL, Tulving E, et al: Functional retrograde amnesia: a quantitative case study. Neuropsychologia 20:523–532, 1982

Schwartz JH, Greenberg SM: Turtles all the way down: some molecular mechanisms underlying long-term sensitization in Aplysia, in Neural Models of Plasticity. Edited by Byrne JH, Berry WO. New York, Academic, 1989, pp 46–57

Scoville WB, Milner B: Loss of recent memory after bilateral hippocampal lesions. J Neurol Neurosurg Psychiatry 20:11–21, 1957

Shallice T, Evans ME: The involvement of the frontal lobes in cognitive estimation. Cortex 14:294–303, 1978

Shimamura AP: Priming in amnesia: evidence for a dissociable memory function. Q J Exp Psychol 38 (A):619–644, 1986

Shimamura AP: Disorders of memory: the cognitive science perspective, in Handbook of Neuropsychology. Edited by Boller F, Grafman J. Amsterdam, Elsevier Sciences, 1989, pp 35–73

Shimamura AP, Squire LR: Paired-associate learning and priming effects in amnesia: a neuropsychological study. J Exp Psychol [Gen] 113:556–570, 1984

Shimamura AP, Squire LR: A neuropsychological study of fact memory and source amnesia. J Exp Psychol [Learn Mem Cogn] 13:464–473, 1987

Shimamura AP, Salmon DP, Squire LR, et al: Memory dysfunction and word priming in dementia and amnesia. Behav Neurosci 101:347–351, 1987

Shimamura AP, Jernigan TL, Squire LR: Korsakoff's Syndrome: radiological, CT findings and neuropsychological correlates. J Neurosci 8:4400–4410, 1988

Shimamura AP, Janowsky JS, Squire LR: Memory for the temporal order of events in patients with frontal lobe lesions and amnesic patients. Neuropsychologia 28: 803–813, 1990

Shimamura AP, Janowsky JS, Squire LR: What is the role of frontal lobe damage in amnesic disorders?, in Frontal Lobe Functioning and Effects of Injury. Edited by Levin HS, Eisenberg HM. Oxford, England, Oxford University Press (in press)

Squire LR: ECT and memory loss. Am J Psychiatry 134: 997–1001, 1977

Squire LR: Comparisons between forms of amnesia: some deficits are unique to Korsakoff's syndrome. J Exp Psychol [Learn Mem Cogn] 8:560–571, 1982

Squire LR: Memory and Brain. New York, Oxford University Press, 1987

Squire LR, Chace P: Memory functions six to nine months after electroconvulsive therapy. Arch Gen Psychiatry 32:1557–1564, 1975

Squire LR, Shimamura AP: Characterizing amnesic patients for neurobehavioral study. Behav Neurosci 100: 866–877, 1986

Squire LR, Zola-Morgan S: Memory: brain systems and behavior. Trends Neurosci 22:170–175, 1988

Squire LR, Zouzounis JA: Self-ratings of memory dysfunction: different findings in depression and amnesia. J Clin Exp Neuropsychol 10:727–738, 1988

Squire LR, Wetzel CD, Slater PC: Memory complaint after electroconvulsive therapy: assessment with a new self-rating instrument. Biol Psychiatry 14:791–801, 1979

Squire LR, Haist F, Shimamura AP: The neurology of memory: quantitative assessment of retrograde amnesia in two groups of amnesic patients. J Neurosci 9:828–839, 1989a

Squire LR, Shimamura AP, Amaral DG: Memory and the hippocampus, in Neural Models of Plasticity: Experimental and Theoretical Approaches. Edited by Byrne JH, Berry WO. New York, Academic, 1989b, pp 208–239

Steif BL, Sackeim HA, Portnoy S, et al: Effects of depression and ECT on anterograde memory. Biol Psychiatry 21:921–930, 1986

Strubb RL, Black FW: The Mental Status Examination in Neurology. Philadelphia, PA, FA Davis, 1977

Swanson LW, Teyler TJ, Thompson RF: Hippocampal long-term potentiation: mechanisms and implications for memory. Neuroscience Research and Progress Bulletin 20:613–765, 1982

Talland GA: Deranged Memory. New York, Academic, 1965

Teyler TJ: Memory: electrophysiological analogs, in Learning and Memory: A Biological View. Edited by Martinez JL Jr, Kesner RP. New York, Academic, 1984, pp 237–265

Teyler TJ, DiScenna P: The hippocampal memory indexing theory. Behav Neurosci 100:147–154, 1986

Victor M, Adams RD, Collins GH: The Wernicke-Korsakoff Syndrome, 2nd Edition. Philadelphia, PA, FA Davis, 1989

Von Cramon DY, Hebel N, Shury U: A contribution to the anatomical basis of thalamic amnesia. Brain 108: 993–1008, 1985

Warrington EK, Weiskrantz L: New method of testing long-term retention with special reference to amnesic patients. Nature 217:972–974, 1968

Warrington EK, Weiskrantz L: The amnesic syndrome: consolidation or retrieval? Nature 228:628–630, 1970

Weingartner H, Miller H, Murphy DL: Mood-state-dependent retrieval of verbal associations. J Abnorm Psychol 86:276–284, 1977

Weingartner H, Cohen RM, Murphy DL, et al: Cognitive processes in depression. Arch Gen Psychiatry 38:42–47, 1981

Weiskrantz L, Warrington EK: Conditioning in amnesic patients. Neuropsychologia 17:187–194, 1979

Wells CE: Pseudodementia. Am J Psychiatry 136:895–900, 1979

Wilson BA: Rehabilitation of Memory. New York, Guilford, 1987

Whitty CWM, Zangwill OL (eds): Amnesia. London, Butterworths, 1977

Whitty CWM, Stores G, Lishman WA: Amnesia in cerebral disease, in Amnesia. Edited by Whitty CWM, Zangwill OL. London, Butterworths, 1977, pp 52–92

Williams M: Memory disorders associated with ECT, in Amnesia. Edited by Whitty CWM, Zangwill OL. London, Butterworths, 1977, pp 183–198

Witter MP, Van Hoesen GW, Amaral DG: Topographical organization of the entorhinal projection to the dentate gyrus of the monkey. J Neurosci 9:216–228, 1989

Zola-Morgan S, Squire LR, Amaral DG: Human amnesia and the medial temporal region: enduring memory impairment following a bilateral lesion limited to field CA1 of the hippocampus. J Neurosci 6:2950–2967, 1986

Section IV

Neuropsychiatric Disorders

Chapter

16

Neuropsychiatric Aspects of Traumatic Brain Injury

Jonathan M. Silver, M.D.
Robert E. Hales, M.D.
Stuart C. Yudofsky, M.D.

MORE THAN 2 MILLION PEOPLE suffer traumatic brain injuries in the United States each year; 500,000 of these persons require hospitalization, and 70,000–90,000 of the survivors are afflicted with the chronic sequelae of such injuries (Department of Health and Human Services 1989). In this population, psychosocial and psychological deficits are commonly the major source of disability to the victims and of stress to their families. The psychiatrist, neurologist, and neuropsychologist are often called on by other medical specialists or the families to treat these patients. In this chapter, we review the role these professionals play in the prevention, diagnosis, and treatment of the cognitive, behavioral, and emotional aspects of traumatic brain injury.

❑ EPIDEMIOLOGY

It is commonly taught in introductory courses in psychiatry that suicide is the second most common cause of death among persons under the age of 35. What is often not stated is that the most common cause is from injuries incurred during motor vehicle accidents. Approximately 70% of automobile-related deaths result from head trauma (Poleck 1967). Traumatic brain injury (including brain trauma and transient and persistent postconcussion syndromes) has an annual incidence of 370 per 100,000 (Kurtzke 1984), a rate that is at least three times greater than that of schizophrenia and a prevalence that is greater than that for the individual prevalences for schizophrenia, mania, and panic disorder (Regier et al. 1988; Silver et al. 1990a). Disorders arising from traumatic injuries to the brain are more common than any other neurological disease, with the exception of headaches (Kurtzke 1984).

Motor vehicle accidents account for approximately one-half of traumatic injuries; other common causes are falls (21%), assaults and violence (12%), and accidents associated with sports and recreation (10%) (Department of Health and Human Services 1989). Head injury related deaths are most frequently caused by motor vehicle accidents (57%), firearms (14%), and falls (12%). Together, these deaths represent 2% of deaths from all causes (Sosin et al. 1989).

Children are highly vulnerable in accidents as passengers and, as pedestrians, to falls, to impact from moving objects (e.g., rocks or baseballs), and to sports injuries (Hendrick et al. 1965). As many as 5 million children sustain head injuries each year, and of this group 200,000 are hospitalized (Raphaely et al. 1980). As a result of bicycle accidents alone, 50,000 children suffer head injuries and 400 children die each year (Department of Health and Human Services 1989). Tragically, among infants, most head injuries are the result of child abuse (64%) (Department of Health and Human Services 1989).

The total economic cost of brain injury is staggeringly high: an estimated $25 billion a year for the United States alone (Department of Health and Human Services 1989). A study of the treatment cost of brain injury conducted in Maryland (MacKenzie et al. 1988) determined that the average total charge for patients with head injuries was $47,274; the total 1-year treatment charges for all patients in Maryland with head injuries was over $29 million. Because the victims of traumatic brain injury most commonly are young adults, they may require prolonged rehabilitation. The costs of 5–10 years of these services can exceed $4 million for each survivor (Department of Health and Human Services 1989).

Statistics form only a piece of the picture of the cost of traumatic brain injury. Mental health professionals must deal with individuals and families who have endured these tragic events. The psychological and social disability after head injury can be dramatic. As with patients who suffer from many psychiatric illnesses, and in distinction to patients with neurological disorders such as stroke and Parkinson's disease, many survivors of traumatic brain injury appear to be physically well (without sensorimotor impairment). Studies examining the psychosocial functioning and adjustment at 1 month, 2 years, or 7 years after severe traumatic brain injury have shown that patients have extreme difficulty in numerous critical areas of functioning, including work, school, familial, interpersonal, and avocational activities (Crawford 1983; McLean et al. 1984; Oddy et al. 1985; Weddell et al. 1980).

❑ NEUROANATOMY AND NEUROCHEMISTRY OF TRAUMATIC BRAIN INJURY

Neuroanatomy

The patient who suffers brain injury from trauma may incur damage through several mechanisms that are listed in Table 16–1. Because they result in both skull fractures and brain wounds, penetrating injuries are associated with a higher incidence of posttraumatic seizures (Salazar et al. 1985). Contusions affect specific areas of the brain and usually occur as the result of low-velocity injuries, such as falls. Courville (1945) examined the neuroanatomical sites of contusions and found that most injuries were in the temporal and frontal lobes. Most of these lesions were the result of the location of bony prominences that surround the orbital, frontal, and temporal areas along the base of the skull. Contrecoup injuries are contusions that occur when the opposite side of the head is struck. A typical example is the patient who falls on the back of his head and injures the frontal and temporal lobes as the result of brain tissue abrading on the bony prominences.

Diffuse axonal injury refers to damage to the axons in cerebral white matter that commonly occurs during acceleration or deceleration injuries. The axon is vulnerable to injury during high-velocity accidents when there is twisting and turning of the brain around the brain stem (as can occur

TABLE 16–1. MECHANISMS OF TRAUMATIC BRAIN INJURY

Penetrating injuries
Contusions
Diffuse axonal injury
Hematomas
(subdural, epidural, intradural, and multifocal)
Hypoxia
Free radical formation

in "whiplash" car accidents). Diffuse axonal injury often results in sudden loss of consciousness and can occur in minor brain injury or "concussion" (Jane et al. 1985; Povlishock et al. 1983). Among cases of traumatic brain injury without diffuse axonal injury, there is a lower incidence of skull fractures, contusions, and intracranial hematomas (Adams et al. 1982).

Subdural hematomas (acute, subacute, and chronic) and intracerebral hematomas have effects that are specific to their locations and degree of neuronal damage. In general, subdural hematomas affect arousal and cognition. During hypoxia, free radicals and excitotoxic neurotransmitters, such as glutamate, are released and result in further damage to neurons (Becker et al. 1988; Faden et al. 1989).

Neurochemistry

There have been several studies of neurochemical changes after traumatic brain injury (Silver et al. 1991). From these studies, it is evident that traumatic brain injury can affect the neurotransmitter systems that mediate mood and affect, including norepinephrine, serotonin, dopamine, and acetylcholine. Two studies (Clifton et al. 1981; Hamill et al. 1987) found markedly elevated plasma norepinephrine levels after acute head injury. Elevated plasma levels of norepinephrine were correlated with more severe injury and poorer clinical outcome.

The results of four studies of serotonin activity after traumatic brain injury are inconsistent. Whereas Vecht et al. (1975) found that lumbar cerebrospinal fluid (CSF) 5-hydroxyindoleacetic acid (5-HIAA) was below normal in conscious patients and normal in patients who were unconscious, Bareggi et al. (1975) found normal 5-HIAA levels in patients after severe traumatic brain injury. Ventricular CSF 5-HIAA levels were elevated in patients within days of severe traumatic brain injury (Bareggi et al. 1975). Patients with frontotemporal contusions and those patients with diffuse contusions were investigated by van Woerkom et al. (1977). Decreased levels of 5-HIAA were found in those patients with frontotemporal contusions, but those with more diffuse contusions had increased 5-HIAA levels.

Two investigators (Bareggi et al. 1975; Vecht et al. 1975) found a decrease in lumbar CSF homovanillic acid (HVA) levels, whereas Porta et al. (1975) demonstrated elevated ventricular CSF HVA after severe traumatic brain injury. Elevated serum dopamine may be related to the severity of the injury and to poor outcome (Hamill et al. 1987). Finally, patients with traumatic brain injury had elevated acetylcholine levels in fluid obtained from intraventricular catheters or lumbar puncture (Grossman et al. 1975).

Specific lesions may deplete norepinephrine and serotonin by interrupting the nerve tracts of these pathways (Morrison et al. 1979). The norepinephrine nerve tracts course from the brain stem anteriorly to curve around the hypothalamus, the basal ganglia, and the frontal cortex. Similarly, the serotonin system has projections to the frontal cortex. Diffuse axonal injury or contusions can affect both of these systems. Secondary neurotoxicity that is caused by excitotoxins and lipid peroxidation may further damage the neuronal systems that mediate norepinephrine and serotonin.

❑ NEUROPSYCHIATRIC ASSESSMENT OF TRAUMATIC BRAIN INJURY

History Taking

Although brain injuries subsequent to serious automobile, occupational, or sports accidents may not result in diagnostic enigmas for the psychiatrist, less severe trauma may first present as relatively subtle behavioral or affective change. Patients may fail to associate the traumatic event with subsequent symptoms. Prototypic examples include the alcoholic man who is amnestic for a fall that occurred while he was inebriated; the 10-year-old boy whose head was hit while falling from his bicycle, but who fails to inform his parents; or the wife who was beaten by her husband, but who is either fearful or ashamed to report the injury to her family physician. Confusion, intellectual changes, affective lability, or psychosis may occur directly after the trauma or as long as many years afterward.

For all psychiatric patients, the clinician must specifically inquire whether the patient has been involved in situations that are associated with head trauma. The practitioner should ask about automobile, bicycle, or motorcycle accidents; falls; assaults; playground accidents; and participation in sports that are associated frequently with brain injury (e.g., football, rugby, and boxing). Patients must be asked whether there was any loss of consciousness after these injuries, whether they were hospitalized, and whether they had posttraumatic symptoms, such as headache, dizziness, irritability, problems with concentration, and sensitivity to noise or light. Most patients will not volunteer this information without direct inquiry.

Because many patients are either unaware of, minimize, or deny the severity of behavioral changes that occur after traumatic brain injury, family members also must be asked about the effects of injury on the behavior of their relative. For example, in evaluating the social adjustment of patients years after severe brain injury, Oddy et al. (1985) compared symptoms reported by both patients and their relatives. Forty percent of relatives of 28 patients with traumatic brain injury reported that their relative behaved childishly. However, this symptom was not reported by patients themselves. Although 28% of the patients complained of problems with their vision after the injury, this difficulty was not reported by relatives.

Family members also are more aware of emotional changes than are the victims of brain injury. Whereas individuals with traumatic brain injury tend to view the cognitive difficulties as more severe than the emotional changes (Hendryx 1989), mood disorders and frustration tolerance are viewed as more disabling than cognitive disabilities by families (Rappaport et al. 1989).

Documentation and Rating of Symptomatology

Symptom rating scales, electrophysiological imaging, and neuropsychiatric assessments should be used to define symptoms and signs that result from traumatic brain injury (Table 16–2). Severity of injury may be measured by several parameters, including duration of unconsciousness, initial score on the Glasgow Coma Scale (GCS; Teasdale and Jennett 1974), and degree of posttraumatic amnesia.

TABLE 16–2. ASSESSMENT OF TRAUMATIC BRAIN INJURY

Behavioral assessment
Structured interviews, such as the Structured Clinical Interview for DSM-III-R Diagnoses (SCID; Spitzer et al. 1986)
Neurobehavioral Rating Scale (NBRS; Levin et al. 1987b)
Positive and Negative Symptom Scale (PANSS; Kay et al. 1987)
Glasgow Coma Scale (GCS; Teasdale and Jennett 1974)
Galveston Orientation and Amnesia Test (GOAT; Levin et al. 1979)
Rancho Los Amigos Cognitive Scale
Rating scales for depression, such as the Hamilton Rating Scale for Depression (Hamilton 1960)
Rating scales for aggression, such as the Overt Aggression Scale (OAS; Yudofsky et al. 1986)
Brain imaging
Computed tomography (CT)
Magnetic resonance imaging (MRI)
Single photon emission computed tomography (SPECT)
Regional cerebral blood flow (rCBF)
Positron-emission tomography (PET)
Electrophysiological assessment
Electroencephalogram (EEG), including special leads (nasopharyngeal and/or anterotemporal)
Computed EEG (CEEG)
Brain electrical activity mapping (BEAM)
Neuropsychological assessment
Attention and concentration
Premorbid intelligence
Memory
Executive functioning
Verbal capacity
Problem-solving skills

The GCS (Table 16–3) is a 15-point scale that documents eye opening, verbal responsiveness, and motor response to stimuli and may be used to measure the depth of coma, both initially and longitudinally. The Galveston Orientation and Amnesia Test (GOAT; Levin et al. 1979) measures the extent of posttraumatic amnesia and can be used serially to document recovery of memory (Table 16–4). Overall cognitive and behavioral recovery may be documented using the Rancho Los Amigos Cognitive Scale (Table 16–5).

Mild head injury is usually defined as loss of consciousness for less than 15–20 minutes, a GCS score of 13–15, brief or no hospitalization, and no prominent residual neurobehavioral deficits. With severe traumatic brain injury, posttraumatic amnesia or loss of consciousness may persist for at least 1 week or longer or, in extreme cases, may last weeks to months. GCS scores for severe traumatic brain injury are less than 10.

The use of structured clinical interviews and rating scales will assist the clinician in the determination of the presence of symptoms and in rating their severity. For example, the Structured Clinical Interview for DSM-III-R Diagnoses (SCID; Spitzer et al. 1986), may be used to evaluate psychiatric diagnoses, whether or not they are associated with brain injury. Scales such as the Neurobehavioral Rating Scale (NBRS; Levin et al. 1987b) and the Positive and Negative Symptom Scale (PANSS; Kay et al. 1987) may be used to document the presence and severity of many emotional and cognitive symptoms. The Overt Aggression Scale (OAS; Yudofsky et al. 1986) can be used to document the frequency and severity of aggressive outbursts that so commonly are associated with brain injury (Silver and Yudofsky 1987b, 1991).

Laboratory Evaluation

Imaging techniques. Brain imaging techniques are frequently used to demonstrate the location and extent of brain lesions. Computed tomography (CT) is now widely available and may document contusions and hematomas. The timing of such imaging is important, because lesions may be visualized months after the injury that cannot be seen during the acute phase. Thus for a significant number of patients with severe brain injury, initial CT evaluations may not detect lesions that are observable on CT scans performed 1 and 3 months after the injury (Cope et al. 1988).

TABLE 16–3. GLASGOW COMA SCALE (GCS)

Eye opening	
1. None	Not attributable to ocular swelling
2. To pain	Pain stimulus is applied to chest or limbs
3. To speech	Nonspecific response to speech or shout; does not imply the patient obeys command to open eyes
4. Spontaneous	Eyes are open, but this does not imply intact awareness
Motor response	
1. No response	Flaccid
2. Extension	"Decerebrate"; adduction, internal rotation of shoulder, and pronation of the forearm
3. Abnormal flexion	"Decorticate"; abnormal flexion, adduction of the shoulder
4. Withdrawal	Normal flexor response; withdraws from pain stimulus with adduction of the shoulder
5. Localizes pain	Pain stimulus applied to supraocular region or fingertip causes limb to move so as to attempt to remove it
6. Obeys commands	Follows simple commands
Verbal response	
1. No response	(Self-explanatory)
2. Incomprehensible	Moaning and groaning, but no recognizable words
3. Inappropriate	Intelligible speech (e.g., shouting or swearing), but no sustained or coherent conversation
4. Confused	Patient responds to questions in a conversational manner, but the responses indicate varying degrees of disorientation and confusion
5. Oriented	Normal orientation to time, place, and person

Source. Adapted from Teasdale and Jennett 1974.

TABLE 16–4. THE GALVESTON ORIENTATION AND AMNESIA TEST (GOAT)

Name ______________________ Date of test ___/___/___/

Age______________ Sex M F Day of the week: s m t w t f s

Date of birth___/___/___/ Time AM PM

Diagnosis______________________ Date of injury ____/____/____/

Galveston Orientation and Amnesia Test (GOAT)	Error points
1. What is your name? (2) ______	____/____/
When were you born? (4) ______	____/____/
Where do you live? (4) ______	____/____/
2. Where are you now? (5) city ______	____/____/
(5) hospital ______ (unnecessary to state name of hospital)	____/____/
3. On what date were you admitted to this hospital? (5) ______	____/____/
How did you get here? (5) ______	____/____/
4. What is the first event you can remember after the injury? (5) ______	____/____/
Can you describe in detail (e.g., date, time, and companions) the first event you can recall after injury? (5) ______	____/____/
5. Can you describe the last event you recall before the accident? (5) ______	____/____/
Can you describe in detail (e.g., date, time, and companions) the first event you can recall before the injury? (5) ______	____/____/
6. What time is it now? ______ (–1 for each ½ hour removed from correct time to maximum of –5)	____/____/
7. What day of the week is it? ______ (–1 for each day removed from correct one)	____/____/
8. What day of the month is it? ______ (–1 for each day removed from correct date to maximum of –5)	____/____/
9. What is the month? ______ (–5 for each month removed from correct one to maximum of –15)	____/____/
10. What is the year ______ (–10 for each year removed from correct one to maximum of –30)	____/____/
Total error points	____/____/
Total GOAT Score (100 points minus total error points)	____/____/

Source. Reprinted from Levin HS, O'Donnell VM, Grossman RG: The Galveston Orientation and Amnesia Test: a practical scale to assess cognition after head injury. J Nerv Ment Dis 167:675–684, 1979. Copyright 1979 by Williams & Wilkins. Used with permission.

TABLE 16–5. RANCHO LOS AMIGOS COGNITIVE SCALE

I.	No response: unresponsive to any stimulus
II.	Generalized response: limited, inconsistent, and nonpurposeful responses; often to pain only
III.	Localized response: purposeful responses; may follow simple commands; may focus on presented object
IV.	Confused, agitated: heightened state of activity; confusion and disorientation; aggressive behavior; unable to do self-care; unaware of present events; agitation appears related to internal confusion
V.	Confused, inappropriate: nonagitated; appears alert; responds to commands; distractible; does not concentrate on task; agitated responses to external stimuli; verbally inappropriate; does not learn new information
VI.	Confused, appropriate: good directed behavior, needs cuing; can relearn old skills as activities of daily living; serious memory problems; some awareness of self and others
VII.	Automatic, appropriate: appears appropriately oriented; frequently robotlike in daily routine; minimal or absent confusion; shallow recall; increased awareness of self and interaction in environment; lacks insight into condition; decreased judgment and problem solving; lacks realistic planning for future
VIII.	Purposeful, appropriate: alert and oriented; recalls and integrates past events; learns new activities and can continue without supervision; independent in home and living skills; capable of driving; defects in stress tolerance, judgment, and abstract reasoning persist; may function at reduced levels in society

Source. Reprinted with permission of Adult Brain Injury Service of the Rancho Los Amigos Medical Center, Downey, California.

Magnetic resonance imaging (MRI) has been shown to detect clinically meaningful lesions in patients with severe brain injury when CT scans have not demonstrated anatomical bases for the degree of coma (Levin et al. 1987a; Wilberger et al. 1987). MRI is especially sensitive in detecting lesions in the frontal and temporal lobes that are not visualized by CT, and these loci are frequently related to the neuropsychiatric consequences of the injury (Levin et al. 1987a).

New techniques in brain imaging, such as regional cerebral blood flow (rCBF) and positron-emission tomography (PET), can detect areas of abnormal function, when even CT and MRI scans fail to show any abnormalities of structure (Langfitt et al. 1987; Ruff et al. 1989). Single photon emission computed tomography (SPECT) also shows promise in documenting brain damage after traumatic brain injury. This technique may soon be available at community hospitals because the technology and equipment involved is relatively inexpensive and often present at these facilities.

Electrophysiological techniques. Electrophysiological assessment of the patient after traumatic brain injury may also assist in the evaluation. Electroencephalography (EEG) can detect the presence of seizures or abnormal areas of functioning. To enhance the sensitivity of this technique, the EEG should be performed after sleep deprivation, with photic stimulation and hyperventilation and with anterotemporal and/or nasopharyngeal leads (Goodin et al. 1990). Computed interpretation of the EEG (CEEG) and brain electrical activity mapping (BEAM) may be useful in detecting areas of dysfunction not shown in the routine EEG.

Neuropsychological testing. Neuropsychological assessment of the patient with traumatic brain injury is essential to document cognitive and intellectual deficits and strengths. Tests are administered to assess the patient's attention, concentration, memory, verbal capacity, and executive functioning. This latter capacity is the most difficult to assess and includes problem-solving skills, abstract thinking, planning, and reasoning abilities. A valid interpretation of these tests includes assessment of the patient's premorbid intelligence and other higher levels of functioning.

Patients' complaints may not be easily or accurately categorized as either *functional* (i.e., primarily due to a psychiatric disorder), or *neurological* (i.e., primarily caused by the brain injury). Nonetheless, outside agencies (e.g., insurance companies and lawyers) may request a neuropsychiatric evaluation to assist with this "differential." In reality, most symptoms result from the interaction of many factors including neurological, social, emotional, educational, and vocational. Because important insurance and other reimbursement decisions may hinge on whether or not disabilities stem from brain injury, the clinician should take care that his or her impressions are based on data and not misapplied to deprive the patient of deserved benefits. For example, mood disorders and cognitive sequelae of brain injury are often miscategorized as "mental illnesses" that are not covered by some insurance policies.

❑ CLINICAL FEATURES

The neuropsychiatric sequelae of traumatic brain injury include problems with attention, concentration, executive functioning, intellectual changes, cognitive dysfunctions, personality changes, affective disorders, anxiety disorders, psychosis, posttraumatic epilepsy, aggression, and irritability. The severity of the neuropsychiatric sequelae of the brain injury has multiple determinants (Table 16–6). Poorer prognoses subsequent to brain injury are associated with impaired bilateral pupillary response, with either physical underactivity or agitation and/or with increased age. The duration of posttraumatic amnesia correlates with subsequent cognitive recovery (Levin et al. 1982). In a study by Sparadeo and Gill (1989), those victims of traumatic brain injury who were using alcohol when they suffered brain injury had increased length of hospitalization, longer duration of agitation, and lower cognitive functioning at the time of discharge from the hospital compared with patients with traumatic brain injury who had no detectable blood alcohol level at the time of hospitalization. Ruff et al. (1990) found that victims of traumatic brain injury who had a history of alcohol abuse had a poorer outcome, including increased mortality, and a higher prevalence of mass lesions.

The presence of total anosmia in a group of patients with closed head injury predicted major vocational problems at least 2 years after these patients had been given medical clearance to return to work (Varney 1988). Posttraumatic anosmia may occur as a result of damage to the olfactory nerve that is located adjacent to the orbitofrontal cortex. Impairment in olfactory naming and recognition frequently occurs in patients with moderate or severe brain injury and is related to frontal and temporal lobe damage (Levin et al. 1985b).

TABLE 16–6. FACTORS DETERMINING SEVERITY OF NEUROPSYCHIATRIC SEQUELAE OF TRAUMATIC BRAIN INJURY

Extent and severity of brain lesion
Anatomical location of brain lesion
Preinjury behavior
Psychosocial conditions
Posttraumatic seizures
Anosmia
Alcohol: history of abuse and intoxication at time of injury

The interaction between the brain injury and the psychosocial factors cannot be underestimated. Preexisting emotional and behavioral problems are exacerbated after injury. Although many victims of traumatic brain injury may not have a previous history of psychiatric problems, a significant percentage of patients have had histories of learning disabilities, attentional deficits, behavioral problems, and drug or alcohol abuse. Social conditions and support networks that existed before the injury affect the symptoms and course of recovery (Brown et al. 1981). Factors such as levels of education, levels of income, and an individual's socioeconomic status are positive factors in the ability to return to work after minor head injury (Rimel et al. 1981).

Personality Changes

Unlike many primary psychiatric illnesses that have gradual onset, traumatic brain injury often occurs suddenly and devastatingly. Although some patients recognize that they no longer have the same abilities and thus potentials that they had before the injury, many others with significant disabilities deny that there have been any changes. Prominent behavioral traits such as disorderliness, suspiciousness, argumentativeness, isolativeness, disruptiveness, and anxiousness often become more pronounced after brain injury.

In a study of children with head injury, Brown et al. (1981) found that disinhibition, social inappropriateness, restlessness, and stealing were associated to injuries in which there was a loss of consciousness extending for more than 7 days. In a survey of the relatives of victims of severe traumatic brain injury, McKinlay et al. (1981) found that 49% of 55 patients developed personality changes 3 months after the injury. After 5 years, 74% of these patients were reported to have changes in their personality (Brooks et al. 1986). More than one-third of these patients had problems of "childishness" and "talking too much" (Brooks et al. 1986; McKinlay et al. 1981).

Thomsen (1984) found that 80% of 40 patients with severe traumatic brain injury had personality changes that persisted 2–5 years, and 65% had changes lasting 10–15 years after the injury. These changes included childishness (60% and 25%, respectively), emotional lability (40% and 35%, respectively), and restlessness (25% and 38%, respectively). Approximately two-thirds of patients had less social contact, and one-half had loss of spontaneity and poverty of interests after 10–15 years.

Because of the vulnerability of the prefrontal and frontal regions of the cortex to contusions, injury to these regions is common and gives rise to changes in personality known as the *frontal lobe syndrome* (Table 16–7). For the prototypic patient with the frontal lobe syndrome, the cognitive functions are preserved while personality changes abound. Psychiatric disturbances associated with frontal lobe injury commonly include impaired social judgment, labile affect, uncharacteristic lewdness, inability to appreciate the effects of one's behavior or remarks on others, a loss of social graces (such as eating manners), a diminution of attention to personal appearance and hygiene, and boisterousness. Impaired judgment may take the form of diminished concern for the future, increased risk taking, unrestrained drinking of alcohol, and indiscriminate selection of food. Patients may appear shallow, indifferent, or apathetic, with a global lack of concern for the consequences of their behavior.

Certain behavioral syndromes have been related to damage to specific areas of the frontal lobe (Auerbach 1986). The orbitofrontal syndrome is associated with behavioral excesses, such as impulsivity, disinhibition, hyperactivity, distractibility, and mood lability. Injury to the dorsolateral frontal cortex may result in slowness, apathy, and perseveration. This may be considered similar to the negative (deficit) symptoms associated with schizophrenia, wherein the patient may exhibit blunted affect, emotional withdrawal, social withdrawal, passivity, and lack of spontaneity (Kay et al. 1987). As with traumatic brain injury, deficit symptoms in patients with schizophrenia are thought to result from disordered functioning of the dorsolateral frontal cortex (Berman et al. 1988). Outbursts of rage and violent behavior occur after damage to the inferior orbital surface of the frontal lobe and anterior temporal lobes.

Patients also develop changes in sexual behavior after brain injury. Kreutzer and Zasler (1989) assessed 21 male patients for the psychosexual consequences of traumatic brain injury. A majority of subjects had decreased sex drive, erectile function, and frequency of intercourse. Kleine-Levin syndrome, characterized by periodic hypersomnolence, hyperphagia, and behavioral disturbances that included hypersexuality, has also been reported to occur subsequent to brain injury (Will et al. 1988).

Intellectual Changes

Problems with intellectual functioning may be among the most subtle manifestations of brain in-

TABLE 16–7. PERSONALITY AND COGNITIVE CHANGES IN PATIENTS WITH FRONTAL LOBE SYNDROME

Social and behavioral changes
- Exacerbation of preexisting behavioral traits such as disorderliness, suspiciousness, argumentativeness, disruptiveness, and anxiousness
- Apathy, loss of interest in social interactions, and global lack of concern for consequences of behavior
- Uncharacteristic lewdness with loss of social graces and inattention to personal appearance and hygiene
- Intrusiveness, boisterousness, increased volume of speech, and pervasive, uncharacteristic profanity
- Increased risk taking, unrestrained drinking of alcoholic beverages, and indiscriminate selection of foods and gluttony
- Impulsivity and distractibility

Affective changes
- Apathy, indifference, and shallowness
- Lability of affect, irritability, and manic states
- Dyscontrol of rage and violent behavior
- Intellectual changes
- Reduced capacity to utilize language, symbols, and logic
- Reduced ability to use mathematics, to calculate, to process abstract information, and to reason
- Diminished ability to focus, to concentrate, and to be oriented in time or place

Source. Adapted from MacKinnon and Yudofsky 1991. Used with permission.

jury. Changes can occur in the capacity to concentrate, use language, abstract, calculate, reason, remember, plan, and process information (Barth et al. 1983; Levin et al. 1985a; Stuss et al. 1985). Mental sluggishness, poor concentration, and memory problems are common complaints of both patients and relatives (Brooks et al. 1986; McKinlay et al. 1981; Thomsen 1984). Several studies have suggested that among the long-term sequelae of brain trauma is Alzheimer's disease (Amaducci et al. 1986; Graves et al. 1990), although other investigators dispute this finding (Chandra et al. 1989).

Children who survive head trauma often return to school with behavioral and learning problems (Mahoney et al. 1983). Even children who have suffered mild head injuries show neuropsychological sequelae when carefully tested (Gulbrandsen 1984). These intellectual changes, even if not perceptible to others, influence the social rehabilitation and adaptation of the patient (Tyerman and Humphrey 1984). In patients who survive moderate to severe brain injury, the degree of memory impairment often exceeds the level of intellectual dysfunction (Levin et al. 1988). The following case example illustrates a typical presentation of an adolescent with traumatic brain injury presenting as behavioral and academic problems.

Case example

A 17-year-old girl was referred by her father for neuropsychiatric evaluation because of many changes that were observed in her personality over the past 2 years. Whereas she had been an "A" student and had been involved in many extracurricular activities during her sophomore year in high school, there had been a substantial change in her behavior during the past 2 years. She was barely able to maintain a "C" average, was "hanging around with the bad kids," and was frequently using marijuana and alcohol. A careful history revealed that 2 years earlier her older brother hit her in the forehead with a rake, which stunned her, but she did not lose consciousness. Although she had had a headache after the accident, no psychiatric or neurological follow-up was pursued.

Neuropsychological testing at the time of evaluation revealed a significant decline in intellectual functioning from her "premorbid" state. Testing revealed poor concentration, attention, memory, and reasoning abilities. Academically, she was unable to "keep up" with the friends she had before her injury, and she began to socialize with a group of students with little interest in academics and began to conceptualize herself as being a rebel. When neuropsychological testing results were explained to the patient and her family as a consequence of the brain injury, she and her family were able to understand the "defensive" reaction to her changed social behavior.

Affective Changes

Overview. The diagnostic issues that must be considered in the evaluation of the patient who appears depressed after traumatic brain injury is reviewed in greater detail elsewhere (Silver et al. 1991). Sadness is a common reaction after traumatic brain injury, as patients describe "mourning" the loss of their "former selves," often a reflection of deficits in intellectual functioning and motoric abilities. Careful psychiatric evaluation is required to distinguish grief reactions, sadness, and demoralization from major depression.

Although scales such as the Hamilton Rating Scale for Depression (Hamilton 1960) or the Beck Depression Inventory (Beck et al. 1961) are useful in evaluating the severity of depression in patients with major depressive disorder, these are not substitutes for careful and thorough clinical evaluation. Patients with depressed mood may not experience the somatic symptoms required for the diagnosis of major depressive disorder. The clinician must distinguish mood lability that occurs commonly after brain injury from major depression. Lability of mood and affect may be caused by temporal limbic and basal forebrain lesions (Ross and Stewart 1987) and have been shown to be responsive to standard pharmacological interventions of depression (discussed below). In addition, apathy secondary to brain injury (which includes decreased motivation and pursuit of pleasurable activities or schizoid behavior) and complaints of slowness in thought and cognitive processing may resemble depression.

The clinician should endeavor to determine whether or not a patient may have been having an episode of major depression before an accident. Traumatic injury may occur as a result of the depression and suicidal ideation. Alcohol use, which frequently occurs with and complicates depressive illness, is also a known risk factor for motor vehicle accidents. One common scenario is depression leading to poor concentration, to substance abuse, and to risk taking (or even overt suicidal behavior), which together contribute to the motor vehicle accident and brain injury.

Prevalence of depression after traumatic brain injury. The prevalence of depression after brain injury has been assessed through self-report questionnaires, rating scales, and assessments by relatives. Related to problems with differential diagnosis discussed above, no consistent results have been found for the rates of depression subsequent to mild or severe traumatic brain injury. For mild traumatic brain injury, estimates of depressive complaints range from 6% to 39% (Rutherford et al. 1977; Schoenhuber et al. 1988). For depression after severe traumatic brain injury, in which patients often have concomitant cognitive impairments, reported rates of depression vary from 10% to 77% (Brooks et al. 1986; Kinsella et al. 1988; Levin and Grossman 1978; Oddy et al. 1985; Tyerman and Humphrey 1984; van Zomeren and van den Burg 1985; Varney et al. 1987; Weddell et al. 1980).

In the only study that used DSM-III diagnostic criteria (American Psychiatric Association 1980) for major depressive disorder, Varney et al. (1987) interviewed 120 patients who had closed head injury and who were referred for neuropsychological evaluation. Duration of loss of consciousness after injury ranged from a few minutes to 8 days. The researchers found that 77% of these patients fulfilled the DSM-III diagnostic criteria for major depressive disorder. Of those patients with depression, 46% believed their the depression did not begin until more than 6 months after the injury.

Studies consistently report increased risk of suicide subsequent to traumatic brain injury. Data from a follow-up study (Brooks 1990) of 42 patients with severe traumatic brain injury showed that 1 year after injury, 10% of those surveyed had spoken about suicide, and 2% had made suicide attempts. Five years after the traumatic event, 15% of the patients had made suicide attempts. In addition, many other patients expressed hopelessness about their condition and that life was not worth living. The medical team, family, and other caregivers must work closely together to gauge suicide risk on a regular and ongoing basis.

The incidence and severity of depression has not been found to be related to the duration of loss of consciousness (Bornstein et al. 1989; Levin and Grossman 1978), to the duration of posttraumatic amnesia (Bornstein et al. 1988), or to the presence or absence of skull fracture (Bornstein et al. 1988). Two studies (Bornstein et al. 1989; Dikmen and Reitan 1977) showed that depression is related to the extent of neuropsychological impairment as documented by neuropsychological testing. Grafman et al. (1986) correlated depression with right-hemisphere damage with penetrating injuries to the brain.

Mania after traumatic brain injury. Manic episodes and bipolar disorders have also been reported to occur after traumatic brain injury, although the occurrence is less frequent than that of depression after brain injury (Bakchine et al. 1989; Bamrah and Johnson 1991; Bracken 1987; Clark and Davison 1987; Nizamie et al. 1988). Predisposing factors for the development of mania after brain injury include damage to the basal region of the right temporal lobe (Starkstein et al. 1990) and right orbitofrontal cortex (Starkstein et al. 1988) in patients who have family histories of bipolar disorder.

Delirium and Psychotic Changes

Psychosis can occur either immediately after brain injury or after a latency of many months of normal functioning. When the psychiatrist is consulted during the time period in which the patient with a brain injury is emerging from coma, the usual clinical picture is one of delirium, with restlessness, agitation, confusion, disorientation, delusions, and/or hallucinations. Although delirium in patients suffering from traumatic brain injury is most often the result of the effects of the injury on brain tissue chemistry, the psychiatrist should be aware that there may be other causes for the delirium (such as side effects of medication, withdrawal, or intoxication from drugs ingested before the traumatic event) and environmental factors (such as sensory monotony). Table 16–8 lists common factors that can result in posttraumatic delirium.

Psychosis that occurs after a span of time subsequent to the trauma is more difficult to diagnose and treat. Lishman (1987) reported schizophrenic-like symptoms of patients after traumatic brain injury that were "indistinguishable" from symptoms

TABLE 16–8. ETIOLOGIES FOR POSTTRAUMATIC DELIRIUM

Fluid and electrolyte imbalance
Infections
Blood disorders (e.g., anemias and coagulopathies)
Decreased oxygenation
Side effects of medications
Drug intoxication or withdrawal
Sensory monotony

of the "naturally occurring" disorder. The psychotic symptoms may persist despite improvement in the cognitive deficits caused by trauma (Nasrallah et al. 1981). Review of the literature (Davison and Bagley 1969) revealed that 1%–15% of schizophrenic inpatients have histories of brain injury. Wilcox and Nasrallah (1987) found that a group of patients diagnosed with schizophrenia had a significantly greater history of brain injury with loss of consciousness before the age of 10 than did patients who were diagnosed with mania or depression or patients who were hospitalized for surgery.

Many patients with schizophrenia may have had brain injury that remains undetected unless the clinician actively elicits a history specific for the occurrence of brain trauma. Homeless mentally ill individuals are also at increased risk for brain injury. We believe that the cognitive deficits subsequent to traumatic brain injury in conjunction with psychosis increase the risk for becoming homeless; in addition, being homeless and living in a shelter carries a definite risk for trauma (Kass and Silver 1990).

Posttraumatic Epilepsy

A varying percentage of patients—depending on the location and severity of injury—will have seizures during the acute period after the trauma. Posttraumatic epilepsy, with repeated seizures and the requirement for anticonvulsant medication, occurs in approximately 12%, 2%, and 1% of patients with severe, moderate, and mild head injuries, respectively, within 5 years of the injury (Annegers et al. 1980). Risk factors for posttraumatic epilepsy include skull fractures and wounds that penetrate the brain.

Salazar et al. (1985) studied 421 Vietnam veterans who had suffered brain-penetrating injuries and found that 53% had posttraumatic epilepsy. In 18% of these patients, the first seizure occurred after 5 years; in 7%, the first seizure occurred after 10 years. In addition, 26% of those patients with epilepsy had an organic mental syndrome as defined in DSM-III. In a study of World War II veterans (Corkin et al. 1984), those patients with brain-penetrating injuries who developed posttraumatic epilepsy had a decreased life expectancy compared with patients with brain-penetrating injuries without epilepsy or compared with patients with peripheral nerve injuries. Patients who develop posttraumatic epilepsy have also been shown to have more difficulties with physical and social functioning and to require more intensive rehabilitation efforts (Armstrong et al. 1990).

Posttraumatic epilepsy is associated with psychosis, especially when seizures arise from the temporal lobes. Brief episodic psychoses may occur with epilepsy; about 7% of patients with epilepsy have persistent psychoses (McKenna et al. 1985). These psychoses exhibited a number of atypical features, including confusion and rapid fluctuations in mood. Psychiatric evaluation of 101 patients with epilepsy revealed that 8% had organic delusional disorder that, at times, was difficult to differentiate symptomatically from schizophrenia (Garyfallos et al. 1988).

Anticonvulsant drugs can result in cognitive and emotional symptoms (Reynolds and Trimble 1985; Rivinus 1982; Smith and Bleck 1991). Phenytoin has more profound effects on cognition than does carbamazepine (Gallassi et al. 1988), and negative effects on cognition have been found in patients who received phenytoin after traumatic injury (Dikmen et al. 1991). Intellectual deterioration in children on chronic treatment with phenytoin or phenobarbital has also been documented (Corbett et al. 1985). Folate deficiency caused by phenytoin may be a significant factor in cognitive decline on prolonged use of this medication. Treatment with more than one anticonvulsant (polytherapy) has been associated with increased adverse neuropsychiatric reactions (Reynolds and Trimble 1985). Hoare (1984) found that the use of multiple anticonvulsant drugs to control seizures resulted in an increase in disturbed behavior in children.

Patients who have a seizure immediately after brain injury often are placed on an anticonvulsant drug for seizure prophylaxis. A recent study (Temkin et al. 1990) showed that the administration of phenytoin acutely after traumatic injury had no prophylactic effect on seizures that occurred subsequent to the first week after injury. Therefore, any patient with traumatic brain injury who is treated with anticonvulsant medication requires regular reevaluations to substantiate continued clinical necessity.

Anxiety Disorders

Several anxiety disorders may develop after traumatic brain injury. Approximately 60% of the relatives of 55 patients with severe traumatic brain injury reported that the patients were tense or anxious within the first year after injury (McKinlay et al. 1981). There is no change in this percentage 5 years after the trauma (Brooks et al. 1986). In 1985 van Zomeren and van den Burg found that 18% of 57 patients complained of anxiety 2 years after severe traumatic brain injury. Two controlled studies (Dikmen et al. 1986; Schoenhuber and Gentili 1988) demonstrated that patients with mild traumatic brain injury do not appear to be at an increased risk for complaints of anxiety.

Because of the potential life-threatening nature of many of the causes of traumatic brain injury, including motor vehicle accidents and assaults, patients are at increased risk of developing posttraumatic stress disorder (PTSD). Typical symptoms of PTSD, according to DSM-III-R (American Psychiatric Association 1987), include reexperiencing the traumatic event, social withdrawal, and autonomic hyperactivity (Table 16–9).

Although rare, cases of obsessive-compulsive disorder subsequent to traumatic brain injury have also been described (Drummond and Gravestock 1988; Jenike and Brandon 1988). Patients may also develop anxiety or phobias related to the situation that caused the injury, such as severe anxiety when driving for a person who was injured in a motor vehicle accident.

Minor Brain Injury (Postconcussion Syndrome)

Patients with "minor" brain injury may present with somatic, perceptual, cognitive, and emotional symptoms that have been characterized as the *postconcussion syndrome* (Table 16–10). By definition, minor brain injury is associated with a brief duration of loss of consciousness (less than 20 minutes) or no loss of consciousness, and the patient usually does not require hospitalization after the injury. The psychiatrist is often called to assess the patient years after the injury, and brain-related symptoms such as depression and cognitive dysfunction may not be associated with the injury. The results of laboratory tests, such as brain imaging studies, often do not reveal significant abnormalities.

Nonetheless, patients with a history of "mild" injury or "brief" loss of consciousness can suffer

TABLE 16–9. DIAGNOSTIC CRITERIA FOR POSTTRAUMATIC STRESS DISORDER[a]

A. Experience of event that is outside the range of usual human experience, and that would be distressing to almost anyone

B. Symptoms of reexperiencing the event (one of the following):
   1. Recurrent and intrusive distressing recollections
   2. Recurrent distressing dreams of the event
   3. Acting or feeling the event recurring (flashbacks)
   4. Psychological distress at exposure

C. Persistent avoidance or numbing of responsiveness (three of the following):
   1. Efforts to avoid thoughts or feelings
   2. Efforts to avoid activities or situations
   3. Psychogenic amnesia of the trauma
   4. Diminished interest in significant activities
   5. Detachment or estrangement
   6. Restricted range of affect
   7. Sense of foreshortened future

D. Increased arousal (two of the following):
   1. Difficulty falling or staying asleep
   2. Irritability or outbursts of anger
   3. Difficulty concentrating
   4. Hypervigilance
   5. Exaggerated startle response

E. Minimum duration of symptoms for 1 month

[a]Adapted from DSM-III-R (American Psychiatric Association 1987).
Source. Reprinted from Silver JM, Sandberg DP, Hales RE: New approaches in the pharmacotherapy of posttraumatic stress disorder. J Clin Psychiatry 51 (10, suppl):33–38, 1990. Copyright 1990, Physicians Postgraduate Press. Used with permission.

TABLE 16–10. SYMPTOMS OF POSTCONCUSSION SYNDROME[a]

Somatic symptoms
Headache
Dizziness
Fatigue
Insomnia
Cognitive symptoms
Memory difficulties
Impaired concentration
Perceptual symptoms
Tinnitus
Sensitivity to noise
Sensitivity to light
Emotional symptoms
Depression
Anxiety
Irritability

[a]Adapted from Lishman (1988).

Source. Reprinted from Silver JM, Hales RE, Yudofsky SC: Psychiatric consultation to neurology, in American Psychiatric Press Review of Psychiatry, Vol 9. Edited by Tasman A, Goldfinger SM, Kaufmann CA. Washington, DC, American Psychiatric Press, 1990, pp 433–465. Used with permission.

from severe cognitive sequelae, possibly from diffuse axonal injury. In the evaluation of neuropsychological deficits in 53 patients who were experiencing postconcussive problems from 1 to 22 months after injury, Leininger et al. (1990) detected significantly poorer performance ($P < .05$) on tests of reasoning, information processing, and verbal learning than that found in a control population. Hugenholtz et al. (1988) reported that significant attentional and information-processing impairment ($P < .01$) occurred in a group of adults after mild concussion. Although there was improvement over time, the patient group continued to have abnormalities 3 months after the injury.

Although there is often substantial resolution of postconcussion symptoms within 3 months after injury, Levin et al. (1987c) found that 22% of 57 patients still complained of diminished energy and dizziness, and 47% of patients complained of headaches. Schoenhuber et al. (1988) found that of 103 patients with minor head injury, 54% complained of irritability, 47% complained of memory loss, and 39% complained of depression after 1 year. Unfortunately, these studies did not include a "control" group to ascertain the prevalence of those symptoms in a population without brain injuries. Compensation and litigation do not appear to affect the course of recovery subsequent to "mild" brain injury (Bornstein et al. 1988), and many patients return to work despite the continuation of psychiatric symptoms (Hugenholtz et al. 1988).

Patients with minor traumatic brain injury usually vividly recall the traumatic event, and this may contribute to the development of PTSD in addition to postconcussive symptoms. There is overlap between these two syndromes, and determining the predominate diagnosis may be difficult (Tables 16–9 and 16–10). In general, postconcussion symptoms should decrease within 3 months, whereas symptoms of PTSD may not diminish until 3–6 months after the trauma. Reexperiencing the traumatic event (e.g., in flashbacks or nightmares) is characteristic of PTSD.

Aggression

Irritability and aggressiveness are major sources of disability to patients with traumatic head injuries and of stress to their families. In a review of 26 patients with severe traumatic closed head injury (Rao et al. 1985), 25 exhibited more than one agitated behavior in the acute period after the trauma; 11 remained agitated during the rehabilitation phase. McKinlay et al. (1981) found that irritability and aggressiveness occur in as many as 70% of the people who experience brain damage from blunt trauma in the first year after injury. After 5 years, 64% of relatives complained that irritability was still problematic (Brooks et al. 1986). Seven years after the injury, 31% of patients stated that they often lost their temper, and 43% of relatives characterized them as impatient (Oddy et al. 1985). Thomsen (1984) found that 48% of patients had irritability 10–15 years after severe injury. For patients with minor brain injury, 54% complained of irritability after 1 year (Schoenhuber et al. 1988).

Explosive and violent behaviors have long been associated with focal brain lesions as well as with diffuse damage to the central nervous system (Elliott 1976). The current DSM-III-R classification of this disorder is *organic personality syndrome, explosive type*. However, most of the criteria in this DSM-III-R category refer to changes that are related to injury to the prefrontal and frontal regions of the brain. Dyscontrol of aggression may occur with damage to many other cortical and subcortical structures, without the associated personality disturbances specified in DSM-III-R (Weiger and Bear 1988).

Table 16–11 summarizes the roles of regions of the brain in eliciting aggression secondary to brain lesions. Because of the prominence of this syndrome, we have proposed a specific diagnostic category of *organic aggressive syndrome* (Table 16–12) (Silver et al. 1987; Yudofsky and Silver 1985; Yudofsky et al. 1989). Organic aggressive syndrome more accurately describes the specific condition of dyscontrol of rage and violence secondary to the brain lesions and avoids reference to the variety of emotional and behavioral changes described in the DSM-III-R classification. Table 16–13 summarizes the characteristic features of organic aggressive syndrome when compared with aggression related to diagnoses not associated with brain injury (Yudofsky et al. 1990).

❑ TREATMENT

There are many useful therapeutic approaches available for people who have brain injuries. Brain-injured patients may develop neuropsychiatric symptoms based on the location of their injury, the emotional reaction to their injury, their preexisting strengths and difficulties, and social expectations and supports. Comprehensive rehabilitation centers address many of these issues with therapeutic strategies that are developed specifically for this population (Ben-Yishay and Lakin 1989; Binder and Rattok 1989; Pollack 1989; Prigatano 1989).

Although these programs meet many of the needs of patients with traumatic brain injury, comprehensive neuropsychiatric evaluation (including the daily evaluation and treatment of the patient by a psychiatrist) is rarely available. Although we propose a multifactorial, multidisciplinary, collaborative approach to treatment, for purposes of exposition we have divided treatment into psychopharmacological, behavioral, psychological, and social interventions.

Psychopharmacological Treatment

Overview. Psychopharmacological agents are commonly prescribed and may be highly effective in the treatment of specific psychiatric syndromes and symptomatologies. A key principle is that patients with brain injury of any type are far more likely to be sensitive to the side effects (and, occasionally, the therapeutic effects) of medications than are patients without brain injury. For example, the sedative and anticholinergic side effects (especially memory impairment) of thioridazine (Mellaril and others) or amitriptyline (Elavil and others) occur at much lower doses for patients with brain injury than for those without brain injury. Therefore, doses of psychotropic medications must be raised and lowered in small increments over protracted periods of time, although patients ultimately may require the same doses and serum levels that are used for patients without brain injury to achieve therapeutic response (Silver et al. 1990a, 1990b, 1991).

Many psychotropic medications affect seizure threshold (Silver and Yudofsky 1988). This can be of concern because of the frequent problem of posttraumatic seizures after traumatic brain injury. Of all the antipsychotic drugs, molindone and fluphenazine have consistently demonstrated the lowest potential for lowering the seizure threshold (Oliver et al. 1982; Silver and Yudofsky 1988). Clozapine treatment is associated with a significant dose-related incidence of seizures (ranging from 1% to 2% of patients who receive doses below 300 mg/day, and 5% of patients who receive 600–900 mg/day). Patients treated with the antidepressants maprotiline and bupropion also possibly have a higher incidence of seizures.

TABLE 16–11. NEUROPATHOLOGY OF AGGRESSION

Locus	*Activity*
Hypothalamus	Orchestrates neuroendocrine response via sympathetic arousal Monitors internal status
Limbic system	
Amygdala	Activates and/or suppresses hypothalamus Input from neocortex
Temporal cortex	Associated with aggression in both ictal and interictal status
Frontal neocortex	Modulates limbic and hypothalamic activity Associated with social and judgment aspects of aggression

TABLE 16–12. DIAGNOSTIC CRITERIA FOR PROPOSED ORGANIC AGGRESSIVE SYNDROME

Persistent or recurrent aggressive outbursts, whether of a verbal or physical nature.
The outbursts are out of proportion to the precipitating stress or provocation.
Evidence from history, physical examination, or laboratory tests of a specific organic factor that is judged to be etiologically related to the disturbance.
The outbursts are not primarily related to the following disorders: paranoia, mania, schizophrenia, narcissistic personality disorder, borderline disorder, conduct disorder, or antisocial personality disorder.

Source. Reprinted from Yudofsky SC, Silver JM, Yudofsky B: Organic personality disorder, explosive type, in Treatments of Psychiatric Disorders: A Task Force Report of the American Psychiatric Association. Washington, DC, American Psychiatric Association, 1989, pp 839–852. Used with permission.

Wroblewski et al. (1990) reviewed the records of 68 patients with traumatic brain injury who received tricyclic antidepressant (TCA) treatment for at least 3 months. The frequency of seizures were compared for the 3 months before, during, and after treatment. Seizures occurred among 6 patients during the baseline period, 16 during TCA treatment, and 4 after treatment. Fourteen patients (19%) had seizures shortly after the initiation of TCA treatment. For 12 of these patients, no seizures occurred after TCA treatment was discontinued. Importantly, 7 of these patients were receiving anticonvulsant medication before and during TCA treatment. The occurrence of seizures was related to greater severity of brain injury. The authors concluded and we concur that TCAs should be used with caution in patients with severe traumatic brain injury. Nonetheless, other investigators found that seizure control did not appear to worsen if psychotropic medications were introduced cautiously and if the patient was on an effective anticonvulsant regimen (Ojemann et al. 1987).

Affective Illness

Depression. Affective disorders related to brain damage are common and can be detrimental to a patient's rehabilitation and socialization. The literature regarding the effects of antidepressant agents in the treatment of patients with brain damage and, specifically, traumatic brain injury is sparse (Silver et al. 1991). Somatic therapies can be effective in the treatment of depression in patients with other neurological diseases. These treatments include antidepressants, stimulants, and electroconvulsive therapy (ECT) (Silver et al. 1990b).

Saran (1985) performed a crossover study of phenelzine and amitriptyline administered at therapeutic doses to patients who had "minor brain injury." No response to medication was observed. Although the patients were "melancholic," they did not have significant weight loss or problems sleeping; therefore we believe there is some question as to the diagnostic categorization of these patients. Varney et al. (1987) found that 82% of 51 patients with major depressive disorder and traumatic brain injury who received treatment with either TCAs or carbamazepine reported at least moderate relief of depressive symptoms. Cassidy (1989) reported on an open trial using fluoxetine with 9 patients with severe traumatic brain injury and associated depression. He found that 2 had marked improvement and 3 had moderate improvement. Interestingly, half the patients experienced sedative side effects, and 3 out of 8 patients reported an increase in the levels of anxiety.

Ross and Rush (1981) reported the case of a 38-year-old woman who had suffered a traumatic

TABLE 16–13. CHARACTERISTIC FEATURES OF ORGANIC AGGRESSIVE SYNDROME

Reactive	Triggered by modest or trivial stimuli
Nonreflective	Usually does not involve premeditation or planning
Nonpurposeful	Aggression serves no obvious long-term aims or goals
Explosive	Buildup is **not** gradual
Periodic	Brief outbursts of rage and aggression; punctuated by long periods of relative calm
Ego-dystonic	After outbursts patients are upset, concerned, and embarrassed, as opposed to blaming others or justifying behavior

Source. Reprinted from Yudofsky SC, Silver JM, Hales RE: Pharmacologic management of aggression in the elderly. J Clin Psychiatry 51 (10, suppl):22–28, 1990. Copyright 1990, Physicians Postgraduate Press. Used with permission.

brain injury with loss of consciousness extending 2–3 weeks after the accident. The authors examined the patient 2 years later and found that she was irritable, had pathological laughing and crying, had gained weight, and had pervasive feelings of sadness and helplessness. CT scanning revealed bilateral prefrontal atrophy. Nonetheless, she had a "remarkable improvement in her behavior, with total resolution of her dysphoria" after treatment with nortriptyline at a dose of 100 mg/day (Ross and Rush 1981).

Antidepressants should be carefully monitored to ensure that the patient receives an adequate dose of medication. The choice of medication depends on the desired side effect profile. For this reason, antidepressants with the fewest sedative, hypotensive, and anticholinergic side effects are preferred. We suggest nortriptyline (initial doses of 10 mg/day), or desipramine (initial doses of 10 mg tid), and a careful plasma monitoring to achieve plasma levels in the therapeutic range for the parent compound and its major metabolites (e.g., nortriptyline levels 50–100 ng/ml; desipramine levels greater than 125 ng/ml) (American Psychiatric Association 1985). If the patient becomes sedated, confused, or severely hypotensive, the dosage of these drugs should be reduced. Fluoxetine (Prozac), with no anticholinergic effects, is also recommended. Occasionally, patients with brain injury and depression may become sedated during treatment with fluoxetine, whereas others become restless and experience insomnia. ECT remains a highly effective and underutilized modality for the treatment of depression overall, and it can be used effectively after acute traumatic brain injury (Ruedrich et al. 1983). We recommend initiating treatment with low-threshold bilateral ECT—using pulsatile currents, increased spacing of treatment (2–5 days between each treatment), and fewer treatments in an entire course (four to six). If there is preexisting memory impairment, nondominant unilateral ECT should be used.

Mania. Manic episodes that occur after traumatic brain injury have been successfully treated with lithium carbonate, carbamazepine (Stewart and Nemsath 1988), valproic acid (Pope et al. 1988), clonidine (Bakchine et al. 1989), and ECT (Clark and Davison 1987). Many of these drugs have neurological side effects.

Lithium has been reported to aggravate confusion in patients with brain damage (Schiff et al. 1982), as well as to induce nausea, tremor, ataxia, and lethargy. A patient with preexisting bipolar disorder who experienced a recurrence of mania after suffering closed head injury was treated with lithium carbonate at previously well-tolerated serum levels (Hornstein and Seliger 1989). The patient then exhibited difficulties in attention and concentration that reversed with the lowering of the lithium dosage. Pleak et al. (1988) described the development of mania, irritability, and aggression with carbamazepine treatment; however, in our own general experience, this reaction is unusual. We have seen one case of increased aggressive behavior in a patient treated with high plasma levels of carbamazepine and valproic acid who responded to lowering of the dosages of these medications. Brain damage increases the susceptibility to neurotoxicity induced by combination therapy with carbamazepine and lithium (Parmelee and O'Shannick 1988). These symptoms frequently include lethargy, confusion, drowsiness, weakness, ataxia, nystagmus, and increased seizures.

For patients with affective disorders following brain injury, we limit the use of lithium to those with mania or with recurrent depressive illness that preceded brain damage. To avoid lithium-related side effects, we begin with low doses (300 mg/day) and assess the response to low therapeutic blood levels (e.g., 0.2–0.5 mEq/L). For patients who have a seizure disorder in addition to mania, carbamazepine or valproic acid should be considered.

Mood lability. Antidepressants can be used to treat the labile mood that often occurs with neurological disease. Schiffer et al. (1985) conducted a double-blind crossover study with amitriptyline and placebo in 12 patients with pathological laughing and crying secondary to multiple sclerosis. Eight patients had a dramatic response to amitriptyline, at a maximum dose of 75 mg/day. Hornstein et al. (1990) reported that patients with "emotional incontinence" secondary to several neurological disorders responded to treatment with fluoxetine. In our experience, antidepressants such as nortriptyline and desipramine can also be effective for this condition. It may be necessary to administer these medications at standard antidepressant dosages to obtain full therapeutic effects.

Cognitive Function and Arousal

Stimulants, such as dextroamphetamine and methylphenidate, and dopamine agonists, such as amantadine and bromocriptine, may be beneficial in treating the patient with apathy and impaired concentration. Evans et al. (1987) reported improvement in verbal memory and learning, attention, and behavior in a 24-year-old man who suffered severe traumatic brain injury with the double-blind administration of dextroamphetamine (0.20 mg/kg body weight bid) or methylphenidate (0.3 mg/kg body weight bid).

Other reports have also indicated that these medications may be beneficial (Lipper and Tuchman 1976; Weinstein and Wells 1981). Gualtieri (1988) recommended stimulant medication for brain-injured patients with attention-deficit disorder with hyperactivity, anergia or apathy, and/or frontal lobe syndrome. These medications are not without side effects: patients may develop agitation and irritability or may become depressed on discontinuation. Therefore, stimulants should never precipitously be discontinued and should always be tapered slowly. When prescribed in usual dosages, stimulants do not appear to lower seizure threshold.

Interestingly, there may be a role for stimulants to increase neuronal recovery after brain injury (Crisostomo et al. 1988). Amantadine, in doses ranging from 100 to 400 mg/day, may have positive effects on arousal (Gualtieri et al. 1989). Naltrexone 50–100 mg/day was administered to two patients with mild traumatic brain injury (Tennant and Wild 1987). Improvement was reported in memory, headaches, temper, and depression. Further studies need to be conducted to confirm these anecdotal reports.

Psychosis

The psychotic ideation resulting from traumatic brain injury is generally responsive to treatment with antipsychotic medications. However, side effects such as hypotension, sedation, and confusion are common. Also, patients with brain injury are particularly subject to dystonias, akathisias, and other parkinsonian side effects—even at relatively low doses of antipsychotic medications. Antipsychotic medications may also impede the neuronal recovery that follows brain injury (Feeney et al. 1982). Therefore, we advise that antipsychotics be used sparingly during the acute phases of recovery after the injury. Haloperidol (Haldol) 0.5 mg bid, or fluphenazine (Prolixin) 0.5 mg bid, may be used as initial treatment. In general, we recommend a low-dose neuroleptic strategy for all patients (Silver and Yudofsky 1988).

Anxiety Disorders and PTSD

We prefer to treat complaints of anxiety in patients with brain injury with supportive psychotherapy and social interventions. When the symptoms are so severe that they require pharmacological intervention, treatment with benzodiazepines or buspirone may be considered. Side effects of benzodiazepines include sedation and memory impairment, which often affect the cognitive performance of patients with brain injury. Benzodiazepines with briefer half-lives may be used, if those agents are indicated. Buspirone has less effect on cognitive functioning than do benzodiazepines, but its therapeutic effects occur after a latency of several weeks. Gualtieri (1991) found that four out of seven patients with postconcussion syndrome experienced decreased anxiety, depression, irritability, somatic preoccupation, inattention, and distractibility after treatment with buspirone.

Patients with brain injury may also develop other anxiety disorders, such as panic disorder, obsessive-compulsive disorder, PTSD, and phobias. Medications, particularly antidepressants, are often indicated for these disorders, with the caveat that these patients are more susceptible to side effects. The most important step in the treatment of the patient with PTSD is the careful assessment and diagnosis of comorbid DSM-III-R Axis I or II conditions. When there is no pervasive comorbid condition, antidepressant medications should be the initial pharmacological treatment. The positive symptoms of PTSD, including reexperiencing of the event and increased arousal, often improve with medication. The negative symptoms of avoidance and withdrawal usually respond poorly to pharmacotherapy. Depending on the response to this initial treatment, several therapeutic strategies are suggested. Figure 16–1 summarizes graphically our approach to the pharmacological treatment of PTSD (Silver et al. 1990c).

Sleep

Sleep patterns of patients with brain damage are often disordered, with impaired rapid-eye-movement (REM) recovery and multiple nocturnal awakenings (Prigatano et al. 1982). Hypersomnia that occurs after severe penetrating head injury most often resolves within the first year after injury, whereas insomnia that occurs in patients with long periods of coma and diffuse injury has a more chronic

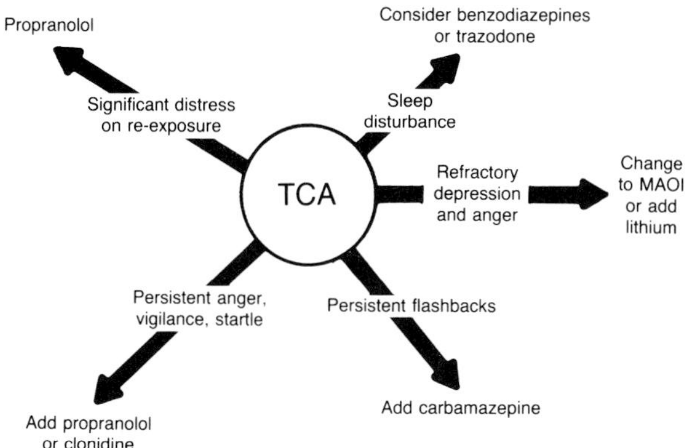

Figure 16–1. Psychopharmacological treatment of posttraumatic stress disorder. TCA = tricyclic antidepressant; MAOI = monoamine oxidase inhibitor. (Reprinted from Silver JM, Sandberg DP, Hales RE: New approaches in the pharmacotherapy of posttraumatic stress disorder. J Clin Psychiatry 51 (10, suppl):33–38, 1990. Copyright 1990 by Physicians Postgraduate Press. Used with permission.)

course (Askenasy et al. 1989). Barbiturates, alcohol, and long-acting benzodiazepines should be prescribed with great caution. These drugs interfere with REM and stage 4 sleep patterns, and may contribute to persistent insomnia (Buysse and Reynolds 1990). Clinicians should advise patients against using over-the-counter preparations for sleeping and for colds because of the prominent anticholinergic side effects of these remedies.

Aggression

Although there is no medication that is approved by the Food and Drug Administration (FDA) specifically for the treatment of aggression, medications are widely used (and commonly misused) in the management of acute aggressive episodes as well as for chronically aggressive patients. Below we discuss specific treatment modalities and their clinical indications for patients with traumatic brain injury.

Before any therapeutic intervention is planned for the treatment of violent behavior, the clinician must have a method for carefully documenting these behaviors. There are spontaneous day-to-day and week-to-week fluctuations in aggression that cannot be correctly interpreted without prospective documentation. In our study (Silver and Yudofsky 1987b, 1991) of over 4,000 aggressive episodes among chronically hospitalized patients, hospital records failed to document 50%–75% of episodes. This study also indicated that aggression—like certain mood disorders—may have cyclic exacerbations. The OAS is an operationalized instrument of proven reliability and validity that can be used for this purpose (Silver and Yudofsky 1991, 1987b; Yudofsky et al. 1986) (Figure 16–2). It is essential that the clinician establish a treatment plan that uses objective documentation of aggressive episodes to monitor the efficacy of interventions and to designate specific time frames for the initiation and discontinuation of pharmacotherapy of acute episodes and the initiation of pharmacotherapy for chronic aggressive behavior. The use of sedation-producing medications must be time limited to avoid the emergence of seriously disabling side effects, ranging from oversedation to tardive dyskinesia.

Treatment of acute aggression—antipsychotic drugs. Antipsychotics are the most commonly used medications in the treatment of aggression. Although these agents are appropriate and effective when aggression is related to active psychosis, the use of neuroleptic agents to treat chronic aggression, especially due to organic brain injury, is often ineffective and entails significant risks for the patient to develop serious complications. In these cases, the sedative side effects, rather than the antipsychotic properties of the drugs, are used to "treat" (i.e., mask) the aggression.

Often, patients develop tolerance to the sedative effects of the neuroleptics and, therefore, require increasing doses. As a result, extrapyramidal and anticholinergic-related side effects occur. Paradoxically (and frequently), because of the development of akathisia, the patient may become more agitated and restless as the dose of neuroleptic is increased, especially when a high-potency antipsychotic is administered. The akathisia is often mistaken for increased irritability and agitation, and a vicious cycle of increasing neuroleptics and worsening akathisias occurs.

Herrera et al. (1988) demonstrated that there was a marked increase in violent behavior when patients with schizophrenia were treated with haloperidol (doses up to 60 mg/day) when compared with the behaviors that occurred during treatment with chlorpromazine (1,800 mg/day) or clozapine (900 mg/day), two drugs that are associated with less akathisia than is haloperidol. Although other investigators have recommended antipsychotic drugs such as haloperidol for the treatment of agi-

OVERT AGGRESSION SCALE (OAS)

Stuart Yudofsky, M.D., Jonathan Silver, M.D., Wynn Jackson, M.D., and Jean Endicott, Ph.D.

IDENTIFYING DATA

Name of Patient	Name of Rater
Sex of Patient: 1 Male 2 Female	Date / / (mo/da/yr) Shift: 1 Night 2 Day 3 Evening

☐ No aggressive incident(s) (verbal or physical) against self, others, or objects during the shift. (check here)

AGGRESSIVE BEHAVIOR (check all that apply)

VERBAL AGGRESSION	PHYSICAL AGGRESSION AGAINST SELF
☐ Makes loud noises, shouts angrily ☐ Yells mild personal insults, e.g., "You're stupid!" ☐ Curses viciously, uses foul language in anger, makes moderate threats to others or self ☐ Makes clear threats of violence toward others or self, (I'm going to kill you.) or requests to help to control self	☐ Picks or scratches skin, hits self, pulls hair, (with no or minor injury only) ☐ Bangs head, hits fist into objects, throws self onto floor or into objects, (hurts self without serious injury) ☐ Small cuts or bruises, minor burns ☐ Mutilates self, makes deep cuts, bites that bleed, internal injury, fracture, loss of consciousness, loss of teeth
PHYSICAL AGGRESSION AGAINST OBJECTS	**PHYSICAL AGGRESSION AGAINST OTHER PEOPLE**
☐ Slams door, scatters clothing, makes a mess ☐ Throws objects down, kicks furniture without breaking it, marks the wall ☐ Break objects, smashes windows ☐ Sets fires, throws objects dangerously	☐ Makes threatening gesture, swings at people, grabs at clothes ☐ Strikes, kicks, pushes, pulls hair (without injury to them) ☐ Attacks others causing mild–moderate physical injury (bruises, sprain, welts) ☐ Attacks others causing severe physical injury (broken bones, deep lacerations, internal injury)
Time incident began: __ __ : __ __ am/pm	Duration of incident: __ __ : __ __ (hours/minutes)

INTERVENTION (check all that apply)

☐ None ☐ Talking to patient ☐ Closer observation ☐ Holding patient	☐ Immediate medication given by mouth ☐ Immediate medication given by injection ☐ Isolation without seclusion (time out) ☐ Seclusion	☐ Use of restraints ☐ Injury requires immediate medical treatment for patient ☐ Injury requires immediate treatment for other person

COMMENTS

Figure 16–2. The Overt Aggression Scale. (Reprinted from Yudofsky SC, Silver JM, Jackson W, et al: The Overt Aggression Scale for the objective rating of verbal and physical aggression. Am J Psychiatry 143:35–39, 1986. Used with permission.)

tation with closed head injury (Rao et al. 1985), we recommend the use of antipsychotic agents only for the management of aggression stemming from psychotic ideation or for the intermittent management of brief aggressive events related to organic dyscontrol (through the sedative effects of neuroleptics). Table 16–14 summarizes the most disabling side effects that occur when neuroleptics are used to treat chronic aggression in patients with traumatic brain injury. Table 16–15 summarizes our prescribing regimen with haloperidol for the management of acute aggression.

Treatment of acute aggression—sedatives and hypnotics. The literature concerning the effects of the benzodiazepines in the treatment of aggression is inconsistent. Reports of increased hostility and paradoxical induction of rage are balanced by reports that this phenomenon is rare and that benzodiazepines may be effective in controlling aggression (Dietch and Jennings 1988; Silver and Yudofsky 1988; Yudofsky et al. 1987). If sedation is necessary in the management of acute aggression, medications such as paraldehyde, chloral hydrate, or diphenhydramine may be preferable to sedative antipsychotic agents.

The sedative properties of benzodiazepines are especially helpful in the acute management of agitation and aggression. Intramuscular lorazepam has been suggested as an effective medication in the emergency treatment of the violent patient (Bick and Hannah 1986). Lorazepam in 1 or 2 mg doses may be administered, if necessary, in combination with a neuroleptic medication (haloperidol, 2–5 mg). Table 16–14 summarizes the problems associated with the use of benzodiazepines, and Table 16–16 summarizes our use of lorazepam to treat acute aggression. Clonazepam may be effective in the long-term management of aggression, although controlled, double-blind studies have not been conducted (Freinhar and Alvarez 1986). We use this medication when aggression and anxiety occur together as pronounced symptoms in patients with brain injury.

Treatment of chronic aggression—buspirone. In preliminary reports, buspirone—a serotonin subtype (5-HT_{1A})—agonist has been reported to be effective in the management of aggression and agitation in patients with head injury (Levine 1988), dementia (Colenda 1988; Tiller et al. 1988), and developmental disabilities (Ratey et al. 1989). We have also noted that some patients become more aggressive when treated with buspirone. Therefore, buspirone should be initiated at low dosages (i.e., 5 mg bid) and increased by 5 mg every 3–5 days. Dosages of 45–60 mg/day may be required before there is improvement in aggressive behavior.

Treatment of chronic aggression—antidepressants. There have been several reports of the use of antidepressants to control aggressive behavior. In open studies, Mysiw et al. (1988) and Jackson et al. (1985) reported that amitriptyline (maximum dose 150 mg/day) was effective in the treatment of patients with recent severe brain injury whose agitation had not responded to behavioral techniques. Slabowicz and Stewart (1990) successfully treated a 43-year-old man with aggressive behavior subsequent to anoxic encephalopathy with amitriptyline 75 mg at bedtime.

Trazodone has also been reported effective in treating aggression that occurs with organic mental disorders (Pinner and Rich 1988; Simpson and Foster 1986). Preliminary reports have been published on the use of fluoxetine (a potent serotonergic antidepressant) in the treatment of aggressive behavior in a patient who suffered brain injury (Sobin et al. 1989), as well as patients with personality disorders (Coccaro et al. 1990). Fluoxetine is started with low

TABLE 16–14. SIDE EFFECTS OF DRUGS USED IN THE MANAGEMENT OF AGGRESSION

Neuroleptics
- Oversedation
- Hypotension (falls)
- Confusion
- Neuroleptic malignant syndrome
- Parkinsonian side effects
- Akathisia
- Dystonia
- Tardive dyskinesia

Benzodiazepines
- Oversedation
- Motor disturbances (poor coordination)
- Mood disturbances
- Memory impairment and confusion
- Dependency, overdoses, and withdrawal syndromes
- Paradoxical violence

Source. Reprinted from Yudofsky SC, Silver JM, Hales RE: Pharmacologic management of aggression in the elderly. J Clin Psychiatry 51 (10, suppl):22–28, 1990. Copyright 1990 by Physicians Postgraduate Press. Used with permission.

TABLE 16–15. USE OF HALOPERIDOL IN THE MANAGEMENT OF AGGRESSION

A. At first, 1 mg po or 0.5 mg iv or im every hour until control of aggression is achieved.
B. Then, 2 mg po or 1 mg iv or im every 8 hours.
C. When patient is not agitated or violent for a period of 48 hours, taper at rate of 25% of highest daily dose.
D. If violent behavior reemerges, reassess etiology and consider changing to a more specific medication to manage chronic aggression.
E. Do not maintain patient on haloperidol for more than 6 weeks—except for aggression secondary to psychosis.

Source. Reprinted from Yudofsky SC, Silver JM, Hales RE: Pharmacologic management of aggression in the elderly. J Clin Psychiatry 51 (10, suppl):22–28, 1990. Copyright 1990 by Physicians Postgraduate Press. Used with permission.

doses (5 mg/day) by diluting the contents of a 20 mg capsule in water, and raising the dose as tolerated every week to doses as large as 80 mg/day.

Treatment of chronic aggression—lithium carbonate. Although lithium is known to be effective in controlling aggression related to manic excitement, many studies have suggested that it may also have a role in the treatment of aggression in selected, nonbipolar patient populations. These include patients with head injury (Haas and Cope 1985), patients with mental retardation who exhibit self-injurious behavior (Luchins and Dojka 1989), and patients with other organic brain syndromes (Silver and Yudofsky 1988; Yudofsky et al. 1987). As mentioned above, patients with brain injury have increased sensitivity to the neurotoxic effects of lithium (Hornstein and Seliger 1989). Because of the potential for neurotoxicity and its relative lack of efficacy in many patients with aggression secondary to brain injury, we recommend the use of lithium in those patients whose aggression is related to manic effects or recurrent irritability related to cyclic mood disorders.

Treatment of chronic aggression—anticonvulsants. Carbamazepine, an anticonvulsant effective for the treatment of bipolar disorders and generalized and complex partial seizures, has been advocated for the control of aggression in both epileptic and nonepileptic populations (Gleason and Schneider 1990; Silver and Yudofsky 1988; Yudofsky et al. 1987). This is a highly effective medication to treat aggression in patients with brain injury, particularly for those patients who have aggressive episodes and seizures or epileptic foci.

Although a specific antiaggressive response to carbamazepine has not yet been demonstrated according to the most strict scientific criteria, a vast amount of clinical experience strongly suggests its efficacy in this area. However, the clinician should be aware of the potential risks associated with carbamazepine treatment, particularly bone marrow suppression (including aplastic anemia) and hepatotoxicity. Complete blood counts and liver function tests should be appropriately monitored (Silver and Yudofsky 1988). Hematologic monitoring (complete blood count and platelet count) should be obtained every 2 weeks for the first 2 months of treatment, and every 3 months thereafter. Liver function monitoring (serum glutamic-oxaloacetic transaminase [SGOT], serum glutamic-pyruvic transaminase [SGPT], lactic dehydrogenase [LDH], and alkaline phosphatase) should be obtained every month for the first 2 months of treatment, and every 3 months

TABLE 16–16. USE OF LORAZEPAM IN THE ACUTE MANAGEMENT OF AGGRESSION

A. At first, 1–2 mg po or im.
B. Then, repeat every hour until patient is calm.
C. Once patient is no longer violent or agitated, maintain at maximum of 2 mg po or im tid.
D. When patient is not agitated or violent for 48 hours, taper at rate of 10% of highest total daily dose.
E. If violent behavior reemerges, reassess etiology and consider changing to a more specific medication to manage chronic aggression.
F. If, after 6 weeks, lorazepam cannot be tapered without reemergence of aggression, reevaluate and revise treatment plan to include a more specific medication to manage chronic aggression.

Source. Adapted from Yudofsky et al. 1990. Used with permission.

thereafter. In our experience and that of others (Giakas et al. 1990), the anticonvulsant valproic acid may also be helpful to some patients with organically induced aggression.

Treatment of chronic aggression—β-blockers. Since the first report of the use of β-adrenergic receptor blockers in the treatment of aggression in 1977, over 25 papers have appeared in the neurological and psychiatric literature reporting experience with over 200 patients (Silver and Yudofsky 1988; Yudofsky et al. 1987). Most of these patients had been unsuccessfully treated with antipsychotics, minor tranquilizers, lithium, and/or anticonvulsants before treatment with β-blockers. The β-blockers that have been investigated include propranolol (a lipid-soluble, nonselective receptor antagonist), nadolol (a water soluble, nonselective receptor antagonist), pindolol (a lipid-soluble, nonselective β-adrenergic receptor antagonist with partial sympathomimetic activity), and metoprolol (a lipid soluble, selective β-adrenergic receptor antagonist). A list of β-blockers and their pharmacological properties is shown in Table 16–17.

A growing body of preliminary evidence suggests that β-adrenergic receptor blockers are effective agents for the treatment of aggressive and violent behaviors, particularly those related to organic brain syndrome. Guidelines for the use of propranolol are listed in Table 16–18. When a patient requires the use of a once-a-day medication because of compliance difficulties, long-acting propranolol (i.e., Inderal LA) or nadolol (Corgard) can be used in once-a-day regimens. When patients develop bradycardia that prevents prescribing therapeutic dosages of propranolol, pindolol (Visken) can be substituted, using one-tenth the dosage. The intrinsic sympathomimetic activity of pindolol stimulates the β-receptor and restricts the development of bradycardia.

Table 16–19 summarizes our recommendations for the use of various classes of medication in the treatment of aggressive disorders. In treating aggression, the clinician, where possible, should diagnose and treat underlying disorders and use, where possible, antiaggressive agents specific for those disorders.

Pharmacotherapy of Recovery of Brain Injury

Historically, pharmacological treatment has been directed towards controlling the resultant symptomatologies (e.g., depression, aggression, and psychosis) that occur after brain injury. Over the past several years, there have been significant developments in the pharmacotherapy of brain injury to limit the extent of damage.

As discussed above, many intracellular events occur during injury, including hypoxia and release of excitotoxic substances, such as glutamate (Albers et al. 1989; Becker et al. 1988). Glutamate binds to

TABLE 16–17. PHARMACOLOGICAL CHARACTERISTICS OF β-ADRENERGIC RECEPTOR ANTAGONISTS

Drug (generic/trade)	*Potency*[a]	*Local anesthetic activity*	*ISA*[b]	*Lipid solubility*	*Plasma half-life (hours)*
Nonselective (β_1- and β_2-adrenergic receptor) antagonists					
Alprenolol/Aptine	0.3–1	+	++	++	2–3
Carteolol/Cartrol	50	0	+	?	6
Nadolol/Corgard	0.5	0	0	0	14–18
Penbutolol/Levatal	4	0	+/–	?	26
Pindolol/Visken	5–10	+/–	++	+	3–4
Propranolol/Inderal	1.0	++	0	++	3–5
Sotalol/Sotalex	0.3	0	0	0	5–12
Timolol/Blocadren	5–10	0	+/–	+	4
Selective (β_1-adrenergic receptor) antagonists					
Acebutalol/Sectral	0.3	+	+	+	3
Atenolol/Tenormin	1.0	0	0	0	6–8
Betaxolol/Kerlone	4	+/–	–	?	14–22
Metoprolol/Lopressor	0.5–2	+/–	0	+	3–7

[a]Propanolol = 1.
[b]ISA = Intrinsic symptomometric activity.
Source. Data from Hoffman and Lefkowitz 1990 and American Medical Association, Department of Drugs, Division of Drugs and Toxicology 1991.

TABLE 16–18. CLINICAL USE OF PROPRANOLOL

1. Conduct a thorough medical evaluation.
2. Exclude patients with the following disorders: bronchial asthma, chronic obstructive pulmonary disease, insulin-dependent diabetes mellitus, congestive heart failure, persistent angina, significant peripheral vascular disease, hyperthyroidism.
3. Avoid sudden discontinuation of propranolol (particularly in patients with hypertension).
4. Begin with a single test-dose of 20 mg/day in patients for whom there are clinical concerns with hypotension or bradycardia. Increase dose of propranolol by 20 mg/day every 3 days.
5. Initiate propranolol on a 20 mg tid schedule for patients without cardiovascular or cardiopulmonary disorder.
6. Increase the dosage of propranolol by 60 mg/day every 3 days.
7. Increase medication unless the pulse rate is reduced below 50 bpm, or systolic blood pressure is less than 90 mmHg.
8. Do not administer medication if severe dizziness, ataxia, or wheezing occurs. Reduce or discontinue propranolol if such symptoms persist.
9. Increase dose to 12 mg/kg of body weight or until aggressive behavior is under control.
10. Doses of greater than 800 mg are not usually required to control aggressive behavior.
11. Maintain the patient on the highest dose of propranolol for at least 8 weeks before concluding that the patient is not responding to the medication. Some patients, however, may respond rapidly to propranolol.
12. Utilize concurrent medications with caution. Monitor plasma levels of all antipsychotic and anticonvulsive medications (Silver et al. 1986).

Source. Adapted from Silver and Yudofsky 1987a. Used with permission.

the *N*-methyl-D-aspartate (NMDA) receptor, and causes neuronal swelling and intracellular calcium entry, leading to further toxicity and cell destruction. In addition, glutamate may lead to the production of free radicals, which also are neurotoxic. NMDA receptor antagonists, such as MK-801 and dextrorphan can block this toxicity. Interestingly, phencyclidine, a potent psychotomimetic agent, is an NMDA antagonist. Lazaroides, such as U74006F, inhibit lipid peroxidation that occurs after injury.

In animal models, U74006F enhances recovery after brain injury (Hall et al. 1988). The administration of nerve growth factor (NGF) to rats after injury has also been shown to increase neuronal survival (Kromer 1987). Stimulants may improve recovery after brain injury that occurs with cerebrovascular accidents (Crisostomo et al. 1988). Although a detailed review of this subject is beyond the scope of this chapter, major advances in this area will certainly occur within this decade. We anticipate that, in the near future, initial treatment of victims of brain trauma will be directed toward minimizing damage rather than treating the neuropsychiatric sequelae of the injury.

Behavioral and Cognitive Treatments

Behavioral treatments are important in the care of patients who have suffered traumatic brain injury. These programs require careful design and execution by a staff well versed in behavioral techniques. Behavioral methods can be used in response to aggressive outbursts and other maladaptive social behaviors (Burke and Lewis 1986). One study (Eames and Wood 1985) found that behavior modification was 75% effective in dealing with disturbed behaviors after severe brain injury.

After brain injury, patients may need specific cognitive strategies to assist with impairments in memory and concentration. As opposed to earlier thoughts that cognitive therapy should "exercise" the brain to develop skills that have been damaged, current therapies involve teaching the patient new strategies to compensate for lost or impaired functions. (For more information on cognitive treatments, see Chapter 31.) We emphasize that, for most patients, treatment strategies are synergistic. For example, the use of β-adrenergic receptor antagonists to treat agitation and aggression may enhance a patient's ability to benefit from behavioral and cognitive treatments.

Psychological and Social Interventions

In the broadest terms, psychological issues involving patients who incur brain injury revolve around four major themes: psychopathology that preceded the injury; psychological response to the traumatic event; psychological reactions to deficits brought

TABLE 16–19. PSYCHOPHARMACOLOGICAL TREATMENT OF AGGRESSION

Agent	*Indications*	*Special clinical considerations*
Acute aggression		
Antipsychotics	Psychotic symptoms Acute management of violence using sedative side effects	Oversedation and multiple side effects
Benzodiazepines	Acute management of violence using sedative side effects	Paradoxical rage
Chronic aggression		
Anticonvulsants		
Carbamazepine (CBZ); valproic acid (VPA)	Seizure disorder	Bone marrow suppression (CBZ) and hepatotoxicity (CBZ and VPA)
Lithium	Manic excitement or bipolar disorder	Neurotoxicity and confusion
Buspirone	Persistent, underlying anxiety and/or depression	Delayed onset of action
Antidepressants	Depression or mood lability with irritability	May need usual clinical doses
Propranolol (and other β-blockers)	Chronic or recurrent aggression	Latency of 4–6 weeks

Source. Adapted from Yudofsky et al. 1990. Used with permission.

about by brain injury; and psychological issues related to potential recurrence of brain injury.

Preexisting psychiatric illnesses are most frequently intensified with brain injury. Therefore, the angry, obsessive patient or the patient with chronic depression will exhibit a worsening of these symptoms after brain injury. Specific coping mechanisms that were used before the injury may no longer be possible because of the cognitive deficits caused by the neurological disease. Therefore, patients need to learn new methods of adaptation to stress. In addition, as mentioned above, the social, economic, educational, and vocational status of the patient—and how these are affected by brain lesions—influence the patient's response to the injury.

The events surrounding brain injury often have far-reaching experiential and symbolic significance for the patient. Such issues as guilt, punishment, magical wishes, and fears crystallize about the nidus of a traumatic event. For example, a patient who suffers brain injury during a car accident may view his injury as punishment for long-standing violent impulses toward an aggressive father. In such cases, reassurance and homilies about his lack of responsibility for the accident are usually less productive than psychological exploration.

A patient's reactions to being disabled by brain damage has "realistic" as well as symbolic significance. When intense effort is required for a patient to form a word or to move a limb, frustration may be expressed as anger, depression, anxiety, or fear. Particularly in cases in which brain injury results in permanent impairment, a psychiatrist may experience countertransferential discomfort that results in failure to discuss directly with the patient and his or her family the implications of resultant disabilities and limitations. Gratuitous optimism, collaboration with denial of the patient, and facile solutions to complex problems are rarely effective and can erode the therapeutic alliance and ongoing treatment.

Tyerman and Humphrey (1984) assessed 25 patients with severe brain injury for changes in self-concept. Patients viewed themselves as markedly changed after their injury but believed that they would regain preexisting capacities within a year. The authors concluded that these unrealistic expectations may hamper rehabilitation and adjustment of both the patient and their relatives. By gently and persistently directing the patient's attention to the reality of the disabilities, the psychiatrist may help the patient begin the process of acceptance and adjustment to the impairment. Clinical judgment will help the psychiatrist in deciding whether and when explorations of the symbolic significance of the patient's brain injury should be pursued. The persistence of anxiety, guilt, and fear beyond the normative stages of adjustment and rehabilitation may indicate that psychodynamic approaches are required.

Families of patients with neurological disorders are under severe stress. The relative with a brain injury may be unable to fulfill his or her previous role or function as parent or spouse, thus significantly affecting the other family members. Oddy et al. (1978) evaluated 54 relatives of patients with brain injury within 1, 6, and 12 months of the traumatic event. Approximately 40% of the relatives showed depressive symptomatologies within 1 month of the event; 25% of the relatives showed significant physical or psychological illness within 6 and 12 months of the brain damage. Mood disturbances, especially anxiety, and social role dysfunction are also seen within this time (Livingston et al. 1985a, 1985b). By treating the psychological responses of relatives to the brain injury, the clinician can foster a supportive and therapeutic atmosphere for the patient as well as significantly help the relative.

For both patients and their families, severe traumatic brain injury results in multifaceted losses including the loss of dreams about and expectations for the future. The psychiatrist may be of enormous benefit in treating the family and patient by providing support, insight, and other points of view. A patient from a high-achieving family who lost his ability to do theoretical physics told an author (SCY), "If I can't go to graduate school in physics at Princeton like my brother and my cousin, I am worthless."

Educational and supportive treatment of families can be therapeutic when used together with appropriate social skills training. Patient advocacy groups, such as the National Head Injury Foundation, can provide important peer support for families. Many patients require clear, almost concrete statements describing their behaviors because insight and judgment may be impaired.

It is a distressing fact that brain injury can and often does recur. With repeated injury, there is an increase in the incidence of neuropsychiatric and emotional symptoms (Carlsson et al. 1987). In fact, trauma from accidents occurs more commonly in patients who have already suffered from such events than in those who have not. Therefore, patients' fears and anxieties about recurrence of injury are more than simply efforts at magical control over terrifying conditions. Therapeutic emphasis should be placed on those actions and activities that will aid in preventing recurrence, including compliance with appropriate medications and abstinence from alcohol and other substances of abuse.

❑ PREVENTION

Motor Vehicle Accidents

The proper use of seat belts with upper torso restraints is 45% effective in preventing fatalities, 50% effective in preventing moderate to critical injuries, and 10% effective in preventing minor injuries when used by drivers and passengers (U.S. Department of Transportation 1984). This would translate to 12,000–15,000 lives saved a year (National Safety Council 1986). Orsay et al. (1988) noted that victims of motor vehicle accidents who wore seat belts had a 60.1% reduction in injury severity. It is calculated that the installation of air bag safety devices in automobiles for drivers and passengers would save from 3,000 to 7,000 lives per year (National Safety Council 1986). Without specific legislation, car restraints are used infrequently (less than 10%) (Haddon and Baker 1981). The recent action by many state legislatures in mandating the use of car restraints has increased the use of safety belts. As of early 1990, 33 states and the District of Columbia had regulations requiring the use of seat belts.

Initial use of seat belts after enactment of those laws is high, but it decreases with time. A 19-city survey in 1989 (Datta and Guzek 1990) revealed that 46% of drivers used safety belts, and 81% of infants were in car seat restraints. Related to these statistics, we strongly advocate laws mandating car manufacturers to build cars with both passive (automatically functioning) seat belt restraints as well as both driver- and passenger-side air bags. Other factors related to increased mortality from motor vehicle accidents include increase in the speed limit and the increased use of utility vehicles and pickup trucks for noncommercial purposes (Baker et al. 1987).

Alcohol dependence is a highly prevalent and destructive illness. In addition, alcohol abuse is a common concomitant of affective and characterological disorders. Alcohol intoxication is frequently found in the patient who has suffered brain injury, whether from violence, falls, or motor vehicle accidents (Brismar et al. 1983). In the United States, it is estimated by the National Safety Council that alcohol ingestion is implicated in more than 50% of all automobile-related fatalities (Haddon and Baker 1981). Alcohol-related deaths among persons aged

19 and 20 can be decreased by over one-third with the increase in minimum drinking age from 18 to 21 (Decker et al. 1988).

Drivers in fatal accidents have a more frequent history of alcohol use, previous accidents, moving traffic violations, psychopathology, stress, paranoid thinking, and depression. They often have less control of hostility and anger, with a decreased tolerance for tension, and a history of increased risk taking (Tsuang et al. 1985). Cigarette smoking, alcohol use, obesity, and physical inactivity were found to be associated with nonuse of seat belts (Goldbaum et al. 1986). Therefore, we strongly advocate that in all psychiatric and other medical histories a detailed inquiry about alcohol use, seat belt use, and driving patterns be present. Examples of driving patterns, accident records, violations, driving while intoxicated, speeding patterns, car maintenance, presence of distractions such as children and animals, and hazardous driving conditions should be included as a complete driving record. The use of illicit substances and medications that may induce sedation, such as antihistamines, antihypertensive agents, anticonvulsants, minor tranquilizers, and antidepressants, should also be assessed and documented. Psychiatric patients are at greater risk for motor vehicle accidents because they often have several of these characteristics (Noyes 1985).

Clearly, motorcycle riding—with or without helmets—and using bicycles for commuting purposes are associated with head injuries, even when safety precautions are taken and when driving regulations are observed. Nonuse of motorcycle helmets is associated with increased accident rates and fatalities (Heilman et al. 1982; McSwain and Petrucelli 1984). The use of bicycle helmets can significantly decrease the morbidity and mortality from bicycle-related head injuries (Thompson et al. 1989).

Significant preventive measures to reduce head trauma include counseling a patient about risk taking; the treatment of alcoholism and depression; the judicious prescription of medications and full explanations of sedation, cognitive impairment, and other potentially dangerous side effects; and public information activities on topics such as the proper use of seat belts, the dangers of drinking and driving, and automobile safety measures.

Prevention of Brain Injury in Children

Beyond nurturance, children rely on their parents or guardians for guidance and protection. Each year in the United States over 1,400 children under age 13 die as motor vehicle passengers; more than 90% of these children were not using car seat restraints (Insurance Institute for Highway Safety 1983). Child safety seats have been found to be 80%–90% effective in the prevention of injuries to children (National Safety Council 1985). In a sample of 494 children younger than 4 years old who had suffered motor vehicle accident trauma (Agran et al. 1985), 70% had been unrestrained, 12% were restrained with seat belts, and 22% were restrained in child safety seats. In general, restrained children tended to sustain less serious injuries than the unrestrained children.

Children younger than 4 years old who are not restrained in safety seats are 11 times more likely to be killed in motor vehicle accidents (National Safety Council 1985). It is not safe for the child to sit on the lap of the parent, with or without restraints, because the adult's weight can crush the child during an accident. Young children traveling with drivers who, themselves, are not wearing seat belts are four times as likely to be left unrestrained (National Safety Council 1985). Legislation in Britain mandating the use of child safety seats has had a significant effect on decreasing fatal and serious injuries to children (Avery and Hayes 1985). In the United States, all 50 states and the District of Columbia have mandatory laws for child safety seats (National Safety Council 1985). Children who ride on bicycle-mounted child seats are highly subject to injuries to the head and face and must wear bicycle helmets (Sargent et al. 1988).

Children are often involved in sports that carry the risk of brain injury. Minor brain injury is not uncommon in football and can result in persistent symptoms and disabilities (Gerberich et al. 1983). Soccer may involve the use of the head with sudden twists to strike the ball that may also result in neuropsychiatric abnormalities (Tysvaer et al. 1989).

The clinician must always be alert to the possibility that patients may be neglectful, may use poor judgment, and may even be directly violent in their treatment of children. Unfortunately, it is not uncommon for head trauma to result from overt child abuse on the part of parents, other adults, and peers. We must always be alert to such possibilities in our patients and, when discovered, take direct actions to address these problems. We encourage direct counseling of patients who do not consistently use infant and child car seats for their children.

❑ CONCLUSIONS

Invariably, brain injury leads to emotional damage in the patient and in the family. In this chapter, we have reviewed the most frequently occurring psychiatric symptomatologies that are associated with traumatic brain injury. We have emphasized how the informed psychiatrist is not only effective but essential both in the prevention of brain injury and, when it occurs, the treatment of its sequelae. We advocate, in addition to increased efforts devoted to the prevention of brain injury, a multidisciplinary and multidimensional approach to the assessment and treatment of neuropsychiatric aspects of brain injury.

❑ REFERENCES

Adams JH, Graham DI, Murray LS, et al: Diffuse axonal injury due to nonmissile head injury in humans: an analysis of 45 cases. Ann Neurol 12:557–563, 1982

Agran PF, Dunkie DE, Winn DG: Motor vehicle accident trauma and restraint usage patterns in children less than 4 years of age. Pediatrics 76:382–386, 1985

Albers GW, Goldberg MP, Choi DW: N-methyl-D-aspartate antagonists: ready for clinical trial in brain ischemia? Ann Neurol 25:398–403, 1989

American Medical Association, Department of Drugs, Division of Drugs and Toxicology: American Medical Association Drug Evaluations, Annual 1991. Chicago, IL, American Medical Association, 1991

Amaducci LA, Fratiglioni L, Rocca WA, et al: Risk factors for clinically diagnosed Alzheimer's disease: a case control study of an Italian population. Neurology 36: 922–931, 1986

American Psychiatric Association: Diagnostic and Statistical Manual of Mental Disorders, 3rd Edition. Washington, DC, American Psychiatric Association, 1980

American Psychiatric Association: Task Force on the Use of Laboratory Tests in Psychiatry: tricyclic antidepressants: blood level measurements and clinical outcome: an APA Task Force Report. Am J Psychiatry 142:155–162, 1985

American Psychiatric Association: Diagnostic and Statistical Manual of Mental Disorders, 3rd Edition, Revised. Washington, DC, American Psychiatric Association, 1987

Annegers JF, Grabow JD, Groover RV, et al: Seizures after head trauma: a population study. Neurology 30:683–689, 1980

Armstrong KK, Sahgal V, Bloch R, et al: Rehabilitation outcomes in patients with posttraumatic epilepsy. Arch Phys Med Rehabil 71:156–160, 1990

Askenasy JJM, Winkler I, Grushkiewicz J, et al: The natural history of sleep disturbances in severe missile head injury. Journal of Neurological Rehabilitation 3: 93–96, 1989

Auerbach SH: Neuroanatomical correlates of attention and memory disorders in traumatic brain injury: an application of neurobehavioral subtypes. Journal of Head Trauma Rehabilitation 1:1–12, 1986

Avery JG, Hayes HRM: Death and injury to children in cars: Britain. Br Med J 291:515, 1985

Bakchine S, Lacomblez L, Benoit N, et al: Manic-like state after bilateral orbitofrontal and right temporoparietal injury: efficacy of clonidine. Neurology 39:777–781, 1989

Baker SP, Whitfield RA, O'Neill B: Geographic variations in mortality from motor vehicle crashes. N Engl J Med 316:1384–1387, 1987

Bamrah JS, Johnson J: Bipolar affective disorder following head injury. Br J Psychiatry 158:117–119, 1991

Bareggi SR, Porta M, Selenati, A, et al: Homovanillic acid and 5-hydroxyindole-acetic acid in the CSF of patients after a severe head injury, I: lumbar CSF concentration in chronic brain post-traumatic syndromes. Eur Neurol 13:528–544, 1975

Barth JT, Macciocchi SN, Giordani B, et al: Neuropsychological sequelae of minor head injury. Neurosurgery 13:529–533, 1983

Beck AT, Ward CH, Mendeson M, et al: An inventory for measuring depression. Arch Gen Psychiatry 4:561–571, 1961

Becker DP, Verity MA, Povlishock J, et al: Brain cellular injury and recovery: horizons for improving medical therapies in stroke and trauma [specialty conference]. West J Med 148:670–684, 1988

Ben-Yishay Y, Lakin P: Structured group treatment for brain-injury survivors, in Neuropsychological Treatment After Brain Injury. Edited by Ellis DW, Christensen A-L. Boston, MA, Kluwer Academic, 1989, pp 271–295

Berman KF, Illowsky BP, Weinberger DR: Physiological dysfunction of dorsolateral prefrontal cortex in schizophrenia, IV: further evidence for regional and behavioral specificity. Arch Gen Psychiatry 45:616–622, 1988

Bick PA, Hannah AL: Intramuscular lorazepam to restrain violent patients (letter). Lancet 1:206, 1986

Binder LM, Rattok J: Assessment of the postconcussive syndrome after mild head trauma, in Assessment of the Behavioral Consequences of Head Trauma. Edited by Lezak MD. New York, Alan R. Liss, 1989, pp 37–48

Bornstein RA, Miller HB, van Schoor T: Emotional adjustment in compensated head injury patients. Neurosurgery 23:622–627, 1988

Bornstein RA, Miller HB, Van Schoor JT: Neuropsychological deficit and emotional disturbance in head-injured patients. J Neurosurg 70:509–513, 1989

Bracken P: Mania following head injury. Br J Psychiatry 150:690–692, 1987

Brismar B, Engstrom A, Rydberg U: Head injury and intoxication: a diagnostic and therapeutic dilemma. Acta Chir Scand 149:11–14, 1983

Brooks N: Personal communication, reported in Eames P, Haffey WJ, Cope DN: Treatment of behavioral disorders, in Rehabilitation of the Adult and Child with Traumatic Brain Injury, 2nd Edition. Edited by Rosenthal M, Griffith ER, Bond MR, et al. Philadelphia, PA, FA Davis, 1990, pp 410–432

Brooks N, Campsie L, Symington C, et al: The five year outcome of severe blunt head injury: a relative's view. J Neurol Neurosurg Psychiatry 49:764–770, 1986

Brown G, Chadwick O, Shaffer D, et al: A prospective study of children with head injuries, III: psychiatric sequelae. Psychol Med 11:63–78, 1981

Burke WH, Lewis FD: Management of maladaptive social behavior of a brain injured adult. Int J Rehabil Res 9:335–342, 1986

Buysse DJ, Reynolds III CF: Insomnia, in Handbook of Sleep Disorders. Edited by Thorpy MJ. New York, Marcel Dekker, 1990, pp 373–434

Carlsson GS, Svardsudd K, Welin L: Long-term effects of head injuries sustained during life in three male populations. J Neurosurg 67:197–205, 1987

Cassidy JW: Fluoxetine: a new serotonergically active antidepressant. Journal of Head Trauma Rehabilitation 4:67–69, 1989

Chandra V, Kokmen E, Schoenberg BS, et al: Head trauma with loss of consciousness as a risk factor for Alzheimer's disease. Neurology 39:1576–1578, 1989

Clark AF, Davison K: Mania following head injury: a report of two cases and a review of the literature. Br J Psychiatry 150:841–844, 1987

Clifton GL, Ziegler MG, Grossman RG: Circulating catecholamines and sympathetic activity after head injury. Neurosurgery 8:10–14, 1981

Coccaro EF, Astill JL, Herbert JL, et al: Fluoxetine treatment of impulsive aggression in DSM-III-R personality disorder patients. J Clin Psychopharmacol 10:373–375, 1990

Colenda CC: Buspirone in treatment of agitated demented patients. Lancet 1:1169, 1988

Cope DN, Date ES, Mar EY: Serial computerized tomographic evaluations in traumatic head injury. Arch Phys Med Rehabil 69:483–486, 1988

Corbett JA, Trimble MR, Nichol TC: Behavioral and cognitive impairments in children with epilepsy: the long-term effects of anticonvulsant therapy. J Am Acad Child Psychiatry 24:17–23, 1985

Corkin S, Sullivan EV, Carr A: Prognostic factors for life expectancy after penetrating head injury. Arch Neurol 41:975–977, 1984

Courville CB: Pathology of the Nervous System, 2nd Edition. Mountain View, CA, Pacific Press, 1945

Crawford C: Social problems after severe head injury. N Z Med J 96:972–974, 1983

Crisostomo EA, Duncan PW, Propst M, et al: Evidence that amphetamine with physical therapy promotes recovery of motor function in stroke patients. Ann Neurol 23:94–97, 1988

Datta TK, Guzek P: Restraint System Use in 19 US Cities: 1989 Annual Report. Washington, DC, U.S. Dept of Transportation, National Highway Traffic Safety Administration, 1990

Davison K, Bagley CR: Schizophrenic-like psychoses associated with organic disorders of the central nervous system: a review of the literature, in Current Problems in Neuropsychiatry: Schizophrenia, Epilepsy, the Temporal Lobe. Edited by Herrington RN. Br J Psychiatry (special publication no 4), 1969

Decker MD, Graitcer PL, Schaffner W: Reduction in motor vehicle fatalities associated with an increase in the minimum drinking age. JAMA 260:3604–3610, 1988

Department of Health and Human Services: Interagency Head Injury Task Force Report. Washington, DC, U.S. Government Printing Office, 1989

Dietch JT, Jennings RK: Aggressive dyscontrol in patients treated with benzodiazepines. J Clin Psychiatry 49: 184–189, 1988

Dikmen S, Reitan RM: Emotional sequelae of head injury. Ann Neurol 2:492–494, 1977

Dikmen S, McLean A, Temkin N: Neuropsychological and psychosocial consequences of minor head injury. J Neurol Neurosurg Psychiatry 49:1227–1232, 1986

Dikmen SS, Temkin NR, Miller B, et al: Neurobehavioral effects of phenytoin prophylaxis of posttraumatic seizures. JAMA 265:1271–1277, 1991

Drummond LM, Gravestock S: Delayed emergence of obsessive-compulsive neurosis following head injury: case report and review of its theoretical implications. Br J Psychiatry 153:839–842, 1988

Eames P, Wood R: Rehabilitation after severe brain injury: a follow-up study of a behavior modification approach. J Neurol Neurosurg Psychiatry 48:613–619, 1985

Elliott FA: The neurology of explosive rage. Practitioner 217:51–59, 1976

Evans RW, Gualtieri CT, Patterson D: Treatment of chronic closed head injury with psychostimulant drugs: a controlled case study and an appropriate evaluation procedure. J Nerv Ment Dis 175:106–110, 1987

Faden AI, Demediuk P, Panter S, et al: The role of excitatory amino acids and NMDA receptors in traumatic brain injury. Science 244:798–800, 1989

Feeney DM, Gonzalez A, Law WA: Amphetamine, haloperidol, and experience interact to affect rate of recovery after motor cortex injury. Science 217:855–857, 1982

Freinhar JP, Alvarez WA: Clonazepam treatment of organic brain syndromes in three elderly patients. J Clin Psychiatry 47:525–526, 1986

Gallassi R, Morreale A, Lorusso S, et al: Carbamazepine and phenytoin: comparison of cognitive effects in epileptic patients during monotherapy and withdrawal. Arch Neurol 45:892–894, 1988

Garyfallos G, Manos N, Adamopoulou A: Psychopathology and personality characteristics of epileptic patients: epilepsy, psychopathology and personality. Acta Psychiatr Scand 78:87–95, 1988

Gerberich SG, Priest JD, Boen JR, et al: Concussion incidences and severity in secondary school varsity football players. Am J Public Health 73:1370–1375, 1983

Giakas WJ, Seibyl JP, Mazure CM: Valproate in the treatment of temper outbursts (letter). J Clin Psychiatry 51: 525, 1990

Gleason RP, Schneider LS: Carbamazepine treatment of agitation in Alzheimer's outpatients refractory to neuroleptics. J Clin Psychiatry 51:115–118, 1990

Goldbaum GM, Remington PL, Powell KE, et al: Failure to use seat belts in the United States: the 1981–1983 behavioral risk factor surveys. JAMA 255:2459–2462, 1986

Prigatano GP: Work, love, and play after brain injury. Bull Menninger Clinic 53:414–431, 1989

Prigatano GP, Stahl ML, Orr WC, et al: Sleep and dreaming disturbances in closed head injury patients. J Neurol Neurosurg Psychiatry 45:78–80, 1982

Rao N, Jellinek HM, Woolston DC: Agitation in closed head injury: haloperidol effects on rehabilitation outcome. Arch Phys Med Rehabil 66:30–34, 1985

Raphaely RC, Swedlow DB, Downes JJ, et al: Management of severe pediatric head trauma. Pediatr Clin North Am 27:715–727, 1980

Rappaport M, Herrero-Backe C, Rappaport ML, et al: Head injury outcome up to ten years later. Arch Phys Med Rehabil 70:885–892, 1989

Ratey JJ, Sovner R, Mikkelsen E, et al: Buspirone therapy for maladaptive behavior and anxiety in developmentally disabled persons. J Clin Psychiatry 50:382–384, 1989

Regier DA, Boyd JH, Burke Jr JD, et al: One-month prevalence of mental disorders in the United States. Arch Gen Psychiatry 45:977–986, 1988

Reynolds EH, Trimble MR: Adverse neuropsychiatric effects of anticonvulsant drugs. Drugs 29:570–581, 1985

Rimel RW, Giordani B, Barth JT, et al: Disability caused by minor head injury. Neurosurgery 9:221–228, 1981

Rivinus TM: Psychiatric effects of the anticonvulsant regimens. J Clin Psychopharmacol 2:165–192, 1982

Ross ED, Rush J: Diagnosis and neuroanatomical correlates of depression in brain-damaged patients. Arch Gen Psychiatry 38:1344–1354, 1981

Ross ED, Stewart RS: Pathological display of affect in patients with depression and right frontal brain damage: an alternative mechanism. J Nerv Ment Dis 176:165–172, 1987

Ruedrich I, Chu CC, Moore SI: ECT for major depression in a patient with acute brain trauma. Am J Psychiatry 140:928–929, 1983

Ruff RM, Buchsbaum MS, Troster AI, et al: Computerized tomography, neuropsychology, and positron emission tomography in the evaluation of head injury. Neuropsychiatry, Neuropsychology, and Behavioral Neurology 2:103–123, 1989

Ruff RM, Marshall LF, Klauber MR, et al: Alcohol abuse and neurological outcome of the severely head injured. Journal of Head Trauma Rehabilitation 5:21–31, 1990

Rutherford WH, Merrett JD, McDonald JR: Sequelae of concussion caused by minor head injuries. Lancet 1:1–4, 1977

Salazar AM, Jabbari B, Vance SC, et al: Epilepsy after penetrating head injury, I: clinical correlates: a report of the Vietnam head injury study. Neurology 35:1406–1414, 1985

Saran AS: Depression after minor closed head injury: role of dexamethasone suppression test and antidepressants. J Clin Psychiatry 46:335–338, 1985

Sargent JD, Peck MG, Weitzman M: Bicycle-mounted child seats: injury risk and prevention. Am J Dis Child 142:765–767, 1988

Schiff HB, Sabin TD, Geller A, et al: Lithium in aggressive behavior. Am J Psychiatry 139:1346–1348, 1982

Schiffer RB, Herndon RM, Rudick RA: Treatment of pathologic laughing and weeping with amitriptyline. N Engl J Med 312:1480–1482, 1985

Schoenhuber R, Gentili M: Anxiety and depression after mild head injury: a case control study. J Neurol Neurosurg Psychiatry 51:722–724, 1988

Schoenhuber R, Gentili M, Orlando A: Prognostic value of auditory brain-stem responses for late postconcussion symptoms following minor head injury. J Neurosurg 68:742–744, 1988

Silver JM, Yudofsky SC: Aggressive behavior in patients with neuropsychiatric disorders. Psychiatric Annals 17:367–370, 1987a

Silver JM, Yudofsky SC: Documentation of aggression in the assessment of the violent patient. Psychiatric Annals 17:375–384, 1987b

Silver JM, Yudofsky SC: Psychopharmacology and electroconvulsive therapy, in The American Psychiatric Press Textbook of Psychiatry. Edited by Talbott JA, Hales RE, Yudofsky SC. Washington, DC, American Psychiatric Press, 1988, pp 767–853

Silver JM, Yudofsky SC: The Overt Aggression Scale: overview and clinical guidelines. Journal of Neuropsychiatry and Clinical Neurosciences 3:S22–S29, 1991

Silver, JM, Yudofsky SC, Kogan M, et al: Elevation of thioridazine plasma levels by propranolol. Am J Psychiatry 143:1290–1292, 1986

Silver JM, Yudofsky SC, Hales RE: Neuropsychiatric aspects of traumatic brain injury, in The American Psychiatric Press Textbook of Neuropsychiatry. Edited by Hales RE, Yudofsky SC. Washington, DC, American Psychiatric Press, 1987, pp 179–190

Silver JM, Hales RE, Yudofsky SC: Psychiatric consultation to neurology, in American Psychiatric Press Review of Psychiatry, Vol 9. Edited by Tasman A, Goldfinger SM, Kaufmann CA. Washington, DC, American Psychiatric Press, 1990a, pp 433–465

Silver JM, Hales RE, Yudofsky SC: Psychopharmacology of depression in neurologic disorders. J Clin Psychiatry 51 (1, suppl):33–39, 1990b

Silver JM, Sandberg DP, Hales RE: New approaches in the pharmacotherapy of posttraumatic stress disorder. J Clin Psychiatry 51 (10, suppl):33–38, 1990c

Silver JM, Yudofsky SC, Hales RE: Depression in traumatic brain injury. Neuropsychiatry, Neuropsychology, and Behavioral Neurology 4:12–23, 1991

Simpson DM, Foster D: Improvement in organically disturbed behavior with trazodone treatment. J Clin Psychiatry 47:191–193, 1986

Slabowicz JW, Stewart JT: Amitriptyline treatment of agitation associated with anoxic encephalopathy. Arch Phys Med Rehabil 71:612–613, 1990

Smith MC, Bleck TP: Convulsive disorders: toxicity of anticonvulsants. Clin Neuropharmacol 14:97–115, 1991

Sobin P, Schneider L, McDermott H: Fluoxetine in the treatment of agitated dementia. Am J Psychiatry 146: 1636, 1989

Sosin DM, Sacks JJ, Smith SM: Head injury-associated deaths in the United States from 1979–1986. JAMA 262: 2251–2255, 1989

Sparadeo FR, Gill D: Effects of prior alcohol use on head injury recovery. Journal of Head Trauma Rehabilitation 4:75–82, 1989

Spitzer R, Williams JB, Gibbon M: Structured Clinical Interview for DSM-III-R. New York, Biometrics Research Department, New York State Psychiatric Institute, 1986

Starkstein SE, Boston JD, Robinson RG: Mechanisms of mania after brain injury: 12 case reports and review of the literature. J Nerv Ment Dis 176:87–100, 1988

Starkstein SE, Mayberg HS, Berthier ML, et al: Mania after brain injury: neuroradiological and metabolic findings. Ann Neurol 27:652–659, 1990

Stewart JT, Nemsath RH: Bipolar illness following traumatic brain injury: treatment with lithium and carbamazepine. J Clin Psychiatry 49:74–75, 1988

Stuss DT, Ely P, Hugenholtz H, et al: Subtle neuropsychological deficits in patients with good recovery after closed head injury. Neurosurgery 17:41–47, 1985

Teasdale G, Jennett B: Assessment of coma and impaired consciousness: a practical scale. Lancet 2:81–84, 1974

Temkin NR, Dikmen SS, Wilensky AJ, et al: A randomized, double-blind study of phenytoin for the prevention of post-traumatic seizures. N Engl J Med 323:497–502, 1990

Tennant FS, Wild J: Naltrexone treatment for postconcussion syndrome. Am J Psychiatry 144:813–814, 1987

Thompson RS, Rivara FP, Thompson DC: A case-control study of the effectiveness of bicycle safety helmets. N Engl J Med 320:1361–1367, 1989

Thomsen IV: Late outcome of very severe blunt head trauma: a 10–15 year second follow-up. J Neurol Neurosurg Psychiatry 47:260–268, 1984

Tiller JWG, Dakis JA, Shaw JM: Short-term buspirone treatment in disinhibition with dementia. Lancet 2:510, 1988

Tsuang MT, Boor M, Fleming JA: Psychiatric aspects of traffic accidents. Am J Psychiatry 142:538–546, 1985

Tyerman A, Humphrey M: Changes in self-concept following severe head injury. Int J Rehabil Res 7:11–23, 1984

Tysvaer AT, Storli OV, Bachen NI: Soccer injuries to the brain: a neurologic and electroencephalographic study of former players. Acta Neurol Scand 80:151–156, 1989

U.S. Department of Transportation: Final Regulatory Impact Assessment on Amendments to Federal Motor Vehicle Safety Standard 208, Front Seat Occupant Protection (Publ DOT HS 806 572). Washington, DC, U.S. Government Printing Office, 1984

van Woerkom TCAM, Teelken AW, Minderhoud JM: Difference in neurotransmitter metabolism in frontotemporal-lobe contusion and diffuse cerebral contusion. Lancet 1:812–813, 1977

van Zomeren A, van den Burg W: Residual complaints of patients two years after severe head injury. J Neurol Neurosurg Psychiatry 48:21–28, 1985

Varney NR: Prognostic significance of anosmia in patients with closed-head trauma. J Clin Exp Neuropsychol 10: 250–254, 1988

Varney NR, Martzke JS, Roberts RJ: Major depression in patients with closed head injury. Neuropsychology 1:7–9, 1987

Vecht CJ, van Woerkom TCAM, Teelken AW, et al: Homovanillic acid and 5-hydroxyindoleacetic acid cerebrospinal fluid levels. Arch Neurol 32:792–797, 1975

Weddell R, Oddy M, Jenkins D: Social adjustment after rehabilitation: a two year follow-up of patients with severe head injury. Psychosom Med 10:257–263, 1980

Weiger WA, Bear DM: An approach to the neurology of aggression. J Psychiatr Res 22:85–98, 1988

Weinstein GS, Wells CE: Case studies in neuropsychiatry: post-traumatic psychiatric dysfunction: diagnosis and treatment. J Clin Psychiatry 42:120–122, 1981

Wilberger JE, Deeb A, Rothfus W: Magnetic resonance imaging in cases of severe head injury. Neurosurgery 20:571–576, 1987

Wilcox JA, Nasrallah HA: Childhood head trauma and psychosis. Psychiatry Res 21:303–306, 1987

Will RG, Young JPR, Thomas DJ: Klein-Levin syndrome: report of two cases with onset of symptoms precipitated by head trauma. Br J Psychiatry 152:410–412, 1988

Wroblewski BA, McColgan K, Smith K, et al: The incidence of seizures during tricyclic antidepressant drug treatment in a brain-injured population. J Clin Psychopharmacol 10:124–128, 1990

Yudofsky SC, Silver JM: Psychiatric aspects of brain injury: trauma, stroke, and tumor, in Psychiatry Update: American Psychiatric Press Annual Review, Vol 4. Edited by Hales RE, Frances AJ. Washington, DC, American Psychiatric Press, 1985, pp 142–158

Yudofsky SC, Silver JM, Jackson W, et al: The Overt Aggression Scale for the objective rating of verbal and physical aggression. Am J Psychiatry 143:35–39, 1986

Yudofsky SC, Silver JM, Schneider SE: Pharmacologic treatment of aggression. Psychiatric Annals 17:397–407, 1987

Yudofsky SC, Silver JM, Yudofsky B: Organic personality disorder, explosive type, in Treatments of Psychiatric Disorders: A Task Force Report of the American Psychiatric Association. Washington, DC, American Psychiatric Association, 1989, pp 839–852

Yudofsky SC, Silver JM, Hales RE: Pharmacologic management of aggression in the elderly. J Clin Psychiatry 51 (10, suppl):22–28, 1990

Chapter

17

Neuropsychiatric Aspects of Seizure Disorders

Vernon M. Neppe, M.D., Ph.D.
Gary J. Tucker, M.D.

BEFORE THE DEVELOPMENT of the electroencephalogram (EEG) by Dr. Hans Berger in the 1930s, all seizure disorders were classified with mental disorders (Berger 1929–1938). Indeed, a strong link between seizures and psychiatry has been known for a century. Even the noted neuropsychiatrist Emil Kraepelin (1922, 1968) recognized three types of psychotic conditions, namely dementia praecox, manic-depressive illness, and the psychoses associated with epilepsy, and epilepsy was still conceived of as a mental disorder until recently in many countries. Today, however, this link is possibly less well recognized: DSM-III-R (American Psychiatric Association 1987) does not even include such a condition (Neppe and Tucker 1988b). Nevertheless, as psychiatrists have become more aware of the multiple physical conditions that can cause behavior change and particularly psychosis, they have become increasingly aware of the behavior changes associated with seizure disorders. The study of seizure disorders for psychiatrists is not only important for diagnostic and treatment purposes, it also has many theoretical implications for the understanding of behavioral disorders in general (Neppe and Tucker 1988b).

Two major historical relationships between epilepsy and psychopathology exist, namely personality and psychosis. There are also several controversies in the psychiatric perception of epilepsy, such as the place of temporal lobe epilepsy and the difficulties of evaluating epilepsy in the modern psychiatric context and the relationship of epilepsy to psychopathology. In this chapter we address all these areas.

We gratefully acknowledge the permission given by the American Psychiatric Association and *Hospital and Community Psychiatry* to reproduce here significant, updated sections from our two-part series on epilepsy and psychiatry (Neppe and Tucker 1988a, 1988b).

❑ EPILEPSY IN MODERN PSYCHIATRY

As noted above, the study of seizure disorders for psychiatrists has not only been important for diagnostic and treatment purposes, it also has many theoretical implications pertinent to the understanding of behavioral disorders. However, seizure disorders have been largely ignored in current psychiatric nosology, and in DSM-III-R there is no diagnosis of epilepsy and related conditions and the entity of *epileptic psychosis* does not exist except as a part of the more general concept of organic delusional disorder. Epilepsy with psychosis generally is classified as *atypical psychosis* or organic hallucinosis or organic delusional state. Even a diagnosis of atypical psychosis will only be disputably correct because DSM-III-R refers to "other nonorganic psychotic disorders," and it is unclear whether or not organic disorders can be included under atypical psychosis.

In general, the person with epilepsy is healthy and does not have any psychiatric stigmata. However, one apparently conservative estimation suggested that about one-fifth of epileptic outpatients have major psychopathology, for which about one-half will require hospitalization (Blumer 1975). There is a substantial increase in psychoses in seizure disorders. The incidence in epileptic populations has been variably cited at frequencies from 2.8% to 27% (with an average of 7%), and the prevalence of epilepsy in psychiatric hospitals is 2%–3%, which is much higher than the general population prevalence rate for seizure disorders of about 1.5% (Pincus and Tucker 1985). These figures would make the lifetime expectancy of psychosis in epilepsy about 10% over a 30-year period, whereas the lifetime risk for schizophrenia in the general population is about 0.8% (McKenna et al. 1985). Consequently, there is no doubt that there is a higher incidence of severe behavior disturbance (which would include psychosis as a major subgroup) among patients with seizure disorders. However, as noted, there is controversy with regard to whether the behavioral disturbance is limited to seizure patients with temporal lobe foci or to patients with seizure disorders in general.

❑ THE "EPILEPSY PLUS" PATIENT

Many epileptologists, neurologists, and psychiatrists perceive the epileptic patient in the context of major psychopathology. The epileptic patients who present to major centers are members of a selected population of patients who are intractable and difficult to manage and have behavior disorders and/or associated organic brain syndromes. They constitute a very small minority of the total numbers of epileptic patients. However, despite constituting only a very small proportion of the total epilepsy population, these patients—with underlying coarse organic neurobehavioral syndromes superimposed on or coexisting with the epilepsy or with behavioral disturbances or psychoses as a consequence of the epilepsy—are the ones most often written about. Difficulties in doing undistorted epidemiological surveys and evaluating members of the population at large in detail make exact proportions for these populations uncertain (Moehle et al. 1984). For example, the midtown Manhattan study (Singer et al. 1976) suggested a substantial proportion of the general population had major psychopathology, and figures of 90%–95% of epileptic patients having no more psychopathology or organic brain pathology than the general population may even be appropriate. These "normal" epileptic patients without additional psychopathology who work well within the community comprise what we call the "epilepsy standard group" as opposed to the "epilepsy plus group" who have these additional organic concomitants or psychotic predispositions. The differentiation is more than academic because associated psychopathology or coarse neurobehavioral syndromes in and of themselves may produce symptoms that may distort interpretations of the psychiatric population with epilepsy when in fact the epilepsy was not causal but only coexisting.

❑ SEIZURE DISORDERS

Seizures and Epilepsy

A person is only epileptic when he or she has seizures recurrently. An epileptic seizure involves paroxysmal cerebral neuronal firing, which may or may not produce disturbed consciousness and/or other perceptual or motor alterations (Neppe 1985a). The diagnosis of epilepsy is made when these seizures are recurrent and in quality. The most classical and most common epileptic seizures are of the *grand mal* or generalized tonic-clonic kind. These usually involve relatively short (10–30 seconds) tonic movements with marked extension or flexion of muscles, but no shaking, and then a longer (15–60 seconds) clonic movement manifesting as rhythmic muscle group shaking. These movements may be associated with a phase of laryngeal stridor due to tonic muscles manifesting as a high-pitched scream sound. Urinary and occasionally fecal incontinence may occur due to sphincteric change, and the seizures are almost invariably followed by headache, sleepiness, and confusion (Neppe and Tucker 1988b). When preceded by perceptual, autonomic, affective, or cognitive alterations, such seizures are secondarily generalized, as opposed to no original locus of firing, producing focal features before the tonic-clonic movements (generalized from the start) (International League Against Epilepsy Commission 1985).

The term *seizure* at times is also applied to other nonepileptic episodic phenomena that do not involve paroxysms of firing of cerebral neurons. The most common nonepileptic seizure is the so-called pseudoseizure or hysterical seizure. The pseudoseizure involves episodic behavioral aberrations that may closely mimic epileptic seizures. The term *seizure* when used alone should be limited to mean epileptic seizures.

Although one epileptic seizure does not make a person epileptic, a single seizure does require evaluation to ensure that underlying treatable, discernible etiologies are not present. These causes are best perceived as either nonprogressive or progressive. Important nonprogressive causes include head injury, encephalitis, birth trauma, hyperpyrexic convulsions, genetic predisposition, medication (e.g., neuroleptics and tricyclic antidepressants [TCAs]), and withdrawal states (e.g., from alcohol). Relevant potentially progressive conditions include tumor, metabolic disease (e.g., hypoglycemia and uremia), endocrine disease, Alzheimer's disease and other dementias, multiple sclerosis, cerebral arteriopathy, and other degenerative or infiltrative conditions. The physician should attempt to establish the underlying causes of seizures, particularly those presenting in adulthood (over age 30) (Pincus and Tucker 1985).

Classification of Seizures

The classification of seizures and epilepsy has been controversial. It has shifted away from terms such as *grand mal* to an attempt to correlate clinical seizure type with EEG ictal (i.e., during the seizure) and interictal (i.e., between the seizure) changes. The latest classification of epileptic seizures, as recognized by the International League Against Epilepsy (ILAE) in 1981, ignores anatomical aspects; for example, the term *temporal lobe epilepsy,* technically no longer exists (International League Against Epilepsy Commission 1981). Furthermore, it ignores attempts at explaining pathology and does not take into account age and sex (Table 17–1). It makes a descriptive attempt at classifying epilepsy as generalized or partial seizures and describes the progression of firing; for example, seizures may begin as simple partial, progress on to complex partial, and then secondarily generalize. The number of permutations is very large. When the kind of seizure is uncertain the term *unclassified* is used (Neppe 1982b). As these seizure types are somewhat perplexing, we describe them here briefly (Neppe and Tucker 1988b).

Generalized seizures. Generalized seizures (or generalized attacks) are epileptic seizures that manifest immediately and spread bilaterally through the cerebral cortex. They are generalized in that subcortical fibers may have been involved and there is simultaneous spread throughout the cerebral cortex.

TABLE 17–1. INTERNATIONAL LEAGUE AGAINST EPILEPSY REVISED CLASSIFICATION OF EPILEPTIC SEIZURES

1. Partial (focal, local) seizures
   - A. Simple: motor, somatosensory, autonomic, or psychic
   - B. Complex
     - a) Impaired consciousness at outset
     - b) Simple partial followed by impaired consciousness
   - C. Partial seizures evolving to generalized tonic-clonic (GTC)
     - a) Simple to GTC
     - b) Complex to GTC

2. Generalized seizures (convulsive or nonconvulsive)
   - A. a) Absence seizures
     - b) Atypical absences
   - B. Myoclonic
   - C. Clonic
   - D. Tonic
   - E. Tonic-clonic
   - F. Atonic
   - G. Combinations

3. Unclassified epileptic seizures

Source. International League Against Epilepsy Commission 1981.

There are no preceding motor or perceptual experiences, and there is almost invariably total loss of consciousness.

Partial (focal) seizures. In partial (focal) seizures (or partial focal attacks), epileptic firing starts in a specific area (focus or locus) of the brain. This evokes the physiological experience that stimulating that focus would produce. When such seizures involve no alteration in consciousness they are *simple partial seizures* (previously called *elementary partial seizures*). When there is a defect in consciousness they are *complex partial seizures* (*CPSs*). Some authors further subdivide CPSs into Type 1 (temporal) and Type 2 (extratemporal).

Tonic-clonic seizures. Tonic-clonic seizures (or grand mal seizures) are the most common form of generalized seizure. They manifest as total consciousness loss with a tetanic muscular phase (i.e., tonic) followed by a phase of repetitive jerking (i.e., clonic). These seizures may be generalized from the start or begin as partial seizures and secondarily generalize.

Partial seizures secondarily generalized are seizures that start as partial seizures. This phase may or may not be remembered. They then spread bilaterally throughout the cerebral cortex producing secondary generalization. (This terminology is different from a previous classification that spoke of *secondary generalized epilepsy,* which referred to a kind of epilepsy generalized from the start with features of a diffuse cerebral pathology).

Petit mal seizures. Petit mal seizures (or typical absence seizure) are a common seizure type (occurring particularly in children) generalized from the start, with loss of consciousness for a few seconds without any motor phase and typical EEG findings (i.e., bilateral, synchronous, 3–4 per second spike wave, and discharge).

Status epilepticus. Status epilepticus involves two or more seizures superimposed on each other without total recovery of consciousness between.

Certain other classifications are emerging in relation to partial seizures. One relates to the development of Type 1 or Type 2 complex partial seizures based on localization of the seizure at either temporal or extratemporal levels. At this point in time, such a classification is defeating the objectives of the ILAE in that an attempt has been made to shift away from the anatomic to the descriptive and classifications based on extratemporal or temporal complicate matters unnecessarily. In this chapter we use the term *temporal lobe epilepsy* in this regard, but we emphasize that the term is used in the descriptive sense implying both complex and simple partial seizures and also including psychomotor automatisms and tonic-clonic seizures that may originate from the temporal lobe. Many such phenomena interpreted to have originated from the temporal lobe may, in fact, be extratemporal.

In addition to the 1981 ILAE classification of seizures, in 1985 the ILAE developed a more esoteric classification of epilepsies and epileptic syndromes (International League Against Epilepsy 1985).

A final term that requires clarification does not refer to epileptic seizures at all: the term *pseudoseizure* is used synonymously with *hystero-epilepsy* and *nonepileptic seizure.* The differentiation of this heterogeneous group from true seizures is at times difficult, and Table 17–2 clarifies the features sug-

TABLE 17–2. GENERAL FEATURES OF NONEPILEPTIC SEIZURES

Setting
- Unconsciously motivated
- Environmental gain (audience usually present)
- Seldom sleep-related
- Often triggered (e.g., by stress)
- Suggestive profile on Minnesota Multiphasic Personality Inventory (Hathaway and McKinley 1989)

Attack
- Atypical movements, often bizarre or purposeful
- Seldom results in injury
- Ends gradually
- Out-of-phase movements of extremities
- Pelvic thrusting or side-to-side movements

Examination
- Restraint accentuates the seizure
- Inattention decreases over time
- Plantar flexor reflexes
- Reflexes intact (corneal, pupillary, and blink)
- Consciousness preserved
- Autonomic system uninvolved
- Autonomically intact

After attack
- No postictal features
- Prolactin normal (after 20–30 minutes)
- No or little amnesia
- Memory exists (hypnosis or Amytal Sodium)

gesting nonepileptic seizures (Neppe and Tucker 1988b).

Temporal Lobe Epilepsy

Although the term *temporal lobe epilepsy* has formally become an anachronism, in practice it is still commonly used in the absence of an adequate alternative. Temporal lobe epilepsy phenomena are not synonymous with its attempted, nonanatomical replacement, *complex partial seizures*, because complex partial seizures are restricted to patients who have focal firing with defects of consciousness (Neppe 1982a).

In practice many patients with temporal lobe epilepsy have no defect of consciousness and have simple partial seizures (e.g., olfactory hallucinations), which may derive from the temporal lobes. In addition, they may have simple partial seizures with psychic symptomatology (e.g., cognitive alterations, such as flashbacks or déjà vu experiences occurring in clear consciousness). Temporal lobe epilepsy may also manifest with the *temporal lobe absence* or behavioral arrest that is associated with a brief loss of consciousness of 10–30 seconds (Neppe 1981b). These episodes may be associated with minor automatisms (e.g., chewing movements) and at times with "drop attacks"—the falling associated with loss of muscle tone. Patients with temporal lobe epilepsy often appear to be staring and after the episode may be aware that there was a loss of consciousness. They may experience postictal features such as headache and sleepiness, but certainly they have a perplexity and disorientation (Neppe 1985a). Thus the temporal lobe absence differs from petit mal as the latter is a shorter episode, without muscle movements and postictal features.

Temporal lobe epilepsy may also manifest with psychomotor automatisms alone, which are no longer regarded as a form of complex partial seizures. Psychomotor automatisms may involve a so-called psychic (or cognitive-affective sensory perceptual) phase followed by a motor phase. The psychic phase may be very brief and not recognized by the patient who may be amnesic for it. It may be associated with many perceptual alterations, such as an auditory buzz or hum, more complex verbalizations, or aphasias. Visual abnormalities include diplopia, perceived movement, and changes in perceived object size or shape. Other alterations include illusional phenomena, tactile distortions, olfactory phenomena (e.g., generally unpleasant, burning, or rotting smells), and gustatory phenomena (e.g., metallic tastes). Flashbacks and illusions of interpretations (so-called jamais vu, depersonalization, derealization, and déjà vu) may occur. These are followed by automatisms of various degrees of complexity. There may be simple buttoning or unbuttoning or masticatory movements, more complex "wandering" fugue states, furor type anger (which is very rare), or speech automatisms (which are far more common than recognized) (Neppe 1981b).

The features of temporal lobe epilepsy are so varied and so protean that it is necessary to classify them. The term *possible temporal lobe symptoms (PTLSs)* has been suggested (Neppe 1983e). These are symptoms that can be induced by stimulating areas of the temporal lobe during neurosurgery (implying a link with the temporal lobe), but without direct EEG confirmation during the episode, they cannot of themselves be demonstrated to derive from the temporal lobe; hence the word *possible.* PTLSs are further subdivided into controversial (dubious), benign (symptoms not of themselves requiring treatment), and disintegrative (symptoms severe enough to require treatment) (Table 17–3). They should be distinguished from nonspecific symptoms such as depersonalization or decreased concentration, which do not of themselves have any localizing value.

Role of the EEG

The ultimate differentiation of epileptic from nonepileptic seizures and of aberrant behavior that may be interpreted as truly epileptic from behavior that is not epileptic is via EEG confirmation. Developments in this regard have been rapid over the past few years with the increasing usage of EEG telemetry. Telemetry involves prolonged monitoring over periods of time varying from 12 hours to 2 weeks while the patient is generally confined to a particular room. Cable telemetry is most commonly used. This involves, for example, a 25-foot cable connected to the EEG montage on the patient's head.

Radio telemetry in which the EEG is picked up in effect by a method akin to radio is now more common, but at this point rather experimental due to its sensitivity and the profound degree of artifact. Thus most clinicians currently prefer cable telemetry. Very often no seizure manifestations are picked up for prolonged periods of time because seizures only occur paroxysmally. Moreover, those patients evaluated in a specialized center with EEG teleme-

TABLE 17–3. POSSIBLE TEMPORAL LOBE SYMPTOMS (PTLSs)

Controversial (dubious) PTLSs (CPTLSs)
- Hypergraphia
- Hyperreligiosity
- Polymodal hallucinatory experience
- Paroxysmal episodes of
  - Profound mood changes within hours
  - Frequent subjective paranormal experiences (e.g., telepathy, mediumistic trance, writing automatisms, visualization of presences or of lights or colors round people, dream extrasensory power, out-of-body experiences, alleged healing abilities, precognition, near-death experiences, and sense of floating)
  - Intense libidinal change
  - Uncontrolled, limited precipitated, directed, nonamnesic aggressive episodes
  - Recurrent nightmares of stereotyped kind
  - Episodes of blurred vision or diplopia
  - Intense ecstasy or religious experience
  - Hyposexuality
  - Unexplained episodes of dizziness
  - Flowery or perfumy smells

Benign PTLSs (BPTLSs) *symptoms not necessarily requiring treatment*
- Paroxysmal episodes of
  - Complex visual hallucinations linked to other qualities of perception such as voices, emotions, or time
  - Olfactory hallucinations with burning, rotting, episodic components or linked to other PTLSs
- Any form of
  - Simple auditory perceptual abnormality
  - Gustatory hallucinations
  - Rotation or disequilibrium feelings linked to other perceptual qualities
  - Unexplained "sinking," "rising," or "gripping" epigastric sensations
  - Flashbacks
  - Illusions of distance, size (micropsia or macroscopy), loudness, tempo, strangeness, unreality, fear, or sorrow
  - Hallucinations of indescribable modality
  - Temporal lobe epileptic déjà vu (has associated ictal or postictal features [e.g., headache, sleepiness, and confusion] linked to the experience in clear or altered consciousness)
  - Any CPTLSs that appear to improve after administration of an anticonvulsant agent such as carbamazepine
  - Depersonalization or derealization linked with other PTLS features
  - Any CPTLSs associated with postevent headache (consistent quality), sleepiness, or confusion or with other PTLSs

Disintegrative PTLSs (DPTLSs) *symptoms requiring treatment*
- Paroxysmal episodes of
  - Epileptic amnesia
  - Lapses in consciousness
  - Conscious "confusion" (apparent clear consciousness but abnormalities of orientation, attention, and behavior)
  - Epileptic automatisms
  - Masticatory-salivatory episodes
  - Speech automatisms
  - "Fear which comes of itself" linked to other disorders (hallucinatory or unusual autonomic)
  - Uncontrolled, unprecipitated, undirected, amnesic aggressive episodes
  - Superior quadrantic homonymous hemianopia
  - Receptive (Wernicke's) aphasia
  - Any CPTLSs or BPTLSs with ictal EEG correlates

Seizure-related features
- Any typical absence, tonic or clonic, tonic-clonic, or bilateral myoclonic seizures in the absence of metabolic, intoxication, or withdrawal-related phenomena

Note. Patients may have more symptoms than those noted above.
Source. Adapted from Neppe 1991.

try are invariably so atypical that the hypothesized seizure originates deep within the brain. Commonly, therefore, these patients have sphenoidal EEG monitoring, which increases enormously the potential for picking up deep mesial temporal lesions (Ebersole and Leroy 1983).

Unfortunately, EEG telemetry is not easily available to most clinicians. The apparatus costs more than $100,000, the costs involved in monitoring patients substantially exceed $1,000 a day, and at times 2 weeks of monitoring are necessary. Instead, EEGs are easily available. EEG technology is still rather primitive, and reflections of brain waves from the perspective of analysis of psychopathology are limited. Nevertheless, the only definitive way to demonstrate that a symptom or physical sign such as an olfactory hallucination is definitely epileptic is to demonstrate correlates of seizure phenomena on EEG, such as spike-wave paroxysms, while the person is having that experience.

It is unusual for a person to have such an experience during an EEG unless their seizure phenomena are relatively uncontrolled. Even in the event of such an experience, the EEG correlate may not necessarily be of a spike kind but of a marked slowing, with a theta rhythm, which is nonspecific and generally of limited help, or a delta rhythm, which is frankly abnormal unless the patient is asleep (theta is 4–7 cycles/second; delta < 4). Moreover, it is extremely difficult to localize such features on scalp EEG even when a firing is occurring because many of these symptoms occur from the mesial temporal areas or deep structures within the brain, and they do not easily manifest on surface EEGs (Neppe 1982a).

Special techniques have been used to overcome the problem. One commonly used technique was nasopharyngeal electrodes. However, the increased yield with nasopharyngeal electrodes is not substantial—some studies indicate less than 10% (Neppe and Tucker 1988b). On the other hand, the yield with sphenoidal electrodes is very greatly increased (Bickford 1979). Unfortunately, however, sphenoidal electrode placement requires time and expertise, and therefore these are not easily available.

A relatively recent suggestion has been the placement of electrodes on the buccal skin surface in the area of the submandibular notch (McKenna et al. 1985). It appears that these placements may entirely eclipse nasopharyngeal electrodes because they are almost as effective in picking up foci as sphenoidal placements (Sadler and Goodwin 1986). Much more definitive, however, is the use of cerebral cortical placements during neurosurgery procedures. These may show firing (e.g., in patients with temporal lobe epilepsy and psychosis) in the region of the hippocampus (Heath 1982). The direct placement of intracranial electrodes shows how commonly spike firing may be occurring in this area with no correlate of any kind on surface EEGs (Gardner and Cowdry 1986).

There are several methods that are used for evoking EEG abnormalities. One very common one is the usage of sleep records. In this method the yield of actual ictal-related events is not substantially increased. However, the potential in terms of picking up a particular focus or focal abnormality may be increased because of the extra synchronization that may be occurring. There are phases of sleep in which there may, in fact, be a raised threshold for inducing seizures (i.e., less potentiality for seizures), but it is during such phases that focal abnormalities may be more evident (Brodsky et al. 1983). This explains the apparent paradox of the usage for many years of barbiturates such as secobarbital sodium in sleep records.

The most logical kind of sleep record is natural induction of sleep. However, in a laboratory situation this is not very easy, and at times (e.g., overnight) the patient is sleep deprived so that no medication need be given. Such a practice is a good one but is not easily applicable in the psychiatric patient who is generally disturbed enough to require some kind of sedative. The alternative is the administration of chloral hydrate 1–3 g as premedication before the sleep record. This induces little change of significance in the EEG and does not prevent the demonstration of focal abnormalities.

Certain medications should be particularly avoided in this regard. The first are those in the benzodiazepine group, which may have by virtue of their very strong antiepileptic effects profound effects in normalizing the EEG. Because such effects at a receptor level may last weeks even with the apparent short-acting benzodiazepines, the yield of demonstrating epilepsy after the patient has had benzodiazepines administered apparently decreases substantially, although adequate data in this regard are not easily available (Neppe 1984). The second medication to be avoided as a nocturnal medication for sleep is L-tryptophan. Adamec and Stark (1983) demonstrated that L-tryptophan has some effect in preventing onset of seizures during electroconvulsive therapy (ECT).

Overall, a sleep EEG record increases the chances of picking up a focal abnormality such as a temporal lobe focus by approximately fourfold. For example, Gibbs and Gibbs (1952) found only 20% interseizure waking EEG abnormalities in temporal lobe epilepsy; this figure went up to 80% in sleep records in a nonhomogeneous neurological population (Reynolds 1967).

Recent advances in EEG technology may ultimately change the whole perspective of its use in psychiatry. Computed EEG monitoring allows breakdown of wave forms and allows correlation with evoked potentials including cognitive evoked potentials. It also facilitates demonstrations of changes in particular areas of the brain that can be easily delineated at a visual level. This should prove to be a useful psychophysiological correlate of psychopathology. Indeed, this may be the beginning of an important new era. However, at this time it is still experimental.

Kindling

Kindling—the pathophysiological process whereby repetitive subthreshold electrical or chemical stimuli to certain brain areas will eventually induce threshold responses (Neppe 1985a)—and related hypotheses have become fashionable and possibly useful ways to explain certain episodic behavioral disturbances. Evidence from animal studies (McNamara et al. 1980; Wada et al. 1974) has shown that repetitive intermittent subthreshold stimuli administered to parts of the brain (e.g., the amygdala, piriform, and hippocampal areas) will induce a permanent threshold change allowing a progression of seizure phenomena. Such changes occur throughout the animal kingdom but are more difficult to induce with higher degrees of encephalization. Behavioral manifestations begin to precede seizure manifestations in cats, as contrasted with rats (Stevens and Livermore 1978).

Although kindling has never been demonstrated definitively in man, there is indirect support for the occurrence of kindling phenomena in man (Adamec et al. 1981) in the development of mirror foci, in epilepsy in the generalization of partial seizure phenomena, and in certain models such as alcohol withdrawal and posttraumatic stress reaction (Neppe 1985b). The major evidence against such a phenomenon is the prolonged duration of time it should take (i.e., years) and the fact that certain behavior disturbances appear to occur almost immediately after seizures and do not take such a long period of time. The most potent limbic antikindling agent available is carbamazepine, which has psychotropic effects, possibly as a consequence of kindling reduction (Albertson et al. 1980; Albright and Burnham 1980; Wada et al. 1976).

The kindling phenomenon, even if it can be applied to human behavior, should not be perceived as a single entity (Neppe 1989b, 1990b; Post and Weiss 1989). Drugs that act against kindling act on a variety of processes. For example, carbamazepine has a potent action on the endpoint of the kindled animal preparation; however, it has very little effect in preventing the kindling phenomenon. On the other hand, the benzodiazepines act early on in preventing kindling-like episodes.

The kindling phenomenon should be differentiated from chemical phenomena that also produce a sensitization (Post and Weiss 1989). These have variably been called "chindling" by Neppe (1989b, 1990b) and "sensitization" by Post and Weiss (1989). Whereas kindling and sensitization are not equivalent, they both describe chemical phenomena whereby changes occur in behavior or seizure-related episodes when, previous to this, no such change has occurred. Chindling is broadly equivalent to the reverse tolerance that is seen with cocaine and amphetamine-related substances (Table 17–4). It is probable that the sensitization that is occurring is an entirely different phenomenon from chemical-related kindling, such as is occurring with local anesthetics such as lidocaine. Cocaine may be a model for both kinds of episodes (Post and Weiss 1989).

The practical implications of such research still require formal conceptualization. However, kindling research may imply that certain anticonvulsants may be better at different stages in behavioral disorders in a single person's illness. For patients with histories of hallucinogen abuse, for example, we find phenytoin preferable at times to carbamazepine, and the patient may be resistant to carbamazepine. On the other hand, relatively early in the process, carbamazepine may be the appropriate drug (Scher and Neppe 1989). The role of valproate in these phenomena is not as clear. Its mechanism is different from those of phenytoin, phenobarbital, and carbamazepine (Neppe 1990b).

TABLE 17–4. SIMPLIFIED MODEL OF DIFFERENCE BETWEEN THE KINDLING PHENOMENON AND SENSITIZATION OR CHINDLING

Variable	*Kindling*	*Sensitization or chindling*
Mechanism	Electrical Chemical possible	Chemical Several mechanisms behavior/reverse tolerance?
Permanence	Permanent (?)	Long to decay
Occurrence in humans	Uncertain	Yes
Chemical links	*N*-methyl-D-aspartate (?)	Cholinergic (?)
Vasopressin	Facilitates	Inhibits
Catecholamines	Inhibits	Facilitates
Responses	Convulsion	Behavioral aberrations
Gradation	Graded seizures	More "all-or-none" phenomenon
Stress	Decrease	Increase
Dose	Subthreshold	High or low doses
Chronicity	Chronic intermittent effects	Acute or chronic effects

Source. Neppe 1989b.

❑ SEIZURES AND PSYCHIATRIC DISORDERS

Controversial Areas

Psychosocial facets of epilepsy. The epileptic patient encounters major psychosocial stressors. First is the stress of having a chronic illness. Studies comparing the epileptic patient with groups of patients with other chronic illnesses such as rheumatic heart disease, diabetes mellitus, and cancer have concluded that each of these conditions has its own special stressors (Dodrill and Batzel 1986). However, when comparing any of these populations to patients with organic brain disease, there are also specific difficulties in that organicity in and of itself has its own problems (Szatmari 1985).

The special difficulty of the epileptic patient is the paroxysmal (or episodic) element of the illness. In between episodes the person with epilepsy may be functioning normally. There is a substantial covert stress leading the person with epilepsy to being afraid of performing normal social activities, like dating with a favored friend of the opposite sex during adolescence. The threat is greater than the occurrence (Neppe 1985a). In addition, the actual tonic-clonic seizure is such a frightening experience for many members of the general population, and there is so much folklore associated with the grand mal seizure, that the visualization of such an episode is said to be far more traumatic for the spectator than for the epileptic patient. The consequence of this is that interpretations of the epilepsy may be distorted thereafter, and even an isolated seizure may have grave consequences at an interpersonal level.

Therefore, the psychosocial stressors encountered by the person with epilepsy are very substantial, but they are additionally based on limitation of particular activities. To indicate that epileptic individuals should not operate dangerous machinery, work in jobs that expose them to great heights, swim alone, or, in some instances, even bathe autonomously is obvious. The trauma of not driving is a very substantial one for the average person with epilepsy. (In a study in France in the 1980s, 90% of epileptic subjects surveyed, who were not supposed to be driving, were noncompliant.)

The functional limitations of epilepsy are substantial, and when they are not adhered to the epileptic individual must conquer his or her guilt. Criminal behavior (e.g., driving) puts the person with epilepsy at a high stress-risk level; he or she needs to deceive to survive, and this is not healthy. Also, the phenomenon of dependency on others is often hard to break in the neuropsychological rehabilitation of the epileptic patient. It is sometimes easier to remain ill than to become seizure free and healthy. The patient has to learn to deal with health (Neppe 1985d).

Within our Western culture, persons with epilepsy are at times perceived as an inferior minority group. However, in certain preliterate subcultures, an epileptic seizure is often regarded as some kind of communication with ancestors and with higher beings, and epileptic individuals may be perceived as having special powers; many of them became sangomas (shamans or witch doctors) and highly respected members of their culture (Neppe and Tucker 1989). Finally, the extent to which the apparent psychological facets may be consequent on interictal firing or related phenomena should not be underestimated (Stevens et al. 1969).

Temporal lobe specificity and psychopathology. A major question about temporal lobe epilepsy is whether behavior disturbances occur more commonly in patients with temporal lobe epilepsy specifically or whether behavior disturbance is related to seizure disorders in general (Neppe and Tucker 1988b).

There are many confounding issues within this issue. For example, more complicated patients gravitate toward university hospitals where the studies are usually done. In Currie's hospital study in London (Currie et al. 1970), for example, 25% of the 2,664 patients seen in a university hospital clinic had a history of psychiatric hospitalization, whereas only 5%–9% of 678 patients in a private clinic in the same city had such a psychiatric hospitalization history. Also confounding is the fact that the age at onset of psychomotor epilepsy is similar to the age at onset of schizophrenia (Neppe 1981c). Moreover, three-quarters of patients with psychomotor or complex partial seizures are over age 16 at the onset of the seizure disorder; Stevens (1975) has discussed such epidemiological flaws in a cogent manner.

Furthermore, the vast majority of patients with seizure disorders have temporal lobe foci on EEG examination at some point during their illness (Pincus and Tucker 1985). Kristensen and Sindrup (1978) compared patients with complex partial seizures and psychosis to complex partial seizure patients without psychosis and could find little difference in the two groups with regard to age at onset, laterality of focus, and interval between epilepsy onset and time of examination. The patients with psychosis had significantly more neurological signs, spike EEGs, a history of brain damage, and no family history of seizure disorders, suggesting that these people may have had other associated organic brain syndromes (Pincus and Tucker 1985). Increased incidence of psychosocial problems in these groups may further confound the relationship to behavior disturbances (Neppe and Tucker 1988b).

Moreover, patients with complex partial seizures and secondary generalization are often more difficult to keep seizure free than those with generalized seizures. Consequently, they are often on high doses of anticonvulsants and/or anticonvulsant polytherapy. Their greater number of seizures and the frequent definite evidence of associated organic brain syndromes confound the relationship to behavior disturbance even further (Neppe and Tucker 1988b).

The incidence of psychoses associated with temporal lobe epilepsy (compared with non-temporal-lobe epilepsy) is usually noted as four to seven times greater, rarely only at twice as much (McKenna et al. 1985; Sengoku et al. 1983). The confounding variables include increased seizures, increased amount of anticonvulsants, and increased numbers of different types of seizures. Additionally, the temporal lobe constitutes 40% of the cerebral cortex anyway, and the age at onset for temporal lobe seizures somewhat resembles that for psychoses (Neppe 1986; Stevens 1988). These factors could variably be perceived as important causal, predisposing, or incidental features. However, patients with temporal lobe epilepsy have increased difficulties with seizure control and medication, and this may be related to the more primitive embryological structure of the archipallium (the relative degree of encephalization here is less than that in other areas of the brain). This primitive structure could predispose to psychopathology. Consequently the linkup is not only correlative, but indirectly causal as well.

Methodological Difficulties

Fundamental definitions. The epidemiological studies of seizures, the temporal lobe, and psychopathology have major difficulties and consequent methodological flaws. These have plagued the literature on epilepsy and psychosis. A major difficulty is fundamental definitions. In the epilepsy psychosis literature, psychosis has often been perceived in a far broader way, including clouded-consciousness patients with hallucinations (Bruens 1971). Psychosis in the context of epilepsy should best be limited to hallucinations, delusions, and thought disorder or other incoherence in clear or altered consciousness, but not defects of consciousness (Neppe 1986). Psychosis can still be diagnosed even when profound depersonalization or derealization with rare amnestic components exist, but not when there are profound, persistent amnesia states (Neppe and Tucker 1989).

Although epilepsy has been defined as a recurrent paroxysmal condition with biochemical and electrical discharges in the brain and association with alterations in consciousness, behavior, cognition, affect, and motoric functions, its clinical operational definition is more difficult. Psychiatric patients particularly are sometimes dubiously labelled as *epileptic* on the basis of previous psychiatric history: they may have histories of a single seizure; their seizures may have been associated with alcohol or other withdrawal; or they may be on anticonvulsant medication for "blackouts." Such cases are difficult to interpret. Operationally, the term *epileptic psychotic patients* should be limited to individuals with psychoses in clear or altered consciousness plus a confirmed history of epilepsy associated with at least two documented seizures not linked to withdrawal phenomena (Neppe and Tucker 1989).

Clinical evaluation. Because of the array of strange behavioral symptoms associated with seizure disorders, patients commonly present to the psychiatrist as opposed to the neurologist, and it is important for the physician to be able to distinguish seizure phenomena from the dissociative states and other conditions that the psychiatrist encounters. It is important that the patient be interviewed carefully for the exact nature of the subjective alterations. Usually these are repetitive and consistent in quality (Neppe and Tucker 1988b). There may be multiple perceptual and cognitive modalities that are involved, but these are usually simple and consistent in each specific patient. In other words the patient will hallucinate the same repetitive voice or have a particular nightmare or forced thought but will usually not have all the symptoms at one time (Tucker et al. 1986).

These phenomena often occur in clear consciousness. They are generally not complicated exotic experiences. A helpful aspect of diagnosis occurs if there is some alteration of state of consciousness, however, or if the automatisms typical of this condition occur. Often a history of amnesia is a clue. Unfortunately, dissociative disorders also produce amnesia. It is also important to note that some memory of the events may occur in patients with seizure disorders, particularly the auras of the experiences (i.e., the psychic kinds of experiences). At times the patient will experience some postictal depression or lethargy, wanting to sleep, developing a headache, and feeling perplexed (Tucker et al. 1986).

In a study using a phenomenological analysis (Neppe 1983d), the simple symptom of déjà vu—so commonly regarded as symptomatic of temporal lobe epilepsy—was demonstrated to have a very special phenomenological quality in patients with temporal lobe epilepsy. This involves its association with postictal features such as sleepiness, headache, and clouded consciousness and its link in time with these features. This association provides an excellent clue to the existence of temporal lobe epilepsy (Neppe 1981a). Déjà vu is a normal phenomenon occurring in 70% of the population and unless such phenomenological detail is obtained, patients' symptomatology may be misinterpreted (Neppe 1983c, 1983d). In a similar study with olfactory hallucinations (Neppe 1983a), a specific type of temporal lobe epilepsy olfactory hallucination could not be demonstrated although there were suggestive features.

A major message, therefore, may be the relevance of adequately assessing the symptomatology of patients presenting with epilepsy. It may be that this is a direction as relevant as EEG (Neppe and Tucker 1989).

Etiological Links of Seizures to Psychopathology

Eight major interconnected elements may be responsible for aberrant behavior in the epileptic patient (Neppe 1985a):

1. *Ictal or subictal firing.* In this instance the behavior reflects an actual epileptic effect. The most common example here would be the so-called psychomotor automatism in which the person is motorically producing deviant behavior as part of the seizure manifestation. In psychiatry this is relatively rare, but it achieves a preeminence in forensic neuropsychiatry.
2. *Medication effects.* Overmedication or incorrect medication may lead to side effects. Unfortunately, the anticonvulsants produce a variety of cognitive, perceptual, and behavioral side effects that may substantially modify the person's behavior, predisposing to a psychiatric presentation.
3. *Other cerebral abnormalities.* The epilepsy may be an epiphenomenon of a psycho-organic syndrome of some kind. The most common example would be mild mental retardation, which may be associated with diffuse organic brain pathology (possibly submicroscopic) and also

with a lowered seizure threshold (i.e., a predisposition to epilepsy). An alternative mechanism for other cerebral abnormalities is the induction of cerebral anoxia secondary to status epilepticus, which may cause organic brain damage. Recent work (Mattson et al. 1989) has suggested that generalized convulsive seizures (e.g., tonic-clonic) may induce microscopic changes in the hippocampal area of the mesial temporal lobe so that structural organic change may occur with seizures.

4. *Psychosocial aspects.* Environmental stressors commonly trigger disorganization, personality disintegration, or decompensation in the person with epilepsy. Moreover, usage of even small amounts of alcohol or substance abuse of any kind may precipitate loss of control of the epileptic condition or aggravate psychopathology. Alternatively, persons with epilepsy may not be coping because of the enormous difficulties they encounter in the community. Their condition is socially stigmatized, and severe limitations are imposed on them functionally and socially. From a psychological perspective they often feel inadequate or paranoid that people may find out about their seizures, and they withdraw into themselves, not having the confidence to interact in a socially appropriate manner.
5. *The site of the focus.* The area at which the firing of the partial seizure originates or through which it passes may or may not play a substantial role in psychopathology. A great body of literature has attempted to show the temporal lobe to be the source of behavioral disturbances (Neppe 1981c; Trimble 1983). Also disputed is the linkup of laterality with psychopathology. For example, dominant hemispheric lesions are sometimes linked to psychosis and personality disorder. Far less robust is the attempt to link nondominant hemispheric lesions to neurotic or affective manifestations.
6. *Predisposition.* Genetic, in utero, or other constitutional or later environmental experiences (e.g., encephalitis, hyperpyrexic convulsions, minor head injury, or drug abuse) may induce, precipitate, or predispose to psychiatric illness in the epileptic patient. All people have an underlying temperament that is molded by the environment to produce their personality, and such personality necessarily interacts with the bio-psycho-familial-socio-cultural world, be they epileptic or not. Epilepsy is a stressful form of this interaction, and psychopathology may be mobilized by such a stressor.
7. *Kindling-like phenomena.* As noted above, kindling is the pathophysiological process whereby repetitive subthreshold electrical or chemical stimuli to certain brain areas will eventually induce threshold responses (Neppe 1985a). These responses are classically in the form of seizures; however, it appears that they may manifest as abnormal behavior before the onset of the seizures (Stevens and Livermore 1978).
8. *As a complication.* Epilepsy may be associated with psychopathology because numerous psychiatric conditions may secondarily be associated with epilepsy (e.g., the Alzheimer's groups of dementias and the cerebral arteriopathies).

Time-Related Links: The Ictus and Psychopathology

Peri-ictal phenomena. Classically, the aberrant behavior in epilepsy is measured with regard to whether or not it is associated with the seizure phenomenon. When it appears to be directly linked to a particular seizure phenomenon the behavior is described as peri-ictal; when the phenomenon seems to be occurring between seizures, the behavior is considered interictal (Neppe 1985a). Unfortunately, all of this terminology is rather simplistic because many patients are unaware of whether or not they have had a seizure, and therefore phenomena that may, in fact, be peri-ictal are called interictal. Alternatively, epileptic patients with poor control of their illness who have a seizure and a day later develop behavioral aberrations may be called peri-ictal by one authority and interictal by a second. The ultimate determining factor is EEG monitoring, and when seizure phenomena are picked up on such monitoring, the manifestation can be described definitely as peri-ictal. Finally, peri-ictal manifestations can be subdivided into events occurring preictally, ictally, or postictally.

Preictal events. Preictal events immediately precede the seizure manifestation. These may have a prodrome quality or be an aura to the actual seizures. The epileptic prodrome is a phase before the onset of the actual seizure that may last several days and occasionally more than a week. It is characterized by changes in the individual's personality, behavior, or emotionality. Emotions such as mild irritability or poor concentration may be the most common but nonspecific manifestations. When such manifestations are of a profound nature (e.g., severe depression), it is theoretically worthwhile directly bringing on the seizure by a single controlled ECT (Post and Uhde 1986). In practice, such an indication is rare and should be carefully considered. Similarly, patients occasionally become thought disordered and overtly psychotic during their epileptic prodrome, which will cease when the seizure occurs.

In contrast the aura to the seizure is short. Patients may describe these as lasting up to half an hour, but usually they occur for periods of seconds before the seizure manifestation.

Ictal events. The ictal manifestation that most commonly presents psychiatrically is the psychomotor automatism. This may involve behavioral aberrations, and in the psychiatric presentation these may be complicated and have marked cognitive manifestations. Episodes of altered consciousness involving marked misinterpretations of reality, profound derealization, and depersonalization, as well as significant paranoid symptomatology, may occur.

Postictal events. Postictal manifestations are important in that there is commonly clouding of consciousness during this phase and patients may manifest a great deal of aggression, which is generally nonspecific and undirected and will occur only if the person is physically handled or their behavior is put under some kind of restraint (Rodin 1973). Occasionally psychotic manifestations occur during this phase with marked delusional and hallucinatory features. Because these hallucinatory features are very often visual and auditory in quality and are associated with a state of impaired consciousness, these patients are best regarded as in a state of "postictal delirium" and not as in a "postictal psychosis."

Postictal features are particularly relevant in differentiating true epileptic seizure phenomena from so-called hysterical seizures (i.e., nonepileptic seizures or pseudoseizures). Patients with hysterical seizures may very closely mimic a generalized seizure or at times appear to be having complex partial seizures but are unaware of the very common concomitants of headache, sleepiness, and clouded consciousness: the classical postictal triad of symptoms.

A recent but important advance has involved measuring blood prolactin levels to differentiate true epileptic seizures from nonepileptic seizures. If the serum prolactin is substantially elevated after a seizure, it is reasonable evidence that, in fact, the person has had an epileptic seizure. Unfortunately, however, a normal prolactin level may occasionally occur in the face of true epileptic seizures, particularly when the seizures were of the simple partial kind. Interpretation of a raised prolactin level is at times difficult and is best done by comparing the peak prolactin level—generally 20–30 minutes after the apparent seizure—with a prolactin level at the same time the following day and also with the prolactin level an hour after the "seizure." If the "seizure" has caused the elevated prolactin level, the 1-hour level should be less than the 30-minute level.

Interpretation is also further complicated in the psychiatric patient because other medications, such as neuroleptics, also elevate the prolactin level. Furthermore, at times results are equivocal where the prolactin elevation may be only slight. A useful rule is that the prolactin elevation should be above the upper limit of normal and should be at least double the level at the same time the following day. Also the prolactin should have fallen an hour after the apparent seizure phenomenon.

Seizures and Psychopathology: Classification

How important seizure disorders are for psychiatry is reflected by the behavior disorders they manifest. In their 1963 landmark article, "The Schizophrenia-like Psychoses of Epilepsy," Slater, Beard, and Glithero demonstrated that the basic symptoms associated with classical schizophrenic disorders are present in patients with seizure disorders. More recently, Perez and Trimble (1980), in a prospective study, and Toone et al. (1982), in a retrospective study, using the standardized Present State Examination (PSE; Wing et al. 1974) demonstrated that psychoses associated with temporal lobe seizure disorders are indistinguishable from schizophrenia. However, such studies analyze specifically positive and particularly Schneiderian symptoms of schizophrenia; the negative symptoms appear different (Neppe 1986).

Epilepsy and psychiatry have distanced themselves partly as a consequence of the inadequacy of current attempts to classify psychopathology in epileptic patients.

Bruens classification. An early classification of psychosis in seizure disorders was that of Bruens (1971) who classified the psychoses into those associated with clouding. The problem with such a conceptualization is that so-called psychoses occurring in clouded consciousness are generally delirium with agitation, delusions, hallucinations, and misinterpretations of reality (Neppe and Tucker 1989). Psychoses occurring in clear consciousness would, on the surface, therefore constitute all the psychoses associated with epilepsy (Neppe and Tucker 1989). However, there are patients who present with profound states of depersonalization, derealization, and misinterpretations of reality and who may have partial amnesia for these episodes and yet appear to be in an altered state of consciousness more than in a clouded state. Because these patients would still be classified as *psychotic*, the delineation is difficult.

Trimble classification. A further attempt at classification was that of Trimble (1985) who emphasized not only level of consciousness but EEG changes and whether or not the events were occurring at a peri-ictal or an interictal level. He grouped the acute "episodic" psychoses as the peri-ictal events and the more chronic psychoses as interictal events. Trimble's classification, therefore, involved a listing of the kinds of psychotic phenomena that occur in the person with epilepsy.

The Tiered Axes for Psychopathology and Epilepsy (TAPE) classification. Using Trimble's approach, we went one step further and applied psychopathology in the epileptic patient along a multiaxial framework with the Neppe Multiaxial Epilepsy Schema (Neppe and Tucker 1988b). This bears some similarity to the DSM-III (American Psychiatric Association 1980) multiaxis approach and has, in fact, been modelled on such approaches. Table 17–5 reflects new updated ideas on this classification, which we now call the Tiered Axes for Psychopathology and Epilepsy (TAPE) (Neppe 1981c, 1986; Neppe and Tucker 1989).

The Axes I through V of the psychopathology tier are amplifications of current DSM-III-R terminology. Axes I and II include descriptive diagnoses as well. A descriptive psychopathological diagnosis, for example, on Axis I may be paranoid hallucinatory psychosis or monodelusional psychosis; this framework can be extended to any form of psychopathology. Axis II relates to personality disorder and developmental problems and in this instance includes personality features. On Axis III of the Psychiatric Tier, we include the symptomatic etiology of the psychopathology (anticipating DSM-IV). We emphasize the importance of Axis IV: the psychosocial stressors predisposing, precipitating, and perpetuating the illness. Under Axis V, we include four levels of DSM-III-R's Global Assessments of Functioning scale: current, the highest in the past year, during the current illness, and expected functioning on recovery. Axis V, therefore, analyzes the level of functionality cross-sectionally. Diagnoses in epileptic patients with psychoses are special enough to require non-DSM-III terminology.

The second tier of the TAPE is the epilepsy tier. On Axis I of this tier, we suggest a listing of the kind of seizure type and epileptic syndrome, if present, as well as extent of control of each seizure type. Axis II lists intelligence and includes mental retardation, an important condition in the "epilepsy plus" patient. Axis III discusses the organic aspects, particularly associated organic brain syndromes and factors predisposing to the epilepsy and complicating the seizure disorder. We emphasize the importance of Axis IV—the core investigations clarifying the diagnosis—namely EEGs, and neuroradiological and nuclear medicine scans, as well as cerebral cortical tests and neuropsychological testing. Axis V analyzes level of functionality based on longitudinal history evaluating deterioration or maintenance of a steady level of functioning.

After attempting unsuccessfully to achieve this with the conventional five axes, we suggest two more axes. Axis VI is the pharmacological response, and Axis VII is the age at onset. These two new axes exist not only on the psychopathology tier, which on Axes I–V closely reflects the DSM-III-R framework, but also on the corresponding epilepsy tier. Axis VI—pharmacological response—can and probably should be applied to any psychopathology. Factors such as compliance, response, blood and other levels, and duration and frequency of all psychotropics, anticonvulsants, and other nonneuropsychiatric medications should be recorded so that pharmacokinetic and dynamic factors are considered. Age at onset of both seizures and the major psychiatric conditions (such as psychotic features) is an important epidemiological consideration for these conditions.

We believe the TAPE classification should be applied as a basic for all patients with seizures and psychopathology. It would unify diagnostic and research frameworks in this area and allow an added appreciation of the similarities and differences between the many conditions that manifest with seizures and psychopathology. The classification can

TABLE 17–5. TIERED AXES FOR PSYCHOPATHOLOGY AND EPILEPSY (TAPE)

Axis	
Psychopathology tier	
I	Psychiatric diagnosis (DSM-III-R; American Psychiatric Association 1987) Descriptive psychopathology diagnosis Severity of episode (mild, moderate, or severe)
II	Personality or developmental disorder (DSM-III-R) Personality description
III	Physical disorders (DSM-III-R) (related or unrelated) Symptomatic etiology of psychopathology
IV	Psychosocial stressors (DSM-III-R)
V	Global assessment of functioning (current, past year, during illness, and expected on recovery)
VI	Pharmacological response of psychopathology Pharmacological compliance Neuroleptic dose, levels and response, duration of treatment, and frequency of dosing Other treatments or medications responsiveness Duration of treatment for each drug Combinations and frequency of dosing
VII	Age at onset of current psychopathology (e.g., psychosis)
Epilepsy tier	
I	Seizure classification Epilepsy syndrome Extent of seizure control (complete, occasional, moderate, or poor)
II	Intelligence (normal or borderline, mild, or moderate mental retardation)
III	Time link of psychopathology and seizures (peri-ictal, interictal, nonictal, or unclear)
IV	Electroencephalographic (EEG) localization EEG seizure features Neuroradiological or nuclear medicine or other brain tests
V	Course (deteriorating or nondeteriorating) Chronicity (single episode, episodic, or chronic)
VI	Pharmacological response of seizures Pharmacological compliance with antiseizure medication Anticonvulsant doses and frequency of dosing and levels Duration of treatment for each drug
VII	Age at onset of seizures

also easily be modified for use in any organic condition or pseudoseizures.

At this point, however, there is no other comparative gold standard by which the utility of such a classification can be assessed. Applying the TAPE involves several elements or attempts to clarify questions such as analyses of the occurrence of psychopathology in the context of whether it is periictal or interictal or whether the relationship to the ictus is not clear. The TAPE correlates certain epilepsy features with the psychiatric disorder, prompting certain questions: Is the psychiatric disorder of the organic kind? Are there major psychosocial elements to it? Is it a direct manifestation of the seizure disorder? Could the site of the lesion be hypothesized to be important? Could kindling be playing some kind of role? Are the anticonvulsants or other medications the patient is taking relevant in this instance?

The TAPE classification also emphasizes looking in detail at the patient's mental status at specific points in time and, particularly when the condition is episodic, the mental status during previous episodes. In the same way, longitudinal historical bases are all important. Using this framework, alternative multiaxial evaluation schemata can also be developed.

Kinds of Epileptic Psychoses

Empirically it appears that there are several different kinds of psychoses associated with epilepsy (Table 17–6) (Neppe 1986; Neppe and Tucker 1989).

TABLE 17–6. EXAMPLES OF "EPILEPTIC PSYCHOSES"

Interictal, clear consciousness psychoses

1. Mild mental retardation, secondary generalized epilepsy, and unfixed unsystematized delusions
2. Temporal lobe epilepsy with paranoid-hallucinatory psychosis
3. Manic-like episodic interictal psychosis
4. Postsurgical (temporal lobe) psychosis
5. Nonorganic "epileptic psychosis"

Peri-ictal psychoses

6. Complex partial seizure and status epilepticus
7. Preictal psychosis
8. Peri-ictal psychosis without clouding but with delusional syndrome
9. Postictal delirium (not in our definition)
10. Psychotic episode (with clear consciousness) after a seizure (? postictal or ? early interictal)

One common kind involves the patient with mild developmental delay who has an underlying brain injury associated with generalized tonic-clonic seizures, diffuse electroencephalographic change (what used to be called *secondary generalized epilepsy*), and a psychosis characterized by a fluctuating, unsystematized delusional system. These patients do not tolerate high doses of neuroleptics and generally the prognosis is poor (Neppe 1986; Neppe and Tucker 1989).

The second group is possibly the most common: the chronic, paranoid hallucinatory psychoses described by many—recently by Diehl (1989). These patients have paranoid persecutory and sometimes a grandiose delusional schema that are relatively systematized, and they require high doses of neuroleptic medication in addition to the anticonvulsant. It is possible that the anatomic site of the lesion, for example, dominant temporal hemisphere or bilateral damage, may be important. This group may, in fact, turn out to be dichotomous: one group having organic disorders, the other nonorganic disorders. Generally, the psychoses are perceived as interictal, but only because they most commonly occur between seizures, not because they may have a special reciprocal relationship to the peri-ictal phenomena.

A similar, related group are patients with episodic manic-like psychoses and epilepsy. Using the same kind of hypothesis, such patients may in fact have nondominant temporal hemisphere damage. However, this is completely unproven. We have called these the *maniform episodic interictal psychoses.*

A fourth, rare group is also associated with prior temporal lobe epilepsy. These are those patients who become psychotic after surgical resection of part of the temporal lobe. Again, an organic etiology is hypothesized that may not necessarily relate to the surgery and these patients occasionally develop very intractable hallucinatory conditions that do not respond to neuroleptics, rather like the leukotomized patients of old (Neppe 1986; Neppe and Tucker 1989).

A fifth group includes the paranoid psychotic patients who appear to have no brain dysfunction of any kind but respond to environmental stressors by developing episodes of brief reactive psychosis. These patients require several dynamic interventions, respond reasonably to neuroleptics, and may have a substantial amount of affect (Neppe and Tucker 1988a).

The next group involves patients who appear to be psychotic but who actually have complex partial seizure manifestations with some defect in consciousness and some amnesia for the episode. Such patients may have profound states of derealization, depersonalization, and apparent delusional misinterpretations of reality. This rare group is managed with high doses of anticonvulsants as the predominant therapy, with no or little neuroleptic (Neppe 1986; Neppe and Tucker 1989). These patients include those in partial status epilepticus.

A difficult group are those who present preictally with profound changes in insight and reality testing and often have marked affective alteration, sometimes a profound depression, and at other times elevations of mood with or without delusional features. These patients may, occasionally, require ECT to induce a seizure as part of their therapy but in general are treated symptomatically (Neppe 1986; Neppe and Tucker 1989).

A difficult to categorize group are those patients who appear to be having episodes of psychoses at the time of the ictus implying that they are "peri-ictal psychoses." This group does not have clouding of consciousness but has an overt delusional syndrome. Such patients are particularly difficult to categorize as to whether they have actual partial seizure phenomena (without consciousness implying simple partial seizures) or postictal phenomena. It is difficult to prove that such an entity actually exists because such psychoses can at times be argued to be unrelated to the ictal events that had occurred coincidentally (Neppe and Tucker 1988a).

The ninth group are those with "postictal psychotic phenomena." It is patients in this group who most commonly are clouded in consciousness and are better considered as having "delirium."

Occasionally, a tenth group occurs with psychosis in clear consciousness presenting after a seizure. The differentiation between these psychotic patients in clear consciousness and an early interictal psychosis is unclear, and there are often other reactive organic elements to this (Wilensky and Neppe 1986).

The ten kinds of psychoses linked to epilepsy can be classified using the Trimble, Bruens, and Neppe systems. However, Bruens' system has the least application because it defines epilepsy with psychosis in the context of absence of clouding of consciousness (thus excluding the ninth group above). Trimble's classification has substantial application; however, difficulties relate to interpretations of both episodic and chronic forms and links to the ictus. The TAPE classification potentially has broader application because of its diminished focus on just the Axis I presentation and the greater emphasis on personality, organic, psychosocial, and functionality frameworks (Neppe and Tucker 1988a).

Moreover, it is extremely difficult to place these ten kinds (and there may be more) of epileptic psychosis in the context of those psychoses that are antagonistic to seizures and those that more commonly occur with seizures. Such a study would require a substantial epidemiological survey in which like conditions were compared with like conditions as opposed to the global single basket kind of approach that has been used in previous epidemiological research (Neppe and Tucker 1988a).

Consequently, the TAPE classification takes into account not only a multiaxial framework but also responses to appropriate pharmacological and other interventions (Neppe 1986; Neppe and Tucker 1989). It is emphasized, however, that none of the classifications (Bruens, Trimble, or the TAPE classification) have been used extensively.

Special Conditions

Depression and seizures. Despite the claims that the incidence of depression is higher among persons with epilepsy than in the general population and, moreover, that patients with complex partial seizures are particularly predisposed to depression, especially if this involves nondominant hemisphere lesions, there is currently little empirical support for such assertions (Stevens 1988). Recent doctoral work by Robertson (see Robertson et al. 1987) has clarified the area somewhat: of 66 patients with epilepsy and depression who were studied, 34 had a family history of psychiatric illness, with depression being the most common condition. The depression generally was moderate and was endogenous-melancholic in approximately two-fifths of the patients. Attendant features were high state and trait anxiety and hostility. The EEGs of the patients and a control group were not significantly different. Patients receiving phenobarbital were more depressed compared with those on carbamazepine. The phenomenology of the depression was not clearly influenced by epilepsy variables. Depression in patients with epilepsy represents the outcome of multiple factors in genetically predisposed individuals (Robertson et al. 1987).

Personality profiles. The consistency of the behavioral symptoms are particularly relevant in the light of modern attempts at developing personality profiles in patients with temporal lobe disorders. For example, Waxman and Geschwind (1975) reported a specific interictal syndrome associated with temporal lobe disorders that consists of hypergraphia, hyposexual activity, and a preoccupation with philosophical and moral concerns. This work was continued in a well-known study by Bear and Fedio (see Bear 1986; Bear et al. 1982), who analyzed the above symptoms and 14 other behavior traits. Their 18-point personality inventory is hypothesized to characterize persons with temporal lobe epilepsy but markedly influenced by intellectual factors and, to some extent, by gender and anticonvulsant drug levels, especially those of carbamazepine. The test in its current form measures overall psychopathology rather than a specific syndrome (Rodin and Schmaltz 1984).

Hermann and Riel (1981) found that four traits (sense of personal destiny, dependence, paranoia, and philosophical interest) were significantly elevated in a temporal lobe epilepsy group. Specific laterality aspects have been hypothesized: left-sided lesion patients showed a paranoid and depressed personality, were guilt-ridden and aggressive, and gave a negative image of themselves, whereas right-sided lesion patients rated themselves in a positive way (Perini 1986). Several studies have been done that do not confirm the original findings of an increased incidence of pathological, behavioral, or personality traits in any of the temporal lobe, left-sided, or even epileptic patients (Mungus 1982; Rodin and Schmaltz 1984). This is true even with specific behavioral symptoms like hyperreligiosity (Tucker et al. 1987).

Some studies have argued against syndrome specificity, showing that traits were also present in the other populations (Stark-Adamec et al. 1985) or that there may be hemisphere differences in control groups (e.g., left-hemisphericity types had greater control over their impulses, were more trusting and imaginative, and viewed themselves in a positive light, whereas right-hemisphericity types were more tense, suspicious, shy, and pragmatic [Vingiano 1989]). As is true of many statistical studies on large populations, many symptoms may occur in any one specific kind of patient, distorting population studies. For example, in a Caucasian African population, hypergraphia was not commonly found among persons with temporal lobe epilepsy, suggesting that it may be culturally and not organically related (Neppe and Tucker 1988b).

It is important to emphasize that the most common sexual abnormality in temporal lobe epilepsy appears to be hyposexuality and that the relationship of altered sexuality in temporal lobe epilepsy is a particularly controversial one (Blumer 1975). Alternatively, Roberts and Guberman (1989) reported a remarkable proportion (involving about half the patients they identified) of religious conversions in their epileptic study population. Many psychiatrists who have seen a large number of such patients argue that a specific personality profile has yet to be identified and point out how many of the apparent traits are actually opposites (Stevens 1983, 1988). However, this does not imply that such traits may not occur with increased prevalence or may not reflect nonspecific personality changes in certain subpopulations of patients with temporal lobe epilepsy (Neppe and Tucker 1988b). Certain other subpopulations (e.g., suicidal epileptic patients) may have a higher prevalence of personality disorders (Mendez et al. 1989).

Psychoses. We now discuss the common aspects of seizure disorders and psychoses, as well as the antagonistic features. This leads us to a broader framework of looking at epilepsy in relation to psychopathology and an attempted classification of psychopathology in epilepsy. We then discuss the management of behavior disturbances in epilepsy-related (possibly) seizure disorders (Neppe and Tucker 1988a).

Many empirical similarities exist between seizure disorders and schizophrenia. Schizophrenia and seizure disorders are both hard to define simply; the genetic frequencies are similar for both conditions, with somewhere between 10% and 13% of the offspring of the parents with these conditions having the condition (Metrakos and Metrakos 1961). They are also both basically clinical diagnoses presenting primarily as behavioral disturbances, and there are generally no pathological changes evident in either of these conditions. Furthermore, the peak age at onset is similar with both being disorders of early to late adolescence, although epilepsy often presents in childhood and may present at any age (Neppe and Tucker 1988a). The neurotransmitter dopamine is somehow related in both conditions as dopamine antagonists are antipsychotic and mildly epileptogenic, and dopamine agonists are psychotogenic and mildly antiepileptic (Trimble 1977). Perhaps most significantly, both conditions need a team to rehabilitate patients.

Despite more than 100 publications in the scientific literature dealing with core issues of epilepsy in relation to psychosis, the area remains particularly poorly explored and ill defined (McKenna et al. 1985). Researchers such as Slater (1963), Krohn (1961), Gudmundsson (1966), Gibbs (1951), Ey (1954), Betts (1974), and Lindsay et al. (1979) have argued for an increased affinity of the two conditions. These diverse studies came from several different countries and range from national surveys of unselected populations to studies of patients in outpatient clinics, as well as mental hospital populations. The most well-known of these studies is the epic study of the Slater-Beard group in London (Slater 1963). A second important study is that of Gudmundsson (1966) because it involved the whole population of Iceland. Such studies suggest that the incidence of psychosis in relation to epilepsy is of an increased rate from 4% (Trimble 1977) through 27% (average about 7%) (Dongier 1959–1960).

The antagonist theory of epilepsy and psychosis is interesting in the face of these apparent increased epidemiological links of the psychoses to epilepsy. The most interesting historical association was the link-up of Muller (see Pincus and Tucker 1985), who noted that psychotic patients who have had seizures often spontaneously improved. This led Von Meduna to initiate convulsive therapy (at that time chemical convulsive therapy) in the treatment of schizophrenia (Fink 1984; Von Meduna 1937). These patients improved substantially after induction of these chemical seizures. ECT with its increasingly sophisticated changes over the decades has replaced chemical seizures (Neppe and Tucker 1988a).

Another important observation was made by Landolt (1958). He described his so-called forced normalization (or drive-in) phenomenon: when the psychosis occurs ("drives in") the epileptic seizures are not predominant, and when epileptic seizures occur in clusters the patient is not psychotic. He noted this inverse relationship, and others noted that this seems to apply particularly to the acute psychoses (Slater 1963). However, only about one-third of such acute psychoses and possibly even fewer chronic psychoses have any inverse relationship with the ictus, and there are a substantial number of patients whose psychoses terminate or are differently linked to major seizure manifestations (Trimble 1985).

❑ PSYCHOPATHOLOGY IN THE NONEPILEPTIC PATIENT

Possibly Related Seizure Disorders

An interesting area of speculation involves the concept of so-called atypical psychosis. Clinicians have often noted that the distinctions made by classification systems often are more distinct in theory than in practice. Consequently, although there are clear cases that few would quibble over as being schizophrenic and similarly cases few would quibble over as being affective disordered, there is a group of patients that we tend to call *schizoaffective* and a further group of atypical psychoses that occupy a middle ground. In an excellent review, Procci (1976) noted that these cases usually have an acute onset, remissions, good premorbid functioning, Bleulerian symptoms of schizophrenia, and affective symptoms, as well as confusion and agitation. Mitsuda (1967) also described a group of atypical psychotic patients while doing a large genetic study of schizophrenia and affective disorder. This may reflect the possibility of another kind of disorder linked with seizures. The schizophrenic patients had few children with atypical psychosis, the manic-depressive patients had a rare occurrence of atypical psychosis in their children, and the atypical psychotic patients seemed to produce exclusively children with atypical psychosis, but with no schizophrenia. Mitsuda also noted that patients with atypical psychosis seem to have marked disturbance in their EEGs and that the incidence of epilepsy was higher among them than among the manic-depressive patients or the schizophrenic patients (Neppe and Tucker 1988a).

Monroe (1982) extended this concept by delineating a group he called "episodic psychotics," and he related this to a limbic ictal disorder that was unresponsive to TCAs and neuroleptics. He noted that these patients also had a psychosis of precipitous onset, intense affects, and intermittent course with symptom-free intervals. As an extension of these studies, Tucker et al. (1986) described a series of patients who had documented temporal lobe dysfunction on EEG and symptomatology very similar to the group described by Procci (1976) and the episodic psychosis described by Monroe (1982). All of the patients described spell-type episodes. They also experienced marked mood lability, often with suicidal ideation and suicide attempts, as well as psychotic phenomena and cognitive changes. All patients returned to normal baseline with symptom-free intervals. It is extremely important that many of these conditions occur in a state of clear consciousness and do not necessarily present themselves with either a clouding of consciousness or symptoms of disorientation (Neppe and Tucker 1988a).

Such studies of patients with possible temporolimbic dysfunction have been continued from other sources (Wells and Duneau 1980), including chronic nonepileptic psychiatric patients with EEG temporal lobe foci (Neppe 1983b), violent refractory schizophrenic patients (Hakola and Laulumaa 1982), patients with borderline personality disorder (Gardner and Cowdry 1986), and patients who become dysphoric on neuroleptics and have abnormal EEGs (Brodsky et al. 1983), suggesting the extended use of anticonvulsant medication, particularly carbamazepine, in such a population (Neppe 1984). Carbamazepine particularly should not be seen as a panacea. When it is used inappropriately some patients appear to deteriorate, and response to anticonvulsants does not imply seizure disorder (Neppe and Tucker 1988a).

Spells

In psychiatry particularly, patients at times have episodes that are extremely difficult to interpret.

These episodes may be very short-lived, lasting seconds or minutes, but on occasion can last for days. Such patients behave out of character and usually exhibit a lability of affect that is profound, with disturbances ranging from depression through mania. They may appear markedly thought disordered, deluded, or hallucinated, and very often these episodes are repetitive and of the same quality each time. These patients may exhibit behavioral alterations perceived as characterological disorders. We have called such episodes *spells* to obviate debate as to whether they are truly ictal (Neppe and Kaplan 1988; Tucker et al. 1986).

In such episodes, EEGs may not reveal any additional information, or these patients may have temporal lobe spikes or at least slowing in the temporal lobe. Such episodes have been labelled *temporal lobe epilepsy* or *atypical complex partial seizures*. The neurologist epileptologists have justifiably debated whether these are "real" seizures. These patients may respond to anticonvulsant medication, and trials of anticonvulsants are needed. In our experience many of these patients respond well to carbamazepine (Tegretol particularly), phenytoin (Dilantin), or valproate (Depakene-Depakote). This may or may not imply that these patients have seizurelike episodes. It is possible that these patients may occasionally respond to short courses of anticonvulsant therapy and not require permanent treatment (Neppe and Kaplan 1988). This is a major transition area between psychiatry and neurology. Table 17–7 outlines our classification for epileptic patients with behavioral abnormality (Blumer et al. 1990).

TABLE 17–7. NEUROBEHAVIORAL DISORDERS OF EPILEPSY

1. Mood disorder (dysphoric, euphoric, rapid cycling, and mixed)
2. Irritable-impulsive disorder
3. Schizophreniform disorder (paranoid, delusional, and hallucinatory)
4. Anxiety disorder (panic, phobic, and generalized)
5. Amnestic-confusional disorder
6. Somatoform disorder (pseudoseizures and pain)
7. Personality disorder (viscous, hyperemotional, and hypersexual)
8. Compound (more than two of the preceding categories)
9. Not otherwise specified

Source. Blumer et al. 1990.

Etiology of Behavioral Symptoms

Behavioral changes in patients with temporal lobe dysfunction have been disputed to be more frequent than in patients with generalized seizure disorders. Alterations of limbic function in animals and in humans are associated with a significant amount of behavioral disturbance. Whether the temporal lobe or limbic system itself is looked at as a way station or as the actual seat of origin of the behavior change is debatable. Whether this is etiologically relevent in seizure disorder also remains in question (Adamec and Stark 1983).

Initially there was concern that the behavior changes of seizure disorders were associated with folate deficiencies due to the interaction with phenytoin, phenobarbital, and other anticonvulsants. However, Reynolds (1967) showed that the psychotic manifestations and behavioral disturbances were equally present in patients with folate deficiencies as in those without such deficiencies. Perhaps the most consistent hypothesis postulates a form of subictal discharges, particularly in the temporal lobe, that leads to behavioral changes. Although there is contradictory evidence, clinically (as described above) there is an inverse relationship at times between the occurrence of seizures and the appearance of psychosis. This has led to hypotheses pertaining to inverse relationships of neurotransmitters as well, such as Trimble's "dopamine bridge" (1977); dopamine antagonists are antipsychotic and mildly epileptogenic, whereas dopamine agonists are mildly antiepileptic and psychotogenic.

The etiology of behavioral features has become more interesting of late with nine studies suggesting that patients with dominant temporal lobe epilepsy have an increased chance of psychotic-type reactions compared with patients with foci in the nondominant hemisphere (see Trimble 1985). However, in our opinion, such results are premature and possibly flawed (Neppe and Tucker 1989).

❑ TREATMENT

Management of Epilepsy With Behavior Disturbance

The management of epileptic patients presenting with behavior disturbance is closely linked to the discussion of epilepsy in relation to psychopathology. The heterogeneity of such conditions implies a heterogeneity of management that is patient based and individually tailored (Neppe and Tucker 1988a).

The single most important principle is anticonvulsant monotherapy. It has been well demonstrated that the degree of seizure control is not increased by increasing the number of anticonvulsant medications (Neppe 1985c). It is more important to achieve adequate anticonvulsant dosage, and therapeutic ranges on blood levels are often helpful indicators. However, the object should be to adequately control all the patient's seizures, and the choice of anticonvulsant is equally important (Table 17–8) (Neppe 1985a, 1985c).

Essential Clinical Pharmacology of Anticonvulsants

Anticonvulsants may induce change in the psychiatric patient by both pharmacokinetic and pharmacodynamic interactions with other medications.

Pharmacokinetic interactions. Anticonvulsant administration is particularly important and particularly difficult by virtue of enzyme induction occurring in the liver. This enzyme induction tends to affect predominantly the P_{450} cytochrome enzyme system in the liver. This implies that both anticonvulsant metabolism—particularly carbamazepine—and the metabolism of other lipid-soluble compounds are accelerated (Neppe et al. 1988).

Three major anticonvulsants, namely phenobarbital, phenytoin, and carbamazepine (in that order), are potent enzyme-inducing agents in the liver. Once induction occurs, theoretically, there should be lowered blood levels and bioavailability of almost all psychotropic agents. This is so as their lipid-solubility implies passage into the brain, but also implies similar hepatic metabolism; in practice however, because of the limited availability of many psychotropic blood levels, we are uncertain. Table 17–9 indicates what is known about some interactions (Bertilsson 1978; Birkhimer et al. 1985; Bramhall and Levine 1988; Dorn 1986; Jann et al. 1985; Kidron et al. 1985; Shukla et al. 1984; Zimmerman 1986).

Blood levels for many of the neuroleptics are difficult to interpret. Lowering of the serum level after treatment with anticonvulsants has been demonstrated with haloperidol (Jann et al. 1985; Kidron et al. 1985).

Pharmacodynamics and indirect effects. Pharmacodynamic interactions are even more complex and difficult. Interactions at receptors in the brain may produce modulatory effects at, for example, dopaminergic, serotonergic, and γ-aminobutyric acid (GABA)-ergic levels.

Phenobarbital. Phenobarbital is the most potent of the enzyme inducers, and when used in combination, other anticonvulsants' levels are very commonly reduced because of the extensive enzyme

TABLE 17–8. CHOICE OF ANTICONVULSANT

Type of seizure	*First choice*	*Alternatives*
	Oral	
Typical absences (petit mal [PM])	Ethosuximide	Valproate Clonazepam
Generalized tonic-clonic (GTC) seizures	Carbamazepine	Phenytoin Valproate
Partial seizures	Carbamazepine	Phenytoin Primidone
PM and GTC seizures	Valproate Carbamazepine	Carbamazepine plus ethosuximide
Atypical absences	Carbamazepine	Phenytoin Phenytoin Primidone
Myoclonus (MC)	Valproate	Clonazepam
Psychiatric overlay (not PM or MC)	Carbamazepine	Clonazepam
	Intravenous	
Status epilepticus	Diazepam Clonazepam	Phenytoin

TABLE 17–9. KNOWN INTERACTIONS BETWEEN CARBAMAZEPINE AND OTHER DRUGS[a]

Increased carbamazepine levels in patients taking both	**Carbamazepine causes**
Isoniazid	Pregnancy test failure
Valproic acid (increased free carbamazepine in vitro)	Escape from dexamethasone suppression
Carbamazepine epoxide only	Oral contraceptive failure
Troleandomycin	
Propoxyphene	**Carbamazepine decreases the effects of**
Erythromycin	Vitamin D, calcium, and folate; causes possible hyponatremia
Nicotinamide	
Cimetidine	Clonazepam
Viloxazine	Dicumarol
	Doxycycline
Decreased carbamazepine levels in patients taking both	Phenytoin
Phenobarbital	Sodium valproate
Phenytoin	Theophylline
Primidone and phenobarbital	Ethosuximide
Carbamazepine itself (autoinduction)	Haloperidol
Alcohol (chronic use)	Isoniazid
Cigarettes	

[a]Because enzyme induction is the mechanism in most of these interactions, one can hypothesize similar effects with phenytoin, phenobarbital, and primidone.

induction. In addition, phenobarbital causes psychological depression, has the potential for addiction (although this is generally low among patients receiving phenobarbital for seizures), and is potentially lethal in overdose. Indeed it was the major cause of death by overdose during the 1950s. It also produces a cognitive impairment, which may explain the rigidity of personality that was at times seen with patients with seizure disorders on phenobarbital.

We see little role for barbiturates in the management of seizure disorders today; their only place may be for patients who are already taking them and do not have any side effects. In our experience most patients have side effects such as central nervous system depression, psychological depression, or cognitive impairments of one kind or another. It is extremely difficult to taper patients off the barbiturates without them having an epileptic seizure whether or not the taper is given by using high loading doses of other anticonvulsants and even when the taper occurs over many months. It is the last few milligrams, the last 50 or even 25 mg of phenobarbital, that are particularly difficult to taper without seizures.

Phenytoin. Although not as problematic as the nearly anachronistic drug phenobarbital, diphenylhydantoin sodium (or phenytoin) is now less popular than it was and has limited use in the neuropsychiatric patient despite being an outstanding anticonvulsant to control generalized tonic-clonic and some partial seizures. Its problem, like phenobarbital, is its side-effect profile (Neppe 1985a, 1985c; Neppe et al. 1991). Mild cognitive impairment occurs, particularly in higher doses. Because phenytoin has a small therapeutic range, patients can easily become drug toxic, and (ironically) one of the side effects of significant toxicity is seizures. Additionally, it can make petit mal seizures worse. Gum hyperplasia is a particular problem with chronic use of phenytoin, producing an appearance that can at times be unsightly (Trimble 1979, 1988). Phenytoin is a potent enzyme inducer but weaker than phenobarbital.

Carbamazepine. The trend in psychiatry has been increasing use of carbamazepine rather than phenytoin, because it is safer, has apparent psychotropic properties, and has proven value in several conditions. Carbamazepine is particularly relevant in the psychiatric context because it appears to include less cognitive, motoric, and affective dysfunction than some of the older anticonvulsants such as phenytoin, phenobarbital, and primidone (Trimble 1979). It is as effective as phenytoin in both generalized tonic-clonic seizures and partial seizures and thus is the drug of choice for such conditions. It is ineffective in petit mal absences where sodium valproate or ethosuximide is generally used.

Carbamazepine, however, also appears to have a substantial psychotropic effect (Neppe 1985c; Trimble 1979). This psychotropic effect may or may not relate to its anticonvulsant structure because it is also structurally similar to both TCAs and phenothiazines (Gagneux 1975).

Carbamazepine therapy has become extremely topical in neuropsychiatry (Neppe 1988). It is particularly frequently used in the management of manic illness and in the prophylaxis of bipolar illness, particularly when lithium cannot be used or is ineffective. A possible further role for carbamazepine is its use in treating nonresponsive psychotic patients or atypical psychotic patients with any EEG temporal lobe abnormalities, with episodic hostility, or with affective lability. Our research in this direction has been extremely promising and has included one double-blind study (Neppe 1983b; Neppe et al. 1991). It appears that this may become a prime indication for carbamazepine in the future. Therapeutic ranges have not been established for anticonvulsants in nonepileptic patients. Only one double-blind study (Neppe 1990b) used fixed-dosed carbamazepine in patients with chronic psychoses who were on adjunct neuroleptics; a therapeutic range in the low anticonvulsant range for seizures, namely 6–9 µg/mole, was suggested. Ranges could also vary with different psychiatric conditions.

Carbamazepine and the other anticonvulsants involved in enzyme induction produce important metabolic and endocrine effects. Patients on oral contraceptives may have their steroid level lowered, with the consequence that they may become pregnant. In addition, by virtue of the lipid solubility of cholecalciferol and consequently increased rate of metabolism, patients may become vitamin D deficient, particularly in cold winter climates. Consequently, alterations in calcium metabolism with mild hypocalcemia might result. Furthermore, by virtue of the enzyme induction, folic acid (as a coenzyme vitamin in hepatic enzyme pathways) may be depleted, with the consequence that patients may require small folic acid supplementation, rather like that occurring in pregnancy (Neppe et al. 1988). Probably 5 mg per day or even per week is sufficient. Finally, there is commonly a slight elevation in hepatic enzyme levels such as γ-glutamyl transferase: this does not imply that these drugs should be stopped.

The rate of onset of the induction process has not been well studied. In our research it appears to be somewhere between 24 and 72 hours for carbamazepine (Neppe and Friel 1987), implying that in that early phase, in fact, patients on neuroleptics placed onto carbamazepine may well have more side effects as a consequence of raised levels and competition at an enzyme system level (Neppe 1990b).

Conversely, the levels of all the anticonvulsants are theoretically raised by psychotropics because of competition at a hepatic level. Consequently, the anticonvulsant doses necessary for monotherapy are lower when given in conjunction with psychotropic agents, partly because of competition and partly because the additive pharmacodynamic effects produce sedation. Most carbamazepine tests interact with thiothixene. Consequently, haloperidol remains the sole neuroleptic to have had this phenomenon empirically tested (Jann et al. 1985; Kidron et al. 1985). There are also surprisingly few studies with TCAs.

In addition to the phenomenon of induction of hepatic enzymes, a second phenomenon of deinduction of hepatic enzyme systems also occurs (Neppe 1990b). We have recently described this in the context of carbamazepine (Neppe 1990b). It is probable that patients going off anticonvulsant medication will experience a reverse process, whereby the liver enzymes will be slowed down, with the consequence that there may be accumulation of higher amounts of psychotropic agent.

These effects imply particular care in medicating patients with or without seizure disorders with anticonvulsants. For example, many of the early studies with carbamazepine suggested a starting dose of 200 mg tid because these patients already had induced enzyme systems from phenytoin and phenobarbital, the two major anticonvulsants that induce enzyme systems. However, in naive subjects, it is better to start off with 100 mg tid or even 200 mg daily because at that stage the long half-life of carbamazepine is generally somewhere between 18 and 70 hours.

In practice, within a week patients require carbamazepine three times a day. Patients receiving the carbamazepine as a once-a-day dose or as a loaded dose at night with a small dose in the morning may therefore not respond in bipolar affective illness. Eighty percent of patients require dosing three times a day (Neppe et al. 1988).

The dosing should be increased approximately 100 mg every 2–3 days. Generally, in combination with TCAs and neuroleptics, the dose required may only be about 200 mg tid. No therapeutic level has been established for psychiatric use as opposed to the anticonvulsant therapeutic range being used in patients with seizure disorders. Therefore, at this stage it is unknown whether the dosage in psychiatric usage should correspond with the therapeutic blood range of 6–12 μg/ml suggested in the management of epilepsy (Neppe 1989b, 1990b).

In our experience, the therapeutic level for psychiatric use may be on the low side of that anticonvulsant range, something between 6 μg/ml and 9 μg/ml (Neppe et al. 1988).

Initial concerns about irreversible hemopoietic complications with carbamazepine have lessened. Such complications occur with the same order of frequency as with some TCAs. Extremely common, unrelated to these irreversible effects, and of no practical immunological significance is a small drop in the white cell count (Neppe et al. 1988).

Valproate. Sodium valproate is a good broad spectrum drug that apparently also has a low incidence of cognitive side effects. The drug is an outstanding anticonvulsant and is particularly useful in combined tonic-clonic and petit mal seizures. It also appears effective against partial epilepsy. The role of valproate is far less proven in the nonepileptic psychiatric context than that of carbamazepine. It has become fashionable to use it as a third-line drug in manic-depressive illness, at times with remarkable success. Still, such success is relatively rare, and in our experience the real role of valproate in affective illness is unproven. An added difficulty is the limited value of valproate serum levels even in the patient with seizure disorders. Because of this, dosing is a "guesstimate" at best.

Valproate does not induce enzymes but metabolically competes; thus theoretically it raises psychotropic levels and has its own level raised. It is safe, relatively nontoxic, and generally well tolerated. The major concern with its use is potentially fatal, rare hepatotoxicity in young children, particularly when they are on other anticonvulsants. This may or may not be linked with a deficiency of carnitine.

Use of Other Psychotropics in Seizure Disorders

Neuroleptics. Often a neuroleptic agent is required in epileptic patients with psychosis. All neuroleptics are epileptogenic. In vitro studies (Larkin 1983) in guinea pig hippocampal slices suggest that some are less so than others. For example, pimozide (Orap) is certainly less so (Neppe 1985c, 1989b; Larkin 1983). Chlorpromazine appears to achieve its highest epileptogenicity mid-dosage and, in fact, in higher doses appears potentially even mildly anticonvulsant. Haloperidol increases in epileptogenicity as the dosage increases, and there is marked synergism of epileptogenicity when combined with chlorpromazine (Remick and Fine 1979).

These findings suggest that preferably neuroleptics should not be combined in patients with epilepsy (Neppe 1989b). At a clinical level, haloperidol has traditionally been used commonly in epileptic patients with good effects. Thiothixene appears to be a good alternative as is thioridazine (Neppe 1989b). Prochlorperazine and chlorpromazine have also been used. A drug that may have potential application but is as yet unproven is pimozide, as based on animal research (Larkin 1983). Pimozide currently is limited in indication according to the *Physicians' Desk Reference* (1991) to those patients nonresponsive to haloperidol and who have Tourette's syndrome. However, it is used in other countries for psychoses, particularly for schizophrenic patients with marked autistic withdrawal. The complications and contraindications to pimozide are similar to those for other neuroleptics. The drug may be underused at present.

A major caution in using neuroleptics is to administer low dosage and to adequately cover the patient in terms of anticonvulsants. In this regard the anticonvulsants carbamazepine, phenytoin, phenobarbital, and primidone will all theoretically lower the level of psychotropic agents because they are all lipid soluble and are metabolized via the P_{450} cytochrome (Gagneux 1975) system in the liver, which the above anticonvulsants induce (Gagneux 1975; Neppe 1985c). Consequently, higher doses of neuroleptics may be required. On the other hand, neuroleptics will increase the levels of these anticonvulsants by competing for this enzyme system. Interactions are more complicated because of differences in protein binding and, unfortunately, from a practical perspective there are insufficient studies to make adequate comments (Neppe 1989b).

Antidepressants. When used in patients with epilepsy, antidepressants are problematic because they lower the seizure threshold (Edwards 1985). Some antidepressants have had very few reported cases of seizure disturbance (e.g., protriptyline), but this may be because of its less frequent usage. The tetracyclic antidepressants, such as maprotiline and possibly mianserin, may be more epileptogenic than the tricyclics (TCAs). One antidepressant commonly used is doxepin. It remains to be established whether this has any special attributes over the other TCAs. Monoamine oxidase inhibitors (MAOIs) appear far less epileptogenic than TCAs. In practice, the TCAs are probably far more epileptogenic than the neuroleptics.

β-Adrenergic blockers and the azaperones. On many occasions, patients with epilepsy are not fully controlled on anticonvulsants, despite apparent adequate medication trials. These patients may give a history of seizures occurring more frequently during or after stress. The use of β-blockers (like propranolol) or azaperones (like buspirone) in seizure patients has not formally been researched, but preliminary evidence based on a few cases suggests that they have promise, apparently diminishing seizure frequency. Clearly, formal controlled studies are necessary.

The most lipid-soluble β-blocker is propranolol, and levels of anticonvulsant may be raised by hepatic competition. Moreover, a breakdown product, propranolol glycol, has some anticonvulsant effect—a potential advantage (Neppe 1989a). Non-lipid-soluble β-blockers, like atenolol and nadolol, should not induce drug interactions, although absorption may be altered (Neppe 1989a).

Buspirone, as the prototype azaperone, also has some promise in anxious epileptic patients. In animal studies (Neppe 1989c, 1990a), the drug has little effects on seizure threshold in therapeutic doses.

Benzodiazepines. We do not recommend the routine use of benzodiazepines. Despite their initial extremely potent anticonvulsant effects, suggesting they may be ideal in these populations, their use for chronic stress is often protracted. It is at times extremely difficult to remove epileptic patients from benzodiazepines without them having seizures, and the long-term efficacy of maintenance benzodiazepine for stress in epileptic patients is unproven. Moreover, the cognitive, psychomotor, and mnestic impairments induced by anticonvulsants could be accentuated.

Nevertheless, a significant proportion of truly intractable epileptic patients with behavior disturbances require benzodiazepines. Many of these patients have been taking them for years and are anticipated to be on them for a lifetime.

Other Pharmacological and Nonpharmacological Perspectives

Management of patients with seizure disorders involves primarily appropriate use of anticonvulsants (Neppe et al. 1988). In addition, however, counselling and the various aspects of psychosocial support—allowing the patient to live as normal a life as possible and to be supported within the framework of the environment—is clearly also very important. At times special techniques such as relief of anxiety using noninvasive medications (e.g., propranolol or buspirone) may be appropriate (Neppe 1989a, 1990a). At other times treatment of underlying problems such as depression with TCAs or very rarely ECT (Robertson and Trimble 1983; Robertson et al. 1987) is required.

Occasionally techniques such as biofeedback may help. An indirect form of biofeedback is being made aware of the onset of seizure, recognizing this, and being able to intervene by consciously performing other techniques. This may abort seizures. These techniques are all useful in the management of patients with seizure disorders.

❑ CURRENT PERSPECTIVES

Psychopathology occurs only in a minority of persons with epilepsy. Attempted etiological explanations like kindling, lateralization, localization, and biochemical changes are all, therefore, explanations for a small proportion of the epileptic population. Medications used to treat seizure disorders often do not alleviate behavior changes, and at times agents such as neuroleptics help behavior change but not seizure disturbances. The exact etiology of these conditions remains to be determined. Perhaps the use of more sophisticated dynamic imaging techniques such as single photon emission computed tomography (SPECT), positron-emission tomography (PET), magnetic resonance imaging (MRI), and computed tomography (CT) will give better ideas of the source of the behavioral changes (Neppe and Tucker 1988a).

❑ REFERENCES

Adamec RE, Stark AC: Limbic kindling and animal behavior: implications for human psychopathology associated with complex partial seizures. Biol Psychiatry 18:269–293, 1983

Adamec RE, Stark-Adamec C, Perrin R, et al: What is the relevance of kindling for human temporal lobe epilepsy? in Kindling 2. Edited by Wada JA. New York, Raven, 1981, pp 303–311,

Albertson TE, Peterson SL, Stark LG: Anticonvulsant drugs and their antagonism on amydalized kindled seizures in rats. Neuropharmacology 19:643–652, 1980

Albright PS, Burnham WM: Development of a new pharmacological seizure model: effects of anticonvulsants on cortical—and amaygdala—kindled seizures in the rat. Epilepsia 21:681–689, 1980

American Psychiatric Association: Diagnostic and Statistical Manual of Mental Disorders, 3rd Edition. Washington, DC, American Psychiatric Association, 1980

American Psychiatric Association: Diagnostic and Statistical Manual of Mental Disorders, 3rd Edition, Revised. Washington, DC, American Psychiatric Association, 1987

Bear DM: Behavioural changes in temporal lobe epilepsy: conflict, confusion challenge, in Aspects of Epilepsy and Psychiatry. Edited by Trimble ME, Bolwig TG. London, John Wiley, 1986, pp 19–29

Bear D, Levin K, Blumer D, et al: Interictal behaviour in hospitalised temporal lobe epileptics: relationship to idiopathic psychiatric syndromes. J Neurol Neurosurg Psychiatry 45:481–488, 1982

Berger H: Ueber das Elektrenkephalogramm des Menschen. Archives of Psychiatry. I–XIV: 87–108, 1929–1938

Bertilsson L: Clinical pharmacokinetics of carbamazepine. Clin Pharmacokinet 3:128–143, 1978

Betts TA: A follow-up study of a cohort of patients with epilepsy admitted to psychiatric care in an English city, in Epilepsy: Proceedings of the Hans Berger Centenary Symposium, Edinburgh, 1973. Edited by Harris P, Mawdsley C. New York, Churchill Livingstone, 1974, Chapter 56

Bickford RG: Activation procedures and special electrodes, in Current Practice of Unusual Electroencephalography. Edited by Kass D, Daly DD. New York, Raven, 1979

Birkhimer LJ, Curtis JL, Jann MW: Use of carbamazepine in psychiatric disorders. Clin Pharm 4:425–434, 1985

Blumer D: Temporal lobe epilepsy and its psychiatric significance, in Psychiatric Aspects of Neurological Disease. Edited by Benson FD, Blumer D. New York, Grune & Stratton 1975, pp 171–198

Blumer D, Neppe V, Benson DF: Diagnostic criteria for epilepsy-related mental changes. Am J Psychiatry 147: 676–677, 1990

Bramhall D, Levine M: Possible interaction of ranitidine with phenytoin. Drug Intelligence and Clinical Pharmacy 22:979–980, 1988

Brodsky L, Zuniga JG, Casenas ER, et al: Refractory anxiety: a masked epileptiform disorder. Psychiatr J Univ Ottawa 8(1):42–45, 1983

Bruens JH: Psychosis in epilepsy. Psychiatry Neurology Neurochirurg 74:175–192, 1971

Currie S, Heathfield RWG, Henson RA, et al: Clinical course and prognosis of temporal lobe epilepsy: a survey of 666 patients. Brain 94:173–190, 1970

Diehl LW: Schizophrenic syndromes in epilepsies. Psychopathology 22(2–3):65–140, 1989

Dodrill CB, Batzel LW: Interictal behavioral features of patients with epilepsy. Epilepsia 27 (suppl 2):S64–S76, 1986

Dongier S: Statistical study of clinical and electroencephalographic manifestations of 536 psychotic episodes occurring in 516 epileptics between clinical seizures. Epilepsia 1:117–142, 1959–1960

Dorn JM: A case of phenytoin toxicity possibly precipitated by trazodone. J Clin Psychiatry 47:89–90, 1986

Ebersole JS, Leroy RJ: Evaluation of ambulatory EEG monitoring. Neurology 33:853, 1983

Edwards JG: Antidepressants and seizures: epidemiological and clinical aspects, in The Psychopharmacology of Epilepsy. Edited by Trimble MR. Chichester, England, John Wiley, 1985

Ey H: Etudes Psychiatriques. Paris, Desclee de Brouwer, 1954

Fink M: Meduna and the origins of convulsive therapy. Am J Psychiatry 141:1034–1041, 1984

Gagneux AR: The chemistry of carbamazepine, in Epileptic Seizures—Behaviour—Pain. Edited by Birkmayer W. Berne, Hans Huber, 1975, pp 120–126

Gardner DL, Cowdry RW: Positive effects of carbamazepine on behavioral dyscontrol in borderline personality disorder. Am J Psychiatry 143:519–522, 1986

Gibbs FA: Ictal and non-ictal psychiatric disorders in temporal lobe epilepsy. J Nerv Ment Dis 113:522–528, 1951

Gibbs FA, Gibbs EL: Atlas of Electroencephalography. Cambridge, MA, Addison-Wesley, 1952

Gudmundsson G: Epilepsy in Iceland. Acta Neurol Scand 43 (suppl 25):1–124, 1966

Hakola HP, Laulumaa VA: Carbamazepine in treatment of violent schizophrenics. Lancet 1:1356, 1982

Hathaway SR, McKinley JC: Minnesota Multiphasic Personality Inventory-2. Minneapolis, MN, University of Minnesota Press, 1989

Heath RG: Psychosis and epilepsy: similarities and differences in the anatomic-physiologic substrate. Advances in Biologic Psychiatry 8:106–116, 1982

Hermann BP, Riel P: Interictal personality and behavioral traits in temporal lobe and generalized epilepsy. Cortex 17:125–128, 1981

International League Against Epilepsy Commission: Proposal for revised clinical and electroencephalographic classification of epileptic seizures. Epilepsia 22:489–501, 1981

International League Against Epilepsy Commission: Proposal for classification of epilepsies and epileptic syndromes. Epilepsia 26:268–278, 1985

Jann MW, Ereshefsky L, Saklad SR, et al: Effects of carbamazepine on plasma haloperidol levels. J Clin Psychopharmacol 5:106–109, 1985

Kidron R, Averbuch I, Klein E, et al: Carbamazepine-induced reduction of blood levels of haloperidol in chronic schizophrenia. Biol Psychiatry 20:219–222, 1985

Kraepelin E: Psychiatre. Leipzig, Johan Abrosiuis Barth, 1922

Kraepelin E: Lecture VI: epileptic insanity, in Lectures in Clinical Psychiatry. Translated by Johnstone T. New York, Hafner, 1968

Kristensen O, Sindrup EH: Psychomotor epilepsy and

psychosis, II: electroencephalographic findings. Acta Neurol Scand 57:370–379, 1978
Krohn W: A study of epilepsy in Northern Norway, its frequency and character. Acta Psychiatr Neurol Scand Suppl 150:215–225, 1961
Landolt H: Serial encephalographic investigations during psychotic episodes in epileptic patients and during schizophrenic attacks, in Lectures on Epilepsy. Edited by Lorentz de Haas AM. London, Elsevier, 1958
Larkin C: Epileptogenic effect of pimozide. Am J Psychiatry 140:372–373, 1983
Lindsay J, Ounstead C, Richards P: Long-term outcome in children with temporal lobe seizures, III: psychiatric aspects in childhood and adult life. Dev Med Child Neurol 21:630–636, 1979
McKenna PJ, Kane JM, Parrish K: Psychotic syndromes in epilepsy. Am J Psychiatry 142:895–904, 1985
McNamara JO, Byrne MC, Dasheiff RM, et al: The kindling model of epilepsy: a review, in Progress in Neurobiology. Edited by Phillis JW, Kerkut G. London, Pergamon, 1980, pp 139–159
Mattson MP, Guthrie PB, Kater SB: Intrinsic factors in the selective vulnerability of the hippocampal pyramidal neurons, in Alzheimer's Disease and Related Disorders. New York, Alan R Liss, 1989, pp 333–351
Mendez MF, Lanska DJ, Manon ER, et al: Causative factors for suicide attempts by overdose in epileptics. Arch Neurol 46:1065–1068, 1989
Metrakos K, Metrakos JD: Genetics of convulsive disorders, II: genetics and encephalographic studies in centrencephalic epilepsy. Neurology 11:474–483, 1961
Mitsuda H: Clinical Genetics in Psychiatry. Bulletin of the Osaka Medical School. (suppl 12), 1967
Moehle KA, Bolter JF, Long CJ: The relationship between neuropsychological functioning and psychopathology in temporal lobe epileptic patients. Epilepsia 25:418–422, 1984
Monroe RR: Limbic ictus and atypical psychoses. J Nerv Ment Dis 170:711–716, 1982
Mungus D: Interictal behavior abnormality in temporal lobe epilepsy. Arch Gen Psychiatry 39:108–111, 1982
Neppe VM: Is deja vu a symptom of temporal lobe epilepsy? S Afr Med J 60(23):907–908, 1981a
Neppe VM: Review Article: symptomatology of temporal lobe epilepsy. S Afr Med J 60(23):902–907, 1981b
Neppe VM: Review article: non-epileptic symptoms of temporal lobe dysfunction. S Afr Med J 60(26):989–991, 1981c
Neppe VM: Differing perspectives to the concept of temporal lobe epilepsy. The Leech 52:6–10, 1982a
Neppe VM: The new classification of epilepsy—an improvement? S Afr Med J 61(7):219–220, 1982b
Neppe VM: Anomalies of smell in the subjective paranormal experiment. Psychoenergetics—Journal of Psychophysical Systems 5:11–27, 1983a
Neppe VM: Carbamazepine as adjunctive treatment in nonepileptic chronic inpatients with EEG temporal lobe abnormalities. J Clin Psychiatry 44(9):326–331, 1983b
Neppe VM: The incidence of deja vu. Parapsychological Journal of South Africa 4(2):94–106, 1983c
Neppe VM: The Psychology of Deja Vu: Have I Been Here Before? Johannesburg, South Africa, Witwatersrand University Press, 1983d
Neppe VM: Temporal lobe symptomatology in subjective paranormal experients. Journal of the American Society for Psychiatric Research 77:1–30, 1983e
Neppe VM: The use of carbamazepine in psychiatry, in Update on Psychiatric Management. Edited by Carlile JB. Durban, South Africa, Medical Association of South Africa, 1984, pp 50–54
Neppe VM: Epilepsy and psychiatry: essential links. Psychiatric Insight 2(2):18–22, 1985a
Neppe VM: The kindling phenomenon implications for animal and human behaviour, in Neuropsychology 2—Proceedings, Second South African Congress of Brain and Behaviour. Edited by Griesel D. Pretoria, South Africa, South African Brain and Behaviour Society, 1985b, pp 47–51
Neppe VM: The management of epilepsy in the psychiatric patient. Psychiatric Insight 2(2):23–26, 1985c
Neppe VM: Non-responsive psychosis: neuropsychological rehabilitation by antikindling agents. in Neuropsychology 2—Proceedings, Second South African Congress of Brain and Behaviour. Edited by Griesel D. Pretoria, South Africa, South African Brain and Behaviour Society, 1985d, pp 52–56
Neppe VM: Epileptic psychosis: a heterogeneous condition. Epilepsia 27:634, 1986
Neppe VM: Carbamazepine use in neuropsychiatry. J Clin Psychiatry 49 (suppl 4):1–64, 1988
Neppe VM: Beta-adrenergic blocking agents: perspectives in psychiatry, in Innovative Psychopharmacotherapy. Edited by Neppe VM. New York, Raven, 1989a, pp 1–34
Neppe VM: Carbamazepine, limbic kindling and non-responsive psychosis, in Innovative Psychopharmacotherapy. Edited by Neppe VM. New York, Raven, 1989b, pp 123–151
Neppe VM: The clinical neuropharmacology of buspirone, in Innovative Psychopharmacotherapy. Edited by Neppe VM. New York, Raven, 1989c, pp 35–57
Neppe VM: Buspirone: an anxioselective neuromodulator, in Innovative Psychopharmacotherapy, Revised. Edited by Neppe VM. New York, Raven, 1990a, pp 35–57
Neppe VM: Carbamazepine in the non affective psychotic and non psychotic dyscontrol, in Carbamazepine and Ox-carbazepine in Psychiatry: International Clinical Psychopharmacology. Edited by Emrich H, Schiwy W, Silverstone T. London, Clinical Neuroscience Publishers, 1990b, pp 43–54
Neppe VM: The Inventory of Neppe of Symptoms of Epilepsy and Temporal Lobe–Manual. Seattle, WA, University of Washington, 1991
Neppe VM, Friel P: Carbamazepine, clinical and pharmacokinetic variation with psychotropics, in Proceedings of Epilepsy International Congress, Jerusalem, Israel , September 1987, p 85
Neppe VM, Kaplan C: Short-term treatment of atypical spells with carbamazepine. Clin Neuropharmacol 11: 287–289, 1988
Neppe VM, Tucker GJ: Modern perspectives on epilepsy in relation to psychiatry: behavioral disturbances of

epilepsy. Hosp Community Psychiatry 39:389–396, 1988a

Neppe VM, Tucker GJ: Modern perspectives on epilepsy in relation to psychiatry: classification and evaluation. Hosp Community Psychiatry 39:263–271, 1988b

Neppe VM, Tucker GJ: Atypical, unusual and cultural psychoses, in Comprehensive Textbook of Psychiatry, 5th Edition. Edited by Kaplan HI, Sadock BJ. Baltimore, MD, Williams & Wilkins, 1989, pp 842–852

Neppe VM, Tucker GJ, Wilensky AJ: Fundamentals of carbamazepine use in neuropsychiatry. J Clin Psychiatry 49 (suppl 4):4–6, 1988

Neppe VM, Bowman B, Sawchuk KSLJ: Carbamazepine for atypical psychosis with episodic hostility: a preliminary study. J Nerv Ment Dis 179:339–340, 1991

Perez MM, Trimble MR: Epileptic psychosis: psychopathological comparison with process schizophrenia. Br J Psychiatry 137:245–249, 1980

Perini GI: Emotions and personality in complex partial seizures. Psychother Psychosom 45(3):141–148, 1986

Physicians' Desk Reference, 45th Edition. Oradell, NJ, Medical Economics, 1991

Pincus JH, Tucker GJ: Behavioral Neurology, 3rd Edition. New York, Oxford University Press, 1985

Post RM, Uhde TW: Anticonvulsants in non-epileptic psychosis, in Aspects of Epilepsy and Psychiatry. Edited by Trimble MR, Bolwig TG. London, John Wiley, 1986, pp 177–212

Post RM, Weiss SR: Sensitization, kindling, and anticonvulsants in mania. J Clin Psychiatry 50 (suppl):23–30, 1989

Procci WR: Schizo-affective psychosis: fact or fiction? a survey of the literature. Arch Gen Psychiatry 33:1167–1178, 1976

Remick PA, Fine SH: Antipsychotic drugs and seizures. J Clin Psychiatry 40:78–80, 1979

Reynolds EH: Schizophrenia-like psychoses of epilepsy and disturbances of folate and vitamin B12 metabolism induced by anticonvulsant drugs. Br J Psychiatry 113: 911–919, 1967

Roberts JK, Guberman A: Religion and epilepsy. Psychiatr J Univ Ottawa 14(1):282–286, 1989

Robertson MM, Trimble MR: Depressive illness in patients with epilepsy: a review. Epilepsia 24 (suppl 2):S109–S116, 1983

Robertson MM, Trimble MR, Townsend HR: Phenomenology of depression in epilepsy. Epilepsia 28:364–372, 1987

Rodin EA: Psychomotor epilepsy and aggressive behavior. Arch Gen Psychiatry 28:210–213, 1973

Rodin EA, Schmaltz S: The Bear-Fedio personality inventory and temporal lobe epilepsy. Neurology 34:591–596, 1984

Sadler M, Goodwin J: The sensitivity of various electrodes in the detection of epilepsy from potential patients with partial complex seizures. Epilepsia 27:627, 1986

Scher M, Neppe V: Carbamazepine adjunct for nonresponsive psychosis with prior hallucinogenic abuse. J Nerv Ment Dis 177:755–757, 1989

Sengoku A, Yagi K, Seino M, et al: Risks of occurrence of psychoses in relation to the types of epilepsies and epileptic seizures. Folia Psychiatry and Neurology of Japan 37:221–225, 1983

Shukla S, Godwin CD, Long LE, et al: Lithium-carbamazepine neurotoxicity and risk factors. Am J Psychiatry 141:1604–1606, 1984

Singer E, Cohen SM, Garfinkel R, et al: Replicating psychiatric ratings through multiple regression analysis: the Midtown Manhattan Restudy. J Health Soc Behav 17:376–387, 1976

Slater E, Beard AW, Glithero E: The schizophrenia-like psychoses of epilepsy. Br J Psychiatry 109:95–150, 1963

Stark-Adamec C, Adamec R, Graham J, et al: Complexities in the complex partial seizures personality controversy. Psychiatr J Univ Ottawa 10:232–236, 1985

Stevens JR: Interictal clinical manifestations of complex partial seizures, in Complex Partial Seizures and Their Treatment (Advances in Neurology Series, Vol 11). Edited by Penry JK, Daly DD. New York, Raven, 1975

Stevens JR: Epilepsy, personality, behavior and psychopathology—the state of the evidence and directions for future research and treatment. Folia Psychiatr Neurol Jpn 37:203–216, 1983

Stevens JR: Psychiatric aspects of epilepsy. J Clin Psychiatry 49 (suppl 4):49–57, 1988

Stevens JR, Livermore AJ: Kindling of the mesolimbic dopamine system: animal model of psychosis. Neurology 28:36–46, 1978

Stevens JR, Mark VH, Erwin F, et al: Deep temporal stimulation in man: long latency, long-lasting psychological changes. Arch Neurol 21:157–169, 1969

Szatmari P: Some methodologic criteria for studies in developmental neuropsychiatry. Psychiatr Dev 3:153–170, 1985

Toone BK, Garralda ME, Ron MA: The psychoses of epilepsy and the functional psychoses: a clinical and phenomenological comparison. Br J Psychiatry 141:256–261, 1982

Trimble MR: The relationship between epilepsy and schizophrenia: a biochemical hypothesis. Biol Psychiatry 12:299–304, 1977

Trimble MR: The effects of anticonvulsant drugs on cognitive abilities. Pharmacol Ther 4:677–685, 1979

Trimble MR: Limbic system disorders in man. in Psychopharmacology of the Limbic System. Edited by Trimble MR, Zarifian E. Oxford, England, Oxford University Press, 1983, pp 110–124

Trimble MR: The psychoses of epilepsy and their treatment, in The Psychopharmacology of Epilepsy. Edited by Trimble MR. Chichester, England, John Wiley, 1985, pp 83–94

Trimble MR: Cognitive hazards of seizure disorders. Epilepsia 29 (suppl 1):S19–S24, 1988

Tucker DM, Novelly RA, Walker PJ: Hyperreligiosity in temporal lobe epilepsy: redefining the relationship. J Nerv Ment Dis 175:181–184, 1987

Tucker GJ, Price TP, Johnson VB, et al: Phenomenology of temporal lobe dysfunction: a link to atypical psychosis—a series of cases. J Nerv Ment Dis 174:348–356, 1986

Vingiano W: Hemisphericity and personality. Int J Neurosci 44(3–4):263–274, 1989

Von Meduna L: Die Konvulsionstherapie der Schizophrenia. Marhold, Germany, Halle, 1937

Wada JA, Sato M, Corcoran ME: Persistent seizure susceptibility and recurrent spontaneous seizures in kindled cats. Epilepsia 15:465–478, 1974

Wada JA, Osawa T, Sato M, et al: Acute anticonvulsant effects of diphenylhydantoin, phenobarbital, and carbamazepine: a combined electroclinical and serum level study in amygdaloid kindled cats and baboons. Epilepsia 17:77–88, 1976

Waxman SG, Geschwind N: The interictal behavior syndrome of temporal lobe epilepsy. Arch Gen Psychiatry 32:1580–1586, 1975

Wells C, Duneau GW: Neurology for Psychiatrists. Philadelphia, PA, FA Davis, 1980

Wilensky AJ, Neppe VM: Acute interictal psychoses in epileptic patients. Epilepsia 27:634, 1986

Wing JK, Cooper JE, Sartorius N: The Measurement and Classification of Psychiatric Symptoms. New York, Cambridge University Press, 1974

Zimmerman AW: Hormones and epilepsy. Neurol Clin 4:853–861, 1986

Chapter

18

Neuropsychiatric Aspects of Sleep

Thomas C. Neylan, M.D.
Charles F. Reynolds III, M.D.
David J. Kupfer, M.D.

THE RELEVANCE OF SLEEP to neuropsychiatry needs little elaboration in that the importance of sleep to mood, cognition, and general health is intuitively obvious. What is particularly exciting is that the recognition of and early intervention in sleep disorders have the potential for preventing recurrent depressions. A recent community-based prospective epidemiological study by Ford and Kamerow (1989) showed that people who had symptoms of insomnia at initial and 1-year follow-up were at a much higher risk of developing a new depression than those without insomnia. The authors suggested that early intervention with the treatment of insomnia may prevent the occurrence of depression. This is consistent with the theory that disordered sleep physiology may precede the development of an affective disturbance (Reynolds and Kupfer 1987).

Although the interest in disorders of sleep dates back to the earliest writings of descriptive medicine, the rapid growth in the scientific study of sleep and sleep-related clinical disorders did not begin until the discovery of rapid-eye-movement (REM) sleep by Aserinsky and Kleitman in 1953. Sleep became understood not as just a passive phenomenon arising from a reduction in wakefulness (Sterman and Shouse 1985), but rather as a dynamic process comprised of two major brain states: REM and non-REM (NREM) sleep. Although there is good evidence that the role of sleep is intrinsically linked to energy and temperature regulation (Rechtschaffen et al. 1989), the essential life-sustaining or homeostatic functions served by sleep remain unknown.

The field of sleep medicine has grown into a unique multidisciplinary enterprise comprised of an improbable marriage of psychiatrists, neurologists, pulmonologists, otolaryngologists, and pediatricians. There are now more than 140 sleep disorder centers in the United States accredited by the Amer-

Supported in part by Grants MN 00295 (to CFR:RSA), MH37869 (to CFR), MH30915 (to DJK), and AG06836 (to CFR).

ican Sleep Disorders Association. The American Board of Sleep Disorders Medicine certifies clinicians trained in sleep medicine. At present there are two periodicals devoted to sleep research and numerous professional organizations including the Association of Professional Sleep Societies, the Academy of Sleep Disorders Medicine, the Association of Polysomnography Technologists, and the Sleep Research Society (Richardson 1990).

❑ CLINICAL MANIFESTATIONS OF SLEEP-WAKE DISORDERS

Approximately 50 million Americans complain of some form of sleep disturbance (Bixler et al. 1979), and each year 10 million seek treatment from physicians for a sleep-related disturbance (Institute of Medicine 1979). Disorders of sleep and wakefulness produce a wide spectrum of symptomatology. In obtaining a clinical history from patients, the entire 24-hour time period should be explored with respect to sleep-wake habits. Patients' chief complaints are usually related to disrupted or too little sleep, excessive sleepiness, or adverse events associated with the sleep period. Patients with insomnia should be questioned about their views as to what constitutes healthy sleep. Very often patients, who by virtue of their constitution are short sleepers, are subjectively distressed by their inability to sleep for the popular standard of 8 hours. The severity of insomnia can only be understood in terms of its impact on daytime function such as mood, fatigue, muscle aches, attention, and concentration.

A 2-week sleep-wake log is invaluable for obtaining history of irregular sleep-wake patterns; napping; use of stimulants, hypnotics, or alcohol; diet; activity during the day; number of arousals; and perceived length of sleep time and its relationship to daytime mood and alertness. The log is an essential component of the evaluation. A thorough medical and psychiatric history is essential for diagnosing conditions that impact on sleep-wake function. Additional history should be obtained from bed partners for events usually not perceived by the patient, such as snoring, respiratory pauses longer than 10 seconds, unusual body movements, or somnambulism. Patients with excessive somnolence should be questioned carefully about falling asleep while driving or performing any other potentially dangerous activity.

Sleepiness relates to the propensity to sleep, such as after sleep deprivation. Daytime sleepiness can be measured objectively with the Multiple Sleep Latency Test (MSLT; Carskadon et al. 1986) or the Maintenance of Wakefulness Test (MWT; Mitler et al. 1982) (also see Chapter 6). Clinically, the severity of sleepiness can be determined as mild if sleep episodes occur during sedentary activity such as watching television; as moderate, if sleep occurs during mild physical activity such as driving; and severe, if sleep occurs during physical activity that requires moderate attention such as talking or eating (American Sleep Disorders Association Diagnostic Classification Steering Committee 1990). Patients should be asked about symptoms of morning headaches, cataplexy, hypnagogic-hypnopompic hallucinations, sleep paralysis, automatic behavior, or sleep drunkenness (Table 18–1). Patients who complain of disturbances associated with the sleep period should be questioned about nocturnal incontinence or polyuria, orthopnea, paroxysmal nocturnal dyspnea, headaches that interrupt sleep, painful nocturnal erections, jaw clenching or bruxism, sleep talking, and somnambulism (Aldrich 1989).

TABLE 18–1. SLEEP DEFINITIONS

apnea cessation of airflow for at least 10 seconds.
cataplexy sudden loss in muscle tone usually precipitated by a sudden emotional response such as fear or laughter.
circadian rhythm a regular pattern of fluctuation in physiology or behavior that is usually linked to the 24-hour light-dark cycle.
diurnal a behavior or physiological variable that is tied to daytime.
hypersomnia excessive sleepiness. Pertains to the propensity to fall asleep.
hypnagogic-hypnopompic hallucinations hallucinations occurring at the beginning or end of sleep that are usually a manifestation of REM sleep.
hypopnea reduction in airflow by at least 50% for at least 10 seconds.
insomnia difficulty with initiating or maintaining sleep.
parasomnia adverse physiological or behavioral event occurring during sleep.
phase advance or delay shift of the sleep or wake cycle to an earlier or later position in the 24-hour day.
polysomnogram the electrophysiological recording of multiple biological parameters during sleep.
Zeitgeber an environmental factor such as the light-dark cycle that helps entrain biological rhythms to a 24-hour time period.

Source. American Sleep Disorders Association Diagnostic Classification Steering Committee 1990.

❑ NORMAL HUMAN SLEEP

Normal sleep consists of recurring 70- to 120-minute cycles of NREM and REM sleep. NREM sleep consists of 4 stages characterized polysomnographically by the electroencephalogram (EEG), the electrooculogram (EOG), and the electromyogram (EMG) (Rechtschaffen and Kales 1968). By convention, the EEG is monitored with either the C3 or C4 lead (Jasper 1958). Eye movements can be detected by the EOG because of an electrical dipole that exists between the cornea and retina. During wakefulness, the EEG is characterized by low-voltage fast activity consisting of a mix of alpha (8–13 Hz) and beta (>13 Hz) frequencies.

Stage 1 of NREM sleep is a transitional stage between wakefulness and sleep during which the predominant alpha rhythm disappears, giving way to the slower theta (4–7 Hz) frequencies. Stage 2 is characterized by a background theta rhythm and the episodic appearance of sleep spindles (brief bursts of 12–14 Hz activity), and K complexes (a K complex is a single high-amplitude, slow-frequency electronegative wave followed by a single electropositive wave). Stages 3 and 4, also called slow-wave or delta sleep, are defined as epochs of sleep consisting of more than 20% and 50%, respectively, of high-amplitude activity in the delta band (0.5–3.0 Hz). Typically, sleep progresses from wakefulness through the 4 stages of NREM sleep until the onset of the first REM period. The length of the first NREM period is referred to as REM latency—an important variable in diagnosing narcolepsy and in research studies of major depression. In the healthy adult, most of the slow-wave sleep occurs in the first two NREM periods (Figure 18–1). In contrast, the REM periods in the first half of the sleep period are brief in duration and lengthen in duration in successive cycles.

REM sleep is a dramatic physiological state in that the brain becomes electrically and metabolically activated with frequencies approaching that of wakefulness accompanied by a 62%–173% increase in cerebral blood flow (Reivich et al. 1968). Perhaps as a defense to preserve sleep, there is a generalized muscle atonia that is detected polysomnographically by the disappearance of EMG activity. There are phasic bursts of rapid eye movements accompanied by fluctuations in respiratory and cardiac rate. There is penile and clitoral engorgement presumed to be mediated by the increase in cholinergic tone associated with the REM state. There is a suspension of normal temperature regulation such that humans become transiently poikilothermic (Parmeggiani 1980). Finally, REM sleep is the stage in which there are the most vivid and often times bizarre dreams.

Ontogeny of Sleep Stages

Infants at birth spend up to 20 hours a day asleep. REM and NREM stages are not fully differentiated until 3–6 months of age, owing to the relative immaturity of neural structures governing sleep. During the first 3 years, the sleep-wake rhythm develops from an ultradian to a circadian pattern with the principal sleep phase occurring at night. Sleep in prepubertal children is characterized by large percentages of REM and high-amplitude slow-wave sleep. During adolescence there is a precipitous drop in slow-wave sleep (Feinberg 1974). Feinberg (1982) has suggested that the reduction in slow-wave sleep is related to the normal senescence of neurons or synaptic pruning that occurs relatively rapidly in adolescence (Huttenlocher 1979). In the third through sixth decades there is a gradual and slight decline in sleep efficiency and total sleep time. With advancing age, sleep becomes more fragmented and lighter in depth. There are more transient arousals, sleep stage shifts, and a gradual disappearance of slow-wave sleep. In addition, the diurnal sleep-wake pattern decays with a redistribution of sleep during the light phase in the form of frequent naps (Reynolds et al. 1989a).

❑ OVERVIEW OF THE INTERNATIONAL CLASSIFICATION OF SLEEP DISORDERS

In 1979, the Association of Sleep Disorders Centers (ASDC) published its first nosology dividing sleep disorders into four major categories: disorders of initiating and maintaining sleep (insomnias); disorders of excessive somnolence; sleep-wake schedule disorders; and parasomnias (Association of Sleep Disorders Centers and the Association for the Psychophysiological Study of Sleep 1979). DSM-III-R (American Psychiatric Association 1987) presented a much simplified nosology deemphasizing the role of polysomnography in making clinical diagnoses and stressing the psychiatric aspects of sleep disorders (Fredrickson et al. 1990). In 1990 the original ASDC nosology was revised through a joint effort of the American Sleep Disorders Association, the

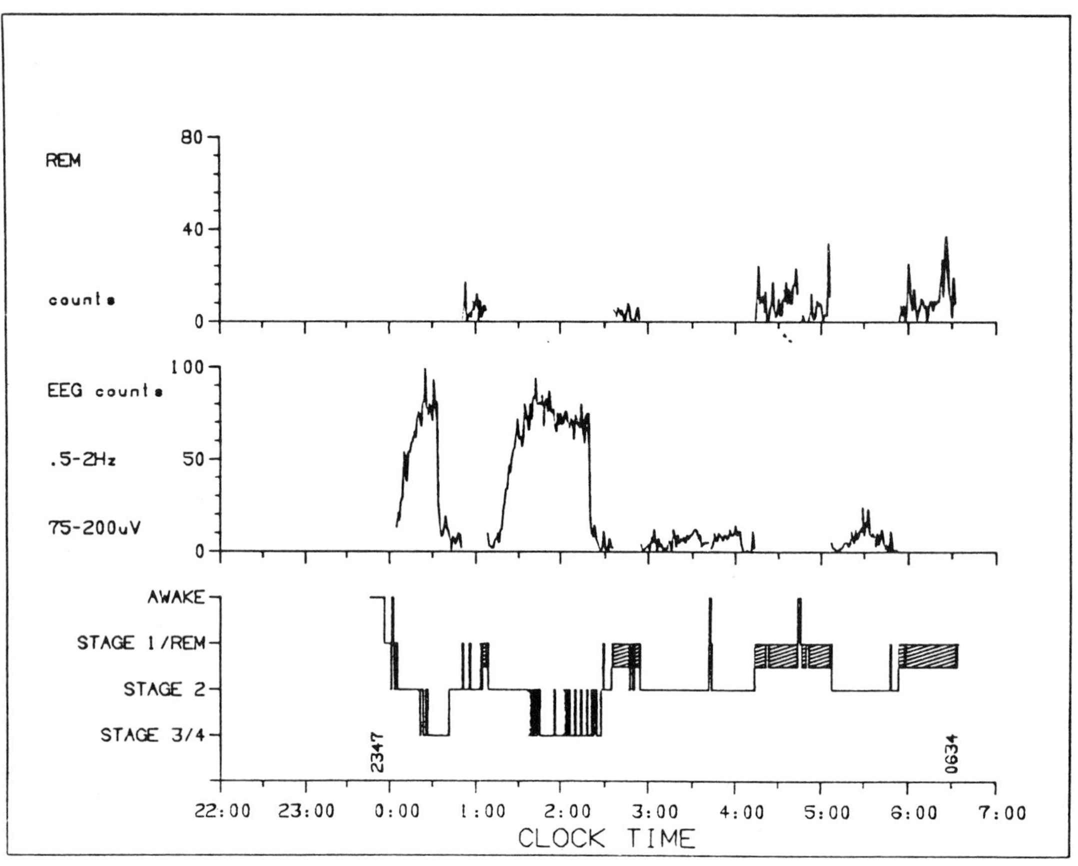

Figure 18–1. Electroencephalogram (EEG) sleep structure in a 22-year-old healthy female control patient. Computed rapid-eye-movement (REM) and delta activity are shown juxtaposed to a sleep histogram derived from visual scoring.

European Sleep Research Society, the Japanese Society of Sleep Research, and the Latin American Sleep Society. The resulting International Classification of Sleep Disorders (ICSD; American Sleep Disorders Association Diagnostic Classification Steering Committee 1990) substantially modified the original ASDC nosology with the introduction of a triaxial diagnostic system. Axis A lists the primary sleep diagnosis, Axis B specifies the procedures used to establish the diagnosis, and Axis C lists relevant nonsleep medical and/or psychiatric diagnoses. The essential change in the revised nosology was that disorders were classified on the basis of presumed pathophysiology as opposed to predominant symptom such as insomnia.

A multicenter field trial of the sleep nosologies in DSM-III-R, ICSD, and the upcoming version of the World Health Organization's International Classification of Diseases (ICD-10) is under way in preparation for DSM-IV (Table 18–2). This study will compare the performance characteristics of the insomnia diagnostic systems with respect to interrater reliability, effects of diagnostic system on interrater reliability, and effects of rater expertise (i.e., sleep specialist versus general psychiatrist) on interrater reliability. In this chapter we present the major sleep-wake disorders organized around the ICSD nosology.

❑ DIFFERENTIAL DIAGNOSIS OF DYSSOMNIAS

The following section provides a brief review of the dyssomnias that cause insomnia and excessive sleepiness (Table 18–3). The ICSD nosology divides the dyssomnias into those caused by so-called in-

TABLE 18–2. PROPOSED DSM-IV CLASSIFICATION OF SLEEP DISORDERS[a]

I. Primary sleep disorders
  A. Dyssomnias
    1. Primary insomnia
    2. Primary hypersomnia
    3. Narcolepsy
    4. Breathing-related sleep disorder
    5. Circadian rhythm sleep disorder
    6. Dyssomnia not otherwise specified (NOS)
  B. Parasomnias
    1. Nightmare disorder
    2. Sleep terror disorder
    3. Sleepwalking disorder
    4. Parasomnia NOS

II. Sleep disorders related to another mental disorder (nonsubstance and/or primary)
  A. Insomnia related to [Axis I or Axis II disorder]
  B. Hypersomnia related to [Axis I or Axis II disorder]

III. Secondary sleep disorder due to an Axis III condition

IV. Substance-induced sleep disorder

[a]Obtained from personal communication with D. J. Kupfer, Chairman of the DSM-IV Workgroup on Sleep Disorders.

TABLE 18–3. INTERNATIONAL CLASSIFICATION OF SLEEP DISORDERS—DYSSOMNIAS

A. Intrinsic sleep disorders
  1. Psychophysiological insomnia
  2. Sleep state misperception
  3. Idiopathic insomnia
  4. Narcolepsy
  5. Recurrent hypersomnia
  6. Idiopathic insomnia
  7. Posttraumatic hypersomnia
  8. Obstructive sleep apnea syndrome
  9. Central sleep apnea syndrome
  10. Central alveolar hypoventilation syndrome
  11. Periodic limb movement disorder
  12. Restless legs syndrome
  13. Intrinsic sleep disorder, not otherwise specified (NOS)

B. Extrinsic sleep disorders
  1. Inadequate sleep hygiene
  2. Environmental sleep disorder
  3. Altitude insomnia
  4. Adjustment sleep disorder
  5. Insufficient sleep syndrome
  6. Limit-setting sleep disorder
  7. Sleep-onset association disorder
  8. Food allergy insomnia
  9. Nocturnal eating (drinking) syndrome
  10. Hypnotic-dependent sleep disorder
  11. Stimulant-dependent sleep disorder
  12. Alcohol-dependent sleep disorder
  13. Toxin-induced sleep disorder
  14. Extrinsic sleep disorder NOS

C. Circadian rhythm sleep disorders
  1. Time zone change (jet lag) syndrome
  2. Shift work sleep disorder
  3. Irregular sleep-wake pattern
  4. Delayed sleep phase syndrome
  5. Advanced sleep phase syndrome
  6. Non-24-hour sleep-wake disorder
  7. Circadian rhythm sleep disorder NOS

Source. American Sleep Disorders Association Diagnostic Classification Steering Committee 1990.

trinsic factors (i.e., originating within the body) and those caused by extrinsic factors (e.g., stimulants or environmental noise that can disrupt sleep). The distinction between intrinsic and extrinsic factors remains controversial given that most sleep disorders are influenced by both. The adaptation of this schema by DSM-IV will depend on the outcome of field trials now under way.

Intrinsic Sleep Disorders

The intrinsic sleep disorders include the majority of disorders treated by sleep specialists: the major insomnias, sleep apnea, myoclonus, and narcolepsy. Two common forms of insomnia not caused by a primary psychiatric disorder are psychophysiological insomnia and idiopathic (childhood-onset) insomnia referred to as *primary insomnia* in DSM-III-R. They share certain features in common in that they can be externally validated by polysomnography (Hauri and Fisher 1986; Hauri and Olmstead 1980). Typical polysomnographic features of these disorders include prolonged latency to sleep onset, decreased sleep efficiency with increased wakefulness after sleep onset, and increased stage 1 sleep indicative of multiple transitions from arousal to sleep.

Psychophysiological insomnia is sometimes referred to as *learned* or *conditioned* insomnia. Typically, it begins during a period of increased stress that manifests in an acute sleep disruption. Normally, the insomnia remits with the passing of the stressful event. However, some individuals may react to the sleep disturbance by struggling harder to sleep. Patient's preoccupation with sleep, usually accompanied by arousal, often become associated with anticipatory anxiety related to expected daytime fatigue and diminished performance. Often environmental cues in the sleeping environment, such as clocks, become associated and paired with arousals thus perpetuating the disorder. Patients with this disorder are often able to sleep better when they are away from home because of the removal of these environmental cues. The disorder can become chronic, persisting over many years, and cause chronic fatigue, muscle aches, and mood disturbance (Hauri and Fisher 1986).

Idiopathic insomnia does not have any psychosocial antecedents and appears to be a trait phenomenon in which the patient has a constitutional predisposition for fragmented sleep. Often the disorder is lifelong, originating in early childhood (Hauri and Olmstead 1980). Although the pathophysiology is unknown, it is presumed to be secondary to a neurochemical or structural disorder involving neural networks governing sleep-wake states. It is difficult to treat and often requires unconventional or innovative pharmacological intervention (Regestein 1987). Hauri and Esther (1990) have recommended low-dose sedating tricyclic antidepressants such as amitriptyline 25–50 mg. A more detailed discussion of the nonpharmacological treatments of insomnias is presented in a subsequent section.

Sleep apnea. Sleep-disordered breathing is an age-related disorder affecting approximately 31% of men and 19% of women over the age of 65 (Ancoli-Israel et al. 1987). Based on a multicenter study of polysomnographic diagnoses made in sleep centers nationwide (Coleman et al. 1982), 43% of all patients with excessive daytime somnolence had a sleep apnea syndrome. Although apnea occasionally causes insomnia, it is typically an occult disorder that causes daytime somnolence, impaired concentration and intellectual functioning, and morning headaches. It is associated with obesity, loud snoring, systemic and pulmonary hypertension, cardiac arrhythmias, and excessive mortality. It can be caused by an impairment in central respiratory drive (central apnea), intermittent upper-airway obstruction (obstructive apnea), or a combination of the two (mixed apnea). Patients with this disorder experience frequent respiratory pauses during sleep associated with oxygen desaturation. The apneic events are terminated by loud gasping, thrashing movements, and EEG arousal. Patients, who usually have no awareness of these events, are often brought to clinical attention by alarmed bed partners (Guilleminault 1982).

Sleep apnea is characterized polysomnographically by measuring oral and nasal airflow with thermistors, which are warmed by exhaled air; respiratory effort, by either thoracic and abdominal strain gauges, diaphragmatic or intercostal EMG, or an esophageal pressure gauge; oxygen saturation with an oximeter; and architecture with a standard sleep montage (EEG, EOG, and EMG) (Figure 18–2). Patients typically have evidence of pathological sleepiness as measured by latencies to sleep onset of less than 5 minutes on the MSLT.

There are various behavioral, medical, pharmacological, and surgical treatments for sleep apnea. Behavioral approaches include weight loss, abstinence from sedative-hypnotics, and training to avoid the supine position during sleep. Mechanical approaches include a variety of tongue-retaining devices and continuous positive airway pressure (CPAP). Medical approaches consist of the use of tricyclic antidepressants, particularly protriptyline, progesterone, and supplemental oxygen. Surgical techniques are currently being refined (Guilleminault et al. 1989) and consist primarily of uvulopalatopharyngoplasty (UPPP) and chronic tracheostomy.

Nocturnal myoclonus and restless legs syndrome. Sleep can be fragmented by the occurrence of periodic leg movements leading to complaints of either insomnia or daytime sleepiness. Nocturnal myoclonus is repetitive, brief leg jerks that occur in regular 20- to 40-second intervals (Figure 18–3). They are frequently associated with transient arousals leading to sleep fragmentation and a predominance of the lighter stages of NREM sleep. Patients are usually unaware of this disorder other than the experience of morning leg cramps and a sense of insufficient sleep.

Nocturnal myoclonus is a common disorder that is seen frequently in association with sleep apnea, narcolepsy, uremia, diabetes, and a variety of disorders affecting the cortex, brain stem, and spinal cord (Coleman et al. 1980). Typically, it is idiopathic with no evidence of gross central nervous system (CNS) pathology. It is a normal phenomenon at birth, disappears in childhood, and frequently reemerges in old age. The emergence of myoclonus is

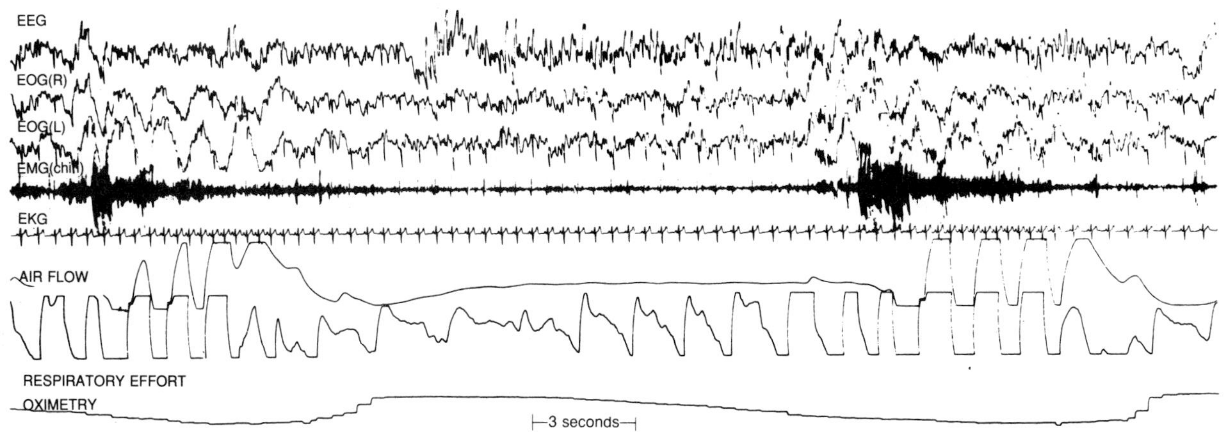

Figure 18–2. Sleep recording from a 25-year-old man with obstructive sleep apnea syndrome. Despite sustained respiratory effector, upper-airway collapse during sleep prevents airflow, resulting in oxyhemoglobin desaturation, electrocardiogram (EKG) bradytachycardia, and electroencephalogram (EEG) microarousals. This pattern recurs hundreds of times nightly. The resulting sleep fragmentation and loss (through repeated arousals necessary for the resumption of breathing) cause excessive daytime sleepiness. EOG(R) = right electrooculogram; EOG(L) = left electrooculogram; EMG(chin) = electromyogram. (Reprinted from Reynolds CF, Kupfer DJ: Sleep disorders, in American Psychiatric Press Textbook of Psychiatry. Edited by Talbott JA, Hales RE, Yudofsky SC. Washington, DC, American Psychiatrc Press, 1988, pp 737–752. Used with permission.)

thought to be secondary to the loss of inhibition of a naturally occurring pacemaker operating at the level of the spinal cord (Lugaresi et al. 1972; Smith 1985). The most common form of treatment for this disorder involves the use of benzodiazepines, particularly clonazepam.

Restless legs syndrome is a disorder that causes sleep-onset insomnia. It is characterized by the presence of deep paresthesias in the calf muscles prompting the urge to keep the legs in motion. It can be extremely distressing and has been linked to suicide. It is associated with uremia, anemia, and pregnancy, as well as to nocturnal myoclonus. There is a familial form of this disorder with an autosomal dominant pattern of transmission. Treatment trials for restless legs syndrome are currently under investigation and include agents such as opioids, carbamazepine, clonidine, benzodiazepines, baclofen, and levodopa (L-dopa).

Narcolepsy. Narcolepsy is a common cause of daytime hypersomnolence in which REM sleep repeatedly and suddenly intrudes into wakefulness. It represents an impairment in the ability to maintain a stable neural state in which REM is no longer segregated in its usual ultradian rhythm during sleep. The clinical phenomenology of narcolepsy is best understood by a consideration of normal REM physiology (e.g., activated EEG, generalized atonia, and dream cognition). Both cataplexy and sleep paralysis involve muscle atonia occurring at a time when the patient is cognizant of the environment and subjectively feels awake. Hypnagogic hallucinations are not well understood but are thought to be related to the dreamlike perceptual phenomenon of REM sleep. Nocturnal sleep is characterized by short REM latency, frequent arousals, and shifts from NREM to REM to wakefulness (Rechtschaffen et al. 1963).

Although the term narcolepsy (literally, "sleep seizure"), as coined by Gelineau (1880), suggests an ictal disorder, the pathophysiology remains unknown. There is convincing evidence of a heritable transmission of the disorder. There is a canine form of narcolepsy that shows an autosomal recessive mode of transmission (Foutz et al. 1979). In humans, there is a close association of the disorder with the human leukocyte antigen (HLA)-DR2 and HLA-DQw1 haplotypes. Although the HLA-DR2 is found in 10%–35% of the general population, in some ethnic groups it has been found to be 100% associated with narcolepsy (Juji et al. 1984; Langdon et al. 1986).

Treatment approaches include the use of REM-suppressing agents such as tricyclic antidepressants to control cataplexy. Stimulants such as methylphe-

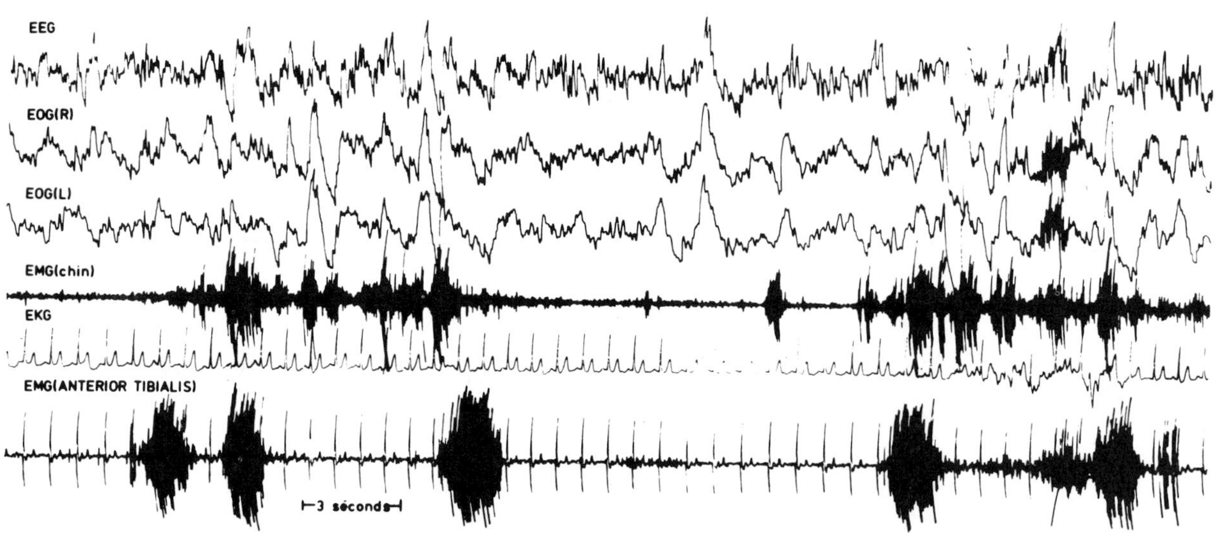

Figure 18–3. Sleep recording from an 84-year-old woman with nocturnal myoclonus. The anterior tibialis electromyogram (EMG) shows frequent bursts of 0.5–2 second muscle activity, which coincide with leg twitches and electroencephalogram (EEG) microarousals. EOG(R) = right electrooculogram; EOG(L) = left electrooculogram. (Reprinted from Reynolds CF, Kupfer DJ: Sleep disorders, in American Psychiatric Press Textbook of Psychiatry. Edited by Talbott JA, Hales RE, Yudofsky SC. Washington, DC, American Psychiatric Press, 1988, 737–752. Used with permission.)

nidate, amphetamine, and pemoline are useful for controlling daytime somnolence. The use of γ-hydroxybutyrate is currently under investigation. An important nonpharmacological approach is the use of scheduled naps throughout the wake period.

Extrinsic Sleep Disorders

Extrinsic sleep disorders are caused by external factors, including behavioral patterns, without which there would be no sleep disturbance. The purest forms of these disorders are altitude insomnia and environmental sleep disorder in which there is a clear easily identifiable external cause for the sleep disturbance. This classification scheme does not exclude the possibility that constitutional or intrinsic factors predispose individuals to be more vulnerable to extrinsic perturbations. However, it suggests that treatment should be directed toward manipulating the external factors.

Several of these sleep disorders are related to ingestion of substances that have direct toxic effects on sleep. Both alcohol- and hypnotic-dependent sleep disorders involve the development of tolerance to the sleep-inducing effects of the agent, as well as increased arousals during withdrawal periods. Stimulants cause sleep-onset insomnia during usage and rebound hypersomnia during withdrawal. Food allergy and toxin-induced sleep disorders presumably involve a direct toxic effect on the physiological substrate regulating sleep. In all of these disorders, careful removal of the offending agent either eliminates the problem or exposes an intrinsic sleep disorder.

Several of these disorders are related to dysfunctional behavior patterns that perturb sleep. In limit-setting sleep disorder, a childhood problem, the sleep disturbance is secondary to parental reluctance to enforce a bedtime, thereby inadvertently reinforcing a child's refusal to go to bed. Sleep-onset association disorder involves a child's inability to fall asleep unless certain exact rituals (e.g., reading a book or taking a bottle) are performed. Often, the child has a normal awakening in the middle of the night and is unable to return to sleep unless the same rituals are repeated. Nocturnal eating (or drinking) syndrome is similar to sleep-onset association disorder in that patients are unable to fall asleep after an arousal unless they ingest something. Insufficient sleep causes daytime fatigue and hypersomnolence by chronic voluntary sleep deprivation often arising in the context of excessive work demands. Adjustment sleep disorder, experienced by most people at some point in their lives, is typically an insomnia related to difficulties adjusting to acute stress such as a school examination. Finally, inadequate sleep hygiene, one of the most common extrinsic sleep disorders, is related to habits such as napping or late-evening exercise that adversely affect sleep. The treatment for these disorders include counselling parents to help them avoid reinforcing their child's maladaptive sleep habits and, for adult patients, the implementation of habits promoting good sleep hygiene (Table 18–4).

Circadian Rhythm Sleep Disorders

The sleep-wake cycle, under the circadian control of endogenous regulators or oscillators, can be disrupted by a misalignment between biological rhythms and external demands on waking behavior. The circadian cycle is under the principal control of the suprachiasmatic nucleus, the destruction of which eliminates any circadian rhythmicity (Moore and Eichler 1972; Rusak and Zucker 1979). Circadian rhythm disorders present with either insomnia or hypersomnolence depending on the juxtaposition of performance demands and the underlying circadian cycle.

Rapid shifts in the sleep-wake schedule cause an acute circadian dysrhythmia. Jet lag is one of the most common of these disorders. Travelers flying across multiple time zones are met with a radical change in the cues called *Zeitgebers*, which help entrain circadian rhythms with respect to both the social schedule and the light-dark cycle. Similarly, workers who rotate on to different shifts experience an acute misalignment in their underlying biological rhythms. Night-shift workers are usually in a state of permanent circadian misalignment because of their tendency to revert to conventional schedules on their days off. Patients with irregular sleep-wake patterns have little to no circadian rhythmicity to their sleep cycle. This disorder is frequently seen in institutionalized geriatric patients who have a polyphasic sleep-wake cycle in which brief periods of wakefulness followed by napping persist throughout the 24-hour day. All of these disorders give rise to sleep-wake complaints, mood disturbance, decreased work performance, and general physical malaise. The general treatment approach is to promote good sleep hygiene with the goal of properly aligning patients' circadian system with their sleep-wake schedule.

Some circadian sleep-wake disorders are related to a diminished capacity to respond to external Zeitgebers. In the non-24-hour sleep-wake disorder, patients are free running with respect to their internal oscillators, typically in a day longer than 24 hours. This has been described in congenitally blind

TABLE 18–4. RULES OF SLEEP HYGIENE

1. Sleep as much as needed to feel refreshed during the following day. Restricting the time in bed seems to solidify sleep, but excessively long times in bed seem related to fragmented and shallow sleep.
2. Get up at the same time each day, 7 days a week. (A regular awake time in the morning leads to regular times of sleep onset.)
3. A steady daily amount of exercise probably deepens sleep.
4. Insulate your bedroom against sounds (carpeting, insulated curtains, and closing the door).
5. Excessively warm rooms may disturb sleep; keep the room temperature moderate.
6. Hunger may disturb sleep. A light snack at bedtime may help sleep.
7. Try to avoid excessive liquids in the evening, in order to minimize the need for nighttime trips to the bathroom.
8. Avoid caffeine-containing beverages in the evening.
9. Avoid alcohol in the evening. Although alcohol helps tense people fall asleep more easily, the ensuing sleep is then broken up.
10. People who feel angry and frustrated because they cannot sleep should not try harder and harder to fall asleep but should turn on the light, leave the bedroom, and do something different like reading a boring book. Don't engage in stimulating activity. Return to bed only when sleepy. Get up at your regular time the next day, no matter how little you slept.
11. The chronic use of tobacco disturbs sleep.
12. If you find yourself waking up and looking at the clock, put the clock under the bed or cover it up.

Note. Adapted from Hauri and Orr 1982.
Source. Reprinted from Reynolds CF, Kupfer DJ: Sleep disorders, in American Psychiatric Press Textbook of Psychiatry. Edited by Talbott JA, Hales RE, Yudofsky SC. Washington, DC, American Psychiatric Press, 1988, pp 737–752. Used with permission.

subjects who are nonresponsive to light as a Zeitgeber (Miles et al. 1977). Of interest, a recent report (Sack et al. 1990) showed that melatonin administration could entrain a free-running blind subject to a conventional sleep-wake schedule. In the delayed sleep phase syndrome, patients—typically young adults—are described as "night owls" with an innate preference to begin sleeping in the late hours of night and to sleep until the late morning or early afternoon. They experience sleep-onset insomnia and morning hypersomnolence when forced to comply with a conventional sleep-wake schedule. Conversely, patients with advanced sleep phase syndrome experience hypersomnolence in the early evening hours and mid-night arousal. Typically these are older patients because there is a tendency for the sleep-wake cycle to advance relative to clock time with age. The treatment for many of these disorders involves the realignment of the sleep-wake schedule with manipulation or augmentation of external Zeitgebers such as the use of bright light therapy.

TABLE 18–5. INTERNATIONAL CLASSIFICATION OF SLEEP DISORDERS—PARASOMNIAS

A. Arousal disorders
   1. Confusional arousals
   2. Sleepwalking
   3. Sleep terrors

B. Sleep-wake transition disorders
   1. Rhythmic movement disorder
   2. Sleep starts
   3. Sleepwalking
   4. Nocturnal leg cramps

C. Parasomnias usually associated with rapid-eye-movement (REM) sleep
   1. Nightmares
   2. Sleep paralysis
   3. Impaired sleep-related penile erections
   4. Sleep-related painful erections
   5. REM sleep-related sinus arrest
   6. REM sleep behavior disorder

D. Other parasomnias
   1. Sleep bruxism
   2. Sleep enuresis

Source. American Sleep Disorders Association Diagnostic Classification Steering Committee 1990.

❑ DIFFERENTIAL DIAGNOSIS OF PARASOMNIAS

Parasomnias are adverse events that occur during sleep (Table 18–5). Many of these disorders are found normally in young children and are labelled as pathological only if they persist into adulthood. With few exceptions they involve a partial arousal from sleep either before, during, or after the event (Karacan 1988). Two common parasomnias occurring as a partial arousal from deep sleep are sleepwalking and sleep terrors. Both disorders occur most frequently during the first third of the night, a period characterized by a predominance of slow-wave sleep. In sleepwalking, subjects become partially aroused and ambulatory. They are typically difficult to awaken and have amnesia for the events. Sleep terrors involve an emergence of intense fear associated with autonomic arousal in which patients are inconsolable, difficult to fully awaken, and unable to assign specific cognitions associated with the anxiety. This is in contradistinction to nightmares, which arise from REM sleep and are characterized by vivid, detailed imagery, associated with good recall. Treatment is directed toward reducing stress, anxiety, and sleep deprivation, all of which are known to exacerbate these disorders. In extreme cases low-dose benzodiazepines are indicated and effective.

Some parasomnias occur during sleep-wake transitions. Head banging, formerly known as *jactatio capitis nocturnus*, is a rhythmic movement disorder that is thought to be a self-soothing behavior in children during the transition from wakefulness to sleep. Sleep starts, or hypnic jerks, are sudden muscle contractions that often occur during sleep onset and are thought to be clinically insignificant.

Several prominent parasomnias are characterized by abnormal motor behavior during sleep. Nocturnal paroxysmal dystonia is characterized by stereotypic and violent movements that can resemble seizure activity (Lugaresi et al. 1986). They can occur multiple times during the night and are associated with NREM sleep. REM-sleep behavior disorder occurs when there is incomplete or absent muscle atonia during REM. The disorder is characterized by violent and dramatic motor activity, which represents the motor expression of dreaming. Several dramatic cases have involved patients who suddenly assaulted their bed partners in response to frightening dreams. Benzodiazepines, particularly clonazepam, are useful in reducing these events (Mahowald and Schenck 1989).

❑ MEDICAL AND/OR PSYCHIATRIC SLEEP DISORDERS

Sleep can be adversely affected by a variety of psychiatric, neurological, and medical disorders (Table 18–6). In each case, the treatment is directed to the underlying disorder. In the following section we highlight some of the more common or better-studied disorders that affect sleep.

Affective Disorders

Perhaps no other neuropsychiatric disorders have been as well studied polysomnographically as the affective disorders. Sleep disturbance is verifiable in 90% of patients with major depression and is characterized by sleep fragmentation, decreased quantity and altered distribution of delta sleep, reduced duration of the first NREM period (e.g., REM latency), redistribution of REM sleep into the first half of the night, and increased density of rapid eye movements (Reynolds and Kupfer 1987; Kupfer and Reynolds, in press). Bipolar patients, in contrast, typically become hypersomnolent during depressive episodes and have comparatively increased sleep efficiency and total sleep time (Detre et al. 1972).

Of all the sleep EEG characteristics associated with depression, no other has received as much scientific scrutiny as the finding of short REM latency as first described by Kupfer and Foster in 1972. Although reduced REM latency is not pathognomonic for major depression, it nevertheless has been found to be a reliable marker for particular state and trait variables, as well as having value in predicting clinical course and treatment outcome.

Multiple studies have shown that REM latency is related to state-dependent factors in major depression. For example, Giles et al. (1986) found that REM latency helped distinguish endogenous versus nonendogenous depression. Short REM latency was related to appetite loss, terminal insomnia, anhedonia, and unreactive mood. In contrast, sleep EEG does not support the biological validity of the diagnoses of primary versus secondary depressions in that their polysomnographic characteristics are similar (Thase et al. 1984). Kupfer has shown, in one of the few longitudinal studies of sleep in depression (Kupfer et al. 1988), that REM latency is shorter during the earlier phases of relapse in recurrent major depression. Short REM latency is more prevalent among depressed inpatients compared with outpatients, suggesting a relationship with the severity of the index episode (Spiker et al. 1978). Finally, delusional depression is distinguishable from the nondelusional subtype because of the higher frequency of sleep-onset REM periods and decreased total REM time (Thase et al. 1986).

In addition, there are intriguing data that suggest that short REM latency may be a vulnerability or trait marker for major depression. Several groups (e.g., Hauri et al. 1974; Rush et al. 1986) have found reduced REM latency in patients after clinical remission of their depressive episodes. First-degree relatives of depressed probands with short REM latency have been found to be at increased risk of developing major depression (Giles et al. 1988). Similarly, first-degree relatives concordant for depression have been found to be concordant for REM latency as well (Giles et al. 1987a).

TABLE 18–6. INTERNATIONAL CLASSIFICATION OF SLEEP DISORDERS—SLEEP DISORDERS ASSOCIATED WITH MEDICAL AND/OR PSYCHIATRIC DISORDERS

A. Associated with mental disorders
   1. Psychoses
   2. Mood disorders
   3. Anxiety disorders
   4. Panic disorder
   5. Alcoholism

B. Associated with neurological disorders
   1. Cerebral degenerative disorders
   2. Dementia
   3. Parkinsonism
   4. Fatal familial insomnia
   5. Sleep-related epilepsy
   6. Electrical status epilepticus of sleep
   7. Sleep-related headaches

C. Associated with other medical disorders
   1. Sleeping sickness
   2. Nocturnal cardiac ischemia
   3. Chronic obstructive pulmonary disease
   4. Sleep-related asthma
   5. Sleep-related gastroesophageal reflux
   6. Peptic ulcer disease
   7. Fibrositis syndrome

Source. American Sleep Disorders Association Diagnostic Classification Steering Committee 1990.

REM latency and other REM measures have been found useful in predicting response to treatment and risk of relapse. Kupfer et al. (1976) showed that the degree of REM latency prolongation and total REM suppression seen during initiation of treatment with amitriptyline predicted clinical response. Similarly, REM suppression by clomipramine has been found to predict response to treatment (Hochli et al. 1986). Short REM latency during an index episode of depression confers a higher risk of relapse after clinical remission (Giles et al. 1987b; Reynolds et al. 1989b).

There have been several attempts to integrate the above findings into a model that explains the association of REM latency to both state and trait characteristics in depression. Kupfer and Ehlers (1989) recently have suggested two subtypes of short REM latency. In type I, there is a heritable predisposition to both depression and short REM latency. In this subtype, REM latency is a trait marker that is abbreviated because of a relatively weak slow-wave sleep process that allows REM to be expressed earlier. In type II, REM latency is responsive to state-dependent phenomena such as arousal or stress. In this subtype, REM latency serves as a state marker that is related to the severity of the episode. Studies exploring the neuroendocrine features of these two subtypes are under way.

Schizophrenia

Sleep has not been as extensively studied in schizophrenia because of practical difficulties in studying drug-free patients. The results are more variable than findings in studies of depressed patients. In addition, studies are difficult to interpret because of the lack of suitable control subjects for confounding variables such as age, presence of centrally active medication, proximity to drug withdrawal, clinical features (e.g., negative and positive symptoms), and state-dependent characteristics such as acute relapse. Nevertheless, schizophrenic patients have been found to have prolonged sleep latencies, sleep fragmentation with multiple arousals, decreased slow-wave sleep, variability in REM latency, and decreased REM rebound after REM-sleep deprivation (Ganguli et al. 1987; Zarcone 1988; Zarcone et al. 1987).

Several investigators have attempted to find correlations between clinical features of schizophrenia and specific sleep variables. For example, the variability in REM latency has been found to be linked to family history of affective disorder (Keshavan et al. 1990), presence of negative symptoms (Tandon et al. 1988), tardive dyskinesia (Thaker et al. 1989), and neuroleptic withdrawal (Neylan et al., in press). Diminished slow-wave sleep, one of the most replicated findings in schizophrenia (Feinberg and Hiatt 1978), has been found to be associated with poor performance on neuropsychological tests of attention (Orzack et al. 1977). Ganguli et al. (1987) and van Kammen et al. (1988) found an inverse relationship between presence of negative symptoms and slow-wave sleep, although this has not been replicated in all studies.

Anxiety Disorders

Sleep in patients with generalized anxiety disorder is similar to that seen in psychophysiological insomnia in that there are prolonged sleep latencies and increased sleep fragmentation. Sleep in patients with anxiety disorders differs from that seen in patients with major depression in the presence of normal REM latencies and decreased REM percent (Reynolds et al. 1983a). The suggestion that patients with symptoms of depression and anxiety may be segregated with respect to sleep variables on the basis of the presence or absence of a family history of depression has been forwarded by Sitaram et al. (1984).

A recent report on sleep and panic disorder by Mellman and Uhde (1989) confirmed that panic attacks can arise during sleep. Six of 13 patients with panic disorder were observed to have panic symptoms during sleep when they were being studied electrographically. Of interest, all panic attacks occurred during NREM sleep, particularly during transitions from stage 2 to delta sleep. This adds further data to the theory that panic attacks can be physiologically provoked. The mild hypercapnia normally found in sleep may predispose patients to sleep panic (Mellman and Uhde 1989), although this needs further testing.

Ross et al. (1989) have recently reviewed what is known about sleep in posttraumatic stress disorder (PTSD). They argued that sleep disturbance, particularly disturbing repetitive dreams, may be the essential feature of the disorder. Moreover, they suggested that dysfunctional REM-sleep physiology may contribute to the pathogenesis of the disorder. Further studies are needed to delineate if intrusive memories of the traumatic event are segregated to any particular sleep stage.

Dementia

Sleep in patients with primary degenerative dementia of the Alzheimer's type (PDDAT) represents an exaggeration of the deterioration of sleep seen in normal aging. Compared to age-matched control subjects, patients with PDDAT have more sleep fragmentation and less delta and REM sleep (Reynolds 1989; Vitiello and Prinz 1988). Reynolds et al. (1985a) and Smirne et al. (1977) showed that patients with dementia have little to no spindle and K complex activity. Stage 2 sleep with a paucity of spindles or K complexes is called indeterminate sleep (Figure 18–4). The amount of indeterminate sleep is positively correlated with the severity of dementia (Reynolds et al. 1985a). In addition, patients with PDDAT have more sleep-related phenomena, such as sundowning and nocturnal wanderings. They spend as much as half of the 24-hour day in bed, which leads to a breakdown in the diurnal pattern of sleep and wakefulness. The inability to have a consolidated period of sleep during the night is often the precipitating factor that provokes families to institutionalize their elderly relatives (Sanford 1975).

There is evidence that the prevalence of sleep apnea is higher in patients with probable Alzheimer's dementia compared with age- and sex-matched control subjects. Furthermore, the severity of dementia is correlated with the severity of apnea (Hoch et al. 1986; Reynolds et al. 1985b). Additional studies needed to confirm these findings are currently under way.

Sleep EEG has been found to accurately distinguish depressed patients with pseudodementia from dementia patients with superimposed depression. Buysse et al. (1988) showed that depressed patients experienced an improvement in mood after sleep deprivation compared with dementia patients who either had a worsening in depressive symptoms or showed no change. Further, depressed patients showed a more robust rebound in REM sleep on recovery nights compared with dementia patients. Interestingly, Hoch et al. (1989) showed that sleep EEG predicted mortality in a sample of patients with mixed symptoms of depression and dementia. Patients who had died during a 2-year follow-up period had significantly longer REM latencies, less REM-sleep rebound after sleep deprivation, and higher indices of sleep-disordered breathing.

Other Neuropsychiatric Conditions

Sleep and seizures. NREM sleep has a well-known activating effect on seizure activity, whereas epileptic discharges usually are suppressed during REM sleep. EEG synchronization may explain the higher prevalence of seizures and interictal discharges seen in NREM sleep (Shouse 1989). Many epileptic patients have their seizures predominantly during sleep or on arousal from sleep (Janz 1962). The clinical course depends on the type and severity of the seizure disorder. Although complaints of insomnia are unusual, sleep can be sufficiently fragmented to cause daytime hypersomnolence.

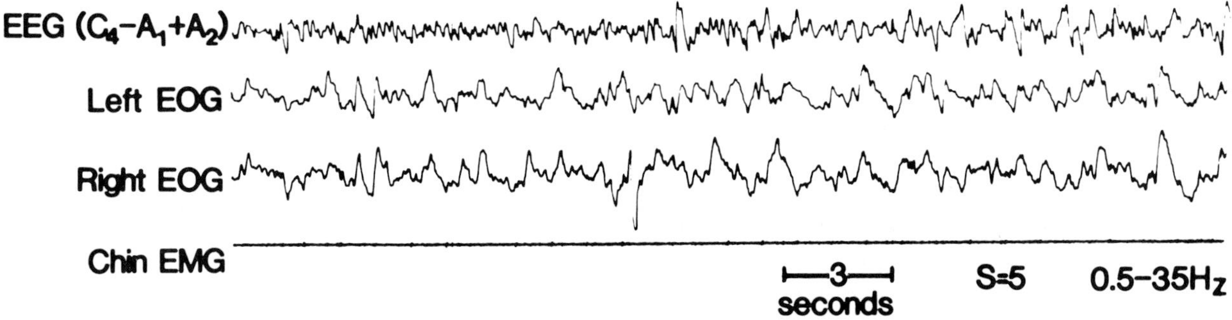

Figure 18–4. Appearance of indeterminate non-rapid-eye-movement (NREM) sleep in a 62-year-old woman with probable Alzheimer's dementia. Sleep has a stage 2 appearance except for the absence of spindles and K complexes. EEG = electroencephalogram; EOG = electrooculogram; EMG = electromyogram.

Unusual nocturnal motor behavior, sleep-related incontinence, or nocturnal tongue biting warrants an evaluation for sleep seizures. Often seizure-related behavior is difficult to distinguish from parasomnias such as enuresis and somnambulism. Family history of either parasomnias or seizure disorder is useful collaborative evidence. Somnambulists usually have more purposeful motor behavior and are easier to redirect. Finally, an all-night EEG may be needed to screen for epileptiform activity.

Sleep in parkinsonism. Sleep disturbance is reported in approximately 75% of patients with parkinsonism. Sleep is characterized by increased number of awakenings, decreased delta and REM sleep, and a scarcity of sleep spindles. The resting tremor usually subsides with the onset of stage 1 sleep but, depending on the severity of the disorder, can persist into stage 2 or reemerge during sleep stage changes (April 1966). The pathophysiology of the sleep disturbance is unclear. Patients with parkinsonism have been shown to have a higher prevalence of sleep disordered breathing (Hardie et al. 1986). Nigrostriatal degeneration may have a direct or indirect impact on the neural substrate regulating sleep. Dopaminomimetic drugs such as L-dopa have dose-dependent effects on sleep with lower doses improving sleep quality and higher doses causing decreased sleep efficiency (Bergonzi et al. 1974).

Kleine-Levin syndrome. A rare form of periodic hypersomnolence is the Kleine-Levin syndrome, which is characterized by intermittent attacks of hypersomnolence and hyperphagia often associated with indiscreet hypersexuality, poor social judgment, mood disturbance, and hallucinations. In between episodes there can be a complete remission of symptoms. It occurs most frequently in males in their late adolescence and early 20s and is followed by a gradual decline in the frequency and duration of the episodes (Critchley 1962). The pathophysiology is postulated to involve an underlying disturbance of limbic and hypothalamic function. Several abnormal laboratory findings have been documented including slowing of background rhythm on EEGs, abnormal growth hormone secretion, and elevated cerebrospinal fluid serotonin and dopamine metabolites (Billiard 1989). Polysomnographic studies have shown diminished delta sleep, increased number of awakenings, and reduced REM latency (Reynolds et al. 1980). In one report (Reynolds et al. 1984), the MSLT revealed the presence of sleep-onset REM periods during the acute attack but not during recovery. Treatment usually involves the use of stimulants for both the hypersomnolence and increased appetite.

❑ NEUROPSYCHIATRIC ASPECTS OF SLEEP DISORDERS

Sleep Deprivation

The study of the neuropsychiatric aspects of sleep deprivation in control subjects helps place into perspective the clinical sequelae of any disorder that fragments sleep. (For an in-depth discussion of the effects of sleep deprivation, see reviews by Horne 1985 and Mendelson 1987.) Short-term effects of 1–2 nights of sleep deprivation include fatigue, irritability, impaired attention with poor performance on dull monotonous tasks, and impairments in short-term memory. Sleep deprivation has well-described mood-elevating effects in more than 50% of endogenous depressive patients (Wu and Bunney 1990) and is increasingly being used by clinicians in the treatment of depression. The deprivation of REM sleep in particular has been postulated as the mechanism by which antidepressants exert their clinical effects (Vogel et al. 1975). Long-term sleep deprivation can lead to reversible perceptual abnormalities, including hallucinations, in a minority of subjects. During his trans-Atlantic crossing, Charles Lindbergh experienced visual hallucinations that remitted permanently after recovery sleep (Gill 1977). Mood disturbance with irritability, transient paranoia, disorientation, and severe fatigue are well-described sequelae of prolonged sleep deprivation.

Sleep Apnea

The clinical impact of sleep apnea is related to two important phenomena: hypoxia and sleep fragmentation. Cerebral hypoxia can lead to the intellectual deterioration, impaired attention and memory, and personality changes seen in apnea patients. (A detailed discussion of the neuropsychology of hypoxia is beyond the scope of this chapter; see review by Berry et al. 1986.)

From a psychosocial perspective, the symptom of hypersomnolence is the most debilitating of symptoms seen in apnea patients. Motor vehicle accidents caused by falling asleep while driving contribute to the excessive mortality seen among apnea patients. Several investigators have attempted to discern if hypersomnolence is related to sleep hypoxia or to sleep fragmentation. Roehrs et al. (1989) reported a study of 466 patients with obstructive sleep apnea in which multiple polysomnographic variables, including EEG arousals and oxygen desaturations, were independently analyzed for prediction of excessive daytime somnolence. Although the number of arousals and hypoxic events covaried significantly, it was the arousal index that best predicted short latencies on the MSLT. This finding supports the hypothesis that daytime somnolence is secondary to the disruption in quantity and quality of sleep.

Narcolepsy

Narcolepsy has been found to affect psychological state as well as cognition. Patients have been found to have more job-related injuries, problems with occupational or academic performance, and a higher prevalence of anxiety and affective disorders (Richardson et al. 1990). Several studies have shown impaired performance in tasks requiring sustained attention as a result of intrusive microsleeps. However, not all performance decrements can be attributed to impaired arousal because attentional deficits have been found in narcoleptic patients during EEG verified wakefulness (for a review, see Mendelson 1987). In one study (Reynolds et al. 1983b), 20% of 25 narcoleptic patients met criteria for major depression, 8% for generalized anxiety disorder, and 12% for alcohol abuse. An unresolved issue is whether the higher prevalence of psychiatric symptomatology is a response to the psychosocial consequences of having a chronic disorder in which existing treatments are often inadequate, or whether the mood and affective disturbance are driven by a common pathophysiology.

Sleep-Wake Schedule Disorders and Effects of Shift Work

Sleep-wake schedule disorders can give rise to various neuropsychiatric and medical symptoms. Rotating-shift workers have been found to have 2–3 times the injury rate compared with co-workers who work stable day, evening, or night shifts (Smith and Colligan 1982). Shift workers have high rates of gastrointestinal, cardiac, and reproductive disorders (Czeisler and Allan 1988). There is a 10% increase in motor vehicle accidents after the switch to daylight saving time in which the day is shortened by 1 hour (Monk 1980). Monk (1989) pointed out that the ability to cope with shift work is related to tolerance for circadian desynchronosis, decreased sleep, and domestic pressures often experienced by those who work unconventional hours.

Cognitive Effects of Sleep Disorders in the Elderly

Studies examining the relationship between sleep, aging, and dementia suggest an important relationship between normal sleep-wake function and cognition. Feinberg et al. (1967) suggested that EEG sleep is an indicator of the functional integrity of the cerebral cortex. An important unanswered question is whether sleep loss in aging is related to cognitive impairment, or whether sleep loss and cognitive impairment emerge secondary to some underlying independent biological process (Reynolds et al. 1989a).

❑ MANAGEMENT OF SLEEP DISORDERS

Given the broad spectrum of pathophysiological processes that affect sleep-wake function, the management of sleep disorders rests on the foundation of the specific diagnosis. Interestingly, during the past few decades in which our knowledge of sleep disorders has greatly increased, the percentage of the general population receiving sedative-hypnotics for sleep has fallen. The clinical history, exam, and sleep diary remain the cornerstone of the initial assessment. Polysomnography is indicated in any patient with complaints of irresistible daytime sleepiness given the high prevalence of sleep apnea and narcolepsy in this population. The use of polysomnography in all patients with insomnia is controversial (and is discussed in further detail in Chapter 6). In general, polysomnography is indicated for insomnia patients when initial attempts to improve sleep hygiene, modify sleep-related habits that elicit arousal, or treat clinical affective disorders are unsuccessful.

Patients who are eventually referred for polysomnography are usually asked to record their sleep-wake habits in a sleep diary for a 2-week period before the sleep study. Ideally, patients should taper off of all psychoactive substances, when clinically feasible, to minimize artifact in the sleep recording. The sleep recording should be obtained during the patient's usual sleep period, which means that the sleep laboratory must be flexible enough to accommodate shift workers. The patient is fitted with the various sensor devices well in advance of the sleep period allowing some time to adjust to the multiple wires (Figure 18–5). The patient is allowed to sleep, read, ambulate, and so on in a comfortable quiet setting. After the recording period, the patient fills out a postsleep questionnaire and gives a subjective rating of the length and quality of sleep. The record is scored manually or by computer using standardized criteria (Rechtschaffen and Kales 1968), and a report is generated.

A detailed discussion of the treatment of sleep disorders secondary to apnea, narcolepsy, nocturnal myoclonus, major depression, parasomnias, and sleep-wake schedule disorders is beyond the scope of this chapter. A broad overview is presented in Table 18–7. (For excellent reviews, see American Psychiatric Association 1989.) In this section we focus on the use of nonpharmacological and pharmacological interventions in patients with insomnia.

Education about healthy sleep habits is potentially a sufficient intervention. However, as Hauri (1989) aptly pointed out, handing patients a list of rules for better sleep hygiene rarely is effective. If patients could readily respond to the admonishment, "Stop smoking, quit drinking alcohol and caffeine-containing beverages, no napping, and start getting regular exercise," the public health benefits would be staggering. Given that patients are usually entrenched in their habits, a more realistic and longer-term approach is needed to help patients gradually make these adjustments.

Various relaxation therapies such as hypnosis, meditation, deep breathing, and progressive muscle

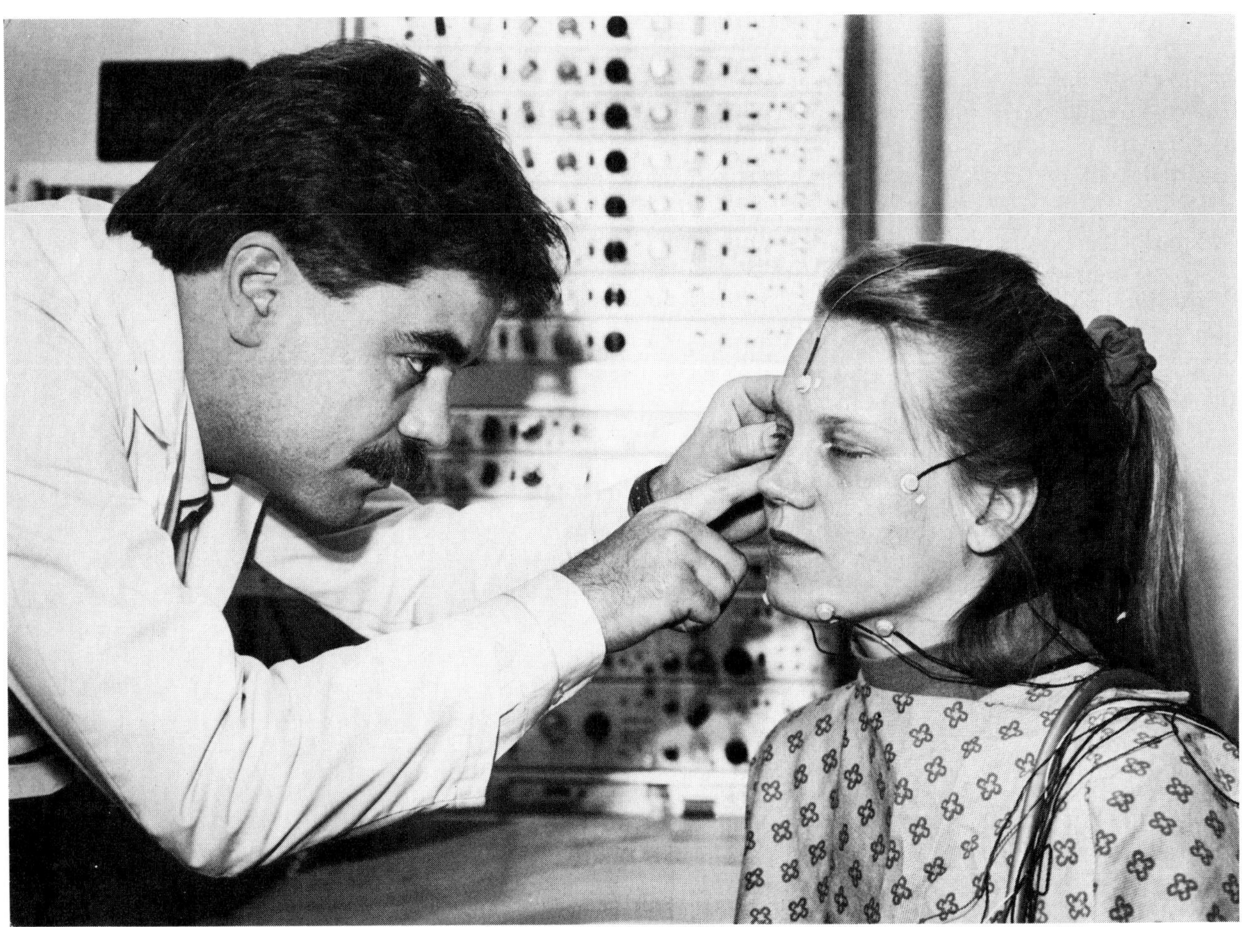

Figure 18–5. The electrodes and sensors are applied before beginning the polysomnographic recording.

TABLE 18–7. SELECTED SLEEP/WAKE DISORDERS: CLASSIFICATION, POLYSOMNOGRAPHIC FINDINGS, AND TREATMENT

DSM-III-R classification	*ICSD classification*	*Polysomnographic findings*	*Primary treatment*
Primary insomnia	Psychophysiological insomnia and idiopathic insomnia	Varies from normal to moderate sleep continuity disturbance	Biofeedback, stimulus control, temporal control, and short-term benzodiazepines
Myclonic sleep disorder	Periodic limb movement disorder	Periodic leg twitches, electroencephalogram (EEG) microarousals	Benzodiazepines
Hypersomnia disorders related to a physical condition	Obstructive sleep apnea syndrome	Mixed or obstructive apneas, EEG microarousals, and electrocardiogram arrhythmias	Weight loss, continuous positive airway pressure, and surgery
	Narcolepsy	Repeated sleep-onset REM periods (multiple sleep latency test)	Stimulants (e.g., methyl-phenidate) and tricyclic antidepressants for cataplexy
Insomnia related to a physical condition, (e.g., sleep apnea)	Central sleep apnea syndrome	Central sleep apneas and microarousals	Continuous positive airway pressure and low-flow oxygen
Sleep-wake schedule disorder, delayed type	Delayed sleep phase syndrome	Normal sleep 4–6 hours later than conventional	Chronotherapy
Parasomnias	Parasomnias	Partial arousal out of slow-wave sleep	Various: behavioral or pharmacological
Dyssomnias related to a mental condition (e.g., major depression)	Sleep disorders associated with mood disorders	Short REM latency, prolonged first REM period, and increased rapid eye movements	Pharmacotherapy and/or psychotherapy for depression (with or without adjunctive benzodiazepines)

Note. DSM-III-R = Diagnostic and Statistical Manual of Mental Disorders, 3rd Edition, Revised (American Psychiatric Association 1987); ICSD = International Classification of Sleep Disorders (American Sleep Disorders Association Diagnostic Classification Steering Committee 1990); REM = rapid eye movement.
Source. Adapted from Reynolds and Kupfer 1988.

relaxation can be helpful. Success depends on a high degree of motivation from patients who must devote considerable time to practicing these techniques. Biofeedback can be helpful in those patients who are not sensitive to their internal state of arousal (Hauri and Esther 1990). Patients are provided an external measure of a biological variable such as EMG or EEG, allowing them a means to influence their own level of arousal.

Stimulus control behavior modification is focused on eliminating environmental cues associated with arousal (Bootzin 1972). This technique is similar to implementing rules for sleep hygiene in that patients are instructed to restrict the use of their bed for sleep and intimacy, to go to bed only when sleepy, to remove clocks from sight, and to adhere to a stable sleep-wake schedule. The goal is to limit the amount of wake time spent in bed, thereby reestablishing the association between the bed and sleep.

Sleep restriction therapy is similarly aimed at reducing the amount of wake time spent in bed (Spielman et al. 1987). Patients are asked to record in a sleep diary the amount of time they estimate they are asleep. They are then instructed to restrict their time in bed commensurate to their estimate of their total sleep time. Patients often have their usual difficulties with sleep fragmentation during the first few nights and become sleep deprived. Sleep deprivation helps consolidate sleep on subsequent nights, thereby improving sleep efficiency. Increases in length of time in bed can subsequently be titrated to the presence of daytime fatigue.

Most sleep clinicians are reluctant to prescribe sedative-hypnotics for patients with chronic insomnia. The brief use of short–half-life benzodiazepines is an effective and benign treatment for the occasional difficult night in young or middle-aged adults. Long–half-life benzodiazepines have been found to impair daytime performance, whereas those with a short half-life are relatively free of daytime "hangover" effects (Johnson and Chernik 1982). Benzodiazepines are not well tolerated in geriatric patients because of cognitive side effects, daytime somnolence, and potentiation of sleep-disordered breathing. In this group, the use of 25–50 mg of trazodone or 20–75 mg of nortriptyline can be quite effective (Reynolds et al. 1987). In younger adults, low-dose amitriptyline is effective and less liable for the development of tolerance compared with benzodiazepines.

Finally, in some nonapneic, nongeriatric patients with chronic insomnia, who have not responded to the interventions mentioned above, the long-term use of benzodiazepines is indicated. Although chronic use of these medications can reduce delta sleep and increase the number of brief arousals, some patients derive long-term benefit without any significant daytime impairment. Rebound insomnia after drug withdrawal, particularly with short–half-life benzodiazepines, is well described and represents an abstinence syndrome (Roehrs et al. 1986). However, with well-motivated patients, this can be easily managed. As has recently been suggested by the American Psychiatric Associations Task Force on benzodiazepines, the abuse potential for these drugs, albeit real, has probably been overstated in the past decade (American Psychiatric Association 1990).

❑ REFERENCES

Aldrich MS: Cardinal manifestations of sleep disorders, in Principles and Practice of Sleep Medicine. Edited by Fryger MN, Roth T, Dement WC. Philadelphia, PA, WB Saunders, 1989, pp 313–319

American Psychiatric Association: Diagnostic and Statistical Manual of Mental Disorders, 3rd Edition, Revised. Washington, DC, American Psychiatric Association, 1987

American Psychiatric Association: Treatment of Psychiatric Disorders: A Task Force Report of the American Psychiatric Association, Vol 3. Washington, DC, American Psychiatric Association, 1989, pp 2419–2453

American Psychiatric Association: Benzodiazepine Dependence, Toxicity, and Abuse: Task Force Report. Washington, DC, American Psychiatric Association, 1990

American Sleep Disorders Association Diagnostic Classification Steering Committee: International Classification of Sleep Disorders: Diagnostic and Coding Manual. Rochester, MN, American Sleep Disorders Association, 1990

Ancoli-Israel S, Kripke DF, Mason W: Characteristics of obstructive and central sleep apnea in the elderly: an interim report. Biol Psychiatry 22:741–750, 1987

April RS: Observations on parkinsonian tremor in all-night sleep. Neurology (NY) 16:720–724, 1966

Aserinsky E, Kleitman N: Regularly occurring periods of eye motility and concomitant phenomena during sleep. Science 118:273–274, 1953

Association of Sleep Disorders Centers and the Association for the Psychophysiological Study of Sleep: Diagnostic classification of sleep and arousal disorders. Sleep 2:1–137, 1979

Bergonzi P, Chiurulla C, Cianchetti C, et al: Clinical pharmacology as an approach to the study of biochemical sleep mechanisms: the action of L-dopa. Confin Neurol 36:5–22, 1974

Berry DT, Webb WE, Block AJ, et al: Nocturnal hypoxia and neuropsychological variables. J Clin Exp Neuropsychol 8:229–238, 1986

Billiard M: The Kleine-Levin syndrome, in Principles and Practices of Sleep Medicine. Edited by Kryger MH, Roth T, Dement WC. Philadelphia, PA, WB Saunders, 1989, pp 377–378

Bixler EO, Kales A, Soldatos CR, et al: Prevalence of sleep disorders in the Los Angeles metropolitan area. Am J Psychiatry 136:1257–1262, 1979

Bootzin RR: A stimulus control treatment for insomnia, in American Psychological Association Proceedings. Washington, DC, American Psychological Association, 1972, pp 395–396

Buysse DJ, Reynolds CF, Kupfer DJ, et al: Electroencephalographic sleep in depressive pseudodementia. Arch Gen Psychiatry 45:568–575, 1988

Carskadon MA, Dement WC, Mitler MM, et al: Guidelines for the Multiple Sleep Latency Test (MSLT): a standard measure of sleepiness. Sleep 9:519–524, 1986

Coleman RM, Pollack CP, Weitzman ED: Periodic movements in sleep (nocturnal myoclonus): relationship to sleep disorders. Ann Neurol 8:416–421, 1980

Coleman RM, Roflwarg HP, Kennedy SJ, et al: Sleep-wake disorders based on a polysomnographic diagnosis: A national cooperative study. JAMA 247:997–1003, 1982

Critchley M: Periodic hypersomnia and megaphagia in adolescent males. Brain 59:494–515, 1962

Czeisler CA, Allan JS: Pathologies of the sleep-wake

schedule, in Sleep Disorders: Diagnosis and Treatment, 2nd Edition. Edited by Williams RL, Karacan I, Moore CA. New York, Wiley, 1988, pp 109–129

Detre TP, Himmelhoch J, Swartzburg M, et al: Hypersomnia and manic-depressive disease. Am J Psychiatry 128:1303–1305, 1972

Feinberg I: Changes in sleep cycle patterns with age. J Psychiatr Res 10:283–306, 1974

Feinberg I: Schizophrenia: caused by a fault in programmed synaptic elimination during adolescence? J Psychiatr Res 17:319–334, 1982

Feinberg I, Hiatt JF: Sleep patterns in schizophrenia: a selective review, in Sleep Disorders: Diagnosis and Treatment. Edited by Williams RC, Karacan I. New York, Wiley, 1978, pp 205–231

Feinberg I, Koresko RL, Heller: EEG sleep patterns as a function of normal and pathological aging in man. J Psychiatr Res 5:107–144, 1967

Ford DE, Kamerow DB: Epidemiologic study of sleep disturbances and psychiatric disorders: an opportunity for prevention? JAMA 262:1479–1484, 1989

Foutz AS, Mitler MM, Cavalli-Sforza LL, et al: Genetic factors in canine narcolepsy. Sleep 1:413–422, 1979

Fredrickson PA, Richardson JW, Esther MS, et al: Sleep disorders in psychiatric practice. Mayo Clin Proc 65: 861–868, 1990

Ganguli R, Reynolds CF, Kupfer DJ: Electroencephalographic sleep in young, never medicated, schizophrenics: a comparison with delusional and nondelusional depressives and with healthy controls. Arch Gen Psychiatry 44:36–44, 1987

Gelineau J: De la narcolepsie. Gaz des Hop (Paris) 53:626–628, 1880

Giles DE, Roffwarg HP, Schlesser MA, et al: Which endogenous depressive symptoms relate to REM latency reductions? Biol Psychiatry 21:473–482, 1986

Giles DE, Roffwarg HP, Rush AJ: REM latency concordance in depressed family members. Biol Psychiatry 22:910–924, 1987a

Giles DE, Jarrett RB, Roffwarg HP, et al: Reduced rapid eye movement latency: a predictor of recurrence in depression. Neuropsychopharmacology 1:33–39, 1987b

Giles DE, Biggs MM, Rush AJ, et al: Risk factors in families of unipolar depression, I: psychiatric illness and reduced REM latency. J Affective Disord 14:51–59, 1988

Gill B: Lindbergh Alone. New York, Harcourt Brace Jovanovich, 1977

Guilleminault C: Sleep and breathing, in Sleep and Waking. Edited by Guilleminault C. Menlo Park, CA, Addison-Wesley, 1982, pp 155–182

Guilleminault C, Riley RW, Poweli NB: Surgical treatment of obstructive sleep apnea, in Principles and Practices of Sleep Medicine. Edited by Kryger MH, Roth T, Dement WC. Philadelphia, PA, WB Saunders, 1989, pp 571–583

Hardie RJ, Efthimiou J, Stern GM: Respiration and sleep in Parkinson's disease. J Neurol Neurosurg Psychiatry 49:1326, 1986

Hauri P: Primary insomnia, in Treatment of Psychiatric Disorders: A Task Force Report of the American Psychiatric Association, Vol 3. Washington, DC, American Psychiatric Association, 1989, pp 2424–2433

Hauri PJ, Esther MS: Insomnia. Mayo Clin Proc 65:869–882, 1990

Hauri P, Fisher J: Persistent psychophysiologic (learned) insomnia. Sleep 9:38–53, 1986

Hauri P, Olmstead P: Childhood-onset insomnia. Sleep 3:59–65, 1980

Hauri P, Orr WC: The Sleep Disorders: A Current Concepts Monograph. Kalamazoo, MI, Upjohn, 1982

Hauri P, Chernik D, Hawkins D, et al: Sleep of depressed patients in remission. Arch Gen Psychiatry 31:386–391, 1974

Hoch CC, Reynolds CF, Kupfer DJ, et al: Sleep disordered breathing in normal and pathologic aging. J Clin Psychiatry 47:498–503, 1986

Hoch CC, Reynolds CF, Houck PR, et al: Predicting mortality in mixed depression and dementia using sleep EEG variables. Journal of Neuropsychiatry and Clinical Neurosciences 1:366–371, 1989

Hochli D, Riemann D, Zulley J, et al: Initial REM sleep suppression by clomipramine: a prognostic tool for treatment response in patients with a major depressive disorder. Biol Psychiatry 21:1217–1220, 1986

Horne JA: Sleep function, with particular reference to sleep deprivation. Ann Clin Res 17:199–208, 1985

Huttenlocher PR: Synaptic density in human frontal cortex: developmental changes and effects of aging. Brain Res 163:195–205, 1979

Institute of Medicine: Report of a Study: Sleeping Pills, Insomnia and Medical Practice. Washington, DC, U.S. National Academy of Medical Sciences, 1979

Janz D: The grand mal epilepsies and the sleeping-waking cycle. Epilepsia 3:69–109, 1962

Jasper NH: The ten-twenty electrode system of the International Federation. Electroencephalogr Clin Neurophysiol 10:371–375, 1958

Johnson LC, Chernik DA: Sedative-hypnotics and human performance. Psychopharmacology 76:101–113, 1982

Juji T, Satake M, Honda Y, et al: HIA antigens in Japanese patients with narcolepsy. Tissue Antigens 24:316–319, 1984

Karacan I: Parasomnias, in Sleep Disorder: Diagnosis and Treatment, 2nd Edition. Edited by Williams RL, Karacan I, Moore CA. New York, Wiley, 1988, pp 131–144

Keshavan MS, Reynolds CF, Kupfer KJ: Electroencephalographic sleep in schizophrenia: a critical review. Compr Psychiatry 30:34–47, 1990

Kupfer DJ, Ehlers CL: Two roads to rapid eye movement latency. Arch Gen Psychiatry 46:945–948, 1989

Kupfer DJ, Foster FG: Interval between onset of sleep and rapid-eye-movement sleep as an indicator of depression. Lancet 2:684–686, 1972

Kupfer DJ, Reynolds CF: Sleep and affective disorders, in Handbook of Affective Disorders, 2nd Edition. Edited by Paykel ES. London, Churchill-Livingstone (in press)

Kupfer DJ, Foster FG, Reich L, et al: EEG sleep changes as predictors in depression. Am J Psychiatry 133:622–626, 1976

Kupfer DJ, Frank E, Grochocinski VJ, et al: Electroencephalographic sleep profiles in recurrent depression: a longitudinal investigation. Arch Gen Psychiatry 45:678–681, 1988

Langdon N, Lock C, Welsh K, et al: Immune factors in narcolepsy. Sleep 9:143–148, 1986

Lugaresi E, Coccagna G, Mantovani M, et al: Some periodic phenomenon arising during drowsiness and sleep in man. Electroencephalogr Clin Neurophysiol 32:701–705, 1972

Lugaresi E, Ciriguotta F, Montagna P: Nocturnal paroxysmal dystonia. J Neurol Neurosurg Psychiatry 49: 375–380, 1986

Mahowald MW, Schenck CH: REM sleep behavior disorder, in Principles and Practices of Sleep Medicine. Edited by Kryger MH, Roth T, Dement WC. Philadelphia, PA, WB Saunders, 1989, pp 389–409

Mellman TA, Uhde TW: Electroencephalographic sleep in panic disorder. Arch Gen Psychiatry 46:178–184, 1989

Mendelson WB: Human Sleep: Research and Clinical Care. New York, Plenum Medical, 1987

Miles LM, Raynal DM, Wilson MA: Blind man living in normal society has circadian rhythms of 24.9 hours. Science 198:421–423, 1977

Mitler MM, Gujavarty KS, Browman CP: Maintenance of wakefulness test: a polysomnographic technique for evaluating treatment efficacy in patients with excessive somnolence. Electroencephalogr Clin Neurophysiol 53:658–661, 1982

Monk TH: Traffic accident increases as a possible indicant of desynchronosis. Chronobiologica 7:527–529, 1980

Monk TH: Shift work, in Principles and Practices of Sleep Medicine. Edited by Kryger MH, Roth T, Dement WC. Philadelphia, PA, WB Saunders, 1989, pp 332–337

Moore RY, Eichler VB: Loss of a circadian adrenal corticosterone rhythm following suprachiasmatic lesions in the rat. Brain Res 42:201–206, 1972

Neylan TC, van Kammen DP, Kelley ME, et al: Sleep in schizophrenic patients on and off haloperidol: clinically stable versus relapse patients. Arch Gen Psychiatry (in press)

Orzack MN, Hartmann EL, Kornetsky C: The relationship between attention and slow wave sleep in chronic schizophrenia. Psychopharm Bull 13:59–61, 1977

Parmeggiani PL: Temperature regulation during sleep: a study in homeostasis, in Physiology in Sleep. Edited by Orem J, Barnes CD. New York, Academic, 1980, pp 98–143

Rechtschaffen A, Kales A (eds): A Manual of Standardized Terminology, Techniques, and Scoring System for Sleep Stages of Human Subjects. Bethesda, MD, U.S. Department of Health, Education, and Welfare, Public Health Service, 1968

Rechtschaffen A, Wolpert EA, Dement WC, et al: Nocturnal sleep of narcoleptics. Electroencephalogr Clin Neurophysiol 15:599–609, 1963

Rechtschaffen A, Bergmann BM, Everson CA, et al: Sleep deprivation in the rat, X: integration and discussion of the findings. Sleep 12:68–87, 1989

Regestein QR: Specific effects of sedative/hypnotic drugs in the treatment of incapacitating chronic insomnia. Am J Med 83:909–916, 1987

Reivich M, Isaacs G, Evarts E, et al: The effect of slow wave sleep and REM sleep on regional cerebral blood flow in cats. J Neurochem 15:301–306, 1968

Reynolds CF: Sleep in dementia, in Principles and Practices of Sleep Medicine. Edited by Kryger MH, Roth T, Dement WC. Philadelphia, PA, WB Saunders, 1989, pp 415–416

Reynolds CF, Kupfer DJ: Sleep research in affective illness: State of the art circa 1987. Sleep 10:199–215, 1987

Reynolds CF, Kupfer DJ: Sleep disorders, in American Psychiatric Press Textbook of Psychiatry. Edited by Talbott JA, Hales RE, Yudofsky SC. Washington, DC, American Psychiatric Press, 1988, pp 737–752

Reynolds CF, Black RS, Coble PA, et al: Similarities in EEG sleep findings for Kleine-Levin syndrome and unipolar depression. Am J Psychiatry 137:116–118, 1980

Reynolds CF, Shaw DH, Newton TF, et al: EEG sleep in generalized anxiety disorder: a preliminary comparison with primary depression. Psychiatry Res 8:81–89, 1983a

Reynolds CF, Christiansen CL, Taska IS, et al: Sleep in narcolepsy and depression: does it all look alike? J Nerv Ment Dis 171:290–295, 1983b

Reynolds CF, Kupfer DJ, Christiansen CL, et al: Multiple sleep latency test findings in Kleine-Levin syndrome. J Nerv Ment Dis 172:41–44, 1984

Reynolds CF, Kupfer DJ, Taska IS, et al: EEG sleep in elderly depressed, demented and healthy subjects. Biol Psychiatry 20:431–442, 1985a

Reynolds CF, Kupfer DJ, Taska LS, et al: Sleep apnea in Alzheimer's dementia: correlation with mental deterioration. J Clin Psychiatry 46:257–261, 1985b

Reynolds CF, Perel JM, Kupfer DJ, et al: Open-trial response to antidepressant treatment in elderly patients with mixed depression and and cognitive impairment. Psychiatry Res 21:95–109, 1987

Reynolds CF, Hoch CC, Monk TH: Sleep and chronobiologic disturbances in the late life, in Geriatric Psychiatry. Edited by Busse EW, Blazer DG. Washington, DC, American Psychiatric Press, 1989a, pp 475–488

Reynolds CF, Perel JM, Frank E, et al: Open-trial maintenance nortriptyline in late-life depression: survival analysis and preliminary data on the use of REM latency as a predictor of recurrence. Psychopharmacol Bull 25:129–132, 1989b

Richardson JW: Mayo sleep disorders update. Mayo Clin Proc 65:857–860, 1990

Richardson JW, Fredrickson PA, Siong-Chi L: Narcolepsy update. Mayo Clin Proc 65:991–998, 1990

Roehrs T, Jorick NJ, Wittig RM, et al: Dose determinants of rebound insomnia. Br J Clin Pharmacol 22:143–147, 1986

Roehrs T, Zorick F, Wittig R, et al: Predictors of objective level of daytime sleepiness in patients with sleep-related breathing disorders. Chest 95:1202–1206, 1989

Ross RI, Ball WA, Sullivan KA, et al: Sleep disturbance as the hallmark of posttraumatic stress disorder. Am J Psychiatry 146:697–707, 1989

Rusak B, Zucker I: Neural regulation of circadian rhythms. Physiology Review 59:449–526, 1979

Rush AJ, Erman MK, Giles DE, et al: Polysomnographic findings in recently drug free and clinically remitted depressed patients. Arch Gen Psychiatry 43:878–884, 1986

Sack RL, Stevenson J, Lewy AJ: Entrainment of a previously free-running blind human with melatonin administration. Sleep Research 19:80, 1990

Sanford JRA: Tolerance of debility in elderly dependents by supports at home: significance for hospital practice. Br Med J 3:471–473, 1975

Shouse MN: Epilepsy and seizures during sleep, in Principles and Practices of Sleep Medicine. Edited by Kryger MH, Roth T, Dement WC. Philadelphia, PA, WB Saunders, 1989, pp 364–376

Sitaram N, Gillin JC, Bunney WE Jr: Cholinergic and catecholaminergic receptor sensitivity in affective illness: strategy and theory, in Neurobiology of Mood Disorders. Edited by Post RM, Ballenger JC. Baltimore, MD, Williams & Wilkins, 1984, pp 629–651

Smirne S, Come G, Franceschi M, et al: Sleep in presenile dementia, in Communications in EEG. International Federation of Societies for Electroencephalography and Clinical Neurophysiology, 9th Congress, 521–522, E271, 1977

Smith M, Colligan M: Health and safety consequences of shift work in the food processing industry. Ergonomics 25:133–144, 1982

Smith RC: Relationship of periodic movements in sleep (nocturnal myoclonus) and the Babinski sign. Sleep 8: 239–243, 1985

Spielman AJ, Saskin P, Thorpy MJ: Treatment of chronic insomnia by restriction of time in bed. Sleep 10:45–56, 1987

Spiker DG, Coble P, Cofsky J, et al: EEG sleep and severity of depression. Biol Psychiatry 13:485–488, 1978

Sterman MB, Shouse MN: Sleep centers in the brain: the preoptic basal forebrain area revisited, in Brain Mechanisms of Sleep. Edited by McGinty DJ, Drucker-Colin R, Morrison A, et al. New York, Raven, 1985, pp 277–299

Tandon R, Shipley JE, Eiser AS, et al: Association between abnormal REM sleep and negative symptoms in schizophrenia. Psychiatry Res 27:359–361, 1988

Thaker GK, Wagman AM, Kirkpatrick B, et al: Alterations in sleep polygraphy after neuroleptic withdrawal: a putative supersensitive dopaminergic mechanism. Biol Psychiatry 25:75–86, 1989

Thase ME, Kupfer DJ, Spiker DG: EEG sleep in secondary depression: a revisit. Biol Psychiatry 19:805–814, 1984

Thase ME, Kupfer KJ, Ulrich RF: EEG sleep in psychotic depression: a valid subtype? Arch Gen Psychiatry 43:886–893, 1986

van Kammen DP, van Kammen WB, Peters J, et al: Decreased slow-wave sleep and enlarged lateral ventricles in schizophrenia. Neuropsychopharmacology 1:265–271, 1988

Vitiello MV, Prinz PN: Aging and sleep disorders, in Sleep Disorders: Diagnosis and Treatment 2nd Edition. Edited by Williams RL, Karacan I, Moore CA. New York, Wiley, 1988, pp 293–312

Vogel GW, Thurmond A, Gibbons P, et al: REM sleep reduction effects on depressive syndromes. Arch Gen Psychiatry 32:765–777, 1975

Wu JC, Bunney WE: The biological basis of an antidepressant response to sleep deprivation and relapse: review and hypothesis. Am J Psychiatry 147:14–21, 1990

Zarcone VP: Sleep and schizophrenia, in Sleep Disorders: Diagnosis and Treatment, 2nd Edition. Edited by Williams RL, Karacan I, Moore CA. New York, Wiley, 1988, pp 165–188

Zarcone VP, Benson KL, Berger PA: Abnormal rapid eye movement latencies in schizophrenia. Arch Gen Psychiatry 44:45–48, 1987

Chapter

19

Neuropsychiatric Aspects of Cerebral Vascular Disorders

Sergio E. Starkstein, M.D., Ph.D.
Robert G. Robinson, M.D.

CEREBROVASCULAR DISEASE represents one of the major health problems in the United States, with an estimated annual incidence for thromboembolic stroke between 300,000 and 400,000 (Wolf et al. 1977). During the past 10 years, however, there has been a steady decline in the incidence of stroke, which is presumed to be related to the improved control of hypertension. Nevertheless, stroke remains the third leading cause (behind heart disease and cancer) of mortality and morbidity in the United States.

The neuropsychiatric complications of cerebrovascular disease include a wide range of emotional and cognitive disturbances. Although studies providing empirical data about individual neuropsychiatric disorders and their relationship to specific types of cerebrovascular disease have begun to emerge only within the last few years, these kinds of investigations are essential before we will have a firm empirical data base for our understanding of the clinical manifestations, treatments, and mechanisms of these disorders.

One of the confounding factors in our understanding of neuropsychiatric disorders associated with cerebrovascular disease is the tendency of investigators to intermix different types of brain disorders when studying emotional problems in patients with brain injury. For example, the early work

This work was supported in part by National Institutes of Mental Health Grants Research Scientist Award MH00163 (to RGR), MH40355, and NS15080; a grant from the National Alliance for the Research on Schizophrenia and Depression Young Investigator Award (to SES), and a grant from the Institute of Neurological Investigation "Dr. Raul Carrea," Buenos Aires, Argentina (to SES). The authors thank Thomas R. Price, John R. Lipsey, Rajesh Parikh, Kenneth L. Kubos, Krishna Rao, and Godfrey D. Pearlson, Lynn Book Starr, and Paula Andrezewski who participated in many of the studies described.

of Babinski (1914) or Denny-Brown et al. (1952), as well as the systematic study of emotional disorders in patients with brain injury by Gainotti (1972), included patients with various types of brain injuries such as traumatic closed head injury, penetrating head injury, thromboembolic stroke, surgical incision, and intracerebral hemorrhage (ICH). Although it is generally assumed that neuronal death produced by a variety of mechanisms will result in similar clinical symptoms, depending on the size and location of the lesion, that is not necessarily the case. Moreover, it is rare that two conditions producing brain injury will result in identical types of lesions. For example, closed head injury generally produces widespread brain injury with multiple small areas of shear or torsion injury, whereas cerebral embolism produces a focal lesion with an area of transient peripheral ischemia. Thus much of the early information about emotional disorders associated with cerebrovascular disease must draw on data obtained from a heterogeneous group of patients, some of whom had cerebrovascular disease and others of whom did not.

We have organized this chapter into four sections: the historical development of concepts in neuropsychiatry related to cerebrovascular disease, the classification of types of cerebrovascular disease, the description and classification of clinical psychiatric disorders associated with cerebrovascular disease, and a more in-depth discussion of the syndromes of depression, mania, and anxiety for which the most empirical data are available.

❑ HISTORICAL PERSPECTIVE

The first reports of emotional reactions following brain damage (usually caused by cerebrovascular disease) were made by neurologists and psychiatrists in case descriptions. Meyer (1904) proposed a relationship between traumatic insanities and specific locations and causes of brain injury. Babinski (1914) noted that patients with right-hemisphere disease frequently displayed the symptoms of anosognosia, euphoria, and indifference. Bleuler (1951) wrote that after stroke "melancholic moods lasting for months and sometimes longer appear frequently" (p. 230). Kraepelin (1921) recognized an association between manic depressive insanity and cerebrovascular disease when he wrote

> The diagnosis of states of depression may, apart from the distinctions discussed, offer difficulties especially when the possibility of arteriosclerosis has to be taken into consideration. It may, at a time, be an accompanying phenomenon of manic depressive disease, but at another time may itself engender states of depression. (p. 271)

The emotional symptoms associated with brain injury have frequently been attributed to the existence of aphasia (Benson 1976). In the middle of the 19th century, Broca (1861) localized the process of speech to the inferior left frontal lobe and deduced that the left brain was endowed with different functions than the right brain. Hughlings-Jackson (1915) regarded language as an extension of brain function existing in two basic forms: the intellectual (conveying content) and the emotional (expressing feeling). He suggested that these components may be separated by disease.

Goldstein (1939) was the first to describe an emotional disorder thought to be uniquely associated with brain disease: the catastrophic reaction. The catastrophic reaction is an emotional outburst involving various degrees of anger, frustration, depression, tearfulness, refusal, shouting, swearing, and sometimes aggressive behavior. Goldstein ascribed this reaction to the inability of the organism to cope when faced with a serious defect in its physical or cognitive functions. In his extensive studies of brain injuries in war, Goldstein (1942) described two symptom clusters: those related directly to physical damage of a circumscribed area of the brain and those related secondarily to the organism's psychological response to injury. Emotional symptoms, therefore, represented the latter category (i.e., the psychological response of an organism struggling with physical or cognitive impairments).

A second emotional abnormality, also thought to be characteristic of brain injury, was the indifference reaction described by Hecean et al. (1951) and Denny-Brown et al. (1952). The indifference reaction, associated with right-hemisphere lesions, consists of symptoms of indifference toward failures, lack of interest in family and friends, enjoyment of foolish jokes, and minimization of physical difficulties.

A third emotional disorder that has been historically associated with brain injury, such as cerebral infarction, is pathological laughter or crying. Ironside (1956) described the clinical manifestations of this disorder. Patients' emotional displays are characteristically unrelated to their inner emotional state. Crying for example may occur spontaneously or after some seemingly minor provocation. This phenomenon has been given various names, such as emotional incontinence, emotional lability, pseudobulbar affect, or pathological emotionalism. Some investigators have differentiated the pseudobulbar disorder in which there are bilateral brain lesions and subjective feelings of being forced to laugh or cry from emotional lability in which there is an easy and sometimes rapid vacillation between laughter and crying. These disorders, however, have never been systematically examined or divided into subcategories based on reliable features such as a characteristic clinical presentation, etiology, or response to treatment.

The first systematic study to contrast the emotional reactions of patients with right- and left-hemisphere brain damage was done by Gainotti (1972). He reported that catastrophic reactions were more frequent among 80 patients with left-hemisphere brain damage, particularly those with aphasia, than were indifference reactions, which occurred more frequently among 80 patients with right-hemisphere brain damage. The indifference reaction was also associated with neglect for the opposite half of the body and space. Gainotti agreed with Goldstein's explanation (1942) of the catastrophic reaction: the desperate reaction of the organism confronted with severe physical disability. The indifference reaction, on the other hand, was not as easy to understand. Gainotti suggested that denial of illness and disorganization of the nonverbal type of synthesis may have been responsible for this emotional symptom.

Despite the assertions by Meyer (1904) and others (e.g., Post 1962) that emotional disorder may be produced directly by focal brain injury, as indicated above, many investigators have adopted "psychological" explanations for the emotional symptoms associated with brain injury. Studies examining the emotional symptoms associated specifically with cerebrovascular disease began to appear in the early 1960s. Ullman and Gruen (1960) reported that stroke was a particularly severe stress to the organism, as Goldstein (1942) had suggested, because the organ governing the emotional response to injury had itself been damaged. Adams and Hurwitz (1963) noted that discouragement and frustration caused by disability could themselves impede recovery from stroke. Fisher (1961) described depression associated with cerebrovascular disease as reactive and understandable because "the brain is the most cherished organ of humanity" (p. 379). Thus depression was viewed as a natural emotional response to a decrease in self-esteem from a life-threatening injury and the resulting disability and dependence.

Systematic studies, however, led other investigators, who were impressed by the frequency of association between brain injury and emotional disorders, to hypothesize more direct causal links. In a study of 100 elderly patients with affective disorder, Post (1962) stated that the high frequency of brain ischemia associated with first episodes of depressive disorder suggested that the causes for atherosclerosis disease and depression may be linked. Folstein et al. (1977) compared 20 stroke patients with 10 orthopedic patients. Although the functional disability in both groups was comparable, more of the stroke patients were depressed. The authors concluded that "mood disorder is a more specific complication of stroke than simply a response to motor disability" (p. 1018). Finklestein et al. (1981) found that depression and failure to suppress serum cortisol after dexamethasone administration were more common among 25 randomly selected stroke patients than among a group of 13 control patients with equally disabling medical illnesses.

In conclusion, there have been two primary lines of thought in the study of emotional disorders that are associated with cerebrovascular disease. One attributes emotional disorders to an understandable psychological reaction to the associated impairment; the other, based on a lack of association between severity of impairment and severity of emotional disorder, suggests a direct causal connection between cerebrovascular disease and neuropsychiatric disorder.

❑ CLASSIFICATION OF CEREBROVASCULAR DISEASE

There are many ways to classify the wide range of disorders that comprise the spectrum of cerebrovascular disease. On the one hand, cerebrovascular disease can be understood as an anatomic-pathological process of the blood vessels that perfuse the central nervous system. This leads to a classification based on the etiologies of underlying anatomic-pathological processes. Such a classification would include an extensive list of diseases, including infectious, connective tissue, neoplastic, hematologic, pharmacological, and traumatic causes. Alternatively, one could examine the mechanisms by which these pathological processes manifested themselves: for example, the interactive effects of systemic hypertension and atherosclerosis on the resilience of large arteries, integrity of vessel lumens, and production of end-organ ischemia; the formation of aneurysmal dilatations or vascular disease; or the effect of cardiac arrhythmias on the propagation of thromboemboli.

From the perspective of schematizing the neuropsychiatric complications of cerebrovascular disease, however, probably the most pragmatic way of classifying cerebrovascular disease is not to focus on the anatomic-pathological process or the interactive mechanisms but to examine the means by which parenchymal changes in the brain occur. The first of these, ischemia, may occur either with or without infarction of parenchyma, and includes transient ischemic attacks (TIAs), atherosclerotic thrombosis, cerebral embolism, and hemorrhage. The last of these, hemorrhage, may cause either direct parenchymal damage by extravasation of blood into the surrounding brain tissue, as in ICH, or indirect damage by hemorrhage into the ventricles, subarachnoid space, extradural area, or subdural area. These changes result in a common mode of expression, defined by Adams and Victor (1985) as a sudden, convulsive, focal neurological deficit—or stroke.

Expanding slightly on this categorization (i.e., the means by which parenchymal changes occur), there are four major categories of cerebrovascular disease (Table 19–1). These include atherosclerotic thrombosis, cerebral embolism, lacunae, and intracranial hemorrhage. In various studies of the incidence of cerebrovascular disease (e.g., Wolf et al. 1977), the ratio of infarcts to hemorrhages has been shown to be about 5:1. Atherosclerotic thrombosis and cerebral embolism each account for approximately one-third of all stroke.

Atherosclerotic Thrombosis

Atherosclerotic thrombosis is often the result of a dynamic interaction between hypertension and atherosclerotic deposition of hyaline-lipid material in the walls of peripheral, coronary, and cerebral arteries. Risk factors in the development of atherosclerosis include hyperlipidemia, diabetes mellitus, hypertension, and cigarette smoking. Atheromatous plaques tend to propagate at the branchings and curves of the internal carotid artery or the carotid sinus, in the cervical part of the vertebral arteries and their junction to form the basilar artery, in the posterior cerebral arteries as they wind around the midbrain, and in the anterior cerebral arteries as they curve over the corpus callosum. These plaques may lead to stenosis of one or more of these cerebral arteries or to complete occlusion. TIAs, defined as periods of transient focal ischemia associated with reversible neurological deficits, almost always indicate that a thrombotic process is occurring. Only rarely is embolism or ICH preceded by transient neurological deficits. Thrombosis of virtually any cerebral or cerebellar artery can be associated with TIAs.

TABLE 19–1. CLASSIFICATION OF CEREBROVASCULAR DISEASE

Ischemic phenomena (85%)
- Infarction
  - Atherosclerotic thrombosis
  - Cerebral embolism
  - Lacunae
  - Other causes (arteritis [e.g., infectious or connective tissue disease], cerebral thrombophlebitis, fibromuscular dysplasia, and venous occlusions)
- Transient ischemic attacks

Hemorrhagic phenomena (15%)
- Intraparenchymal hemorrhage
  - Primary (hypertensive) intracerebral hemorrhage
  - Other causes (hemorrhagic disorders [e.g., thrombocytopenia and clotting disorders] and trauma)
- Subarachnoid or intraventricular hemorrhage
  - Ruptured saccular aneurysm or arteriovenous malformation
  - Other causes
- Subdural or epidural hematoma

TIAs, therefore, although not listed among the main causes of stroke, may precede, accompany, or follow the development of stroke or may occur by themselves without leading to complete occlusion of a cerebral or cerebellar artery. Most commonly, TIAs have a duration of 2–15 minutes, with a range from a few seconds to up to 12–24 hours. Whereas the neurological examination between successive episodes of this thrombotic process is entirely normal, the permanent neurological deficits of atherosclerotic thrombosis indicate that infarction has occurred. The progression of events leading to the completed thrombotic stroke, however, can be quite variable.

Cerebral Embolism

Cerebral embolism, which similarly accounts for approximately one-third of all strokes, is usually caused by a fragment breaking away from a thrombus within the heart and travelling up the carotid artery. Less commonly, the source of the embolism may be from an atheromatous plaque within the lumen of the carotid sinus or from the distal end of a thrombus within the internal carotid artery, or it may represent a fat, tumor, or air embolus within the internal carotid artery. The causes of thrombus formation within the heart can include cardiac arrhythmias, congenital heart disease, infectious processes (e.g., syphilitic heart disease, rheumatic valvular disease, and endocarditis), valve prostheses, postsurgical complications, or myocardial infarction with mural thrombus. Of all strokes, those due to cerebral embolism develop most rapidly. In general, there are no warning episodes; embolism can occur at any time. A large embolus may occlude the internal carotid artery or the stem of the middle cerebral artery producing a severe hemiplegia. More often, however, the embolus is smaller and passes into one of the branches of the middle cerebral artery, producing infarction distal to the site of arterial occlusion, characterized by a pattern of neurological deficits consistent with that vascular distribution, or producing a transient neurological deficit that resolves as the embolus fragments and travels into smaller, more distal arteries.

Lacunae

Lacunae, accounting for nearly one-fifth of strokes, are the result of occlusion of small penetrating cerebral arteries. They are infarcts that may be so small as to produce no recognizable deficits, or, depending on their location, they may be associated with pure motor or sensory deficits. There is a strong association between lacunae and both atherosclerosis and hypertension, suggesting that lacunar infarction is the result of the extension of the atherosclerotic process into small diameter vessels.

Hemorrhage

Intracranial hemorrhage is the fourth most frequent cause of stroke. The main causes of intracranial hemorrhage that present as acute strokes include ICH, usually associated with hypertension; rupture of saccular aneurysms or arteriovenous malformations (AVMs); a variety of hemorrhagic disorders of assorted etiology; and trauma producing hemorrhage. Primary (hypertensive) ICH occurs within the brain tissue. The extravasation of blood forms a roughly circular or oval-shaped mass that disrupts and displaces the parenchyma. Adjacent tissue is compressed, and seepage into the ventricular system usually occurs, producing bloody spinal fluid in more than 90% of the cases. ICHs can range in size from massive bleeds of several centimeters in diameter to petechial hemorrhages of a millimeter or less, most commonly occurring within the putamen, in the adjacent internal capsule, or in various portions of the white matter underlying the cortex. Hemorrhages of the thalamus, cerebellar hemispheres, or pons are also common. Severe headache is generally considered to be a constant accompaniment of ICH, but this occurs in only about 50% of cases. The prognosis for ICH is grave, with 70%–75% of patients dying within 1–30 days (Adams and Victor 1985).

Finally, there are several less common types of cerebrovascular disease. These may lead to intraparenchymal damage, but frequently bleeds on the surface of the brain (e.g., subdural hematoma) do not produce permanent parenchymal damage.

Aneurysms and AVMs

Ruptured aneurysms and AVMs are the next most common type of cerebrovascular disease after thrombosis, embolism, lacunae, and ICH. Aneurysms are usually located at arterial bifurcations and are presumed to result from developmental defects in the formation of the arterial wall; rupture occurs when the intima bulges outward and eventually breaks through the adventitia. AVMs consist of a tangle of dilated vessels that form an abnormal communication between arterial and venous systems. They are developmental abnormalities consisting of embryonic patterns of blood vessels. Most AVMs are clinically silent but will bleed ultimately. Hemorrhage from aneurysms or AVMs may occur within the subarachnoid space, leading to an identifiable presentation as a bleeding vessel anomaly, or may occur within the parenchyma, leading to hemiplegia or even death.

Subdural and Epidural Hematomas

Although it could be contended that subdural hematomas (SDH) and epidural hematomas do not represent forms of cerebrovascular disease, nonetheless their behavior as vascular space-occupying lesions that produce many of the signs and symptoms of stroke warrants a brief description here.

Chronic SDHs are frequently (60%), but not exclusively, caused by head trauma, followed by a gradual progression of signs and symptoms during the subsequent days to weeks. Traumatic chronic SDH may be caused by tears of bridging veins in the subdural space. Nontraumatic causes include ruptured aneurysms or AVMs of the pial surface or rapid deceleration injuries. The most common symptom of chronic SDH is headache, with a variety of neuropsychiatric manifestations paralleling the gradual increase in intracranial pressure, confusion, inattention, apathy, memory loss, drowsiness, and coma. Chronic SDH is also one of the many conditions in the differential diagnosis of treatable causes of dementia. Fluctuations in the level of consciousness predominate over any focal or lateralizing signs, which may include hemiparesis, hemianopsia, cranial nerve abnormalities, aphasia, or seizures. Chronic SDH may continue to expand, if left unchecked, or may reabsorb spontaneously.

Acute SDH and epidural hematomas, although frequently manifested by similar changes in level of consciousness and focal neurological deficits (as in chronic SDH), are associated with severe head trauma, may occur simultaneously or in combination with cerebral laceration or contusion, and progress rapidly over a period of a few hours to days, rather than days to weeks. Epidural hematomas usually follow a temporal or parietal skull fracture that causes a laceration or avulsion of the middle meningeal artery or vein or a tear of the dural venous sinus; acute SDH is usually caused by the avulsion of bridging veins or laceration of pial arteries. Both conditions produce loss of consciousness or a brief period of lucidity followed by a loss of consciousness, hemiparesis, cranial nerve palsies, and death, usually secondary to respiratory compromise, if the hematoma is not emergently evacuated.

Other Types of Cerebrovascular Disease

One of the other causes of cerebrovascular disease is fibromuscular dysplasia, which leads to narrowed arterial segments caused by degeneration of elastic tissue, disruption and loss of the arterial muscular coat, and an increase in fibrous tissue. Inflammatory diseases of the arterial system can also lead to stroke; these include meningovascular syphilis, pyogenic or tuberculous meningitis, temporal arteritis, and systemic lupus erythematosus.

There are many other less common causes of cerebrovascular disease that have not been cited here due to lack of space. It appears obvious, however, that examining the many causes and types of cerebrovascular disease in relation to specific neuropsychiatric disorders is a very formidable task. Studies that have compared traumatic with thromboembolic stroke, or hemorrhagic versus ischemic infarcts (Robinson and Szetela 1981; Robinson et al. 1983b), have found that the associated mood disorders are the same, depending on the size and location of the lesion and the time elapsed since injury. As indicated previously, however, the type or pattern of neuronal damage may be different, depending on the cause of the cerebrovascular disease. Resultant neuropsychiatric disorders must be systematically examined.

❑ CLINICAL PSYCHIATRIC DISORDERS ASSOCIATED WITH CEREBROVASCULAR DISEASE

Various emotional disorders have been associated with cerebrovascular disease (Table 19–2). As indicated above, Goldstein (1939) described the catastrophic reaction in the 1930s, and Hecaen et al. (1951) and Denny-Brown et al. (1952) described the indifference reaction in the early 1950s. Davison and Kelman (1939) and others have identified pathological laughing and crying. In addition, we have described two types of depressive disorders (major depression and minor depression), mania with or

least two syndromes of dementia have been identified: multi-infarct dementia (associated with cortical infarcts) and Binswanger's subcortical encephalopathy (associated with infarcts of the subcortical white matter). Space does not permit a full discussion of these interesting disorders here. (For a more in-depth discussion, see Cummings and Benson 1992.)

In summary, there are numerous emotional disorders associated with cerebrovascular disease, and they are probably intermixed to some degree (e.g., major depression and emotional lability frequently coexist). The syndromes that have been investigated, using systematic empirical studies, are detailed in the following section.

❑ SYNDROMES OF DEPRESSION, MANIA, AND ANXIETY

Poststroke Depression

By far, the most common emotional disorders associated with cerebrovascular disease are depressions, which occur in between 30% and 50% of patients after acute stroke (Robinson et al. 1983b).

Diagnosis. Although most studies of emotional disorders associated with cerebrovascular disease have not used strict diagnostic criteria (Sinyor et al. 1986b), recent studies have used structured interviews and diagnostic criteria defined by DSM-III (American Psychiatric Association 1980). DSM-III as well as the revised edition (DSM-III-R; American Psychiatric Association 1987), however, categorize all mood disorders associated with brain injury that manifest certain signs and symptoms as organic affective mood disorders. The problem with this categorization is that the diagnostic symptoms are quite nonspecific. For example, an organic mood syndrome (depressed) is diagnosed based on the existence of a prominent depressed mood, evidence of a "specific" organic factor (i.e., "judged" to be etiologically related to the disturbance), and occurrence not limited to the course of delirium. These criteria lack enough specificity to allow the study of phenomenologically different groups of poststroke depression (PSD) patients. Therefore, most recent studies (Eastwood et al. 1989; Morris et al. 1990; Robinson et al. 1983a) have used DSM-III criteria for major depressive disorder and dysthymic disorder or Research Diagnostic Criteria (RDC; Spitzer et al. 1975) for major depression and minor depression, even though an organic factor was present.

Phenomenology. Robinson and colleagues have carried out two studies examining the phenomenology of PSD. In the first (Lipsey et al. 1986), the frequency of depressive symptoms was compared between a group of 43 patients with major PSD and a group of 43 age-matched patients with "functional" (i.e., no known brain pathology) depression. The main finding was that both groups showed almost identical profiles of symptoms including symptoms that were not part of the diagnostic criteria. More than 50% of those patients who met diagnostic criteria for major PSD reported sadness, anxiety, tension, loss of interest and concentration, sleep disturbances with early morning awakening, loss of appetite with weight loss, difficulty concentrating and thinking, and thoughts of death.

In the second study (Fedoroff et al. 1991), depressive symptoms among stroke patients were assessed for their relationship to physical impairments (i.e., the frequency of depressive symptoms that were the consequence of the medical illness was compared with the frequency of depressive symptoms in depressive syndrome). Alternatively, it was also determined whether the medical condition was masking depressive symptoms that would result in a failure to diagnose depression. A consecutive series of 85 stroke patients who acknowledged the presence of a depressed mood (no other symptom was required) were compared with 120 stroke patients without a depressed mood. Groups were comparable for important variables, such as age and duration of illness. They also were comparable in terms of lesion location and volume. The study found that, except for early morning awakening, all the affective and autonomic symptoms of depression were significantly more frequent among patients with a depressed mood than among patients without a depressed mood ($P < .01$) (Figure 19–1). Moreover, the presence of nonspecific symptoms of depression (i.e., the frequency of depressive symptoms in the nondepressed group) may have led to false-positive diagnoses in only 3% of patients, and only 5% of patients had all the symptoms necessary for a diagnosis of major depression except for feelings of sadness (i.e., possible false-negative cases). Therefore, the use of DSM-III criteria in an acutely medically ill population does not appear to produce

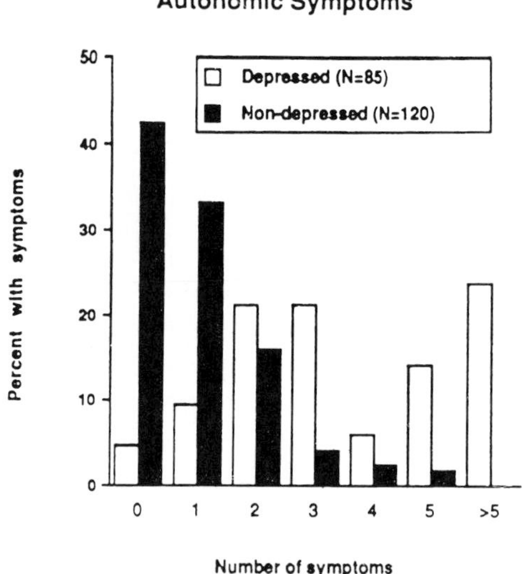

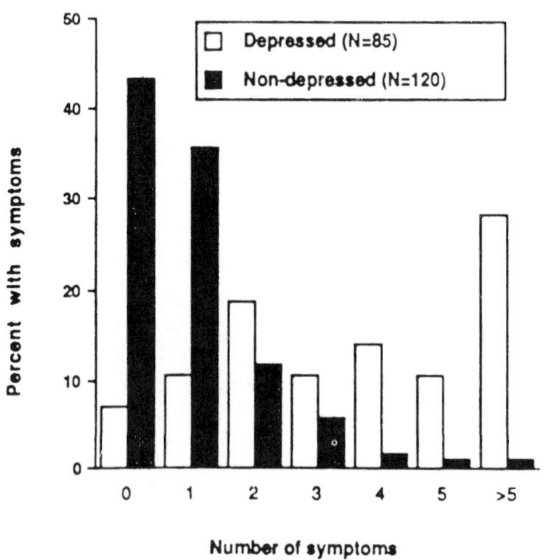

Figure 19–1. Autonomic and psychological symptoms of depression among patients with depressed mood after stroke. (Reprinted from Fedoroff UP, Starkstein SE, Parikh RM, et al: Are depressive symptoms non-specific in patients with acute stroke? Am J Psychiatry 148:1172–1176, 1991. Used with permission.)

significant numbers of false-positive or false-negative cases.

In summary, the phenomenology of depressive disorder in stroke patients appears to be virtually identical to that found in patients with functional mood disorders. In addition, the presence of an acute cerebral infarction does not appear to lead to a significant number of incorrectly diagnosed cases of depression.

Prevalence. In a study of 103 patients with acute cerebrovascular lesions, Robinson et al. (1983b) found that 26% of patients who could reliably respond to a verbal interview had the symptom cluster of major depression, and that 20% showed the symptom cluster of dysthymic depression. Others (Eastwood et al. 1989; Ebrahim and Nouri 1987; Sinyor et al. 1986b; Wade et al. 1987) have reported a similar prevalence of depression in stroke patients in a variety of settings, such as rehabilitation centers, general hospitals, and outpatient clinics.

Thus about 40%–50% of patients may develop depression within the first few months after an acute stroke. Approximately half of them will show the symptom cluster of major depression, whereas the other half will show the symptom cluster of minor depression.

Duration. At present, only two groups of investigators (Robinson and colleagues and Morris and colleagues) have examined the longitudinal course of PSD. In an outpatient stroke clinic, Robinson and Price (1982) found that almost one-third of 103 patients were depressed at the time of the initial interview. At the time of the follow-up evaluations (8–9 months after the initial evaluation), 67% of the patients who were depressed initially remained depressed. One year after the initial evaluation, however, none of the patients seen for follow-up remained depressed.

In a second longitudinal study (Robinson et al. 1987), a consecutive series of 103 acute stroke patients were prospectively studied over a 2-year course. At the time of the initial in-hospital evaluation, 26% of the patients had the symptom cluster of major depression, whereas 20% had the symptom cluster of minor depression. Although both major and minor depressive disorders lasted for prolonged periods, patients with in-hospital major depression fully recovered between 1 and 2 years poststroke. Patients with minor depression had a less favorable prognosis, with only 30% having recovered by 2 years poststroke. In addition, about 30% of patients who were not depressed in-hospital became depressed after discharge. Thus the natural course of major depression appeared to be approximately 1 year, whereas the duration of minor depression was more prolonged and in many cases fulfilled the 2-year duration requirement for dysthymic disorder.

Morris et al. (1990) found that among a group of 99 patients in a stroke rehabilitation hospital in Australia, those with major depression had a duration of major depression of 40 weeks, whereas those with adjustment disorders (minor depression) had a duration of depression of only 12 weeks. These findings confirm the approximately 1-year duration of major depression but suggest that less severe depressive disorders may be more variable in their duration.

Two factors have been identified that can influence the natural course of PSD. One is treatment of depression with antidepressant drugs (discussed below). The second factor is lesion location. In a recent study, Starkstein et al. (1988f) compared two groups of depressed patients: one group ($n = 6$) had recovered from depression by the 6th month poststroke, whereas the other group ($n = 10$) remained depressed at this time point. There were no significant between-group differences in important demographic variables, such as age, sex, and education, and both groups had similar social functioning and degree of cognitive dysfunction. There were, however, two significant between-group differences. One was lesion location: the recovered group had a higher frequency of subcortical and cerebellar/brain stem lesions; the nonrecovered group had a higher frequency of cortical lesions ($P < .01$). Impairments in activities of daily living (ADLs) were also significantly different between the two groups: the nonrecovered group had significantly more severe impairments in ADLs in-hospital than did the recovered group ($P < .01$).

In summary, the available data suggest that PSD is not a transient but a long-standing disorder with a natural course of approximately 1 year for major depression and, although perhaps more variable, a course of more than 2 years for some minor depressions. Lesion location and severity of impairments in ADLs may influence the longitudinal evolution of PSD.

Biological markers. The dexamethasone suppression test (DST; Carroll et al. 1981) has been investigated as a possible biological marker for functional melancholic depression. Several studies have demonstrated that although there is a statistical association between major PSD and failure to suppress serum cortisol in response to administration of dexamethasone, the specificity of the test is insufficient to allow it to be diagnostically useful (Finklestein et al. 1981; Lipsey et al. 1985; Olsson et al. 1989; Reding et al. 1985). For example, in a study of 65 patients whose acute strokes had occurred within the preceding year, Lipsey et al. (1985) found that 67% of the patients with major depression failed to suppress serum cortisol, compared to 25% of patients with minor depression, and 32% of nondepressed patients. The sensitivity of the DST for major depression was 67%, but the specificity was only 70%. False-positive tests, found in 30% of patients, seemed to be related to large lesion volumes. Similarly, Reding et al. (1985) reported a sensitivity of 47% and a specificity of 87%, with the more extensive strokes more likely to lead to an abnormal DST response.

A recent study by Barry and Dinan (1990) examined growth-hormone response to desipramine as a biological marker of PSD. They found that growth-hormone responses were significantly blunted in patients with PSD, suggesting that diminished α_2-adrenergic receptor function may be an important marker for PSD. The sensitivity of the test was 100%, and the specificity was 75%. Future studies may further examine the validity of the growth-hormone response to desipramine as a marker of PSD.

Relationship to lesion variables. In a study of a consecutive series of patients admitted to a hospital after the acute onset of stroke, Robinson et al. (1984) found that major or minor depression occurred in 14 of 22 patients with a left-hemisphere injury, but in only 2 of 14 patients with a right-hemisphere lesion ($\chi^2 = 9.4$, df = 1, $P < .01$). The intrahemispheric location of the lesion was also an important determinant of the presence of depression: 6 of 10 patients with left anterior (frontal) lesions had depression, as compared to 1 of 8 patients with left posterior lesions ($\chi^2 = 4.4$, df = 1, $P < .05$). Moreover, there also was a significant correlation between the distance of the anterior border of the lesion from the frontal pole and severity of depression ($r = -.92$, $P < .05$).

Three other investigators have also systematically examined the association between anterior or posterior lesion location and PSD. First, Sinyor et al. (1986b) found a significant inverse correlation between depression scores and distance of the lesion from the frontal pole for both left- and right-hemisphere lesions ($r = -.47$, $P < .05$). Thus although it was smaller, the correlation was in the same direction as that of the Robinson et al. (1984) study, but was not specific to patients with left-hemisphere lesions. Differences in demographic characteristics of the samples, the time since stroke, and the lack of standardized diagnoses in Sinyor et al.'s study may underlie the difference in results between the studies. A more comprehensive discussion of methodological factors is provided elsewhere (Robinson and Starkstein 1990).

In more recent studies, Eastwood et al. (1989) examined a consecutive series of patients with stroke lesions who had been admitted to a rehabilitation center. They found that among patients with left-hemisphere lesions, scores on a depression-rating scale were significantly correlated with the distance of the lesion to the frontal pole ($r = -.74$, $P < .01$). On the other hand, among patients with right-hemisphere lesions, depression scores were not significantly correlated with lesion location ($r = -.04$, NS). Similarly, Morris et al. (in press) found that after controlling for family history of mood disorder patients with single left-hemisphere lesions (but not with right-hemisphere lesions) showed a significant ($r = -.87$, $P < .0001$) inverse correlation between distance of the lesion from the frontal pole and severity of depression.

In summary, several studies conducted by different investigators support the hypothesis that depressive disorders after stroke are more severe the closer the lesion is to the frontal pole and that left frontal lesions are usually the most likely lesions to show this relationship. Thus the location of the lesion along the anterior-posterior dimension is an important variable in the severity of depression following stroke.

Cortical and subcortical lesions. In a recent study of 45 patients with single lesions restricted to either cortical or subcortical structures in the left or right hemisphere, Starkstein et al. (1987b) found that 44% of patients with left cortical lesions ($n = 16$) were depressed, whereas 39% of patients with left subcortical lesions ($n = 13$), 11% of patients with right cortical lesions ($n = 9$), and 14% of patients with right subcortical lesions ($n = 7$) were depressed. Thus although the frequencies of depression between patients with left cortical versus left subcortical lesions or right cortical versus right subcortical lesions were not significantly different, patients who had lesions in the left hemisphere had significantly higher rates of depression than patients with right-hemisphere lesions, regardless of the cortical or subcortical location of the lesion (χ^2 Yates = 4.0, df = 1, $P < .05$).

When patients were further divided into those with anterior lesions and posterior lesions, all five patients with left cortical lesions involving the frontal lobe had depression, as compared to 2 of the 11 patients with left cortical posterior lesions (χ^2 Yates = 6.7, df = 1, $P < .01$). Moreover, 4 of the 6 patients with left subcortical posterior lesions had depression, as compared to 1 of 7 patients with left subcortical posterior lesions. Finally, correlations between depression scores and the distance of the lesion from the frontal pole were significant for both patients with left cortical lesions ($r = -.52$, $P < .05$), and patients with left subcortical lesions ($r = -.68$, $P < .05$). These relationships were not significant for patients with right-hemisphere lesions.

In a subsequent study (Starkstein et al. 1988a), the relationship between lesions of specific subcortical nuclei and depression was examined. Basal ganglia (caudate and/or putamen) lesions produced major PSD in 7 of the 8 patients with left-sided lesions, in only 1 of 7 patients with right-sided lesions, and in none of the patients with left ($n = 6$) or right ($n = 4$) thalamic lesions ($\chi^2 = 17.0$, df = 3, $P < .001$).

In summary, the preponderance of evidence suggests that the frequency of depression is higher among patients with left anterior hemisphere lesions than among patients with right-hemisphere lesions. When other confounding factors are removed (e.g., prior lesions and family or personal history of mood disorder) left dorsal lateral frontal cortical and left basal ganglia lesions produce a similar high frequency of major depression that is greater than that for any other lesion location.

Middle cerebral circulation versus posterior circulation lesions. Starkstein et al. (1988d) compared 37 patients with posterior circulation lesions to 42 patients with middle cerebral artery lesions. Patients with posterior circulation lesions were further subdivided into those with hemispheric lesions (temporo-occipital), and those with cerebellar/brain stem lesions. Major or minor depression occurred in 48% of the patients in the middle cerebral artery lesion group and in 35% of patients with cerebellar/brain stem lesions. At 6-months follow-up, frequencies of depression among the patients with in-hospital depression were 82% and 20%, respectively. At follow-up 1 to 2 years poststroke, frequencies of depression were 68% and zero, respectively

(Figure 19–2). Thus patients with lesions in the cerebellar/brain stem region had a significantly shorter course of depression. These findings suggest that the mechanism of depression after middle cerebral artery lesions may differ from the mechanism of depression after cerebellar/brain stem lesions. Starkstein et al. (1988d) speculated that the shorter duration of depression after cerebellar/brain stem lesions may be related to their smaller size and to the possibility that the cerebellar/brain stem lesions produce less injury to the biogenic amine pathways that have been proposed to play an important role in the modulation of emotions.

In summary, depressions associated with cerebellar/brain stem lesions appear to be somewhat less frequent and shorter in duration that depressions associated with middle cerebral artery lesions. This may indicate differences in the mechanism of depression associated with these two lesion locations.

Right-hemisphere lesions. In a consecutive series of 93 patients with acute right-hemisphere lesions, Starkstein et al. (1989a) reported that, of 54 patients with positive computed tomography (CT) scans, 6 of 9 patients (66%) with major depression, and 5 of 8 patients (63%) with minor depression had lesions that involved the parietal lobe, compared to 9 of 25 patients (36%) without mood changes and 1 of 12 patients (8%) with undue cheerfulness ($\chi^2 = 9.6$, df = 3, $P < .05$). In addition, similar results were reported by Finset (1988), who found that patients with lesions in the parietal white matter had a higher frequency of depression than patients with lesions in any other location in the right hemisphere.

Premorbid risk factors and depression. Although a significant proportion of patients with left anterior or right posterior lesions develop PSD, not every patient with a lesion in these locations develops a depressive mood. That raises the questions of why clinical variability occurs and why some but not all patients with lesions in these locations develop depression.

Starkstein et al. (1988e) examined these questions by comparing 13 patients with major PSD to 13 stroke patients without depression, who had lesions of the same size and location. Eleven pairs had left-hemisphere lesions, and 2 pairs had right-hemisphere lesions. Damage was cortical in 10 pairs and subcortical in 3 pairs. The groups did not differ on important demographic variables, such as age, sex, socioeconomic status, or education. They also did not differ on family or personal history of psy-

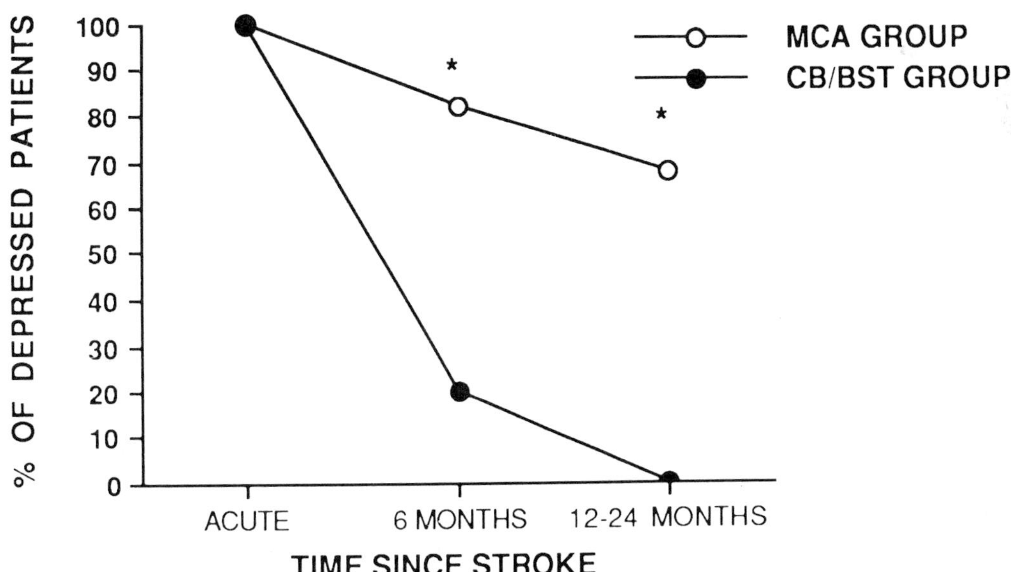

Figure 19–2. Duration of depression for patients with cerebellar/brain stem (CB/BST) lesions and patients with middle cerebral artery (MCA) lesions. (Reprinted from Starkstein SE, Robinson RG, Berthier ML, et al: Depressive disorders following posterior circulation compared with middle cerebral artery infarcts. Brain 111:375–387, 1988. Used with permission.)

chiatric disorders or neurological deficits. Patients with major PSD, however, had significantly more subcortical atrophy ($P < .05$), as measured both by the ratio of third ventricle to brain (i.e., the area of the third ventricle divided by the area of the brain at the same level), and the ratio of lateral ventricle to brain (i.e., the area of the lateral ventricle contralateral to the brain lesion divided by the brain area at the same level). Because most patients' CT scans were obtained immediately after the stroke, it is likely that the subcortical atrophy preceded the stroke. Thus a mild degree of subcortical atrophy may be a premorbid risk factor that increases the risk of developing major depression following a stroke.

In the previously described study of patients with right-hemisphere lesions, Starkstein et al. (1989a) found that patients who developed major depression after a right-hemisphere lesion had a significantly higher frequency of family history of psychiatric disorders than did either nondepressed patients with a right-hemisphere lesion (χ^2 Yates = 4.09, df = 1, $P < .05$) or patients with major depression after left-hemisphere lesions (χ^2 Yates = 4.44, df = 1, $P < .05$). This suggests that a genetic predisposition for depression may play an important role in the development of major depression after right-hemisphere lesions. Eastwood et al. (1989) and Morris et al. (1990) have also reported that depressed patients were more likely than nondepressed patients to have either a previous personal history or a family history of psychiatric disorders.

In summary, lesion location is not the only factor that influences the development of PSD. Subcortical atrophy that probably precedes the stroke and a family or personal history of affective disorders also seem to play an important role in determining whether patients develop depression after a stroke.

Relationship to physical impairment. Both Robinson et al. (1983b) and Eastwood et al. (1989) have reported a low but significant correlation between depression and functional physical impairment (i.e., activities of daily living). This association, however, can be construed as either the functional impairment producing depression or depression influencing the severity of functional impairment. Two recent studies lend support to the latter suggestion.

Sinyor et al. (1986a) reported that although nondepressed stroke patients showed a slight increase or no change in functional status over time, depressed patients had significant decreases in function during the first month after the stroke ($P < .05$). In another recent study, Parikh et al. (1990) compared a consecutive series of 63 stroke patients with major or minor depression to nondepressed stroke patients during a 2-year period after the stroke. Although both groups had similar impairments in ADLs during the time they were in-hospital, the depressed patients had significantly less improvement by 2 years follow-up than the nondepressed patients ($P < .05$). This finding held true after controlling for important variables such as the type and extent of in-hospital and rehabilitation treatment, the size and location of the lesion, the patients' demographic characteristics, the nature of the stroke, the occurrence of another stroke during the follow-up period, and medical history.

In summary, although the correlation between depression and physical impairment after a stroke is not strong, the two variables do appear to interact. There is little evidence to support the idea that physical impairment is a major cause of PSD. However, if depression develops, the patient's physical recovery tends to be retarded for 2 years or more. Moreover, the negative effect of depression on physical recovery, especially on ADLs, lasts even after the depression has subsided (i.e., major depression tends to spontaneously resolve in about 1 year).

PSD and cognitive impairments. Numerous investigators have reported that elderly patients with functional major depression have intellectual deficits that improve with treatment of depression (Wells 1979). This issue was first examined in patients with PSD by Robinson et al. (1986). Patients with major depression after a left-hemisphere infarct were found to have significantly lower (i.e., more impaired) scores ($P < .05$) on the Mini-Mental State Exam (MMSE; Folstein et al. 1975) than a comparable group of nondepressed patients. Both the size of the patients' lesions and their depression scores independently correlated with the severity of cognitive impairment.

In a second study (Starkstein et al. 1988e), stroke patients with and without major depression were matched for lesion location and volume. Ten of the 13 patients with major PSD had an MMSE score lower than that of their matched control subject, 2 had the same score, and only 1 patient had a higher score ($\chi^2 = 14.7$, df = 1, $P < .001$). Thus even when patients were matched for lesion size and location, depressed patients were more cognitively impaired.

In a more recent study, Bolla-Wilson et al. (1989) administered a comprehensive neuropsychological battery and found that patients with major depression and left-hemisphere lesions had significantly greater cognitive impairments than nondepressed patients with comparable left-hemisphere lesions ($P < .05$). These cognitive deficits primarily involved tasks of temporal orientation, language, executive motor, and frontal lobe functions. On the other hand, among patients with right-hemisphere lesions, patients with major depression did not differ from nondepressed patients on any of the measures of cognitive impairment.

In summary, major depression associated with a left-hemisphere stroke appears to produce significant cognitive impairments. Whether these cognitive impairments will improve with treatment of the depression remains to be determined.

PSD and aphasia. In a study of depression among patients with fluent or nonfluent aphasias, Robinson and Benson (1981) found that 9 of 17 aphasic patients (53%) were depressed. These findings are similar to the frequencies of major and minor depression among nonaphasic stroke patients (Robinson and Benson 1981). They also found that patients with nonfluent aphasias had a significantly higher frequency of depression than patients with fluent or global aphasia (71% versus 44% versus 22%, respectively) ($P < .05$). Signer et al. (1989) have recently reported similar findings; depression was present in 63% of their nonfluent aphasic patients, as compared to 16% of their fluent aphasic patients.

Although it may be suggested that the higher frequency of depression among nonfluent aphasic patients is related to their greater awareness of their impairment, in a recent study, Starkstein and Robinson (1988) concluded that lesion location was the important variable in the association between PSD and nonfluent aphasia. In other words, the association between nonfluent aphasia and PSD is explained by the fact that the lesion that is producing nonfluent language may also produce depression.

Another important issue is how to diagnose depression among patients with severe comprehension deficits. Some authors diagnose depression based only on observed behaviors, such as diminished sleep and food intake, restlessness and agitation, or retarded or tearful behavior (Ross et al. 1986). However, the sensitivity and specificity of using behavioral observations for the diagnosis of PSD have not been demonstrated. Most investigators have, therefore, excluded patients with severe comprehension deficits.

In conclusion, patients with left-hemisphere lesions that produce aphasia have a frequency of depression similar to that of patients with left-hemisphere lesions that do not produce aphasia. Although nonfluent aphasia and PSD do not appear to be causally related, they are both produced by lesions of similar anatomical location (anterior areas of the left hemisphere). Thus patients with nonfluent aphasia are at higher risk of developing PSD than patients with other types of aphasia.

Mechanism of PSD. Although the cause of PSD remains unknown, one of the mechanisms that has been hypothesized to play an etiological role is dysfunction of the biogenic amine system. The noradrenergic and serotonergic cell bodies are located in the brain stem and send ascending projections through the median forebrain bundle to the frontal cortex. The ascending axons then arc posteriorly and run longitudinally through the deep layers of the cortex, arborizing and sending terminal projections into the superficial cortical layers (Morrison et al. 1979). Lesions that disrupt these pathways in the frontal cortex or the basal ganglia may affect many downstream fibers. Based on these neuroanatomical facts and the clinical findings that the severity of depression correlates with the proximity of the lesion to the frontal pole, Robinson et al. (1984) suggested that PSD may be the consequence of severe depletions of norepinephrine and/or serotonin produced by frontal or basal ganglia lesions.

In support of this hypothesis, laboratory investigations in rats have demonstrated that the biochemical response to ischemic lesions is lateralized. Right-hemisphere lesions produce depletions of norepinephrine and spontaneous hyperactivity, whereas comparable lesions of the left hemisphere do not (Robinson 1979). More recently, a similar lateralized biochemical response to ischemia in human subjects was reported by Mayberg et al. (1988). Patients with stroke lesions in the right hemisphere had significantly higher ratios of ipsilateral-to-contralateral spiperone binding (presumably 5-HT_2 [serotonin] receptor binding) in noninjured temporal and parietal cortex than patients with comparable left-hemisphere strokes ($P < .05$). Patients with left-hemisphere lesions, on the other hand, showed a significant inverse correlation between the amount of spiperone binding in the left temporal cortex and depression scores (i.e., higher depression scores were associated with lower serotonin receptor binding) ($P < .05$).

Thus a greater depletion of biogenic amines in patients with right-hemisphere lesions as compared with those with left-hemisphere lesion could lead to a compensatory upregulation of receptors that might protect against depression. On the other hand, patients with left-hemisphere lesions may have moderate depletions of biogenic amines but without a compensatory upregulation of 5-HT receptors and, therefore, a dysfunction of biogenic amine systems in the left hemisphere. This dysfunction ultimately may lead to the clinical manifestations of depression.

Treatment of PSD. Despite anecdotal reports of the efficacy of tricyclic antidepressants or stimulant medications in the treatment of PSD (Finklestein et al. 1987), only two randomized double-blind treatment studies on the efficacy of antidepressant treatment of PSD have been published. The first study (Lipsey et al. 1984) examined 14 patients treated with nortriptyline and 20 patients given placebo. The 11 patients treated with nortriptyline who completed the 6-week study showed significantly greater improvement in their scores on the Hamilton Rating Scale for Depression (Hamilton 1960) than did 15 placebo-treated patients ($P < .01$). Successfully treated patients had serum nortriptyline levels between 50 and 150 ng/ml. Three patients experienced side effects (including delirium, confusion, drowsiness, and agitation) that were severe enough to require the discontinuation of nortriptyline.

The second double-blind, controlled study was conducted by Reding et al. (1986). Depressed patients taking trazodone were found to have greater improvement in Barthel ADL scores (Granger et al. 1979) than were the placebo-treated control subjects. This trend became statistically significant when the depressed group was restricted to patients with abnormal dexamethasone suppression tests ($P < .05$).

Electroconvulsive therapy (ECT) has also been reported to be effective for treating PSD (Murray et al. 1987). It causes few side effects and no neurological deterioration. Finally, psychological treatment, including group and family therapy, has also been reported to be useful (Oradei and Waite 1974; Watziawick and Coyne 1980). However, controlled studies for these treatment modalities have not been conducted.

Rehabilitation in PSD. Psychosocial adjustment after stroke is an important issue to consider. Thompson et al. (1989) examined 40 stroke patients as well as their caregivers an average of 9 months poststroke. They found that a lack of meaningfulness in life and overprotection by the caregiver were independent predictors of depression. They also found that psychosocial factors could predict depression and motivation in stroke patients. The authors suggested that both cognitive adaptation and social support theories may be useful approaches to understand people's ability to cope after a stroke.

Poststroke Anxiety

Studies of patients with functional (i.e., no known neuropathology) depression have demonstrated that it is important to distinguish depression associated with significant anxiety symptoms (i.e., agitated depressions) from depression without these symptoms (i.e., retarded depressions) because their cause and course may be different (Stravakaki and Vargo 1986). This finding not only raises questions about the frequency and correlates of anxiety in stroke victims, but also raises questions about the nature of the relationship between anxiety and depression among patients with brain injury.

Starkstein et al. (1990a) have recently reported the results of a study examining a consecutive series of patients with acute stroke lesions for the presence of both anxiety and depressive symptoms. Slightly modified DSM-III criteria for "generalized anxiety" disorder were used for the diagnosis of anxiety disorder. The presence of anxious foreboding and excessive worry were required, as were one or more symptoms of motor tension (i.e., muscle tension, restlessness, and easy fatigability), one or more symptoms of autonomic hyperactivity, and one or more symptoms of vigilance and scanning (i.e., feeling keyed up or on edge, difficulty concentrating because of anxiety, trouble falling or staying asleep, and irritability). Of a consecutive series of 98 patients with first episode acute stroke lesions, only 6 met the criteria for generalized anxiety disorder in the absence of any other mood disorder. On the other hand, 23 out of 47 patients with major depression also met the criteria for generalized anxiety disorder. Patients were then divided into those with anxiety only ($n = 6$), anxiety and depression ($n = 23$), depression only ($n = 24$), and no mood disorder ($n = 45$).

The only significant between-group difference in demographic variables was the presence of higher frequency of alcoholism in patients with anxiety only ($P < .05$). No significant between-group differences were found in neurological examination. Examination of patients with positive CT scans revealed that anxious-depressed patients had a significantly higher frequency of cortical lesions (16 of 19) than did either the depression only group (7 of 15; $\chi^2 = 5.40$, df = 1, $P < .05$), or the control group (13 of 27; $\chi^2 = 6.22$, df = 1, $P < .05$). On the other hand, the depression only group showed a significantly higher frequency of subcortical lesions compared with the anxious-depressed group ($\chi^2 = 7.4$, df = 1, $P < .01$).

Subcortical lesions have frequently been associated with abulia, apathy, and indifference (Graff-Radford et al. 1984). On the other hand, lesions of the left frontal cortex have been reported to produce severe anxiety reactions (Gainotti 1972). Moreover, Gur et al. (1987) showed a linear decrease in cortical metabolic rate (i.e., lower cortical metabolism) with increased anxiety. Thus these findings as well as the findings in poststroke anxiety suggest that the integrity of subcortical structures may be necessary for the generation and/or expression of anxious features in depressed patients with cortical lesions and that abulia and apathy are the clinical outcome when the basal ganglia structures are damaged (Starkstein et al. 1990a).

Poststroke Mania

Although mania occurs less frequently than depression (we have only observed three cases among a consecutive series of more than 300 stroke patients), a manic syndrome may be precipitated by brain injury.

Phenomenology of secondary mania. Starkstein et al. (1988a) examined a series of 12 consecutive patients who met DSM-III criteria for an organic affective syndrome, manic type. These patients, who developed mania after a stroke, traumatic brain injury, or tumors, were compared with patients with functional (i.e., no known neuropathology) mania (Starkstein et al. 1987a). Both groups of patients showed similar frequencies of elation, pressured speech, flight of ideas, grandiose thoughts, insomnia, hallucinations, and paranoid delusions. Thus the symptoms of mania that occur after brain damage (secondary mania) appear to be the same as those found in mania without brain damage (primary mania).

Lesion location. Cummings and Mendez (1984) reported two patients who developed mania after right thalamic stroke lesions. After a review of the literature, they suggested a specific association between secondary mania and lesions in the limbic system or limbic-related areas of the right hemisphere.

Robinson et al. (1988) reported on 17 patients with secondary mania. Most of the patients had right-hemisphere lesions involving either cortical limbic areas, such as the orbitofrontal cortex and the basotemporal cortex, or subcortical nuclei, such as the head of the caudate and the thalamus. The frequency of right-hemisphere lesions was significantly different than that for patients with major depression, who tended to have left frontal or basal ganglia lesions.

These findings have recently been replicated in another series of eight patients with secondary mania (Starkstein et al. 1990b). All eight patients had right-hemisphere lesions (seven unilateral and one bilateral injury). Lesions were either cortical (basotemporal cortex in four cases and orbitofrontal cortex in one case) or subcortical (frontal white matter, head of the caudate, and anterior limb of the internal capsule, in three cases, respectively). Positron-emission tomography (PET) scans with [^{18}F]fluorodeoxyglucose (FDG) were carried out in the three patients with purely subcortical lesions. They all showed a focal hypometabolic deficit in the right basotemporal cortex.

In summary, several studies of patients with brain damage have found that patients who develop secondary mania have a significantly greater frequency of lesions in the right hemisphere than patients with depression or no mood disturbance. The right-hemisphere lesions that lead to mania tend to be in specific right-hemisphere structures that have connections to the limbic system. The right basotemporal cortex appears to be particularly important because direct lesions as well as distant hypometabolic effects (diaschisis) of this cortical region are frequently associated with secondary mania.

Risk factors. Not every patient with a lesion in limbic areas of the right hemisphere will develop secondary mania. Therefore, there must be risk factors for this disorder.

In one study (Robinson et al. 1988), patients with secondary mania were compared to patients with secondary major depression. Results indicated that patients with secondary mania had a significantly higher frequency of positive family history of affective disorders than did depressed patients or patients with no mood disturbance ($P < .05$). Therefore, it appears that genetic predisposition to affective disorders may constitute a risk factor for mania.

In another study (Starkstein et al. 1987a), patients with secondary mania were compared with patients with no mood disturbance who were matched for size, location, and etiology of brain lesion. The groups were also compared with patients with primary mania and control subjects. No significant between-group differences were found either in demographic variables or neurological evaluation. Patients with secondary mania, however, had significantly greater degree of subcortical atrophy, as measured by the bifrontal and the third ventricular to brain ratio ($P < .001$). Moreover, of the patients who developed secondary mania, those who had a positive family history of psychiatric disorders had significantly less atrophy than those without such a family history ($P < .05$), suggesting that genetic predisposition to affective disorders and brain atrophy may be independent risk factors.

In summary, the relatively rare occurrence of mania after stroke suggests that there are premorbid risk factors that impact on the expression of this disorder. Studies thus far have identified two such factors. One is a genetic vulnerability for affective disorder; the other is a mild degree of subcortical atrophy. The subcortical atrophy probably preceded the stroke, but its cause remains unknown.

Mechanism of secondary mania. Several studies have demonstrated that the amygdala (located in the limbic portion of the temporal lobe) has an important role in the production of instinctive reactions and the association between stimulus and emotional response (Gloor 1986). The amygdala receives its main afferents from the basal diencephalon (which in turn receives psychosensory and psychomotor information from the reticular formation), and the temporopolar and basolateral cortices (which receive main afferents from heteromodal association areas) (Beck 1949; Crosby et al. 1962). The basotemporal cortex receives afferents from association cortical areas and the orbitofrontal cortex and sends efferent projections to the entorhinal cortex, hippocampus, and amygdala. By virtue of these connections, the basotemporal cortex may represent a cortical link between sensory afferents and instinctive reactions (Goldar and Outes 1972).

The orbitofrontal cortex may be subdivided into two regions: a posterior one, which is restricted to limbic functions and should be considered part of the limbic system, and an anterior one, which exerts a tonic inhibitory control over the amygdala by means of its connection through the uncinate fasciculus with the basotemporal cortex (Nauta 1971). Thus the uncinate fasciculus and the basotemporal cortex may mediate connections between psychomotor and volitional processes generated in the frontal lobe and vital processes and instinctive behaviors generated in the amygdala (Starkstein and Robinson, in press).

It may be hypothesized that, through orbitotemporo-amygdala connections, cognitive functions may influence limbic activity. Thus a lesion in the orbitofrontal cortex, uncinate fasciculus, or basotemporal cortex may release the tonic inhibition exerted by the frontal lobe on the amygdala, which in turn results in emotional disinhibition. The loss of frontolimbic connections may release emotions from intellectual control, and this dissociation results in the cluster of symptoms we identify as secondary mania (Goldar and Outes 1972).

As discussed above, most of the patients with secondary mania have lesions of the right hemisphere. In a rat model of focal brain injury, Starkstein et al. (1988b) found that right, but not left frontolateral cortical lesions produced locomotor hyperactivity as well as bilateral increases in dopaminergic turnover in the nucleus accumbens. Thus it is possible that in the presence of specific risk factors for secondary mania (e.g., subcortical atrophy) increases in biogenic amine turnover produced by right- but not left-hemisphere lesions may play an important role in the production of secondary mania. This biogenic amine dysfunction may also be most pronounced in the basotemporal cortex, which is one of the cortical regions with the highest concentration of serotonergic terminals from the raphe nuclei.

Finally, a recent case report (Starkstein et al. 1989b) suggested that the mechanism of secondary mania is not related to the release of transcallosal inhibitory fibers (i.e., the release of left limbic areas from tonic inhibition due to a right-hemisphere lesion). A patient who developed secondary mania after bleeding from a right basotemporal arteriovenous malformation, underwent a Wada test before the therapeutic embolization of the malformation. Amytal injection in the left carotid artery did not abolish the manic symptoms (which would be the expected finding if the "release" theory were correct).

In summary, although the mechanism of secondary mania remains unknown, both lesion studies and metabolic studies suggest that the right basotemporal cortex may play an important role. A combination of biogenic amine system dysfunction and release of tonic inhibitory input into the basotemporal cortex and lateral limbic system may lead to the production of mania.

Treatment of secondary mania. Although no systematic treatment studies of secondary mania have been conducted, one recent report suggested several potentially useful treatment modalities. Bakchine et al. (1989) carried out a double-blind, placebo-controlled treatment study in a single patient with secondary mania. Clonidine (600 µg/day) rapidly reversed the manic symptoms, whereas carbamazepine (1200 mg/day) was associated with no mood changes, and levodopa (375 mg/day) was associated with an increase in manic symptoms. Other treatment modalities, such as anticonvulsants (valproate and carbamazepine), neuroleptics, and lithium therapy, have been reported to be useful in treating secondary mania (Robinson and Starkstein, in press). None of these treatments, however, have been evaluated in double-blind, placebo-controlled studies.

Poststroke Bipolar Disorder

Although some patients have one or more manic episodes after brain injury, other manic patients also have depression after brain injury. In an effort to examine which factors are crucial in determining which patients have bipolar as compared with unipolar disorder, Starkstein et al. (1991) examined 19 patients with the diagnosis of secondary mania. The bipolar (manic-depressive) group consisted of patients who, after the brain lesion, met the DSM-III-R criteria for organic mood syndrome, manic, followed or preceded by organic mood syndrome, depressed. The unipolar mania (mania only) group consisted of patients who met the criteria for mania described above, not followed or preceded by depression. All the patients had CT scan evidence of vascular, neoplastic, or traumatic brain lesion, and no history of other neurological, toxic, or metabolic conditions.

Background information revealed no significant between-group differences in age, sex, race, education, handedness, or personal history of psychiatric disorder. Also, no significant between-group differences were found on the neurological examination.

On psychiatric examination, which was carried out during the index manic episode, no significant between-group differences were observed in the type or frequency of manic symptoms. The bipolar group, however, showed a significantly greater intellectual impairment as measured by MMSE scores (25.2 ± 4.7 vs. 28.6 ± 1.8; $t = 2.21$, df = 1, $P < .05$). The longitudinal evolution of bipolar and unipolar patients is shown in Figure 19–3. Almost half of the bipolar patients had recurrent episodes of depression, whereas recurrent episodes of mania occurred in approximately one-fourth of patients in both the unipolar and bipolar groups.

Lesion location. Six of the 7 patients with bipolar disorder had lesions restricted to the right hemisphere, which involved the head of the caudate (2 patients), thalamus (3 patients), and head of the caudate, dorsolateral frontal cortex, and basotemporal cortex (1 patient). The remaining patient developed a bipolar illness after surgical removal of a pituitary adenoma. In contrast to the primarily subcortical lesions in the bipolar group, 8 of 12 patients in the unipolar mania group had lesions restricted to the right hemisphere, which involved the basotemporal cortex (6 patients), orbitofrontal cortex (1 patient), and head of the caudate (1 patient). The remaining 4 patients had bilateral lesions involving the orbitofrontal cortex (3 patients), and the orbitofrontal white matter (1 patient).

Thus 6 of the 7 bipolar patients had subcortical lesions, and 1 had a cortical-subcortical lesion. On the other hand, 9 of the unipolar patients had cortical lesions, 1 had a cortical lesion with subcortical extension, and 2 had subcortical lesions. A hypothesis of unequal frequency of bipolar compared with unipolar disorder based on the presence of cortical or subcortical lesions was statistically substantiated (Fisher test, $P < .005$). Patients with unipolar mania also had significantly larger lesion volumes than the patients in the bipolar group ($P < .05$). On the other hand, a hypothesis of unequal frequency of bipolar or unipolar mania based on the presence of unilateral or bilateral lesions was not statistically substantiated.

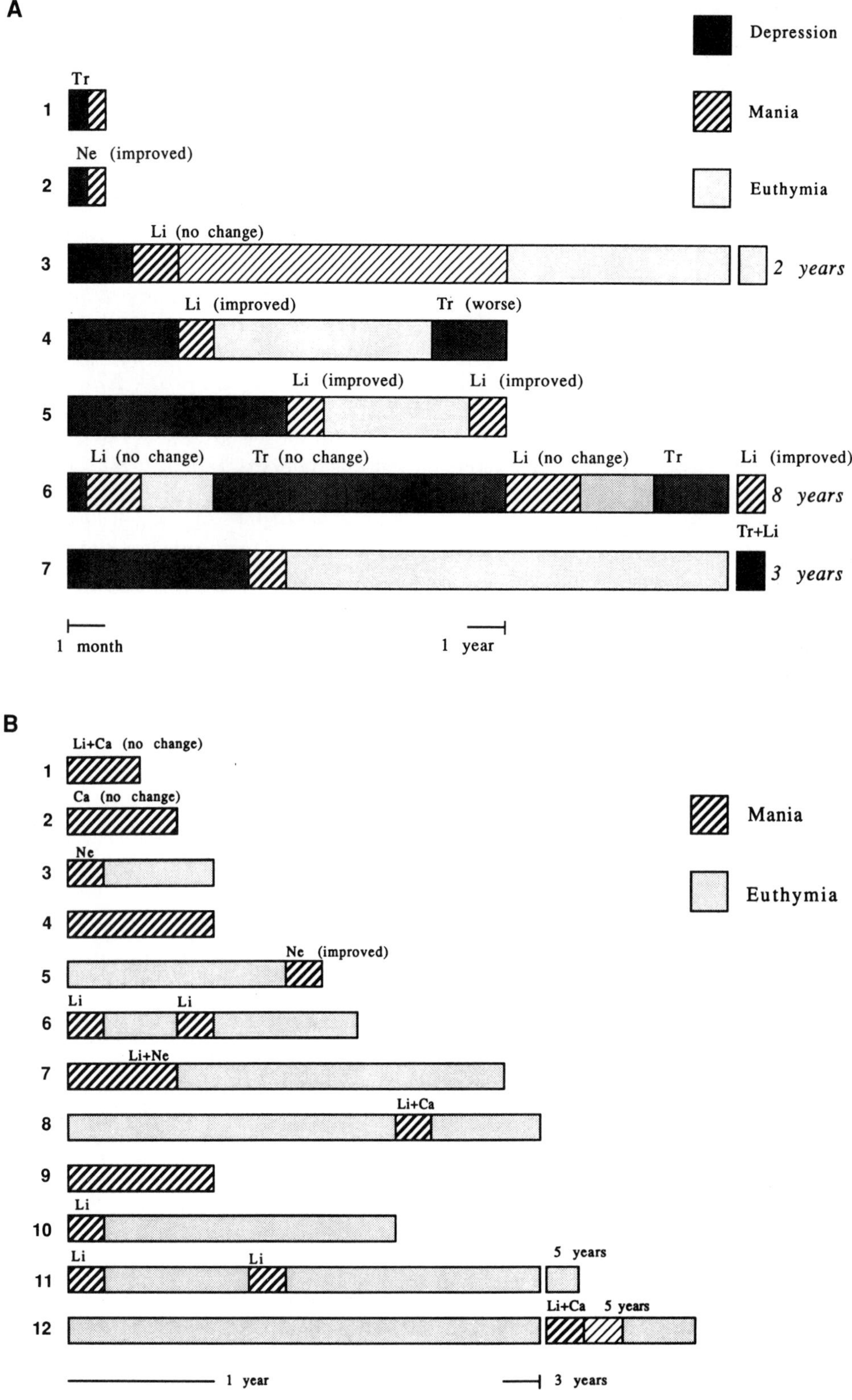

Figure 19–3. *Panel A:* Longitudinal evolution of mood disorder for individual patients with bipolar disorder. *Panel B:* Longitudinal evolution of mood disorder for individual patients with unipolar mania. Tr = tricyclic antidepressant; Ne = nortryptyline; Li = lithium; Ca = carbamazepine.

In summary, this study suggests that among patients with secondary mania, a prior episode of depression may have occurred in about one-third of them. Patients with bipolar disorder tend to have subcortical lesions (mainly involving the right head of the caudate or the right thalamus), whereas patients with pure mania tend to show a higher frequency of cortical lesions (particularly in the right orbitofrontal and right basotemporal cortex). Finally, bipolar patients tend to have greater cognitive impairments than do patients with unipolar mania, which may either reflect differences in lesion location or suggest that the presence of a previous episode of depression may produce residual cognitive effects.

Mechanism. A possible mechanism by which right orbitofrontal and basotemporal cortex may produce mania is discussed above. The question that now arises is how subcortical lesions might produce a bipolar disease. Subcortical lesions have been reported to produce hypometabolic effects in widespread regions including contralateral brain areas (i.e., crossed-hemisphere and crossed-cerebellar diaschisis) (Pappata et al. 1987). Thus it is possible that subcortical lesions may have induced metabolic changes in left frontocortical regions, which (as noted above) are associated with depression. Mania may develop at a later stage, when these metabolic changes become restricted to the orbitofrontal and/or basotemporal cortices of the right hemisphere.

❑ CONCLUSIONS

Depression occurs in about 40% of patients with acute stroke lesions, and its natural evolution is from 1 to 2 years, although patients with subcortical or brain stem lesions may show shorter duration depressions. Both intrahemispheric and interhemispheric lesion location appear to contribute to the development of depression. Major depression is significantly more frequent among patients with left-hemisphere lesions involving anterior cortical (frontal) or subcortical (basal ganglia) regions than any other lesion location. On the other hand, depressions following right-hemisphere lesions are usually associated with a genetic vulnerability and frontal and parietal lobe damage. Finally, an important risk factor for the development of PSD is the presence of subcortical atrophy before the stroke lesion.

Generalized anxiety disorder in the absence of other psychiatric problems is a rare complication of stroke lesions and is frequently associated with a prior history of alcohol abuse. On the other hand, almost 50% of patients with major PSD also meet DSM-III criteria for generalized anxiety disorder. Patients with both major depression and generalized anxiety disorder tend to have cortical lesions, whereas patients with major PSD without anxiety tend to have subcortical lesions.

Mania that develops after brain injury has a phenomenology similar to that of mania without known neuropathology. Secondary mania, however, is almost always the consequence of lesions in the right hemisphere, involving cortical (orbitofrontal or basotemporal) or subcortical (head of the caudate or thalamus) limbic-related regions. Among these areas, dysfunction of the basotemporal cortex seems to be particularly important to the development of secondary mania, and basotemporal dysfunction may be produced by direct or indirect (diaschisis) damage.

In the future, the development of clinical techniques or laboratory markers highly specific to major depression may add to our ability to recognize and treat affective disorders among patients who cannot presently be examined. Because patients with comprehension deficits cannot be reliably interviewed, assessments of frequency of depression or response to treatment cannot be reliably made.

❑ REFERENCES

Adams GF, Hurwitz LJ: Mental barriers to recovery from strokes. Lancet 2:533–537, 1963

Adams RD, Victor M: Principles of Neurology, 3rd Edition. New York, McGraw-Hill, 1985, pp 569–640

American Psychiatric Association: Diagnostic and Statistical Manual of Mental Disorders, 3rd Edition. Washington, DC, American Psychiatric Association, 1980

American Psychiatric Association: Diagnostic and Statistical Manual of Mental Disorders, 3rd Edition, Revised. Washington, DC, American Psychiatric Association, 1987

Babinski J: Contribution a l'etude des troubles mentauz dans l'hemiplegie organique cerebrale (Anosognosie). Rev Neurol (Paris) 27:845–848, 1914

Bakchine S, Lacomblez L, Benoit N, et al: Manic-like state after orbitofrontal and right temporoparietal injury: efficacy of clonidine. Neurology 39:777–781, 1989

Barry S, Dinan TG: Alpha-2 adrenergic receptor function in post-stroke depression. Psychol Med 20:305–309, 1990

Beck E: A cytoarchitectural investigation into the boundaries of cortical areas 13 and 14 in the human brain. J Anatomy 83:145–157, 1949

Benson DF: Psychiatric aspects of aphasia. Br J Psychiatry 123:555–566, 1976

Bleuler EP: Textbook of Psychiatry. New York, Dover Publications, 1951

Bolla-Wilson K, Robinson RG, Starkstein SE, et al: Lateralization of dementia of depression in stroke patients. Am J Psychiatry 146:627–634, 1989

Broca P: New finding of aphasia following a lesion of the posterior part of the second and third frontal convolutions. Bulletin de la Societe Anatomique 6:398–407, 1861

Carroll BJ, Feinberg M, Gredent JF: A specific laboratory test for the diagnosis of melancholia: standardization, validation and clinical utility. Arch Gen Psychiatry 38: 15–22, 1981

Crosby E, Humphrey T, Lauer E: Correlative Anatomy of the Nervous System. New York, Macmillan, 1962

Cummings JL, Benson DF: Dementia: A Clinical Approach, 2nd Edition. Stoneham, MA, Butterworth-Heineman, 1992

Cummings JL, Mendez MF: Secondary mania with focal cerebrovascular lesions. Am J Psychiatry 141:1084–1087, 1984

Davison C, Kelman H: Pathological laughing and crying. Archives of Neurology and Psychiatry 42:595–643, 1939

Denny-Brown D, Meyer JS, Horenstein S: The significance of perceptual rivalry resulting from parietal lesions. Brain 75:434–471, 1952

Eastwood MR, Rifat SL, Nobbs H, et al: Mood disorder following cerebrovascular accident. Br J Psychiatry 154: 195–200, 1989

Ebrahim S, Nouri N: Affective illness after stroke. Br J Psychiatry 151:52–56, 1987

Fedoroff UP, Starkstein SE, Parikh RM, et al: Are depressive symptoms non-specific in patients with acute stroke? Am J Psychiatry 148:1172–1176, 1991

Finklestein S, Benowitz LI, Baldessarini RJ: Mood, vegetative disturbance, and dexamethasone suppression test after stroke. Ann Neurol 12:463–468, 1981

Finklestein SP, Weintraub RJ, Karmouz N: Antidepressant drug treatment for poststroke depression: retrospective study. Arch Phys Med Rehabil 68:772–776, 1987

Finset A: Depressed mood and reduced emotionality after right hemisphere brain damage, in Cerebral Hemisphere Function in Depression. Edited by Kinsbourne M. Washington, DC, American Psychiatric Press, 1988, pp 49–64

Fisher S: Psychiatric considerations of cerebral vascular disease. Am J Cardiol 7:379, 1961

Folstein MF, Folstein SE, McHugh PR: Mini-Mental State: a practical method for grading the cognitive state of patients for the clinician. J Psychiatr Res 12:189–198, 1975

Folstein MF, Maiberger R, McHugh PR: Mood disorder as a specific complication of stroke. J Neurol Neurosurg Psychiatry 40:1018–1020, 1977

Gainotti G: Emotional behavior and hemispheric side of the brain. Cortex 8:41–55, 1972

Gloor P: Role of the human limbic system in perception, memory and affect: lessons for temporal lobe epilepsy, in The Limbic System: Functional Organization and Clinical Disorders. Edited by Doane BK, Livingstone KE. New York, Raven, 1986

Goldar JC, Outes DL: Fisiopatologia de la desinhibicion instintiva. Acta Psiquiatrica y Psicologica de America Latina 18:177–185, 1972

Goldstein K: The Organism: A Holistic Approach to Biology Derived from Pathological Data in Man. New York, American Books, 1939

Goldstein K: After-Effects of Brain Injuries in War. New York, Grune & Stratton, 1942

Graff-Radford NR, Eslinger PJ, Damasio AR: Nonhemorrhagic infarction of the thalamus: behavioral, anatomic and physiologic correlates. Neurology 34:14–23, 1984

Granger CV, Denis LS, Peters NC, et al: Stroke rehabilitation: analysis of repeated Barthel Index measures. Arch Phys Med Rehabil 60:14–17, 1979

Gur RC, Gur RE, Resnick SM, et al: The effect of anxiety on cortical cerebral blood flow and metabolism. J Cereb Blood Flow Metab 7:173–177, 1987

Hamilton M: Rating depressive patients. J Clin Psychiatry 41:21–24, 1960

Hecaen H, Ajuriaguerra J de, Massonet J: Les troubles visoconstructifs par lesion parieto occipitale droit. Encephale 40:122–179, 1951

Hughlings-Jackson J: On affections of speech from disease of the brain. Brain 38:106–174, 1915

Ironside R: Disorders of laughter due to brain lesions. Brain 79:589–609, 1956

Kraepelin E: Manic Depressive Insanity and Paranoia. Edinburgh, Livingstone, 1921

Lipsey JR, Robinson RG, Pearlson GD, et al: Nortriptyline treatment for post-stroke depression: a double-blind trial. Lancet 1:297–300, 1984

Lipsey JR, Robinson RG, Pearlson GD: Dexamethasone suppression test and mood following strokes. Am J Psychiatry 142:318–323, 1985

Lipsey JR, Spencer WC, Rabins PV, et al: Phenomenological comparison of poststroke depression and functional depression. Am J Psychiatry 143:527–529, 1986

Mayberg HS, Robinson RG, Wong DF, et al: PET imaging of cortical S_2, serotonin receptors after stroke: lateralized changes and relationship to depression. Am J Psychiatry 145:937–943, 1988

Meyer A: The anatomical facts and clinical varieties of traumatic insanity. American Journal of Insanity 60: 373, 1904

Morris PLP, Robinson RG, Raphael B: Prevalanece and course of post-stroke depression in hospitalized patients. Int J Psychiatry Med 20:349–364, 1990

Morris PLP, Robinson RG, Raphael B: Lesion characteristics and post-stroke depression: evidence of a specific relationship in the left hemisphere. J Neuropsychiatry Behavioral Neurology (in press)

Morrison JH, Molliver ME, Grzanna R: Noradrenergic innervation of the cerebral cortex: widespread effects of local cortical lesions. Science 205:313–316, 1979

Murray GB, Shea V, Conn DK: Electroconvulsive therapy for poststroke depression. J Clin Psychiatry 47:258–260, 1987

Nauta WJH: The problem of the frontal lobe: a reinterpretation. Journal of Psychological Research 8:167–187, 1971

Olsson T, Astrom M, Eriksson S: Hypercotisolism revealed by the dexamethasone suppression test with acute ischemic stroke. Stroke 20:1685–1690, 1989

Oradei DM, Waite NS: Group psychotherapy with stroke patients during the immediate recovery phase. Am J Orthopsychiatry 44:386–395, 1974

Pappata S, Dinh ST, Baron JC, et al: Remote metabolic effects of cerebrovascular lesions: magnetic resonance and positron tomography imaging. Neuroradiol 29:1–6, 1987

Parikh RM, Robinson RG, Lipsey JR, et al: The impact of poststroke depression on recovery in activities of daily living over a 2-year follow-up. Arch Neurol 47:785–789, 1990

Post F: The Significance of Affective Symptoms in Old Age (Maudsley Monograph No. 10). London, Oxford University Press, 1962

Rabins PV, Starkstein SE, Robinson RG: Risk factors for developing atypical (schizophreniform) psychosis following stroke. Journal of Neuropsychiatry and Clinical Neurosciences 3:6–9, 1991

Reding MJ, Orto LA, Willenski P: The dexamethasone suppression test: an indicator of depression in stroke but not a predictor of rehabilitation outcome. Arch Neurol 42:209–212, 1985

Reding MJ, Orto LA, Winter SW: Antidepressant therapy after stroke: a double-blind trial. Arch Neurol 43:763–765, 1986

Robinson RG: Differential behavioral and biochemical effects of right and left hemispheric cerebral infarction in the rat. Science 205:707–710, 1979

Robinson RG, Benson DF: Depression in aphasic patients: frequency, severity and clinical pathological correlations. Brain Lang 14:282–291, 1981

Robinson RG, Price TR: Poststroke depressive disorders: a follow-up study of 103 patients. Stroke 13:635–641, 1982

Robinson RG, Starkstein SE: Current research in affective disorders following stroke. Journal of Neuropsychiatry and Clinical Neurosciences 2:1–14, 1990

Robinson RG, Szetela B: Mood change following left hemispheric brain injury. Ann Neurol 9:447–453, 1981

Robinson RG, Kubos KL, Starr LB, et al: Mood changes in stroke patients: relationship to lesion location. Compr Psychiatry 24:555–566, 1983a

Robinson RG, Starr LB, Kubos KL, et al: A two-year longitudinal study of poststroke mood disorders: findings during the initial evaluation. Stroke 14:736–741, 1983b

Robinson RG, Kubos KL, Starr LB, et al: Mood disorders in stroke patients: importance of lesion location. Brain 107:81–93, 1984

Robinson RG, Bolla-Wilson K, Kaplan E, et al: Depression influences intellectual impairment in stroke patients. Br J Psychiatry 148:541–547, 1986

Robinson RG, Bolduc PL, Price TR: Two-year longitudinal study of post-stroke mood disorders: diagnosis and outcome at one and two years. Stroke 18:837–843, 1987

Robinson RG, Boston JD, Starkstein SE: Comparison of mania with depression following brain injury causal factors. Am J Psychiatry 145:172–178, 1988

Ross ED, Mesulam MM: Dominant language functions of the right hemisphere: prosody and emotional gesturing. Arch Neurol 36:144–148, 1979

Ross ED, Rush AJ: Diagnosis and neuroanatomical correlates of depression in brain damaged patients. Arch Gen Psychiatry 38:1344–1354, 1981

Ross ED, Gordon WA, Hibbard M, et al: The dexamethasone suppression test, post-stroke depression, and the validity of DSM-III–based diagnostic criteria. Am J Psychiatry 38:1344–1354, 1986

Signer S, Cummings JL, Benson DF: Delusions and mood disorders in patients with chronic aphasia. Journal of Neuropsychiatry and Clinical Neurosciences 1:40–45, 1989

Sinyor D, Amato P, Kaloupek P: Poststroke depression: relationship to functional impairment, coping strategies, and rehabilitation outcome. Stroke 17:1102–1107, 1986a

Sinyor D, Jacques P, Kaloupek DG: Post-stroke depression and lesion location: an attempted replication. Brain 109:537–546, 1986b

Spitzer R, Endicott J, Robins E: Research Diagnostic Criteria (RDC) for a Group of Functional Disorders. New York, Biometrics Research Division, New York Psychiatric Institute, 1975

Starkstein SE, Robinson RG: Aphasia and depression. Aphasiology 2:1–20, 1988

Starkstein SE, Robinson RG: Affective disorders and cerebral vascular disease. Br J Psychiatry 154:170–182, 1989

Starkstein SE, Robinson RG: The role of the frontal lobes in affective disorder following stroke, in Frontal Lobe Function and Injury. Edited by Levin HS, Eisenberg HM. Oxford, England, Oxford University Press (in press)

Starkstein SE, Pearlson GD, Boston JD, et al: Mania after brain injury: a controlled study of causative factors. Arch Neurol 44:1069–1073, 1987a

Starkstein SE, Robinson RG, Price TR: Comparison of cortical and subcortical lesions in the production of poststroke mood disorders. Brain 110:1045-1059, 1987b

Starkstein JE, Boston JD, Robinson RG: Mechanisms of mania after brain injury: 12 case reports and review of the literature. J Nerv Ment Dis 176:87–100, 1988a

Starkstein SE, Moran TH, Bowersox JA, et al: Behavioral abnormalities induced by frontal cortical and nucleus accumbens lesions. Brain Res 473:74–80, 1988b

Starkstein SE, Robinson RG, Berthier ML, et al: Differential mood changes following basal ganglia vs thalamic lesions. Arch Neurol 45:725–730, 1988c

Starkstein SE, Robinson RG, Berthier ML, et al: Depressive disorders following posterior circulation compared with middle cerebral artery infarcts. Brain 111:375–387, 1988d

Starkstein SE, Robinson RG, Price TR: Comparison of patients with and without post-stroke major depression matched for size and location of lesion. Arch Gen Psychiatry 45:247–252, 1988e

Starkstein SE, Robinson RG, Price TR: Comparison of spontaneously recovered versus non-recovered patients with poststroke depression. Stroke 19:1491–1496, 1988f

Starkstein SE, Robinson RG, Honig MA, et al: Mood changes after right-hemisphere lesions. Br J Psychiatry 155:79–85, 1989a

Starkstein SE, Berthier PL, Lylyk A, et al: Emotional behavior after a Wada test in a patient with secondary mania. Journal of Neuropsychiatry and Clinical Neurosciences 1:408–412, 1989b

Starkstein SE, Cohen BS, Fedoroff P, et al: Relationship between anxiety disorders and depressive disorders in patients with cerebrovascular injury. Arch Gen Psychiatry 47:246–251, 1990a

Starkstein SE, Mayberg HS, Berthier ML, et al: Mania after brain injury: neuroradiological and metabolic findings. Ann Neurol 27:652–659, 1990b

Starksteln SE, Fedoroff P, Berthier ML, et al: Manic-depressive and pure manic states after brain lesions. Biol Psychiatry, 29:149–158, 1991

Stravakaki C, Vargo B: The relationship of anxiety and depression: a review of the literature. Br J Psychiatry 149:7–16, 1986

Thompson SC, Sobolew-Shobin A, Graham MA, et al: Psychosocial adjustment following a stroke. Soc Sci Med 28:239–247, 1989

Ullman M, Gruen A: Behavioral changes in patients with strokes. Am J Psychiatry 117:1004–1009, 1960

Wade DT, Legh-Smith JE, Hewer RA: Depressed mood after stroke: a community study of its frequency. Br J Psychiatry 141:200–205, 1987

Watziawlck P, Coyne JC: Depression following stroke: brief, problem-focused family treatment. Family Treatment 19:13–18, 1980

Wells CE: Pseudodementia. Am J Psychiatry 136:895–900, 1979

Wolf PA, Dawber TR, Thomas HE, et al: Epidemiology of stroke, in Advances in Neurology, Vol 16. Edited by Thompson RA, Green JR. New York, Raven, 1977, pp 5–19

Chapter

20

Neuropsychiatric Aspects of Brain Tumors

Trevor R. P. Price, M.D.
Kenneth L. Goetz, M.D.
Mark R. Lovell, Ph.D.

TUMORS INVOLVING THE central nervous system (CNS) are common. With an annual incidence of 30 per 100,000 and a point prevalence of 80 per 100,000 people, they account for an estimated 10% of all neoplasms and 2% of cancer-related deaths (Gilroy and Holliday 1982; Kurtzke 1984). In adults, brain tumors are typically classified according to whether they are primary or metastatic, as well as according to location and histological cell type. Eighty percent of brain tumors in adults are primary and 20% are metastatic, with the reverse being the case in children. Seventy percent are supratentorial, whereas 30% are infratentorial with distribution by lobe as indicated in Figure 20–1. This distribution is influenced to some degree by tumor histology (Figure 20–2). Gliomas and meningiomas are the most common histological types of primary brain tumors; the most common metastatic lesions are from lung and breast primaries (Tables 20–1 and 20–2). A substantial proportion of CNS tumors are associated with psychiatric symptomatology and/or neuropsychological deficits.

Although the above classifications may eventually turn out to be important in understanding the occurrence of various neuropsychiatric symptoms associated with brain tumors, large-scale detailed studies carefully examining the correlations between clinical phenomenology and various tumor parameters have not as yet been done.

Thus our knowledge of the neuropsychiatric and neuropsychological aspects of brain tumors is based on a relatively small number of clinical case reports and larger, uncontrolled case series from the older neurological and neurosurgical literature. Much of the discussion that follows draws on this data base.

The authors wish to acknowledge the assistance of Olga Petruska in the preparation of this manuscript.

❑ FREQUENCY OF NEUROPSYCHIATRIC SYMPTOMS IN PATIENTS WITH BRAIN TUMORS

Keschner et al. (1938) noted psychiatric symptoms in 78% of their 530 cases, and Schlesinger (1950) found behavioral changes in 51% of his series of 591 patients with brain tumors. Although complex neuropsychiatric symptoms may occur in conjunction with focal neurological signs and symptoms, frequently they may be the first clinical indication of a tumor, as was the case in 18% of patients examined by Keschner et al. (1938).

An interesting point was made by Minski (1933), who studied 58 patients with cerebral tumors. In addition to reporting that the psychiatric symptomatology of 25 of these patients simulated "functional psychoses," he noted that 19 of his patients actually attributed the onset of their behavioral symptoms to a number of stresses, including financial worries and the deaths of relatives. This underscores the difficulty clinicians face in making an appropriate diagnosis early on, as it may be impossible on purely clinical grounds to determine the organic basis of the patient's complaints until progression of the tumor has resulted in the emergence of more typical neurological signs and symptoms.

Fortunately, despite the high prevalence of psychiatric symptoms in patients with brain tumors, the risk of an occult neoplasm in patients presenting with purely psychiatric complaints is much lower. One survey of all patients discharged from an acute psychiatric hospital over a 30-year period found that only 34 of approximately 17,000 patients had been diagnosed as having "psychosis due to brain tumor" during their stay (Remington and Robert 1962). Ten of those 34 patients were known to have had tumors on admission. The other 24 were therefore initially hospitalized for psychiatric complaints that were later found to be brain tumor related.

Selecki (1965) summarized autopsy material from patients in state hospitals (where the incidence of brain tumors ranged from 1% to 13.5%) and noted that, on average, 55% of the tumors had gone unrecognized before the patient's death. Klotz (1957) reviewed over 44,000 autopsy cases of psychiatric patients and found that 2.1% had had brain tumors, 45% of which had also gone unrecognized before death.

These and other similar data support the notion that as many as 1%–2% of patients given a psychiatric diagnosis may actually have undiagnosed CNS tumors. This figure is, of course, significantly higher than the prevalence of brain tumors in the general population and therefore emphasizes the fact that psychiatrists and other mental health professionals

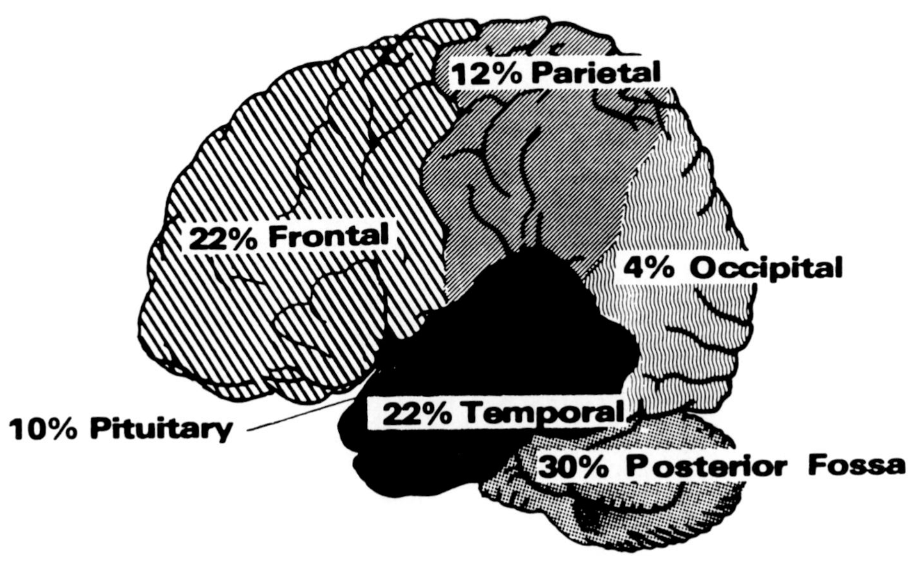

Figure 20–1. Relative frequency of intracranial brain tumors according to location in the adult. (Reprinted from Lohr JB, Cadet JL: Neuropsychiatric aspects of brain tumors, in The American Psychiatric Press Textbook of Neuropsychiatry. Washington, DC, American Psychiatric Press, 1987, p 355. Used with permission.)

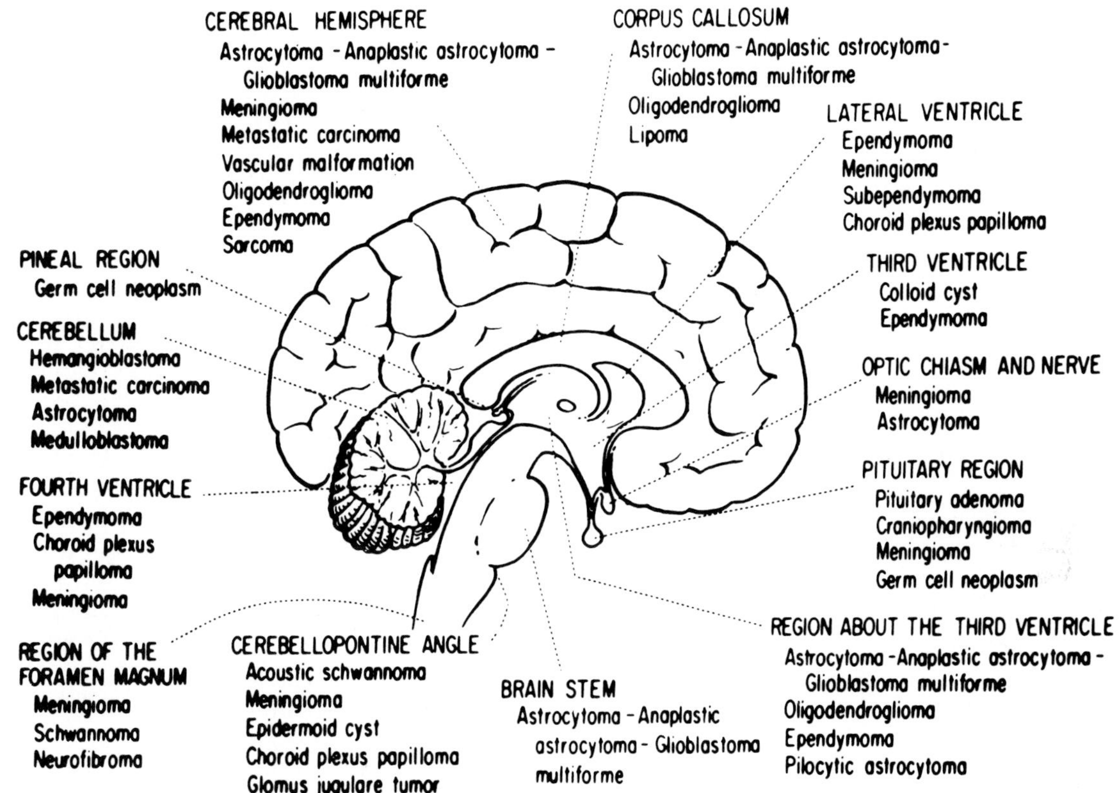

Figure 20–2. Topographic distribution of intracranial tumors in the adult. (Reprinted from Burger PC, Scheithauer BW, Vogel FS: Surgical Pathology of the Nervous System and Its Coverings, 3rd Edition. New York, Churchill Livingstone, 1991, p 195. Copyright 1991 by Churchill Livingstone. Used with permission.)

need to be keenly aware of the broad spectrum of neuropsychiatric manifestations with which brain tumors may be associated.

❑ GENERAL NEUROPSYCHIATRIC AND NEUROPSYCHOLOGICAL CONSIDERATIONS IN RELATION TO BRAIN TUMORS

General Neuropsychiatric Considerations

CNS tumors can present with mental symptoms virtually identical to those found in primary functional psychiatric disorders, running the gamut from major depression and schizophrenia to personality disorders and conversion disorders. Over the years, many clinicians and researchers have hypothesized the existence of a predictable relationship between tumor location and observed neuropsychiatric phenomenology. Unfortunately, the association between tumor location and neuropsychiatric symptom formation does not appear to be nearly as strong as many might have wished. For example, two of the larger studies evaluating psychiatric symptoms in patients with brain tumors (Keschner et al. 1938; Selecki 1965) concluded that the observed behavioral changes were of no localizing value and that there were no mental syndromes that were strictly characteristic of lesions located in specific areas of the brain.

In truth, the nature and severity of psychiatric dysfunctions that accompany tumors are determined by a number of other factors that are of as great or even greater importance than anatomical location. One reason for this may be the fact that neuroanatomical substrates of particular behaviors tend not to be localized to single lobes or specific anatomical locations. The best examples of this are behaviors mediated by tumors involving the limbic

TABLE 20–1. RELATIVE FREQUENCIES OF COMMON HISTOLOGICAL TYPES OF BRAIN TUMORS

Tumor type	*Frequency (%)*
Primary	
Gliomas	40–50
Astrocytomas	10–15
Glioblastomas	20–25
Others	10–15
Meningiomas	10–20
Pituitary adenomas	10
Neurilemmomas (mainly acoustic neuromas)	5–8
Medulloblastomas and pinealomas	5
Miscellaneous primary tumors	5
Metastatic	15–25

Source. Reprinted from Lohr JB, Cadet JL: Neuropsychiatric aspects of brain tumors, in The American Psychiatric Press Textbook of Neuropsychiatry. Washington, DC, American Psychiatric Press, 1987, p 356. Used with permission.

system, which includes the temporal lobes and portions of the frontal lobes, the hypothalamus, and the midbrain. Tumors affecting any of these structures may produce similar psychopathology. Furthermore, even lesions outside the limbic system may produce similar behavioral changes, attributable to limbic release or disinhibition. Limbic tumors have been frequently associated with depression, affective flattening, apathy, agitation, assaultive behavior, and even a variety of psychotic symptoms. One study (Malamud 1967) of patients with tumors in or near limbic system structures who had initially been admitted to psychiatric hospitals found that the patients shared similar psychopathology regardless of the actual structures involved.

A study of patients who developed mania after a variety of brain lesions (Starkstein et al. 1988), including tumors, also exemplifies the difficulty of trying to associate specific kinds of psychiatric symptoms with the anatomical location of tumors. Although there was an overall predominance of right-sided involvement, lesions occurred in the frontal, temporoparietal, and temporo-occipital lobes, as well as in the cerebellum, thalamus, and pituitary. The authors concluded that the unifying aspect in all of these lesions was not anatomical location but rather the interconnection of the involved structures with the orbitofrontal cortex.

Other factors may also influence presenting symptoms and thereby diminish the localizing value of a particular observed behavioral change. Increased intracranial pressure (ICP) is a nonspecific consequence of CNS tumors in general and has been implicated in behavioral changes such as apathy, depression, irritability, agitation, and changes in consciousness. For example, in a study of lesions involving the occipital lobes, Allen (1930) concluded that the majority of observed mental changes were due to increases in ICP rather than to focal effects of the tumors themselves.

Another factor is the patient's premorbid level of functioning, which often has a significant impact on the nature of the clinical presentation. Tumors frequently cause an exaggeration of the individual's previous predominant character traits and coping styles. Also, once a brain tumor is discovered, the behavioral changes noted may often represent a complex combination of premorbid psychiatric status, tumor-associated organic mental symptoms, and the patient's adaptive psychological responses to the stress of the recently made diagnosis.

It has also been noted that rapidly growing tumors are more commonly associated with severe, acute psychiatric symptoms such as agitation or psychosis, as well as with more obvious cognitive dysfunctions. Slow-growing tumors are more likely to present with vague personality changes, apathy, or depression, often without associated cognitive changes. Additionally, compared with single lesions, multiple tumor foci tend to produce behavioral symptoms with greater frequency.

The relationship between tumor type and neuropsychiatric symptoms is also unclear. Several

TABLE 20–2. RELATIVE FREQUENCIES OF METASTATIC BRAIN TUMORS BY SITE OF THE PRIMARY LESION

Tumor	*Frequency (%)*
Lung	35–45
Breast	10–20
Kidney	5–10
Gastrointestinal tract	5–10
Melanoma	2–5
Others (including thyroid, pancreas, ovary, uterus, prostate, testes, bladder, and sarcoma)	25–30

Source. Reprinted from Lohr JB, Cadet JL: Neuropsychiatric aspects of brain tumors, in The American Psychiatric Press Textbook of Neuropsychiatry. Washington, DC, American Psychiatric Press, 1987, p 356. Used with permission.

large studies (e.g., Frazier 1935; Keschner et al. 1938) have noted no association between the histological type of tumor and associated behavioral changes. Davison and Bagley (1969) reviewed the literature on numerous patients with psychosis secondary to brain tumors and found little predominance of one tumor type over another. This should not be surprising given the variability of tumor classification systems used by different pathologists (Reitan and Wolfson 1985). Schirmer and Bock (1984) found no differences in symptoms when comparing primary brain tumors and intracranial metastases. Others (e.g., Lishman 1978), however, have suggested that gliomas may be more likely than benign tumors to produce behavioral changes, possibly because of the rapidity of growth or the multiplicity of tumor sites.

Conversely, there have been reports that meningiomas most commonly produce neuropsychiatric symptoms, in spite of the greater overall frequency of gliomas (McIntyre and McIntyre 1942). Patton and Sheppard (1956) noted a greater incidence of meningiomas among psychiatric patients compared with general hospital patients, whereas gliomas were equally common in both groups. Perhaps this is because of the greater predilection for meningiomas to occur in proximity to the frontal lobes, lesions of which often are associated with behavioral changes. Furthermore, because of their location and slow growth, meningiomas often produce few focal signs and less obvious symptomatology, tend to be neurologically silent, and therefore are associated with an increased likelihood that the patient will first present to a psychiatrist. For the most part, however, tumor type seems to be far less important than other factors in determining the presence and quality of neuropsychiatric symptoms.

In general, the factors that most significantly influence symptom formation appear to include the extent of tumor involvement, the rapidity of its growth, and its propensity to cause increased ICP. Additionally, the patient's premorbid psychiatric history, level of functioning, and characteristic psychological defense mechanisms may play a significant contributing role in determining the nature of the particular symptoms the patient manifests. Lesion location often, in fact, plays a relatively minor role.

Nonetheless, there remains among many physicians a tendency to search for certain neuropsychiatric syndromes that are characteristic of lesions located in specific neuroanatomical regions. One reason for this may be the fact that much of what we now know about tumors and their associated psychopathology is based on retrospective, uncontrolled, single case reports and clinical series. These studies often describe the type and range of symptoms associated with mass lesions occurring in particular locations, rather than prospectively comparing the relative frequencies of behavioral changes associated with tumors occurring in various regions of the brain. Notably, when one large study (Keschner et al. 1936) examined the comparative types of psychiatric symptoms in patients with frontal and temporal lobe tumors, few differences were found (Figure 20–3). Of course, this should not be very surprising given the intimate anatomical interconnections between these two lobes. Nonetheless, most large comparative studies have supported the conclusion that the range of behavioral changes tends to be similar regardless of the specific anatomical brain region involved (Keschner et al. 1936; Schlesinger 1950; Selecki 1965).

Lesion location may therefore not be the most important factor in determining the occurrence of specific types of neuropsychiatric symptoms. However, there have been some reports that brain lesions in certain locations may be associated with an increased frequency of certain kinds of psychiatric symptoms. For example, although Keschner et al. (1936) noted no overall difference in the types of symptoms found in association with frontal and temporal lobe tumors, they did find that to a small degree complex visual and auditory hallucinations were more common among patients with temporal lobe tumors and "facetiousness" was more frequently found among those with frontal lobe tumors. Perhaps more significantly, they found that mental changes were twice as likely to occur among patients with supratentorial tumors compared with those with infratentorial lesions (Keschner et al. 1938). Likewise, mental changes tended to be early symptoms in 18% of the patients with supratentorial tumors but in only 5% of those with infratentorial tumors. Additionally, psychiatric disturbances were more commonly associated with frontal lobe and temporal lobe tumors than with parietal or occipital lobe tumors.

Psychotic symptoms tend to be particularly frequent in patients with tumors of the temporal lobes and pituitary gland and much less commonly seen in those with occipital and cerebellar tumors, although this finding seems to depend, to some extent, on the particular study being reviewed (Davi-

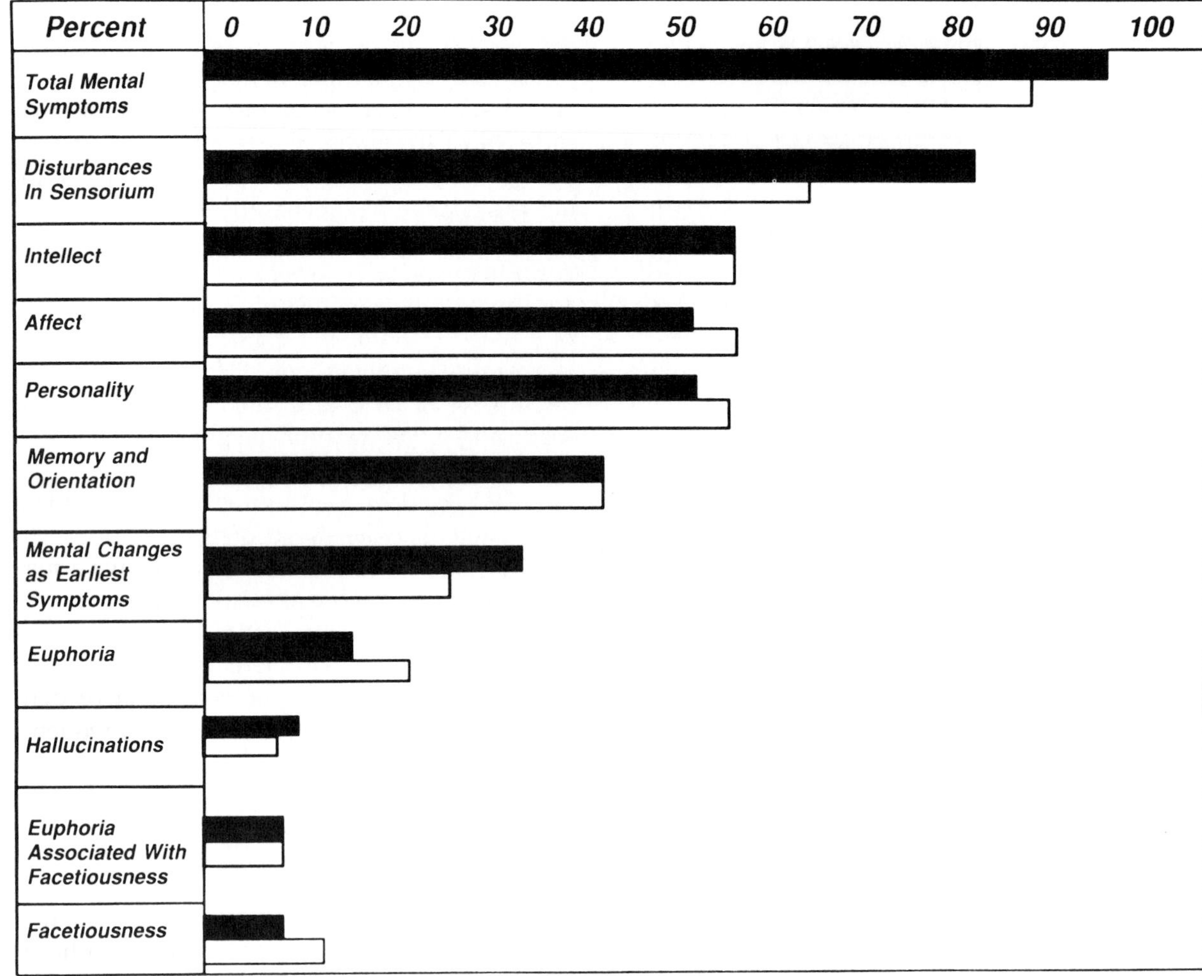

Figure 20–3. Comparison of incidence of mental symptoms in 110 cases of tumor of the temporal lobe (*solid bars*) and in 64 cases of tumor of the frontal lobe (*open bars*). (Reprinted from Keschner M, Bender MB, Strauss I: Mental symptoms in cases of tumor of the temporal lobe. Archives of Neurology and Psychiatry 35:572–595, 1936. Copyright 1936 by American Medical Association. Used with permission.)

son and Bagley 1969). This underscores one of the major difficulties in comparing clinical series, especially when they were collected during different time periods. Most of the available literature antedates the development of our current diagnostic system for classifying psychiatric clinical phenomenology, and thus significant methodological problems result when one attempts to compare the conclusions of such older series to either each other or more recent studies.

Despite these limitations, the literature taken as a whole seems to support a higher frequency of behavioral changes among patients with lesions of the frontal and temporal lobes, as well as with lesions involving deep midline structures. Similarly, bilateral tumors and those with multifocal involvement generally appear to be more frequently associated with the occurrence of neuropsychiatric symptoms.

General Neuropsychological Considerations

Neuropsychological testing is often useful in patients with CNS neoplasms. Although neuropsychological testing was initially used to provide diagnostic information about the location and nature of brain tumors, the current widespread availability of computed tomography (CT) and magnetic resonance imaging (MRI) and their greater capacity for precise anatomical localization have lessened the use of neuropsychological testing for diagnostic purposes. Currently, such testing is most often requested to determine the extent of cognitive dysfunction associated with a tumor, to provide a preoperative baseline measure of cognitive functioning, or as a means of monitoring the efficacy and progress of cognitive rehabilitation efforts after treatment.

Brain tumors can have a wide range of effects on cognitive functioning, and it is important to emphasize that patients with brain tumors rarely present with a circumscribed cognitive deficit in one area without more diffuse dysfunction elsewhere (Lezak 1983). The nature and severity of neuropsychological dysfunctions that accompany tumors are determined by several factors (Bigler 1984).

For instance, the histological type of the tumor and the rate of growth may affect the expression of symptoms. For example, a rapidly growing tumor such as a glioblastoma multiforme is likely to result in obvious cognitive dysfunction, whereas patients with slower-growing tumors such as meningiomas may demonstrate subtle personality changes but no obvious cognitive changes or focal neurological deficits (Reitan and Wolfson 1985). This may be due to the individual's ability to compensate better for less severe, more gradually developing cognitive deficits (Golden 1983). With slower-growing tumors, the degree to which cognitive deficits will be clinically apparent is substantially affected by the individual's premorbid level of intelligence. Thus patients with higher IQs tend to have a broader range of coping and adaptive skills, which allows them to more successfully compensate for and conceal emerging cognitive impairment.

In general, younger patients are likely to manifest less striking cognitive and behavioral deficits than are older patients (Bigler 1984). The size of the tumor is also likely to have a significant impact on the expression of cognitive dysfunction. Larger tumors generally give rise to both more clinically apparent, focal cognitive abnormalities directly reflecting the anatomical location of the lesion and more diffuse, less obvious, nonspecific manifestations secondary to the effects of cerebral edema, compression of adjacent brain tissue, or elevation of ICP.

In addition to the diffuse disruption of cognitive functioning secondary to cerebral edema, elevated ICP, and compression of brain tissue, other factors may result in cognitive deficits that do not reflect the anatomic location of the tumor. According to Lezak (1983), several types of "distance effects" may be important in determining the types of deficits found on neuropsychological testing. First, *diaschisis* refers to the depression of neural activity in a functionally related but often distant region of the brain (von Monakow 1914). Second, *disconnection* of a given region of the brain from a more distant region by a structural lesion can also affect the cognitive expression of the symptom, as has been dramatically demonstrated in patients who have undergone surgical sectioning of the corpus callosum as a treatment for intractable seizures (Sperry 1974).

The location of a tumor can also have a major impact on the type of cognitive dysfunction manifested. Although, as stressed above, the cognitive sequelae of tumors often do not reflect the specific site of the tumor, the particular cognitive deficit demonstrated by the patient may, not infrequently, have some localizing value.

Summary

Despite methodological flaws and other limitations, the large body of descriptive literature that has examined neuropsychiatric and neuropsychological symptoms associated with brain tumors over the past several decades clearly documents the broad array of behavioral and cognitive changes that can accompany tumors of the brain. Thus it underscores the need for the psychiatrist to at least consider the possibility of an organic mental disorder due to a brain tumor when initially evaluating any psychiatric patient. It also helps the psychiatrist to better understand, evaluate, and treat the known brain tumor patient with neuropsychiatric and neuropsychological symptoms. Finally, despite the generally weak association between lesion location and specific psychiatric, behavioral, and cognitive symptoms, the literature does describe certain constellations of neuropsychiatric symptoms suggestive of the involvement of particular CNS regions. Recognition of these "syndromes," when they occur, may be helpful in leading one to suspect organic pathology and thereby perhaps diagnose a previously unsuspected brain tumor.

❑ SPECIFIC NEUROPSYCHIATRIC AND NEUROPSYCHOLOGICAL SYMPTOMATOLOGY AND BRAIN TUMOR LOCATION

The discussion that follows reviews the range of neuropsychiatric and neurophysiological concomitants that have been described in association with brain tumors occurring in the following anatomical locations: frontal lobes, temporal lobes, parietal lobes, occipital lobes, the diencephalon, the corpus callosum, the pituitary, and the posterior fossa.

Frontal Lobe Tumors

Neuropsychiatric and behavioral manifestations. As noted above, tumors of the frontal lobe are frequently associated with neuropsychiatric symptoms, with some studies reporting mental changes in as many as 90% of cases (Strauss and Keschner 1935). In the study by Strauss and Keschner (1935), 43% of 85 patients with frontal lobe tumors manifested behavioral changes early in the course of their illnesses. This is not surprising when one considers the higher level "executive" and cognitive functions carried out by this region of cortex. Rather than being homogeneous and unidimensional in their function, the frontal lobes appear to consist of a variety of functionally distinct subregions. These areas are involved in a number of both related and unrelated tasks, such as the mediation of problem-solving behavior, the regulation of attentional processes, the temporal organization of behavior, and the modulation of affective states (McAllister and Price 1987).

Injuries to the frontal lobes have been associated with three different kinds of clinical syndromes (Cummings 1985) (Table 20–3). The orbitofrontal syndrome is typically characterized by behavioral disinhibition with emotional lability, irritability, and socially inappropriate behavior. Cognitively, patients with this syndrome often demonstrate poor judgment and a lack of insight into their behavior. These patients have sometimes been referred to as *pseudopsychopathic* (McAllister and Price 1987).

In contrast to the symptoms associated with orbitofrontal syndrome, patients with injuries to the frontal convexities, or the so-called convexity syndrome, often present with apathy, indifference, and psychomotor retardation. Cognitively, such patients demonstrate difficulty initiating or persisting in behavioral activities, have problems with sustained attention and/or sequencing, or may demonstrate perseverative behavior (Goldberg 1986). These latter deficits may not be especially apparent on standard intellectual or neuropsychological assessments, but usually become obvious on more specific tests of executive functioning, such as the Wisconsin Card Sorting Test (Goldberg 1986). This syndrome has been referred to as a *pseudodepressed* state (McAllister and Price 1987).

Finally, the medial frontal syndrome has also been described. Patients with this syndrome are predominantly akinetic, with frequent mutism and failure to respond to commands.

TABLE 20–3. CLINICAL CHARACTERISTICS OF THE THREE PRINCIPAL FRONTAL LOBE SYNDROMES

Orbitofrontal syndrome (disinhibited)
- Disinhibited, impulsive behavior (pseudopsychopathic)
- Inappropriate jocular affect and euphoria
- Emotional lability
- Poor judgment and insight
- Distractibility

Frontal convexity syndrome (apathetic)
- Apathetic (pseudodepressed)
- Occasional brief angry or aggressive outbursts common
- Indifference
- Psychomotor retardation
- Motor perseveration and impersistence
- Loss of set
- Stimulus boundedness
- Discrepant motor and verbal behavior
- Motor programming deficits
  - Three-step hand sequence
  - Alternating programs
  - Reciprocal programs
  - Rhythm tapping
  - Multiple loops
- Poor word-list generation
- Poor abstraction and categorization
- Segmented approach to visuospatial analysis

Medial frontal syndrome (akinetic)
- Paucity of spontaneous movement and gesture
- Sparse verbal output (repetition may be preserved)
- Lower extremity weakness and loss of sensation
- Incontinence

Source. Reprinted from Cummings JL: Clinical Neuropsychiatry. Orlando, FL, Grune & Stratton, 1985, p 58. Used with permission of Allyn and Bacon.

Despite the occurrence of these three syndromes as distinct entities with other types of organic frontal lobe disorders, most patients with frontal lobe tumors present with a mixture of symptoms. This is probably in part due to the fact that frontal tumors are rarely confined to a single subregion of the frontal lobes and may have effects on other areas through pressure effects and edema, as well as through mechanisms such as diaschisis and disconnection. It is therefore difficult to find clear descriptions of these three syndromes in pure form when reviewing the literature on frontal lobe neoplasms. Nonetheless, all of the symptoms noted above have been reported in patients with tumors involving the frontal areas.

Affective symptoms are certainly common and can include depression, irritability, apathy, and euphoria. Symptoms of depression are often similar to those seen in patients with functional psychiatric disturbances. Frequently psychomotor retardation, with aspontaneity, hypokinesia or akinesia, or inertia is present. In one study of 25 patients with frontal lobe tumors (Direkze et al. 1971), 5 patients had initially presented to psychiatric units with a variety of mood disturbances. In their study of 85 patients, Strauss and Keschner (1935) reported affective disturbances in 63% of the patients, with 30% presenting with euphoria and 4% presenting with hypomania. Although Strauss and Keschner (1935) found no correlation between clinical presentation and laterality of the lesion, Belyi (1987) noted a tendency for right frontal lesions to present with euphoria and left frontal lesions to present with akinesia, abulia, and depressed affect.

Changes in personality have been found in as many as 70% of patients with frontal lobe tumors (Strauss and Keschner 1935). These changes have been noted by some authors (e.g., Pincus and Tucker 1978) to be "characteristic" of frontal lobe disease. They include irresponsibility, childishness, facetiousness, disinhibition, and indifference toward others, as well as inappropriate sexual behavior. The term *Witzelsucht* has been used to describe the tendency of patients with frontal lobe lesions to make light of everything. Frequently, however, this humorous bent tends to have an angry, cutting quality to it. Although these behaviors are consistent with descriptions of the characteristic features of the orbitofrontal syndrome, it should be noted that similar "frontal lobe" personality changes have been described in patients with both temporal lobe and diencephalic lesions, again probably partly as a result of the close temporal-limbic-frontal interconnections.

Psychotic symptoms also occur with some regularity in patients with frontal lobe tumors, with incidence reports of approximately 10% for frank delusions and another 10% for hallucinations (Strauss and Keschner 1935). Other reported psychotic manifestations have included vague paranoid ideation or ideas of reference.

Hypersomnolence has also been reported (Frazier 1935). A careful psychiatric assessment and evaluation of mental status may be needed to clearly differentiate this symptom from the lethargy and fatigue frequently encountered in patients with major depression.

Neuropsychological manifestations. Cognitively, patients with tumors of the frontal region of the brain, and of the prefrontal area in particular, often present with significant behavioral changes in the absence of obvious intellectual decline or focal neurological dysfunction. In such patients previously acquired cognitive skills are often preserved and the patient may perform quite adequately on formal intelligence testing. However, more sophisticated neuropsychological assessment often reveals profound deficits in the individual's ability to organize, initiate, and direct personal behavior (Teuber 1972). These deficits in executive functioning are often the most devastating type of cognitive dysfunction encountered in neurological, neurosurgical, and psychiatric patients, disrupting the very core of the individual's drive, initiative, and integration of critical cognitive functions (Luria 1980).

Tumors of the frontal lobes can also result in significant deficits in attentional processes (Luria 1973). Additionally, posterior frontal lobe tumors can lead to expressive (Broca's) aphasia when the lesion is localized to the dominant hemisphere (Benson 1979), or aprosody when localized to the nondominant hemisphere.

Temporal Lobe Tumors

Neuropsychiatric and behavioral manifestations. It is important to distinguish ictal from interictal phenomena when discussing the neuropsychiatry of temporal lobe tumors, given the high frequency of seizure disorders seen in such patients. Ictal phenomena are discussed in Chapter 17. Here we confine ourselves to interictal phenomena associated with temporal lobe tumors.

A high likelihood of schizophrenic-like illnesses has been noted with temporal lobe tumors. Malamud (1967) reported that 6 of 11 patients with temporal lobe tumors initially presented with a diagnosis of schizophrenia. Selecki (1965) also reported that an initial diagnosis of schizophrenia had been made in 2 of his 9 patients with temporal lobe tumors, and he reported auditory hallucinations in 5 of them.

Again, one must bear in mind that these studies were published before the advent of DSM-III-R diagnostic criteria (American Psychiatric Association 1987) and therefore may have had a tendency to overdiagnose schizophrenia. On closer reading, many of Malamud's case descriptions (1967) do not indicate that the patients had clear evidence of psychotic symptoms such as delusions, hallucinations, or formal thought disorder.

In fact, patients with temporal lobe dysfunction generally tend to present with psychotic symptoms somewhat atypical for classical schizophrenia. Frequently these patients present with episodic mood swings, suicidal ideation or suicide attempts, and visual, olfactory, and tactile hallucinations, as well as with the more typical auditory hallucinations seen in schizophrenia (Tucker et al. 1986). Patients with temporal lobe diseases very often complain of "spells" consisting of dreamlike episodes or report "staring" or "dazed feelings" (Tucker et al. 1986). Also, unlike schizophrenic patients who have notably flat or inappropriate affect and markedly diminished capacity to interact with and relate appropriately to others, patients with temporal lobe diseases often retain appropriate, broad affective ranges and interact interpersonally in a relatively normal fashion. Nonetheless, regardless of the similarities and differences between functional psychiatric disorders and temporal lobe disease, Davison and Bagley (1969) reviewed 77 psychotic patients with known brain tumors and found the temporal lobe to be the region of the brain most frequently involved.

Other studies, however, have not confirmed this apparent high frequency of interictal psychosis in patients with temporal lobe tumors. Keschner et al. (1936) studied 110 such patients and found that only 2 had complex hallucinations. In another study (Mulder and Daly 1952), only 4 of a group of 100 temporal lobe tumor patients had evidence of psychosis. Strobos (1953) noted complex auditory hallucinations in only 1% of his 62 temporal lobe tumor patients. He did, however, report complex visual hallucinations in 8% and simple olfactory or gustatory hallucinations in approximately 30% of his patients, although these almost invariably preceded the onset of seizures.

Regardless of the prevalence of psychosis, temporal lobe tumors are commonly associated with behavioral changes. Neuropsychiatric symptoms associated with temporal lobe tumors often tend to be very similar to those noted in patients with frontal lobe tumors and may include depressed mood with apathy and irritability or mania, hypomania, or euphoria. As noted above, this is probably a result of the complex interconnections between the frontal lobes, the temporal lobes, and other related structures of the limbic system.

Personality changes have been described in more than half of temporal lobe tumor patients and may often be an early manifestation of a previously unsuspected tumor (Keschner et al. 1936). Previous research (Bear and Fedio 1977) suggested that characteristic interictal personality traits occurred in patients with temporal lobe epilepsy and further suggested that the presence or absence of certain traits depended on whether the seizure focus was right or left sided. However, more recent studies (Mungas 1982; Rodin and Schmaltz 1984) have failed to confirm these initial findings. Thus there do not appear to be specific interictal personality traits characteristic of temporal lobe lesions. Frequently, patients present with an intensification of their previous character traits, predominant coping mechanism, or adaptive styles or, again, with symptoms similar to those seen with frontal lobe tumors. Organic personality syndromes with episodic behavioral dyscontrol and/or affective instability are also frequently encountered.

Anxiety symptoms appear to be quite commonly associated with temporal lobe tumors. Mulder and Daly (1952) noted anxiety in 36% of their 100 patients. Two cases of panic attacks in patients with right temporal lobe tumors have been reported (Drubach and Kelly 1989; Ghadirian et al. 1986), though the number of cases is obviously too small to draw any conclusions about the influence of laterality on the appearance of such phenomena. However, these case reports are consistent with work by Reiman et al. (1986) that demonstrated abnormally low ratios of left-to-right parahippocampal blood flow in panic disorder patients vulnerable to lactate-induced panic. The authors suggested that this asymmetry could be secondary to increases in neuronal activity or anatomical asymmetry or to an increase in blood-brain barrier permeability in the right parahippocampal region. Such mechanisms could also conceivably be associated with temporal lobe tumors.

Neuropsychological manifestations. Tumors of the temporal lobe can also result in neuropsychological and cognitive deficits. First, verbal or nonverbal memory functioning may be affected, depending on the cerebral hemisphere involved. Dominant temporal lobe dysfunction is often associated with deficits in the patient's ability to learn and remember information of a verbal nature, whereas nondominant temporal lobe dysfunction is often associated with deficits in acquiring and retaining nonverbal (i.e., visuospatial) information (Butters 1979). Tumors of the dominant temporal lobe may also result in receptive (Wernicke's) aphasia, whereas nondominant tumors may lead to disruption of the discrimination of nonspeech sounds (Spreen et al. 1965).

Because of the high incidence of seizure disorders with tumors of the temporal lobes (Strobos 1953), cognitive dysfunction may result from the occurrence of seizure activity, which may induce dysfunction in other areas of the brain, or from the administration of certain anticonvulsants used to treat the seizures, especially when used in high doses, for long time periods, or in multidrug regimens.

Parietal Lobe Tumors

Neuropsychiatric and behavioral manifestations. Tumors of the parietal lobe are generally less likely to cause behavioral changes. This has been well documented in large, comparative studies examining psychiatric and behavioral phenomenology as a function of anatomic location. Schlesinger (1950) found affective symptomatology in only 16% of 31 patients with parietal lobe tumors. Affective symptoms present in these patients tended to reflect predominantly depression and apathy, rather than euphoria or mania, a finding Keschner et al. (1938) had previously noted in their series. Psychotic symptoms also appear to be considerably less common in parietal lobe tumor patients, although Selecki (1965) reported episodes of "paranoid psychosis" in 2 of the 7 patients in his series.

Neuropsychological manifestations. Of greater significance than the psychiatric and behavioral symptoms associated with parietal lobe tumors are the various complex sensory and motor abnormalities that may be seen. In fact, tumors localized in the parietal lobes are considerably more likely to result in cognitive as opposed to psychiatric symptoms. Depending on the location of the neoplasm within the parietal lobe, a variety of deficits may be observed.

Tumors of the anterior parietal lobe may result in abnormalities of sensory perception in the contralateral hand. Inability of the individual to perceive objects placed in the hand (astereognosis) is common and may have localizing value to the contralateral parietal cortex of the cerebral hemisphere. Difficulty in the recognition of shapes, letters, and numbers drawn on the hand (agraphesthesia) is also seen and may aid in localizing the neoplasm. Apraxias may be present. Tumors of the parietal lobe may also affect the patient's ability to decipher visuospatial information, particularly when the tumor is localized to the nondominant hemisphere (Warrington and Rabin 1970).

Dominant parietal lobe tumors may lead to dysgraphia, acalculia, finger agnosia, and right-left confusion (Gerstmann's syndrome) and may often affect reading and spelling. Individuals with parietal lobe tumors may also present with a marked lack of awareness or even frank denial of their neurological and/or neuropsychiatric difficulties, even in the face of rather obvious organic dysfunction (i.e., denial of hemiparesis) (Critchley 1964a). Such phenomena are sometimes referred to as anosognosia or the so-called neglect syndromes. Because of the often bizarre neurological complaints and atypical symptoms that may accompany tumors in this area, such patients are frequently initially thought to have psychiatric problems and are diagnosed as having either a conversion disorder or some other type of somatization disorder (Critchley 1964b).

Occipital Lobe Tumors

Neuropsychiatric and behavioral manifestations. Occipital lobe tumors may present with psychiatric symptoms, but, like tumors involving the parietal lobes, they appear less likely to do so than tumors of the frontal or temporal lobes (Keschner et al. 1938). However, Allen (1930) examined a large series of such cases (N = 40) and found psychiatric symptoms in 55% of his patients. In fact, in 17% of these patients, behavioral symptoms were the presenting complaint. The most characteristic finding appears to have been visual hallucinations, which were present in 25% of his patients. These generally tended to be unformed and were often frequently merely flashes of light. In only two patients were there complex visual hallucinations.

Other changes seen included agitation, irritability, suspiciousness, and fatigue, though Allen (1930) felt that many of the changes (apart from the visual hallucinations) were nonspecific effects of increased ICP. Keschner et al. (1938) noted affective symptoms in 5 of 11 patients with occipital tumors. Three of these 5 patients were predominantly dysphoric, whereas 2 presented with euphoria or facetiousness.

Neuropsychological manifestations. Tumors of the occipital lobe tend to cause significant and characteristic difficulties in cognitive and perceptual functions. Therefore, a typical finding in patients who have neoplasms localized to the occipital lobe is a homonymous hemianopsia, the loss of one-half of the visual field in each eye. The inability to recognize items visually (visual agnosia) may also be seen (Lezak 1983). The inability of the patient to recognize familiar faces, prosopagnosia, may also accompany lesions in the occipital lobes, particularly when there is bilateral involvement (Meadows 1974).

Diencephalic Tumors

Neuropsychiatric and behavioral manifestations. Tumors of deep midline structures, such as the thalamus, hypothalamus, and the areas surrounding the third ventricle, typically involve regions that are part of or closely contiguous with the limbic system. Not surprisingly then, these lesions are very frequently associated with psychiatric symptoms. For example, in addition to a diagnosis of schizophrenia in 6 of 11 temporal lobe tumor patients, Malamud (1967) reported similar diagnoses in 4 of 7 patients with tumors near the third ventricle. Cairns and Mosberg (1951) reported "emotional instability" and psychosis in patients with colloid cysts of the third ventricle. Burkle and Lipowski (1978) also reported depression, affective flattening, and withdrawal in a patient with a colloid cyst of the third ventricle. Personality changes similar to those seen with frontal lobe disease have also been reported (Alpers 1937), as has akinetic mutism (Cairns et al. 1941).

Hypothalamic tumors have been associated with disorders in eating behavior, including hyperphagia and symptoms indistinguishable from anorexia nervosa (Climo 1982; Coffey 1989; Reeves and Plum 1969). Additionally, lesions of the hypothalamus can present with hypersomnia and daytime somnolence.

Neuropsychological manifestations. Neoplasms originating in subcortical brain regions often have their most dramatic effect on memory, resulting in significant impairments in new learning, whereas other aspects of cognitive functioning may remain relatively intact (Lishman 1978). Tumors in this area may also lead to more diffuse, generalized cognitive dysfunction by interfering with the normal circulation of cerebral spinal fluid, thereby causing hydrocephalus.

Corpus Callosum Tumors

Tumors of the corpus callosum have been associated with behavioral symptoms in as many as 90% of patients (Selecki 1964). Such symptoms appear to be most common with tumors of the genu and splenium (Schlesinger 1950), probably because of involvement of adjacent structures (i.e., the frontal lobes and deep midline and limbic structures). A broad array of behavioral changes has been found. These changes range from depression and apathy to psychotic symptoms, as well as organic personality features similar to those typically seen with frontal lobe tumors.

In a recent comparison of five patients with corpus callosal tumors with eight patients with other types of tumors, significantly more depression was found in the corpus callosum group (Nasrallah and McChesney 1981). One of these patients had in fact received a trial of tricyclic antidepressants (TCAs) for a presumed primary affective disorder before emerging neurological symptoms led to the correct diagnosis. Psychotic symptoms were also noted in two of these patients, although such symptoms appeared equally likely to occur in patients with other types of tumors. Although interesting, these reported differences between callosal and non-callosal tumors cannot be considered other than suggestive, given the small sample size involved.

Pituitary Tumors

Pituitary tumors frequently present with behavioral changes resulting from upward extension of the tumor to involve other structures, particularly those in the diencephalon. This may be most common with craniopharyngiomas, which sometimes present with disorders of sleep or temperature regulation, clinical phenomena otherwise more commonly seen with tumors of the hypothalamus.

Additionally, tumors of the pituitary can result in endocrine disturbances, which can produce neuropsychiatric symptoms. Basophilic adenomas are commonly associated with Cushing's syndrome, which is likewise frequently associated with affective lability, depression, or even psychosis. Acidophilic adenomas frequently present with acromegaly, which has been associated, although infrequently, with both anxiety and depression (Avery 1973).

As with most brain tumors in other anatomic locations, the whole gamut of psychiatric symptoms from depression and apathy to paranoia has been reported with pituitary tumors. One review of five patients with such lesions reported delusions and hallucinations in three (White and Cobb 1955). In Russell and Pennybacker's study (1961), 33% of 24 patients had mental disturbances severe enough to dominate their clinical picture, and 13% had initially presented to psychiatric hospitals for diagnosis and treatment. This broad and unpredictable spectrum of symptoms undoubtedly reflects the multiplicity of ways in which pituitary tumors can effect diencephalic and hypothalamic structures as well as the various endocrine functions involved.

Posterior Fossa Tumors

As noted earlier, infratentorial tumors present much less frequently with psychiatric symptoms. Moreover, an evaluation of the infrequent behavioral changes that are associated with such tumors again underscores the difficulty of localizing lesions on the basis of specific typology of associated psychiatric symptoms. Though observed less frequently overall, virtually every behavioral change that has been described with supratentorial tumors has also been reported with infratentorial lesions.

In fact, mental symptoms have, in some series, been found in as many as 76% of such patients and have included paranoid delusions and affective disorders (Wilson and Rupp 1946). Cases of mania have also been noted (Greenberg and Brown 1985). Posterior fossa tumors have been associated, albeit infrequently, with irritability, apathy, and hypersomnolence. Auditory hallucinations have also been reported (Cairns 1950). Once again, however, no convincing or clear-cut correlation between tumors of particular anatomic structures in the posterior fossa and specific psychiatric or behavioral symptomatology has been established.

❑ LATERALITY OF BRAIN TUMORS AND CLINICAL MANIFESTATIONS

Despite the fact that many older, larger studies reported no consistent differences in the psychiatric and behavioral symptoms associated with left- and right-sided tumors, more recent work appears to raise questions about this. Flor-Henry (1969) proposed that schizophrenia-like psychoses are more common with left-hemisphere lesions, whereas affective psychoses are more common with right-hemisphere lesions. More recent work with unilateral frontal tumors (Belyi 1987) suggests that left frontal tumors are more commonly associated with akinesia and depression, whereas right frontal tumors often present with euphoria and an underestimation of the seriousness of one's illness.

The importance of cerebral hemispheric lateralization was elegantly demonstrated by Robinson et al. (1984) in their work with stroke patients. This work indicated an increased frequency of depression in patients with left anterior lesions and a tendency toward inappropriate cheerfulness in patients with right anterior lesions. Although there have been few reports confirming these findings in patients with brain tumor, studies reviewing cases of mania secondary to CNS lesions, including tumors, have found a preponderance of right-hemisphere lesions (Cummings and Mendez 1984; Jamieson and Wells 1979; Starkstein et al. 1988).

This work suggests that lesion laterality may indeed have a larger impact on symptom formation than had previously been thought. It also implies that we may need to reevaluate tumor location and its implications for neuropsychiatric and neuropsychological symptomatology, from a different, more topographic, perspective. We will need to take into consideration not only specific anatomic location, but factors such as laterality, anterior/posterior and cortical/subcortical localization, and afferent and efferent projections between the region involved with the tumor and distant anatomic regions. Perhaps more importantly, it provides a clinically pertinent, although certainly more complex, theoretical framework from which to begin to study the psychopathology associated with brain tumors. Systematic future research with brain tumors patterned after that of Robinson et al. (1984) may further enhance our understanding not only of these secondary psychiatric and behavioral symptoms and syndromes, but also of the substrates of many primary, functional psychiatric disorders.

❑ CLINICAL DIAGNOSIS AND TREATMENT

General Clinical Characteristics of Brain Tumors

For the clinician, especially the psychiatrist, the prompt and accurate diagnosis of a brain tumor rests on a thorough awareness of the many clinical manifestations such tumors may produce. Both a high index of suspicion and a willingness to vigorously pursue appropriate diagnostic evaluations and consultations are critical to early diagnosis.

The most characteristic clinical aspect of CNS tumors is that they cause the progressive appearance of focal neurological signs and symptoms, as well as neuropsychiatric symptoms, such as personality changes, changes in affect or sensorium, and neuropsychological deficits. (The specific constellation of clinical phenomena encountered and the rapidity of its progression depend, to a large extent, on the size of the tumor, its location, its rate of growth, whether it is benign or malignant, and the presence or absence of associated cerebral edema, increased ICP, and hydrocephalus.)

Several typical neurological signs and symptoms commonly associated with brain tumors include headaches (25%–35%), nausea and vomiting (33%), seizures (20%–50%), and visual changes including field cuts, diplopia, and papilledema. Focal motor and sensory changes may also be of considerable value in localizing the tumor (Table 20–4).

When to Suspect a Brain Tumor in a Psychiatric Patient

Although recognition of a brain tumor presenting with characteristic focal neurological signs and symptoms should not be especially problematic, a brain tumor presenting with predominantly psychiatric and behavioral symptoms may be quite difficult to promptly and accurately diagnose. However, the occurrence of one or more of the five following complaints in a known psychiatric patient or in a patient presenting for the first time with psychiatric symptoms should heighten the clinician's index of suspicion of the possible presence of a brain tumor:

1. Seizures: especially if of new onset in an adult and especially if partial seizures, with or without secondary generalization; seizures may be the initial neurological manifestation of a tumor in as many as 50% of cases.
2. Headaches: especially if generalized and dull (i.e., nonspecific), if of new onset, if of increasing severity and/or frequency, or if positional, nocturnal, or present immediately on awakening.
3. Nausea and vomiting: especially if occurring in conjunction with headaches.
4. Sensory changes: visual changes such as loss or diminution of vision, visual field defects, or diplopia; auditory changes such as tinnitus or hearing loss, especially when unilateral; and vertigo.
5. Other focal neurological signs and symptoms: localized weakness, localized sensory loss, paresthesias or dysesthesias, ataxia, and incoordination.

The clinician should, of course, bear in mind that nausea and vomiting, visual field defects, papilledema, and other focal neurological signs and symptoms frequently are not seen early on in the course of many brain tumors and may not be seen until very late with "silent" tumors, such as meningiomas or tumors occurring in relatively "silent" locations (see below).

The Diagnostic Evaluation

It is clear that a comprehensive, careful, and detailed history of the nature and time course of both psychiatric and neurological clinical signs and symptoms is the cornerstone of diagnosis. This of course must be supplemented by physical and neurological examinations, appropriate brain imaging and electrodiagnostic studies, and bedside neurocognitive as well as formal neuropsychological testing.

Physical and neurological examinations. All psychiatric patients, and particularly those in whom the psychiatrist is considering a brain tumor in the differential diagnosis, should have full and careful physical, neurological, and mental status examinations. Brain tumor patients often manifest focal neurological findings as well as abnormalities in cognitive functioning on careful bedside testing. Table

TABLE 20–4. NEUROLOGICAL AND NEUROPSYCHOLOGICAL FINDINGS THAT HAVE LOCALIZING VALUE

Brain region	*Neurological and neuropsychological findings*
Frontal lobes	
Prefrontal	Contralateral grasp reflex, executive functioning deficits (inability to formulate goals, to plan, and to effectively carry out these plans), decreased oral fluency (dominant hemisphere), decreased design fluency (nondominant hemisphere), motor perserveration or impersistence, and inability to hold set
Posterior	Contralateral hemiparesis, decreased motor strength, speed and coordination, and Broca's aphasia
Temporal lobes	Partial complex seizures, contralateral homonymous inferior quadrantanopsia, Wernicke's aphasia, decreased learning and retention of verbal material (dominant hemisphere), decreased learning and retention of nonverbal material (nondominant hemisphere), amusia (nondominant hemisphere), and auditory agnosia
Parietal lobes	Partial sensory seizures, agraphesthesia, astereognosis, anosognosia, Gerstmann's syndrome (acalculia, agraphia, finger agnosia, and right-left confusion), ideomotor and ideational apraxia, constructional apraxia, agraphia with alexia, dressing apraxia, prosopagnosia, and visuospatial problems
Occipital	Partial sensory seizures with visual phenomena, homonymous hemianopsia, alexia, agraphia, prosopagnosia, color agnosia, and construction apraxia
Corpus callosum	Callosal apraxia
Thalamus	Contralateral hemisensory loss and pain
Basal ganglia	Contralateral choreoathetosis, dystonia, rigidity, motor perseveration, and parkinsonian tremor
Pituitary and hypothalamus	Bitemporal hemianopia, optic atrophy, hypopituitarism, and diabetes insipidus
Pineal	Loss of upward gaze (Parinaud's syndrome)
Cerebellum	Ipsilateral hypotonia, ataxia, dysmetria, intention tremor, and nystagmus toward side of tumor
Brain stem	
Midbrain	Pupillary and extraocular muscle abnormalities and contralateral hemiparesis
Pons	Sixth and seventh nerve involvement (diplopia and ipsilateral facial paralysis)

Source. Reprinted from Lohr JB, Cadet JL: Neuropsychiatric aspects of brain tumors, in The American Psychiatric Press Textbook of Neuropsychiatry. Washington, DC, American Psychiatric Press, 1987, p 354. Used with permission.

20–4 highlights some of the more important and common localizing neurological findings that are found in association with brain tumors in various locations. It is important to be aware of the fact, however, that even despite very careful clinical examination, some brain tumors are not clinically apparent until relatively late in their course. Such tumors frequently involve the anterior frontal lobes, the corpus callosum, the nondominant parietal and temporal lobes, and posterior fossa: so-called silent regions. Thus despite negative clinical examinations for focal neurological signs, other diagnostic studies are necessary to rule out conclusively the presence of a tumor.

CT scans. In the 1970s, the CT scan largely replaced plain skull films, radioisotope brain scans, electroencephalography (EEG), echoencephalography, and pneumoencephalography in the diagnosis of brain tumors, predominantly because it provided far greater resolution in the delineation of anatomic brain structures. The CT scan's capacity to detect neoplasms can be even further enhanced by the concomitant use of intravenous contrast material, which often highlights tumors when present. In addition, CT scans can indirectly suggest the presence of tumors by revealing calcifications, cerebral edema, obstructive hydrocephalus, a shift in midline structures, or other changes in the ventricular system. Although extremely useful, CT scans may not reveal very small tumors, tumors in the posterior fossa, tumors that are isodense with respect to brain tissue and/or cerebrospinal fluid, or tumors diffusely involving the meninges (i.e., carcinomatosis).

MRI scans. In general, MRI is superior to CT scanning in the diagnosis of brain tumors and other soft tissue lesions in the brain because of a higher degree of resolution and a resultant greater capacity to detect very small lesions (Figures 20–4 and 20–5). In addition, MRI does not entail exposure to radiation. The chief drawbacks with it are the cost and the fact that it does not adequately image calcified lesions. It also cannot be used in patients in whom ferrometallic foreign objects are present. Enhancement of MRI scans with gadolinium further increases their diagnostic sensitivity (Figure 20–6).

Cisternography. CT cisternography is a technique for evaluating the ventricular system, subarachnoid spaces, and basilar cisterns, which may be helpful in the differential diagnosis of intraventricular and pituitary tumors as well as hydrocephalus. This technique has largely replaced pneumoencephalography, which was frequently very poorly tolerated by patients.

Skull films. Plain skull films are no longer routinely used in the diagnosis of brain tumors, although tomographs of the sella turcica may be helpful in the diagnosis of pituitary tumors, craniopharyngiomas, and the so-called empty sella syndrome. Plain skull films may be helpful in the diagnosis of bone (skull) metastases, but bone scans are generally superior in this regard.

Cerebral angiography. In certain circumstances cerebral angiography may be helpful in delineating the vascular supply to a tumor before surgery.

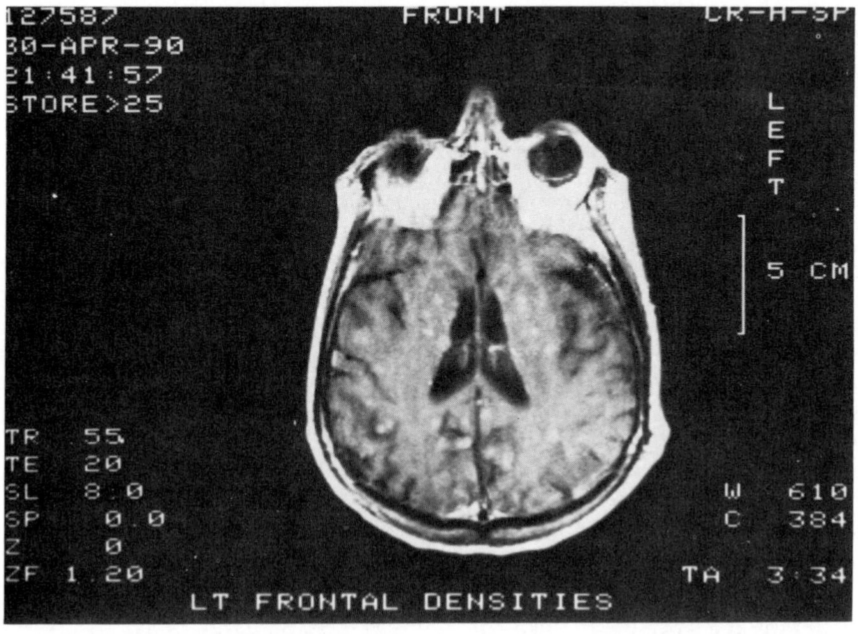

Figure 20–4. Diffuse metastatic disease (small cell carcinoma of the lung) in a 66-year-old man, as seen with magnetic resonance imaging (MRI). A computed tomography (CT) scan had not shown any metastatic lesions. (Courtesy of A. Goldberg, Allegheny General Hospital, Department of Radiology.)

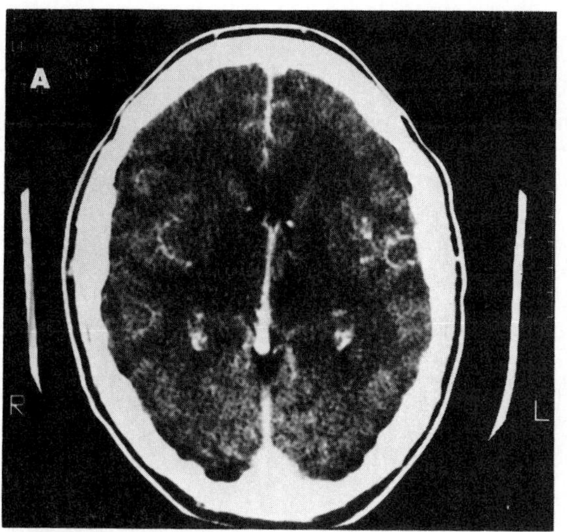

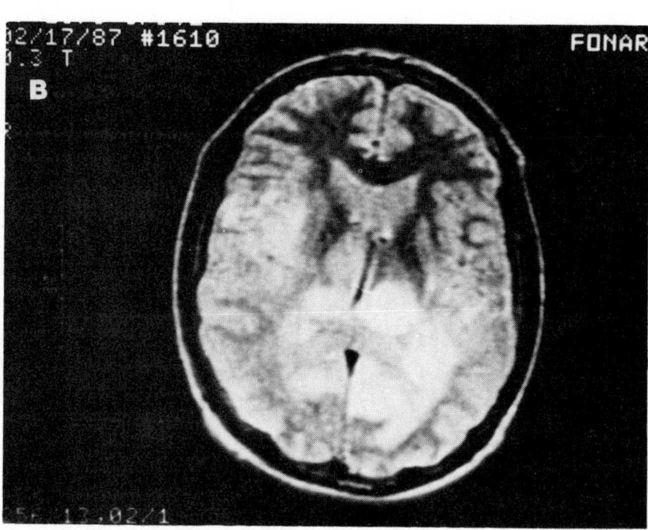

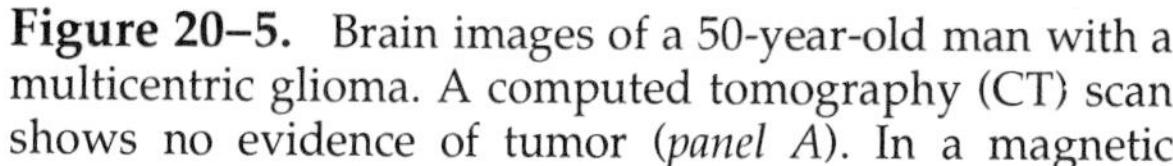

Figure 20–5. Brain images of a 50-year-old man with a multicentric glioma. A computed tomography (CT) scan shows no evidence of tumor (*panel A*). In a magnetic resonance imaging (MRI) scan the tumor is clearly evident (*panel B*). (Courtesy of A. Goldberg, Allegheny General Hospital, Department of Radiology.)

Neuropsychological testing. As mentioned above, before the advent of CT and MRI, neuropsychological testing was often used in the diagnosis and localization of brain tumors. Although no longer used very much for these purposes, it still plays an increasingly important role in the overall management of cerebral tumors. It can be very helpful in determining the extent of tumor-associated cognitive dysfunctions and providing baseline, preoperative measures of cognitive functioning. It may also be very helpful in assessing and monitoring the efficacy of both surgery and postoperative cognitive rehabilitation efforts with respect to premorbid tumor-associated cognitive and neuropsychological dysfunction.

Lumbar puncture. Given the range of other more sensitive, specific, and less invasive diagnostic studies currently available, lumbar punctures (LPs) are now used much less frequently in the diagnosis of brain tumors than in the past. Brain tumors may be associated with elevated cerebrospinal fluid protein and increased ICP, but these findings are diagnostically nonspecific; in the presence of the latter, there is a potential danger of herniation after an LP. Therefore, before proceeding, the eyegrounds should be examined for papilledema and a CT or MRI scan should be done.

With certain specific types of neoplastic diseases of the CNS, such as meningeal carcinomatosis and leukemia, however, an LP may be quite helpful diagnostically when other neurodiagnostic studies have been unrevealing.

EEG. EEG in patients with brain tumors may reveal nonspecific electrical abnormalities, such as spikes and slow waves, either diffuse or focal, paroxysmal or continuous. However, frequently in such patients, the EEG may be normal. Given this, it is neither a very specific nor sensitive test, and thus not very helpful in the differentiation of brain tumors from other localized structural cerebral lesions.

Others. Single photon emission computed tomography (SPECT), positron-emission tomography (PET), and brain electrical activity mapping (BEAM) are newly emerging, quantitative, computer-based techniques for evaluating various aspects of brain structure, as well as brain metabolic and electrical functioning. At present, none of them appears to have major advantages over the more standard approaches discussed above in the diagnostic evaluation of brain tumors, but as our experience with them accumulates this may change.

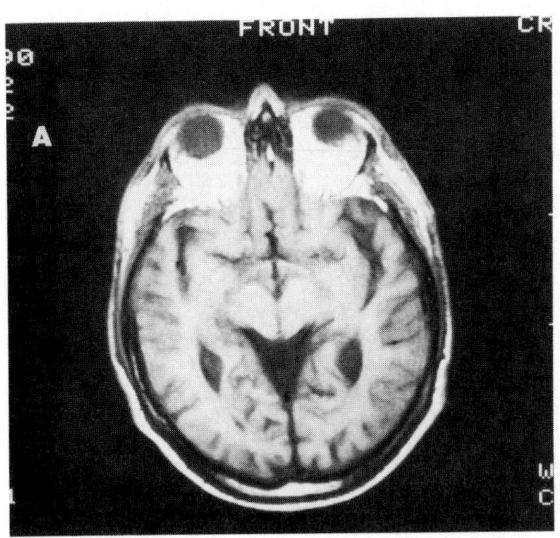

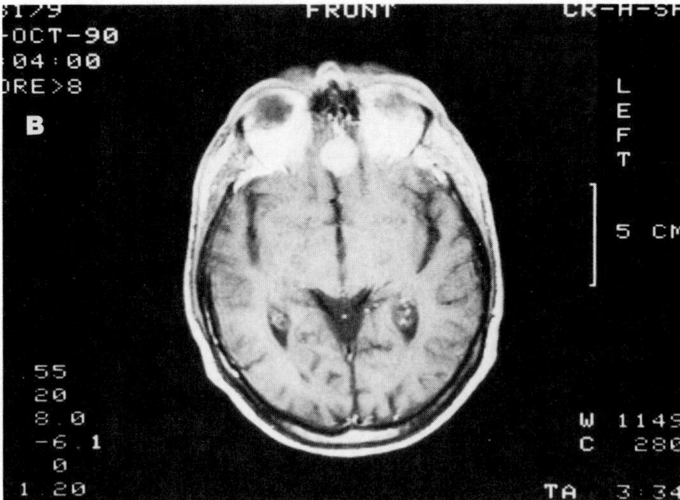

Figure 20–6. A 70-year-old man with a meningioma seen clearly with a gadolinium-enhanced magnetic resonance imaging (MRI) scan (*panel B*). This tumor was not evidenced on an unenhanced MRI scan (*panel A*). (Courtesy of A. Goldberg, Allegheny General Hospital, Department of Radiology.)

❑ TREATMENT OF PSYCHIATRIC AND BEHAVIORAL SYMPTOMS ASSOCIATED WITH CEREBRAL TUMORS

General Considerations

Because psychiatric and behavioral symptoms may sometimes be eliminated with complete removal of the cerebral tumor with which they are associated, this is the first goal of treatment. When this is not possible, as is frequently the case, decreasing the size or slowing the growth of the tumor through surgery, chemotherapy, or radiation therapy (alone, in combination, or sequentially) may significantly ameliorate the severity of associated behavioral symptoms. Furthermore, improvement in cognitive and behavioral symptoms may be rapid and dramatic with treatments that diminish increased ICP or relieve hydrocephalus associated with a brain tumor.

In cases where neuropsychiatric or behavioral symptoms persist or worsen after optimal surgical and nonsurgical interventions, psychopharmacological, psychotherapeutic, and psychosocial interventions become a major focus. The persistence of such psychiatric and behavioral symptoms should lead the neurosurgeon or neurologist caring for the patient to seek psychiatric consultation. It is at this juncture that the psychiatrist or neuropsychiatrist can be of greatest value to the patient and family, by recommending specific somatic treatments for psychiatric symptoms and by providing supportive psychotherapeutic interventions.

Working closely with the attending neurosurgeon, the consulting psychiatrist may contribute significantly to the patient's level of functioning and overall quality of life. Ameliorating the disabling dysphoria and anergia of a severe depression, alleviating the distress caused by overwhelming anxiety, or simply providing consistent supportive contacts to fearful patients and their families may make an enormous difference to them. Often such interventions also lead to greater overall treatment efficacy through increased patient motivation and improved treatment compliance, which simplify and enhance the neurosurgeon's clinical management.

Although patients with cerebral tumors frequently have psychiatric symptoms, only a portion of these are a direct manifestation of the organic mental syndrome caused by the tumor. Others may be persistent or recurrent symptoms of affective or anxiety disorders that were present premorbidly and were uncovered or exacerbated by the stress of the brain tumor. Early in the course of the illness, such symptoms may arise de novo as a result of the patient's psychological reactions to the diagnosis of a brain tumor, concerns about how it will be treated, and fears about its long-term prognosis. Other reactive psychiatric symptoms may emerge later in the context of difficulties adjusting to disabilities or functional changes that result from the tumor or the therapeutic interventions brought to bear on it, such as surgery, radiation therapy, or chemotherapy. It is important for the consulting psychiatrist to differentiate as precisely as possible among symptoms that are specifically tumor related (i.e., symptoms reflecting an organic mental syndrome); those that result from preexisting, primary psychiatric disorders; and those that are predominantly reactive in nature and secondary to psychological stresses, because optimal pharmacological and psychotherapeutic interventions are often quite different for each.

Pharmacological Management of Preexisting Primary Psychiatric Disorders

The psychopharmacological management of patients with preexisting primary psychiatric illnesses that persist or recur in conjunction with the diagnosis and treatment of cerebral tumors should follow the same general therapeutic principles that apply to tumor-free patients with similar disorders. However, it is important for the psychiatrist to be cognizant of the potential need to make downward adjustments in medication dose and to use drugs that are less likely to cause delirium in brain tumor patients, as a result of their increased susceptibility to it. This is especially true of patients who are in the immediate postoperative period or those who are receiving chemotherapy or radiation therapy. Lithium, low-potency antipsychotic drugs, tertiary amine TCAs, and antiparkinsonian agents all have significant, dose-related deliriogenic potential when given alone and even more when given in combination with other potentially deliriogenic agents. Thus these agents should be used with care in such patients.

It may therefore be necessary to substitute haloperidol, carbamazepine, valproate, and/or a benzodiazepine like lorazepam or clonazepam for lithium in a brain tumor patient with mania, a "newer generation" heterocyclic or secondary amine TCA for a tertiary amine TCA in a brain tumor patient with depression, or a high-potency for a low-potency neuroleptic in a brain tumor patient with schizophrenia.

Another significant concern is the potential for precipitating seizures when using these drugs, especially in brain tumor patients in whom seizures are more likely to occur anyway. Neuroleptics, antidepressants, and lithium all have the property of lowering seizure threshold, though to variable degrees. Although the available data are inconclusive, molindone, fluphenazine, and possibly haloperidol are among the antipsychotic drugs believed to carry the smallest risk for seizures. Among the antidepressants, maprotiline and bupropion appear to have the greatest seizure-inducing potential, but the evidence is unclear as to which antidepressants carry the smallest risk. In acutely manic brain tumor patients, for whom lithium would otherwise be the drug of choice, carbamazepine, valproic acid, lorazepam, or clonazepam might be preferable.

The psychiatrist should also bear in mind that brain tumor patients with psychiatric disorders who are also taking anticonvulsants for a known seizure diathesis should be monitored carefully for the adequacy of their anticonvulsant blood levels and have the dose of their anticonvulsant increased or decreased as indicated when psychotropic agents are added. This is because of the direct epileptogenic effects of such medications, as well as their potential for decreasing or increasing anticonvulsant blood levels through drug-drug interactions with a resultant reappearance of previously well-controlled seizures or the development of signs of anticonvulsant toxicity.

Psychotherapeutic Management of Syndromes Associated With Brain Tumors

Supportive psychotherapy geared to the patient's current overall functional status, cognitive capacities, and emotional needs is a very important element in the treatment of any brain tumor patient. The psychological stress of undergoing treatment for a brain tumor can trigger both recurrences of symptoms of antecedent primary psychiatric disorders and the de novo appearance of reactive psychiatric symptoms as the patient attempts to cope with the stress of the illness and its treatment. In either case, supportive psychotherapy can be very important and beneficial, and should play a major role in the patient's overall clinical management.

Supportive psychotherapy ideally involves both the patient and the family and revolves around concrete, reality-based, cognitive, and psychoeducational issues such as diagnosis and prognosis, impact of the illness on the patient's functional status, its effect on the family, coping with actual or anticipated disability, and dealing with anticipatory grief related to potential losses and eventual death.

Not surprisingly, patients with cerebral tumors worry a great deal about anticipated changes in mental and intellectual functioning, physical disability and incapacity, and ultimately death. Patients vary widely in their capacity to adjust to and deal with the potentially devastating consequences of brain tumors, with the success of their adjustment depending largely on the adaptiveness of their previous coping mechanisms. Although some patients may appear to be little affected, others may experience severe and at times overwhelming symptoms of anxiety and depression. Consequently, they may experience great difficulty continuing to function normally in their usual work and family roles.

Denial as a defensive coping mechanism is common and is frequently both effective and desirable in helping patients allay their fears and anxieties, especially in the early stages of a life-threatening illness such as a brain tumor. On the other hand, during the later stages of an illness, it can result in the failure of patients or their families to comply with optimal treatment measures or to deal appropriately and in a timely fashion with important legal, family, or other reality-based issues and obligations that need to be addressed. When denial is producing such negative effects, the clinician may need to directly, though in a sensitive and supportive manner, encourage the patient and family to begin to address such painful issues as increasing disability, growing incapacity, and even impending death.

Though there are no clear-cut, generally accepted guidelines for the optimal nature and timing of discussions of prognosis with brain tumor patients, most clinicians believe that they and their families should be given realistic prognostic information in a time frame that will allow them sufficient time to make well-considered decisions and appropriate plans. Such prognostic information should, of course, be conveyed by the physician in as sensitive and supportive a fashion as possible. This is another juncture where the supportive psychotherapeutic input of the consulting psychiatrist may be quite useful in helping the patient and family process such information.

Some patients who have been completely cured may still manifest significant psychiatric symptoms, including anxiety, fear, and depression. They, like other brain tumor patients with predominantly reactive psychiatric symptoms, may benefit from psychiatric treatment. Unless the psychiatric symptoms are causing functional disability, are very severe and distressing to the patient, persist over extended periods of time, or evolve into an autonomous psychiatric syndrome, psychotherapy rather than pharmacotherapy is generally the preferred treatment approach. Short-term targeted pharmacotherapy can, however, be a useful adjunct even if the major emphasis is on supportive psychotherapy.

It should be kept in mind that psychodynamically focused, insight-oriented psychotherapy, which is frequently used with some primary psychiatric syndromes and requires intact higher-level cognitive and abstracting capacities, is often relatively contraindicated in psychiatrically ill patients with brain tumors. This is because such patients often have some degree of impairment in these intellectual realms as a result of the effects of the tumor or of the neurosurgery, chemotherapy, or radiotherapy the patient may have undergone. When such impairments are present, not only will psychodynamically oriented therapies yield little additional benefit compared with supportive approaches, they may also cause significant psychic distress in patients who are being confronted with mental tasks and cognitive demands that they can no longer carry out.

Somatic Treatment of Organic Mental Disorders

As with primary psychiatric disorders, the psychopharmacological treatment of behavioral symptoms secondary to organic mental syndromes caused by cerebral tumors, whether characterized by psychotic, affective, anxiety, or cognitive disturbances, follows the same general principles as those of phenomenologically similar symptoms resulting from primary functional psychiatric illnesses.

In treating such secondary psychiatric symptoms, some important caveats must be borne in mind. Patients with psychiatric symptoms that are a direct consequence of a brain tumor, like other patients with organic brain disorders, frequently require and tolerate significantly lower doses of psychotropic medication. Thus the side effect profiles of psychotropic drugs being considered in the treatment of such patients need to be very carefully evaluated, especially with regard to sedative, extrapyramidal, deliriofícient, and epileptogenic effects, as well as the potential for drug-drug interactions. The latter three factors are especially important when selecting psychotropic medication for patients with brain tumors.

Drug Treatment of Tumor-Associated Organic Psychoses

Standard antipsychotic medications may be beneficial in treating the hallucinations, delusions, and thought disturbances that frequently accompany tumor-associated organic psychotic syndromes. High-potency agents, which have fewer nonneurological side effects, are generally preferable to lower-potency antipsychotics. Of course, the former more frequently cause extrapyramidal symptoms that may also be more severe and persistent when they do occur. In organic psychotic disorders the therapeutically effective dose is often lower than that required in the treatment of primary functional psychoses. Thus as little as 1–5 mg/day, compared with 10–20 mg/day, of haloperidol may be effective. As is the general rule with the use of other psychotropics in such patients, initiating treatment with neuroleptics in brain tumor patients should "start low and go slow." This is especially true in the elderly, in whom effective neuroleptic doses are often as much as 25%–50% lower than they are in younger patients.

Antiparkinsonian agents such as benztropine, trihexyphenidyl, and orphenadrine are effective in the treatment of extrapyramidal side effects resulting from the use of neuroleptics in brain tumor patients. However, in brain tumor patients these agents are especially likely to cause or contribute to an anticholinergic delirium when used in combination with low-potency neuroleptics and/or tertiary amine TCAs. Thus their use should generally be avoided unless there is a clear-cut indication, and when they are used the dose should be minimized. Diphenhydramine or amantadine for dystonic and parkinsonian symptoms and benzodiazepines for akathisia are effective alternatives and have less deliriofìcient potential.

Treatment of Organic Mood Syndromes

Antidepressant medications are often effective in the treatment of organic mood syndromes of the depressed type in brain tumor patients. Standard TCAs are useful, though currently the newer-generation heterocyclic or secondary amine TCAs are often used preferentially because of their lesser anticholinergic activity and sedating effects and consequently improved patient tolerance. In recent years methylphenidate has been shown to be effective in secondary depressions related to medical and neurological disorders, including brain tumors. Because it is generally well tolerated and does not lower the seizure threshold, this agent is now being used more widely.

Monoamine oxidase inhibitors (MAOIs) may be effective when other antidepressants are not. They do not ordinarily pose an undue risk in brain tumor patients, but, of course, the clinician must bear in mind that the cognitive impairment that often occurs in such patients may interfere with their ability to maintain a tyramine-free diet, thereby increasing the risk associated with the use of the MAOIs.

If single antidepressant medication regimens are ineffective, various combinations may work, and when pharmacological treatments have failed, electroconvulsive therapy (ECT) should be given serious consideration. Previously, brain tumors were thought to be an absolute contraindication to ECT, especially when associated with increased ICP. However, Zwil et al. (1990) recently reviewed a number of cases of refractory depression associated with brain tumors without associated evidence of increased ICP that were treated with ECT. In these cases ECT was not associated with any untoward effects and had positive therapeutic results.

Organic mood disorders of the manic type due to brain tumors, though rare, generally respond to lithium in the usual therapeutic range of 0.8–1.4 mEq/L. However, where seizures have been a part of the clinical picture, carbamazepine, valproate, lorazepam, or clonazepam are probably preferable alternatives, because they do not have lithium's epileptogenic potential.

Treatment of Organic Anxiety Syndromes

Anxiety symptoms associated with a brain tumor, whether indirectly or directly related to it, should not be treated with neuroleptics unless psychotic features are present for reasons noted previously as well as the fact that neuroleptics are generally not effective with such symptoms and often result in dysphoria in nonpsychotic patients.

The benzodiazepines, on the other hand, are often efficacious and have the added benefit of possessing anticonvulsant properties. Thus they are frequently used. However, benzodiazepines (particularly long-acting types) may induce delirium in patients with organic brain disease, including brain tumors, when used in high doses and in older age groups. This argues for the preferential use of short-acting agents in lower doses, especially in older patients. Other disadvantages of benzodiazepines include their abuse potential and the occasional propensity (especially with the long half-life varieties) to cause seemingly paradoxical reactions, characterized by increased anxiety, agitation, and hostility. Thus buspirone, which is free of these potentially negative effects, should be considered an alternative to the benzodiazepines. Its main drawbacks are its delayed onset and only modest degree of anxiolytic action. Vistaril, or low doses of tertiary amine TCAs such as doxepin or amitriptyline, may also have beneficial anxiolytic effects in some patients. Finally, panic attacks associated with temporal lobe tumors may respond to carbamazepine, valproate, or primidone, as well as to the usual antidepressant and antianxiety drugs.

Treatment of Delirium

Delirium in brain tumor patients may be associated with a wide variety of psychiatric and behavioral symptoms, in addition to the characteristic organic and cognitive impairments. Hallucinations, especially visual, and delusions are frequently seen and often respond to interim symptomatic treatment with low doses of haloperidol or other high-potency neuroleptics while the underlying causes of the delirium are being sought out and treated.

Treatment of Organic Personality Syndromes

Mood lability may be a manifestation of an organic personality disorder due to a brain tumor and may respond to lithium or carbamazepine. Some patients with frontal lobe syndromes will respond to carbamazepine, as will some patients with temporal lobe tumors who present with associated interictal aggression and violent behavior. Brain tumor patients with impulse dyscontrol and rageful explosiveness, like other patients with organically based intermittent explosive disorders, may respond to anticonvulsants, such as carbamazepine, as well as to lithium, β-blockers, high-potency neuroleptics, and/or stimulants.

Cognitive Rehabilitation

In addition to psychopharmacological and psychotherapeutic treatments, cognitive rehabilitation can be very helpful for patients whose tumors, or the treatments they receive for them, have produced behavioral or cognitive sequelae. Such sequelae can be identified and quantified by comparing postoperative with preoperative test results using the Halstead-Reitan (Reitan 1955), Luria-Nebraska (Golden et al. 1978), or other comparable neuropsychological batteries. Serial testing at intervals during the patient's postoperative rehabilitation allows for objective documentation of neuropsychological deficits and monitoring of cognitive recovery. Thus, in general, neuropsychological testing should be a standard part of the brain tumor patient's preoperative evaluation and postoperative follow-up.

Used alone or in combination with other therapies, cognitive rehabilitation strategies can be developed that will address deficits in intellectual, language, visuospatial, and memory functioning resulting from a brain tumor. In addition, behavioral techniques have been successfully applied to problematic behaviors resulting from insults to the brain. (For a more detailed discussion of these techniques, see Chapter 31.)

❑ CONCLUSIONS

Brain tumors are frequently associated, and may occasionally even present, with a broad range of psychiatric and/or neuropsychological symptoms. The differential diagnosis of any patient who displays acute or progressive changes in behavior, personality, or cognitive function, should include a brain tumor, especially if there are any associated focal neurological signs and symptoms. In addition to assessing psychiatric and behavioral symptoms, a full neuropsychiatric evaluation should include physical, neurological, and mental status examinations; appropriate brain imaging and other neurodiagnostic studies; and formal neuropsychological testing, particularly when there is any question or evidence of cognitive dysfunction on bedside mental status testing.

The nature, frequency, and severity of psychiatric symptoms observed with brain tumors depend on the combined effects of a number of clinical factors including the type, location, size, rate of growth, and malignancy of the tumor. In general, psychiatric and behavioral symptoms associated with smaller, slower-growing, less aggressive tumors are most likely to be misdiagnosed as being psychiatric in origin, particularly when they occur in "silent" regions of the brain, which do not give rise to focal neurological signs or symptoms.

Although frontal lobe, temporal lobe, and diencephalic brain tumors appear to be most commonly associated with psychiatric and behavioral symptoms, the variation in symptoms that may occur with each is exceedingly broad. In general, the correlation between the occurrence of a particular neuropsychiatric symptom and the anatomic location of its causative brain tumor is not very robust.

Optimal treatment of tumor-associated psychiatric, neuropsychiatric, and neuropsychological dysfunctions should be multifaceted and is dependent on the coordinated interventions of a multidisciplinary treatment team. The psychopharmacological treatment of such psychiatric and behavioral syndromes should follow the same general principles as those of corresponding primary functional psychiatric disorders. However, the choice of drug and/or dosage may require modification because many of the psychotropic agents induce seizures or delirium, and brain tumor patients are more sensitive to these and other side effects.

Adjunctive, supportive psychotherapy for both the patient and the family is very important, as are psychosocial and psychoeducational interventions tailored to their needs. Such psychotherapeutic and psychosocial interventions must be carefully integrated with psychopharmacological, cognitive, physical rehabilitative, and behavioral treatment approaches. In turn, all of these must be coordinated with the neurosurgeon's ongoing clinical care to optimize the patient's overall medical management. With well-planned integration and coordination of these disparate therapeutic approaches, both the quantity and the quality of the brain tumor patient's life may be substantially enhanced.

❑ REFERENCES

Allen IM: A clinical study of tumors involving the occipital lobe. Brain 53:194–243, 1930

Alpers BJ: Relation of the hypothalamus to disorders of personality. Archives of Neurology and Psychiatry 38: 291–303, 1937

American Psychiatric Association: Diagnostic and Statistical Manual of Mental Disorders, 3rd Edition, Revised. Washington, DC, American Psychiatric Association, 1987

Avery TL: A case of acromegaly and gigantism with depression. Br J Psychiatry 122:599–600, 1973

Bear DM, Fedio P: Quantitative analysis of interictal behavior in temporal lobe epilepsy. Arch Neurol 34:454–467, 1977

Belyi BI: Mental impairment in unilateral frontal tumors: role of the laterality of the lesion. Int J Neurosci 32:799–810, 1987

Benson DF: Aphasia, Alexia, and Agraphia. New York, Churchill Livingstone, 1979

Bigler ED: Diagnostic Clinical Neuropsychology. Austin, TX, University of Texas Press, 1984

Burger PC, Scheithauer BW, Vogel FS: Surgical Pathology of the Nervous System and Its Coverings, 3rd Edition. New York, Churchill Livingstone, 1991

Burkle FM, Lipowski ZJ: Colloid cyst of the third ventricle presenting as psychiatric disorder. Am J Psychiatry 135:373–374, 1978

Butters N: Amnestic disorders, in Clinical Neuropsychology. Edited by Heilman KM, Valenstein E. New York, Oxford University Press, 1979, pp 439–474

Cairns H: Mental disorders with tumors of the pons. Folia Psychiatrica Neurologica Neurochirurgica 53:193–203, 1950

Cairns H, Mosberg WH: Colloid cysts of the third ventricle. Surg Gynecol Obstet 92:545–570, 1951

Cairns H, Oldfield RC, Pennybacker JB, et al: Akinetic mutism with an epidermoid cyst of the 3rd ventricle. Brain 64:273–290, 1941

Climo LH: Anorexia nervosa associated with hypothalamic tumor: the search for clinical-pathological correlations. Psychiatric Journal of the University of Ottawa 7:20–25, 1982

Coffey RJ: Hypothalamic and basal forebrain germinoma presenting with amnesia and hyperphagia. Surg Neurol 31:228–233, 1989

Critchley M: The problem of visual agnosia. J Neurol Sci 1:274–290, 1964a

Critchley M: Psychiatric symptoms and parietal disease: differential diagnosis. Proceedings of the Royal Society of Medicine 57:422–428, 1964b

Cummings JL: Clinical Neuropsychiatry. Orlando, FL, Grune & Stratton, 1985

Cummings JL, Mendez MF: Secondary mania with focal cerebrovascular lesions. Am J Psychiatry 141:1084–1087, 1984

Davison K, Bagley CR: Schizophrenia-like psychoses associated with organic disorders of the central nervous system: a review of the literature, in Current Problems in Neuropsychiatry: Schizophrenia, Epilepsy, the Temporal Lobe (British Journal of Psychiatry Special Publication No 4). Edited by Harrington RN. London, Headley Brothers, 1969, pp 126–130

Direkze M, Bayliss SG, Cutting JC: Primary tumors of the frontal lobe. Br J Clin Pract 25:207–213, 1971

Drubach DA, Kelly MP: Panic disorder associated with a right paralimbic lesion. Neuropsychiatry, Neuropsychology, and Behavioral Neurology 2:282–289, 1989

Flor-Henry P: Schizophrenic-like reactions and affective psychoses associated with temporal lobe epilepsy etiological factors. Am J Psychiatry 126:400–404, 1969

Frazier CH: Tumor involving the frontal lobe alone: a symptomatic survey of 105 verified cases. Archives of Neurology and Psychiatry 35:525–571, 1935

Gilroy J, Holliday PL: Basic Neurology. New York, Macmillan, 1982

Ghadirian, AM, Gauthier S, Bertrand S: Anxiety attacks in a patient with a right temporal lobe meningioma. J Clin Psychiatry 47:270–271, 1986

Goldberg E: Varieties of perseverations: comparison of two taxonomies. J Clin Exp Neuropsychol 6:710–726, 1986

Golden CJ: Cerebral tumors, in Clinical Neuropsychology: Interface With Neurologic and Psychiatric Disorders. Edited by Golden CJ, Moses JA, Coffman JA, et al. New York, Grune & Stratton, 1983, pp 3–20

Golden CJ, Hammeke T, Purisch A: Diagnostic validity of the Luria Neuropsychological Battery. J Consult Clin Psychol 46:1258–1265, 1978

Greenberg DB, Brown GL: Mania resulting from brain stem tumor: single case study. J Nerv Ment Dis 173: 434–436, 1985

Jamieson RC, Wells CE: Manic psychosis in a patient with multiple metastatic brain tumors. J Clin Psychiatry 40: 280–283, 1979

Keschner M, Bender MB, Strauss I: Mental symptoms in cases of tumor of the temporal lobe. Archives of Neurology and Psychiatry 35:572–596, 1936

Keschner M, Bender MB, Strauss I: Mental symptoms associated with brain tumor: a study of 530 verified cases. JAMA 110:714–718, 1938

Klotz M: Incidence of brain tumors in patients hospitalized for chronic mental disorders. Psychiatr Q 31:669–680, 1957

Kurtzke JF: Neuroepidemiology. Ann Neurol 16:265–277, 1984

Lezak MD: Neuropsychological Assessment. New York, Oxford University Press, 1983

Lishman WA: Organic Psychiatry: The Psychological Consequences of Cerebral Disorder. New York, Oxford University Press, 1978

Lohr JB, Cadet JL: Neuropsychiatric aspects of brain tumors, in The American Psychiatric Press Textbook of Neuropsychiatry. Washington, DC, American Psychiatric Press, 1987, pp 351–364

Luria AR: The Working Brain: An Introduction to Neuropsychology. New York, Basic Books, 1973

Luria AR: Higher Cortical Functions in Man. New York, Basic Books, 1980

McAllister TW, Price TRP: Aspects of the behavior of psychiatric inpatients with frontal lobe damage: some implications for diagnosis and treatment. Compr Psychiatry 28:14–21, 1987

McIntyre HD, McIntyre AP: The problem of brain tumor in psychiatric diagnosis. Am J Psychiatry 98:720–726, 1942

Malamud N: Psychiatric disorder with intracranial tumors of limbic system. Arch Neurol 17:113–123, 1967

Meadows JC: The anatomical basis of prosopagnosia. J Neurol Neurosurg Psychiatry 37:489–501, 1974

Minski L: The mental symptoms associated with 58 cases of cerebral tumor. Journal of Neurology and Psychopathology 13:330–343, 1933

Mulder DW, Daly D: Psychiatric symptoms associated with lesions of temporal lobe. JAMA 150:173–176, 1952

Mungas D: Interictal behavior abnormality in temporal lobe epilepsy: a specific syndrome or non-specific psychopathology? Arch Gen Psychiatry 39:108–111, 1982

Nasrallah HA, McChesney CM: Psychopathology of corpus callosum tumors. Biol Psychiatry 16:663–669, 1981

Patton RB, Sheppard JA: Intracranial tumors found at autopsy in mental patients. Am J Psychiatry 113:319–324, 1956

Pincus JH, Tucker GJ: Behavioral Neurology, 2nd Edition. New York, Oxford University Press, 1978, p 131

Reeves AG, Plum F: Hyperphagia, rage, and dementia accompanying a ventromedial hypothalamic neoplasm. Arch Neurol 20:616–624, 1969

Reiman EM, Raichle ME, Robins E, et al: The application of positron-emission tomography to the study of panic disorder. Am J Psychiatry 143:469–477, 1986

Reitan RM: An investigation of the validity of Halstead's measures of biological intelligence. Archives of Neurology and Psychiatry 73:28–35, 1955

Reitan RM, Wolfson D: Neuroanatomy and Neuropathology for Neuropsychologists. Tucson, AZ, Neuropsychology Press, 1985, pp 167–192

Remington FB, Robert SL: Why patients with brain tumors come to a psychiatric hospital: a thirty-year survey. Am J Psychiatry 119:256–257, 1962

Robinson RG, Kubos KL, Starr LB, et al: Mood disorders in stroke patients: importance of location of lesion. Brain 107:81–93, 1984

Rodin E, Schmaltz S: The Bear-Fedio personality inventory and temporal lobe epilepsy. Neurology 34:591–596, 1984

Russell RW, Pennybacker JB: Craniopharyngioma in the elderly. J Neurol Neurosurg Psychiatry 24:1–13, 1961

Schirmer M, Bock WJ: The primary symptoms of intracranial metastases, in Advances in Neurosurgery, Vol 12. Edited by Piotrowski W, Brock M, Klinger M. Berlin, Heidelberg, Springer-Verlag, 1984, pp 25–29

Schlesinger B: Mental changes in intracranial tumors and related problems. Confinia Neurologica 10:225–263, 1950

Selecki BR: Cerebral mid-line tumours involving the corpus callosum among mental hospital patients. Med J Aust 2:954–960, 1964

Selecki BR: Intracranial space-occupying lesions among patients admitted to mental hospitals. Med J Aust 1: 383–390, 1965

Sperry RW: Lateral specialization in the surgically separated hemispheres, in The Neurosciences: 3rd Study Program. Edited by Worden OF, Worden FG. Cambridge, MA, MIT Press, 1974, pp 5–19

Spreen O, Benton A, Fincham R: Auditory agnosia without aphasia. Arch Neurol 13:84, 1965

Starkstein SE, Boston JD, Robinson RG: Mechanisms of mania after brain injury: 12 case reports and review of the literature. J Nerv Ment Dis 176:87–100, 1988

Strauss I, Keschner M: Mental symptoms in cases of tumor of the frontal lobe. Archives of Neurology and Psychiatry 33:986–1005, 1935

Strobos RRJ: Tumors of the temporal lobe. Neurology 3: 752–760, 1953

Teuber HL: Unity and diversity of frontal lobe functions. Acta Neurobiol Exp 32:615–656, 1972

Tucker GJ, Price TRP, Johnson VB, et al: Phenomenology of temporal lobe dysfunction: a link to atypical psychosis: a series of cases. J Nerv Ment Dis 174:348–356, 1986

von Monakow C: Die Lokalisation im Grossheim und der Abbav der Funktion durch Kortikale Herde. Weisbaden, JF Bergmann, 1914

Warrington EK, Rabin P: Perceptual matching in patients with cerebral lesions. Neuropsychologia 8:475–487, 1970

White J, Cobb S: Psychological changes associated with giant pituitary neoplasms. Archives of Neurology and Psychiatry 74:383–396, 1955

Wilson G, Rupp C: Mental symptoms associated with extra medullary posterior fossa tumors. Transactions of the American Neurological Association (New York) 71:104–107, 1946

Zwil AS, Bowring MA, Price TRP, et al: ECT in the presence of a brain tumor: case reports and a review of the literature. Convulsive Therapy 6:299–307, 1990

Chapter

21

Effects of Human Immunodeficiency Virus on the Central Nervous System

John C. Markowitz, M.D.
Samuel W. Perry, M.D.

IN THIS CHAPTER WE PROVIDE an overview of the spectrum of neuropsychiatric disorders associated with the acquired immunodeficiency syndrome (AIDS) and its etiological agent, human immunodeficiency virus (HIV). Neuropsychiatric deficits may be *primary* (i.e., directly induced by HIV), *secondary* (i.e., as when immunodeficiency leads to opportunistic infections or tumors systemically or within central nervous system [CNS]), or *iatrogenic* (i.e., resulting from treatment of HIV or its sequelae). We review these deficits and their treatments. We also discuss current controversies in the literature, particularly that surrounding early neuropsychological impairment in HIV-seropositive patients.

❑ HUMAN IMMUNODEFICIENCY VIRUS

Epidemiology

HIV has been spreading in the United States since the 1970s. The blood-borne virus is transmitted through unprotected sexual contact, use of blood-contaminated needles or other drug paraphernalia, receiving tainted blood or blood product transfusions, or intrauterine infection. The course of HIV infection is highly variable but generally chronic, with a mean duration of roughly 10 years between

Supported in part by Grants MH-19069, 42277, and 46250 from the National Institute of Mental Health.

inoculation and the development of physical symptoms. Most of the estimated one million adults in the United States infected by HIV are currently asymptomatic, and their serological status is generally unreported even when known. Prevalence of HIV infection thus must be extrapolated from subpopulations that have been screened (e.g., military recruits and other personnel who undergo mandatory testing and serologically tested blood donors) (Centers for Disease Control 1989). Simply considering the number of patients with AIDS (Centers for Disease Control [CDC] stage IV) is misleading, because many cases go unreported and the number of these cases comprises a small fraction of the population already infected.

Given this proviso, the available data document changing trends in the epidemic. The majority of adults with AIDS are still homosexual or bisexual men (62%), but the percentage of infected intravenous-drug abusers continues to rise (27% versus 13%–17% in the early 1980s). Also increasing have been the percentage of female and heterosexual cases (4%) and the number of children with AIDS, nearly half of whom were diagnosed in 1988. On the other hand, U.S. cases due to hemophilia and transfusions (4%) are proportionately declining. AIDS is the leading cause of death among intravenous-drug abusers and hemophiliac patients (Heyward and Curran 1988). For an individual with known risk factors it is difficult to predict his or her chance of having acquired HIV.

Neuropsychiatric Effects

HIV attacks the CNS (Price et al. 1988) as well as the immune system (Fauci 1988). It is important to keep in mind that AIDS, being a syndrome rather than a discrete disorder, involves complex, multietiological mental changes resulting both from HIV itself and from the host of secondary disease states it unleashes.

It is generally believed (Janssen et al. 1989; Price et al. 1990), albeit not conclusively demonstrated, that HIV invades the brain shortly after systemic infection, when macrophages bearing HIV cross the blood-brain barrier (Resnick et al. 1988). Release of virus within the CNS causes an acute or subclinical meningoencephalitis. Newly infected patients, not yet having been immunocompromised by chronic destruction of T4 lymphocytes, can generally contain this initial infection. As immunocompetence wanes over months or years, however, viral replication within the CNS escapes the mastery of immune defenses. Progressive multifocal leukoencephalopathy may occur. Different strains of HIV and constitutional and environmental cofactors may explain differences in CNS pathology. Although HIV directly damages a variety of organ systems, the importance of the CNS magnifies its pathology there.

Histopathology

Postmortem CNS findings in HIV-seropositive patients are diffuse and variable (Gray et al. 1988; Petito 1988), complicated by systemic disease and the diversity of potential CNS lesions. HIV most prominently affects subcortical areas, including central white matter and deep gray structures such as the basal ganglia, thalamus, and brain stem. By contrast, the cerebral cortex is relatively spared: hence the term *subcortical dementia.* White matter pallor may be accompanied by astrocytic reaction and marked atrophy, or there may be few inflammatory changes and little pallor.

When encephalitis exists, reactive infiltrates of multinucleated cells, parenchymal and perivascular foamy macrophages, lymphocytes, and microglia are found. Oligodendrocytes and neurons are generally preserved. The minimal neuronal lysis suggests that rather than HIV being "neurotropic," its neurotoxicity results either from an autoimmune response, from HIV synergy with other pathogens, or from release of toxic substances from the viral genes themselves or from adjacent infected cells. Spinal cord involvement may consist of inflammatory changes but usually consists of "vacuolar myelopathy" due to swelling of myelin sheaths.

Psychiatric Differential Diagnosis

Organic mental disorders (OMDs) occur frequently among hospitalized patients with AIDS (Perry and Tross 1984; Price and Brew 1988), may occur in the absence of systemic symptomatology (Marotta and Perry 1989; Navia and Price 1987), and may mimic functional psychiatric disorders. Whether seeing patients on a consultation-liaison service or in a private office, psychiatrists should consider HIV-spectrum disease in the differential diagnosis of psychiatric presentations, particularly in patients with high-risk behaviors and in cases with atypical presentations. Several organic etiologies may coincide with one another or with a superimposed functional disorder.

❑ PRIMARY NEUROPSYCHOLOGICAL IMPAIRMENT BY HIV

By 1987, a variety of evidence suggested that organic mental changes at least occasionally preceded physical signs and symptoms of HIV infection. Case reports (Marotta and Perry 1989; Perry and Marotta 1987) and anecdotal clinical experience indicated that some HIV-seropositive adults who had not yet developed AIDS experienced subjective mental slowing, forgetfulness, apathy, lethargy, social withdrawal, avoidance of complex tasks, and personality change. Although these symptoms initially appeared to be "functional" or psychological, thorough clinical evaluation suggested a "subcortical dementia" (Blumer 1983; Cummings and Benson 1984; Manuelidis and Manuelidis 1989). Other HIV-seropositive patients initially presented with acute psychosis (Perry and Jacobsen 1986; Rundell et al. 1986), delirium (Levy et al. 1985; Perry and Jacobsen 1986), amnesia (Beresford et al. 1986), depression (Beresford et al. 1986; Navia and Price 1987; Perry and Jacobsen 1986), or mania (Boccellari et al. 1989a; Kermani et al. 1985; Price and Forejt 1986; Schmidt and Miller 1988). HIV, like syphilis long before, might be deemed "the great imitator" for its myriad psychiatric presentations (Perry and Marotta 1987).

There was evidence that HIV entered the CNS shortly after systemic infection (Resnick et al. 1988). McArthur et al. (1988) found HIV in the cerebrospinal fluid (CSF) of asymptomatic homosexual men with 6–24 months of known seropositivity. Early presence of HIV, pleocytosis, and elevated protein in CSF, as well as isolation of HIV from neural tissue (Gabuzda et al. 1986; Gartner et al. 1986; Stoler et al. 1986), strongly implied that HIV could affect the CNS before any physical manifestations of disease. HIV-specific antigens and immunoglobulins were also discovered in spinal fluid of both symptomatic and asymptomatic infected patients (Andersson et al. 1988; Brew et al. 1989; Bukasa et al. 1988; Ceroni et al. 1988; Elovaara et al. 1988; Grimaldi et al. 1988).

HIV-seropositive children lag in achieving motor and intellectual milestones and subsequently regress on cognitive measures. Because these phenomena seemed unrelated to concomitant physical illnesses (Epstein et al. 1988; Ultmann et al. 1985), they provided further evidence that HIV itself affected the CNS.

Similarly, brain abnormalities appeared on computed tomography (CT), magnetic resonance imaging (MRI), and electroencephalogram (EEG) of patients with AIDS and AIDS-related complex in the absence of CNS opportunistic infections and malignancies. CT scans showed marked atrophy and enlarged ventricles, MRI showed scattered parenchymal lesions and calcification (Levy et al. 1986; Olsen et al. 1988; Sze et al. 1987), and EEG showed slow alpha rhythms and diffuse theta waves (Jordan et al. 1985; Koppel et al. 1985). Neuropathological studies (Gray et al. 1988; Petito et al. 1988) described subcortical involvement consistent with subtle, noncognitive mental changes, which could explain vague, seemingly psychological symptoms in the absence of intellectual ("cortical") impairment (Blumer 1983; Manuelidis and Manuelidis 1989). These changes suggested insidious CNS damage anteceding the onset of systemic symptoms.

Pilot neuropsychological studies compared seronegative control subjects with subjects who met diagnostic criteria for AIDS but were "currently free of illness" (Joffe et al. 1986), and with those having AIDS-related complex or "early AIDS" (Ayers et al. 1987). These early reports found more neuropsychological impairment among the (physically) relatively asymptomatic HIV-seropositive groups.

❑ NOSOLOGICAL AND DIAGNOSTIC ISSUES

HIV Staging

Many investigators are now researching early neuropsychological impairment among diverse groups of HIV-seropositive adults who have yet to develop other AIDS-related symptoms. Most studies use the staging system for HIV infection developed by the CDC (Council of State and Territorial Epidemiologists, AIDS Program, Center for Infectious Diseases 1987) (Table 21–1).

Stage I indicates acute infection: some individuals may develop a transient syndrome akin to flu or mononucleosis; or, more rarely, acute meningoencephalitis that may prove fulminant and fatal (Carne et al. 1985). Excepting recipients of infected blood products, however, most individuals in stage I cannot specify when they contracted HIV. Stage II encompasses the generally lengthy period of latent infection, a mean 9 years or longer (Centers for Disease Control 1989), when individuals are infectious but lack HIV-related medical complaints. Stage III differs from its predecessor in the development of

TABLE 21–1. CENTERS FOR DISEASE CONTROL (CDC) STAGING FOR HUMAN IMMUNODEFICIENCY VIRUS (HIV) INFECTION

CDC stage	*Description*
I	Acute HIV infection Asymptomatic Viral syndrome Meningoencephalitis
II	Latent infection
III	Chronic lymphadenopathy
IV-A	Constitutional symptoms Weight loss Fever Chronic diarrhea
IV-B	HIV-induced neuropathology Dementia Myelopathy Peripheral neuropathy
IV-C	Opportunistic infections
IV-C1	Secondary infectious diseases, including Pneumocystis carinii pneumonia, toxoplasmosis, and cryptococcosis
IV-C2	Other secondary infectious diseases, including oral hairy leukoplakia, multidermatomal herpes zoster, tuberculosis, and oral candidiasis (thrush)
IV-D	HIV-associated tumors
IV-E	Other conditions, including chronic lymphoid interstitial pneumonitis

Source. Adapted from Centers for Disease Control 1987.

persistent lymphadenopathy at two or more extrainguinal sites; but the virus otherwise remains quiescent.

Stage IV-A describes constitutional symptoms such as weight loss, persistent fever, or chronic diarrhea. Stage IV-B, of particular interest to psychiatrists, indicates HIV-induced neuropathology including dementia, peripheral neuropathy, and myelopathy. Stage IV-C represents the wide spectrum of opportunistic infections arising secondary to immunosuppression. Stage IV-D delineates tumors indicative of defective cell-mediated immunity, including Kaposi's sarcoma, non-Hodgkin's lymphoma, and primary lymphoma of the CNS. Stage IV-E is a miscellany of diseases not listed elsewhere that are attributable to or complicated by HIV infection, such as anemia or chronic lymphoid interstitial pneumonitis.

The CDC classification discards "AIDS-related complex" and "pre-AIDS," imprecise clinical terms that might correspond to stages III, IV-A, and milder opportunistic infections now classified under stage IV-C2. The CDC staging does not describe prognosis or severity. For example, patients in stages I through IV-A sometimes deteriorate rapidly. By contrast, patients with "frank AIDS" (stages IV-B through IV-E) may have relatively mild Kaposi's sarcoma or have recovered long ago from an opportunistic infection and may live for years with minimal physical debility. Longevity and chronicity of the syndrome have increased since the advent of early therapeutic intervention and chemoprophylaxis with maintenance medications such as zidovudine (or AZT), pentamidine, trimethoprim and sulfamethoxazole, diaminodiphenylsulfone, and interferon (Markowitz and Perry 1990).

No classification system has yet been universally accepted. Alternative systems (Haverkos et al. 1985; Redfield et al. 1986), although less widely used, offer certain research advantages by combining immunological and clinical markers to chart the widely variable course of HIV infection.

Neuropsychological Impairment and Clinical Diagnosis

In reviewing studies, mental health professionals should ponder the relationship between neuropsychological impairment and the popular term *AIDS dementia complex* in HIV-related OMDs. DSM-III-R (American Psychiatric Association 1987) defines OMDs as disorders due to a specific and known brain dysfunction, in distinction to disorders that are responses to psychological or social factors (e.g., adjustment disorders) and those where a specific organic factor has not yet been clearly established (e.g., schizophrenia) (Perry and Markowitz 1988; also see Chapter 9). The diagnosis of OMD embraces a wide range of neuropsychiatric pathology. Organic etiologies may be multiple in an individual, with manifestations ranging from dementia, delirium, delusions, and hallucinosis to subtle but clinically significant changes in cognitive functioning, mood, personality, and impulse control.

Neuropsychological impairment is a test result, **not** a diagnosis. "Impairment" implies that scores are abnormal (assuming normative data exist) or fall beneath a cutoff (usually two standard deviations below the sample mean), but the results of neuropsychological testing are not disease specific. In general, the more sensitive the test, the more likely it lacks specificity (Sidtis and Price 1990). The relationship among neuropsychological impairment, OMD, and social and vocational function remains unclear for HIV-seropositive individuals (Marotta and Perry 1989). Test batteries may find neuropsychological impairment in patients who do not meet criteria for a DSM-III-R OMD; conversely, OMD may coexist with a normal neuropsychological examination. For example, a neuropsychological test may be insufficiently sensitive to detect a mild but clinically significant organic mood, anxiety, or personality disorder. Or a once high-functioning individual with significant cognitive slippage may still score within a group normative range. Lacking premorbid neuropsychological data, clinicians cannot rely on such "normal" findings.

AIDS Dementia Complex

The relationship between AIDS dementia complex and OMD according to DSM-III-R also bears examination. Neurologists invented the former term to describe medical inpatients with AIDS whose loss of mentation and motor function was not attributable to CNS tumors, opportunistic infection, or systemic disease (Navia et al. 1986). Antedating the isolation of HIV and recognition of its neurotoxicity, the etiological rubric was inevitably "AIDS" rather than HIV. The population originally studied had advanced neurological symptoms including significant intellectual deficits—hence "dementia"—as well as a "complex" of motoric and behavioral manifestations including poor ambulation and coordination, agitation, and hallucinations.

Studying a wider range of patients at different stages of HIV infection has expanded understanding of HIV-induced mental status changes and suggested that each word in "AIDS dementia complex" is inexact. Patients may have HIV-related mental status changes before developing "AIDS." Early cognitive and behavioral changes tend not to predominantly involve higher cortical function and are therefore not characteristic of "dementia." And the "complex" triad of cognitive, motor, and behavioral impairment is not invariably present (Perry and Tross 1984; Sadler et al. 1989a). The coiners of the phrase have amended and defended their definition, explaining that AIDS dementia intimates an acquired dysfunction clinically distinct from disorders such as Alzheimer's disease (Sidtis and Price 1990). They have also developed a staging system (Price and Brew 1988) delineating deterioration from minimal cognitive or motor impairment to the vegetative state of severe dementia.

❑ STUDIES OF PRIMARY NEUROPSYCHOLOGICAL IMPAIRMENT

Differences in the meanings of neuropsychological impairment, AIDS dementia complex, and DSM-III-R diagnoses should be kept in mind in reviewing studies of potential neuropsychological deficits in HIV-infected subjects. Thirty-one studies have been either published or presented at medical symposia: 18 of them reported neuropsychological impairment before the onset of systemic AIDS, but 13 did not find meaningful early impairment (Perry 1990). A box score tally is misleading, inasmuch as these studies varied broadly in site of recruitment, sample selection, size, design, extent of neuropsychological testing, data analysis, and interpretation of results.

The largest studies to date derive from the Multicenter AIDS Cohort Study of homosexual and bisexual men recruited in Baltimore, Chicago, Los Angeles, and Pittsburgh (McArthur et al. 1989a; Miller et al. 1990; Selnes et al. 1990; Visscher et al. 1989). Visscher et al. (1989) administered a 25-minute neuropsychological battery to 838 subjects with CDC stages II and III—122 of whom had recently seroconverted—and to 767 seronegative subjects. No significant differences were found between the two groups.

The lack of differential impairment in the HIV-seropositive group may have been attributable both to selection bias and insensitivity of the brief neuropsychological testing, yet this research was important in reassuring the public that most asymptomatic HIV-seropositive individuals do not suffer severe cognitive deficits. Neurological evaluation, MRI, and more extensive neuropsychological testing of a subsample with abnormalities on screening (McArthur et al. 1989a), as well as a follow-up study (Selnes et al. 1990) finding no deterioration in neuropsychological performance among 238 subjects remaining asymptomatic on 1-year follow-up, corroborated these initial findings.

By contrast, studies using more exhaustive neuropsychological test arrays on generally smaller patient samples (Grant et al. 1987; Perry et al. 1989; Saykin et al. 1989; Tross et al. 1988) have found HIV-seropositive subjects with CDC stages II and III scoring below cutoffs on subtests at higher rates than seronegative control subjects. These results have been interpreted (Grant et al. 1987; Perry et al. 1989) as evidence that a small subgroup may have HIV-induced neuropsychological impairment before developing AIDS. Others (Dilley et al. 1989a; Saykin et al. 1989; Tross et al. 1988) contend that such inference is premature given the absence of appropriate statistical correction for multiple test comparisons.

Drawing Conclusions About Neuropsychological Impairment

The debate over early neuropsychological impairment will continue until the accumulation and convergence of research data permit critical consensus. Given the complexity of potentially confounding factors in this research, the reader in the interim should consider four questions in analyzing reports:

1. *What are the extent and quality of neuropsychological testing?* Because HIV can produce diverse, subtle subcortical effects, abbreviated batteries are probably not adequately sensitive to neuropsychological impairment. Despite attempts to develop screening instruments for HIV-related neuropsychological impairment (e.g., Boccellari et al. 1989a), there remains no substitute for the lengthy, labor-intensive neuropsychological evaluations that assess multiple faculties, emphasize timed rather than open-ended tasks, and require concentration, attention, and precise, rapid motor performance (Sidtis and Price 1990). These extensive batteries may yield subtests that frequently identify early neuropsychological impairment, and these subtests may in turn correlate with brain function and anatomy. Discriminant function analyses may identify tests that both differentiate cortical from subcortical deficits (Brouwers et al. 1989) and correlate highly with standardized diagnostic ratings of OMD, imaging abnormalities, and other criteria.
2. *What correlative data supplements the neuropsychological assessments?* Longitudinal anamnestic, physical, laboratory, and imaging data can assist in early diagnosis and correlating neuropsychological impairment with subjective or objective impairment in daily living and occupational performance. Whether the neuropsychological impairment suspected among a small subgroup of seropositive adults is clinically significant takes on profound consequences when applied to the million seropositive adults in the United States who have not yet developed systemic AIDS (Centers for Disease Control 1989).
3. *How were subjects selected and screened, and how well were the inclusion criteria defined?* If a study aims to determine whether HIV-related neuropsychological impairment precedes any secondary manifestations of HIV infection, included subjects must not simply be currently asymptomatic, but must also lack generalized lymphadenopathy (CDC stage III), a history of constitutional symptoms (stage IV-A), and subtle OMD caused by an insidious opportunistic infection (stage IV-C1) or tumor (stage IV-D) of the CNS. To limit the effects of fatigue, boredom, and frustration, subjects undergoing neuropsychological testing must not be overburdened by extended research protocols (Sidtis and Price 1990). Ideally, screening should match pairs of HIV-seropositive and -seronegative subjects to control for gender, age, premorbid intelligence (e.g., by vocabulary subscale), education, and handedness and exclude or stratify for such potential biopsychosocial confounds as major psychiatric disorders, substance abuse, and severe medical illness unrelated to HIV (Marotta and Perry 1989). Even with these safeguards, the selection factors leading patients to volunteer for or drop out of studies may bias findings (Sidtis and Price 1990).
4. *How were findings analyzed and interpreted?* The biostatistical literature abounds in argument over how conservative statistical procedures should be in limiting Type I errors, weighing this against the potentially valuable findings that more liberal analyses might find "significant." The importance of statistically significant results emerging from a study that has not corrected for testing scads of battery subscales should not be overstated. What is statistically significant may also prove clinically trivial.

Summary. Although dementia as a late sequela is not uncommon, it is rare as an initial presentation of HIV infection. Most HIV-seropositive subjects do **not** meet diagnostic criteria for or show overt signs of dementia. According to the CDC (Stern et al. 1989), only 3.0% of 38,666 adults and 3.3% of 666 children presented with HIV encephalopathy as the first manifestation of AIDS. These epidemiological data corroborate clinical studies that found that between 6% and 14% of HIV-seropositive patients present to medical clinics with dementia as their initial problem (Abos et al. 1989; Navia and Price 1987). The percentage of psychiatric outpatients and inpatients with manifestations of early HIV-related OMD is unknown; it is assumed that such patients are more likely to present initially to mental health professionals than to nonpsychiatric physicians. The frequency of case reports in the psychiatric literature (Marotta and Perry 1989) may reflect this sampling bias.

❑ DIAGNOSING EARLY HIV-INDUCED OMD

If it remains unclear how frequently clinically significant neuropsychological impairment occurs before physical manifestations of HIV infection, it is certain that early mental status changes can be subtle (Fauci 1988; Faulstich 1987; Perry and Marotta 1987). Emotional, behavioral, and personality changes may be mistakenly diagnosed as functional disorders or attributed to the stress of living with an incurable, stigmatizing, ineluctably lethal infection. No single clinical finding, neuropsychological test, or procedure has proven sufficiently sensitive and specific to diagnose neuropsychological impairment. As with other organic mental disorders (Perry and Markowitz 1988), diagnosis usually depends on clinical judgment of all available data (see Chapter 9). The patient's complaint, mental status examination, physical examination, and laboratory measures have been found to contribute imperfectly to detection of early neuropsychological impairment and HIV-induced OMD (HIV-OMD) in seropositive patients.

Subjective Complaints of Cognitive Impairment

Three studies have corroborated early clinical impressions (Perry et al. 1989) that HIV-seropositive patients do not reliably report presence or absence of early neuropsychological impairment. Temoshok et al. (1989a) found that the severity of cognitive complaints reported by 102 homosexual men with at least one HIV-related physical symptom did not correlate highly with neuropsychological impairment. Herns et al. (1989) reported that whereas 77 homosexual men in CDC stages II or III had more subjective complaints about cognitive functioning than did 32 seronegative control subjects, the seropositive group had no greater actual neuropsychological impairment. Kocsis et al. (1989), using a questionnaire, found that 75 patients with AIDS perceived their deterioration in cognitive performance inaccurately but that caregiving partners provided more valid ratings.

One explanation for the poor correspondence between subjective complaints and measurable neuropsychological impairment is that seropositive patients, especially those aware of the eventuality of HIV-related dementia (Perry et al. 1989), develop situational anxiety that impairs their concentration and memory and which they then attribute to HIV-related organic dysfunction. Correlation of measures of distress with perceived cognitive complaints (Herns et al. 1989; Kocsis et al. 1989; Temoshok et al. 1989a) supports this hypothesis. Alternatively, it may be that some patients correctly recognize mental deterioration. Their apparently exaggerated complaints might then reflect insensitivity of the instruments with which they were tested or lack of premorbid baseline ratings to demonstrate actual decline from a superior to a normal range. Marder et al. (1989) compared 118 seropositive men without AIDS to 42 seronegative control subjects and concluded that the HIV-infected subjects had more subjective memory and attentional complaints, but that the groups did not differ in objective mental status and neurological findings. Yet the protocol lacked the extensive neuropsychological testing that might have revealed subtle impairment linked to the subjective complaints. Conversely, some patients may underestimate early deficits if their impairment is mild enough to escape subjective recognition or if their self-report batteries survey only gross cognitive changes. A 55-item HIV Dementia Checklist designed to confront this possibility successfully differentiated 55 seropositive subjects from 23 seronegative subjects, finding moderate correlations ($r = 0.24 - 0.43$) between checklist and neuropsychological scores (Boccellari et al. 1989b).

Mental Status Examination

Three studies have suggested that standardized mental status examinations are insufficiently sensitive to early neuropsychological impairment. Dilley et al. (1989b) administered the Mini-Mental State Exam (MMSE; Folstein et al. 1975) to 50 hospitalized patients with AIDS. Although 78% of the subjects had abnormal scores on at least 6 of 10 neuropsychological tests, only 8% were below the standard cutoff of the MMSE. Another study of a smaller group of patients corroborated the instrument's lack of sensitivity (Van Gorp et al. 1989)—hardly a surprise, inasmuch as the MMSE was designed to assess cortical dementia. Similarly, the Neurobehavioral Cognitive Status Examination (Northern California Neurobehavioral Group 1988) indicated that 31 patients with AIDS had greater neuropsychological impairment than 39 control subjects, but scores on this test did not reliably correlate with this dysfunction (Kobayashi et al. 1989).

Based on current evidence, we conclude that a clinical mental status examination, standardized or unstructured, is unlikely to uncover neuropsychological impairment unless a dramatic change emerges from repeated inquiries over time.

Distinction From Mood Disorder

Several authors have warned that HIV-OMD may be misdiagnosed as "functional" depression (Perry and Marotta 1987; Rundell et al. 1986), yet research suggests the processes are usually clinically distinct. Associations have been reported between neuropsychological impairment and self-reported distress (Syndulko et al. 1989a) and hostility (Temoshok et al. 1989a), but only one study has uncovered even a weak correlation between neuropsychological impairment and depressive measures (Herns et al. 1989), and most have found none at all (Grant et al. 1989a; Heaton et al. 1989; Martin et al. 1989; Perry et al. 1989). These results are limited by low depression scores: few of the subjects studied scored in the range associated with clinical depression. Furthermore, the research generally failed to distinguish cognitive from noncognitive impairment. Had subcortical dysfunction alone been considered, it might have correlated more strongly with depression. On the whole, however, these results support the perception (Navia and Price 1987; Perry and Jacobsen 1986) that neuropsychological impairment due to early HIV-OMD—apathy, mental slowing, avoidance of complex tasks, and social withdrawal—is clinically distinguishable from the poor self-esteem, irrational guilt, pessimism, and other symptoms of depression.

Individuals at risk for AIDS have high rates of current and lifetime mood disorders (Atkinson et al. 1988; Perry et al. 1990a). Thus the clinician must always consider that mood disorders and HIV-OMD may be concomitant. Although advances in neurochemistry may eventually explain the phenomenological overlap between comorbid "subcortical dementia" and depression (Blumer 1983; Cummings and Benson 1984), the two studies to date are contradictory. One (Britton et al. 1989) found reduced levels of serotonin metabolites in the CSF of 15 seropositive subjects, whereas the other (Keilp et al. 1989) found no relationship between subjective mood rating and blood and CSF levels of the serotonin precursor tryptophan in 45 seropositive individuals.

Neurological Examination

Neurological findings are not pathognomonic of HIV-OMD. Peripheral neuropathies or vacuolar myelopathy due to HIV may produce motor weakness and sensory abnormalities yet cause no clinically significant mental status changes (Berger 1988; Cornblath and McArthur 1988; Grafe and Wiley 1989; Lange et al. 1988; McArthur et al. 1989a). Ataxia (Fauci 1988; Navia et al. 1986), motor slowing (Fitzgibbon et al. 1989), and autonomic dysfunction with orthostatic hypotension (Cohen and Laudenslager 1989) are other indications of HIV-related neurological impairment that can occur in the absence of cognitive and psychological changes. Conversely, mental status changes may precede focal neurological signs (Navia and Price 1987; Price and Brew 1988).

Laboratory Measures

CSF levels. Various studies have correlated CSF abnormalities with serum immunosuppression (McArthur et al. 1989b), and CSF p24 antigen levels with neurological signs (Brown et al. 1989; Portegies et al. 1989), but not CSF abnormalities with neuropsychological impairment. On the contrary, physically asymptomatic seropositive individuals frequently have CSF pleocytosis, elevated protein, immunoglobulins, and HIV antibodies and antigens (Appleman et al. 1988; McArthur et al. 1988; Marshall et al. 1988; Resnick et al. 1988). Thus CSF measures cannot diagnose HIV-OMD. Nonetheless, lumbar puncture is indicated for any HIV-seropositive patient whose change in mental status could reflect meningoencephalitis due to tuberculosis, toxoplasmosis, cryptococcosis, syphilis, other secondary infections, or CNS lymphoma (Markowitz and Perry 1990).

Lymphocyte studies. Neuropsychological impairment has been associated with lymphocyte cell subsets in some studies (Berger et al. 1989; Boccellari et al. 1989a; Perry et al. 1989; Price and Brew 1988), but not others (Chave et al. 1989; Fernandez et al. 1989a; Martin et al. 1989). Even positive studies have generally found only weak correlations. Reduced total T4 lymphocyte count does not reliably indicate neuropsychological impairment and should not be used to screen for vocational competence (Perry et al. 1989).

Electrophysiological measures. EEG abnormalities have been found in 21%–44% of patients with CDC stage II (Arendt et al. 1989; Koralnik et al. 1989; Parisi et al. 1989a), stages III and IV-A (Riedel et al. 1989; Schnurbus et al. 1989), and stages IV-B through IV-E (Koppel et al. 1985; Levy et al. 1986). Yet slowed alpha rhythms and diffuse theta waves often appear in the absence of clinical signs of mental change and neuropsychological impairment (Parisi et al. 1989b; Smith et al. 1988). It has been suggested that the EEG detects early HIV damage to the CNS more sensitively than clinical measures.

Seropositive patients without AIDS also have abnormalities on computed eye tracking (Otto et al. 1988), auditory (Egan et al. 1989; Otto et al. 1988) and somatosensory (McAllister et al. 1989; Smith et al. 1988) evoked potentials, vibratory threshold (Franzblau et al. 1989), perception of transcutaneous stimulation (Katims et al. 1989), centrally mediated motor dysfunction (Arendt et al. 1989), and cortical stimulation (Moglia et al. 1989). These electrophysiological abnormalities again relate uncertainly to diagnosis of early HIV-OMD; their sensitivity and specificity are unclear. Two studies (Cahn et al. 1989; Syndulko et al. 1989b) found abnormal evoked potentials did not reliably correlate with neuropsychological impairment. A brief screening measure for marked impairment among hospitalized patients with AIDS found that a bedside eye movement test correlated linearly with abnormal mental status and form and color sorting tests (Currie et al. 1989).

Imaging. The imaging story is similar to that of other tests: many studies (Koppel et al. 1985; Levy et al. 1985, 1986; Navia et al. 1986; Olsen et al. 1988; Sze et al. 1987) have described MRI and CT abnormalities in patients with AIDS, but their correlation with clinical pathology is frequently low (Grant et al. 1987; Janssen et al. 1988; McArthur et al. 1989a). Mild cerebral atrophy on CT did not correlate with neuropsychological impairment (Aronow et al. 1989); sulcal widening on MRI was not associated with neurological and CSF abnormalities (Koralnik et al. 1989). Of 107 patients with HIV-induced CNS disease, 31 (29%) had normal CT and MRI scans (Henkes et al. 1989). Arendt et al. (1989) reported that EEG was more sensitive than MRI in detecting HIV pathology of the CNS. Tozzi et al. (1989) decided that MRI abnormalities were suggestive but not diagnostic of neuropsychological impairment. As with the EEG, CNS imaging is indicated in HIV-seropositive patients to explore the differential diagnosis of OMD due to treatable opportunistic infections or tumors, not to assess HIV-OMD, per se.

Mild cerebral atrophy on CT and lucent areas on MRI bear no consistent relationship to clinical findings (Awad et al. 1987; Jarvik et al. 1988). Collier et al. (1989) found that 18 of 41 subjects in CDC stages II or III had abnormal MRI results; diffuse white matter abnormalities correlated with abnormal CSF results, but not with neuropsychological impairment. When organic mental syndrome is suspected and both CT and MRI are unremarkable, either enhanced MRI (Henkes et al. 1989) or single photon emission computed tomography (SPECT) (Pigorini et al. 1989; Pohl et al. 1988) may be more sensitive and specific in detecting a lesion. In a longitudinal study (Grant et al. 1989b), development of neuropsychological impairment was predicted by initial MRI findings of high cortical fluid levels and subcortical hyperdensities. This result is consistent with the neuropsychological and laboratory findings discussed above, namely, that various tests indicating CNS involvement may be harbingers of later development of HIV-OMD.

Summary

The mental status examination is insufficiently sensitive to detect noncognitive dysfunction (Faustman et al. 1990). Subjective complaints, neurological signs, brain imaging studies, and laboratory findings do not reliably correspond with early HIV-induced neuropsychological impairment, whose manifestations are frequently subtle.

❑ PROGRESSION OF HIV-OMD

Case reports (Morgan et al. 1988) have described rapid mental decline in some HIV-seropositive subjects, whereas other subjects have a protracted and fluctuant course (Berger and Mucke 1988). The mean rate of deterioration is under study. Sidtis et al. (1989) found that of 132 patients initially diagnosed as having equivocal or subclinical AIDS, about 25% developed clinically significant dementia within 9 months, and another 25% did so within a year.

Many investigators have noted that risk of neuropsychological impairment increases with disease progression (Chave et al. 1989; Collier et al. 1989; Franzblau et al. 1989; Grant et al. 1987; Saykin et al. 1989; Tross et al. 1988), but this is not inevitably the case. Stern et al. (1989) found no worsening of neuropsychological impairment across CDC stages, and Fernandez et al. (1989a) could not distinguish 39 patients with CDC stage IV-A from 41 patients with stages IV-B through IV-E by their neuropsychological impairment. Selnes et al. (1989) found that 26 asymptomatic patients who attained criteria for AIDS over a 12-month period had no more neuropsychological impairment than a comparison sample of HIV-seronegative subjects. O'Dowd et al. (1988) similarly found no increase in neuropsychological impairment over a 7-month follow-up of seropositive intravenous-drug abusers in a methadone program. Temoshok et al. (1989b) found that 23% of 103 patients with AIDS had clear evidence of neuropsychological deterioration over 6 months, whereas 38% showed a marked improvement that was unrelated to zidovudine. Research (Sadler et al. 1989b) has suggested that this improvement was not an artifact of repeated testing.

The largest longitudinal study (Selnes et al. 1990) found no decline in neuropsychological performance among 238 men remaining in CDC stages II and III for approximately 1 year. The analysis excluded 50 subjects who developed AIDS-related complex or AIDS, and hence did not consider progression of neuropsychological impairment across the gamut of HIV disease (Sidtis and Price 1990). Longitudinal studies of progressive neuropsychological impairment must consider concurrent development of systemic disease, opportunistic infections and malignancies of the CNS, and side effects of medications, all of which can cause OMD not directly caused by HIV itself. The development of any CNS complication, regardless of etiology, markedly decreases survival time (Wilson et al. 1989).

❑ TREATMENT

Treatment of HIV-OMD must be tailored to each patient. Strategies include psychoeducation, psychosocial support, evaluation of suicide potential, and pharmacotherapy (Faulstich 1987; Perry and Jacobsen 1986; Perry and Markowitz 1986).

Psychoeducation should ideally begin before patients develop neuropsychological impairment or HIV-OMD. This provides them the opportunity to make informed decisions about their lives while they still possess time, competence, and judgment to do so. Neuropsychological impairment should not be explained in an alarming manner. The clinician can honestly assert that HIV-related mental changes are not inevitable and are unlikely to be dramatic unless the patient has become severely ill. It is important to differentiate HIV-neuropsychological impairment and OMD from Alzheimer's dementia, with which the patient may confuse them. Sexual partners and family members may also be counseled about the risk of cognitive changes, preferably before but in any case promptly after their onset. Although presently incurable, HIV-OMD should not be presented as untreatable: to do so conveys therapeutic nihilism, damages hope, and impedes acceptance of effective psychosocial and pharmacological interventions (Perry and Markowitz 1988).

Psychosocial treatments for patients with severe neuropsychological impairment include those measures generally undertaken for dementia: titration of external stimuli, repeated correction of misperceptions and distortions, maintenance of a familiar environment, and structuring of the environment to prevent impulsive behavior, including HIV transmission (Forrest 1987; Ostrow et al. 1988; also see Chapter 26). Despite the hopelessness and frustration that an ineluctably fatal course may evoke, interpersonal support can dramatically aid patients and those surrounding them, who often feel isolated by this stigmatizing illness and have limited resources for problem solving.

Assessment of suicidal risk is a necessary component of treating AIDS-related OMD. Marzuk et al. (1988) found the odds ratio for suicide in 20- to 50-year-old male New Yorkers who had AIDS to be 36 times that of those without AIDS. In California, Kizer et al. (1988) found the suicide rate of 29- to 39-year-old men with AIDS to be 21 times that of the matched population without AIDS. Inasmuch as knowledge of HIV infection does not seem to increase suicidal ideation or intent, per se (Perry et al. 1990b), these increased rates may be related to premorbid mood disorders or substance abuse (Atkinson et al. 1988), psychosocial stressors (Faulstich 1987), systemic illness (Cross and Hirschfeld 1985; Whitlock 1986), depression and delirium secondary to medication (Abramowicz 1986; Marzuk et al. 1988), or perhaps to the development of HIV-OMD. It is known that CNS disorders increase suicidal risk (Black et al. 1985; Schoenfeld et al. 1984). The lower levels of CSF serotonin metabolites found in some HIV-seropositive subjects (Britton et al. 1989) have been associated with impulsive violent behavior, including suicide (Mann et al. 1986).

Pharmacotherapy for HIV-OMD includes antiviral and symptomatic neurological, analgesic, and psychotropic medication. Patients with OMD often have decreased pain tolerance and may express their discomfort through disruptive behavior. Analgesia alleviates agitation, irritability, and anger both in patients and their caretakers (Perry and Marotta 1987).

Psychopharmacology for secondary mood and behavioral disorders is under study. Psychostimulants have demonstrated efficacy in treating the apathy, lethargy, and withdrawal of patients with AIDS (Fernandez et al. 1988). Depressed subjects with AIDS-related complex responded better to antidepressants than those with AIDS, perhaps because OMD was more prevalent among the latter (Fernandez et al. 1989b). It is not clear whether HIV infection induces hypersensitivity to the anticholinergic side effects of tricyclic antidepressants; nevertheless, they should be dosed cautiously in seropositive patients. High-potency neuroleptics appear more likely to produce severe dystonia and neuroleptic malignant syndromes (Breitbart et al. 1988; Swenson et al. 1989) in patients with HIV-related delirium and psychosis. Midbrain effects of HIV may underlie these adverse responses; lower-potency neuroleptics or benzodiazepines may be more effective in producing acute sedation. Electroconvulsive therapy (ECT) has been safely administered to patients with AIDS (Schaerf et al. 1989).

❑ SECONDARY CNS DISEASE IN HIV-SEROPOSITIVE PATIENTS

As we have done elsewhere (Markowitz and Perry 1990), we now briefly review common sequelae of HIV infection that affect the CNS. As HIV progressively cripples the immune response to infection, patients become vulnerable to infection both from without and from within. Usually nonpathogenic organisms in the external environment and once harmless internal flora now have the "opportunity" to attack the defenseless patient. Previously suppressed syphilitic or tubercular infections may recrudesce. In the absence of immune surveillance, HIV-infected patients are much more susceptible to a wide array of malignancies.

Disorders often overlap in a patient: more than one opportunistic infection, cancer, or neurological disorder may arise simultaneously, and symptoms overlap for many of the opportunistic infections. In addition, treatments for these illnesses are often themselves toxic; patients debilitated by HIV may be particularly sensitive to medication side effects. As relapses are common, internists struggle to balance prophylaxis of infection with minimizing the toxicity of medications. Thus the overall medical picture is frequently complex, requiring the expertise of many medical specialists. The following outline of common infections and tumors is hardly exhaustive and is intended simply to familiarize the psychiatrist with diseases that were extraordinarily rare until the AIDS epidemic began (Table 21–2).

Pneumocystis Carinii Pneumonia

Pneumocystis is a commensal organism residing in alveoli. PCP is a hallmark of AIDS, the initial opportunistic infection in 60% of cases and a complication in more than 80% overall (Glatt et al. 1988). PCP often begins with apparently benign symptoms: an unproductive cough and mild dyspnea on exertion. It may take several weeks before the patient develops fever, weight loss, and respiratory distress severe enough to require hospitalization. Chest roentgenogram may be unremarkable, but usually shows a diffuse granular infiltrate radiating

TABLE 21–2. COMMON SECONDARY HUMAN IMMUNODEFICIENCY VIRUS (HIV)-ASSOCIATED DISEASE

Etiology	*Neuropsychiatric symptoms*	*Treatments*
Pneumocystis carinii pneumonia (PCP)	Cough, dyspnea, fever, and weight loss	Pentamidine Trimethoprim and sulfamethoxazole Diaminodiphenylsulfone
Toxoplasma gondii	Headache, fever, delirium, and coma; seizures, mental status changes, and focal neurological findings	Pyrimethamine Sulfadiazine
Cryptococcus	Encephalitis, organic mood disorder, and mental status changes	Amphotericin B Flucytosine Fluconazole
Candida	Thrush and systemic infection	Local Nystatin Ketoconazole Clotrimazole troches Systemic Ketoconazole Amphotericin B
Gastrointestinal *Fiosospora* *Cryptosporidium*	Diarrhea	Symptomatic
Cytomegalovirus (CMV)	Meningoencephalitis; pneumonia, retinitis, and colitis	Dihydroxypropoxymethylguanine (DHPG)
Herpes zoster virus	Multidermatomal shingles	Acyclovir
Herpes simplex virus	Encephalitis; mucocutaneous ulceration	Acyclovir
Atypical mycobacteria	Cough, fever, weight loss, and night sweats	(Antitubercular medication until *Mycobacterium tuberculosis* has been ruled out)
Kaposi's sarcoma	Violaceous lesions of skin and internal organs	Cosmetics Topical cryo- or radiotherapy α-Interferon and chemotherapy for advanced lesions
Central nervous system lymphoma	Focal neurological findings; mental status changes	Chemotherapy; surgery

symmetrically from the hilum. Diagnosis is confirmed by bronchoscopic washings or biopsy. Treatment of PCP has improved considerably: hospitalizations are shorter and survival rates higher, increasing overall life expectancy of patients with AIDS. Common medications are trimethoprim and sulfamethoxazole (Bactrim), diaminodiphenylsulfone (Dapsone), α-difluromethylornithine (DFMO), and intravenous pentamidine isethionate. In at least half of PCP cases, medication side effects limit treatment (Kaplan et al. 1987). Seropositive individuals, even if asymptomatic or without history of PCP, are often prophylactically given aerosolized pentamidine, Bactrim, or Dapsone; pentamidine appears least toxic and can be self-administered (Montgomery et al. 1987).

Zidovudine (formerly azidothymidine [AZT]) decreases recurrence of PCP. Zidovudine inhibits reverse transcriptase, the retroviral enzyme crucial for HIV replication. In double-blind (Fischl et al. 1987) and open (Creagh-Kirk et al. 1988) trials, the drug increased longevity and quality of life for patients with AIDS and provided some protection against opportunistic infections; it may also improve HIV-induced mental changes, at least in children (Pizzo et al. 1988). Unfortunately, zidovudine has significant side effects, particularly macrocytic anemia and granulocytopenia (Richman et al. 1987), but also mania, coma, or fatal neurotoxicity in rare instances. Administering zidovudine in conjunction with dideoxycytidine (Yarchoan et al. 1988), another viral enzyme blocker, may maximize antiviral effect with less toxicity. Psychiatrists should note that zidovudine itself can cause fatigue and a depression-like syndrome that is often difficult to distinguish from psychological factors, direct effects of HIV, and secondary systemic and CNS illnesses. Given its toxicity, it is unclear whether (or which) physically asymptomatic patients without severe immunosuppression should receive maintenance zidovudine therapy.

Toxoplasma Gondii

Toxoplasma gondii is a protozoan that principally affects the CNS by causing an encephalitis with headache, fever, delirium, and coma (Luft et al. 1984), or mass lesions in the brain that produce seizures, mental changes, and focal neurological findings. Mass lesions can be diagnosed either by CT or MRI. Treatment requires pyrimethamine and sulfadiazine for at least 6–8 weeks (Wong et al. 1984), although alternative protocols are being studied (Kaplan et al. 1987). Treatment response is judged by clinical status rather than by antibody titers, which are insensitive markers of improvement. HIV-infected patients should avoid handling raw meat and cat litter boxes, prime sources of *Toxoplasmas*.

Cryptococcus

Cryptococcus is a fungus that can cause fulminant and multisystemic infection. Psychiatrists should also recognize that encephalitic patients may present with subtle mental changes, including depression, in the absence of meningeal signs or focal findings (Dismukes 1988). Diagnosis is made by lumbar puncture. Amphotericin B is the principal treatment, with flucytosine added if the patient does not have bone marrow suppression; fluconazole may also be effective. Because relapse rates are high, treatment now generally persists for more than 6 weeks (Zuger et al. 1986).

Candida

This fungus often causes a discomfiting albeit not dangerous oral thrush (candidiasis), enveloping the tongue and oral cavity in white. Often an early sign of immune dysfunction, thrush responds to topical nystatin, clotrimazole troches, or oral ketoconazole, which is continued for life. Candidal infection of the esophagus, trachea, bronchi, lungs, and systemic dissemination are more worrisome. Systemic involvement is confirmed by biopsy and treated with ketoconazole or amphotericin B.

Gastrointestinal Pathogens

Unrecognized as a human pathogen before the AIDS epidemic, *cryptosporidium* causes severe, chronic, watery, and ultimately fatal diarrhea. There are no effective treatments either for infection by *cryptosporidium* or a similar infection by *Fiosospora*. Symptomatic management consists of hydration, electrolyte replacement, and opiate control of bowel motility. Management is often further complicated when *Giardia lamblia*, amoebae, or other protozoans are present, as may frequently occur in sexually active gay men.

Viral Pathogens

More than 95% of homosexual men are seropositive for cytomegalovirus (CMV) (Felsenstein et al. 1985). In HIV-infected patients CMV can cause pneumonia, meningoencephalitis, and retinitis leading to blindness. Previously considered untreatable, CMV retinitis and colitis show some response to the experimental drug dihydroxypropoxymethylguanine (DHPG), although the drug causes marrow suppression and relapse is common (Felsenstein et al. 1985).

Herpes zoster virus can cause severe, multidermatomal "shingles." Even the usually milder herpes simplex virus (HSV) may exceed its typical self-limited episodes, producing gastrointestinal and CNS disease. Local mucocutaneous HSV lesions may progress to chronic, enlarging perianal ulcers, particularly in homosexual males with AIDS. Oral acyclovir for 10 days effectively treats mucocutaneous lesions and has relatively few side effects; used for prophylaxis, it may also help prevent HIV immune impairment (Strauss et al. 1984). Intravenous acyclovir is sometimes required for severe herpes zoster.

Other Pathogens

HIV-infected patients may suffer reactivation of previously treated *Mycobacterium tuberculosis* (MTB). Early symptoms such as cough, fatigue, weight loss, fevers, and night sweats may be misattributed to HIV or PCP before pulmonary or miliary spread make secondary MTB infection evident. For this reason, skin testing of HIV- infected patients is advisable, perhaps followed by isoniazid prophylaxis (Pitchenik et al. 1986). HIV-infected patients are also susceptible to infection with atypical mycobacteria, most commonly *Mycobacterium avium cellulare* (MAI): indeed, half of AIDS patients carry this infection or, more rarely, *Mycobacterium Kansasii.* Because prodromal symptoms of fever, weight loss, and malaise mimic HIV and other infections, MAI may be missed as the cause until severe abdominal pain, diarrhea, and malabsorption occur. Standard antitubercular drugs have been used, but their toxicity is high and their effectiveness doubtful (Hawkins et al. 1986). Yet patients with mycobacterial infections should be treated at least until the organism is subtyped, because MTB is responsive to isoniazid, rifampin, ethambutol, and other medications.

Patients with a history of documented, adequate treatment for syphilis may have recurrence with immunosuppression, developing the otherwise rare stigmata of secondary and tertiary lues. Other pathogens include *Coccidioides* and *Histoplasma* (especially in endemic geographic regions), *Salmonella septicemia,* and, in children, the agent causing lymphoid interstitial pneumonitis.

HIV-Related Malignancies

Various types of malignancies have been reported in association with HIV, of which two are especially noteworthy to psychiatrists. Kaposi's sarcoma (KS), a previously rare disorder that had comprised only 0.02% of all malignancies in the United States (Robbins and Cotran 1979), was among the first clinical markers identifying AIDS to physicians. Before AIDS, KS was understood as an indolent, slowly progressive tumor manifested in small, superficial, violaceous plaques on the legs of middle-aged European men. KS associated with HIV is much more aggressive and disseminated. It invades the entire body surface, including the face, mouth, and viscera, particularly the lungs and gastrointestinal tract. Once seen, large skin lesions are easily diagnosed by their characteristic purplish color and absence of blanching when pressed. Smaller early skin lesions or suspected lung lesions require biopsy for diagnosis. For unclear reasons, KS has occurred almost exclusively among seropositive gay men. Equally mysterious is its decrease in incidence from nearly half of all early cases of AIDS to roughly 16% of the current United States caseload.

KS alone is not usually lethal and may linger chronically before suddenly increasing internal and external lesions produce severe disfigurement and respiratory compromise. Vincristine and other highly toxic oncotherapeutic regimens are then employed. α-Interferon and other agents (Kaplan et al. 1987) have been approved for palliative treatment. Although the physical effects of KS can be relatively benign, it can be psychologically devastating both as a cosmetic problem and a stigma of the disease (the "scarlet letter of AIDS"). Before lesions multiply, many patients find cover-up lotions or topical cryotherapy or radiotherapy emotionally helpful. The second neoplasm relevant to psychiatry is lymphoma of the brain, which can cause mental changes before diagnosis. Prognosis for these tumors is worse than that for cancer patients without HIV infection.

❑ CONCLUSIONS

HIV is responsible either directly or indirectly for a complex, symptomatically overlapping series of disorders. Most HIV-seropositive individuals are physically asymptomatic, and it is unclear how prevalent and significant neuropsychiatric impairment is in this population. No single clinical or laboratory finding is pathognomonic either of HIV-induced neuropsychiatric impairment or of OMD directly caused by HIV itself. The clinician assessing patients who are seropositive or at risk for HIV must keep in mind the great variability of presentations and comorbidities accompanying the virus.

❑ REFERENCES

Abos J, Graus F, Alom J, et al: Incidence of the AIDS dementia complex as the first manifestation of AIDS: a prospective study, in Abstracts of the Fifth International Conference on AIDS. Montreal, Quebec, Canada International Development Research Centre, 1989, p 448

Abramowicz M (ed): Drugs that cause psychiatric symptoms. Med Lett Drugs Ther 28:9–18, 1986

American Psychiatric Association: Diagnostic and Statistical Manual of Mental Disorders, 3rd Edition, Revised. Washington, DC, American Psychiatric Association, 1987

Andersson MA, Bergstrom TB, Blomstrand C, et al: Increasing intrathecal lymphocytosis and immunoglobulin G production in neurologically asymptomatic HIV-1 infection. J Neuroimmunol 19:291–304, 1988

Appleman ME, Marshall DW, Brey RL, et al: Cerebrospinal fluid abnormalities in patients without AIDS who are seropositive for the human immunodeficiency virus. J Infect Dis 158:193–199, 1988

Arendt G, Hefter H, Elsing C, et al: Motor dysfunction and cognitive disturbances in 50 clinically asymptomatic HIV-infected patients with normal MRI scans, in Abstracts of the Fifth International Conference on AIDS. Montreal, Quebec, International Development Research Centre, 1989, p 460

Aronow H, Keilp JG, Krol G, et al: Cerebral atrophy in HIV-1 infected patients: relationship to neurological and neuropsychological measures, in Abstracts of the Fifth International Conference on AIDS. Montreal, Quebec, International Development Research Centre, 1989, p 458

Atkinson JH, Grant I, Kennedy J, et al: Prevalence of psychiatric disorders among men infected with human immunodeficiency virus. Arch Gen Psychiatry 45:859–864, 1988

Awad IA, Spetzler RF, Hodak JA, et al: Incidental lesions on magnetic resonance imaging of the brain: prevalence and clinical significance in various age groups. Neurosurgery 20:222–227, 1987

Ayers MR, Abrams DI, Newell TG, et al: Performance of individuals with AIDS on the Luria-Nebraska Neuropsychological battery. International Journal of Clinical Neuropsychology 9:101–105, 1987

Beresford TP, Blow FC, Hall RCW: AIDS encephalitis mimicking alcohol dementia and depression. Biol Psychiatry 21:394–397, 1986

Berger JR: The neurological complications of HIV infection. Acta Neurol Scand 116:40–76, 1988

Berger JR, Mucke L: Prolonged survival and partial recovery in AIDS-associated progressive multifocal leukoencephalopathy. J Neurol 38:1060–1065, 1988

Berger JR, McCarthy M, Resnick L, et al: T4 lymphocyte counts and the presence of abnormalities on neurological examination in asymptomatic HIV seropositive subjects, in Abstracts of the Fifth International Conference on AIDS. Montreal, Quebec, International Development Research Centre, 1989, p 459

Black DW, Warrick G, Winokur G: The Iowa Record Linkage Study: excess mortality among patients with organic mental disorders. Arch Gen Psychiatry 42:78–81, 1985

Blumer DF: Subcortical dementia: a clinical approach, in The Dementias. Edited by Mayeux R, Rosen WG. New York, Raven, 1983

Boccellari A, Davis A, Dilley W: The development of a brief screening battery to detect cognitive deficits in patients with AIDS, in Abstracts of the Fifth International Conference on AIDS. Montreal, International Development Research Centre, 1989a, p 390

Boccellari A, Dilley JW, Davis A, et al: Preliminary findings on a screening symptom checklist for HIV dementia, in Abstracts of the Fifth International Conference on AIDS. Montreal, International Development Research Centre, 1989b, p 390

Breitbart W, Marotta RF, Call P: AIDS and neuroleptic malignant syndrome. Lancet 2:1488–1489, 1988

Brew BJ, Bhalla RB, Fleisher M, et al: Cerebrospinal fluid beta 2 microglobulin in patients infected with human virus. Neurology 39:830–834, 1989

Britton CB, Kranzler S, Naini A, et al: Serotonin metabolite deficiency in HIV infection and AIDS, in Abstracts of the Fifth International Conference on AIDS. Montreal, Quebec, International Development Research Centre, 1989, p 453

Brouwers P, Mohr E, Hendricks M, et al: Multivariate statistical determination of incidence and character of cognitive impairments in HIV patients, in Abstracts of the Fifth International Conference on AIDS. Montreal, Quebec, International Development Research Centre, 1989, p 450

Brown C, Quinn T, Lubakin J, et al: Blood and cerebrospinal fluid lymphocyte phenotyping and HIV-1 p24 antigen detection in HIV-1 infected Zairians with and without neurological signs, in Abstracts of the Fifth International Conference on AIDS. Montreal, Quebec, International Development Research Centre, 1989, p 443

Bukasa KS, Sincic CJ, Bodeus M, et al: Anti-HIV antibodies in the CSF of AIDS patients: a serological and immunoblotting study. J Neurol Neurosurg Psychiatry 51:1063–1068, 1988

Cahn P, Mangone C, Perez H, et al: Subclinical neuropsychological and peripheral abnormalities in HIV positive patients, in Abstracts of the Fifth International Conference on AIDS. Montreal, Quebec, International Development Research Centre, 1989, p 450

Carne CA, Smith A, Elkington SG, et al: Acute encephalopathy coincident with seroconversion for anti-HTLV-III. Lancet 2:1206–1208, 1985

Centers for Disease Control: Revision of the CDC surveillance case definition for acquired immunodeficiency syndrome. MMWR 36:3S–15S, 1987

Centers for Disease Control: AIDS and human immunodeficiency virus infection in the United States: 1988 update. MMWR 38:1–38, 1989

Ceroni M, Minoli L, Di Perri G, et al: Detection of HTLV-III specific IgG bands in the CSF from a patient with AIDS and encephalitis. J Neurol 38:143–144, 1988

Chave JP, Thuillard F, Assal G, et al: Neuropsychological manifestations of HIV infection: a prospective study, in Abstracts of the Fifth International Conference on AIDS. Montreal, Quebec, International Development Research Centre, 1989, p 451

Cohen JA, Laudenslager M: Autonomic nervous system involvement in patients with human immunodeficiency virus infection. Neurology 39:1111–1112, 1989

Collier A, Marra C, Coombs R, et al: Central nervous system findings and neurologic correlates of HIV infection in men with CDC Group II/III disease, in Abstracts of the Fifth International Conference on AIDS. Montreal, Quebec, International Development Research Centre, 1989, p 460

Cornblath DR, McArthur JC: Predominantly sensory neuropathy in patients with AIDS and AIDS-related complex. J Neurol 38:794–796, 1988

Council of State and Territorial Epidemiologists, AIDS Program, Center for Infectious Diseases: Revision of the CDC surveillance case definition for acquired immunodeficiency syndrome. MMWR 36 (suppl 1):1S–15S, 1987

Creagh-Kirk T, Doi P, Andrews E, et al: Survival experience among patients with AIDS receiving zidovudine. JAMA 260:3009–3015, 1988

Cross CK, Hirschfeld RM: Epidemiology of disorders in adulthood: suicide, in Psychiatry, Vol 3. Edited by Cavenar JO Jr, Michels RH, Brodie HKH, et al. Philadelphia, PA, JB Lippincott, and New York, Basic Books, 1985, Chapter 20

Cummings JL, Benson DF: Subcortical dementia: review of an emerging concept. Arch Neurol 41:874–879, 1984

Currie JN, Benson EM, Ramsden MB, et al: Clinical validation of a bedside antisaccadic test for the assessment of AIDS dementia, in Abstracts of the Fifth International Conference on AIDS. Montreal, Quebec, International Development Research Centre, 1989, p 465

Dilley JW, Boccellari A, Davis A, et al: Relationship between neuropsychological and immune variables in HIV positive asymptomatic men, in Abstracts of the Fifth International Conference on AIDS. Montreal, Quebec, International Development Research Centre, 1989a, p 384

Dilley JW, Boccellari A, Davis A: The use of the Mini-Mental State Exam as a cognitive screen in patients with AIDS, in Abstracts of the Fifth International Conference on AIDS. Montreal, Quebec, International Development Research Centre, 1989b, p 384

Dismukes WE: Cryptococcal meningitis in patients with AIDS. J Infect Dis 157:624–628, 1988

Egan V, Chiswick A, Goodwin G, et al: Correlation of p300 auditory evoked potentials and tests of cognitive funciton in HIV positive drug users, in Abstracts of the Fifth International Conference on AIDS. Montreal, Quebec, International Development Research Centre, 1989, p 390

Elovaara I, Seppala I, Poutiainene E, et al: Intrathecal humoral immunologic response in neurologically symptomatic and asymptomatic patients with human immunodeficiency virus infection. J Neurol 38:1455–1456, 1988

Epstein LG, Sharer LR, Goudsmit J: Neurological and neuropathological features of human immunodeficiency virus infection in children. Ann Neurol 23 (suppl):S19–S23, 1988

Fauci AS: The human immunodeficiency virus: infectivity and mechanisms of pathogenesis. Science 239:617–622, 1988

Faulstich ME: Psychiatric aspects of AIDS. Am J Psychiatry 144:551–556, 1987

Faustman WO, Moses JA, Csernansky JG: Limitations of the Mini-Mental State Examination in predicting neuropsychological functioning in a psychiatric sample. Acta Psychiatr Scand 81:126–31, 1990

Felsenstein D, D'Amico DJ, Hirsch MS, et al: Treatment of cytomegalovirus retinitis with O-[2-hydroxy-1-(hydroxymethyl) ethoxymethyl] guanine. Ann Intern Med 103:377–380, 1985

Fernandez F, Adams F, Levy JK, et al: Cognitive impairment due to AIDS-related complex and its response to psychostimulants. Psychosomatics 29:38–46, 1988

Fernandez F, Levy JK, Pirozzolo FP: Neuropsychological and immunological abnormalities in advanced HIV infection, in Abstracts of the Fifth International Conference on AIDS. Montreal, Quebec, International Development Research Centre, 1989a, p 384

Fernandez F, Levy JK, Mansel PWA: Response to antidepressant therapy in depressed persons with advanced HIV infection, in Abstracts of the Fifth International Conference on AIDS. Montreal, Quebec, International Development Research Centre, 1989b, p 383

Fischl MA, Richman DD, Grieco MH, et al: The efficacy of azidothymidine (AZT) in the treatment of patients with AIDS and AIDS-related complex. N Engl J Med 317:185–191, 1987

Fitzgibbon ML, Cella DF, Mumfleet G, et al: Motor slowing in asymptomatic HIV infection. Percept Mot Skill 68:1331–1338, 1989

Folstein MF, Folstein SE, McHugh PR: Mini-Mental State: a practical method for grading the cognitive state of patients for the clinician. J Psychiatr Res 12:189–198, 1975

Forrest DV: Psychosocial treatment in neuropsychiatry, in The American Psychiatric Press Textbook of Neuropsychiatry. Edited by Hales RE, Yudofsky SC. Washington, DC, American Psychiatric Press, 1987, pp 387–409

Franzblau A, Letz RE, Hershman D, et al: Quantitative vibration threshold testing and computer-based neurobehavioral testing of persons infected with HIV, in Abstracts of the Fifth International Conference on AIDS. Montreal, Quebec, International Development Research Centre, 1989, p 462

Gabuzda DH, Ho DD, de la Monte SM, et al: Immunohistochemical identification of HTLV-III antigen in brains of patients with AIDS. Ann Neurol 20:289–295, 1986

Gartner S, Markovits P, Markovitz DM, et al: Virus isolation from and identification of HTLV-III/LAV-producing cells in brain tissue from a patient with AIDS. JAMA 256:2365–2367, 1986

Glatt AE, Chirgwin K, Landesman SH: Treatment of infections associated with human immunodeficiency virus. N Engl J Med 318:1439–1448, 1988

Grafe MR, Wiley CA: Spinal cord and peripheral nerve pathology in AIDS: the roles of cytomegalovirus and human immunodeficiency virus. Ann Neurol 25:561–566, 1989

Grant I, Atkinson JH, Hesselink JR, et al: Evidence for early central nervous system involvement in AIDS and other HIV infections. Ann Intern Med 107:828–836, 1987

Grant I, Olshen R, Atkinson H, et al: Discriminating depression from cognitive impairment in HIV illness, in

Abstracts of the Fifth International Conference on AIDS. Montreal, Quebec, International Development Research Centre, 1989a, p 390

Grant I, Heaton RK, Jernigan T, et al: Neuropsychological changes in CDC II, III, and IV persons after 6 to 12 months: evidence for decline, in Abstracts of the Fifth International Conference on AIDS. Montreal, Quebec, International Development Research Centre, 1989b, p 459

Gray F, Gherardi R, Keohane C, et al: Pathology of the central nervous system in 40 cases of acquired immunodeficiency syndrome (AIDS). Neuropathol Appl Neurobiol 14:365–380, 1988

Grimaldi LM, Castagna A, Lazzarin A, et al: Oligoclonal IgG bands in cerebrospinal fluid and serum during asymptomatic human immunodeficiency virus infection. Ann Neurol 24:277–279, 1988

Haverkos HW, Gotlieb MS, Killen JY, et al: Classification of HTLV-III/LAV-related diseases (letter). J Infect Dis 152:1095, 1985

Hawkins CC, Gold JMW, Whimbey E, et al: Mycobacterium avium complex infections in patients with acquired immunodeficiency syndrome. Ann Intern Med 105:184–188, 1986

Heaton R, Atkinson H, Grant I, et al: Relating depression to neuropsychological impairment, in Abstracts of the Fifth International Conference on AIDS. Montreal, Quebec, International Development Research Centre, 1989, p 390

Henkes H, Schorner W, Jochens R, et al: MR imaging of intracranial manifestations of AIDS: unenhanced and GD-DTPA enhanced studies, in Abstracts of the Fifth International Conference on AIDS. Montreal, Quebec, International Development Research Centre, 1989, p 215

Herns M, Newman S, McAllister R, et al: Mood state, neuropsychology and self-reported cognitive deficits in HIV infection, in Abstracts of the Fifth International Conference on AIDS. Montreal, Quebec, International Development Research Centre, 1989, p 382

Heyward WL, Curran JW: The epidemiology of AIDS in the U.S. Sci Am 259(4):72–81, 1988

Janssen RS, Saykin AJ, Kaplan JE, et al: Neurological complications of human immunodeficiency virus infection in patients with lymphadenopathy syndrome. Ann Neurol 23:49–55, 1988

Janssen RS, Cornblath DR, Epstein LG, et al: Human immunodeficiency virus (HIV) infection and the nervous system: report from the American Academy of Neurology AIDS Task Force. Neurology 39:119–122, 1989

Jarvik JG, Hesselink JR, Kennedy C, et al: Acquired immunodeficiency syndrome: magnetic resonance patterns of brain involvement with pathologic correlation. Arch Neurol 45:731–736, 1988

Joffe RT, Rubinow DR, Squillace K, et al: Neuropsychiatric aspects of AIDS. Psychopharmacol Bull 22:684–688, 1986

Jordan BD, Navia BA, Petito C: Neurological syndromes complicated by AIDS. Front Radiat Ther Oncol 19:82–87, 1985

Kaplan LD, Wofsy CB, Volberding PA: Treatment of patients with acquired immunodeficiency syndrome and associated manifestations. JAMA 257:1367–1373, 1987

Katims JJ, Taylor DN, Wallace JI, et al: Current perception threshold in HIV positive patients, in Abstracts of the Fifth International Conference on AIDS. Montreal, Quebec, International Development Research Centre, 1989, p 463

Kermani EJ, Borod JC, Brown PH, et al: New psychopathologic findings in AIDS: case report. J Clin Psychiatry 46:240–241, 1985

Keilp JG, Brew BJ, Heyes M, et al: Tryptophan levels are unrelated to disturbances of mood in HIV-1 infected patients, in Abstracts of the Fifth International Conference on AIDS. Montreal, Quebec, International Development Research Centre, 1989, 384

Kizer KW, Green M, Perkins CI, et al: AIDS and suicide in California (letter). JAMA 260:1881, 1988

Kobayashi J, Heaton R, Thompson L, et al: A comparison of neuropsychological testing and mental status exam in AIDS patients, in Abstracts of the Fifth International Conference on AIDS. Montreal, Quebec, International Development Research Centre, 1989, p 382

Kocsis AE, Church J, Vearnals S, et al: Personality, behavior, and cognitive changes in AIDS as rated by patients and their careers and as related to neuropsychological test results, in Abstracts of the Fifth International Conference on AIDS. Montreal, Quebec, International Development Research Centre, 1989, p 385

Koppel BS, Wormer GP, Tuchman AJ, et al: Central nervous system involvement in patients with acquired immune deficiency syndrome (AIDS). Acta Neurol Scand 71:337–353, 1985

Koralnik I, Beaumanoir A, Hausler R, et al: Abnormalities of EEG and otoneurologic tests in asymptomatic HIV infected homosexuals: a prospective controlled study, in Abstracts of the Fifth International Conference on AIDS. Montreal, Quebec, International Development Research Centre, 1989, p 462

Lange DJ, Britton CB, Younger DS, et al: The neuromuscular manifestations of human immunodeficiency virus infections. Arch Neurol 45:1084–1088, 1988

Levy RM, Bredesen DE, Rosenblum ML: Neurological manifestations of the acquired immunodeficiency syndrome (AIDS): experience at UCSF and review of the literature. J Neurosurg 62:475–495, 1985

Levy RM, Rosenbloom S, Perret LV: Neuroradiologic findings in AIDS: a review of 200 cases. AJR 147:977–983, 1986

Luft BJ, Brooks RG, Conley FK, et al: Toxoplasmic encephalitis in patients with the acquired immunodeficiency syndrome. JAMA 252:913–915, 1984

McAllister RH, Harrison MJG, Griffin GB, et al: Prospective neurological and neurophysiological assessment in a cohort of homosexual men, in Abstracts of the Fifth International Conference on AIDS. Montreal, Quebec, International Development Research Centre, 1989, p 463

McArthur JC, Cohen BA, Farzedegan H, et al: Cerebrospinal fluid abnormalities in homosexual/bisexual men with and without neuropsychiatric findings. Ann Neurol 23 (suppl):S34–S37, 1988

McArthur JC, Cohen BA, Selnes OA, et al: Low prevalence

of neurological and neuropsychological abnormalities in otherwise healthy HIV-1-infected individuals: results from the Multicenter AIDS Cohort Study. Ann Neurol 26:601–611, 1989a

McArthur JC, McArthur JH, Herman C, et al: Increasing CSF abnormalities in HIV-1 infected individuals with declining systemic immune status, in Abstracts of the Fifth International Conference on AIDS. Montreal, Quebec, International Development Research Centre, 1989b, p 463

Mann JJ, Stanley M, McBride PA, et al: Increased serotonin-2 and beta-adrenergic receptor binding in the frontal cortices of suicide victims. Arch Gen Psychiatry 43:954–959, 1986

Manuelidis EE, Manuelidis L: Suggested links between different types of dementias: Creutzfeldt-Jakob disease, Alzheimer disease, and retroviral CNS infections. Alzheimer Dis Assoc Disord 3:100–109, 1989

Marder K, Bell K, Dooneief G, et al: Absence of neurological disease early in HIV infection, in Abstracts of the Fifth International Conference on AIDS. Montreal, Quebec, International Development Research Centre, 1989, p 459

Markowitz J, Perry S: AIDS: a medical overview for psychiatrists, in American Psychiatric Press Review of Psychiatry, Vol 9. Edited by Tasman A, Goldfinger SM, Kaufmann CA. Washington, DC, American Psychiatric Press, 1990, pp 574–592

Marotta R, Perry S: Early neuropsychological dysfunction caused by the human immunodeficiency virus. Journal of Neuropsychiatry and Clinical Neurosciences 1:225–235, 1989

Marshall DW, Brey RL, Cahill WT, et al: Spectrum of cerebrospinal fluid findings in various stages of human immunodeficiency virus infection. Arch Neurol 45:949–953, 1988

Martin A, Salazar AM, Kampen D, et al: Patterns of neuropsychological dysfunction in a select group of HIV positive individuals in comparison to psychiatric controls, in Abstracts of the Fifth International Conference on AIDS. Montreal, Quebec, International Development Research Centre, 1989, p 463

Marzuk PM, Tierney H, Tardiff K, et al: Increased risk of suicide in patients with AIDS. JAMA 259:1333–1337, 1988

Miller EN, Selnes OA, McArthur JC, et al: Neuropsychological performance in HIV-1-infected homosexual men: the multicenter AIDS Cohort Study (MACS). Neurology 40:197–203, 1990

Moglia A, Zandrini C, Alfonsi E, et al: Electrophysiological investigation of central and peripheral nervous system in HIV-infected patients, in Abstracts of the Fifth International Conference on AIDS. Montreal, Quebec, International Development Research Centre, 1989, p 215

Montgomery AB, Debs RJ, Luce JM, et al: Aerosolised pentamidine as sole therapy for pneumocystis carinii pneumonia in patients with acquired immunodeficiency syndrome. Lancet 2:480–483, 1987

Morgan MK, Clark ME, Hartman WL: AIDS-related dementia: a case report of rapid cognitive decline. J Clin Psychiatry 44:1024–1028, 1988

Navia BA, Price RW: The acquired immunodeficiency syndrome dementia complex as the presenting or sole manifestation of human immunodeficiency virus infection. Arch Neurol 44:65–69, 1987

Navia BA, Jordan BD, Price RW: The AIDS dementia complex, I: clinical features. Ann Neurol 19:517–524, 1986

Northern California Neurobehavioral Group: Test Booklet for the Neurobehavioral Cognitive Status Examination. Fairfax, CA, Northern California Neurobehavioral Group, 1988

O'Dowd MA, McKegney FP, Selwyn PA, et al: Comparison of neuropsychologic function in HIV seropositive intravenous drug abusers in a methadone maintenance program, in Abstracts of the Fourth International Conference on AIDS, Stockholm, Sweden. Washington, DC, BioData, 1988, p 399

Olsen WL, Longo FM, Mills CM, et al: White matter disease in AIDS: findings at MR imaging. Radiology 169:445–448, 1988

Ostrow D, Grant I, Atkinson H: Assessment and management of the AIDS patient with neuropsychiatric disturbances. J Clin Psychiatry 49:S14–S22, 1988

Otto D, Hudnell K, Boyes W, et al: Electrophysiological measures of visual and auditory function as indices of neurotoxicity. Toxicology 49:205–218, 1988

Parisi A, Strosselli M, Di Perri G, et al: Electroencephalography in the early diagnosis of HIV-related subacute encephalitis: analysis of 185 patients. J Clin Electroencephalogr 20:1–5, 1989a

Parisi A, Di Perri G, Strosselli M, et al: Usefulness of computerized electroencephalography in diagnosing, staging, and monitoring AIDS-dementia complex. AIDS 3:209–213, 1989b

Perry SW: Organic mental disorders caused by HIV: update on early diagnosis and treatment. Am J Psychiatry 147:696–710, 1990

Perry SW, Jacobsen P: Neuropsychiatric manifestations of AIDS-spectrum disorders. Hosp Community Psychiatry 37:135–142, 1986

Perry SW, Markowitz J: Psychiatric interventions for AIDS-spectrum disorders. Hosp Community Psychiatry 37:1001–1006, 1986

Perry SW, Markowitz J: Organic mental disorders, in The American Psychiatric Press Textbook of Psychiatry. Edited by Talbott JA, Hales RE, Yudofsky SC. Washington, DC, American Psychiatric Press, 1988, pp 279–311

Perry S, Marotta R: AIDS dementia: a review of the literature. Alzheimer Dis Assoc Disord 1:221–235, 1987

Perry SW, Tross S: Psychiatric problems of AIDS inpatients at The New York Hospital: a preliminary report. Public Health Rep 99:200–205, 1984

Perry S, Belsky-Barr D, Barr WB, et al: Neuropsychological function in physically asymptomatic, HIV-seropositive men. Journal of Neuropsychiatry and Clinical Neurosciences 1:296–302, 1989

Perry S, Jacobsberg LB, Fishman B, et al: Psychiatric diagnosis before serological testing for the human immunodeficiency virus. Am J Psychiatry 147:89–93, 1990a

Perry S, Jacobsberg L, Fishman B: Suicidal ideation and HIV testing. JAMA 263:679–682, 1990b

Petito CK: Review of central nervous system pathology in human immunodeficiency virus infection. Ann Neurol 23 (suppl):S54–S57, 1988

Pigorini F, Pau FM, Galgani S, et al: Single photon emission computed tomography findings in HIV infection, in Abstracts of the Fifth International Conference on AIDS. Montreal, Quebec, International Development Research Centre, 1989, p 458

Pitchenik AE, Burr J, Cole CH: Tuberculin testing for persons with positive serologic studies for HTLV-III (letter). N Engl J Med 314:447, 1986

Pizzo PA, Eddy J, Falloon J, et al: Effect of continuous infusion of zidovudine (AZT) in children with symptomatic HIV infection. N Engl J Med 319:889–896, 1988

Pohl P, Vogl G, Fill H, et al: Single photon emission computed tomography in AIDS dementia complex. J Nucl Med 29:1382–1386, 1988

Portegies P, Epstein LG, Hun ST, et al: Human immunodeficiency virus type 1 antigen in cerebrospinal fluid: correlation with clinical neurologic status. Arch Neurol 46:261–264, 1989

Price RW, Brew BJ: The AIDS dementia complex. J Infect Dis 158:1079–1083, 1988

Price RW, Brew B, Sidtis J, et al: The brain in AIDS: central nervous system HIV-1 infection and AIDS dementia complex. Science 239:586–591, 1988

Price RW, Brew BJ, Rosenblum M: The AIDS Dementia Complex and HIV-1 brain infection: a pathogenic model of virus-immune interaction, in Immunological Mechanisms in Neurological and Psychiatric Disease. Edited by Waksman BH. New York, Raven, 1990

Price WA, Forejt J: Neuropsychiatric aspects of AIDS: a case report. Gen Hosp Psychiatry 8:7–10, 1986

Redfield RR, Wright DC, Tramont EC: The Walter Reed staging classification for HTLV-III/LAV infection. N Engl J Med 314:131–132, 1986

Resnick L, Berger JR, Shapshak P, et al: Early penetration of the blood-brain barrier by HIV. Neurology 38:9–14, 1988

Richman DD, Fischl MA, Grieco MH, et al: The toxicity of azidothymidine (AZT) in the treatment of patients with AIDS and AIDS-related complex. N Engl J Med 317:191–197, 1987

Riedel RR, Clarenbach P, Bulau P, et al: Neurological and neuropsychological deficits in 240 HIV-seropositive hemophiliacs in WR2-6, in Abstracts of the Fifth International Conference on AIDS. Montreal, Quebec, International Development Research Centre, 1989, p 210

Robbins SL, Cotran RS (eds): Pathologic Basis of Disease. Philadelphia, PA, WB Saunders, 1979

Rundell JR, Wise MG, Ursano RJ: Three cases of AIDS-related psychiatric disorders. Am J Psychiatry 143:777–778, 1986

Sadler AE, Keilp JG, Dorfman D, et al: Neuropsychological performance as a function of AIDS dementia complex, in Abstracts of the Fifth International Conference on AIDS. Montreal, Quebec, International Development Research Centre, 1989a, p 395

Sadler AE, Keilp JG, Thaler H, et al: Test-retest performance on neuropsychological tests in a group of HIV-1 seropositive patients, in Abstracts of the Fifth International Conference on AIDS. Montreal, Quebec, International Development Research Centre, 1989b, p 394

Saykin AJ, Janssen R, Sprehn G, et al: Neuropsychological and psychosocial function in two cohorts of gay men: relation to stage of HIV-1 infection in Abstracts of the Fifth International Conference on AIDS. Montreal, Quebec, International Development Research Centre, 1989, p 389

Schaerf FW, Miller RR, Lipsey JR, et al: ECT for major depression in four patients infected with human immunodeficiency virus. Am J Psychiatry 146:782–784, 1989

Schmidt U, Miller D: Two cases of hypomania in AIDS. Br J Psychiatry 152:839–842, 1988

Schnurbus R, Konneke J, Schleuler W, et al: Comparison of EEG findings in HIV-infected and non-infected patients in outpatient and inpatient follow-ups, in Abstracts of the Fifth International Conference on AIDS. Montreal, Quebec, International Development Research Centre, 1989, p 461

Schoenfeld M, Myers RH, Cupples LH, et al: Increased rate of suicide among patients with Huntington's disease. J Neurol Neurosurg Psychiatry 47:1283–1287, 1984

Selnes OA, Miller EN, McArthur JC, et al: Neuropsychological follow-up in patients who have progressed to AIDS, in Abstracts of the Fifth International Conference on AIDS. Montreal, Quebec, International Development Research Centre, 1989, p 449

Selnes OA, Miller E, McArthur J, et al: HIV-1 infection: no evidence of cognitive decline during the asymptomatic stages. Neurology 40:204–208, 1990

Sidtis JJ, Price RW: Early HIV-1 infection and the AIDS dementia complex. Neurology 40:323–326, 1990

Sidtis JJ, Thaler H, Brew BJ, et al: The interval between equivocal and definite neurological signs and symptoms in the AIDS dementia complex, in Abstracts of the Fifth International Conference on AIDS. Montreal, Quebec, International Development Research Centre, 1989, p 215

Smith T, Jakobsen J, Gaub J, et al: Clinical and electrophysiological studies of human immunodeficiency virus-seropositive men without AIDS. Ann Neurol 23: 295–297, 1988

Stern Y, Sano M, Goldstein S, et al: Neuropsychological manifestations of HIV infection in gay men, in Abstracts of the Fifth International Conference on AIDS. Montreal, Quebec, International Development Research Centre, 1989, 383

Stoler MH, Eskin TA, Benn S, et al: Human T-cell lymphotropic virus type III infection of the central nervous system: a preliminary in situ analysis. JAMA 256:2360–2364, 1986

Strauss SE, Seidlin M, Takiff H, et al: Oral acyclovir to suppress recurring herpes simplex virus infections in immunodeficient patients. Ann Intern Med 100:522–524, 1984

Swenson JR, Erman M, Labell J, et al: Extrapyramidal reactions: neuropsychiatric mimics in patients with AIDS. Gen Hosp Psychiatry 11:248–249, 1989

Syndulko K, Singer E, Ruane B, et al: Neuro-performance

measurement and memory profiles of disability in HIV seropositive individuals, in Abstracts of the Fifth International Conference on AIDS. Montreal, Quebec, International Development Research Centre, 1989a, p 464

Syndulko K, Singer E, Ruane B, et al: Latency P300 and pattern visual evoked potential are not sensitive to early HIV related neurologic disease, in Abstracts of the Fifth International Conference on AIDS. Montreal, Quebec, International Development Research Centre, 1989b, p 464

Sze G, Brant-Zawadzki MN, Norman D, et al: the neuroradiology of AIDS. Semin Roentgenol 22:42–53, 1987

Temoshok L, Canick JP, Sweet DM: Cognitive dysfunction and psychosocial factors in symptomatic seropositive men, in Abstracts of the Fifth International Conference on AIDS. Montreal, Quebec, International Development Research Centre, 1989a, p 385

Temoshok L, Drexler M, Canick JP, et al: Neuropsychological change on longitudinal assessment: prevalence and pattern in HIV spectrum disorders, in Abstracts of the Fifth International Conference on AIDS. Montreal, Quebec, International Development Research Centre, 1989b, p 210

Tozzi V, Ciciani R, Galgani S, et al: Brain magnetic resonance imaging findings in HIV infection, in Abstracts of the Fifth International Conference on AIDS. Montreal, Quebec, International Development Research Centre, 1989, p 458

Tross S, Price RW, Navia B, et al: Neuropsychological characterization of the AIDS dementia complex: a preliminary report. AIDS 2:81–88, 1988

Ultmann MH, Belman AL, Ruff HA, et al: Developmental abnormalities in infants and children with acquired immune deficiency syndrome (AIDS) and AIDS-related complex. Dev Med Child Neurol 27:563–571, 1985

Van Gorp W, Miller E, Satz P, et al: Neuropsychological performance in HIV-1 immunocompromised patients, in Abstracts of the Fifth International Conference on AIDS. Montreal, Quebec, International Development Research Centre, 1989, p 464

Visscher BR, Miller E, Satz P, et al: Neuropsychological followup of 1,787 participants in the Multicenter AIDS Cohort Study, in Abstracts of the Fifth International Conference on AIDS. Montreal, Quebec, International Development Research Centre, 1989, p 449

Whitlock FA: Suicide in physical illness, in Suicide. Edited by Roy A. Baltimore, MD, Williams & Wilkins, 1986, pp 151–170

Wilson MJ, Lemp GF, Neal D, et al: The epidemiology of AIDS-related neurologic diseases, in Abstracts of the Fifth International Conference on AIDS. Montreal, Quebec, International Development Research Centre, 1989, p 449

Wong B, Gold JWM, Brown AE, et al: Central nervous system toxoplasmosis in homosexual men and parenteral drug abusers. Ann Intern Med 100:36–42, 1984

Yarchoan R, Mitsuya H, Broder S: AIDS therapies. Sci Am 259(4):110–119, 1988

Zuger A, Louie E, Holzman RS, et al: Cryptococcal disease in patients with the acquired immunodeficiency syndrome. Ann Intern Med 104:234–240, 1986

Chapter

22

Neuropsychiatric Features of Endocrine Disorders

Morris B. Goldman, M.D.

IN THIS CHAPTER I REVIEW those hormonal deficiencies and excesses most clearly associated with neuropsychiatric syndromes. The gonadal axis is not addressed. Releasing factors and anterior pituitary trophic hormones are discussed with their prime target hormones, whereas panhypopituitarism is discussed in the section on adrenal insufficiency (which it frequently mimics).

The discussion on each hormone excess and deficiency includes 1) the clinical picture (etiology, epidemiology, and presenting nonneuropsychiatric signs and symptoms); 2) diagnostic issues (preliminary laboratory workup of endocrinopathy, differential diagnosis from primary psychiatric conditions and other disorders frequently seen in psychiatric patients, and diagnosis when endocrinopathy and psychiatric disorder coexist); 3) details of neuropsychiatric features (the alterations in affect, cognition and reality testing, and the relationship of these alterations to the severity of the endocrinopathy and to other risk factors); 4) mechanism (mechanism of neuropsychiatric symptom induction and its possible relevance to primary psychiatric disorders); and 5) treatment (response of neuropsychiatric syndrome to correction of the endocrinopathy and to psychotropic drugs).

Neuropsychiatric symptoms are prominent in many endocrine disorders, and in some cases the first medical contact may be the psychiatrist (Table 22–1). In most cases, prompt treatment of the endocrinopathy leads to resolution of the neuropsychiatric signs and symptoms; whereas prolonged delays are associated with unsatisfactory outcomes. To promote expedient diagnosis, psychiatrists should familiarize themselves with the characteristic symptoms and signs (Table 22–2) and the preliminary screening studies.

The author wishes to acknowledge Jeff Bennett for assistance in preparing this chapter; Mary B. Dratman, Daniel J. Luchins, and Ned Weiss for their constructive reviews; and Lela Louis for secretarial assistance.

Although the neuropsychiatric features vary both within and between the different endocrinopathies, some generalizations can be cautiously made. Different endocrinopathies of similar severity and duration tend to share similar neuropsychiatric features. Thus mild to moderately severe abnormalities lasting weeks to months often manifest a combination of affective and anxiety symptoms (Table 22–1). Most patients with such abnormalities have mild cognitive impairments. In some cases the prominence of cognitive or physical symptoms and the erratic nature or absence of the core features of a primary psychiatric illness point to an organic etiology. Other endocrinopathies, however, are often "dead ringers" for primary psychiatric disease. In contrast, longstanding mild to moderately severe endocrinopathies are more likely to present with personality changes characterized by apathy or dementia (Table 22–3).

Acute severe disease, or longstanding disease that progresses to a severe disorder, is likely to induce an acute delirium, which may herald a catastrophic outcome (Table 22–4). In some cases the delirium is clearly linked to secondary metabolic disturbances. Psychotic symptoms most often occur with delirium. Some severe (and occasionally moderate) endocrinopathies induce automatisms, depersonalization, or heightened sensory awareness. In these cases, the patient may be incorrectly diagnosed with temporal lobe epilepsy or somatoform disorder.

The suspicion of an underlying endocrinopathy should be high in several situations. These include treatment-resistant atypical affective or anxiety syndromes in which vegetative or cognitive complaints appear out of proportion to the other symptoms. Also late-onset personality disorders characterized by apathy, "neurasthenia," depersonalization, or automatisms warrant an endocrine assessment. Finally, treatment-resistant or atypical psychotic patients and all patients presenting with dementia should have an endocrine disorder excluded. Table 22–5 summarizes the endocrinopathies that should be considered in the differential diagnosis of common primary psychiatric disorders. The screening tests for each (described below) are uncomplicated, except for that for hypocortisolism. Abnormal results are defined for the screening tests, but may vary with the technique used and laboratory.

The mechanism of the neuropsychiatric symptoms in endocrinopathies is unknown. Some syndromes seem tied to changes in small molecules and ionic constituents that are fundamentally involved in neuroregulation (i.e., sodium, calcium, and glucose), whereas others appear to involve secondary alterations in neurotransmitters implicated in psychiatric disease. Mild forms of endocrine disorders are frequently seen in psychiatric patients, particularly those with primary affective illness. Many be-

TABLE 22–1. SYMPTOMS OF MILD OR MODERATE ENDOCRINOPATHIES LASTING WEEKS TO MONTHS

Endocrinopathy	*Anxious*	*Depressed*	*Impaired cognition*[a]	*Mimics psychiatric disorder*
Hyperthyroidism	++	+	C, M	++
Hypothyroidism	+	++	C, M	++
Hypercortisolism	++	++	C, M, H	++
Hypocortisolism	+	++		++
Panhypopituitarism[b]	+	++		++
Hyperparathyroidism	+	++	M	++
Hypoparathyroidism	++	+	?	++
Hyperinsulinism	++		H, C	++
Hypoinsulinism			C	
Excessive vasopressin			C, M	+[c]
Deficient vasopressin			M	+[d]
Hyperprolactinemia	+	++[e]		+

Note. + = sometimes; ++ = often.
[a]C = concentration; M = memory; H = higher order functions (e.g., abstract thinking).
[b]Function of affected hormones.
[c]May mimic psychotic exacerbation in psychiatric patient.
[d]Psychogenic polydipsia.
[e]Females more than males.

TABLE 22–2. NONPSYCHIATRIC SYMPTOMS AND SIGNS OF ENDOCRINOPATHIES

Endocrinopathy	*Symptoms*	*Signs*
Hyperthyroidism	Diaphoresis Heat intolerance Oligomenorrhea	Tachycardia Tremor Proptosis
Hypothyroidism	Cold intolerance Menorrhagia Muscle cramps	Goiter Reflex delay Myxedema
Hypercortisolism	Oligomenorrhea Easy bruising Weakness	Hirsutism Moon facies Hypertension
Hypocortisolism	Nausea Weakness	Hypotension Hyperpigmentation
Panhypopituitarism[a]	Nausea Weakness	Hypotension
Hyperparathyroidism	Nausea Polyuria Abdominal pain	Hypertension
Hypoparathyroidism	Muscle spasms Paresthesias	Choreiform movements
Hyperinsulinism	Diaphoresis Hunger	Tachycardia
Hypoinsulinism	Polydipsia Polyuria Polyphagia	Neuropathy
Excessive vasopressin	Nausea Headache Weakness	Ataxia Tremor Weight gain
Deficient vasopressin	Polydipsia Polyuria	Fever dehydration
Hyperprolactinemia	Galactorrhea[b] Amenorrhea Impotence[c]	Gynecomastia Osteoporosis

[a]Function of affected hormones.
[b]In females.
[c]In males.

lieve, based on evidence summarized below, that these endocrine disturbances are fundamentally linked to psychiatric illness.

❑ THYROID HORMONE

Many patients with thyrotoxicosis exhibit an organic anxiety syndrome or an organic personality syndrome (with prominent emotional lability), whereas elderly patients are often apathetic. The term *hyperthyroidism* is sometimes limited to excessive hormone production by the thyroid gland, but it is used here to mean thyrotoxicosis of any etiology.

Hypothyroidism in adults may present as an organic mood disorder, delirium, dementia, or rarely an organic delusional syndrome. Congenital hypothyroidism results in profound intellectual and developmental deficits (i.e., cretinism).

Hyperthyroidism

Clinical picture. Thyrotoxicosis is usually caused by chronic thyroid gland overproduction of hormone, thyroid glandular inflammatory disorders, and nonthyroidal sources of thyroid hormone. Graves' disease is included in the first category; chronic thyroiditis in the second; and ingested hormone (thyrotoxicosis factitia), functioning metastatic thyroid cancer, and ovarian tumors in the third. Graves' disease occurs commonly in women in their third to fourth decade. Lithium has been associated with hyperthyroidism, but the link may be coincidental (Yassa et al. 1988).

TABLE 22–3. SYMPTOMS OF MILD OR MODERATELY SEVERE LONGSTANDING ENDOCRINOPATHIES

Endocrinopathy	*Apathy*	*Dementia*	*Other personality changes*[a]	*Cyclical course*
Hyperthyroidism	++		L	
Hypothyroidism	++	+		
Hypercortisolism				+
Hypocortisolism	+	+	P	
Panhypopituitarism[b]	+	+		
Hyperparathyroidism	++	++[c]	I	
Hypoparathyroidism	?	+++		
Hyperinsulinism	++	+	D,L	+
Hypoinsulinism		?		
Excessive vasopressin	+			
Deficient vasopressin				
Hyperprolactinemia	+[d]			

Note. + = usually mild; ++ = usually moderate; +++ = usually prominent.
[a]L = labile; P = paranoia; D = dementia; I = irritable.
[b]Function of affected hormones.
[c]Predominantly elderly; may be of short duration.
[d]Males.

Symptoms of hyperthyroidism include fatigue, weakness, oligomenorrhea, frequent bowel movements, excessive sweating, and heat intolerance. Sympathetic nervous system hyperactivity is responsible for anxiety, tachycardia, tremor, hyperreflexia, lid lag, and diminished blinking. Goiter is present in most cases of overproduction and some cases of thyroid inflammatory disease. Patients with Graves' disease may exhibit prominent proptosis and dermopathy, which may progress independently of the hyperthyroidism.

Diagnostic issues. Table 22–6 shows the laboratory studies and cutoff values to diagnose thyrotoxicosis. Free (i.e., unbound) thyroxine (T-4) levels are preferred over total T-4 or the free T-4 index, but the latter (an indirect measure of unbound serum T-4, based on total T-4 levels and competitive binding of serum T-4 to a resin) is acceptable. In rare cases of Graves' disease, free T-4 may be normal and only triiodothyronine (T-3) elevated (i.e., T-3 toxicosis). Thus it is appropriate in suspected cases of thyrotoxicosis to order total T-4, total T-3, and a

TABLE 22–4. OTHER NEUROPSYCHIATRIC FEATURES OF SEVERE ENDOCRINOPATHIES

Endocrinopathy	*Psychosis plus delirium*	*Psychosis without delirium*	*Other*[a]
Hyperthyroidism	+		
Hypothyroidism	++		I
Hypercortisolism	++		D, I
Hypocortisolism	++		H
Panhypopituitarism[b]	++		H
Hyperparathyroidism	++	++	
Hypoparathyroidism	++		A
Hyperinsulinism	++		A, D
Hypoinsulinism	+		
Excessive vasopressin	+		
Deficient vasopressin	+		
Hyperprolactinemia			

Note. + = sometimes present; ++ = often present.
[a]H = heightened sensory acuity; I = impaired sensory acuity; A = automatisms; D = depersonalization.
[b]Function of affected hormones.

TABLE 22–5. ENDOCRINOPATHIES RESEMBLING PRIMARY PSYCHIATRIC DISORDERS

Anxiety disorders	Hyperthyroidism[a] Hypercortisolism Panhypopituitarism Hypoparathyroidism Hyperinsulinism
Affective disorders	Hyperthyroidism[b] Hypothyroidism Hypocortisolism Hypercortisolism Panhypopituitarism Hyperparathyroidism Hyperprolactinemia[a]
Anorexia nervosa	Hypocortisolism Panhypopituitarism
Somatoform disorder	Hypothyroidism Hypercortisolism Hypoparathyroidism Hyperinsulinism
Psychotic disorders	Hypothyroidism Hypercortisolism Hypocortisolism[a] Panhypopituitarism[a] Hyperparathyroidism Hypoparathyroidism[a] Hyperinsulinism[a]
Dementia	Hypothyroidism Hyperparathyroidism[b] Hypoparathyroidism[a] Hyperinsulinism[a]

[a]Can usually be distinguished from primary psychiatric disturbance by careful history.
[b]In elderly.

free T-4 index. A blunted thyrotropin (TSH) response to thyrotropin-releasing hormone (TRH) stimulation is diagnostic in borderline cases of hyperthyroidism. The new TSH immunometric assay, which is accurate down to very low TSH levels, may eliminate the need for TRH stimulation tests.

About 10% of psychiatric inpatients (regardless of diagnosis) show transient elevations of total serum T-3, T-4, and free T-4 index, apparently because of pituitary or hypothalamic stimulation (Rose 1985). Thus psychiatric inpatients who have elevated thyroid hormone levels on admission should have tests repeated 2 weeks later. Acute drug intoxication, particularly with psychostimulants, can closely mimic hyperthyroidism and may also produce transient hyperthyroidism.

TABLE 22–6. DIAGNOSIS OF THYROTOXICOSIS

Total T-4	> 12 μg/dl
Total T-3	> 190 μg/dl
Free T-4	> 3.5 μg/dl
Free T-4 index	> 1.5
TSH response 20 minutes after 500 μg iv TRH	> 5 μU/ml above baseline
TSH (immunometric assay)	< .1 μU/ml

Note. T-4 = thyroxine; T-3 = triiodothyronine; TSH = thyrotropin; TRH = thyrotropin-releasing hormone.

Patients with hyperthyroidism may be distinguished from those with primary anxiety disorders by warm rather than cold skin, increased appetite, and a reported inability to associate anxiety to specific ideas or concerns (Jefferson and Marshal 1981). Hyperthyroidism can usually be distinguished from mania by decreased energy and activity levels. On the other hand, hyperthyroidism in bipolar patients is easily missed, because hyperthyroidism may precipitate mania, and subsequent lithium treatment may lead to a partial response (by its antithyroid and antimanic actions).

Details of neuropsychiatric features. Pervasive anxiety, insomnia, and tense dysphoria are common. Patients may be tearful and crying and baffled about why. Depression may occur but is rarely prominent in younger patients. Psychological testing, although confirming the presence of increased anxiety and depression, rarely fits prescribed patterns of psychiatric illnesses (Bauer et al. 1987). The elderly, however, who are often apathetic, may exhibit classic melancholia.

Diminished concentration and memory are frequent complaints in all hyperthyroid patients and can be confirmed by standard psychological batteries. Many of these symptoms are seen in control subjects given thyroid hormone (Bauer et al. 1987).

Psychosis is occasionally seen as part of a delirium, and may herald the potentially fatal thyroid storm. Psychosis was diagnosed more frequently in the past, perhaps because of a higher prevalence of severe endocrinopathy or overly zealous use of the term *psychosis*.

Mechanism. For many years, hyperthyroidism was considered the prototypical psychosomatic illness. Reports (e.g., Bennett and Cambor 1961) attested to thyrotoxicosis after life stresses and linked it to a particular personality style: one with unmet dependency needs, "pseudomaturity," and the inability to express hostility. Although subsequent studies (Bauer et al. 1987) found no difference in premorbid personality between thyrotoxic patients and control subjects, some studies (e.g., Voth et al. 1970) suggest that radioactive iodine uptake is increased in asymptomatic patients who are dependent and pseudomature. The validity and significance of this finding has not been pursued, probably because this kind of psychosomatic approach has fallen into disfavor.

Despite similar symptoms, patients with primary anxiety disorders do not have increased levels of thyroid hormone, although the immunometric TSH assay and TSH response to TRH have not been applied. On the other hand, a blunted TSH response to TRH is seen in about 25% of depressed patients, and some show diminished levels of immunometric TSH (Kirkegaard et al. 1990), suggesting that some depressed patients have mild hyperthyroidism.

Treatment. Neuropsychiatric symptoms (including the putative personality syndrome) usually reverse with antithyroid treatment, but a year may be needed for complete recovery (Bauer et al. 1987). Psychosis may occur or be exacerbated by antithyroid medication, and haloperidol and perphenazine may induce a syndrome resembling thyroid storm and neuroleptic malignant syndrome in psychotic hyperthyroid patients (Bauer et al. 1987). Available evidence suggests low-potency neuroleptics are tolerated in hyperthyroid patients and thus should be prescribed if indicated.

Hypothyroidism

Clinical picture. Most cases of overt hypothyroidism result from a diseased thyroid gland (primary hypothyroidism); only a small minority are caused by pituitary or hypothalamic disease (secondary hypothyroidism). Thyroid gland disease is commonly caused by 1) ablation (caused by surgery, ionizing radiation, or radioactive iodine), 2) autoimmune disorders, or 3) drugs (e.g., lithium).

Lithium interferes with hormone biosynthesis and release and may accelerate autoimmune thyroiditis. Hypothyroidism occurs in about 10% of patients on lithium and is more common in those with diminished thyroid reserve, particularly women and rapid cyclers. It can occur early or after several years of therapy (Erhardt and Goldman 1991).

Rapid withdrawal of thyroid hormone therapy (e.g., when used as adjuvant treatment for depression) can induce acute hypothyroidism due to endogenous suppression of hormone production. Common symptoms of adult-onset thyroid deficiency include lethargy, constipation, cold intolerance, muscle cramping, menorrhagia, and weight gain. Goiter may be detectable, and there is usually a measurable delay in the relaxation phase of deep tendon reflexes. In more longstanding disease, the patient may appear myxedematous and exhibit cardiovascular impairments.

Newborns with thyroid hormone deficiency classically present with persistent jaundice, a hoarse cry, somnolence, and feeding problems. However, because the diagnosis may be difficult to make, T-4 and TSH levels are routinely obtained at birth in most Western medical centers.

Diagnostic issues. Patients with primary hypothyroidism have been divided into three groups corresponding to grades of severity of symptoms and hormone deficiency (Table 22–7). These distinctions may prove to be important for psychiatry because patients with mild ("subclinical") hypothyroidism (i.e., grade III) may present solely with psychiatric

TABLE 22–7. GRADES OF HYPOTHYROIDISM

Grade	*Severity*	*Physical symptoms*	*Psychiatric symptoms*	*Free T-3, T-4*	*TSH*	*TRH stimulation*[a]
I	Severe	++	++	Decrease	Increase	Increase
II	Moderate	+	++	Normal	Increase	Increase
III	Mild		+?	Normal	Normal	Increase

Note. T-3 = triiodothyronine; T-4 = thyroxine; TSH = thyrotropin; TRH = thyrotropin-releasing hormone; + = usually mild or moderate; ++ = usually prominent.
[a]TRH stimulation = TSH response to TRH.

symptoms (Extein and Gold 1988). Grade III hypothyroidism can only be diagnosed by measuring the TSH response to TRH because thyroid hormone levels and TSH are normal.

Table 22–8 lists the diagnostic studies and cutoff values for the different measures of thyroid hypofunction. Generally, TSH is obtained as the routine screening test for hypothyroidism. Although total T-4 is diminished in severe cases of hypothyroidism, it may be normal in moderate cases, which still require thyroid replacement (i.e., grade II).

Because moderate hormone deficiency can closely mimic primary anxiety and depression (and particularly postpartum disorders), it is reasonable routinely to order TSH levels in these instances. Routine TRH testing (to rule out grade III hypothyroidism) in patients with affective disorders cannot be recommended until the incidence and significance of these mild disturbances and the benefits of thyroid replacement therapy (or any treatment different from standard antidepressant regimens) has been more clearly established.

Details of neuropsychiatric features. Acute and especially longstanding hypothyroidism are associated with changes in cognition and affective state. Changes in cognition may occur alone and seem more pervasive than mood disturbances (Loosen 1986).

Affective disturbances ranging from mild depression to psychosis and suicidality occur in more than one-half of patients with grade I hypothyroidism (Bauer et al. 1987). Depression, and to a lesser extent anxiety, may occur as early as 3 weeks after the onset of hypothyroidism, particularly in patients with histories of affective disorders (Denicoff et al. 1990). Marked irritability, emotional lability, and insomnia are frequently seen. Patients have a reduced amount of stage 3 and stage 4 sleep, similar to that seen in depression.

Changes in concentration may be apparent as early as 3 weeks after the onset of the hypothyroid state, before other cognitive functions are altered (Denicoff et al. 1990). A progressive slowing of mental processing follows, characterized by diminished initiative and impaired memory and concentration (easily identified by asking the patient to perform serial subtractions) (Jefferson and Marshal 1981). Many patients report losing things and making "stupid" mistakes. Although initially very frustrated, ultimately the patient becomes indifferent. Longstanding disease induces marked dementia (Bauer et al. 1987). Diminished taste, visual acuity, and hearing are common.

Psychosis, brought into public knowledge by A. J. Cronin's description of myxedema madness in *The Citadel* (Cronin 1937), occurs in about 10% of patients with grade I hypothyroidism, but may rarely be seen in milder cases. The quality of the psychosis is nonspecific and usually is part of a delirium.

Hypothyroidism in infancy produces profound mental retardation unless treated early. In the full-blown syndrome, the infant is lethargic and may be deaf. Hypothyroidism that manifests later in childhood presents with signs and symptoms intermediate between those of the infant and those of the adult.

Mechanism. Hypothyroidism is known to critically influence the development of the maturing brain, but the mechanism by which it induces changes in adult cognition and affective state is unknown. Previously these and other changes in central nervous system (CNS) function (e.g., evoked responses) were attributed to gross changes in cerebral metabolism or blood flow. Evidence now suggests that thyroid hormone plays a much more direct role in adult brain homeostasis. Thus thyroid hormone levels in the brain are usually maintained despite marked peripheral hypothyroidism; thyroid hormone is metabolized and concentrated in discreet neural tissues (Dratman and Crutchfield 1989), may help maintain adult brain structure, and may regulate central adrenergic neurotransmission; and, lastly, even minor changes in thyroid hormone may induce marked affective disturbances, particularly in patients with rapid cycling disorder (Bauer and Whybrow 1990).

Evidence suggests that 1) mild disturbances in thyroid hormone regulation seem to be common in patients with affective disease, 2) thyroid hormone appears to accelerate the response to standard antidepressant treatments, and 3) thyroid hormone is a useful adjuvant in the treatment of refractory affective illness (although not necessarily correlated with

TABLE 22–8. DIAGNOSIS OF HYPOTHYROIDISM

Total T-4	< 5.0 μg/dl
TSH	> 5.0 μU/ml
TSH response 20 minutes after 500 μg iv TRH	> 30 μU/ml

Note. T-4 = thyroxine; TSH = thyrotropin; TRH = thyrotropin-releasing hormone.

chemical evidence of hypothyroidism) (Bauer et al. 1990). The significance of the relationship between thyroid hormone disturbance and primary affective disorders remains unclear and may require measures of central thyroid hormone activity because peripheral and central regulation may be independent of each other, particularly in disease states (Bauer et al. 1990).

Treatment. Nearly complete recovery of cognitive and affective deficits can be anticipated with thyroid replacement in adult patients with grade I hypothyroidism. Neuropsychiatric symptoms may be the first to resolve, with patients recovering completely over the course of a few days with just thyroid hormone replacement, although complete recovery can take up to 6 months. Moderate doses of neuroleptics (e.g., 2–4 mg of haloperidol) are usually well tolerated, although patients who become psychotic may not fully recover. Many believe that affective symptoms are resistant to treatment with antidepressants alone.

Thyroid hormone relieves physical symptoms in patients with grade II hypothyroidism. However, definitive studies have not yet established whether affective disorders associated with grade II or grade III hypothyroidism preferentially respond either to thyroid hormone alone or in combination with standard antidepressant therapy.

Hypothyroidism must be corrected slowly because acute cardiac or neuropsychiatric decompensation (Bauer et al. 1987) can occur with rapid replacement, particularly in the elderly. Finally, hypothyroidism in patients receiving lithium may spontaneously resolve. If it does not, replacement therapy with T-4 should be instituted, and T-4 and TSH should be monitored to exclude both excessive and inadequate treatment.

❑ CORTISOL

Cushing's syndrome may present as an organic mood, anxiety, or personality syndrome or with delirium. Iatrogenic Cushing's syndrome, and occasionally other causes of Cushing's syndrome, can induce an organic delusional syndrome or organic hallucinosis. Neuropsychiatric changes, particularly depression or personality changes, may be the exclusive presenting symptoms.

Adrenal insufficiency may be accompanied by an organic personality or mood syndrome. Delirium may presage adrenal crisis. In both hypercortisolism and adrenal insufficiency, periods of neuropsychiatric symptoms may be punctuated by return to premorbid function.

Hypercortisolism

Clinical picture. The term *Cushing's disease* has traditionally been reserved for corticotropin (adrenocorticotropic hormone [ACTH])-producing, nonmalignant pituitary tumors, whereas other types of hypercortisolism are referred to as *Cushing's syndrome*. Cushing's disease is most common among women in their third or fourth decade. Nonendocrine sources of ACTH (e.g., malignancies) and cortisol-secreting adrenal adenomas and carcinomas are not uncommon. Drug-induced Cushing's syndrome occurs with either illicit or prescribed steroid consumption.

Symptoms and signs of hypercortisolism include fatigue, muscle weakness, decreased libido, oligomenorrhea, moon facies, buffalo hump, plethora, hirsutism, central adiposity, ecchymosis, violaceous striae, hyperglycemia, and hypertension. Some of the more characteristic features (e.g., moon facies) may also be observed in persons without hypercortisolism.

Diagnostic issues. Table 22–9 summarizes screening studies and cutoffs to diagnose hypercortisolism. An overnight dexamethasone test is the most common screening study, but because of the high incidence of abnormal results in psychiatric patients, a follow-up standard low-dose test (.5 mg every 6 hours) is often needed to establish a definitive diagnosis and exclude most other causes (Aron et al. 1981).

Patients with Cushing's syndrome may look similar to persons with alcoholism, who, on the other hand, may have all the physical and biochemical signs of Cushing's syndrome. Because the depression in Cushing's syndrome may be cyclical

TABLE 22–9. DIAGNOSIS OF HYPERCORTISOLISM

8:00 A.M. cortisol after 11:00 P.M. dexamethasone (1 mg)	> 5.0 μg/dl
24-hour urinary free cortisol	> 100 μg
Cortisol on second day after .5 mg dexamethasone po every 6 hours	> 5.0 μg/dl

(Reus 1987) and occur in the absence of physical symptoms (Starkman et al. 1986b), it can closely resemble a primary affective disease.

Corticosteroid abuse cannot be diagnosed by measuring basal steroid levels (because endogenous production is suppressed, and the oral agents are present in small quantities), but it can be suspected if the patient shows no evidence of adrenal insufficiency yet has a diminished cortisol response to ACTH stimulation (see Table 22–10).

Details of neuropsychiatric features. Depression and anxiety (with or without panic attacks) are seen in about half the patients with Cushing's syndrome. Cognitive changes are equally common, though less pronounced, and may be a consequence of depression (Starkman et al. 1986b).

Patients usually emphasize sadness, decreased libido, insomnia, somatic preoccupation, depersonalization, and impaired concentration (Reus 1987). Unlike most patients with primary major affective disorders, though, many Cushing's syndrome patients note mood lability and deny anhedonia, inappropriate guilt, and hopelessness (Starkman et al. 1986a). Pure mania or hypomania is infrequent (except with oral corticosteroids), and instead the picture resembles that of a mixed manic and depressed state. Suicidal preoccupation or action is not unusual (Jefferson and Marshal 1981). The severity of depression has been related to levels of steroid production (Starkman et al. 1986a).

The cognitive disturbance is most marked in spatial and visual ideation, but many areas are affected. Serial 7s and the recall of three cities are together a fairly sensitive means of screening for cognitive changes (Starkman et al. 1986b). Diminished hearing, vision, and smell have also been noted.

Psychosis occurs in up to 20% of cases. A delirium is often present and may be a result of electrolyte disturbances, congestive heart failure, hypertensive encephalopathy, or uncontrolled diabetes.

TABLE 22–10. DIAGNOSIS OF HYPOCORTISOLISM

Cortisol level 30 and 60 minutes after 0.25 mg iv ACTH	< 7 μg/dl above baseline or absolute < 18 μg/dl

Note. ACTH = adrenocorticotropic hormone (corticotropin).

Either manic or depressive symptoms may accompany paranoia, auditory, and visual hallucinations and disorientation. Patients frequently complain of sensory flooding and may become mute.

Neuropsychiatric symptoms may occur in patients treated with prednisone > 40 mg/day for several days (Reus 1987) and are related to dose and duration of treatment. Acute response seen in most patients includes a mild euphoria, increased appetite, insomnia, irritability, and restlessness. Patients may become depressed on steroid withdrawal, leading to continued elicit use. Psychosis, with or without altered consciousness and cognition, has been reported in up to 20% of patients receiving prednisone 80 mg/day or more and may be more common in women. The course is uneven, with periods of lucidity alternating with periods of psychosis. For unclear reasons, mania seems to occur more frequently with steroid treatment than with other causes of Cushing's syndrome. Hypomania does not necessarily presage a more serious course. Neither the type of steroid preparation, the underlying illness, nor the psychiatric history has been clearly able to predict the occurrence of serious neuropsychiatric symptoms (Reus 1987).

Mechanism. The similarities of hypercortisolism and depression have led investigators to posit a fundamental link between the two disorders (Table 22–11). A popular hypothesis, that excess corticotropin-releasing factor (CRF) causes hypercortisolism and depression in primary psychiatric illness (De Jong and Roy 1990; Nemeroff 1989), could not, however, account for the neuropsychiatric symptoms in Cushing's disease because CRF is presumably suppressed (Gold et al. 1986).

Treatment. Neuropsychiatric symptoms improve in parallel with normalization of urinary free cortisol, although complete recovery may take months to years (Starkman et al. 1986a). Diminished libido lags behind the recovery of other symptoms.

The treatment of neuropsychiatric symptoms in patients with iatrogenic Cushing's' syndrome is often challenging because of the likelihood of relapse of the underlying condition on steroid withdrawal and the frequent difficulty of identifying the cause of neuropsychiatric exacerbations (i.e., Is it steroid intoxication, steroid withdrawal, or the underlying disease?). If possible, patients should be on alternative-day therapy, receiving medication in the morn-

TABLE 22–11. SIMILARITIES BETWEEN HYPERCORTISOLISM AND PRIMARY DEPRESSION

Feature	*Hypercortisolism*	*Depression*
Basal cortisol	Increase	Increase
Overnight DST[a]	Increase	Increase
CRH stimulation[b]	Increase	Decrease
Family history of depression	+(?)	+
Central noradrenergic turnover	Decrease	Decrease(?)

Note. DST = dexamethasone suppression test; CRH = corticotropin-releasing hormone.
[a]Cortisol response to single dose of dexamethasone.
[b]Corticotropin (adrenocorticotropic hormone [ACTH]) response to corticotropin-releasing hormone.

ing to simulate the diurnal pattern and to minimize insomnia.

Tricyclic antidepressants may exacerbate depression secondary to hypercortisolism, particularly if the patient is psychotic. The optimal treatment of depression has not been determined, although electroconvulsive therapy may help. Lithium carbonate and neuroleptics appear to be effective in preventing or treating mania (Reus 1987).

Hypocortisolism

Clinical picture. Adrenal insufficiency occurs with progressive adrenocortical destruction (Addison's disease), pituitary failure, or acute adrenal failure. Progressive adrenocortical destruction historically was a consequence of granulomatous disease, but now is often a result of autoimmune disorders. Pituitary failure is usually a result of panhypopituitarism or iatrogenic suppression. Acute adrenal failure usually follows physical stress occurring in the context of chronic insufficiency, adrenal hemorrhage, or rapid withdrawal of exogenous glucocorticoids.

Weakness, anorexia, nausea, vomiting, and weight loss are the classic presenting symptoms of adrenal insufficiency. Patients may have hypotension and hyperpigmentation. "Chronic fatigue syndrome," characterized by at least 6 months of fatigue, fever, myalgias, arthralgias, and depression after an acute infection, has also recently been linked in preliminary reports to adrenal insufficiency (Demitrack et al. 1990).

Panhypopituitarism often presents with signs and symptoms of adrenal insufficiency (except for easy tanning). It is usually caused by pituitary or hypothalamic damage and less frequently by ischemic necrosis (e.g., postpartum), aneurysms, or radiation. Although apathy and weakness are usually the prominent symptoms, the disorder may present as hypogonadism or hypothyroidism (Smith et al. 1972). Rarely, anterior pituitary failure may also be accompanied by posterior pituitary failure with loss of vasopressin secretion leading to diabetes insipidus. The actual presentation is a function of the age of the patient, the nature of the underlying disorder, the rapidity of onset, and the affected hormones.

Diagnostic issues. Primary adrenal insufficiency cannot be excluded by obtaining basal steroid levels, but only by measuring cortisol response to ACTH stimulation (Table 22–10). The diagnosis of pituitary failure may require giving metyrapone (which blocks cortisol production), because cortisol response to ACTH may be normal in these cases.

Patients with adrenal insufficiency may very closely resemble patients with major depression or anorexia nervosa, and the correct diagnosis is easily missed. Recent onset of easy, prolonged tanning; gastrointestinal distress; hypotension; other medical disorders (e.g., tuberculosis, amyloidosis, and carcinoma); and particularly autoimmune diseases may be helpful clues.

Details of neuropsychiatric features. Fluctuating anxiety, depression, and suspiciousness are seen in about half of the patients with hypocortisolism. In almost all cases of anxiety, depression is also present. The patient may have anorexia nervosa, and the voice may be weak and whiny (Jefferson and Marshal 1981). Intellectual function has not been carefully assessed. Occasionally the history is that of a progressive dementia. Patients often show (but rarely are aware of) heightened sensory acuity, which has been linked to diminished latency of the evoked responses (Reus 1987). Such changes may contribute to the occasional diagnosis of somatoform disorder. Diminished slow-wave sleep (stages 3 and 4) has been documented. Finally, frank psychosis usually occurs in the context of a delirium, with visual hallucinations, paranoia, bizarre posturing, and catatonia described (Jefferson and Marshal 1981).

Mechanism. In some cases the neuropsychiatric symptoms, particularly psychosis, can be attributed to secondary metabolic impairments; however, complete recovery does not occur until glucocorticoids have been replaced (Reus 1987). Increased axonal conductivity; elevated CRF, ACTH, and endorphins; and diminished CNS perfusion all have been cited as responsible for neuropsychiatric changes (Johnstone et al. 1990).

Treatment. The use of psychotropic drugs and the normalization of affective state following glucocorticoid replacement have not been adequately studied (Jefferson and Marshal 1981). Persistence of neuropsychiatric symptoms may indicate other concurrent endocrinopathies (e.g., hypothyroidism) (Johnstone et al. 1990).

Patients with hypocortisolism are notoriously sensitive to CNS depressants and are particularly susceptible to drugs that induce hypotension. Lithium may alter the requirements for mineralocorticoid replacement, and it may be difficult to maintain stable lithium levels.

❑ PARATHYROID AND SERUM CALCIUM REGULATION

Hypercalcemia can present as an organic personality or mood syndrome, dementia, or delirium. It is more likely than other endocrinopathies to present with an organic delusional syndrome (i.e., with clear consciousness). As with hypothyroidism, hypercortisolism, and hypocortisolism, neuropsychiatric changes occur early on and may be the only prominent symptoms. This is particularly true in the elderly, in whom minimal changes can induce reversible dementia. Hypocalcemia may be a chronic disorder with prominent neuropsychiatric, but minimal neuromuscular symptoms. Patients with hypocalcemia may appear histrionic or may develop an organic anxiety or mood syndrome, delirium, or dementia.

Hyperparathyroidism and Hypercalcemia

Clinical picture. There are many causes of hypercalcemia. Primary hyperparathyroidism is caused by a benign adenoma in most cases. The disorder is characterized by an insidious onset after the third decade of life and is more common among women than among men. Lithium induces mild increases in parathyroid hormone (PTH) in about 80% of patients within the first month of treatment, but significant increases may occur and are related to dose and duration of treatment (Mallette and Eichhorn 1986). Malignant neoplasms may release PTH-like substances that cause syndromes indistinguishable from those caused by PTH excess. Thyrotoxicosis, immobilization, excessive ingestion or abnormal production of vitamin D (e.g., granulomatous diseases), thiazide diuretics, and increased calcium and antacid intake (milk-alkali syndrome) are other common causes of hypercalcemia.

Most patients with hypercalcemia appear asymptomatic and are identified on routine laboratory screening. The classic symptoms include nausea, vomiting, constipation, anorexia, polyuria, muscle weakness, and symptoms related to recurrent kidneys stones and peptic ulcer disease. About half of the patients with hypercalcemia have hypertension.

Diagnostic issues. Serum calcium is the initial screening study (Table 22–12). If the level is at the upper limit of normal, ionized calcium (a more sensitive measure) should be considered. Follow-up PTH levels will usually distinguish hyperparathyroidism (PTH elevated) from other causes of hypercalcemia (PTH depressed). The normal range of PTH varies with the assay. Because hypercalcemia is common and can mimic many neuropsychiatric conditions and because calcium levels are inexpensive and easily obtained, the disorder should be excluded in most psychiatric diagnostic evaluations.

Details of neuropsychiatric features. Neuropsychiatric symptoms are found in 66% of hyperparathyroid patients in prospective studies (G. G. Brown et

TABLE 22–12. DIAGNOSIS OF HYPERCALCEMIA

Total calcium	> 10.5 mg/dl
Ionized calcium	> 5.6 mg/dl

al. 1987). Fatigue, apathy, diminished appetite, concentration, and depression occur in about half the patients. Suicidality is not uncommon, and several completed suicides have occurred. A personality change may occur over the course of years, and a previously active and sociable person may become progressively withdrawn, incapacitated, and depressed. The symptoms are similar in quality, but diminished in intensity, to those of primary depression (Linder et al. 1988). Cognitive testing reveals impaired verbal memory, although it is unclear if this is related to depression or other effects of hypercalcemia (G. G. Brown et al. 1987).

Acute psychotic paranoid states, with or without depression, have occurred with clear sensorium. Patients may become extremely violent and homicidal (R. S. Brown et al. 1987). Delirium with prominent hallucinations and delusions occurs with high levels of serum calcium (> 16 mg/dl). Calcium levels > 19 mg/dl generally induce coma (Petersen 1968). The elderly are very sensitive to hypercalcemia and may develop dementia with very mild increases in serum calcium (Joborn et al. 1986). Electroencephalographic (EEG) changes are not a sensitive diagnostic tool (Cooper and Schapira 1973).

Mechanism. Neuropsychiatric symptoms in hyperparathyroidism appear to be mediated primarily by serum calcium rather than PTH, per se, although both vitamin D and PTH have been postulated to have effects on behavior (Joborn et al. 1988). Furthermore, hypomagnesemia and hypophosphatemia frequently accompany hypercalcemia and may themselves induce neuropsychiatric symptoms.

Calcium serves a fundamental role in neurotransmission, regulating maintenance and termination of action potentials and synthesis, release, and receptor responsiveness of many neurotransmitters (Dubovsky et al. 1989). Thus there are many ways in which altered calcium activity could induce neuropsychiatric symptoms. For example, diurnal changes in cortisol secretion and cerebrospinal fluid (CSF) levels of the serotonin metabolite, 5-hydroxyindoleacetic acid (5-HIAA), are similar in hyperparathyroid patients and those with primary depression (Joborn et al. 1988; Linder et al. 1988). Levels of both substances were correlated with severity of depression and were normalized after successful surgery. It is unclear if these findings can be directly attributed to changes in CNS calcium levels, however, because CSF calcium is insensitive to changes in peripheral levels (Fraser and Arieff 1987).

As with cortisol and thyroid hormone, many have speculated that altered calcium metabolism is fundamentally associated with affective illness based on 1) an apparent increase in intracellular (Dubovsky et al. 1989) and CSF (Jimerson et al. 1979) calcium levels; 2) efficacy of psychotropic drugs that also modulate calcium transport; and 3) efficacy of calcium channel blockers (Dubovsky et al. 1989).

Treatment. If the disorder is not chronic, cognitive and affective symptoms are generally reversed by normalizing serum calcium. In particular, elderly patients with dementia who also have hyperparathyroidism usually show considerable improvement if surgery is done within the first 2 years of the illness (Joborn et al. 1986). Improvement is evident within a matter of days and appears to plateau by 3–6 months.

Appropriate treatment of middle-aged, mildly hypercalcemic, "asymptomatic" hyperparathyroid patients is controversial, although most would operate on younger, healthy patients based on the inconvenience of lifetime monitoring. Clearly, if patients complain of fatigue and muscle weakness they are likely to benefit from surgery. The response of other symptoms, such as depression and anxiety, is not predictable (Heath 1989; McAllion and Paterson 1989). Several cases of a delayed, self-limited, postparathyroidectomy psychosis with altered consciousness have been described (Mikkelsen and Reider 1979) and related to the rapid drop in serum calcium that occurs in patients with hypercalcemia and secondary bone disease.

Patients on lithium who become hypercalcemic should first have a lithium level obtained, to rule out lithium toxicity (the two cations are handled similarly by the kidney). If asymptomatic, the patient may be followed, or given another antimanic agent. In either case, calcium levels should be rechecked because lithium may induce, or accelerate, the growth of parathyroid adenomas. Lithium may be restarted after parathyroidectomy (Mallette and Eichhorn 1986).

Hypoparathyroidism and Hypocalcemia

Clinical picture. The causes of hypocalcemia include autoimmune or postsurgical hypoparathyroidism, hypomagnesemia, chronic renal failure, and conditions that diminish vitamin D activity.

Hypomagnesemia occurs with chronic alcoholism or malabsorption; diminished vitamin D activity occurs with reduced intake, deficient exposure to sunlight, malabsorption, and anticonvulsant therapy.

Neuromuscular symptoms, including muscle spasms, carpopedal spasm, and facial grimacing, usually predominate but are not present in all cases. Patients often note fatigue, weakness, and paresthesias. Increased intracranial pressure and calcifications of the basal ganglia occur in some patients with longstanding disease.

Diagnostic issues. Serum calcium and inorganic phosphorous should be obtained in suspected cases of hypocalcemia and followed up with ionized calcium and PTH if further workup is indicated (Table 22–13). Referral of patients with undiagnosed mild cases of hypocalcemia (partial parathyroid insufficiency) to psychiatrists for treatment-resistant anxiety is not unusual. Anxious hypocalcemic patients may have panic disorder, causing them to hyperventilate and develop tetany (Fourman et al. 1967). Thus hypocalcemia should be excluded in all cases of hyperventilation-induced tetany. Rarely the picture resembles bipolar disorder (Denko and Kaelbling 1962).

Hypocalcemic patients who exhibit choreiform movements, paresthesias, and atypical seizures may be referred to psychiatry for "histrionic behavior." These patients may exhibit no symptoms of tetany, and the EEG may be normal (Fonseca and Calverley 1967).

Details of neuropsychiatric features. The neuropsychiatric features of hypocalcemia have not been as carefully studied as those of other endocrinopathies. Neuropsychiatric symptoms, particularly anxiety and dementia, are common. In addition, patients may appear depressed, parkinsonian, or have choreiform movements. Typical and atypical seizures are frequent. Progressive intellectual decline is particularly common in hereditary hypoparathyroidism and pseudohypoparathryoidism.

TABLE 22–13. DIAGNOSIS OF HYPOCALCEMIA

Total calcium	< 9.0 mg/dl
Ionized calcium	< 2.3 mg/dl
Inorganic phosphorous	> 4.5 mg/dl

Mechanism. The mechanism of neuropsychiatric symptoms has not been studied; specifically the effects of increased intracranial pressure and soft tissue calcification have not been separated from other changes. Parkinsonism and choreiform movements, however, are not necessarily caused by basal ganglia calcification (Fonesca and Calverley 1967). Efforts to implicate hypocalcemia in the etiology of primary anxiety disorders have thus far been unfruitful (Liebowitz et al. 1986).

Treatment. Patients with mild hypocalcemia and no symptoms other than anxiety and depression may have "partial parathyroid insufficiency," which benefits from calcium supplementation (Fourman et al. 1967). With severe hypocalcemia, delirium may take 1–3 months to clear and may recur periodically during the recovery period despite "normocalcemia." Because serum calcium is usually maintained in the low-normal range (to prevent kidney stones), the recurrences may actually be secondary to hypocalcemia. Dementia tends to respond poorly.

Seizures and anxiety respond poorly to anticonvulsant and antianxiety agents, respectively (Carlson 1986). Hypocalcemic patients are reported to be more susceptible to the development of extrapyramidal syndrome (EPS) when given neuroleptic medication, although calcium levels (within the normal range) do not appear to influence EPS (Pratty et al. 1986).

❑ INSULIN

The neuropsychiatric effects of hyperinsulinism include organic anxiety, personality, amnestic, or delusional syndrome; delirium and dementia; and other organic mental syndromes characterized by dissociative symptoms and automatisms. Hyperglycemia may predispose to subtle deficits in higher cognitive functions. The two major metabolic complications of diabetes mellitus (diabetic ketoacidosis [DKA] and nonketotic hyperosmolar syndrome) induce delirium and coma.

Hyperinsulinism and Hypoglycemia

Clinical picture. The most common cause of hypoglycemia is insulin treatment of diabetes mellitus, particularly in patients with tight control of their blood glucose levels (Blackman et al. 1990). Hypoglycemia may also result from bowel dysfunction associated with gastric surgery, idiopathic postprandial hypoglycemia, insulin-secreting tumors, other large tumors, various endocrine deficiencies, cirrhosis, or drugs (including alcohol, propranolol, insulin, and the sulfonylureas). Lithium has insulin-like effects, but these are rarely, if ever, of clinical significance in diabetic patients.

Premature neonates are also frequently hypoglycemic. Several fatal cases of hypoglycemia have occurred in anorexia nervosa (Rich et al. 1990), and irreversible complications occurred not infrequently in schizophrenic patients who received insulin shock therapy.

If the hypoglycemia occurs abruptly (as in postsurgical situations and the controversial idiopathic postprandial syndrome), adrenergic symptoms of anxiety, tremor, diaphoresis, and tachycardia tend to predominate, along with hunger and weakness. In cases of chronic hypoglycemia (e.g., insulinoma), "neuroglyclopenic" symptoms, including loss of concentration, confusion, emotional lability, automatisms, and amnesia, are more prominent.

Diagnostic issues. The diagnosis of hypoglycemia requires 1) demonstration of hypoglycemia with fasting (Table 22–14) or after meals similar to those inducing symptoms (if postprandial); 2) the presence of symptoms consistent with hypoglycemia; and 3) improvement with normalization of glucose levels.

Many hypoglycemic patients, some of whom have treatable primary anxiety or affective disorders (Jefferson and Marshal 1981), seek medical advice because of postprandial adrenergic symptoms and are found to have an "abnormal" (i.e., blood glucose < 50 mg/dl) 5-hour glucose tolerance test. These patients may be given a diagnosis of hypoglycemia even though they never become hypoglycemic with normal meals, and many nonhypoglycemic subjects have similar glucose levels but no symptoms. Psychological testing suggests that many of these patients have a somatoform disorder (Jefferson and Marshal 1981). The mechanism of the symptoms and their relationship to hypoglycemia are controversial.

TABLE 22–14. DIAGNOSIS OF HYPOGLYCEMIA

Blood glucose after 24-hour fast	< 50 mg/dl (men) < 45 mg/dl (women)
Blood glucose during hypoglycemia attack	< 50 mg/dl

Factitious hypoglycemia caused by surreptitious administration of insulin occurs most frequently in medical personnel, family members of diabetic patients, or the diabetic patients themselves. In the first two groups, the diagnosis can be made by measuring C peptide levels (levels are depressed). However, the diagnosis can be very difficult to make in diabetic patients (Grunberger et al. 1988). Case reports have suggested that these patients usually have serious personality disturbances (Toth 1990) and respond poorly to psychotherapy (Grunberger et al. 1988).

On the other hand, patients with hypoglycemia may be mistakenly diagnosed as hysteric, epileptic, or intoxicated because they exhibit a combination of dissociative states, automatisms, and rage (Jefferson and Marshal 1981). In many cases hypoglycemic patients have appeared assaultive and paranoid and hence given a primary psychiatric diagnosis. In retrospect, however, these patients had clear signs of delirium: either waxing consciousness or disorientation (Steinberg and Mackenzie 1989). In instances of recurrent episodic hypoglycemia (e.g., islet cell tumor), the diagnosis may be challenging indeed.

Many patients with abrupt onset of hypoglycemia due to insulin treatment have anxiety attacks that are difficult for the patient and physician to distinguish from a primary anxiety disorder. Furthermore, patients with diabetes seem prone to develop anxiety disorders because of the stress of the illness and as a "conditioned" response to prior episodes of hypoglycemia (Steel et al. 1989).

Details of neuropsychiatric features. Unchecked lowering in blood glucose may cause excitement, overactivity, automatisms, muscular spasms, and finally decerebrate rigidity. In control subjects, neurophysiological changes (increased latency of the P300 component of the event-related brain potential) and subtle cognitive impairment are apparent at plasma glucose levels in the range of 45–70 mg/dl and increase in proportion to further reduction in blood glucose levels (Table 22–15) (Blackman et al. 1990; De Feo et al. 1988). Attention and memory seem less impaired than do higher order cognitive functions (Widom and Simonson 1990).

The neuropsychiatric response of patients with diabetes mellitus (whether or not they are in good glycemic control) is similar to that of nondiabetic individuals. In particular, even though basal glucose

TABLE 22–15. NEUROPSYCHIATRIC RESPONSE TO HYPOGLYCEMIA

Blood glucose (mg/dl)	*P300*[a]	*Cognition*	*Attention*	*Amnesia*	*Activity*	*Automatism*	*Decorticate*
45–70	Increase						
30–45	Increase	Decrease					
20–30	NM	Decrease[b]	Decrease	+	Increase		
10–20	NM	Decrease[b]	Decrease[b]	+	Increase or decrease[b]	Increase	
10	NM	(coma)	(coma)	+	Decrease[b]		+

Note. NM = not measurable; + = present.
[a]Latency of P300 component of evoked potential.
[b]Markedly decreased.

levels modulate the threshold for the adrenergic and other hormones involved in the counterregulatory response to hypoglycemia (i.e., lower the threshold for hormone release for those in tight control and raise it for those who are hyperglycemic), the neuroglycopenic threshold is unrelated to basal glucose (Widom and Simonson 1990). Many diabetic patients lose the adrenergic behavioral response entirely, or it may occur at progressively lower blood glucose levels (Widom and Simonson 1990). Thus these patients may depend on neuroglycopenic signals to identify hypoglycemia. If, however, confusion is the primary symptom, the patient may be unable to react appropriately. Elderly patients, and perhaps those with chronic mental disorders (Fishbain and Rotundo 1988), also appear to lose their adrenergic behavioral response.

Recurring episodes of moderate hypoglycemia may produce irreversible neurophysiological and cognitive changes in neonates (Lucas et al. 1988), in children, and to a lesser extent in adults (Ryan 1988). The first finding may be particularly significant because it was previously thought that the neonatal brain was relatively insensitive to hypoglycemia. Age at onset of diabetes is also a risk factor for cognitive impairment. Children whose illness began before age 5 show slower reaction times and may have lower verbal IQs. It is difficult to be certain if these changes are a direct consequence of hypoglycemia or a consequence of other behavioral or personality factors associated with the illness (Ryan 1988). Finally, severe chronic hypoglycemia produces a progressive dementia with or without extrapyramidal or cerebellar signs.

Mechanism. Unlike other organs, the brain's sole energy substrates are glucose or ketone bodies. Unfortunately, the shift from glucose to ketone bodies requires a number of hours, making the brain particularly vulnerable to acute hypoglycemia. In the absence of energy substrate the brain cells metabolize their lipid and protein components, leading to irreversible damage. Considerable controversy surrounds the issue of whether the adrenergic response to hypoglycemia is centrally or peripherally generated (De Feo et al. 1988).

Treatment. Although recovery from moderate levels of hypoglycemia is usually complete (except for amnesia for the incident), recovery from the so-called medullary phase (i.e., blood glucose < 10 mg/dl) is often prolonged and incomplete. Chronic hypoglycemia and multiple episodes of symptomatic hypoglycemia cause irreversible deficits. In modest hypoglycemia, full cognitive recovery lags reestablishment of euglycemia by about 1 hour (Blackman et al. 1990).

Hypoinsulinism and Hyperglycemia

Clinical picture. The major causes of hypoinsulinism are type I (insulin-dependent) and type II (non-insulin-dependent) diabetes mellitus. In type II diabetes, the insulin levels are not actually low, but out of phase and insufficient for the levels of blood glucose reached postprandially. Pancreatic disease, endocrine excesses, catastrophic illness, several medications, and genetic syndromes are also associated with hypoinsulinism or hyperglycemia. The common symptoms are polydipsia, polyuria, and polyphagia, although patients may first present with severe metabolic complications or, rarely, degenerative complications such as neuropathy.

Diagnostic issues. The diagnosis of hyperglycemia is generally not difficult to make (Table 22–16), but the physician must remain alert. In particular, symptoms of polyuria or polyphagia in psychiatric patients should not be attributed to medication side effects or psychogenic polydipsia until diabetes mellitus has been excluded.

Details of neuropsychiatric features. In adults, a history of poorly controlled diabetes (as assessed by retinopathy or glycosylated hemoglobin [HbA_{1c}] values) appears to impair learning, but the impairment is usually of little clinical significance (Ryan 1988). Longstanding disease is associated with micro- and macrocerebrovascular changes, which can cause multiple neuropsychiatric deficits. The severe metabolic complications of diabetes mellitus are DKA and hyperosmolar coma. Both present as a delirium, progressing to coma. Patients with hyperosmolar coma frequently convulse and may exhibit focal neurological signs.

TABLE 22–16. DIAGNOSIS OF HYPERGLYCEMIA	
Fasting blood glucose on two occasions	> 140 mg/dl
Glucose after ingestion of 75 g glucose (at 2 hours and one other time point)	> 200 mg/dl

❑ VASOPRESSIN

Arginine vasopressin, the antidiuretic hormone, is secreted by the posterior pituitary (neurohypophysis) in response to increases in plasma sodium concentration and plasma osmolality. The hormone acts on the distal nephron to increase water reabsorption and is the major means by which the body regulates water content. The regulatory centers for vasopressin secretion and thirst appear to lie adjacent to each other in the hypothalamus.

Excessive vasopressin may induce hyponatremia and water intoxication; whereas vasopressin deficiency causes polyuria and a secondary polydipsia. If water intake does not keep up with water loss, the patient becomes hypernatremic and delirious.

Excessive Vasopressin and Hyponatremia

Clinical picture. Excessive vasopressin secretion or action occurs with pulmonary lesions (especially oat cell carcinoma), adrenal insufficiency, disorders of the neurohypophysis, and medications like carbamazepine. In addition, 3%–5% of chronic psychiatric patients have elevated vasopressin levels (Illowsky and Kirch 1988). These patients exhibit both increased vasopressin secretion and enhanced vasopressin action. The mechanism(s) have not been established (Goldman et al. 1988). Renal, cardiac, and hepatic disease; reduced sodium intake; thiazide diuretics; and other causes of volume contraction may impair water excretion with normal vasopressin function.

Besides the aforementioned abnormalities in vasopressin secretion, impaired water excretion in psychiatric patients is often attributable to antidepressant- induced hypotension (particularly in the elderly) (Abbot 1983; Emsley et al. 1990). Current evidence suggests that neuroleptics rarely play a role (Lawson et al. 1985; Raskind et al. 1987).

Hyponatremia occurs when water intake exceeds water loss and plasma thus becomes dilute. It usually does not occur unless the patient has both increased fluid intake (e.g., psychogenic polydipsia) and impaired water excretion (e.g., increased arginine vasopressin) because the normal kidney (with appropriately depressed vasopressin) can excrete > 20 L of water a day. The signs and symptoms of severe hyponatremia (i.e., water intoxication) include nausea, vomiting, headache, tremor, ataxia, lethargy, delirium, seizures, and coma. Mortality rates of up to 50% have been reported in medical patients with symptomatic hyponatremia, although death is fairly rare in otherwise healthy psychiatric patients (Illowsky and Kirch 1988).

Diagnostic issues. Serum or plasma sodium levels may be substituted for osmolality in diagnosing plasma dilution, except in hyperosmolar conditions such as hyperglycemia (Goldman 1991) (Table 22–17). The syndrome of inappropriate antidiuresis (SIAD) can then be inferred from evidence that the

TABLE 22–17. DIAGNOSIS OF HYPONATREMIA AND INAPPROPRIATE ANTIDIURESIS	
Hyponatremia	< 130 mEq/L
Hypoosmolality	< 265 mOsm/kg
Urine osmolality during hyponatremia	> 100 mOsm/kg
Blood urea nitrogen (BUN)	< 10 mg/dl

patient is fully hydrated (i.e., low-normal blood urea nitrogen [BUN] levels, not orthostatic); has normal adrenal, thyroid, cardiac, renal, and hepatic function; and is not taking a medication such as a thiazide diuretic that impairs water excretion. A concurrent urine osmolality of > 100 milliosmols (mOsm)/kg is helpful in diagnosing SIAD, but urine may be maximally dilute in some variants. Definitive diagnosis may require measuring excretion of an oral water load (Goldman et al. 1988; Robertson 1988). Rarely hyponatremic patients have normal water excreting capacity.

Many times the diagnosis of hyponatremia is missed, and instead psychiatric patients with seizures secondary to water intoxication are erroneously given the diagnosis of idiopathic epilepsy and maintained on anticonvulsant medication (which probably does not reduce the incidence of seizures) (Erhardt and Goldman 1991; Illowsky and Kirch 1988). Water intoxication (along with other secondary causes) should always be excluded after diagnosing a seizure disorder in a psychotic patient, particularly if the seizure is followed by a massive diuresis or the patient has a history of polydipsia, vomiting, or prior alcohol abuse (Ripley et al. 1989). Because patients may be normonatremic between episodes, the diagnosis may require measuring diurnal weight changes over a 1- to 2-week period (Godleski et al. 1989) and taking a careful history focusing on latent symptoms of water intoxication (Goldman 1991).

In patients with severe psychiatric disturbances, hyponatremia is usually the result of marked polydipsia, combined with fairly minor impairments in water excretion (i.e., urine osmolality during hyponatremia rarely exceeds 150 mOsm/kg) (Goldman et al. 1988). Other causes, however, must be excluded, particularly if the urine concentration exceeds 150 mOsm/kg during hyponatremic episodes. Special care should be taken to exclude lung cancer because psychiatric patients are usually heavy smokers.

Details of neuropsychiatric features. In control subjects, mild hyponatremia induces altered taste sensation, nausea, muscle cramps, fatigue, and apathy. Moderate acute hyponatremia (120–130 mEq/L) impairs cognition but does not produce affective disturbances or psychosis (Gehi et al. 1981). In psychiatric patients, however, aggression may occur as a result of hyponatremia (Koczapski and Millson 1989).

Signs and symptoms of hyponatremia develop as a function of the rapidity of the fall of serum sodium. Thus a drop in sodium level of 10 mEq/L over a few hours may produce symptoms (Koczapski and Millson 1989), whereas markedly diminished levels (i.e., 30 mEq/L below normal) produce no obvious symptoms if they occur over days or weeks. Symptoms may progress with an acute fall in sodium level, or the patient may be asymptomatic but then convulse suddenly. Asymmetrical neurological findings have been described (Fraser and Arieff 1987).

Mechanism. Acute neuropsychiatric symptoms may be related to brain swelling and increased intracranial pressure. With chronic hyponatremia, brain cells show lower levels of sodium and potassium ions, thereby reducing brain swelling. The diminished levels of these ions, however, may impair neurotransmitter release (Fraser and Arieff 1987). Reports of increased levels of vasopressin in acute nonmedicated psychotic patients and evidence that inappropriate vasopressin secretion waxes and wanes with the severity of psychosis and cannot be accounted for by changes in "stress" have led some to propose that vasopressin regulation may be altered as a result of psychosis, per se (Goldman et al. 1988; Illowsky and Kirch 1988).

Treatment. Patients on antidepressants should have orthostatic blood pressure determined and, if indicated, should be switched to another structural class not associated with orthostatic hypotension. Patients requiring treatment for hypertension should be switched from thiazide diruretics to another agent, such as a calcium channel blocker. Patients on carbamazepine may show spontaneous resolution of hyponatremia, or resolution, if the dose is lowered or lithium is added (because it blocks vasopressin's actions). Nicotine, a potent stimulant for arginine vasopressin release, contributes to some cases of hyponatremia (Allon et al. 1990), and thus regulating smoking may help. Patients on thorazine may do better when switched to another neuroleptic with less potential to induce orthostasis.

In some cases of asymptomatic or episodic mild hyponatremia, the clinician may do nothing more than educate the patient and family about early signs and symptoms of water intoxication. Voluntary water restriction may work in medical patients with symptomatic hyponatremia but rarely succeeds with psychiatric patients. If reversible factors are not present, water intoxication in psychiatric inpatients can be prevented by monitoring acute changes in body weight and imposing fluid restriction if weight precipitously increases (Goldman and Luchins 1987; Goldman et al. 1989). Demeclocycline, an expensive tetracycline antibiotic, blocks arginine vasopressin and may also help to normalize serum sodium (Vieweg et al. 1988).

In nonedematous, markedly symptomatic (i.e., with seizure, coma, or delirium) patients who fail to show a prompt diuresis after fluid restriction, hypertonic saline should be given so that plasma sodium increases at a rate of no more than 2 mEq/hour. The infusion should be continued so that sodium level in the first day rises to 125 mEq/L or 20 mEq/L above baseline, whichever is lower (Fraser and Arieff 1987). This rate appears to minimize the morbidity and mortality from acute hyponatremia, as well as to prevent the delayed appearance of central pontine myelinolysis, a frequently irreversible and potentially fatal disorder related to rapid correction or overcorrection of hyponatremia (Cheng et al. 1990; Laureno and Karp 1988).

Deficient Vasopressin and Hypernatremia

Clinical picture. Deficient central vasopressin is caused by hypothalamic tumors, pituitary surgery, head trauma, and idiopathic diabetes insipidus. Renal disease, glycosuria, hypercalcemia, and several medications (notably lithium) also cause polyuria by interfering with renal conservation of water despite an adequate vasopressin response. Lithium causes polyuria in about 40% of patients.

Continued water loss without adequate water intake may lead to hypernatremia, but this only occurs if the thirst mechanism is impaired or the person is unable to obtain water (i.e., as with infants, the elderly, extremely ill patients, and mentally retarded patients) (Macdonald et al. 1989; Phillips et al. 1984). Rarely, psychotic psychiatric patients become hypernatremic when they refuse to drink (Phillips and Gabow 1990).

Symptoms of diminished vasopressin secretion are thirst, polydipsia, and polyuria. Signs of hypernatremia are dehydration, lethargy, stupor, and coma. Hypernatremic infants are irritable, have a high-pitched cry, and increased muscle tone. Fatalities are frequent in all cases because symptoms may not occur until very late in the disorder and may be brought on by brain hemorrhaging.

Diagnostic issues. Although 24-hour urine collections are the ideal means of diagnosing polyuria, they are often unreliable in psychiatric patients. Preliminary evidence suggests that polyuria can be inferred by obtaining afternoon urine creatinine concentrations, which are highly correlated to 24-hour urine volumes ($r^2 > 0.90$, $P < .00001$) (M. B. Goldman, D. J. Luchins, R. C. Marks, unpublished observations, February 1991) (Table 22–18). Urinary creatinine concentration appears to be more valid than other measures of spot dilution, presumably because creatinine is excreted at a fairly constant rate. Vasopressin deficiency (versus psychogenic polydipsia or nephrogenic diabetes insipidus; see below) can usually be diagnosed by imposing a fluid restriction. After urine osmolality has become stabilized (< 30 mOsm/kg increase over 3 hours), the patient receives a subcutaneous injection of vasopressin. Patients with psychogenic polydipsia may take a long time after restriction is imposed to attain a stable urine osmolality, but generally increase their urine osmolality above plasma levels and then show little further increase with vasopressin. Urine osmolality in patients with central diabetes insipidus and nephrogenic diabetes insipidus generally plateaus at levels below plasma and only in central diabetes insipidus does it increase further after vasopressin. Fluid-restricted patients must be observed carefully to prevent symptomatic hypernatremia. In occasional cases, measurement of concurrent plasma osmolality and vasopressin are necessary to make a definitive diagnosis (Robertson 1988).

It may be difficult without performing the above test to determine whether the polyuria in psychiatric patients is from psychogenic polydipsia, central diabetes insipidus, or (in certain instances) lithium-induced nephrogenic diabetes insipidus, which may take over a year to resolve after the drug is discontinued. "Psychogenic" polydipsia is exceedingly common among psychiatric patients, oc-

TABLE 22–18. DIAGNOSIS OF POLYURIA AND DEFICIENT VASOPRESSIN

24-hour urine collection	> 3 L
4 P.M. urine creatinine	< 70 mg/dl (men) < 35 mg/dl (women)
Urine osmolality 60 minutes after 5 U sq vasopressin	< 9% above baseline

curring in all diagnostic classes and up to 70% of chronic psychotic patients. Because central diabetes insipidus is much less common than primary polydipsia in psychiatric patients, clinicians normally assume the polydipsia is not secondary to a defect in vasopressin secretion. However, the clinician's index of suspicion should be raised if 1) the patient does not have a serious psychiatric disorder, or polyuria is present when other psychiatric symptoms are in complete remission; 2) the serum is hypertonic (i.e., plasma osmolality exceeds 290 mOsm/kg, or sodium exceeds 145 mEq/L); 3) the patient has a history of head trauma, CNS surgery, or infection; 4) the patient has a family history of polyuria or diabetes insipidus; 5) the water intake or output seems to vary little day-to-day; or 6) the patient has anorexia nervosa (which is associated with deficient vasopressin). Lithium-induced polyuria rarely exceeds 8 L/day, whereas patients with psychogenic polydipsia may produce twice that amount.

Details of neuropsychiatric features. Hypernatremia in control subjects induces extreme thirst, weakness, and impaired cognition. Impaired consciousness may occur late. The symptoms are rarely confused for a psychiatric disturbance.

Mechanism. Acute cell shrinkage from water loss causes mechanical traction on cerebral vessels, leading to vascular damage (Fraser and Arieff 1987). Chronic hypernatremia is associated with generation of intracellular solute (idiogenic osmols), which allows the brain to maintain adequate volume but places the patient at risk of brain edema if hypernatremia is corrected too quickly.

Central vasopressin may contribute to memory consolidation in control subjects; and central vasopressin deficiency has been proposed to contribute to the memory impairments in affective disorders, Alzheimer's disease (Smith and Nemeroff 1987), and putative minor defects in congenital diabetes insipidus (Laczi et al. 1987).

The etiology of psychogenic polydipsia is unknown. Although most of these patients do not complain of thirst, there is subtle evidence of thirst dysregulation (Goldman et al. 1988). Other cases of primary polydipsia do appear to be related to hypothalamic thirst dysregulation (i.e., so-called dipsogenic diabetes insipidus).

Treatment. Lithium-induced nephrogenic diabetes insipidus usually responds to lowering the lithium dose, changing to a single daily dose, or adding amiloride with or without a thiazide diuretic (Erhardt and Goldman 1991). Care should be taken to reduce the lithium dose if a diuretic is added.

Vasopressin deficiency rarely is responsible for the polyuria in psychiatric patients. If a trial of vasopressin is considered, extreme caution must be used to prevent water intoxication. There are no effective treatments for psychogenic polydipsia, although several interventions have been tried (Goldman 1991). Although the anticholinergic properties of the various psychotropic medications do not appear to make a large contribution to the polydipsia (via dry mouth), polydipsic patients should be treated with drugs with minimal anticholinergic effects.

❑ PROLACTIN

Hyperprolactinemia in women may induce an organic mood syndrome; in men it can induce apathy.

Hyperprolactinemia

Clinical picture. Prolactin-secreting tumors are fairly common, and occur much more frequently in women than in men. The most common cause of hyperprolactinemia in psychiatric patients is neuroleptic medication. Even low doses of neuroleptic drugs can produce the full syndrome of hyperprolactinemia (Erhardt and Goldman 1991). Other causes of hyperprolactinemia include hypothalamic or parasellar neoplasms, stress, pregnancy, oral contraceptives, several systemic illnesses (e.g., renal failure, hypothyroidism, and cirrhosis), and idiopathic disease.

Hyperprolactinemic women may present with amenorrhea, galactorrhea, gynecomastia, breast tenderness, diminished libido, or hirsutism. Men may present with obesity, impotence, and diminished libido.

Diagnostic issues. Hyperprolactinemia should be based on at least two levels in the absence of stress (e.g., level drawn 90 minutes after catheter insertion) or pregnancy (Table 22–19). Hyperprolactinemia may mimic depression, but symptoms of prolactin excess are nearly always present. Neuroleptics rarely raise prolactin levels above 100 ng/dl. Higher

TABLE 22–19. DIAGNOSIS OF HYPERPROLACTINEMIA

Prolactin	> 20 mg/dl (women) > 15 mg/dl (men)

levels suggest the presence of a prolactin-secreting adenoma.

In patients taking neuroleptic medication who consistently show elevated levels, a drug holiday should be employed, if possible, to assess whether prolactin levels fall. One report (Gangbar and Swinson 1983) suggested that 4 days off noninjectable neuroleptic is adequate for drug-induced elevations to normalize.

Details of neuropsychiatric features. Women with hyperprolactinemia tend to be depressed, with symptoms of increased hostility, anxiety, and diminished self-esteem (Kellner et al. 1984; Koppelman et al. 1987). Although the severity of these symptoms on self-reports may be severe (Kellner et al. 1984), patients rarely seek psychiatric treatment (Koppelman et al. 1987; Mattox et al. 1986).

Men often present with more advanced disease, complaining of headache and visual field defects (Cohen et al. 1984). Apathy is the predominant neuropsychiatric symptom, which may contribute to the delay in seeking treatment.

Mechanism. The mechanism of the diminished mood and libido is unknown, but it does not appear attributable to the physical symptoms or disturbances in other endocrine systems (Buckman and Kellner 1985).

Treatment. Depression is ameliorated with bromocriptine (Buckman and Kellner 1985; Koppelman et al. 1987). The salutary effects are apparent within 4 weeks, are maintained over long periods, and are unrelated to recurrence of menses; depression reoccurs with drug withdrawal (Mattox et al. 1986).

Both amantadine and bromocriptine are effective in treating symptoms of hyperprolactinemia caused by neuroleptic medication (Erhardt and Goldman 1991). Psychotic exacerbations are rare as long as the patient is maintained on an antipsychotic. Because of lower cost and fewer side effects, amantadine is preferred.

❑ REFERENCES

Abbott R: Hyponatremia due to antidepressant medications. Ann Emerg Med 12:708–710, 1983

Allon M, Allen HM, Deck LV, et al: Role of cigarette use in hyponatremia in schizophrenic patients. Am J Psychiatry 147:1075–1077, 1990

Aron DC, Tyrrell JB, Fitzgerald PA, et al: Cushing's syndrome: problems in diagnosis. Medicine 60:25–35, 1981

Bauer MS, Whybrow PC: Rapid cycling bipolar affective disorder, II: treatment of refractory rapid cycling with high-dose levothyroxine: a preliminary study. Arch Gen Psychiatry 47:435–440, 1990

Bauer MS, Droba M, Whybrow PC: Disorders of the thyroid and parathyroid, in Handbook of Clinical Psychoneuroendocrinology. Edited by Nemeroff CB, Loosen PT. New York, Guilford, 1987, pp 41–70

Bauer MS, Whybrow PC, Winokur A: Rapid cycling bipolar affective disorder, I: association with grade I hypothyroidism. Arch Gen Psychiatry 47:427–431, 1990

Bennett A, Cambor C: Clinical study of hyperthyroidism: comparison of male and female characteristics. Arch Gen Psychiatry 4:160–165, 1961

Blackman JD, Towle VL, Lewis GF, et al: Hypoglycemic thresholds for cognitive dysfunction in humans. Diabetes 39:828–835, 1990

Brown GG, Preisman RC, Kleerekoper M: Neurobehavioral symptoms in mild primary hyperparathyroidism: related to hypercalcemia but not improved by parathyroidectomy. Henry Ford Hospital Medical Journal 34:211–215, 1987

Brown RS, Fischman A, Showalter CR: Primary hyperparathyroidism, hypercalcemia, paranoid delusions, homicide, and attempted murder. J Forensic Sci 32: 1460–1463, 1987

Buckman MT, Kellner R: Reduction of distress in hyperprolactinemia with bromocriptine. Am J Psychiatry 142:242–244, 1985

Carlson RJ: Longitudinal observations of two cases of organic anxiety syndrome. Psychosomatics 27:529–531, 1986

Cheng JC, Zikos D, Skopicki HA, et al: Long-term neurologic outcome in psychogenic water drinkers with severe symptomatic hyponatremia: the effect of rapid correction. Am J Med 88:561–566, 1990

Cohen LM, Greenberg DB, Murray GB: Neuropsychiatric presentation of men with pituitary tumors (the "four A's"). Psychosomatics 25:925–928, 1984

Cooper AF, Schapira K: Case report: depression, catatonic stupor, and EEC changes in hyperparathyroidism. Psychol Med 3:509–515, 1973

Cronin AJ: The Citadel. London, V Gollancz, 1937

De Feo P, Gallai V, Mazzotta G, et al: Modest decrements in plasma glucose concentration cause early impairment in cognitive function and later activation of glucose counterregulation in the absence of hypoglycemic symptoms in normal man. J Clin Invest 82:436–444, 1988

De Jong JA, Roy A: Relationship of cognitive factors to CSF corticotropin-releasing hormone in depression. Am J Psychiatry 147:350–352, 1990

Demitrack MA, Dale JK, Laue L, et al: Hypothalamic-pituitary-adrenal activity in patients with chronic fatigue syndrome. Neuroendocrinology Letters 12:343, 1990

Denicoff KD, Joffe RT, Lakshmanan MC, et al: Neuropsychiatric manifestations of altered thyroid state. Am J Psychiatry 147:94–99, 1990

Denko JD, Kaelbling R: The psychiatric aspects of hypoparathyroidism. Acta Psychiatr Scand 38 (suppl 164):1–70, 1962

Dratman MB, Crutchfield FL: Thyroxine, triiodothyronine, and reverse triiodothyronine processing in the cerebellum: autoradiographic studies in adult rats. Endocrinology 125:1723–1733, 1989

Dubovsky SL, Christiano J, Daniell LC, et al: Increased platelet intracellular calcium concentration in patients with bipolar affective disorders. Arch Gen Psychiatry 46:632–638, 1989

Emsley RA, Van Der Meer H, Aalbers C, et al: Inappropriate antidiuretic state in long-term psychiatric inpatients. S Afr Med J 77:307–308, 1990

Erhardt VR, Goldman MB: Drug-induced endocrine dysfunction, in Drug-Induced Dysfunction in Psychiatry: Diagnosis and Management. Edited by Keshavan MS, Kennedy J. Washington, DC, Hemisphere Publications, 1991, pp 295–310

Extein IL, Gold MS: Thyroid hormone potentiation of tricyclics. Psychosomatics 29:166–174, 1988

Fishbain DA, Rotundo D: Frequency of hypoglycemic delirium in a psychiatric emergency service. Psychosomatics 29:346–348, 1988

Fonseca OA, Calverley JR: Neurological manifestations of hypoparathyroidism. Arch Intern Med 120:202–206, 1967

Fourman P, Rawnsley K, Davis RH, et al: Effect of calcium on mental symptoms in partial parathyroid insufficiency. Lancet 2:914–915, 1967

Fraser CL, Arieff AL: Metabolic encephalopathy associated with water, electrolyte, and acid-base disorders, in Clinical Disorders of Fluid Electrolyte Metabolism. Edited by Maxwell MH, Kleeman C, Narins R. New York, McGraw-Hill, 1987, pp 1153–1196

Gangbar R, Swinson RP: Hyperprolactinemia and psychiatric illness. Am J Psychiatry 140:790–791, 1983

Gehi MM, Rosenthal RH, Fizette NB, et al: Psychiatric manifestations of hyponatremia. Psychosomatics 22: 739–743, 1981

Godleski LS, Vieweg WVR, Hundley PL, et al: Day-to-day case of chronic schizophrenic patients subject to water intoxication. Annals of Clinical Psychiatry 1:179–185, 1989

Gold PW, Loriaux DL, Roy A, et al: Responses to corticotropin-releasing hormone in the hypercortisolism of depression and Cushing's disease. N Engl J Med 134:1329–1334, 1986

Goldman MB: A rational approach to disorders of water balance in psychiatric patients. Hosp Community Psychiatry 42:488–494, 1991

Goldman MB, Luchins DJ: Prevention of episodic water intoxication with target weight procedure. Am J Psychiatry 144:365–366, 1987

Goldman MB, Luchins DJ, Robertson GL: Mechanisms of altered water metabolism in psychotic patients with polydipsia and hyponatremia. N Engl J Med 318:397–403, 1988

Goldman MB, Luchins DJ, Robertson GL: Treatment of hyponatremia secondary to water overload. Lancet 1: 328–329, 1989

Grunberger G, Weiner JL, Silverman R, et al: Factitious hypoglycemia due to surreptitious administration of insulin. Ann Intern Med 108:252–257, 1988

Heath DA: Primary hyperparathyroidism. Endocrinol Metab Clin North Am 18:631–646, 1989

Illowsky BP, Kirch DG: Polydipsia and hyponatremia in psychiatric patients. Am J Psychiatry 145:675–683, 1988

Jefferson JJ, Marshal JR: Endocrine disorders, in Neuropsychiatric Features of Medical Disorders. New York, Plenum, 1981, pp 133–177

Jimerson DC, Post RM, Carman JS, et al: CSF calcium: clinical correlates in affective illness and schizophrenia. Biol Psychiatry 14:37–51, 1979

Joborn C, Hetta J, Frisk P, et al: Primary hyperparathyroidism in patients with organic brain syndrome. Acta Med Scandanavia 219:91–98, 1986

Joborn C, Hetta J, Rastad J, et al: Psychiatric symptoms and cerebrospinal fluid monoamine metabolites in primary hyperparathyroidism. Biol Psychiatry 23:149–158, 1988

Johnstone PA, Rundell JR, Esposito M: Mental status changes of Addison's disease. Psychosomatics 31:103–107, 1990

Kellner R, Buckman MT, Fava GA, et al: Hyperprolactinemia, distress, and hostility. Am J Psychiatry 141:759–763, 1984

Kirkegaard C, Korner A, Faber J: Increased production of thyroxine and inappropriately elevated serum thyrotropin levels in endogenous depression. Biol Psychiatry 27:472–476, 1990

Koczapski AB, Millson RC: Individual differences in serum sodium levels in schizophrenic men with self-induced water intoxication. Am J Psychiatry 146:1614–1615, 1989

Koppelman MCS, Parry BL, Hamilton JA, et al: Effect of bromocriptine on affect and libido in hyperprolactinemia. Am J Psychiatry 144:1037–1041, 1987

Laczi F, Laszlo FA, Kovacs GL, et al: Differential effect of desglycinamide 9-(Arg 8)-vasopressin on cognitive functions of diabetes insipidus and alcoholic patients. Acta Endocrinol (Copenh) 115:392–398, 1987

Laureno R, Karp BI: Pontine and extrapontine myelinolysis following rapid correction of hyponatremia. Lancet 1:1439–1440, 1988

Lawson WB, Karson CN, Bigelow LB: Increased urine volume in chronic schizophrenic patients. Psychiatry Res 14:323–331, 1985

Liebowitz MR, Gorman JM, Fyer A, et al: Possible mechanisms for lactate's induction of panic. Am J Psychiatry 143:495–501, 1986

Linder J, Brismar K, Granberg PO, et al: Characteristic changes in psychiatric symptoms, cortisol and melatonin but not prolactin in primary hyperparathyroidism. Acta Psychiatr Scand 78:32–40, 1988

Loosen PT: Hormones of the hypothalamicpituitary thyroid axis: a psychoneuroendocrine perspective. Pharmacopsychiatry 19:401–415, 1986

Lucas A, Morley R, Cole TJ: Adverse neurodevelopmental outcome of moderate neonatal hypoglycaemia. Br Med J 297:1304–1308, 1988

McAllion SJ, Paterson CR: Psychiatric morbidity in primary hyperparathyroidism. Postgrad Med J 65:628–631, 1989

Macdonald NJ, McConnell KN, Stephen MR, et al: Hypernatraemic dehydration in patients in a large hospital for the mentally handicapped. Br Med J 299:1426–1429, 1989

Mallette LE, Eichhorn E: Effects of lithium carbonate on human calcium metabolism. Arch Intern Med 146: 770–776, 1986

Mattox JH, Buckman MT, Bernstein J, et al: Dopamine agonists for reducing depression associated with hyperprolactinemia. J Reprod Med 31:694–698, 1986

Mikkelsen EJ, Reider AA: Post-parathyroidectomy psychosis: clinical and research implications. J Clin Psychiatry 40:352–358, 1979

Nemeroff CB: Clinical significance of psychoneuroendocrinology in psychiatry: focus on the thyroid and adrenal. J Clin Psychiatry 50 (suppl):13–20, 1989

Petersen P: Psychiatric disorders in primary hyperparathyroidism. Journal of Clinical Endocrinology 28:1491–1495, 1968

Phillips MG, Gabow PA: Psychogeneic adipsia in a patient with psychotic depression. Am J Kidney Dis 15:592–594, 1990

Phillips PA, Rolls BJ, Ledingham JGG, et al: Reduced thirst after water deprivation in healthy elderly men. N Engl J Med 311:753–759, 1984

Pratty JS, Ananth J, O'Brien JE: Relationship between dystonia and serum calcium levels. J Clin Psychiatry 47: 418–419, 1986

Raskind MA, Courtney N, Murburg MM, et al: Antipsychotic drugs and plasma vasopressin in normals and acute schizophrenic patients. Biol Psychiatry 22:453–462, 1987

Reus VI: Disorders of the adrenal cortex and gonads, in Handbook of Clinical Psychoneuroendocrinology. Edited by Nemeroff CB, Loosen PT. New York, Guilford, 1987, pp 71–84

Rich LM, Caine MR, Findling JW, et al: Hypoglycemic coma in anorexia nervosa. Arch Intern Med 150:894–895, 1990

Ripley TL, Millson RC, Koczapski AB: Self-induced water intoxication and alcohol abuse. Am J Psychiatry 146: 102–103, 1989

Robertson GL: Differential diagnosis of polyurias, in Annual Review of Medicine, Vol 39. Edited by Creger WP. Palo Alto, CA, Annual Reviews, 1988, pp 425–442

Rose RM: Psychoendocrinology, in Williams Textbook of Endocrinology, 7th Edition. Edited by Wilson JD, Foster DW. Philadelphia, PA, WB Sanders, 1985, pp 653–681

Ryan CM: Neurobehavioral complications of type 1 diabetes. Diabetes Care 11:86–93, 1988

Smith CK, Barish J, Correa MD, et al: Psychiatric disturbance in endocrinologic disease. Psychosom Med 34: 69–86, 1972

Smith MA, Nemeroff CB: Behavioral effects of nonopioid peptides in humans, in Handbook of Clinical Psychoneuroendocrinology. Edited by Nemeroff CB, Loosen PT. New York, Guilford, 1987, pp 399–416

Starkman MN, Schteingart DE, Schork MA: Cushing's syndrome after treatment: changes in cortisol and ACTH levels, and amelioration of the depressive syndrome. Psychiatry Res 19:177–188, 1986a

Starkman MN, Schteingart DE, Schork MA: Correlation of bedside cognitive and neuropsychological tests in patients with Cushing's syndrome. Psychosomatics 27: 508–511, 1986b

Steel JM, Masterton G, Patrick AW, et al: Hyperventilation or hypoglycaemia? Diabetic Med 6:820–821, 1989

Steinberg PI, Mackenzie R: A patient with insulinoma presenting for psychiatric assessment. Can J Psychiatry 34:68–69, 1989

Toth EL: Factitious hypoglycemia and the multiple personality disorder (letter). Ann Intern Med 112:76, 1990

Vieweg VWR, Wilkinson EC, David JJ, et al: The use of demeclocycline in the treatment of patients with psychosis, intermittent hyponatremia, and polydipsia (PIP syndrome). Psychiatr Q 59:62–68, 1988

Voth HM, Holzman P, Katz J, et al: Thyroid "hot spots": their relationship to life stress. Psychosom Med 32:561–568, 1970

Widom B, Simonson DC: Glycemic control and neuropsychologic function during hypoglycemia in patients with insulin-dependent diabetes mellitus. Ann Intern Med 112:904–912, 1990

Yassa R, Saunders A, Nastase C, et al: Lithium-induced thyroid disorders: a prevalence study. J Clin Psychiatry 49:14–16, 1988

Chapter

23

Neuropsychiatric Aspects of Poisonous and Toxic Disorders

Lawrence S. Gross, M.D.
Robert M. Nagy, M.D.

IN MODERN SOCIETY WE are exposed to a variety of substances with potential neurotoxic effects. Exposure may occur in the workplace, in the home, by ingesting contaminated food, by breathing contaminated air, or by envenomation via bites. *Toxins* have been defined as substances derived from the tissues of a plant, animal, or microorganism that have a deleterious effect on another plant or animal; *poisons* are substances that, in relatively small amounts, produce death or serious dysfunction of tissues or organs (Russell 1980). In this chapter we use the terms interchangeably and address selected industrial and biological toxicities with prominent neuropsychiatric symptomatology.

Industrialization has led to the availability of many products designed to improve our quality of life, yet the manufacturing processes and the products themselves may produce serious health consequences, including neuropsychiatric ones.

❑ METAL POISONING

Although many metals are ubiquitous in nature, their presence in toxic forms and concentrations in the environment has increased significantly since the Industrial Revolution. The neurotoxic effects of certain heavy metals are well documented and are summarized in Table 23–1. These are described in the following discussion with the exception of lithium, which is included in the discussion of psychopharmacological agents. Other metals have been less prominently associated with neurotoxicity and are listed in Table 23–2.

Lead

Background. Lead accumulates in the human body throughout life after exposure, which may occur from a variety of environmental sources. The

TABLE 23–1. SELECTED METALS WITH PROMINENT NEUROTOXIC EFFECTS

Metal	*Delirium*	*Dementia*	*Mood changes*	*Psychosis*	*Personality changes*	*Seizures*	*Peripheral neuropathy*	*Comments*
Aluminum		X			X	X		Dialysis dementia; association with Alzheimer's disease, amyotrophic lateral sclerosis, and parkinsonism—dementia (Guam).
Arsenic	X	X	X	X	X	X	X	Large acute arsenic ingestions and acute arsine gas poisoning are frequently fatal.
Lead	X	X	X	X	X	X	X	Subtle subclinical changes.
Lithium	X					X	X	Parkinsonian syndrome, movement disorders, tremor, paralysis, stupor, coma; symptoms may appear at therapeutic as well as toxic levels.
Manganese	X	X	X	X	X			"Manganese madness"; parkinsonism.
Mercury	X	X	X		X	X	X	Intention tremor, ataxia, visual field disturbances; organic mecurials quite neurotoxic.
Thallium	X	X	X	X		X	X	Acute ingestions frequently fatal.

TABLE 23–2. SELECTED METALS WITH REPORTED NEUROTOXIC EFFECTS

Metal	*Neuropsychiatric symptoms*
Barium	Progressive flaccid paralysis
Copper	Lethargy and coma with severe toxicity
Gold	Encephalopathy with gold therapy
Iron	Lethargy, coma and seizures in severe toxicity
Magnesium	Central nervous system depression, paralysis, and hyporeflexia
Phosphorus	
Yellow phosphorus	Lethargy, stupor, coma, restlessness, hypotension, and shock
Phosphine gas	Headache, fatigue, paresthesias, ataxia, intention tremor, weakness, and diplopia
Platinum	
Cisplatin	Peripheral neuropathy, memory loss, and intention tremor
Potassium	Weakness, paresthesias, hyporeflexia, and paralysis
Selenium	Fatigue, irritability, hyperreflexia, muscle tenderness, and tremor
Tin	
Organic tin compounds	Headache, paresthesias, visual disturbances, tinnitus, deafness, memory loss, disorientation, aggressive behavior, psychosis, movement disorder, and coma
Zinc	Lethargy, ataxia, and writing difficulty

Source. Ellenhorn and Barceloux 1988.

abnormal oral ingestion (pica) of lead-based paints from old houses is a common cause of lead intoxication in children; 70%–90% of children with serious lead poisoning have a history of pica (Feldman 1986). In addition, ingestion of other lead-containing objects as well as contaminated food, water, air, dust, and soil can contribute to pediatric lead toxicity (Chisolm and Barltrop 1979). Adults are most commonly exposed to lead via inhalation in occupations where lead is used in manufacturing and processing. Nonoccupational sources of lead poisoning include ingestion of home-distilled whiskey, eating from unfired pottery, retention of bullets, and gasoline sniffing (Cullen et al. 1983; Louria 1988).

Adults absorb 5%–10% of an ingested lead load, whereas children have increased gastrointestinal absorption (almost 40%). Absorption after inhalation is 50%–70% if the particle size is small enough to reach the alveoli. Inorganic lead does not pass through the skin, but organic lead gasoline additives, such as tetraethyl lead, may be absorbed through intact skin as well as through the lungs. Decreased iron, calcium, and zinc levels increase lead absorption.

In the circulation, 95% of lead is in the red blood cells, but, because of distribution into soft tissue or bone stores, blood levels may not reflect the total body lead burden. Ninety percent of total body lead is contained in bone, where lead is principally stored and has a half-life of 20–30 years (Ellenhorn and Barceloux 1988).

Action. Lead interferes with enzyme systems throughout the body, which leads to diffuse effects. In children, severe central nervous system (CNS) symptomatology is thought to be due to lead's easier passage through the blood-brain barrier and disruption of mitochondrial function (Ellenhorn and Barceloux 1988).

Neuropsychiatric manifestations. Lead toxicity in adults may involve both the CNS and the peripheral nervous system. Early manifestations are often nonspecific and include abdominal pain, fatigue, arthralgia, decreased libido, headache, irritability, impotence, depression, and anorexia. Encephalopathy is rare among adults, with most of the reported cases associated with the ingestion of illicit whiskey. Seizures are the most commonly reported symptom (75%), but obtundation, confusion, focal motor dysfunction, papilledema, headaches, and optic neuritis are also described. Cerebrospinal fluid (CSF) changes include elevated opening pressure, increased protein, and slight pleocytosis. Chelation therapy was reported to be helpful in treating the encephalopathy, but the long-term outcome was often complicated by coexisting alcoholism (Cullen et al. 1983).

In contrast to adults, children are more likely to develop acute lead encephalopathy, the most severe clinical manifestation of lead poisoning. It occurs most commonly during summer months in children under the age of 3 years. As in adults, early CNS symptoms are often nonspecific ones such as anorexia, apathy, irritability, abdominal pain, vomiting, headache, emotional lability, incoordination, sleep disturbance, and memory lapses. Persistent exposure leads to the rapid development of signs of encephalopathy such as disorientation, psychosis, ataxia, syncope, focal neurological signs, delirium, and lethargy progressing to stupor, seizures, blindness, and coma. Pathologically, the syndrome is characterized by massive cerebral edema with associated vasculopathy.

Chelation therapy has reduced the mortality to less than 5%, but when the therapy is begun after the symptoms of acute encephalopathy appear 25%–50% of patients show permanent neuropsychiatric sequelae such as seizures, blindness, hemiparesis, and mental retardation (Chisolm and Barltrop 1979).

Peripheral nerve involvement occurs much more often in adults than in children; peripheral neuropathy is the most common neurological manifestation of lead toxicity in adults. The neuropathy is typically motor with wrist drop and foot drop seen most frequently. Severe intoxication has been associated with decreased motor nerve conduction velocities from segmental demyelination. The appearance of clinical neuropathy seems to be related to the magnitude and duration of lead exposure. Sensory and cranial nerve involvement and a syndrome similar to amyotrophic lateral sclerosis (ALS) have been less frequently described (Cullen et al. 1983).

Psychiatric symptomatology, such as organic affective illness, has been associated with lead intoxication (Schottenfeld and Cullen 1984). Signs of chronic lead intoxication may be confused with depression (Cullen et al. 1983). Organic lead intoxication from inhaling gasoline fumes may cause insomnia, irritability, nervousness, euphoria, delusions, hallucinations, and seizures.

There is increasing evidence of "subclinical" nervous system effects of lead in both children and adults who are found to have increased lead absorption but display no symptoms or only mild nonspecific symptoms of lead intoxication. It has been estimated that between 3 and 4 million American children have blood lead levels above 15 μg/dl, a level previously considered to be safe; prenatal and postnatal exposure to lead at this level has been associated with undesirable health effects in young children (Agency for Toxic Substances and Disease Registry 1988). Descriptions include reduced gestational age, reduced birth weight, and impaired neurobehavioral development (Davis and Svendsgaard 1987); slowed motor nerve conduction velocity (J. Schwartz et al. 1988); and disturbances in attention, learning, and classroom behavior in school children (Needleman 1983). Mean reductions in IQ scores of 4–7 points have been demonstrated in children exposed to lead compared with control groups, with a resultant decreased number of lead-exposed children in the superior range (IQ greater than 125) and an increased number in the below-average range (IQ less than 80) (Needleman 1989). Eleven-year follow-up of children exposed to lead has shown academic and cognitive deficits persisting into young adulthood (Needleman et al. 1990).

Future research needs to further address the role of potentially confounding variables such as individual, family, and socioeconomic factors to clarify the subtle effects of lead in children (Ruff and Bijur 1989). Reports of subclinical CNS effects in adults with increased lead absorption document a high prevalence of nonspecific symptoms such as fatigue, irritability, insomnia, nervousness, headache, and weakness along with abnormalities in neuropsychological testing (Cullen et al. 1983). Some subclinical lead-induced neuropsychiatric deficits may be reversible with reduced exposure (Baker et al. 1985; Yokoyama et al. 1988).

Diagnosis. Often the most important diagnostic information is the identification of a history of lead exposure. The whole blood lead level is the best measure of recent exposure. In children, a whole blood level of 25 μg/dl is considered evidence of increased lead absorption (Centers for Disease Control 1985). This threshold level is the result of downward revision in recent years as symptomatology has been demonstrated at progressively lower levels. For adults, a whole blood level of more than 40 μg/dl indicates excessive absorption. Blood concentration of 60 μg/dl or more is indicative of definite lead poisoning in children (Louria 1988); symptoms of lead intoxication appear at slightly higher blood levels in adults. The current allowable industrial concentration is 50 μg/dl; levels above this require removal from the work place until they decrease to below 40 μg/dl (Ellenhorn and Barceloux 1988).

Elevated blood lead levels are accompanied by increases in urinary δ-aminolevulinic acid and coproporphyrin levels. Measurement of blood levels of free erythrocyte protoporphyrin (FEP) is the best screening for chronic lead intoxication. Asymptomatic increased body lead burdens can be detected by measuring urinary lead excretion after administration of calcium disodium edetate ($CaNa_2EDTA$ mobilization test), described elsewhere (Ellenhorn and Barceloux 1988).

Treatment and prognosis. Patients must be removed from the source of lead exposure. Parenterally administered chelating agents dimercaprol (also known as British anti-lewisite; BAL) and $CaNa_2EDTA$ are usually administered in combination to bind lead and promote tissue excretion in symptomatic poisoning. Penicillamine is a commercially available oral chelating agent, but its use in lead poisoning remains investigational (Ellenhorn and Barceloux 1988). The U.S. Food and Drug Administration (FDA) recently approved an oral chelator succimer, also known as 2,3-dimercaptosuccinic acid (DMSA), for the treatment of lead poisoning in children with blood lead levels above 45 μg/dl (McNeil Consumer Products Company 1991). Although clinical experience is limited, DMSA appears to be safe, effective, and simple to administer (Graziano et al. 1988). General guidelines for chelation treatment are described elsewhere (Ellenhorn and Barceloux 1988; McNeil Consumer Products Company 1991; Piomelli et al. 1984). Initial clinical improvement from the reduction of blood lead levels may be followed by reemergence of symptoms requiring further chelation therapy as lead is mobilized from bone. Treatment response of neuropsychiatric manifestations is often slow and incomplete, so early detection and prevention of lead exposure are essential to minimize permanent damage.

Mercury

Background. Mercury has been used for centuries in medicine and industry. The historical use of mercurials for medicinal purposes (e.g., as diuretics and cathartics and in the treatment of syphilis) has largely been discarded. Poisoning from skin absorption of inorganic mercury salts used in the felting process was common during the 19th century among felt hat workers, leading to expressions such as "the mad hatter" (Sunderman 1988). Industrialization has led to increased environmental exposure to mercury via mining, smelting, and the burning of fossil fuels. Mercury is used in dental amalgams and in a variety of industries.

Mercury exists in three forms: elemental mercury, inorganic mercury, and organic mercury. Occupational exposure to elemental and inorganic mercury occurs among miners, smelters, jewelers, photographers, dentists, dental assistants, and makers of mirrors, batteries, and instruments (Landrigan 1982). At environmental temperatures elemental mercury is in liquid form and easily vaporizes; it is poorly absorbed through the gastrointestinal tract but well absorbed via inhalation with a predilection for the CNS. Inorganic mercury has moderate gastrointestinal absorption and may be absorbed through the lungs and skin as well. Organic mercury compounds fall into two types: 1) the alkyl mercury group (e.g., methyl mercury), which is quite lipid soluble and has extensive gastrointestinal absorption and neurotoxicity, and 2) phenyl mercury and methoxyethyl mercury, which are less extensively absorbed through the gastrointestinal tract and undergo biotransformation to release inorganic mercury with symptoms resembling inorganic mercury toxicity. Mercury from industrial waste and environmental sources usually settles in the aquatic environment and is concentrated in the food chain (Ellenhorn and Barceloux 1988). Organic mercury compounds, used as fungicides and pesticides, have been associated with occupational exposure but more extensively with community outbreaks of poisoning from eating contaminated fish or grains (Landrigan 1982).

Action. The toxicity of mercury is thought to result from its high affinity for sulfhydryl groups leading to inhibition of various enzymes and disruption of membrane functions (Landrigan 1982). Methyl mercury inhibits choline acetyltransferase, the enzyme that catalyzes the final step in the synthesis of acetylcholine (Elhassani 1983).

Neuropsychiatric manifestations. Acute toxic exposure to elemental mercury vapor results primarily in encephalopathy; rarely, seizures occur (Ellenhorn and Barceloux 1988). Mild exposure to inhaled elemental mercury vapor is associated with subtle symptomatology such as insomnia, nervousness, mild tremor, headache, emotional lability, fatigue, decreased sexual drive, depression, and impaired judgment, coordination, and cognition; these early manifestations have been referred to as *micromercurialism* (Louria 1988). Toxic symptoms from chronic occupational exposure to elemental mercury involve problems in the oral cavity (e.g., gingivitis, salivation, and stomatitis); tremor (intention tremor that disappears with sleep); and prominent neuropsychological changes (e.g., emotional lability, shyness, and loss of sleep, appetite, and memory) (Ellenhorn and Barceloux 1988). Workers exposed to elemental mercury vapors have shown prolonged motor and sensory distal latencies on nerve conduction testing (Levine et al. 1982). Thirty percent of a group of dentists with high tissue mercury levels showed electrophysiological evidence of a subclinical polyneuropathy (Shapiro et al. 1982).

Toxicity from chronic inorganic mercury exposure is usually occupational and clinically resembles that from chronic inhalation of mercury vapor. The symptoms include dermatitis, gingivitis, stomatitis, tremor, and neuropsychiatric dysfunction termed *erethism,* which is a syndrome consisting of irritability, pathological shyness, and impairment of memory, attention span, and intellect (Landrigan 1982).

Methyl mercury is the most neurotoxic of the short-chain alkyl mercury compounds and serves as the model for organic mercury poisoning. Epidemics throughout the world have resulted from the ingestion of fish or grain contaminated with methyl mercury used as a fungicide. Early symptoms include paresthesias of the limbs, nose, and lips. Motor incoordination, ataxic gait, and loss of position sense are accompanied by dysarthria, constriction of visual fields, hearing defects, and muscle rigidity or spasticity with hyperreflexia. Epidemics have been associated with significant death rates and permanent neurological sequelae. Neuropsychiatric symptoms that have been reported include headache, sleep disturbances, dizziness, irritability, emotional instability, mania, and depression (Elhassani 1983). Methyl mercury easily crosses the blood-brain barrier, exerting a permanent effect on the nervous system, particularly the cerebellum. It also passes through the placenta, with higher concentrations demonstrated in fetal blood compared with maternal blood. Established embryotoxic effects include microcephaly and cerebral palsy. Infants born shortly before maternal exposure and exposed to methyl mercury solely via breast milk have demonstrated hyperreflexia and delayed motor and speech development (Elhassani 1983).

Diagnosis. Classic findings on physical examination and a history of exposure are often sufficient to identify cases of mercury poisoning, but determining the type and level of mercury in samples of blood, urine, hair, and food will help confirm the diagnosis. Care must be taken in the collection of these samples to avoid false-positive results from outside contamination (Elhassani 1983). The correlation between blood and urine mercury measurements and clinical symptoms depends on the form and duration of mercury exposure. Normal concentration of mercury in the blood is less than 3–4 μg/dl; concentrations greater than 4 μg/dl are considered abnormal in adults. Normal urinary mercury excretion is less than 25 μg/L (Klaassen 1985a). Mild cases of poisoning may present with subjective complaints. Routine medical screening of exposed workers may not detect subtle symptomatology, suggesting that more sensitive measures be used to detect workplace toxicity and prevent progression to more serious illness (Rosenman et al. 1986).

Treatment and prognosis. After acute inorganic and organic mercury ingestion, treatment should be initiated with the induction of emesis or gastric lavage along with the administration of activated charcoal and cathartics. The use of chelating agents such as dimercaprol (BAL), BAL derivatives, and penicillamine has been helpful in elemental and inorganic mercury poisoning, but these agents have little or no effect in organic intoxication. Dimercaprol is contraindicated in the treatment of organic mercury poisoning because it increases methyl mercury levels in laboratory animals; polythiol resins may be more effective than penicillamine in removing methyl mercury compounds from the body (Klaassen 1985a).

Hemodialysis may be helpful in treating acute inorganic mercury poisoning in patients with renal impairment. Conventional hemodialysis is of little use in the treatment of methyl mercury intoxication because of its concentration in erythrocytes, but the use of L-cysteine has been effective in complexing methyl mercury into a more dialyzable form (Klaassen 1985a). Diaphoresis has been used for centuries in the therapy of mercury poisoning (Sunderman 1988). Mercury is sequestered in lysosomal dense bodies in neurons and persists in the brain for long periods of time (Cavanagh 1988). Damage to the central and peripheral nervous systems appears to be permanent, but physical therapy has been associated with clinical improvement in less severely poisoned patients. Administration of neostigmine has been reported to improve motor strength in patients with methyl mercury intoxication (Elhassani 1983).

Arsenic

Background. Infamous for its long history as a homicidal poison, arsenic is a tasteless, odorless metal found naturally in the environment and used in a variety of industries. Accidental, suicidal, and homicidal ingestions continue to occur. Used in the past to treat a number of infectious bacterial and parasitic illnesses, arsenic compounds have largely been eliminated from modern medicine, although arsenicals are still found in some veterinary medicines and homeopathic preparations.

Arsenic is used in pesticides, herbicides, rodenticides, ant paste, glassware, paints, metal alloys, pigments, wood preservatives, and cosmetics (Ellenhorn and Barceloux 1988; Schoolmeester and White 1980; Zaloga et al. 1985). Workplace exposure occurs in the above industries and has been reported among chemical workers, pesticide formulators, pesticide applicators, and carpenters working with treated woods. Community exposure has resulted through airborne emissions from smelters and from well water contaminated by natural arsenic deposits (Landrigan 1982). Transformation by microorganisms leads to accumulation in seafood (Ellenhorn and Barceloux 1988). Significant amounts of arsenic are found in natural and processed foods, which may be the result of industrial pollution, the use of arsenic-containing agricultural products, and arsenic's natural presence in water and soil. The average daily ingestion of arsenic has been estimated to be about 1 mg (Schoolmeester and White 1980).

Arsenic is present in three toxic forms in the environment: pentavalent salts, trivalent salts, and arsine gas. The pentavalent form (arsenate) is found in the earth's crust and in most foods and is water soluble, rapidly absorbed through mucous membranes, and less toxic than the trivalent form (arsenite) which is more lipid soluble, has greater skin absorption, and accumulates in the body (Louria 1988; Schoolmeester and White 1980). Fine powders have more effective gastrointestinal absorption than do coarser forms. Inhalation of arsenic compounds can result in significant absorption. Colorless, odorless arsine gas used in the semiconductor industry is released when acid is added to arsenic compounds and is extremely toxic (Ellenhorn and Barceloux 1988).

After absorption, arsenic in the bloodstream is initially localized in erythrocytes and bound to proteins with minimal penetration of the blood-brain barrier. Within 24 hours, arsenic redistributes mainly into liver, kidney, heart, and lungs with lesser amounts in muscle and nervous tissue; 2–4 weeks after ingestion, deposition of arsenic begins in the sulfhydryl-rich keratin of hair, skin, and nails where it remains for years. Long-term incorporation also takes place into bones and teeth. Excretion of arsenic is mainly through the kidney. Carcinogenicity of arsenic is controversial. Arsenic that crosses the placenta has been associated with neonatal death; fetal damage has been reported but epidemiological confirmation of teratogenicity is lacking (Klaassen 1985a; Schoolmeester and White 1980).

Action. The most clinically significant toxic effect is thought to be the reversible combination of arsenic with sulfhydryl groups. This leads to the inhibition of many enzyme systems. Blockage of the Krebs cycle and interference with oxidative phosphorylation lead to depletion of cellular energy stores, disruption of multiple metabolic systems, and cell death. A secondary mechanism disrupting oxidative phosphorylation is termed *arsenolysis,* in which arsenic is substituted for phosphate (Schoolmeester and White 1980).

Neuropsychiatric manifestations. Ingestion of large amounts of arsenic in homicide or suicide attempts frequently results in acute intoxication. Initial symptoms of a metallic taste and garlic breath odor begin within 30 minutes to several hours after ingestion and progress to profound gastrointestinal inflammation and varying degrees of circulatory collapse from generalized vasodilation. CNS symptoms include drowsiness, headache, vertigo, stupor, encephalopathy, delirium, convulsions, and coma

(Landrigan 1982; Schoolmeester and White 1980; Zaloga et al. 1985). Neuropathologically, it is thought that capillary damage leads to cerebral edema and focal microhemorrhages (Schoolmeester and White 1980) with multiple symmetrical foci of hemorrhagic necrosis present in both the gray and white matter (Klaassen 1985a). Less common manifestations of acute toxicity include optic atrophy and CNS depression without gastrointestinal symptoms (Schoolmeester and White 1980) and prolonged encephalopathy and/or psychosis (Louria 1988). In severe arsenic exposures, death usually occurs within 1–4 days from circulatory collapse (Ellenhorn and Barceloux 1988).

A symmetrical sensorimotor polyneuropathy is the most prominent feature after the first week of acute intoxication (Louria 1988) and is a hallmark of chronic arsenic poisoning (Schoolmeester and White 1980). The lower extremities are affected first. Sensory symptoms predominate initially and include paresthesias, numbness, and pain in a stocking-glove distribution. Motor involvement may progress from weakness to muscle atrophy with loss of reflexes to paralysis in prolonged poisoning. Microscopically, demyelination and axonal degeneration progress to nerve atrophy and perineural fibrosis in chronic poisoning (Schoolmeester and White 1980).

Cranial nerves are usually spared in chronic arsenic intoxication, but visual changes, optic neuritis, vestibular toxicity, and facial nerve palsy have been reported (Schoolmeester and White 1980; Zaloga et al. 1985). Encephalopathy may be a rare initial presentation of chronic poisoning; headache, personality changes, seizures, or coma may occur but are much more common in acute intoxication. Neurosis or psychosis may be present, and the encephalopathy may resemble the Wernicke-Korsakoff syndrome secondary to arsenic's interference with thiamine metabolism (Schoolmeester and White 1980). Cases of both acute and chronic encephalopathies have been reported with occupational exposure to arsenic (Beckett et al. 1986; Morton and Caron 1989).

Acute arsine gas poisoning is frequently fatal from hemolysis and/or renal failure. Associated neuropsychiatric features may include headache, paresthesias, and encephalopathy characterized by agitation and disorientation (Klaassen 1985a; Louria 1988). Survivors may develop signs of chronic arsenic intoxication.

Diagnosis. A history of arsenic exposure and recognition of clinical signs are extremely important. Severe abdominal pain with bloody diarrhea, albuminuria, and a garlic breath odor are commonly seen in acute arsenic poisoning. Chronic intoxication is often insidious and overlooked diagnostically; it should be considered in patients with combinations of neuropathy, skin rash, and gastrointestinal and blood disturbances (Schoolmeester and White 1980).

Aldrich-Mee's lines are transverse whitish bands from arsenic deposits in fingernails and may be seen in acute and chronic poisoning. Because of arsenic's short half-life in blood, blood levels may be helpful only for same-day exposure. Urine levels are more accurate for recent exposures (1–2 days); dietary contamination of foods with arsenic must be ruled out. Normally, urine levels are less than 50 µg/L. Levels between 100 µg/L and 200 µg/L suggest arsenic intoxication, and levels greater than 200 µg/L indicate significant exposure; elevated urine levels may persist for 1–2 months after absorption (Ellenhorn and Barceloux 1988).

Analysis of arsenic in hair may confirm chronic toxicity but does not discriminate between internally and externally deposited arsenic. Screening tests for the presence of arsenic in urine (Gutzeit test) and in gastric contents (Reinsch's test) are described elsewhere (Schoolmeester and White 1980).

Treatment and prognosis. If the patient presents within the first few hours after acute arsenic ingestion, attempts should be made to remove arsenic by emesis, gastric lavage, activated charcoal, and a cathartic; hemodialysis may be helpful as an adjunct only in the presence of renal failure and is otherwise not indicated (Schoolmeester and White 1980). Exposed skin surfaces should be thoroughly cleaned. Care must be taken to maintain intravascular volume with intravenous fluids; pressor agents may be added if necessary.

Topical dimercaprol may be helpful in dermal exposures. Chelation with parenteral dimercaprol is indicated in symptomatic acute arsenic exposures except for arsine gas and should be administered as early as possible to minimize systemic toxicity. The benefit of dimercaprol in chronic poisoning is unclear; it may be helpful for hematologic disturbances, but it usually does not affect the neurological symptoms (Schoolmeester and White 1980). Penicillamine is used adjunctively in serious acute intoxications, but oral penicillamine alone may be sufficient after chronic arsenic exposure (Klaassen 1985a). The length of chelation therapy depends on the patient's clinical condition and periodic monitoring of urinary arsenic levels.

In arsine gas poisoning, initial decontamination and supportive measures are followed by exchange transfusions and forced alkaline diuresis. Dimercaprol has not been shown to be effective and is not recommended (Klaassen 1985a).

Accurate diagnosis, removal from exposure, and early institution of dimercaprol therapy for acute arsenic intoxication may be helpful in preventing neuropathy (Zaloga et al. 1985). As mentioned above, chelation therapy does not usually help the manifestations of chronic poisoning. These may slowly resolve completely, or there may be permanent neurological sequelae, ranging from mild to severe (Louria 1988).

Aluminum

Background. Aluminum is one of the most abundant elements in the earth's crust. In the environment it exists in the oxidative state in combination with other elements. Despite its environmental abundance, healthy persons are at little risk for developing aluminum toxicity. Aluminum is poorly absorbed through the gastrointestinal tract and once absorbed is bound to protein. Both biliary and renal elimination takes place. Accumulation of aluminum in the body tends to occur when either the gastrointestinal absorption barrier is bypassed (e.g., parenteral introduction) or renal excretion is impaired; patients with renal failure are particularly at risk. Medical sources of aluminum exposure include aluminum-containing antacids and phosphate-binding gels, as well as contaminated dialysis solutions, total parenteral nutrition (TPN) solutions, and human serum albumin used in plasmapheresis (Monteagudo et al. 1989). Occupational exposure occurs in the aluminum production industry.

Action. The exact mechanism for aluminum neurotoxicity is unknown. Aluminum has been shown to alter the function of the blood-brain barrier by affecting membrane function, and it has been postulated that many of aluminum's effects on the CNS and peripheral tissues can be explained by its actions as a membrane toxin (Banks and Kastin 1989).

Neuropsychiatric manifestations. Reports of neurotoxicity in aluminum workers have been isolated and inconclusive (Ellenhorn and Barceloux 1988). Intraneuronal aluminum accumulation has been demonstrated in patients with ALS and parkinsonism dementia of Guam—one of three western Pacific regions (the others being southern West New Guinea and the Kii Peninsula of Japan) with unusually high incidences of these disorders (Perl et al. 1982). Senile dementia of the Alzheimer type (SDAT) is associated with the intranuclear presence of aluminum in neurons with neurofibrillary changes but not in adjacent normal appearing neurons (Perl and Brody 1980). Total body aluminum levels appear to be normal in Alzheimer's patients (Alfrey 1983); reports of elevated aluminum in the brains of these patients may reflect an age-associated phenomenon because other studies have shown no difference in the aluminum concentration between SDAT patients and age-matched control subjects (Wisniewski and Sturman 1989). Despite the association between the presence of aluminum and these degenerative nervous system disorders, no etiologic role for aluminum has been established.

Dialysis dementia is a progressive encephalopathy described in patients on long-term renal dialysis. Initial symptoms include speech difficulties and electroencephalographic (EEG) changes (e.g., generalized slowing, periodic bursts of delta activity, and occasional spike and wave complexes). Over a period of months these initial manifestations are followed by the development of dyspraxia, asterixis, tremor, myoclonus, memory loss, and personality changes. In the late stages, seizures and progressive deterioration of speech and motor coordination are frequently followed by death, which usually occurs within 6–9 months of the initial symptoms (Wisniewski and Sturman 1989).

Increased aluminum in the brain gray matter of patients who died of this syndrome led Alfrey et al. (1976) to propose aluminum intoxication as the etiology. This remains the commonly accepted theory resulting from exposure to aluminum-containing dialysis solutions and phosphate-binding gels. Unlike Alzheimer's dementia, patients dying from dialysis encephalopathy do not demonstrate neurofibrillary degeneration; aluminum accumulates in the cytoplasm and lysosomes of histologically normal-appearing neurons throughout the central gray matter, and brain and total body aluminum levels are markedly increased (Alfrey 1983; Wisniewski and Sturman 1989).

Diagnosis. Identifying a history of exposure in patients at risk (e.g., those with renal failure) is extremely important. Because aluminum is highly protein bound, serum levels may not reflect total body burden. Average serum aluminum levels are less than 10 µg/ml; asymptomatic dialysis patients may have levels up to 50 µg/ml. Levels greater than 60 µg/ml are indicative of increased absorption. Toxicity may appear at levels above 100 µg/ml, and serum aluminum concentrations greater than 200 µg/ml are usually associated with clinical symptoms (Ellenhorn and Barceloux 1988).

Treatment and prognosis. The management of aluminum toxicity begins with identifying the source of aluminum exposure and eliminating it if possible. Removing aluminum from water used for dialysis has reduced the incidence and morbidity of dialysis encephalopathy. Elimination or reduction of aluminum-containing medications and phosphate-binding gels should be attempted if the patient's clinical situation will permit. Calcium carbonate may be substituted as it has been shown to effectively bind phosphate in both adults and children with chronic renal failure (Monteagudo et al. 1989). Chelation of aluminum with deferoxamine has been helpful in the treatment of dialysis dementia, but the best mode of administration, optimum dose, and duration of treatment are not clearly established; potential side effects include anaphylactic reactions, visual disturbances, ototoxicity, opportunistic infections, and depletion of other trace metals (Monteagudo et al. 1989). Successful renal transplantation early in the course of dialysis encephalopathy has been associated with gradual although often incomplete recovery. Because transplantation late in the course of the disease does not halt the downhill progression, diagnosis at an early, potentially reversible stage is essential (Parkinson et al. 1981).

Manganese

Background. Manganese is an essential trace element used in the production of metal alloys, dry-cell batteries, and various chemicals. It is found in paints, ceramics, glass, inks, dyes, matches, pigments, welding rods, fungicides, fertilizers, and antiknock gasoline additives. Toxic exposure is strictly occupational, with most cases reported in the mining and processing of manganese ores; intoxication has also been reported in metal workers and persons working in fertilizer preparation and the dry-cell battery industry (Emara et al. 1971; Hine and Pasi 1975; Wang et al. 1989). Recently, exposure to a manganese-containing pesticide was reported as a possible source of CNS manganese intoxication in agricultural workers (Ferraz et al. 1988). Due to the low solubility of inorganic manganese, gastrointestinal absorption and dermal absorption are negligible. Toxicity results from chronic inhalation of dust and fumes containing mainly manganese dioxide. Symptoms usually follow months to years of exposure.

Action. The exact mechanism of manganese neurotoxicity is unknown. The similarity between the clinical features of manganese intoxication and Parkinson's disease has implicated dopamine in the pathophysiology and has led to numerous hypotheses (Huang et al. 1989; Parenti et al. 1988).

Neuropsychiatric manifestations. Chronic manganese intoxication (manganism) begins insidiously, often with complaints of anorexia, apathy, sleep disturbance, and impaired motor performance. Manganese miners, but not manufacturers, may present with a transient psychiatric disturbance characterized by psychomotor agitation, hallucinations, emotional lability, compulsions, and aberrant behavior; this syndrome has been termed *manganese madness* and lasts from 1 to 3 months whether the miner is removed from the mine or not (Cook et al. 1974; Huang et al. 1989).

Other symptoms of chronic manganese intoxication include malaise, somnolence, gait imbalance, decreased libido, impotence, speech difficulty, impaired fine motor movements, and limb stiffness. Less frequent complaints are tremor, paresthesias, cramps, memory loss, dysphagia, urinary urgency or incontinence, lumbosacral pain, metallic taste, nervousness, and anorexia (Cook et al. 1974).

Neurological signs in chronic poisoning include bradykinesia, gait disturbance, postural instability, impaired arising ability, masked facies, disordered speech, rigidity, tremor, micrographia, and dystonia. Psychiatric abnormalities also occur, such as depression, anxiety, emotional lability, compulsive acts, inappropriate affect, pathological laughter, and impaired memory and calculation ability (Cook et al. 1974; Hine and Pasi 1975).

The extensive extrapyramidal symptomatology described above results in a clinical picture of parkinsonism. However, unlike in Parkinson's disease, neuropathological changes in autopsy specimens of patients with manganese intoxication have shown degeneration of the medial segment of the globus pallidus, frequently of the caudate nucleus and the putamen, and rarely of the substantia nigra (Huang et al. 1989).

Diagnosis. The diagnosis of chronic manganese intoxication depends on the presence of clinical signs and symptoms along with a positive history of manganese exposure. There are no specific diagnostic tests, although elevated manganese levels in blood and urine may confirm an increased level of exposure. Normal manganese levels are 2–8 μg/dl in blood and 0.1–0.8 μg/dl in urine (Hine and Pasi 1975). Chelation with $CaNa_2EDTA$ may lead to increased manganese excretion in nonexposed control subjects as well as intoxicated patients; whereas urinary excretion after EDTA is not useful as a diagnostic test, improvement in clinical symptoms after administration of EDTA may suggest a diagnosis of manganese intoxication (Cook et al. 1974).

Treatment and prognosis. Manganese workers who develop symptoms and signs of intoxication should be removed from further exposure. If this is done early in the course of the illness, some signs may slowly resolve. In most cases the disability stabilizes after removal, but occasionally the symptoms progress. Speech deficits and tremor may improve with time; gait disturbances show little change (Cook et al. 1974). Chronic psychosis has been reported (Emara et al. 1971). Young patients and those with shorter durations of exposure have a better prognosis, with reports of complete recovery (Hine and Pasi 1975). Treatment with levodopa (L-dopa) and $CaNa_2EDTA$ have been associated with some improvement, but their therapeutic benefit remains inconsistent and controversial (Cook et al. 1974; Hine and Pasi 1975; Huang et al. 1989).

Thallium

Background. Thallium sulfate is recognized as a deadly poison. Historically, thallium was used in the late 19th century as a treatment for venereal disease, gout, dysentery, and tuberculosis and in the early 20th century as a treatment for ringworm of the scalp and as a dermatologic depilatory agent. Significant and sometimes fatal side effects led to its abandonment in medicinal compounds. More recently, thallium sulfate was used as an insecticide and rodenticide, but numerous cases of toxicity and death from accidental and suicidal ingestions resulted in restricted use and, since 1965, the total prohibition of thallium use in the United States. However, thallium-containing compounds are still available in other countries, including Mexico, and isolated cases of thallotoxicosis continue to appear (J. G. Schwartz et al. 1988).

Thallium is well absorbed from the gastrointestinal tract and can be absorbed via the skin and lungs. It is widely distributed intracellularly and is eliminated primarily via the feces, although renal excretion does occur (Ellenhorn and Barceloux 1988).

Action. The exact mechanism of thallium toxicity is uncertain. Like other heavy metals, it has an affinity for mitochondrial sulfhydryl groups and interferes with a variety of enzyme reactions, including oxidative phosphorylation (Ellenhorn and Barceloux 1988).

Neuropsychiatric manifestations. Acute thallium poisoning, often from the ingestion of large amounts of thallium-containing rat poisons, is frequently fatal. Initial symptoms are gastrointestinal, and they usually begin within 12–24 hours after ingestion. Neurological manifestations appear in 2–5 days and include paresthesias, muscle weakness, delirium, hallucinations, cranial nerve palsies, blindness, seizures, and coma; death due to respiratory paralysis may result in 5–7 days after large ingestions (Goldblatt 1984; Reed et al. 1963; Wainwright et al. 1988).

Oral or dermal exposure to smaller amounts of thallium-containing compounds may result in chronic thallium intoxication. Alopecia and neurological symptoms predominate, and the onset is often insidious. Hair loss begins about 10 days after thallium ingestion and reaches a maximum after about 1 month (Reed et al. 1963). Both the peripheral and central nervous systems may be involved. Paresthesias, particularly of the lower extremities, and hyperesthesias of the palms and soles may progress to a combined sensorimotor polyneuropathy (Ellenhorn and Barceloux 1988; Reed et al. 1963). CNS effects include tremor, chorea, athetosis, myoclonus, and ataxia; encephalopathy may be reflected by alterations in consciousness, delirium, seizures, and coma. Mental abnormalities include confusion, psychosis, paranoia, depression, and retardation (Reed et al. 1963; Thompson et al. 1988). A case of severe deterioration in intellectual function, particularly in memory and performance abilities, has been described (Thompson et al. 1988).

Examination of affected peripheral nerves has revealed demyelination as well as axonal and neuronal degeneration. CNS changes in thallium poisoning include engorgement of cortical blood vessels, edema of the pial and arachnoid membranes, and swelling and various degrees of degeneration of neurons in the brain and spinal cord (Reed et al. 1963).

Diagnosis. Thallium is not detected by routine heavy metal or other toxicology screens. Intoxication should be considered in patients with alopecia and a burning peripheral neuropathy (J. G. Schwartz et al. 1988). Measurement of thallium in the blood confirms exposure, with blood levels greater than 30 μg/dl indicating serious ingestion. Urine levels are less helpful because of the extensive fecal elimination of thallium (Ellenhorn and Barceloux 1988).

Treatment and prognosis. Emesis, gastric lavage, activated charcoal, and cathartics may be used to attempt to remove thallium from the gastrointestinal tract within the first few hours of exposure, but their benefit may be limited because of the usual delay in onset of clinical symptoms. Serial doses of activated charcoal may be helpful in acute overdose as most of the thallium initially remains in the gut. Although not approved by the FDA, Prussian blue, the crystal blue lattice of potassium ferricyanoferrate, binds thallium and increases fecal excretion by exchanging thallium for potassium (Ellenhorn and Barceloux 1988). Orally administered Prussian blue and laxatives and forced diuresis with potassium chloride loading are advocated for the treatment of acute thallium poisoning; hemodialysis may be helpful if there are high serum levels or impairment in renal function (Wainwright et al. 1988).

Large acute thallium ingestions have been associated with significant mortality. Follow-up studies in thallium poisoning are limited. In a retrospective study of 72 children with thallotoxicosis (Reed et al. 1963), there was a 13% mortality rate, and 54% of the 48 patients who survived and were followed for an average of 4 years demonstrated neurological disturbances. Mental abnormalities (retardation and psychosis) were the most common findings, followed by abnormal reflexes, ataxia, tremors, seizures, muscle weakness or paralysis, movement disorders, and visual disturbances. More recent reports have indicated neurological sequelae of flaccid paraparesis, cerebellar ataxia, and intellectual impairment in a patient 1 year after acute thallium poisoning (Thompson et al. 1988; Wainwright et al. 1988).

❑ ORGANOPHOSPHATES

Background. Organophosphates are anticholinesterases that were used first as insecticides and later for chemical warfare (nerve gas). The first synthesis was of tetraethyl pyrophosphate (TEPP) in 1854. More than 50,000 organophosphates have been synthesized with 36 currently in commercial use. Generally, exposure occurs via contact with pesticides. Occupational exposure, which can be chronic, is commonly dermal or pulmonary. In suicidal or homicidal presentations, exposure is usually by oral ingestion (Taylor 1985). In 1982 there were 1,400 reported cases of work-related illness secondary to pesticides in California; it has been estimated that less than 1% of such cases are actually reported (Kahn 1976).

Action. Organophosphates act as hemisubstrates, which bind to the anticholinesterase enzyme, creating a stable, generally irreversible, inactive compound. This leads to accumulation of acetylcholine in the neuronal gap. Acute intoxication is due to muscarinic, nicotinic, and CNS effects. Muscarinic symptomatology is due to potentiation of postganglionic parasympathetic activity mostly on smooth muscle sites. Nicotinic action results from accumulation of acetylcholine at the motor end plate and autonomic ganglion, which leads to depolarization of skeletal muscles. CNS effects cause initial stimulation and later depression of all activity and coma (Worrell 1975). There is also described a delayed neurotoxicity with a Wallerian degeneration of axons, which starts focally in large myelinated fibers (Barret and Oehme 1985).

Neuropsychiatric manifestations. In a study of 236 patients (Lerman et al. 1984), 40% presented with CNS symptoms. These included giddiness, subjective tension, anxiety, restlessness, labile mood, insomnia, headache, tremor, nightmares, increased dreaming, apathy, withdrawal and depression, drowsiness, confusion, slurred speech, ataxia, generalized weakness, and coma with absence of reflexes.

Onset of action can be quite sudden (5 minutes) in massive ingestion. Usual presentation is 4–12 hours after exposure. Exceptions are the highly lipophilic organophosphates, which have mild initial symptoms followed by severe cholinergic symptoms 48 hours later. Duration depends on severity of exposure; mild to moderate acute symptoms usually resolve within 1 month.

Chronic effects include both polyneuropathies and neurobehavioral changes. The polyneuropathies include delayed sensorimotor peripheral neuropathies that occur 8–14 days after exposure and are not necessarily preceded by acute cholinergic symptoms (Barret and Oehme 1985). Persistent neuropsychiatric symptoms include drowsiness, lability, depression, fatigue, anxiety, and irritability (Tabershaw and Cooper 1966). One study (Savage et al. 1980) showed that the subject's assessment of impairment was much greater than the assessment by their relatives. In other studies (Levin et al. 1976; Rodnitzky et al. 1975), pesticide applicators showed higher anxiety scales but no visuomotor or memory problems. An older study of 16 patients (Gershon and Shaw 1961) showed memory and concentration deficits that interfered with work and reading ability. Most of the persistent symptoms that develop from acute exposure resolve in less than a year.

Diagnosis. Diagnosis is usually made by obtaining a history of exposure to pesticides. A garlic odor from either the patient or the container can sometimes aid in the diagnosis. Inhibition of acetylcholinesterase is a confirming test in conjunction with history of exposure. The red blood cell cholinesterase is the preferred marker because it measures the same enzyme active in nervous tissue. With acute exposure, there can be a 50% decrease in baseline cholinesterase levels. In mild to moderate exposure, there is return to normal levels in several weeks (Ellenhorn and Barceloux 1988).

Treatment and prognosis. The first response must be to stabilize any vital sign abnormalities. Atropine will noncompetitively antagonize both muscarinic and CNS effects. Decontamination procedures include removing contaminated clothing and washing exposed skin surfaces. Because of possible potentiation of the organophosphates, the use of phenothiazines, antihistamines, tricyclics, and anticholinergics should be avoided; CNS depressants can increase the possibility of respiratory depression.

Full resolution is expected of acute CNS symptoms if appropriate and prompt treatment is rendered. However, persistent CNS effects (irritability, fatigue, lethargy, poor memory, depression, and psychosis) have been seen in a few survivors (Ellenhorn and Barceloux 1988).

❑ ORGANIC SOLVENTS

Background and action. Organic solvents are found in a variety of substances. Selected solvents with neuropsychiatric toxicities are listed in Table 23–3.

Toluene is found in plastic cement, airplane model cement, lacquer thinner, ink, liquid shoe polish, cleaning fluid, and other industrial solvents; it is also used as a replacement for benzene. Acetone is contained in fingernail polish remover and plastic cement (Ellenhorn and Barceloux 1988).

Benzene, tolulene, propylene glycol, and ethylene glycol act like CNS depressants. Benzene exposure can occur via ingestion or breathing. Ethylene glycol is absorbed only by ingestion; propylene glycol has low oral and dermal toxicity.

Most of the halogenated hydrocarbons such as carbon tetrachloride, trichlorethylene, and trichloroethane are lipid soluble and metabolically stable. Thus they are easily absorbed via the gastrointestinal tract, skin, or respiratory surfaces. Most of the aliphatic hydrocarbons act as CNS depressants (Klaassen 1985b). Organic lead found in gasoline causes the neuropsychiatric sequelae in chronic gasoline abuse (discussed above).

Of the alcohol solvents, isopropyl alcohol (isopropanol) is prominent for universality in industrial and home settings. It is found in large concentrations in such items as frost remover, windshield washer solvent, antifreeze, rubbing alcohol, dog repellent, rust preventive, and gasket cement (Lacouture et al. 1983). Poisoning occurs from ingestion

TABLE 23–3. SELECTED ORGANIC SOLVENTS WITH NEUROPSYCHIATRIC TOXICITIES

Alcohols	**Glycols**
Isopropanol	Ethylene glycol
Methanol	Propylene glycol
Aliphatic hydrocarbons	**Halogenated hydrocarbons**
Hexane	Carbon tetrachloride
Aromatic hydrocarbons	Trichloroethane
Benzene	Trichloroethylene
Toluene	**Ketones**
Xylene	Acetone

and inhalation. The toxic oral dose of isopropyl alcohol in adults is 1 ml/kg body weight, but symptoms are possible at 0.5 ml/kg body weight. As few as three swallows of 70% isopropyl alcohol can produce symptoms in children (Ellenhorn and Barceloux 1988). Isopropyl alcohol is a CNS depressant, and its metabolite acetone is believed to contribute to the symptoms.

Methyl alcohol (methanol) is found in 95% concentration in antifreeze and 35%–95% in windshield washer fluid. As little as 10 ml of 40% methyl alcohol can cause serious neurological effects. Methyl alcohol itself has CNS depressant effects, and poisoning occurs when its metabolites formaldehyde and formic acid are created. Formaldehyde is rapidly converted to formic acid, which acts to inhibit intracellular oxidation. The level of toxicity correlates best with the production of formic acid (Ellenhorn and Barceloux 1988).

Neuropsychiatric manifestations. The hydrocarbons act as CNS depressants and can lead to dizziness and incoordination. Hexane has been noted to cause a reversible polyneuropathy.

Toluene exposure can lead to three syndromes, one of them being a neuropsychiatric syndrome (Streicher et al. 1981). The symptoms include headache, dizziness, vertigo, syncope, sensorimotor neuropathy, cerebellar signs, hallucinations, emotional lability, personality changes, lethargy, and coma (Ellenhorn and Barceloux 1988).

Mild acute exposure to benzene presents with dizziness, weakness, euphoria, and headache, whereas severe acute exposure can cause blurred vision, tremor, and unconsciousness. Chronic exposure leads to loss of appetite, drowsiness, and nonspecific anxiety (Klaassen 1985b).

Acetone and xylene exposure can lead to initial CNS excitement. With acetone this is often followed by lethargy, stupor, or coma. Chronic xylene exposure can cause cerebral and cerebellar degeneration.

Ethylene glycol has a three-stage presentation of intoxication, the first of which has prominent neuropsychiatric symptoms. Within the first 12 hours after ingestion, transient excitation occurs followed by convulsions, myoclonic jerks, nystagmus, and ophthalmoplegia. Further CNS depression is caused by cerebral edema (Ellenhorn and Barceloux 1988). Propylene glycol, besides acting as a CNS depressant, can also cause seizures and hypoglycemia (Demey et al. 1984).

Various visual symptoms have been described in methyl alcohol poisoning, including blurred vision and photophobia as well as signs such as retinal edema, fixed pupils, and constricted visual fields (Swartz et al. 1981). Mild intoxication can cause headache, vertigo, lethargy, and confusion. Higher levels can lead to coma and convulsions via cerebral edema. Putamen necrosis and a permanent Parkinson-like syndrome have also occurred (Ellenhorn and Barceloux 1988).

Treatment and prognosis. Stabilization and supportive care are the primary treatment goals. The solvent must be identified, and metabolic complications associated with that solvent must be assessed. Electrolyte disturbances and acute tubular necrosis require aggressive treatment. If mouth-to-mouth resuscitation is required, the possibility of transfer of the inhalant to the rescuer should be noted (Ellenhorn and Barceloux 1988). With isopropyl alcohol ingestions, gut decontamination, elimination enhancement via dialysis, and supportive care can quickly reduce the effects. The primary antidote for methyl alcohol poisoning is ethyl alcohol, which inhibits the enzyme alcohol dehydrogenase from creating formaldehyde and formic acid. Folic acid is also given as a cofactor to facilitate the conversion of formic acid to carbon dioxide (Ellenhorn and Barceloux 1988). Despite prompt therapy, 25% of visual defects do not resolve (Swartz et al. 1981).

With both ethylene glycol and propylene glycol intoxications, supportive care and decontamination are the mainstays for treatment. Ethyl alcohol infusion is used with ethylene glycol poisoning to block the enzymatic formation of toxic metabolites (Gabow et al. 1986). The cofactors pyridoxine and thiamine are given to promote the conversion of ethylene glycol to nontoxic products (Ellenhorn and Barceloux 1988).

❑ CARBON MONOXIDE

Background. Carbon monoxide is a colorless, tasteless, and generally undetectable gas that is formed from incomplete combustion of organic matter. It is the leading cause of poisoning deaths in the United States (3,500–4,000 a year) (Ellenhorn and Barceloux 1988). Many deaths occur from automobiles or inadequate venting of furnaces. From 15% to 40% of persons with serious nonlethal carbon monoxide poisoning develop neuropsychiatric symptoms, which can appear after apparent recovery (Ginsburg and Pomano 1976).

The average concentration of carbon monoxide in the atmosphere is about 0.1 parts per million (ppm). An automobile can produce concentrations of up to 115 ppm, with underground garages and tunnels having levels greater than 100 ppm for extended periods of time. Catalytic converters have decreased carbon monoxide emissions considerably (Klaassen 1985b).

Cigarette smoking is another significant source of carbon monoxide. Endogenous production of carbon monoxide results in a blood carboxyhemoglobin (COHb) level of 0.4%–0.7%. A one-pack-a-day smoker has a COHb level of 5%–6%, and a two- to three-pack-a-day smoker has a COHb level of 7%–9% (Ellenhorn and Barceloux 1988). Passive inhalation of carbon monoxide can occur (with secondhand smoke).

Heating equipment such as charcoal grills, kerosene space heaters, and hibachis can give off carbon monoxide in closed spaces. Paint removers can be another source of carbon monoxide from in vivo conversion of methylene chloride. COHb levels of up to 50% have been recorded after methylene chloride exposure (Fagin et al. 1980). Any survivor of a fire is especially at risk for carbon monoxide exposure.

Action. Carbon monoxide combines with hemoglobin to form COHb. Hemoglobin in this form cannot perform its primary function of carrying oxygen. The affinity of hemoglobin for carbon monoxide is more than 200 times greater than that for oxygen. This high affinity makes carbon monoxide potent and very dangerous. The amount of oxygen available to the tissues is also affected by the inhibitory influence of COHb on the dissociation of any oxyhemoglobin. The concentration of the gas in the air, the duration of exposure, the respiratory minute volume, the cardiac output, the oxygen demand of the tissues, preexisting cerebral vascular disease, and anemia will help determine the toxicity of carbon monoxide (Klaassen 1985b). The increased metabolic activity of children makes them more susceptible than adults to the effects of carbon monoxide.

Neuropsychiatric manifestations. The presentation can look very similar to that of hypoxia. High concentrations of carbon monoxide may give no warning before producing loss of consciousness; however, there are often preliminary signs of transient weakness and dizziness.

At 20% COHb, one can see headaches with throbbing temples. This headache is characteristically bandlike. At 30% COHb, there is irritability, disturbed judgment, fatigue, dizziness, and dimming of vision. At 40%–50% COHb, there is increasing confusion and collapse. At 60%–70% COHb, the patient can present with unconsciousness, convulsions, and death if exposure is prolonged (Winter and Miller 1976). The severe headache following exposure to carbon monoxide is believed to be caused by cerebral edema and increased intracranial pressure from excessive transudation across capillaries. Gross pathological changes in the brain show congestion and/or edema, petechiae, hemorrhagic focal necrosis, and perivascular infarct. Bilateral necrosis of the globus pallidus is the characteristic lesion of carbon monoxide toxicity. Other vulnerable gray matter areas include the substantia nigra, hippocampus, cerebral cortex, and cerebellum (Ginsberg 1985). These histopathological changes are hard to differentiate from etiologies such as cardiorespiratory arrest, hypoglycemia, cyanide poisoning, and hypoxia (Ginsburg and Pomano 1976). The anoxic leukoencephalopathy has a "motheaten" appearance in the gray matter of the cerebral cortex, globus pallidus, thalamus, and cerebellar cortex (Garland and Pearce 1967). Other studies have shown extensive demyelination of the white matter, bilateral necrosis of the globus pallidus, and necrotic lesions of Ammon's horn (Brucher 1967; Lapresle and Fardeau 1967).

After initial recovery from carbon monoxide exposure, patients may develop neurological symptoms of apathy, mutism, amnesia, irritability, personality changes, confusion, memory loss, and visual changes within 2–4 weeks of exposure (Myers et al. 1985). Cerebellar signs are unusual. A recent case was reported of a 39-year-old man who suffered carbon monoxide poisoning and developed anterograde and retrograde amnesia, bulimia, hypersexuality, and placidity (Starkstein et al. 1989). After approximately 3 weeks, the placidity and anterograde amnesia continued along with new symptoms of akinesia and abnormal involuntary movements. A computed tomography (CT) scan showed bilateral low-density lesions involving the globus pallidus.

Diagnosis. Laboratory tests are generally not helpful. Clinical features are at best roughly correlative with COHb levels. As mentioned above, environmental factors and patient susceptibility have strong influences.

Abnormal EEG findings are common and can reflect the progression of hypoxic encephalopathy. EEGs are not thought to have much predictive value because patients with markedly abnormal EEGs may show complete recovery (Ellenhorn and Barceloux 1988). Common EEG findings include low-voltage waves and diffuse slow waves.

Treatment and prognosis. The first step should be transfer from the contaminated environment to fresh air. Control of airway, support of breathing with high oxygen concentration (preferably 100%), and cardiac monitoring should also be initiated. Supplemental oxygen should be continued until COHb is significantly reduced (Ellenhorn and Barceloux 1988).

The use of hyperbaric oxygen is controversial. There have been no large prospective clinical studies to show that hyperbaric oxygen therapy is superior to high concentrations of oxygen. In a series of almost 3,000 patients hospitalized for acute carbon monoxide poisoning (Min 1986), 2.7% developed delayed neuropsychiatric symptoms. Of these patients, 37% received hyperbaric oxygen following the acute exposure.

Rates of complete recovery from carbon-monoxide–induced hypoxic unconsciousness are inversely related to the age of the patient (Bokorjic 1963).

The level of consciousness on initial evaluation has some correlation with subsequent development of gross neuropsychiatric sequelae (Smith and Brandon 1973). However, loss of consciousness is not necessary for developing delayed neurological problems (Min 1986). Up to 75% of the neuropsychiatric sequelae, except memory deficits and gait disturbances, resolve after 1 year (Lee 1978).

❑ BIOLOGICAL TOXINS

Biological toxins are found in abundance throughout the animal and plant kingdoms. Table 23–4 lists various food-borne neurotoxins and their sources. The brief discussion of selected toxicities that follows is provided to illustrate the variety of causes and neuropsychiatric manifestations of these illnesses. The more "classic" botulism toxin is presented in detail, followed by two marine toxins with particular neuropsychiatric sequelae and a discussion of poisonous snake envenomation.

Botulinum Toxin

Background. Botulinum toxin, produced by *Clostridium botulinum*, is the most potent natural poison by weight known to man. There are seven distinct botulinum toxins of which three (A, B, and E) can

TABLE 23–4. NEUROPSYCHIATRIC EFFECTS OF SELECTED FOOD-BORNE NEUROTOXINS

Source	*Neurotoxin*	*Symptoms and signs*
Contaminated home-canned food, preserved fish, and meat products	Enterotoxin *Clostridium botulinum*	Cranial nerve palsy (blurred vision and diplopia), bulbar palsy (dysarthria and dysphagia), and descending paralysis
Contaminated large reef fish (snapper, grouper, and barracuda)	Ciguatoxin *Gambierdiscus toxicus*	Paresthesias, heat-cold sensation reversal, and depression
Contaminated mussels	Domoic acid *Nitzchia pungens*	Confusion, disorientation, and anterograde amnesia
Contaminated scombroid fish (tuna, mackerel, and albacore)	Histamine	Headache and dizziness
Puffer fish	Tetrodotoxin	Paresthesias, lightheadedness, and feeling of impending doom
Paralytic shellfish	Neurotoxin	Paresthesias, dysphagia, and respiratory paralysis

Sources. Bartlett 1988; Ellenhorn and Barceloux 1988; Lipkin 1989; Morrow et al. 1991; Teitelbaum et al. 1990.

cause human toxicity. Home-canned foods are the most common source of the toxin. The clostridium spores are heat resistant and can survive boiling to produce toxin in food that was initially cooked and then kept at ambient temperature (Corzine et al. 1985).

Action. The heat-labile toxin binds irreversibly to the neuromuscular junction and impairs the presynaptic release of acetylcholine. This causes nerve conduction to be blocked and results in weakness (Centers for Disease Control 1981).

Neuropsychiatric manifestations. Gastrointestinal symptoms are the first to appear 24–36 hours after ingestion with complaints of nausea, dry mouth, constipation, and sore throat, as well as malaise and generalized weakness (Hughes et al. 1981). Neurological symptoms are delayed, appearing 3–7 days after exposure. Cranial nerve involvement presents with diplopia, ptosis, blurred vision, and lateral rectus palsy. Respiratory failure often follows soon after oculomotor weakness (Terranova et al. 1979). Mental status changes do not frequently occur. Other associated signs include dysarthria, dysphagia, and bilateral descending symmetrical weakness (Ellenhorn and Barceloux 1988).

Diagnosis. *Clostridium botulinum* can be found in stool cultures, whereas the neurotoxin can be isolated from blood or gastric contents.

Treatment and prognosis. If treatment occurs within 24 hours, lavage, emesis, or charcoal are indicated. Equine antitoxin neutralizes toxin in the blood and stops progression of poisoning but does not reverse existing neurological deficits. Patients with a pulmonary vital capacity reduced to 30% should be intubated. Aminoglycosides and polymyxins are contraindicated because of enhanced neuromuscular blockade (Ellenhorn and Barceloux 1988).

Ciguatoxin

Background. The dinoflagellate *Gambierdiscus toxicus,* which produces ciguatoxin, is found attached to algae on tropical reefs and ingested by small herbivorous fish. Larger, predator fish consume the small fish, which concentrates the toxin up the food chain. It then is eaten by humans in the form of barracuda, grouper, snapper, and other large reef fish. The toxin is heat stable, acid stable, tasteless, and odorless, making it very difficult to recognize contaminated fish.

Action. The exact mechanism leading to the toxin's neurological effect is unclear. However it does appear to interact at sodium channels along nerve cell membranes involved with action potentials.

Neuropsychiatric manifestations. Gastrointestinal symptoms including watery diarrhea, nausea, and vomiting occur 6–24 hours after ingestion. Neurological symptoms follow and present with numbness and paresthesias of the extremities, dysphonia, perioral paresthesia, dysphagia, tremor, athetosis, ataxia, headache, dizziness, and blurred vision. A nearly pathognomonic sign is dysesthesia reflecting a heat-cold sensation reversal. The gastrointestinal symptoms resolve in a few days, but the neurological complaints can last for months or even years. There is one report (Lipkin 1989) of major depression with "somatization" felt to be secondary to ciguatera poisoning.

Diagnosis. There are no laboratory tests for identifying ciguatoxin in humans. Diagnosis is by history of ingestion of reef fish followed by the symptoms mentioned above.

Treatment and prognosis. Treatment is mostly supportive. There have been several reports of alleviation of neurological and psychiatric symptoms with amitriptyline (Davis and Villar 1986; Lipkin 1989).

Domoic Acid

Domoic acid is a heat-stable, amino-acid–like neurotoxin created by *Nitzchia pungens*, a pennate phytoplanktonic diatom. Domoic acid has biochemical properties similar to those of kainic acid and glutamic acid, which are both neuroexcitatory.

One recent outbreak of domoic acid toxicity occurred after ingestion of contaminated mussels (Perl et al. 1990; Teitelbaum et al. 1990). Intoxicated individuals experienced confusion and disorientation within 3 days that progressed to agitation, somnolence, or coma. Follow-up of some patients 4–6 months after the ingestion showed individuals with anterograde amnesia, but preservation of other cognitive function. There was also evidence of pure motor or sensorimotor neuropathy. EEGs revealed mild to moderate generalized slowing. Positron-emission tomography (PET) in several patients demonstrated decreased metabolic activity in the cerebral cortex as well as in the amygdala and hippocampus. The autopsy of three patients revealed neuronal necrosis and astrocytosis in the hippocampus and amygdaloid nucleus. At this time, there is no specific treatment.

Snake Envenomation

Background. Poisonous snake bites cause significant morbidity and mortality in certain areas of the world. It has been estimated that more than 30,000 people worldwide die annually from snake bites, with death most commonly occurring from paralysis, followed by shock. In the United States 12–15 fatalities result from approximately 7,000–8,000 bites per year; most of these American deaths are from rattlesnake bites (Nelson 1989).

There are five families of venomous snakes (Table 23–5). Colubridae, Viperidae, and Crotalidae bites usually cause local symptoms and may result in systemic bleeding problems. Hydrophidae bites cause paralysis and myolysis, and Elapidae bites commonly cause neurological symptoms (Nelson 1989).

Action. Venoms are complex mixtures of enzymes and proteins, the composition of which varies between species and results in different symptomatology. Syndromes may include combinations of coagulopathy and bleeding, edema, myonecrosis, shock, renal failure, pituitary failure, and neurotoxicity (Nelson 1989). Both presynaptic and postsynaptic neurotoxins have been identified in sea snake venoms (Tu 1987).

Neuropsychiatric manifestation. Neurotoxicity from elapid and hydrophid envenomation results in serious symptomatology and death in India, Africa, Southeast Asia, and Australia. Symptoms include ptosis, impaired vision, dysarthria, dysphagia, hypersalivation, and paresthesias; muscle weakness may progress to respiratory distress, paralysis, and death (Nelson 1989). Bites from the Eastern coral snake in the United States make up only a small percentage of elapid envenomations; local effects are usually minimal, and presenting symptoms may be delayed as long as 12 hours or more. Up to 25% of bites do not involve envenomation. In a recent series of 39 cases in the United States (Kitchens and Van Mierop 1987), there were no deaths; but neurological symptoms were common, and severe envenomation did occur, resulting in 2 cases of bulbar paralysis that required endotracheal intubation.

Treatment and prognosis. Treatment includes local wound care, supportive measures, tetanus prophylaxis, and antibiotics. Although there is some controversy in the United States, administration of

TABLE 23–5. POISONOUS SNAKE ENVENOMATION

Family	*Geographic distribution (and examples)*	*Prominent toxicity*
Elapidae	Asia (cobras and kraits) Australia (death adders and tiger snake) Americas (coral snakes) Africa (cobras and mambas)	Neurotoxicity
Colubridae	Africa (boomslang and bird snake)	Local effects and anticoagulation
Hydrophidae	Indo-Pacific and west coast of South America (sea snakes)	Neurotoxicity and rhabdomyolysis
Viperidae	Africa, Europe, Mid-East, Asia (vipers and puff adder)	Local symptoms and systemic anticoagulation
Crotalidae	Worldwide (pit vipers) North America (rattlesnakes, copperhead, and cottonmouth)	Local symptoms and systemic coagulopathy

Sources. Nelson 1989; Russell 1980.

Chapter

24

Alcohol-Induced Organic Mental Disorders

John E. Franklin, Jr., M.D.
Richard J. Frances, M.D.

ALCOHOLISM IS ONE OF THE leading public health problems in the United States, directly affecting 14 million people (West et al. 1984). Robins et al. (1984) found that substance abuse disorders rank first among 15 DSM-III (American Psychiatric Association 1980) diagnoses, and lifetime prevalence of alcohol abuse or dependence is 13.6%. The cost to society of alcoholism was estimated to be $136.3 billion for 1990 (Harwood et al. 1985). Mass media campaigns have increased public awareness of the problem. Medical schools and residency programs are becoming increasingly aware of the importance of educating future health care providers about alcoholism. Attention has focused on early identification and prevention in high-risk populations, the search for biological markers, and improvement of legal control and public education. Family history of alcoholism increases the risk of developing alcoholism four- or fivefold in both sexes (Goodwin 1985). Recently, using restriction fragment length polymorphism (RFLP) as a genetic tool, Blum et al. (1990) found allelic association of the human dopamine receptor gene to confer susceptibility to at least one form of alcoholism. An active search using a variety of probes is under way for one or more genes that contribute to susceptibility to alcoholism.

Pathological neuropsychiatric findings in alcoholism are prevalent (Table 24–1). Problems range from transient organic brain syndromes during intoxication to permanent dementia and memory difficulty. Psychiatric and neuropsychological assessment is important in treatment selection and implementation. Effective recognition and treatment of signs and symptoms of alcoholism require knowledge of its major neuropathological findings.

❑ ALCOHOL INTOXICATION

Alcohol intoxication is a common, time-limited, organic condition precipitated by varying amounts of alcohol use. Stages of intoxication can range from

TABLE 24–1. PATHOLOGICAL NEUROPSYCHIATRIC SIGNS AND SYMPTOMS

Syndrome	*Key signs and symptoms*	*Key neuropsychiatric signs and symptoms*	*Time of onset of syndrome*	*Treatment (medication)*
Alcohol intoxication	Disinhibition, sedation at high doses	Acute organic brain syndrome	Rapid; depends on tolerance of individual	Time, protective environment
Alcohol idiosyncratic intoxication	Marked aggressive or assaultive behavior	Absence of focal neurological signs and symptoms	Erratic occurrence	None
Alcohol withdrawal	Tremulousness, irritability, nausea, vomiting, insomnia, malaise, autonomic hyperactivity	Transient sensory disturbances possible	Several hours; peak symptoms 24–48 hours after last drink or relative drop-in level	See Table 24–3
Alcohol seizures	Grand mal seizures in bursts of 2–6 seizures; rarely status epilepticus	Loss of consciousness, tonic-clonic movements, urinary incontinence, post-ictal confusion; look for focal signs	7–38 hours after cessation of alcohol	Diazepam, phenytoin; maintenance phenytoin if underlying seizure disorder is present; prevent by chlordiazepoxide detoxification
Alcohol withdrawal delirium	Confusion, disorientation, fluctuating consciousness, perceptual disturbances, autonomic hyperactivity	Marked variations in levels of consciousness and disorientation; may be fatal	Gradual onset 2–3 days after cessation of alcohol; peak intensity at 4–5 days	Chlordiazepoxide detoxification; haloperidol 2–5 mg po bid for psychotic symptomatology may be added if necessary
Alcohol hallucinosis	Vivid auditory hallucination with affect appropriate to content (often threatening)	Clear sensorium	Usually within 48 hours or less of last drink; may last several weeks	Haloperidol 2–5 mg po bid for psychotic symptoms
Wernicke's	Oculomotor disturbances, cerebellar ataxia	Mental confusion	Abrupt onset; ataxia may precede mental confusion	Thiamine 100 mg iv with $MgSO_4$ 1–2 ml in 50% solution should be given before glucose loading
Korsakoff's	Alcohol stigmata possible	Retrograde and anterograde amnesia; confabulation early; intellectual functioning generally spared	Several days following occurrence of Wernicke's	No effective treatment; institutionalization often needed
Alcohol dementia	Absence of other causes for dementia	Nonprogressing dementia if alcohol free	Associated with greater than 10-year history of drinking	None

mild inebriation to anesthesia, coma, respiratory depression, and (rarely) death. Pathological ramifications include acute delirium, seizures, pathological or idiosyncratic intoxication, and blackouts. Alcohol is a central nervous system depressant that, in low amounts, disinhibits higher cortical activity, producing clinical excitement (Adams and Victor 1981). A direct depressant action on cortical neurons produces sedation at higher blood levels.

Early manifestations of intoxication are believed to result from the preferential involvement of polysynaptic neuronal pathways in the reticular formation of the brain stem, cerebral cortex, and cerebellum (Klemm 1979). Positron-emission tomography (PET) is being used to examine metabolic changes during acute alcohol consumption (Eckardt et al. 1988b). Phenomenological presentations of intoxication depend not only on absolute blood levels but also on the rate of rise of blood alcohol level, duration of consumption, and the tolerance of the individual involved. Women have higher blood alcohol levels than do men after consuming comparable amounts of alcohol, even with allowances for differences in size. Recently, the "first pass" metabolism by gastric tissue has been found to be lower in women alcoholic patients compared with men and this may explain the increased bioavailability of alcohol in women and increased rates of hepatic injury (Frezza et al. 1990).

In nonhabituated persons, alcohol blood levels of 30 mg/dl can lead to mild euphoria, and 50 mg/dl can cause mild coordination problems. Ataxia is present at 100 mg/dl. Confusion and decreased consciousness can occur at 200 mg/dl. Blood levels of 500 mg/dl may produce anesthesia, coma, and even death (Adams and Victor 1981). Minion et al. (1989) reported on a series of 204 consecutive patients in an emergency room setting. The average blood alcohol concentration (BAC) was 467 mg/dl with a range of 400–719 mg/dl. Strikingly, 88% of the patients were oriented to time, person, and place. This is consistent with other reports that find that BACs above 400 mg/dl are common, especially in urban areas, and may not be associated with as serious a morbidity and mortality as previously thought. Due to tolerance, persons with chronic alcoholism consume larger quantities and reach proportionally higher blood levels without obvious signs of drunkenness. When alcohol levels are raised very slowly by gradual consumption or reduced absorption, few symptoms may appear in nonhabituated individuals. An increased degree of neuronal adaptation to alcohol has been proposed as an explanation, but the neurochemical basis is not clearly delineated (Adams and Victor 1981). Acute alcohol intoxication produces deficits in functions associated with prefrontal and temporal lobes (Peterson et al. 1990). Tolerance to alcohol may involve adaptive changes in membrane lipids, neuromodulators, neurotransmitter receptors, ion channels, G proteins, and intracellular second messengers that serve to counteract the short-term effects of ethanol (Charness et al. 1989).

Alcohol intake modifies γ-aminobutyric acid (GABA)-activated inhibitory neurotransmission by stimulating ion flux through chloride channels activated by GABA and dissolves into plasma membrane causing disruption of membrane lipids and proteins (Glowa et al. 1989). The *N*-methyl-D-aspartate (NMDA) receptor of glutamate, an excitatory neurotransmitter, may contribute to cognitive impairments associated with alcohol intoxication. Alcohol affects components of the second messengers system (i.e., adenylate cyclase [AC]) (Tabakoff and Hoffman 1987). Many different neurotransmitter-receptor complexes may be affected by acute intake of alcohol through action on the second messenger system. Alcohol intoxication has also been related to release of epinephrine. Dopaminergic activity may be involved in the reinforcing properties of alcohol, and tolerance has been associated with changes in neuronal calcium channels (Dolin and Little 1989). Inhibition of monoamine oxidase by alcohol may be correlated with excessive alcohol consumption or predisposition to alcoholism (Tabakoff et al. 1988).

Inebriation can produce exhilaration, excitement, and gregariousness, often described by patients with alcoholism as a "glow." Other manifestations are impaired motor performance with poor muscular control, increased risk taking, slurred speech, and ataxia. Thinking is slowed, with impaired concentration, reasoning, attention, judgment, and ability to form word associations (Lishman 1978). Fairly consistent psychophysiological symptoms occur with intoxication: an increase in heart rate, nystagmus, electromyographic (EMG) and electroencephalographic (EEG) changes, and slowed reaction times (Cohen et al. 1983).

Some evidence exists that, as measured by brain electrical activity mapping (BEAM), ethanol induces rapid and widespread increases in EEG alpha activity, which may be associated with the reinforcing properties of ethanol (Lukas et al. 1989). Severe intoxication may contribute to emotional lability, personality changes, and loss of control. The consequences of these states may result in driving while intoxicated, physical assault, and increased suicidal or homicidal behavior (Frances et al. 1987). Individual and cultural variations of tolerance may influence the manifestation of intoxication. For example, an "alcohol flush" reaction (caused by an inborn variation of alcohol dehydrogenase enzyme, which causes increased acetaldehyde) may contribute to a lower rate of alcoholism among Asians (Schwittes et al. 1982).

Treatment of Intoxication

Intoxication is a time-limited condition. General management principles include decreasing threatening external stimuli, interrupting alcohol ingestion, and, when necessary, protecting individuals from damaging themselves and others. There is no effective method of hastening ethanol removal, except in potentially fatal cases, in which hemodialysis has been attempted. Several experimental amethystic agents have been suggested. These include α_2-adrenergic receptor agonists such as atipamezole (Linnoila 1989) and naloxone in reversing ethanol-induced coma and respiratory depression (Liskow and Goodwin 1987).

Zimelidine, a serotonin reuptake blocker, and ibuprofen have shown reversal in some alcohol-induced cognitive deficits, and lithium has attenuated the subjective sense of intoxication. The inverse benzodiazepine receptor agonist Ro 15-4513 has been shown to antagonize specific biochemical and behavioral effects of alcohol, blocking some of alcohol's anxiolytic and intoxicating properties (Liebowitz et al. 1990; Lister and Nutt 1989). Unfortunately, because Ro 15-4513 causes anxiety and seizures, it is unlikely to be clinically useful. Fluvoxamine, fluoxetine, citalopram, and buspirone have shown promise in reducing alcohol consumption (Collins and Myers 1987; Naranjo et al. 1986). There is a possibility that therapeutic drugs may be developed in the future to modify alcohol tolerance (Liebowitz et al. 1990). In patients with alcoholism, prevention of severe intoxication requires total abstinence because of a tendency toward loss of control. In the nonalcoholic population, teaching more sensible patterns of alcohol use, especially among young people, may prevent unfortunate and sometimes disastrous consequences.

Blackouts

Alcohol blackouts are transient episodes of amnesia that accompany varying degrees of intoxication. These phenomena are characterized by relatively dense retrograde amnesia for events and behavior during periods of intoxication, even though the state of consciousness is not grossly abnormal as observed by others. Behavior during these episodes may be relatively benign or grossly abnormal. A blackout is a symptom indicative of impaired functioning in the DSM-III-R (American Psychiatric Association 1987) criteria for alcohol dependence. Blackouts can occur in isolated episodes of drinking in persons who never become alcoholic as well as at any time in the course of the disease of alcoholism (Adams and Victor 1981). In general, blackouts occur relatively late in the course of the illness and are directly correlated with severity and duration (Goodwin et al. 1969). The sharpness of the rise and fall of the blood alcohol level has been proposed as an associated factor, although the etiological mechanism of this phenomenon is not clear or well studied (Lishman 1978).

Explanations of pathogenesis have ranged from psychological repression to organic etiologies such as deep seizures and problems in capacity for laying down long-term memory during these episodes (Ballenger and Post 1984; Lishman 1978). There is evidence that some memories may be recovered when prompted by others, but classically there is a complete amnesia for the period during intoxication. More recent theories have proposed decreased central serotonin neurotransmission and disruption at excitatory neurotransmitter synapses (Tabakoff et al. 1990). Low plasma tryptophan levels and blackouts in male alcoholic patients suggest a specific relationship between memory problems and serotonergic activity (Branchey et al. 1985).

❑ ALCOHOL IDIOSYNCRATIC INTOXICATION

Alcohol idiosyncratic intoxication (DSM-III-R) or pathological intoxication, has been a controversial concept that is associated with blind unfocused assaultive and destructive behavior with intoxication. DSM-III-R defines alcohol idiosyncratic intoxication as a marked aggressive or assaultive behavioral change, with drinking, that is not typical of the person when sober. In susceptible individuals, this reaction occurs with small amounts of alcohol ingestion, insufficient to induce intoxication in most people. Differentiation of idiosyncratic intoxication from severe intoxication, frank epileptic phenomena, delirium tremens (DTs), compromised brain function from trauma, or hysterical phenomena may be difficult. There may be certain individuals with a genetic vulnerability and possible subclinical epileptic focus, but these phenomena have not been well studied and cases are anecdotal. Workup includes an EEG and a computed tomography (CT) scan if focal neurological signs or symptoms are present.

❑ ALCOHOL WITHDRAWAL SYMPTOMS

Alcohol withdrawal symptoms can occur after cessation of alcohol in patients with chronic alcoholism or secondary to a relative drop in blood levels. Therefore, clear-cut withdrawal symptoms may be present during a period of continuous alcohol consumption. Alcohol withdrawal proper (DSM-III-R) may precede or accompany more pathological withdrawal phenomena such as DTs, seizures (rum fits), and alcohol hallucinosis. A pattern of pathological use of alcohol, which can include withdrawal or tolerance symptoms, has been defined in DSM-III-R as alcohol dependence. Increased duration of drinking and binge patterns of alcohol ingestion are clearly tied to an increase in withdrawal phenomena. By far, the most common and earliest symptoms are tremulousness, general irritability, nausea, and vomiting occurring several hours after the last drink or, frequently, the next morning. Persons going through withdrawal may use a drink to "calm the nerves." Peak symptoms occur 24–48 hours after the last drink and, in uncomplicated cases, subside in 5–7 days, even without treatment, although mild irritability and insomnia may last 10 days or longer. It is helpful to educate patients about the time course of withdrawal because a rapid return to drinking may be precipitated by these residual withdrawal symptoms.

The generalized tremor is coarse, is of low frequency (5–7 cycles/second), can worsen with motor activity or emotional stress, and is most likely observed when the tongue or the hands are extended. Often patients complain only of feeling shaky inside. In addition, patients manifest malaise and autonomic hyperactivity, tachycardia, increased blood pressure, sweating, and orthostatic hypotension. Careful attention should be given to vital signs in patients suspected of having alcoholism. Individuals may complain of disturbed sleep with nightmares, transitory illusions, or hallucinations. Extrapyramidal symptoms were found to occur in susceptible highly dependent individuals after an intensive brief binge of days' duration (Shen 1984).

Several studies have tried to explain withdrawal. Because of the observed autonomic hyperactivity during withdrawal mediated by the sympathetic nervous system, neurochemical studies have focused on the noradrenergic system. Increased cerebrospinal fluid (CSF) norepinephrine has been associated with intensity of withdrawal symptoms (Fujimato et al. 1983). Downregulation of α_2-adrenergic receptor sensitivity has also been reported (Nutt 1987). Alcohol by-products, including acetaldehyde, may have an inhibitory effect on the adrenergic receptors. Increased cyclic adenosine monophosphate (cAMP) in neurons with long-term alcohol exposure may increase norepinephrine receptor sensitivity and increase norepinephrine turnover (Hawley et al. 1981). Monoamine oxidase (MAO), which is low in platelets of patients with alcoholism, is increased during withdrawal (Alexopoulos et al. 1981; Black et al. 1980).

Ballenger and Post (1984) proposed a "kindling model," in which repeated mild withdrawal from alcohol increases presumed subcortical nerve spiking. First demonstrated in rat studies (Hunter et al. 1973), repeated mild withdrawal from alcohol increases presumed subcortical nerve spiking serving as a kindling focus for limbic, hypothalamic, and thalamic areas, increasing severity of withdrawal. Early studies (Greenberg and Pearlman 1967) reported a decrease in rapid-eye-movement (REM) sleep during alcohol use and REM rebound during abstinence. Besson and Glen (1985) reported an increase in brain water content during withdrawal and a decrease during intoxication in nuclear magnetic resonance imaging (MRI) studies of the brain. Berglund and Risberg (1981) reported a decrease in regional cerebral blood flow in the first 2 days of withdrawal. This is associated with a decrease in clear sensorium and is correlated positively with duration of drinking.

Alcohol Withdrawal Seizures

Seizures are associated with cessation of long-term use of alcohol. Ninety percent of such seizures occur

7–38 hours after last use, with peak incidence somewhat greater than 24 hours (Adams and Victor 1981; Holloway et al. 1984; Sellers and Kalant 1976). In some series (Espir and Rose 1987), 10% of patients with chronic alcoholism have recurrent seizures, and a considerably higher number have solitary seizures. Half of these occur in bursts of two to six grand mal seizures. Less than 3% develop status epilepticus, which can be a life-threatening condition unless interrupted (Adams and Victor 1981). Focal seizures suggest a focal lesion, which may be the result of trauma or idiopathic epilepsy.

Seizures can be precipitated during a short bout of drinking by lowering seizure threshold. These alcohol-precipitated seizures usually occur after the period of acute intoxication (Adams and Victor 1981). Ng et al. (1988) concluded, however, that alcohol in a dose-related fashion can independently induce seizures outside the normal withdrawal period. Devetag et al. (1983) found that in patients with alcohol withdrawal seizures the amount and years of drinking are increased. Alcohol-induced epilepsy can occur with less than 5 years of steady drinking (Brennan and Lyttle 1987).

EEG findings in nonepileptic individuals can be abnormal during withdrawal, with occurrences of brief periods of dysrhythmia that usually result in a normal EEG with clearance. Victor and Brausch (1967) did EEGs on 130 of 241 alcohol-related seizure patients and found 109 had normal EEGs. Status epilepticus could result from the combination of discontinuation of phenytoin, which is often unnecessarily prescribed, and alcohol withdrawal (Aminoff and Simon 1980). In a study of nonaddicted adults, Zilm et al. (1981) reported that evoked potentials are sensitive to tolerance and withdrawal. Two studies of alcoholic seizure patients (Feussner et al. 1981; Tarter et al. 1983) reported that 50% had abnormal CT scans. In a study of patients with no other indication of a major intracranial process (Earnest et al. 1988), 16% had significant intracranial lesions on CT. Feussner et al. (1981) found that 39% had generalized cerebral atrophy and 15% had focal structural lesions. Focal neurological signs were found in 30% of those with a focal deficit on CT scan versus 6% of those without a focal deficit. A careful neurological examination may predict those who may need a CT scan.

Hypomagnesemia, respiratory alkalosis, hypoglycemia, and increased intracellular sodium have been associated with alcohol seizures, and the seizures may be the result of hyperexcitability of the neuronal systems caused by these conditions (Victor and Wolfe 1973). Upregulation of the NMDA-receptor–calcium-ion-channel complex might contribute to production of withdrawal seizures (Hoffman et al. 1989).

These seizures have an important prognostic value in predicting a complicated withdrawal period. Approximately one-third of patients with generalized seizures secondary to alcohol withdrawal go on to develop alcoholic withdrawal DTs (Adams and Victor 1981). Tarter et al. (1983) reported that alcoholic patients who experience withdrawal seizures do not suffer decreased intellectual or neuropathological performances on tests and that seizures are not a marker for severity of alcoholism.

Alcohol Withdrawal Delirium (DTs)

Alcohol's association with DTs was first described in the 18th century, but it was not until 1955 that Isbell related it specifically to sudden withdrawal from alcohol (see Isbell et al. 1955). DTs are distinguished from uncomplicated withdrawal symptoms by a characteristic delirium. Confusion, disorientation, fluctuating or clouded consciousness, and perceptual disturbances may all be present. The syndrome includes delusions, vivid hallucinations, agitation, insomnia, mild fever, and marked autonomic arousal that can appear suddenly, but more usually appear gradually, 2–3 days after cessation of drinking, with peak intensity on the fourth or fifth day. Terror, agitation, and primarily visual hallucinations of insects, small animals, or other perceptual distortions are classic, although a wide variation in presentation can occur.

The clinical picture can vary from quiet confusion, agitation, and peculiar behavior lasting several weeks to marked abnormal behavior, vivid terrifying delusions, and hallucinations. Hallucinations may be auditory and of a persecutory nature, or they may be kinesthetic, such as a tactile sensation of crawling insects. Hallucinations may be systematized or unsystematized. The level of consciousness may fluctuate widely.

Approximately one-half of cases present in an atypical manner (Victor and Adams 1953). The syndrome is often modified by illness, therapeutic medications such as sedatives or analgesics, or trauma. Patients may show similar patterns of behavior each time they withdraw from alcohol (Turner et al. 1989). During the height of delirium, the rhythms show moderate increases in fast frequencies or EEGs in the normal range. In most cases, the DTs are benign and short lived. Less commonly, the delirious state may be characterized by several relapses separated by lucid intervals. Most cases subside after 3 days of full-blown DTs, although DTs may last as long as 4–5 weeks. When cases are complicated by medical conditions, it has been reported that up to 20% may end fatally (Victor 1966). More recent reports (Gessner 1979), however, have found overall fatality may be less than 1%. Deaths due to DTs may be related to infections, fat emboli, or cardiac arrhythmia associated with hyperkalemia, hypokalemia, hyponatremia, hypophosphatemia, alcoholic ketoacidosis, hyperpyrexia, poor hydration, rhabdomyolysis, and hypertension. Other complications include pancreatitis, gastritis, upper gastrointestinal bleeds, and hepatitis.

DTs generally occur in alcoholic individuals with 5–15 years of heavy drinking who decrease their blood alcohol levels and who have a major physical illness, such as infection, trauma, liver disease, or metabolic disorders. Useful predictors of DTs include a past history of DTs or seizures (Cushman 1987). Only 1%–10% of alcoholic patients hospitalized for detoxification develop DTs (Holloway et al. 1984). There is some evidence that the severity of DTs is related to the severity of the acute drinking bout before admission, the amount of insomnia, and gastrointestinal disturbance. Other associated factors that have been discussed include hypocalcemia, hypophosphatemia, and hypokalemia. Although hypomagnesemia has been associated with seizures, it is probably not an associated agent in DTs (Kramp and Hemmingsen 1984; Tonnesen 1982).

Alcohol Hallucinosis

Alcohol hallucinosis is described in DSM-III-R as a vivid auditory hallucination, occurring shortly after the cessation or reduction of heavy ingestion of alcohol. Differential diagnoses include DTs, withdrawal syndrome, paranoid psychosis, other drug abuse, and borderline transient psychotic episodes. Withdrawal-induced hallucinosis is not a predictor of DTs (Holloway et al. 1984). In contrast to delirium, the hallucinations usually occur in a clear sensorium. A paucity of autonomic symptoms also differentiates the syndrome from withdrawal syndrome. The hallucinations may range from sounds such as clicks, roaring, humming, ringing bells, or chanting to frank voices of friends or enemies, which often are threatening or maligning (Lishman 1978). A single derogatory remark may proceed to a relentless persistence of auditory accusations by several voices and auditory commands. Patients usually respond appropriately with fear, anxiety, and agitation. These symptoms may resemble paranoid schizophrenia (Surawicz 1980). However, the diagnosis is usually made on the basis of heavy alcohol use, lack of formal thought disorder, and lack of schizophrenia or mania in past or family history.

The onset is classically after cessation of drinking, but onset during drinking bouts has been reported. In the great majority of cases, the symptoms recede in a few hours to days, with patients fully realizing that the voices were imaginary. A small percentage of patients may proceed to develop a quiet, chronic paranoid delusional state or frank schizophrenia (Sellers and Kalant 1976). A period of 6 months has been reported as a cutoff point beyond which remission is not expected (Lishman 1978).

Treatment of the Withdrawal Syndrome

Treatment and prevention of complications from the cessation of alcohol use in an alcohol-dependent individual depend on recognition of patterns of alcohol abuse and a careful evaluation of the stage of the illness, complicating medical problems, and flexibility in the use of treating medications. Alcohol-related medical disorders are often not detected as such and are evident in approximately 23% of general hospital admissions (Beresford 1979). These disorders can include gastritis, ulcers, pancreatitis, liver disease, cardiomyopathy, anemia, neurological complications, sexual dysfunction, and cancer. Withdrawal symptoms are most dangerous when accompanied by medical illness such as pneumonia, liver failure, and subdural hematomas. A high index of suspicion is needed to treat target symptoms in individuals undergoing withdrawal. Denial is a major defense mechanism in alcoholism, and the magnitude of an individual's drinking may not be evident until withdrawal phenomena appear.

Inpatient Versus Outpatient Treatment

The choice of setting for treatment of withdrawal symptoms depends on the severity of symptoms, medical complications, the use of other substances, and the patient's cooperation, ability to follow instructions, social support systems, and past history.

Patients with organic brain syndrome, low intelligence, Wernicke's encephalopathy, dehydration, history of trauma, neurological symptoms, medical complications, psychopathology that may require psychotropic medications, DTs, alcoholic seizures, or alcoholic hallucinosis are probably best treated in an inpatient setting. Supervision, observation, and proper medical backup are often required. A past history of withdrawal seizures, DTs, or poor compliance also warrants withdrawal in an inpatient setting. Concomitant use of other substances (e.g., barbiturates and benzodiazepines) may complicate alcohol withdrawal. Concomitant opiate addiction may require cautious use of more than one agent for detoxification.

In a randomized, prospective study of lower-socioeconomic veterans, Hayshida et al. (1989) found outpatient detoxification effective, safe, and low-cost for patients with mild to moderate alcohol withdrawal who have good transportation and voluntarily seek treatment.

TABLE 24–2. MEDICAL WORKUP FOR ALCOHOL WITHDRAWAL

Medical history and complete physical examination
Routine laboratory tests
Complete blood count with differential
Serum electrolytes
Liver function tests (including bilirubin)
Blood urea nitrogen
Creatinine
Fasting blood glucose
Prothrombin time
Cholesterol
Triglycerides
Calcium
Magnesium
Albumin with total protein
Hepatitis B surface antigen
B_{12} folic acid levels
Stool guaiac
Urinalysis
Urine drug and alcohol screen
Chest X ray, electrocardiogram
Ancillary tests
Electroencephalogram
Head computed tomography
Gastrointestinal series

General Management of Inpatient Treatment

If inpatient treatment is deemed necessary for withdrawal, an atmosphere that avoids overstimulation and that is well structured is preferable. A closed unit with good lighting, minimal noise, frequent orientation, and a nonthreatening approach is recommended. A good medical history and physical and neurological examinations are required. Standard laboratory tests are listed in Table 24–2. An EEG, head CT scan, and gastrointestinal (GI) series are frequent ancillary tests. An EEG may rule out metabolic or focal seizure focus. A CT scan helps rule out structural deficits and masses. GI series are helpful to rule out peptic ulcers or esophageal varices. Vital signs should be routinely taken every 8 hours, and the patient should be observed closely.

Patients with alcoholism are often nutritionally deficient. Deficiencies in thiamine, vitamin B_{12}, and folic acid levels are commonly found. For patients who are not severely debilitated, daily oral thiamine 100 mg, folic acid 1 mg, and one multivitamin plus adequate nutrition are sufficient to prevent Wernicke-Korsakoff syndrome and to replenish vitamin stores if given throughout the hospitalization. In patients suspected of very poor nutrition, thiamine 100–200 mg iv should be administered and immediately followed by 100 mg/day po. Thiamine should be given before any situation in which glucose loading is required, because glucose infusion can further exhaust stores of thiamine. Recently, some have suggested that beverage companies fortify alcoholic beverages with thiamine to prevent thiamine deficiencies (Reuler et al. 1985). However, high levels of thiamine (7.5 mg/L) would be necessary to overcome malabsorption, and thiamine would be detectable in taste (Meilgaard 1985). Attention to the total protein, albumin, and prothrombin time may determine if hyperalimentation or vitamin K (5–10 mg parenterally) should be given. Hyperalimentation is rarely needed for alcoholic malnutrition.

Magnesium sulfate 1 g (2 mg in 50% solution) im every 6 hours for 2 days should be given to any individual with a past history of alcohol withdrawal seizures. In mild to moderate withdrawal, dehydration is usually not a problem that requires parenteral intravenous fluids, and overhydration may occur. In severe cases where autonomic hyperarousal, sweating, and fever cause considerable dehydration, careful rehydration and attention to electrolyte replacement should be done with medical supervision.

Inpatient Nonpharmacological Treatment

In mild uncomplicated cases of withdrawal, nonpharmacological withdrawal can be attempted. Many alcoholic patients have had the experience of stopping alcohol rather suddenly and tolerating withdrawal symptoms without complication. However, there is some evidence that nonpharmacological withdrawal may hasten cognitive decline (Linnoila 1989). Femino and Lewis (1982) described withdrawing patients nonpharmacologically in a secure hospital setting over 2–7 days, observing for any complications. They suggested this approach may help provide the alcoholic patient with the experience of nonpharmacological control. Several other studies have reported supportive care being sufficient for the vast majority of withdrawing alcoholic patients (Shaw 1981; Whitfield et al. 1978). In our experience, convenience and legal issues have limited the use of this technique.

Pharmacological Treatment

The rationale for pharmacological treatment of withdrawal symptoms is to relieve discomfort secondary to autonomic symptoms and to prevent complications such as seizures and DTs. An ideal medication is currently unavailable, although numerous medications have been tried. An ideal medication for withdrawal would produce adequate sedation, abort autonomic hyperarousal, be easy to administer, provide a good therapeutic safety index, be without primary liver metabolism, and be nonaddicting. Numerous medications have been reported to be effective for uncomplicated withdrawal symptoms, such as alcohol, paraldehyde, chloral hydrate, antihistamines, barbiturates, chlormethiazole, major tranquilizers, phenytoin, propranolol, piracetam, and benzodiazepines. Some experimental studies suggest that lithium has the potential to suppress withdrawal symptoms (Miller et al. 1988).

Cross-tolerance with alcohol and sedation have been the main rationales for these medications. On these alternatives, several medications have been found to be efficacious when properly used. Recommendations have been made on the basis of safety, ease, and comfort of administration and clinical experience. Moskowitz et al. (1983) reviewed 81 therapeutic trials in 2,313 randomized patients and found only four deaths. The studies reviewed generally lacked either clear endpoints, proper handling of dropouts, or adequate details of side effects. No definite conclusion other than the efficacy of benzodiazepines could be ascertained.

General principles of pharmacological detoxification providing the maximum degree of safety include the adequate sedation of the patient and the gradual withdrawal of blood levels of a medication cross-tolerant with alcohol. Alcohol itself is often used by alcoholic patients as a weaning device. Clinically, its disadvantages include short half-life, gastric irritation, excessive sedation, and confusion about the abstinence message for the patient.

Antihistamines have been used in mild withdrawal and provide sedation but no cross-tolerance or prevention against DTs or seizures. Chlormethiazole has similar effects, but it is not available in the United States and has not been well studied. Propranolol can decrease anxiety, tremor, mild hypertension, tachycardia, and subjective symptoms. The relationship of a central versus peripheral mechanism is unclear. In severe withdrawal, propranolol up to 160 mg/day may decrease tremor but provides no protection from seizures or DTs (Sellers and Kalant 1976). A recent randomized clinical trial of atenolol (a β-blocker) during alcohol withdrawal (Horowitz et al. 1989) showed beneficial effects compared with placebo; atenolol also seemed to be associated with a reduction in craving. Major tranquilizers do produce sedation but are not cross-tolerant with alcohol: they have the disadvantages of causing hypotension and lowering seizure threshold.

Carbamazepine is an anticonvulsant, antikindling drug that has demonstrated efficiency in treating withdrawal. In a double-blind controlled trial comparing carbamazepine and oxazepam (Malcolm et al. 1989), carbamazepine exhibited equal efficacy and a suggestion of a role in treating psychiatric sequelae of repeated withdrawal. Clonidine has been reported to be as effective as chlordiazepoxide in relieving the subjective symptoms of withdrawal and more effective in reducing systolic blood pressure and heart rate (Baumgartner and Rowen 1987). Lofexidine, another α_2-adrenergic agonist, also had successful clinical trials (Cushman et al. 1985). Successful use of high-potency antipsychotics in controlling the agitated psychotic symptoms associated with delirium has been reported (Holloway et al. 1984). This may be due to their general sedating effects.

Chloral hydrate is not cross-tolerant. It has a relatively short half-life of 6–8 hours, can only be given orally or rectally, and intramuscular use is limited because of possible nerve damage, risks of sterile abscess, and fat embolization. One group (Embry and Lippmann 1987) has advocated the use of magnesium to decrease the need for benzodiazepines during withdrawal; however, a controlled double-blind study found no indication for magnesium for withdrawal without a seizure history (Wilson and Vulcano 1984).

Barbiturates and benzodiazepines are both cross-tolerant. The major advantage of cross-tolerance is the prevention of seizure activity during withdrawal. Barbiturates have had a decreased popularity in recent years, secondary to high incidence of respiratory depression and a low therapeutic safety index compared with those of benzodiazepines. In the presence of severe liver disease, oversedation is a danger with the use of barbiturates because of their decreased liver metabolism. Longer-acting barbiturates such as phenobarbital are preferable over short-acting medications and can be used with equivalent doses of benzodiazepines. Barbital, a long-acting barbiturate, is used widely in Denmark and reportedly is not metabolized by the liver (Hemmingsen et al. 1979).

Benzodiazepines are clearly the medication of choice for withdrawal symptoms because of a relatively high therapeutic safety index, oral and intravenous administration, anticonvulsant properties, and good prevention of DTs. Disadvantages include poor intramuscular absorption (except for lorazepam), primary liver metabolism, high cost, and abuse potential. There are no clear advantages to any one benzodiazepine, although special circumstances may favor one over another. Short-acting benzodiazepines such as triazolam should generally be avoided. Rapidly fluctuating blood levels may promote withdrawal seizures. In patients with severe liver disease and in the elderly, intermediate-acting benzodiazepines such as lorazepam or oxazepam can be used. Oxazepam has the added advantage of renal versus liver excretion. Intermediate-acting benzodiazepines must be given at short intervals and must be carefully tapered. Lorazepam 1–4 mg po every 6–8 hours and oxazepam 15–60 mg every 6–8 hours are standard doses.

Diazepam and chlordiazepoxide, longer-acting benzodiazepines, are comparable in length of action, with half-lives of 24–36 hours. The onset of action is slow, thus rapid loading doses are often needed. Chlordiazepoxide and diazepam have the advantage of smooth induction and gradual decline in blood levels so that there are fewer symptoms on discontinuation of low dosages. Chlordiazepoxide may be preferable because of its greater sedation. In severe withdrawal cases with a history of seizures, and in cases of cross-addiction with other depressant drugs, diazepam is used because of its greater anticonvulsant effect. Diazepam 10 mg is the eqivalent of chlordiazepoxide 25 mg.

Outpatient Management

For the majority of people with mild withdrawal symptoms, an outpatient medical detoxification is possible. Close follow-up, including daily visits, is essential to assure adequate sedation and observation for complications. This method has the advantages of leaving the patients in their own work and social settings and of fostering a positive therapeutic alliance with the treating outpatient therapist.

In uncomplicated outpatient withdrawal, chlordiazepoxide 25–50 mg po qid should be prescribed on the first day, with a 20% decrease in dose over a 5-day period and with daily visits to assess symptoms (Table 24–3). The advantage of inpatient detoxification is the security of being able to assess subjective and objective symptomatology rapidly and to adjust the dose properly.

Inpatient Detoxification

For inpatient withdrawal, generally 100–400 mg of chlordiazepoxide is given the first day in quarterly divided dosages (Table 24–3). This generally provides adequate sedation and control of autonomic

TABLE 24–3. STANDARD TREATMENT REGIMEN FOR ALCOHOL WITHDRAWAL

Outpatient
- Chlordiazepoxide 25–50 mg po qid on first day; 20% decrease in dose over a 5-day period
- Daily visits to assess symptoms

Inpatient
- Chlordiazepoxide 25–100 mg po qid on first day; 20% decrease in dose over 5–7 days
- Chlordiazepoxide 25–50 mg po qid prn for agitation, tremors, or change in vital signs
- Thiamine 100 mg po qid
- Folic acid 1 mg po qid
- Multivitamin one per day
- Magnesium sulfate 1 g im every 6 hours for 2 days (if status postwithdrawal seizures)

symptoms, although chlordiazepoxide may not take away all the subjective discomforts of withdrawal. Skilled staff should be available to assess adequacy of dosage and give prn doses if objective signs are present. Countertransference problems may lead staff to over- or undermedicate withdrawal symptoms secondary to fears of promoting addiction or anger at the patient.

Our standard inpatient detoxification is chlordiazepoxide 25–100 mg po qid with 25–50 mg every 2 hours prn for agitation, tremulousness, or change of vital signs. If some sedation is not achieved 1 hour after the first dose, chlordiazepoxide 25 mg can be prescribed hourly until the patient is sedated. Sellers and Kalant (1976) suggested that higher levels of chlordiazepoxide may be necessary for cigarette smokers. The total 24-hour dose on the first day should be tapered over 5–7 days in equally divided dosages per day. Holloway et al. (1984) suggested that if 600 mg is used over a 24-hour period, the entire situation should be reevaluated. A patient may have mild chronic withdrawal symptoms that may last for several weeks. Kolin and Linet (1981) found equal efficacy comparing alprazolam and diazepam in subacute withdrawal symptoms (5–21 days after last drink).

Treatment of Withdrawal Seizures

Single withdrawal seizures do not require anticonvulsant medication. Alcohol withdrawal seizures are generally self-limited and only require supportive care.

Treatment of Status Epilepticus

Patients with known idiopathic or traumatic epilepsy may require the additional anticonvulsant properties of phenytoin, but it is not indicated in uncomplicated withdrawal or seizures (Chan 1985). Status epilepticus is a major neurological emergency. Diazepam 10 mg iv usually aborts status epilepticus; however, phenytoin loading 1,000 mg iv slowly over 20 minutes (50 ml/minute) in glucose-free solution may be necessary. Patients with abnormal EEGs repeated 2–3 weeks after withdrawal may require maintenance phenytoin 100 mg po tid with follow-up blood levels. Calcium channel blocking agents may play a role in management of withdrawal seizures (Koppi et al. 1987; Little et al. 1986).

Treatment of DTs

The best care for DTs is preventive treatment. There is evidence that once DTs occur the course may not be significantly altered by available treatment (Victor and Wolfe 1973). The chief aims are sedation and supportive care. Sedation is necessary in cases of extreme agitation. Diazepam can be used 5–10 mg iv every 5 minutes until the patient is awake, but calm. Oversedation should be avoided. In less extreme agitation oral or intravenous benzodiazepine of long or short half-lives, depending on age or liver status, can be used. Restraints should be used only if necessary and in most cases should be four-point restraints. Restraints in paranoid patients may increase agitation. A quiet environment with minimal stimulation will help diminish delusional material. Correction of metabolic derangements and vitamin supplementation are parts of the supportive care. High-potency neuroleptics such as haloperidol may be helpful in patients who are psychotic with marked perceptual changes.

Treatment of Alcohol Hallucinosis

Patients with alcohol hallucinosis should receive the same basic appropriate withdrawal treatment. For those patients with hallucinosis and extreme agitation, a potent antipsychotic such as haloperidol 2–5 mg po bid successfully decreases symptoms. Medication should not be continued indefinitely and reassessment should take place shortly after cessation of symptoms.

❑ WERNICKE-KORSAKOFF SYNDROME

Wernicke-Korsakoff syndrome is a spectrum neurological disorder associated with thiamine deficiency. It is most often associated with alcoholism, but it can occur in any condition that causes thiamine deficiency, such as malabsorption syndrome, severe anorexia, upper GI obstruction, prolonged intravenous feeding, thyrotoxicosis, and hemodialysis. Repeated bouts of marginal thiamine deficiency could lead to the same pathological changes induced by a single episode of severe thiamine deficiency (Harper 1983). It has been estimated that Wernicke-Korsakoff syndrome constitutes 3% of all alcohol-related disorders (Nakada and Knight 1984). Again, it is a spectrum disease in which Wernicke's encephalopathy can evolve into a Korsakoff permanent memory disorder. However, Wernicke's encephalopathy is not the inevitable forerunner of Korsakoff's syndrome.

Wernicke's Encephalopathy

Classically, Wernicke's encephalopathy has an abrupt onset with oculomotor disturbances, cerebellar ataxia, and mental confusion. Several authors (e.g., Brew 1986) have suggested that the diagnosis of Wernicke's encephalopathy should not rely on the presence of all three criteria and that the presence of two of the three criteria is suggestive of limited forms of the disorder. Autopsy studies (Harper et al. 1986) confirm that there is a high rate of mental confusion (82%) but lower rates of ataxia (23%) and oculomotor disturbances (29%). The oculomotor disturbances range from various types of nystagmus to complete gaze palsy. The ataxia is truncal, and these conditions may precede the mental confusion by days. A general confusional state with disorientation, in addition to slow response, may proceed to frank stupor and coma in 10%–80% of cases (Nakada and Knight 1984).

Wernicke's encephalopathy should be suspected in any unexplained case of coma. It has a 17% mortality rate and should be considered a medical emergency. Thiamine deficiency produces a diffuse decrease in the use of glucose, and the neurotoxicity may be due to release of excitatory neurotransmitters such as glutamic acid. If a patient does not respond quickly (within 48–72 hours) to treatment, the development of Korsakoff's psychosis (also known as Korsakoff's syndrome or Korsakoff's disease) is likely. Approximately 80% of patients with Wernicke's encephalopathy who survive develop Korsakoff's psychosis (Reuler et al. 1985).

Alcohol Amnestic Disorder (Korsakoff's Psychosis)

Korsakoff's psychosis is classically a chronic condition, with both retrograde and anterograde amnesia. The period of retrograde amnesia may cover up to a few years before the onset of the illness. Confabulation may be typical in the early stages, but it is not always present. Korsakoff's psychosis can also show changes in behavior indicative of frontal lobe damage (e.g., apathy, inertia, and loss of insight). Numerous studies have outlined some of the neuropathological aspects of the disorder. Selzer and Benson (1974) confirmed the classic Korsakoff memory problem in which recent, well-known public events were poorly remembered compared with remote events. Albert et al. (1979) also reported retrograde amnesia in Korsakoff's psychosis and suggested that it was not related to the difficulty of the fact to be remembered. Zola-Morgan and Oberg (1980) suggested the need to study Korsakoff patients in more naturalistic settings to get a better view of their functional memory difficulties. Sensory, motivational, and visuospatial difficulties have also been found in Korsakoff's psychosis, but intellectual functioning is generally spared.

Korsakoff patients may have faulty memory retrieval due to increased reactive inhibition; they can encode semantically, and some association mechanisms can help them remember (Mattis et al. 1981). Butters (1985) reviewed studies that indicated that Korsakoff patients present with an inability to acquire new information because of interference from previously learned material (perseveration of response).

Structural and neurochemical findings have also characterized Wernicke-Korsakoff syndrome. Punctate lesions in the periventricular, periaqueductal regions of the brain stem and diencephalon have been found on brain autopsy (Victor et al. 1989). Periventricular lesions of the thalamus, hypothalamus, mammillary bodies, the reticular activating system, periaqueductal areas of the midbrain, and floor of the fourth ventricle have been found and may relate to the memory problems and various states of consciousness (Victor et al. 1989). MRI brain images demonstrate loss of tissue in the area of the mammillary bodies (Charness and DeLaPaz 1987). CT scans of Wernicke patients have correlated with postmortem findings (Figures 24–1, 24–2, and 24–3). Edema has been found in the mammillary bodies around the third ventricle and the aqueductal floor of the fourth ventricle (Mensing et al. 1984).

Weingartner et al. (1983) suggested that the memory pathology in Korsakoff's psychosis may be based on a disruption of the functional anatomic linkages between the reward-reinforcement and memory systems. Because the patients may have access to semantic memory, unlike Alzheimer's disease patients, psychobiological mechanisms have been proposed. Decreases in CSF levels of norepinephrine, dopamine, and serotonin have been found,

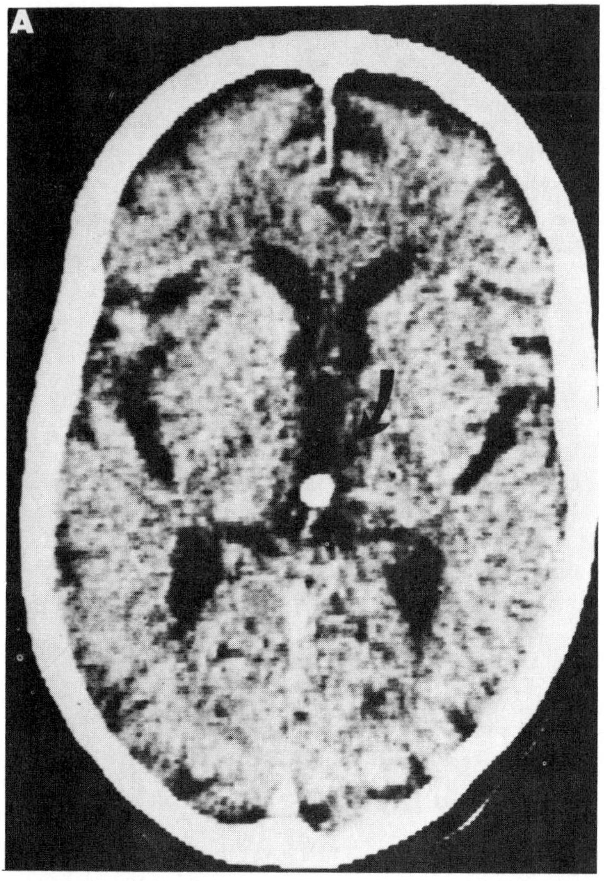

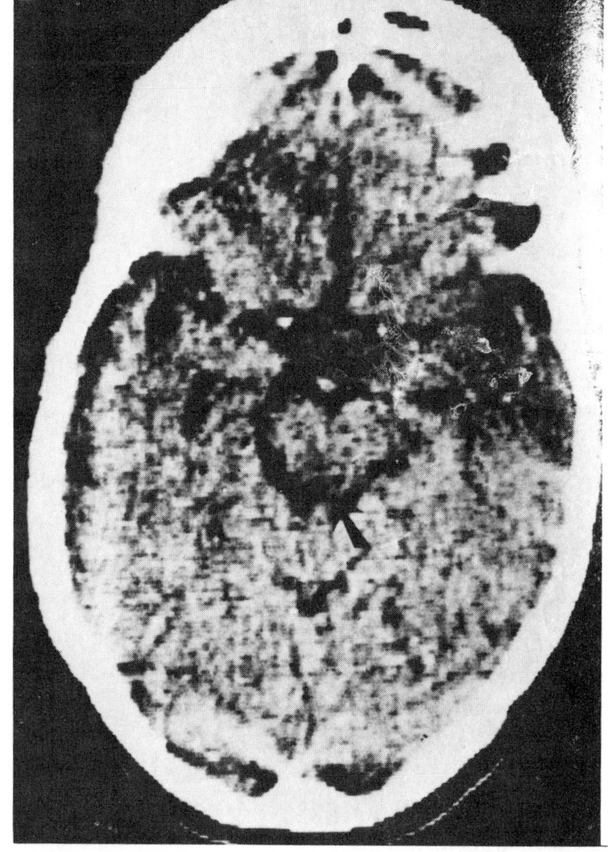

Figure 24–1. Computed tomography (CT) scan of a patient with Wernicke's encephalopathy, made 1 day after admission. *Panel A*: CT scan shows poor definition of the walls of the third ventricle and an adjacent hypodense area (*curved arrow*). *Panel B*: CT scan shows a poorly defined hypodense area around the aqueduct, near the quadrigeminal plate (*arrow*). These changes, typically arranged around the midline of the brain, strongly suggest Wernicke's encephalopathy. (Reprinted from Mensing JW, Hoogland PH, Slooff JL: Computed tomography in the diagnosis of Wernicke's encephalopathy: a radiological-neuropathological correlation. Ann Neurol 16:363–365, 1984. Used with permission.)

with the greatest decrease in norepinephrine levels. Negative studies have also been reported (McEntee and Mair 1978). The hypothesis is that norepinephrine systems are selectively damaged in Korsakoff's psychosis, producing memory deficits but not global dementia. Others (Butters 1985) have reported deficits in the acetylcholine system, suggesting a milder form of damage to the basalis of Meynert compared to what is found in Alzheimer's disease. Direct alcohol neurotoxicity to the basalis of Meynert may also play a role (Arendt et al. 1988). Cholinergic blockade produces anterograde amnesia similar to the pattern seen in Alzheimer and Korsakoff patients (Kopelman and Corn 1988). Butters (1985) characterized this as a basal forebrain rather than a diencephalon amnesia. At this time, Korsakoff's psychosis cannot be attributed to damage of any one structure.

Abnormalities in the metabolism of thiamine have been postulated as a contributory factor in the development of severe thiamine deficiency. Transketolase activity in the muscle fibroblasts of Wernicke-Korsakoff patients has been found to be decreased, but the expression of the syndrome may not become evident unless there is a thiamine-deficient diet (Blass and Gibson 1977). A report of monozygotic twins (Leigh et al. 1981), both having a decrease in erythrocyte transketolase activity, with

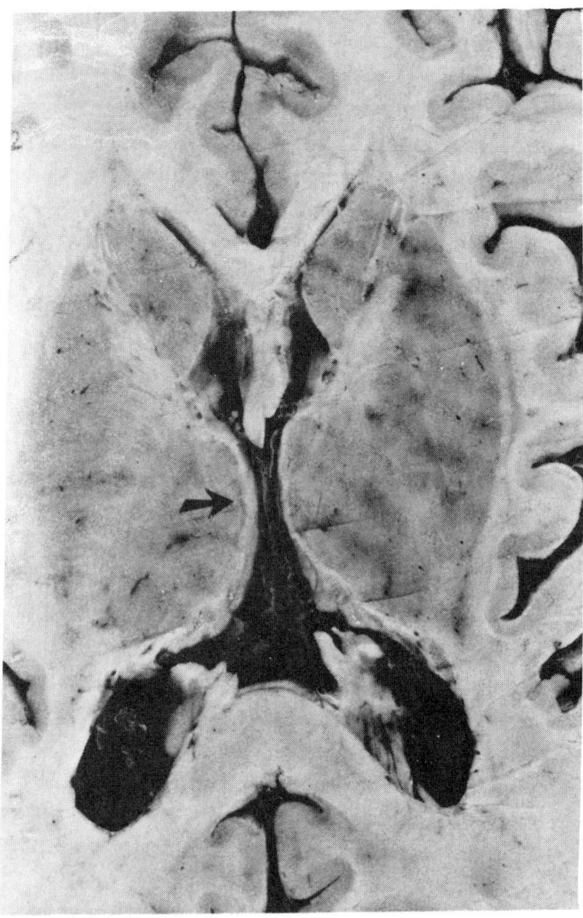

Figure 24–2. Postmortem slide of brain tissue from a patient with Wernicke's encephalopathy, showing smooth walls of the third ventricle, with an adjacent small discolored zone (*arrow*). (Reprinted from Mensing JW, Hoogland PH, Slooff JL: Computed tomography in the diagnosis of Wernicke's encephalopathy: a radiological-neuropathological correlation. Ann Neurol 16:363–365, 1984. Used with permission.)

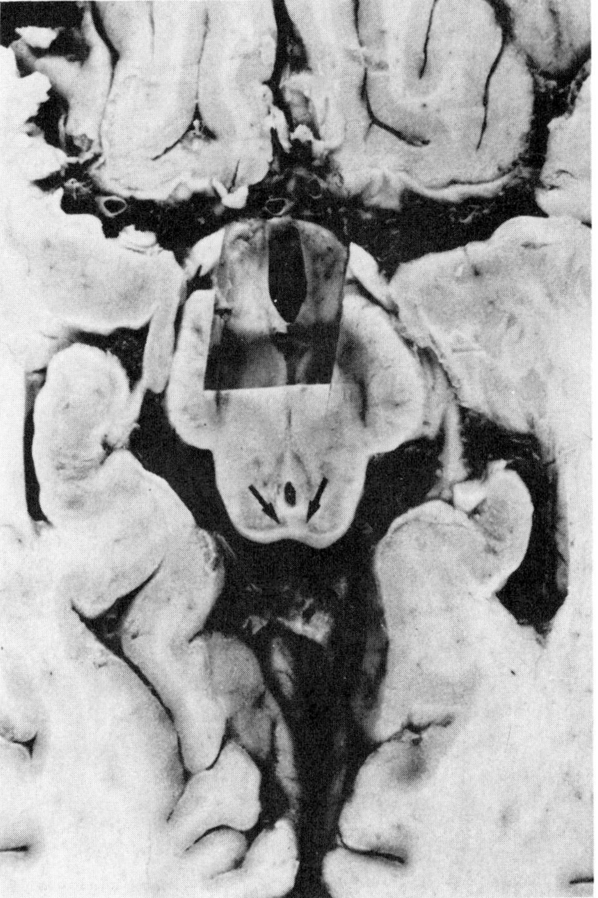

Figure 24–3. Postmortem slide of brain tissue from a patient with Wernicke's encephalopathy, showing discolored zone near the quadrigeminal plate (*arrows*). (Reprinted from Mensing JW, Hoogland PH, Slooff JL: Computed tomography in the diagnosis of Wernicke's encephalopathy: a radiological-neuropathological correlation. Ann Neurol 16:363–365, 1984. Used with permission.)

one developing Wernicke-Korsakoff syndrome secondary to alcoholism, suggested a possible genetic basis, although this is currently speculative.

Treatment of Wernicke's Encephalopathy

Wernicke's encephalopathy is a life-threatening condition; treatment should be considered a medical emergency. Treatment consists of parenteral thiamine 100 mg with titration of thiamine upward until ophthalmoplegia has been resolved. Resistance to thiamine replacement may result from hypomagnesemia because magnesium is a cofactor for thiamine transketolase. Magnesium sulfate 1–2 ml im in 50% solution should be administered. Thiamine should be given before any glucose loading. Ophthalmoplegia usually responds fairly quickly, but truncal ataxia may persist.

Treatment of Korsakoff's Psychosis

Korsakoff's psychosis can be a devastating illness that often requires institutionalization. Korsakoff's psychosis and alcoholic dementia may occur in combination and may be difficult to separate clinically. Clonidine, an α-norepinephrine agonist, has been reported (0.3 mg bid) to improve recent memory and recall, perhaps as a result of hypothesized damage to the ascending norepinephrine-containing neurons in the brain stem and diencephalon (McEntee et al. 1981). Propranolol, up to 20 mg/kg body weight per day, has been used for rage attacks in Korsakoff's psychosis (Yudofsky et al. 1984). This points to a chronic catecholamine supersensitivity. More recently, fluvoxamine has shown some promise in reducing memory deficits, hypothesized to occur through its serotonergic effects (Martin et al. 1989). Unfortunately, none of these pharmacological approaches is terribly effective. Thiamine replacement is not effective in established Korsakoff's psychosis.

Neuropsychological Changes With Alcohol Abuse

Alcohol's neurotoxicity is the result of years of alcohol abuse and occurs independently of thiamine deficiency. Impaired abstracting ability, verbal reasoning, face-name recognition, problem solving, tactile and spatial performance, visual perception, olfactory acuity, visual learning, and memory have all been reported in alcoholic patients (Drejer et al. 1985; Parsons 1977; Schaeffer and Parsons 1987; Yohman and Parsons 1987). Basic intellectual functioning is generally spared in a substantial number of patients with chronic alcoholism (Parsons 1977); however, a small number of patients do manifest general cognitive deficits and have a dementia-like picture. Determining what processes are impaired, when in the course of the drinking history problems become evident, and permanent versus temporary deficits becomes important in establishing prognosis, appropriateness of treatment, and discharge plans.

Duration and quantity of drinking, sensitivity of tests, patterns of drinking, and length of abstinence are factors that affect neuropsychological studies. Selection of patients may be fundamental in determining results in neuropsychological testing. Age, length of drinking, history of poor nutrition, genetic background, trauma, and other drug abuse will vary outcome. Increased age is an important variable in poor neuropsychological performance, and it may not correlate with abstinence. Alcohol has greater effects in older individuals because their brains are more sensitive to the toxic effects of alcohol, they are more likely to have had longer drinking histories, and their vulnerability increases with age. Social drinking in the elderly may produce decreases in cognitive functioning, but the hypothesis that alcohol leads to premature aging has not been supported by the data (Ryan 1982).

Porjesz and Begleiter (1982) found very different evoked potentials between elderly individuals and alcoholic patients. In studies of young alcoholic men versus nonalcoholic control subjects, there was no difference in psychological findings (Grant et al. 1974). There is a significant difference between middle-aged alcoholic individuals and elderly nonalcoholic individuals. Reversibility of cognitive deficits also argues against the premature aging hypothesis. Drinking may diminish in older age groups due to changes in neurotransmitters, cognitive impairment, decreased rate of alcohol metabolism, decrease in body water, and increased brain sensitivity to alcohol (Nordstrom and Berglund 1987). Some studies (Acker 1986) have suggested that women alcoholic patients, despite significantly shorter drinking histories at peak alcohol consumption, perform as poorly on cognitive tests.

Patterns of drinking may affect neuropsychological findings. Alcoholic patients with more than 10 years of heavy drinking show greater cognitive deficits. Binge drinking may be more neurotoxic. Repeated withdrawal may also be associated with cortical-related neurological damage. Social drinkers show greater decrease in cognitive performance when larger amounts are consumed at one time rather than spread out over time (Parker and Noble 1977).

Various studies have stressed the importance of the length of sobriety on neuropsychological testing. Page and Schaub (1977) studied 51 recovering alcoholic patients and found no further improvement of their specific intellectual functions after 3 weeks. At 7 weeks, Yohman et al. (1985) still found verbal memory, abstracting ability, problem solving, perceptual motor skills, and learning deficits, which cleared at 13 months of abstinence. Large-scale studies of sober alcoholic patients over longer periods of time (e.g., 3 years) are needed to characterize permanent deficits. The general wisdom is that most neuropsychological findings will clear in most alcoholic patients after several weeks. In others, a more permanent, although limited deficit may be evident.

Brain shrinkage is detectable by CT scanning in many patients with chronic alcoholism, and prolonged abstinence results in reversibility in some patients (Lishman 1990). Correlation of damage between CT findings, drinking history, and neuropsychological deficits is not linear. PET scan studies (Eckardt et al. 1988a) have suggested that glucose utilization may be decreased in the frontal lobe area and is correlated with severity of clinical dementia. Brain shrinkage may be due to reduction in extent of dendritic domain. Linnoila (1989) hypothesized that repeated bouts of elevated cortisol during withdrawal may result in hippocampal damage and the development of cognitive deficits. Alcoholic patients have a significantly altered hypothalamic-pituitary-adrenal axis 3 weeks after cessation of drinking (Adinoff et al. 1990). Pharmacological withdrawal mutes elevated cortical levels. These findings may argue against the use of psychosocial detoxification in patients with moderate to severe alcoholism. Alcohol's effect at the NMDA receptor may also impair memory and learning (Lister et al. 1987).

In short-term (21–28 days) rehabilitation programs, educational efforts may be hampered by cognitive deficits. There is evidence that cognitive impairment may be predictive of poor treatment outcome (Caster 1977). Kupke and O'Brien (1985) found neuropsychological test scores predictive of completion of inpatient program, outpatient attendance, future drinking episodes, work behavior, and behavior while in the program. Recidivism is higher among patients with greater neuropsychological deficit (Abbott and Gregson 1981). Donovan et al. (1984) found no prediction of success of abstinence at 6 months, but found decreased employment with poor neuropsychological scores. Focusing efforts at behavioral change or insight in treatment programs may be hampered by cognitive deficits. Programs need to take these problems into account in designing treatment. Patients are more fragile and less open to treatment when cognitive problems are most likely to affect judgment, learning, and attention.

Two hypotheses have been raised to explain these neuropsychological findings. One states that deficits are the consequence of prolonged drinking; the other states that cognitive deficits in individuals predispose one to develop alcoholism. A prospective longitudinal study of sons of alcoholic patients at high risk for developing alcoholism (Drejer et al. 1985) revealed relatively poorer vocabulary and worse performance on categorizing ability, organization, and planning compared with control subjects. Minimal brain dysfunction symptoms have been associated with primary alcoholism and poor neuropsychological testing. A history of these symptoms in childhood may be associated with later impairment in neuropsychological testing (De Obaldia and Parsons 1984). Tarter and Alterman (1984) suggested that minimal brain dysfunction or, more specifically, hyperactive temperament may predispose individuals toward alcoholism. In the families of alcoholic individuals, abstracting and problem-solving deficits have been found, suggesting that learning and memory problems may antedate alcoholism and that alcoholism plus neuropsychological deficits may have additive effects in susceptible individuals.

Begleiter et al. (1983) described a characteristic P300 wave attenuation on the evoked potential found in alcoholic patients and sons of alcoholic patients that may provide a trait marker for alcoholism. The P300 wave is thought to be characteristic of the decreased reaction to novel experience related to a hippocampal deficit. Studies of teenage offspring of alcoholic fathers who are not drinking abusively display P300 abnormalities (Whipple et al. 1988).

There are some similarities between neuropsychological findings in long-term alcoholic patients and Korsakoff patients, although there are also important differences. Both have impairments with visual perception and problem solving, which are both association cortex tasks. Ryback (1971) suggested that there is a continuum of decrease in function from abstinent individuals to persons who drink moderately to chronically and Korsakoff patients. However, recent evidence has not supported the notion that Korsakoff's psychosis is at the extreme end of the spectrum of alcohol dementia (Butters 1985). Compared with Korsakoff patients, long-term alcoholic patients have less learning impairment, dissimilar memory impairment processes, and less verbal memory impairment.

❑ ALCOHOL DEMENTIA

Alcohol dementia is dementia presumably caused by long-term alcohol use. Because it may be difficult to separate the effects from subacute Wernicke-Korsakoff syndrome, trauma, and hepatic encephalopathy, careful exclusion criteria may decrease the reported incidence of this entity. Impaired neuropsychological testing is evident in 50%–70% of sober alcoholic patients (Charness et al. 1989). Cala and Mastaglia (1981) reviewed the literature on CT scans in patients with chronic alcoholism. There is positive evidence for cortical shrinkage but no direct correlation between CT atrophy and neuropsychological deficits, except in the frontal lobe areas. This accompanies findings in Alzheimer's disease in which cortical atrophy does not necessarily predict level of dementia. Reversal of cortical atrophy can follow a prolonged period of abstinence, suggesting that neuronal fallout is not the only factor responsible for alcohol brain atrophy. Advances in the use of PET scans now provide a potential for further study of alcohol's functional metabolic effect on the brain.

❑ OTHER NEUROLOGICAL COMPLICATIONS

Alcoholic polyneuropathy is characterized by stocking-glove paresthesia, with decreased reflexes and autonomic nerve dysfunctions such as impotence, orthostatic hypotension, and bowel or bladder difficulties (Nakada and Knight 1984). It is nerve damage that may be partially improved by vitamin B supplementation. Folic acid deficiency may contribute to the development of alcoholic polyneuropathy (Gimsing et al. 1989).

Hepatic encephalopathy is a reversible neurological deficit often caused by severe alcohol liver disease. Clinical symptoms range from mild confusion, decreased attention, and irritability to coma. Simple cognitive exams, like a trail making test, can detect early stages. There is generally good correlation between clinical stage of hepatic encephalopathy and degree of abnormality of the EEG; however, there is not a good correlation between ammonia levels and degree of hepatic encephalopathy. Behavioral and electrophysiological manifestations of hepatic encephalopathy may be due to functional increase in GABAergic tone in the brain (Gammal and Jones 1989).

Acquired (non-Wilsonian) hepatocerebral degeneration is a chronic, largely irreversible hepatocerebral syndrome frequently developing after several episodes of hepatic coma. Symptoms may include tremor, dysarthria, ataxia, choreoathetosis, and dementia, usually in the context of classic signs of cirrhosis. The syndrome may resemble Wilson's disease; however, there are no Kayser-Fleischer rings, and cerebral lesions tend to be more cortical.

Trauma-induced acute and chronic subdural hematoma are not uncommon in alcoholic patients who are exposed to falls and blunt head injury. Acute subdural hematomas are often confused with cerebral contusion and laceration. CT scans are particularly effective in diagnosis. Chronic subdural hematomas may reveal little in the way of focal signs. Disturbances in mentation, concentration, mood, or thought processes are more common.

Alcohol cerebellar degeneration is a slowly evolving condition encountered along with longstanding history of excessive alcohol use. It affects the cerebellar midline structures and produces truncal ataxia and gait disturbance. The exact course is unknown, but typical symptoms, alcoholic history, and supporting CT findings may make the diagnosis. Etiology may be related to thiamine deficiency or electrolyte abnormalities, but is not correlated with alcohol consumption.

Central pontine myelinolysis, Marchiafava-Bignami disease, and nutritional amblyopia are rare neurological conditions associated with chronic alcoholism. Pontine dysfunction evident in central pontine myelinolysis is of unknown etiology and often causes death. Proposed etiologies include rapid changes of water content and hyponatremia correction (Illowsky and Laureno 1987). Signs and symptoms include paraparesis and quadriparesis, dysarthria, dysphagia, and "locked in" syndrome. Marchiafava-Bignami disease is a rare demyelinating disease of the corpus callosum, whose etiology is totally unknown. The course may be acute or chronic and is associated with dementia, spasticity, and gait disturbance (Victor et al. 1989). A nutritional amblyopia is associated with alcohol and tobacco use and is treated with B complex vitamins.

Alcoholism is also associated with an increased risk of stroke, possibly due to hyperlipidemia, hypertension, or blood flow abnormalities. There is a positive correlation between moderate alcohol consumption and hemorrhagic stroke and possible excess risk of ischemic stroke at high levels of alcohol consumption and protection from ischemic stroke at moderate levels of use (Gorelick 1989).

❑ CONCLUSIONS

Alcohol can have acute and chronic effects that can lead to neuropsychiatric impairment, making diagnosis difficult. Intoxication, withdrawal, and temporary and lasting brain effects require careful history taking, mental status evaluation, selective laboratory testing, and treatment planning. Frequently these problems become complicated by interactions of alcohol-related organic brain syndromes with psychiatric, medical, and neurological conditions. Further research is needed to establish the specific pathogenesis of these neuropsychiatric problems. New approaches such as PET scanning and tools for study of neurotransmitters, receptor sites, ion channels, and second messenger systems may help us understand these effects better. Ultimately, prevention and early diagnosis are the best ways to minimize the devastating consequences of alcohol abuse and dependence.

❑ REFERENCES

Abbott W, Gregson RAM: Cognitive dysfunction in the prediction of relapse in alcoholics. J Stud Alcohol 42: 230–245, 1981

Acker C: Neuropsychological deficits in alcoholics: the relative contributions of gender and drinking history. Br J Addict 81:395–403, 1986

Adams RD, Victor M: Principles of Neurology. New York, McGraw-Hill, 1981

Adinoff B, Martin PR, Bone GHA, et al: Hypothalamic-pituitary-adrenal axis functioning and cerebrospinal fluid corticotropin-releasing hormone and corticotropin levels in alcoholics after recent and long-term abstinence. Arch Gen Psychiatry 47:325–330, 1990

Albert MS, Butters N, Levin J: Temporal gradients in the retrograde amnesia of patients with alcoholic Korsakoff's disease. Arch Neurol 36:211–216, 1979

Alexopoulos GS, Lieberman KW, Frances R, et al: Platelet MAO during the alcohol withdrawal syndrome. Am J Psychiatry 138:1254–1255, 1981

American Psychiatric Association: Diagnostic and Statistical Manual of Mental Disorders, 3rd Edition. Washington, DC, American Psychiatric Association, 1980

American Psychiatric Association: Diagnostic and Statistical Manual of Mental Disorders, 3rd Edition, Revised. Washington, DC, American Psychiatric Association, 1987

Aminoff NJ, Simon RP: Status epilepticus: causes, clinical features and consequences in 98 patients. Am J Med 69:657–666, 1980

Arendt T, Allen Y, Sinden J, et al: Cholinergic-rich brain transplants reverse alcohol-induced memory deficits. Nature 332:448–450, 1988

Ballenger JC, Post RM: Carbamazepine in alcohol withdrawal syndromes and schizophrenic psychoses. Psychopharmacol Bull 20:572–584, 1984

Baumgartner GR, Rowen RC: Clonidine vs. chlordiazepoxide in the management of acute alcohol withdrawal syndrome. Arch Intern Med 147:1223–1226, 1987

Begleiter H, Porjesz B, Chou CL, et al: P_3 and stimulus incentive value. Psychophysiology 1:95–101, 1983

Beresford TP: Alcoholism consultation and general hospital psychiatry. Gen Hosp Psychiatry 1:293–300, 1979

Berglund M, Risberg J: Regional cerebral blood flow during withdrawal. Arch Gen Psychiatry 38:351–355, 1981

Besson JA, Glen AI: Brain water in alcoholics (letter). Lancet 2:50, 1985

Black RF, Hoffman RL, Tabakoff B: Receptor-mediated dopaminergic function after ethanol withdrawal. Alcoholism 4:294–297, 1980

Blass JP, Gibson GE: Abnormality of a thiamine requiring enzyme in patients with Wernicke-Korsakoff syndrome. N Engl J Med 297:1367–1370, 1977

Blum K, Noble EP, Sheridan PJ, et al: Allelic association of human dopamine D_2 receptor gene in alcoholism. JAMA 263:2055–2060, 1990

Branchey L, Branchey M, Zucker D, et al: Association between low plasma tryptophan and blackouts in male alcholic patients. Alcoholism 9:393–395, 1985

Brennan FN, Lyttle JA: Alcohol and seizures: a review. J R Soc Med 9:571–573, 1987

Brew BJ: Diagnosis of Wernicke's encephalopathy. Aust N Z J Med 16:676–678, 1986

Butters N: Alcoholic Korsakoff's syndrome: some unresolved issues concerning etiology: neuropathology and cognitive deficits. J Clin Exp Neuropsychol 7:181–210, 1985

Cala LA, Mastaglia FL: Computerized tomography in chronic alcoholics. Alcoholism (N Y) 5:283–294, 1981

Caster DU: The treatment of the recidivist alcoholic. Alcoholism (N Y) 1:87–90, 1977

Chan AW: Alcoholism and epilepsy. Epilepsia 26:323–333, 1985

Charness ME, DeLaPaz RL: Mamillary body atrophy in Wernicke's encephalopathy: antemortem identification using magnetic resonance imaging. Ann Neurol 22: 595–600, 1987

Charness ME, Simon RP, Greenberg DA: Ethanol and the nervous system. N Engl J Med 321:442–454, 1989

Cohen MJ, Schandler SL, Naaliboff BD: Psychophysiological measures from intoxicated and detoxified alcoholics. J Stud Alcohol 44:271–282, 1983

Collins DM, Myers RD: Buspirone attenuates volitional alcohol intake in chronically drinking monkey. Alcohol 4:49–56, 1987

Cushman P Jr: Delirium tremens: update on an old disorder. Postgrad Med 82(5):117–122, 1987

Cushman P Jr, Forbes R, Lerner W, et al: Alcohol withdrawal syndromes: clinical management with lofexidine. Alcoholism (N Y) 9:103–108, 1985

De Obaldia R, Parsons OA: Relationship of neuropsychological performance to primary alcoholism and self-reported symptoms of childhood minimal brain dysfunction. J Stud Alcohol 45:386–392, 1984

Devetag F, Mandich G, Zaiotte G, et al: Alcoholic epilepsy: review of a series and proposed classification and etiopathogenesis. Ital J Neurol Sci 3:275–284, 1983

Dolin SJ, Little HJ: Are changes in neuronal calcium channels involved in ethanol tolerance. J Pharmacol Exp Ther 250:985–991, 1989

Donovan DM, Kivlahann DR, Walker RD: Clinical limitations of neuropsychological testing in predicting treatment outcome among alcoholics. Alcoholism (N Y) 8:470–475, 1984

Drejer K, Theilgaard A, Teasdale TW, et al: Prospective

study of young men at high risk for alcoholism: neuropsychological assessment. Alcoholism 6:498–502, 1985

Earnest MP, Feldman F, Marx JA, et al: Intracranial lesions shown by CT scans in 259 cases of first alcohol-related seizures. Neurology 38:1561–1565, 1988

Eckardt MJ, Campbell GA, Marietta CA, et al: Acute ethanol administration selectively alters localized cerebral glucose metabolism. Brain Res 444:53–58, 1988a

Eckardt MJ, Rohrbaugh JW, Rio D, et al: Brain imaging in alcoholic patients. Adv Alcohol Subst Abuse 7:59–71, 1988b

Embry CK, Lippmann S: Use of magnesium sulfate in alcohol withdrawal. Am Fam Physician 35:167–170, 1987

Espir ML, Rose FC: Alcohol, seizures, and epilepsy. J R Soc Med 9:542–543, 1987

Femino J, Lewis DC: Clinical Pharmacology and Therapeutics of the Alcohol Withdrawal Syndrome (Report 0372). Rockville, MD, National Institute on Alcohol Abuse and Alcoholism, 1982

Feussner J, Linfus E, Blessing C, et al: CAT scanning in ETOH withdrawal syndromes: value of the neurological exam. Ann Intern Med 94:519–522, 1981

Frances RJ, Franklin JE, Flavin DK: Suicide and alcoholism. Am J Drug Alcohol Abuse 13:327–341, 1987

Frezza M, Di Padova G, Pozzato G, et al: High blood alcohol levels in women: the role of decreased gastric alcohol dehydrogenase activity and first-pass metabolism. N Engl J Med 322:95–99, 1990

Fujimato A, Nagaao T, Ebara T, et al: Cerebrospinal fluid monoamine metabolite during alcohol withdrawal syndrome and recovered state. Biol Psychiatry 18: 1141–1152, 1983

Gammal SH, Jones EA: Hepatic encephalopathy. Med Clin North Am 73:793–813, 1989

Gessner PK: Drug withdrawal therapy of the alcohol withdrawal syndrome, in Biochemistry and Pharmacology of Ethanol, Vol 2. Edited by Majchowicz E, Moble E. New York, Plenum, 1979, pp 375–435

Gimsing P, Melgaard B, Andersen K, et al: Vitamin B-12 and folate function in chronic alcoholic men with peripheral neuropathy and encephalopathy. J Nutr 119:416–424, 1989

Glowa JR, Crawley J, Suzdak PD, et al: Ethanol and the GABA receptor complex: studies with the partial inverse benzodiazepine receptor agonist RO 15-4513. Pharmacol Biochem Behav 3:767–772, 1989

Goodwin DW: Alcoholism and genetics. Arch Gen Psychiatry 42:171–174, 1985

Goodwin DW, Crane JB, Guze SB: Alcoholic blackouts: a review and clinical study of 100 alcoholics. Am J Psychiatry 126:174–177, 1969

Gorelick PB: The status of alcohol as a risk factor for stroke. Stroke 20:1607–1610, 1989

Grant I, Adams K, Reed R: Normal neuropsychological abilities of alcoholic men in their late thirties. Am J Psychiatry 136:1263–1269, 1974

Greenberg P, Pearlman C: Delirium tremens and dreaming. Am J Psychiatry 124:133–142, 1967

Harper C: The incidence of Wernicke's encephalopathy in Australia: a neuropathological study of 131 cases. J Neurol Neurosurg Psychiatry 46:593–598, 1983

Harper CG, Giles M, Finlay-Jones R: Clinical signs in the Wernicke-Korsakoff complex: a retrospective analysis of 131 cases diagnosed at necropsy. J Neurol Neurosurg Psychiatry 49:341–345, 1986

Harwood HJ, Kristiansen P, Rachal JV: Social and economic costs of alcohol abuse and alcoholism (Issue Report No 2). Research Triangle Park, NC, Research Triangle Institute, 1985

Hawley BJ, Major LF, Schulman EA, et al: CSF levels of norepinephrine during alcohol withdrawal. Arch Neurol 38:289–292, 1981

Hayshida M, Alterman AI, McLellan AT, et al: Comparitive effectiveness and costs of inpatient and outpatient detoxification of patients with mild to moderate alcohol withdrawal syndrome. N Engl J Med 320:358–365, 1989

Hemmingsen R, Kramp P, Rafaelsen OJ: DTs and related clinical states: etiology, pathophysiology and treatment. Acta Psychiatr Scand 59:337–369, 1979

Hoffman PL, Rabe CS, Moses F, et al: *N*-methyl-D-aspartate receptors and ethanol: inhibition of calcium flux and cyclic gMP production. J Neurochem 52:1937–1940, 1989

Holloway HC, Hales RE, Wantanabe HK: Recognition and treatment of acute alcohol withdrawal syndrome. Psychiatr Clin North Am 7:729–743, 1984

Horowitz RI, Gottlieb LD, Kraus ML: The efficacy of atenolol in the outpatient management of the alcohol withdrawal syndrome. Arch Intern Med 149:1089–1093, 1989

Hunter BE, Boast CA, Walker DW: Alcohol withdrawal syndrome in rats: neural and behavioral correlates. Pharmacol Biochem Behav 1:719–725, 1973

Illowsky BP, Laureno R: Encephalopathy and myelinolysis after rapid correction of hyponatraemia. Brain 110: 855–867, 1987

Isbell H, Fraser HG, Winkler A, et al: An experimental study of the etiology of "rum fits" and delirium tremens. Quarterly Journal of the Study of Alcohol 16:1–13, 1955

Klemm WR: Effects of ethanol on nerve impulse activity, in Biochemistry and Pharmacology of Ethanol. Edited by Majchrowicz E, Noble EP. New York, Plenum, 1979, pp 243–267

Kolin IS, Linet OT: Double blind comparison of alprazolam and diazepam for subchronic withdrawal from alcohol. J Clin Psychiatry 42:169–173, 1981

Kopelman MD, Corn TH: Cholinergic "blockade" as a model for cholinergic depletion. Brain 111:1079–1110, 1988

Koppi S, Eberhardt G, Haller R, et al: Calcium-channel-blocking agent in the treatment of acute alcohol withdrawal: cavoreine versus meprobamate in a randomized double-blind study. Neuropsychobiology 17: 49–52, 1987

Kramp P, Hemmingsen R: Delirium tremens and related clinical sites: changes in calcium and inorganic phosphate concentrations in plasma and cerebrospinal fluid. Acta Psychiatr Scand 69:250–258, 1984

Kupke T, O'Brien W: Neuropsychological impairment and behavioral limitation exhibited within an alcoholic treatment program. J Clin Exp Neuropsychol 7:292–304, 1985

Leigh D, McBurney A, McIlwain H: Wernicke-Korsakoff syndrome in monozygotic twins: a biochemical peculiarity. Br J Psychiatry 139:156–159, 1981

Liebowitz NR, Kranzler HR, Meyer RE: Pharmacologic approaches to alcoholism treatment, in Alcohol and Health (Seventh Special Report to the U.S. Congress from the Secretary of Health and Human Services). Washington, DC, U.S. Department of Health and Human Services, 1990 pp 144–153

Linnoila M: Alcohol withdrawal syndrome and sympathetic nervous system function. Alcohol Health and Research World 13:355–357, 1989

Lishman WA: Organic Psychiatry. Philadelphia, PA, JB Lippincott, 1978

Lishman WA: Alcohol and the brain. Br J Psychiatry 156: 635–644, 1990

Liskow BI, Goodwin DW: Pharmacological treatment of alcohol intoxication, withdrawal and dependence: a critical review. J Stud Alcohol 48:356–370, 1987

Lister RG, Nutt DJ: Antagonizing the behavioral effects of ethanol using drugs that act at the benzodiazepine/GABA receptor macromolecular complex. Pharmacol Biochem Behav 31:731, 1989

Lister RG, Eckardt M, Weingarter H: Ethanol intoxication and memory: recent developments and new directions, in Recent Developments in Alcoholism, Vol 5. Edited by Galanter M. New York, Plenum, 1987, pp 111–125

Little HJ, Dolin SJ, Halsey MJ: Calcium channel antagonists decrease the ethanol withdrawal syndrome. Life Sci 39:2059–2065, 1986

Lukas SE, Mendelson JH, Woods BT, et al: Topographic distribution of EEG alpha activity during ethanol-induced intoxication in women. J Stud Alcohol 50:176–185, 1989

McEntee WJ, Mair RG: Memory impairment in Korsakoff's psychosis: a correlation with brain norepinephrine activity. Science 202:905–907, 1978

McEntee WJ, Mair RG, Langlais PJ: Clonidine in Korsakoff disease: pathophysiologic and therapeutic implications. Prog Clin Biol Res 71:211–223, 1981

Malcolm R, Ballenger JC, Sturgis ET, et al: Double-blind controlled trial comparing carbamazepine to oxazepam treatment of alcohol. Am J Psychiatry 146:617–621, 1989

Martin PR, Adinoff B, Eckardt MJ, et al: Effective pharmacotherapy of alcoholic amnestic disorder with fluvoxamine. Arch Gen Psychiatry 46:617–621, 1989

Mattis S, Kovner R, Gartner J, et al: Deficits in retrieval of category exemplars in alcoholic Korsakoff patients. Neuropsychologia 19:357–363, 1981

Meilgaard MC: Wernicke's encephalopathy (letter). N Engl J Med 313:637–638, 1985

Mensing JW, Hoogland PH, Slooff JL: Computed tomography in the diagnosis of Wernicke's encephalopathy: a radiological-neuropathological correlation. Ann Neurol 16:363–365, 1984

Miller SI, Frances RJ, Holmes DJ: Use of psychotropic drugs in alcoholism treatment: a summary. Hosp Community Psychiatry 39:1251–1252, 1988

Minion GE, Slovis CM, Boutiette L: Severe alcohol intoxication: a study of 204 consecutive patients. Clinical Toxicology 27:375–384, 1989

Moskowitz G, Chalmers TG, Sacks HS, et al: Deficiencies of clinical trials of alcohol withdrawal. Alcoholism (N Y) 7:42–46, 1983

Nakada T, Knight RT: Alcohol and the central nervous system. Med Clin North Am 68:121–131, 1984

Naranjo CA, Sellers EM, Lawrin MO: Modulation of ethanol intake by serotonin uptake inhibitors. J Clin Psychiatry 47 (Apr suppl):16–22, 1986

Ng SKC, Hauser WA, Brust JCM, et al: Alcohol consumption and withdrawal in new-onset seizures. N Engl J Med 319:666–673, 1988

Nordstrom G, Berglund M: Ageing and Recovery from Alcoholism. Br J Psychiatry 151:382–388, 1987

Nutt D: Alpha-2 adrenoceptor function during ethanol withdrawal (NIH Conference report: Alcohol Withdrawal and Noradrenergic Function. Moderated by Linnoila M). Ann Intern Med 107:880–884, 1987

Page RD, Schaub LH: Intellectual functioning in alcoholics during six months abstinence. J Stud Alcohol 38:1240–1246, 1977

Parker ES, Noble E: Alcohol consumption and cognitive functioning in social drinkers. J Stud Alcohol 38:1224–1232, 1977

Parsons O: Neuropsychological deficits in chronic alcoholics: facts and fantasies. Alcoholism (N Y) 1:51–56, 1977

Peterson JB, Rothfleisch J, Zelazo PD, et al: Acute alcohol intoxication and cognitive functioning. J Stud Alcohol 51:114–122, 1990

Porjesz B, Begleiter H: Evoked brain potential deficits in alcoholism and aging. Alcoholism (N Y) 6:53–63, 1982

Reuler JB, Girard DE, Cooney TG: Wernicke's encephalopathy. N Engl J Med 312:1035–1039, 1985

Robins LN, Helzer JE, Weissman MM, et al: Lifetime prevalence of specific psychiatric disorders in three sites. Arch Gen Psychiatry 41:949–958, 1984

Ryan C: Alcoholism and premature aging: a neuropsychological perspective. Alcoholism (N Y) 6:22–30, 1982

Ryback R: The continuum and specificity of the effects of alcohol on memory. Quarterly Journal of the Study of Alcohol 32:995–1016, 1971

Schaeffer KW, Parsons OA: Learning impairment in alcoholics using an ecologically relevant test. J Nerv Ment Dis 175:213–218, 1987

Schwittes SY, Johnson RC, McGlean GE, et al: Alcohol use and the flushing response in different rural and ethnic groups. J Stud Alcohol 43:1254–1262, 1982

Sellers EM, Kalant H: Alcohol intoxication and withdrawal. N Engl J Med 294:757–762, 1976

Selzer B, Benson DF: The temporal pattern of retrograde amnesia in Korsakoff's disease. Neurology 24:527–530, 1974

Shaw JM: Development of optimal treatment tactics for alcohol withdrawal. J Clin Psychopharmocol 1:382–389, 1981

Shen WW: Extrapyramidal symptoms associated with alcohol withdrawal. Biol Psychiatry 19:1037–1043, 1984

Surawicz FG: Alcoholic hallucinosis: a missed diagnosis: differential diagnoses and management. Can J Psychiatry 1:57–63, 1980

Tabakoff B, Hoffman PL: Biochemical pharmacology of alcohol, in Psychopharmacology: The Third Generation of Progress. New York, Raven, 1987, pp 1521–1526

Tabakoff B, Hoffman PL, Lee JM, et al: Differences in platelet enzyme activity between alcoholics and nonalcoholics. N Engl J Med 318:134–139, 1988

Tabakoff B, Hoffman PL, Peterson RC: Advances in neurochemistry, in Alchohol and Health (Seventh Special Report to the U.S. Congress from the Secretary of Health and Human Services). Washington, DC, U.S. Department of Health and Human Services, 1990, pp 109–160

Tarter RE, Alterman AL: Neuropsychological deficits in alcoholics: etiological considerations. J Stud Alcohol 45:1–9, 1984

Tarter RE, Goldstein G, Alterman A, et al: Alcoholic seizures: intellectual and neuropsychological sequelae. J Nerv Ment Dis 171:123–125, 1983

Tonnesen E: Delirium tremens and hypokalemia (letter). Lancet 2:97, 1982

Turner RG, Lichstein PR, Peden JG, et al: Alcohol withdrawal syndromes: a review of pathophysiology, clinical presentation and treatment. J Gen Intern Med 4: 432–444, 1989

Victor M: Treatment of alcohol intoxication and the withdrawal syndrome: a critical analysis of the use of drugs and other forms of therapy. Psychosom Med 28:636–650, 1966

Victor M, Adams RD: The effect of alcohol on the nervous system. Res Publ Assoc Res Nerv Ment Dis 32:526–573, 1953

Victor M, Brausch C: The role of abstinence in the genesis of alcohol epilepsy. Epilepsia 8:1–20, 1967

Victor M, Wolfe SM: Causation and treatment of the alcohol withdrawal syndrome, in Alcoholism: Progress in Research and Treatment. Edited by Bourne PG, Fox R. New York, Academic, 1973, pp 137–166

Victor M, Adams RD, Collins GH: The Wernicke-Korsakoff Syndrome and Related Neurologic Disorders Due to Alcoholism and Malnutrition (Contemporary Neurology Series, Vol 3). Philadelphia, PA, FA Davis, 1989

Weingartner H, Groifman J, Boutelle W, et al: Forms of memory failure. Science 221:380–383, 1983

West LJ, Maxwell DS, Noble EP, et al: Alcoholism. Ann Intern Med 100:405–416, 1984

Whipple SW, Parker ES, Nobel EP: Atypical neurocognitive profile in alcoholic fathers and their sons. J Stud Alcohol 49:240–244, 1988

Whitfield GL, Thompson G, Lamb A, et al: Detoxification of 1,024 alcoholic patients with psychoactive drugs. JAMA 239:1409–1410, 1978

Wilson A, Vulcano B: A double-blind, placebo-controlled trial of magnesium sulfate in the ethanol withdrawl syndrome. Alcoholism 8:542–545, 1984

Yohman JR, Parsons OA: Verbal reasoning deficits in alcoholics. J Nerv Ment Dis 175:219–223, 1987

Yohman JR, Parsons OA, Leber WR: Lack of recovery in male alcoholics: neuropsychological performance one year after treatment. Alcoholism (N Y) 9:114–117, 1985

Yudofsky SC, Stevens L, Silver J, et al: Propranolol in the treatment of rage and violent behavior associated with Korsakoff's psychosis. Am J Psychiatry 141:114–115, 1984

Zilm DH, Kaplan HC, Capell H: Electroencephalographic tolerance and abstinence phenomena during repeated alcohol ingestion by nonalcoholics. Science 212:1175–1177, 1981

Zola-Morgan SM, Oberg RG: Recall of life experience in an alcoholic Korsakoff patient: a naturalistic approach. Neuropsychologia 18:549–557, 1980

Chapter

25

Neuropsychiatric Aspects of Degenerative Dementias Associated With Motor Dysfunction

Peter J. Whitehouse, M.D., Ph.D.
Robert P. Friedland, M.D.
Milton E. Strauss, Ph.D.

THE DEGENERATIVE DEMENTIAS associated with motor system dysfunction are a diverse group of disorders that present a particular challenge to the neuropsychiatrically oriented clinician. Depending on where the pathology occurs in the motor system (basal ganglia, cerebellum, or motor neuron), the motor symptoms can include abnormal movements, incoordination, or weakness. In this chapter, we review Huntington's disease (HD), Parkinson's disease (PD), and other rarer degenerative conditions characterized by dementia and movement disorders (Table 25–1). Primary degenerative dementias, particularly Alzheimer's disease (AD) and Pick's disease—in which motor signs are found more rarely than in the conditions we consider here and often only in the later stages of the disease—are addressed in Chapter 26.

As degenerative disorders, the dementias included in this chapter are characterized by gradual loss of function caused by progressive loss of neurons in specific regions of the brain associated with pathological hallmarks that are characteristic of the individual diseases. The specific etiologies of these diseases are often unknown, and biological interventions are limited in effectiveness. There are many rare conditions in this category, and features fre-

The authors wish to thank Monisha Pasupathi and Jan Martin for assistance in the preparation of this chapter.

quently overlap among different conditions, making a clear nosology difficult. These conditions are particularly stressful for patient, family, and professional caregiver because the combinations of motor, cognitive, and behavioral abnormalities cause significant impairment in quality of life. Although in some conditions, drugs are available to treat the motor symptoms, these drugs frequently contribute to the cognitive and behavioral dysfunction. The motor impairments themselves create special difficulties in neuropsychiatric and neuropsychological testing of the cognitive and psychiatric dysfunction.

The classification of the dementias included in this chapter and their nosological relationships to those considered in Chapter 26 are controversial. Ideally, classification should be based on better understanding of essential clinical and biological features. Our understanding of the relationships between brain changes and behavioral alterations in these disorders, however, is limited. Many attempts have been made to define subtypes of dementia; for example, age at onset has been used to characterize different forms of AD, HD, and PD. One attempt to develop a classification of dementia based on an understanding of biology has been the development of the concept of cortical and subcortical dementia (Albert et al. 1974; McHugh and Folstein 1975). AD and Pick's disease are thought to represent cortical dementias in which the predominant pathology is found in the neocortex and the clinical symptoms are believed to reflect this cortical pathology (e.g., aphasia, apraxia, and agnosia).

It has been suggested that the clinical picture of the dementias considered in this chapter is due to primary pathology in subcortical structures and includes dysfunction in affect, speed of processing, and memory (Cummings 1990). This attempt to categorize dementias into these two superordinate categories has stimulated research and debate concerning nosology. Many authors have come to the conclusion that all dementias cannot be classified easily into these two large categories and, for example, that the dementias of HD and PD are as clinically different from one another as they are different from AD. (For a review, see Brown and Marsden 1988; Mayeux et al. 1983; Whitehouse 1986; cf., Cummings 1990.)

In the following sections we focus on specific diseases, briefly reviewing general features of the disease including defining features, epidemiology, etiology, and biology and discussing the motor system abnormalities occurring in the disease. The bulk of each section is devoted, however, to a discussion of the cognitive impairments in each condition, followed by a discussion of the accompanying behavioral and psychiatric pathology and treatment.

TABLE 25–1. DEGENERATIVE DEMENTIAS ASSOCIATED WITH MOTOR SYSTEM DYSFUNCTION

Extrapyramidal diseases
- Parkinson's disease
- Huntington's disease
- Progressive supranuclear palsy
- Thalamic dementias
- Wilson's disease
- Hallervorden-Spatz disease
- Fahr's disease

Cerebellar diseases
- Olivopontocerebellar atrophy
- Friedreich's ataxia

Motor neuron diseases
- Motor neuron disease with dementia
- Amyotrophic lateral sclerosis/parkinsonism-dementia complex

Other
- Normal-pressure hydrocephalus

❑ HUNTINGTON'S DISEASE

HD is a genetically transmitted, progressive neuropsychiatric disorder that can appear at any time in life. The peak period of onset is in the fourth and fifth decade. Because of their clinical prominence and central place in Huntington's description (1872), dyskinesias, particularly chorea, are usually considered the first sign of the disease. However, clinical presentation is quite variable in early stages of HD, and cognitive and psychiatric symptoms are often evident well before the movement disorder begins (Folstein 1989). Depression, irritability, and impulsive or erratic behavior are the most common psychiatric symptoms. Memory and concentration difficulties are cognitive symptoms that appear early (Folstein 1989; Martin and Gusella 1986).

Epidemiology

HD is an autosomal dominant disorder with variable age at onset. Presentation differs in juvenile-onset and adult-onset cases. Chorea is the cardinal motor symptom in adult-onset HD. In the 3%–9% of cases in which onset occurs before adolescence, rigidity, myoclonus, or dystonic movements are characteristic. Early onset is typically associated with paternal transmission and has a more rapid course (Folstein 1989; Martin and Gusella 1986). In adult-onset cases, death usually occurs after 16–20 years (Folstein 1989). Rate of decline may be slower in patients with onset after the fifth decade of life (Martin and Gusella 1986). Age at onset is earlier among persons of African ancestry compared with those of European ancestry (Folstein et al. 1987; Hayden et al. 1980).

Estimates of the prevalence of HD vary widely. Folstein (1989) concluded that the best estimate of point prevalence among Caucasians is 5–7 cases per 100,000. There are pockets of isolated populations of European origin in which the rates are much higher. In some instances, the elevated rates may be artifacts of the instability of estimates based on small samples, but they may also be the consequence of reproductive isolation. These isolated populations are invaluable for genetic studies, as illustrated in the location of the chromosome carrying the HD gene using a Venezuelan population with a very high prevalence of the disease (Gusella et al. 1983).

As Folstein (1989) reviewed, there are sometimes large differences among ethnic groups (e.g., blacks, northern Europeans, and Japanese) in prevalence, but these must be considered with caution. It is difficult to evaluate the reliability of the racial and/or ethnic differences that have been reported because of differences in survey and diagnostic methods as well as the errors of estimation inherent in statistical surveys.

Etiology

George Huntington (1872) was fortunate to practice medicine in the same location as his father, for it afforded him ample opportunity to observe the familial transmission of this disease. He correctly concluded that the familial transmission was hereditary and, although the concepts were not yet developed, appreciated that it was a dominant, fully penetrant, autosomal condition (Folstein 1989).

The gene for HD is as yet unknown, but genetic linkage analysis has identified its location as at the distal end of the short arm of chromosome 4 (Gusella et al. 1983). The same locus has been implicated in unrelated families of different ethnic and/or racial background and with varying clinical presentations. The uniformity of the linkage suggests a single genetic locus for the disease. However, it is not clear whether there is allelic homogeneity as well. Allelic heterogeneity has been suggested by the findings of family-related and race-related differences in age at onset (Farrer and Conneally 1985; Folstein et al. 1987; Hayden et al. 1982). Familial aggregation of major affective disorder with HD in some families has been suggested as evidence of allelic heterogeneity as well (Folstein et al. 1983b, 1984). The mutation rate in HD is very low. The persistence of the disease is due to its onset typically after the peak period of reproduction (Folstein 1989).

Because of the complete penetrance of the HD gene, there has been considerable interest in identifying preclinical indicators of the disease in persons at genetic risk. Neuropsychological tests have been explored for this purpose, but are not useful for clinical prediction (Lyle and Gottesman 1979; Strauss and Brandt 1986). Genetic testing for HD in the family members of affected persons is now possible in many cases because of the development of multiple genetic linkage markers for the HD gene (Gilliam et al. 1987; Gusella et al. 1983; Wasmuth et al. 1988). However, because the test is for genetic linkage rather than for the gene itself, available tests may be inconclusive for presymptomatic testing. (For a discussion of the methods and clinical context of genetic testing, see Brandt et al. 1989; Martin and Gusella 1986.)

Diagnosis and Clinical Features

As Folstein (1989) noted in her recent monograph, "In principle, the diagnosis of HD is straightforward: it is a clinical-pathological entity defined by involuntary movements and abnormalities of voluntary motor control.... Most patients also suffer from nonaphasic dementia and emotional symptoms, particularly irritability and depression.... There is almost always a history of an affected parent" (p. 125). Nonetheless, there can be considerable diagnostic inaccuracy in cross-sectional assessment of patients.

One reason for diagnostic inaccuracy is the variability in presentation early in the disease. Nearly half of HD cases initially present with emotional or cognitive symptoms. These can be very diverse and include depression, irritability, hallucinations, and apathy. Motor symptoms, if present, may be mild rigidity, restlessness, or ticlike jerks that are easily attributable to another disorder (Folstein 1989). Conditions such as PD, Sydenham's chorea, ataxias, cerebrovascular disease, other dementias, schizophrenia, affective disorder, thyroid disease, acanthocytosis, and alcoholism are also considerations in the differential diagnosis. However, when there is a positive family history, HD is a very likely explanation of these symptoms. Folstein (1989) suggested that a second reason the diagnosis of HD may be missed is the failure to take an adequate family history. A positive family history strongly implicates HD as a diagnosis given the clinical pictures described above. It is difficult to make the diagnosis unequivocally during life without family history because of the variety of presentation and course (Martin and Gusella 1986).

Neurobiology

The most obvious gross pathology in HD occurs in the basal ganglia. The striatum is consistently affected in this disease, with degeneration beginning in the medial caudate and proceeding laterally to the putamen and then occasionally to the globus pallidus (Folstein 1989). γ-Aminobutyric acid (GABA), the most abundant neurotransmitter of the spiny output neurons, and acetylcholine, the principal neurotransmitter of Type I aspiny interneurons, are especially affected in this disease (Folstein 1989; Martin and Gusella 1986). There are many other neurotransmitter changes in HD. The hope that a selective neurotransmitter deficit would be identified that would lead to a corrective therapy has not yet been realized (Martin and Gusella 1986). The alterations in absolute neurotransmitter concentrations and relative balance among different systems may account for some of the symptoms of HD (Folstein 1989). In caudate, for example, somatostatin levels increase because of the selective survival of Type II spiny interneurons (Folstein 1989). In an animal model, injection of somatostatin into the caudate increases dopamine turnover, offering a possible explanation of the utility of neuroleptics in the control of chorea in HD (Martin and Gusella 1986).

There are rich interconnections between the striatum and the prefrontal and parietal cortices (Folstein 1989; Folstein et al. 1990). Alexander et al. (1986) summarized evidence that there are five distinct, parallel corticostriatal circuits that subserve distinct neurobehavioral functions including eye movements, motor behavior, emotion, and cognitive functions. Except for the motor circuit that involves the putamen, the others are caudate-frontal circuits. Interestingly, lesions at any of the segments of the circuit produce similar functional consequences.

Degree of caudate atrophy correlates with cognitive dysfunction including intelligence, memory, and visuospatial deficits (Bamford et al. 1989; Sax et al. 1983) (Figure 25–1). Caudate atrophy is generally more robustly correlated than measures of frontal atrophy, with "executive" functions typically considered to be evidence of prefrontal cortical pathology (Bamford et al. 1989; Starkstein et al. 1988). Similar associations between functional impairments and caudate pathology have been reported with positron-emission tomography (PET) (Bamford et al. 1989). With the development of more sensitive radiographic measures, cortical atrophy may be detected earlier than it is now, leading to some reevaluation of these conclusions. However, at present the deterioration in neuropsychological functions in HD appears to derive principally from disruptions in neural circuits caused by basal ganglia pathology (Bamford et al. 1989; Folstein et al. 1990).

Motor Abnormalities

Both involuntary movements and abnormal voluntary movements occur in HD (Folstein 1989; Folstein et al. 1983a; Leigh et al. 1983) (Table 25–2). The earlier name of the disease in the United States, Huntington's chorea, emphasized the prominence of sudden jerky movements of the limbs, face, or trunk. These are less abrupt and of longer duration and involve more muscle groups than Sydenham's chorea (Paulson 1979). Unlike tics, choreic movements in HD are not repetitive or periodic. They can occur while the patient is at rest or in the course of planned movement (e.g., walking and reaching), although they appear to be absent during sleep. Stress, such as that experienced during cognitive challenges (e.g., serial 7s and mental calculation), can increase choreic movements. Patients can generally suppress them for only short periods of time. Motor restlessness may occur before chorea, and dystonia, in the absence of chorea, is frequent in juvenile-onset (Westphal variant) cases (Folstein 1989).

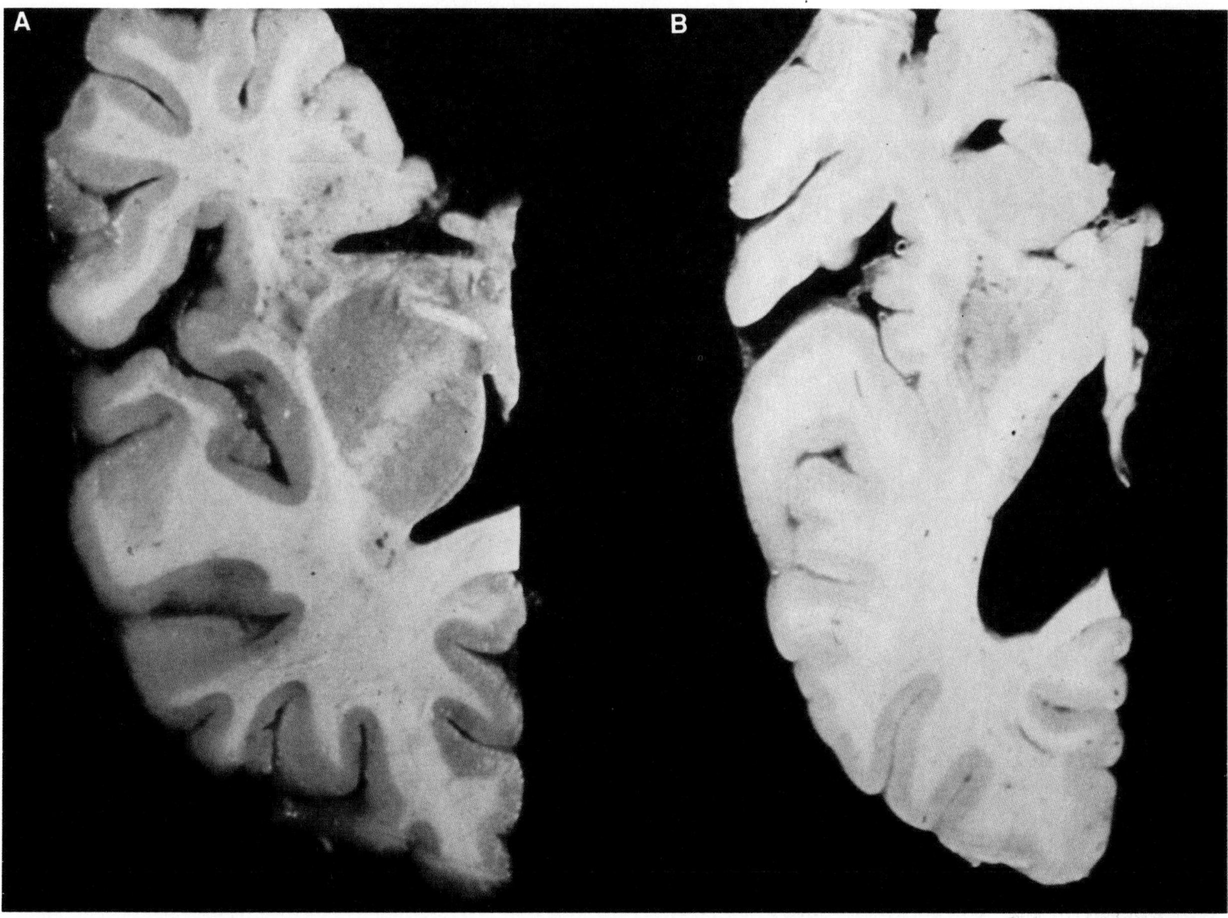

Figure 25–1. Caudate atrophy in Huntington's disease (coronal section). *Panel A*: control subject; *panel B*: Huntington's disease patient.

Because they have been seen as less central to the diagnosis of the disease, abnormalities in voluntary movement have received less attention clinically than has chorea. However, abnormalities in voluntary motor movements are universal in HD, even in the absence of chorea. As summarized by Folstein (1989), abnormalities exist in initiation and inhibition of eye movements, coordination of limb movements, and articulation. Although nonspecific features of the illness, they are important to assess because of their more robust relationship than severity of chorea to intellectual impairment, memory disorder, and capacity for activities of daily living (Brandt et al. 1984; Folstein 1989). A standardized neurological examination that provides independent assessments of chorea and voluntary motor impairment in HD has been developed (Folstein et al. 1983a).

Cognitive Abnormalities

Cognitive deficits appear early in the course of HD and are progressive (Caine et al. 1977) (Table 25–2). If of sufficient severity, they can be detected and coarsely evaluated in brief, formal mental status testing, such as with the Mini-Mental State Exam (MMSE; Folstein et al. 1975). Detailed neuropsychological evaluation of patients with HD is often useful because of the range of deficits that may be encountered and the variability in the course of this dementia.

Very early in the disease, intelligence may be normal, but deficits in memory and verbal fluency can be detected on neuropsychological testing (Butters et al. 1978). Intellectual impairment is a major contribution to disability even early in the illness (Mayeux et al. 1986b). Dementia of the same clini-

TABLE 25–2. CLINICAL FEATURES OF HUNTINGTON'S DISEASE

Motor symptoms
- Involuntary movement abnormalities
  - Chorea, consisting of nonrepetitive, nonperiodic, jerky movements of limbs, face, or trunk
  - Exacerbated by stress
  - Absent during sleep
  - May be consciously suppressed only for short periods
- Voluntary movement abnormalities
  - Initiation and inhibition of eye movements
  - Coordination of limb movements
  - Articulation

Neuropsychological deficits
- Declarative memory, with greater impairment for retrieval of information from memory than in recognition
- Procedural memory
- Verbal fluency
- Visuospatial skills
- Sustained concentration
- Executive functions (i.e., mental planning, organization of sequential actions, and mental flexibility)
- Language functions relatively preserved

Psychiatric features
- Common symptoms
  - Apathy
  - Irritability
  - Dysphoria
  - Anxiety
- Common syndromes
  - Mood disorders (especially symptomatic major depression and bipolar disorder)
  - Intermittent explosive disorder
  - Schizophreniform disorder
  - Atypical psychosis

cally assessed level of severity (e.g., by MMSE) may be due to different disabilities in different illnesses. Brandt et al. (1988) demonstrated that at any given level of dementia the pattern of failure for specific items is different in HD as compared with AD. At mild levels of dementia (MMSE scores 20–24), for example, HD patients are more impaired than AD patients in the serial subtraction of 7 from 100, whereas AD patients are less likely than HD patients to recall three items learned earlier in the examination. Object naming is relatively preserved on the MMSE even in advanced stages of HD (Brandt et al. 1988). Naming and other language functions appear to be relatively preserved in HD (Butters et al. 1978; Cummings and Benson 1988; Smith et al. 1988), but not invariably.

The cognitive deficits of HD include—in addition to those of memory and verbal fluency—difficulties in tasks requiring sustained concentration (e.g., mental arithmetic) and visuospatial skills. The deficits in visuospatial tasks are most easily seen on tests measuring constructional ability (e.g., the Wechsler Adult Intelligence Scale-Revised [WAIS-R; Wechsler 1981] Block Design and Object Assembly), but can be detected on tasks that do not require coordinated motor activity as well (Fedio et al. 1979). HD patients also have difficulty identifying or using their position in space relative to some fixed point (Folstein et al. 1990). Although cognitive deficits occur very early in the disease, neuropsychological abnormalities appear not to be detectable before clinical signs in individuals with a high probability (> .95) of having the HD gene (Strauss and Brandt 1990).

Planning, organizing, and mental flexibility—the "executive" functions that are typically impaired in patients with pathology of the frontal cortex—have been studied in HD as well. Such deficits are seen early in HD (Brandt and Butters 1986; Caine et al. 1978), but the "frontal" or "executive" dysfunctions of HD patients are less severe than in AD or Korsakoff's disease (KD; also known as Korsakoff's psychosis) patients (Butters 1984, 1985). These cognitive deficits of HD patients are most prominent in tasks that require keeping track of several things at once, discovering rules, or frequently changing mental set (Bylsma et al. 1990; Fedio et al. 1979; Starkstein et al. 1988; Wexler 1979).

The memory deficits of HD are the best characterized neuropsychological feature of the disease. To more clearly delineate the specific aspects of memory most impaired, HD patients are often compared with AD and KD patients. Early studies of learning and memory in HD (e.g., Butters et al. 1976; Weingartner et al. 1979; for a review, see Brandt and Butters 1986) suggested major deficits in the elaborative encoding or storage of new information. The pattern of memory deficits in HD changes in the course of the disease, and many early studies did not estimate severity or duration of disease (Brandt et al. 1984). More recent studies attend to this factor and suggest that, although present, encoding deficits are not the most prominent memory dysfunction. Retrieval of information from memory and the acquisition of skill-based (procedural) memory appear to be more pronounced deficits in this disease (Folstein et al. 1990).

HD patients are better able to recognize than recall information to which they have recently been exposed and are able to make use of verbal mediators to improve their memory performance. The dissociation between recognition and recall memory and the ability to make use of verbal mediators are not seen in AD or KD patients (Butters et al. 1983; Folstein 1989; Martone et al. 1984). The relative sparing of recognition memory may be limited to verbal material and reflect HD patients' more relatively intact language abilities (Josiassen et al. 1982). Moss et al. (1986) found that recognition memory for designs, colors, or the positions of objects on a board were as impaired in HD patients as in AD and KD patients. Only recognition memory for words was comparable to that of control subjects. HD patients do not benefit from increased encoding opportunities and do not show a gradient of retrograde amnesia, such that more recent memories are more difficult to retrieve than are events from the more distant past. Benefits of increased encoding opportunities and a sharp temporal gradient for recall of past events are seen in KD, which is principally a disorder of new learning. This also suggests that encoding deficits are not a principal feature of HD (Folstein et al. 1990). The greater impairment in retrieval and skill-acquisition processes than in the laying down of new memories may be more apparent in early stages of the disease in which functional capacity is relatively preserved (Folstein 1989).

Psychiatric Abnormalities

Psychiatric symptomatology is common in HD and is often the first sign of the disorder. Insanity with a tendency to suicide was one of the three cardinal features of the disease noted by Huntington (1872). A schizophrenia-like syndrome was thought to be the most common psychiatric manifestation of HD (Garron 1973), although mood disorders were emphasized by some early workers as well (McHugh and Folstein 1975). More recent research, using explicit diagnostic criteria and more standardized methods, has suggested that a symptomatic affective disorder and intermittent explosive disorder are the more prevalent psychiatric conditions in HD (Folstein 1989; Folstein et al. 1990).

In earlier decades of this century, many HD patients were referred to state hospitals, and, still today, HD patients' initial contact with physicians is often a psychiatric consultation. Consequently, it is important to evaluate the incidence and distribution of psychiatric syndromes and symptoms in HD in samples of patients not specifically referred to psychiatric settings. There appear to be three studies that meet this criterion.

Folstein et al. (1979) reported on 11 HD patients seen in either the medical genetics clinic or neurology clinics of Johns Hopkins Hospital over an 18-month period. None had come seeking psychiatric consultation, but on direct examination five of the 11 met criteria for manic-depressive disorder. Two had auditory hallucinations, but did not otherwise meet research criteria for schizophrenia. The symptoms of apathy and irritability were seen in most patients, including those without psychotic symptoms.

In a series of 30 patients at the National Institute of Mental Health and the Neurology Department at the University of Rochester, Caine and Shoulson (1983) evaluated psychopathology using standardized methods. Nineteen patients met DSM-III (American Psychiatric Association 1980) criteria for specific psychiatric disorders and an additional 5 had significant psychiatric symptomatology but did not meet specific diagnostic criteria. The most common syndromes were dysthymia or major depression, which were diagnosed in a total of 10 patients. Schizophrenia or atypical psychosis was seen in 5 patients. Ratings were made of the severity of psychopathology to capture impairing symptoms that did not meet syndromic criteria. Functional capacity was correlated with severity of psychopathology as well as with degree of dementia.

Folstein (1989) summarized the results of the only population-based study of psychiatric symptoms in HD (Folstein et al. 1983b, 1987) as well as the experience of the research clinic for HD at Johns Hopkins Hospital. Affective disorder, meeting DSM-III criteria, was diagnosed in nearly 40% of the 186 patients, and intermittent irritability (described as approximating the intermittent explosive disorder of DSM-III) was diagnosed in 31%. Schizophrenia, although less frequent (6%), occurred at a higher rate than would be expected in the general population. It is likely that the appearance of a very high rate of schizophrenia in earlier literature was due to ascertainment through mental hospitals and a bias to more severe cases. Schizophrenia syndromes may be more common in more advanced cases of HD, but earlier in the disease disorders of affect are more prevalent (Folstein 1989; Folstein et al. 1983b). The Johns Hopkins Hospital group has also reported aggregation of major affective disorder in conjunction with HD in some families, as well as much less psychiatric morbidity among black patients than among white patients (Folstein et al. 1983b).

Although it has been believed that alcoholism is frequent among HD patients, Folstein et al. (1983b, 1987) did not find an elevated rate. Other psychiatric symptoms are common in HD, even in the absence of diagnosable disorders. These symptoms include irritability, often precipitated by the kinds of events that previously had not provoked such reactions, and anxiety. Irritability and aggressive behavior are rarely reported by the patient but must be inquired about from the caregiver and are more common in patients with such traits earlier in life (Folstein 1989).

The dysphoria that is often seen in HD patients can be seen as an understandable reaction to the degenerative neurological disorder (Caine and Shoulson 1983). However, there are a number of lines of evidence suggesting an intrinsic association between HD and affective disorder, at least in some families. As noted above, Folstein et al. (1983b) found familial aggregation for affective disorder and HD in families identified by a proband with both disorders. The rate of affective disorder in families of probands with HD but no affective disorder was much lower. Affective disorder preceded the onset of HD by nearly a decade in this series. In an earlier study, Folstein et al. (1979) found emotional disorder to precede onset of chorea in 6 of the 10 cases in which the determination could be made.

Although depression is more common, mania is seen in conjunction with HD. Finally, Mindham, working with the Hopkins group (Mindham et al. 1985), reported that psychiatric disorders, especially mood disorders, tend to occur more often before the onset of HD than that of AD. This suggests that mood disorder is not merely a prodrome of any dementia.

Treatment

HD is preventable but, as yet, incurable. There are no effective treatments for influencing the course of the disease (Folstein 1989; Martin and Gusella 1986). Numerous medical treatments have been used palliatively to manage concurrent psychiatric disorder and chorea.

Early in the course of the disease, chorea can be treated with low-dose neuroleptic pharmacotherapy. Folstein (1989) has recommended withholding treatment until involuntary movements become disabling because of the dysphoria and feeling of cognitive dulling that they can induce; she noted a preference for using fluphenazine because it is less likely than haloperidol to produce dysphoria. Later in the disease larger doses may be helpful, as may a combination of presynaptic and postsynaptic dopamine blockers (Folstein 1989). Treatment is not always effective (Caine and Shoulson 1983), and use of neuroleptics brings with it the risk of tardive dyskinesia (Folstein 1989). Differential effectiveness of various neuroleptics has not been established (Girotti et al. 1984). Further, there are no adequate controlled trials of the treatment of involuntary movements in HD.

Efforts have been made to affect the deterioration in functional capacity that occurs in HD with drugs that address specific neurotransmitter depletions. Cholinergic and GABAergic drugs have proved of no marked benefit (Gram and Bentsen 1985; Martin and Gusella 1986; Nutt 1983). A recently completed trial of baclofen, thought to inhibit release of glutamate and aspartate, also proved ineffective in treating the progression of the disease (Shoulson et al. 1989). There will likely be other trials of drugs selected on the basis of current excitotoxin and oxidative stress hypotheses (Folstein 1989).

Treatment of the emotional symptoms of HD can be more successful at times. Tricyclic antidepressants are often effective in the treatment of depressive symptoms (Caine and Shoulson 1983; Folstein 1989). Improvement may be greater for the somatic-vegetative aspects of the syndrome than for the subjective elements of depression (Caine and Shoulson 1983). The lessened responsivity of helplessness and hopelessness to pharmacotherapy is understandable. Monoamine oxidase inhibitors (MAOIs) were reported useful in several cases by Ford (1986) and have been found clinically useful by Folstein's group (Folstein 1989), as has electroconvulsive therapy (ECT). Ford (1986) as well as Caine and Shoulson (1983) reported loss of therapeutic effectiveness in some cases. Psychotic symptoms, especially hallucinations, are often responsive to neuroleptic therapy (Caine and Shoulson 1983; Folstein 1989), as are manic symptoms (Folstein et al. 1979; McHugh and Folstein 1975).

Irritability and aggressive outbursts can be major problems in the management of HD patients in the home. Often irritability can be decreased by reduction in environmental complexity and the institution of unchanging routines. Neuroleptics can also be effective here (Folstein 1989). Successful treatment with the β-adrenergic blocker propranolol has been reported for three patients with aggressive outbursts that had limited response to neuroleptics (Stewart et al. 1987). A paradoxical response in HD to a β-adrenergic blocking agent has also been reported (von Hafften and Jensen 1989), however, and effective pharmacological control of irritable outbursts in HD awaits development.

Environmental management is important in the care of HD patients, particularly to minimize incontinence and the risk of dehydration (Folstein 1989). Social support along with case management can be very important in the adaptation of the family to the diagnosis of HD and the management of the illness within the family (Shoulson 1982). Because of the inevitable progression of the disease, families need to prepare for chronic and more intensive care of patients. Referral to the Huntington's Disease Society is helpful to provide educational material and psychological support.

Shoulson (1982) has suggested dividing the loss of functional capacity into five stages of illness reflecting the progressive decline in competence to engage in work, handle finances, and manage domestic responsibilities and self-care. Folstein and colleagues (see Folstein 1989) have developed an informant report form for characterizing the HD patient's abilities to manage self-care; household, work, and financial matters; social relationships; and communication. It is easily used by family members and may be useful in monitoring the course of disease and planning of long-term care.

❑ PARKINSON'S DISEASE

In 1817 James Parkinson described a new disorder he referred to as "paralysis agitans," which we now refer to as *idiopathic Parkinson's disease*. The cardinal neurological features of the syndrome of parkinsonism, which is most commonly caused by PD but can be caused by other diseases, include tremor, muscle rigidity, bradykinesia, and postural instability. We now know that neuropsychiatric symptoms, particularly dementia and depression, are frequently associated with PD.

Epidemiology

PD affects perhaps one million individuals in North America and shows dramatic age-related increases in incidence and prevalence. The prevalence of PD is approximately 150/100,000, increasing after age 65 to nearly 1,100/100,000 (Kessler 1972). Of interest, some studies (e.g., Martilla and Rinne 1980) have reported a protective effect of smoking, although sampling artifacts may explain this association. Although cases of familial PD have been reported (Mjones 1949; Pollock and Hornabrook 1966), a low concordance rate in identical twins does not support a strong role for genetics in this disorder (Ward et al. 1983). Prevalence studies have estimated that dementia occurs in 10%–30% of patients with PD. Sample differences probably explain most of this variability, with early studies demonstrating the highest estimates (Lieberman et al. 1979; Martilla and Rinne 1976; Rajput et al. 1984; Sutcliffe 1985). Mayeux et al. (1988) suggested that the best overall estimate is that 10%–15% of PD patients will develop dementia (Girotti et al. 1988). In a recent whole-population cohort study in Scotland (Ebmeier et al. 1990), 24% of patients were found to have dementia. Another recent study (Mayeux 1990) has suggested that cumulative incidence of dementia in PD may be as high as 60% by age 88. In addition to age, family history for dementia is a risk factor for developing dementia in PD (Hofman et al. 1989; Marder et al. 1990). The most common concomitant psychiatric condition in PD is depression, which occurs in 15%–30% of patients (Mayeux et al. 1986a).

Etiology

The primary cause of the most common form of parkinsonism, PD, is unknown. PD fits into the category of diseases referred to as *degenerative* because of its progressive clinical course in association with neuronal loss. The association between PD and arteriosclerosis has been controversial (Celesia and Wanamaker 1972; Martilla and Rinne 1976; Pollock and Hornabrook 1966), although most authors agree that infarcts can cause parkinsonism. Postencephalitic parkinsonism is now rare. The second most common cause of PD now is probably the administration of phenothiazines or related dopamine receptor blocking agents for the treatment of psychiatric symptoms. A description of PD being induced in drug abusers by the intravenous use of 1-methyl-

4-phenyl-1,2,3,6-tetradropyridine (MPTP) (Langston et al. 1983) led to speculation that the idiopathic disease may result from subclinical exposure to toxic agents (Calne et al. 1986).

Neurobiology

In several brain regions, the neuronal loss in PD is accompanied by the formation of Lewy bodies, which are hyaline inclusion bodies and were first described in the pigmented cells of the dorsal vagus nucleus and the substantia nominata or nucleus basalis of Meynert. Lewy bodies can also be seen in the brain stem nuclei, particularly the locus coeruleus and substantia nigra (Jellinger 1986). The loss of dopaminergic cells in the substantia nigra is thought to relate most directly to the motor abnormalities, particularly the bradykinesia and rigidity, and can be partially compensated for by the administration of levodopa (L-dopa) or dopamine agonists. Neuronal loss in the nucleus basalis of Meynert occurs to a small degree in all patients with idiopathic PD but not postencephalitic PD (Arendt et al. 1983; Tagliavini et al. 1984; Whitehouse et al. 1983). Cortical cell loss also occurs and abnormalities have been reported in two neurotransmitters that are thought to be present in cortical interneurons: somatostatin (Epelbaum et al. 1983) and corticotropin-releasing factor (Whitehouse et al. 1987).

In addition to neurotransmitter concentration changes, alterations also occur in neurotransmitter receptors. Ruberg et al. (1982) reported increases in muscarinic cholinergic receptors in PD with dementia, whereas most studies show few changes in AD with the exception of a possible increase in presynaptic muscarinic receptors. (For a review, see Whitehouse et al. 1988.) Nicotinic cholinergic receptors are reduced in both AD and PD (Perry et al. 1987; Whitehouse et al. 1988). Some types of serotonin receptors are also affected in both disorders (Perry et al. 1984). PET studies of dopaminergic function in PD using the catecholamine reuptake blocker nomifensine labeled with carbon-11 have demonstrated reduced dopamine reuptake sites in the putamen contralateral to the most involved extremity (Tedroff et al. 1988). Reduced fluorine-18 6-fluoro-L-dopa uptake in the contralateral putamen has also been observed (Brooks et al. 1990; Leenders et al. 1986; Nahmias et al. 1985).

The relationships among this cellular and neurochemical pathology and the neuropsychiatric symptoms are unclear. Some but not all dementia patients with PD develop senile plaques and neurofibrillary tangles identical to those found in AD (Boller et al. 1980; Chui et al. 1986; Hakim and Mathieson 1979). Others show evidence of more widespread Lewy body formation or loss of neurons without specific stigmata. The strongest correlation between neuronal loss and cognitive symptoms has been between loss of cortical cholinergic markers and dementia (Perry et al. 1983; Ruberg et al. 1982). Neuronal loss occurs in cholinergic basal forebrain to a greater extent in patients who have dementia than in those who do not. Neuronal loss in the dopaminergic cells of midbrain, particularly in the ventral tegmental area, may also relate to cognitive impairment (Javoy-Agid and Agid 1980; Rinne et al. 1989; Uhl et al. 1985). Others have proposed that alterations in the locus coeruleus may contribute to the cognitive disabilities, particularly the slowness of mentation or bradyphrenia (Mayeux 1990). Mayeux et al. (1984) associated raphe pathology with depression by providing evidence of loss of serotonergic markers in cerebrospinal fluid that correlate with the presence of affective symptoms. It is also possible that alterations in noradrenaline and corticotropin-releasing factor may relate to psychiatric symptoms as well.

Motor Symptoms

The most disabling motor features of PD are frequently the bradykinesia and rigidity (Table 25–3). The patient has difficulty initiating movements, and when movement is started it occurs slowly. Poverty of automatic movements (such as movement of the arms when walking) is characteristic. Lack of facial expression reflects hypokinesia of facial musculature. Rigidity (which affects all muscle groups, proximal and distal, agonist and antagonist) can occur asymmetrically. Tremor is the presenting feature in most cases and is slow (5–10 beats/second), often distal, and occurring most often at rest. Other tremors exacerbated by motion such as so-called action tremors also occur. Postural instability, associated with a characteristic flexion at the trunk and neck, occurs and can lead to serious falls.

Cognition

Many patients with PD show cognitive impairment even though the impairment may not be severe enough to warrant the label *dementia* (Table 25–3). In one study (Pirozzolo et al. 1982), 93% of patients

TABLE 25–3. CLINICAL FEATURES OF PARKINSON'S DISEASE

Motor
- Bradykinesia
- Tremor
- Rigidity
- Postural instability

Neuropsychological deficits
- Bradykinesia
- Verbal and visual memory
- Visuospatial skills
- Executive dysfunction (e.g., sequencing and switching set)
- Language difficulties (e.g., naming)

Psychiatric features
- Possible premorbid personality characteristics
- Affective disorder
- Psychosis—often medication induced

with PD showed some form of cognitive impairment. Certain neuropsychological abnormalities seem to be more characteristic of the dementia in PD (Growdon and Corkin 1986; Mortimer et al. 1985). Subtypes of PD have been defined based on presence and patterns of cognitive impairment (Mortimer et al. 1987).

A large literature exists describing problems in visuospatial impairment including spatial capacities, facial recognition, body schema, pursuit tracking, spatial attention, visual analysis, and judgments concerning position in space (Boller et al. 1984; Growdon and Corkin 1986; Levin 1990). "Visuospatial function" comprises many separate abilities that are difficult to isolate and test separately (Brown and Marsden 1986). Visual analysis is impaired in PD (Levin et al. 1990; Pirozzolo 1982; Villardita et al. 1982). Similarly, operating on objects in physical space (i.e., constructional praxis) is affected in PD, perhaps partly because of problems with spatial attention. (For a review, see Levin 1990.)

Abnormalities in memory involving verbal and nonverbal tasks with stimuli presented in different modalities occur. Recently, Levin et al. (1989) showed early problems with verbal memory. The communication difficulties of PD are mostly due to speech abnormalities including hypophonia and dysarthria; however, language impairments can also occur and include reduced verbal fluency and naming difficulties (Matison et al. 1982). Abnormalities in syntax have been reported in PD (Cummings et al. 1988), although most studies have focused on semantics, comprehension, and naming (Bayles 1990). Few studies of phonology or pragmatics have been undertaken. Executive and attentional abnormalities have also been reported that are similar to deficits attributed to frontal lobe dysfunction (Freedman 1990). These deficits include sequencing voluntary motor activities, difficulties in maintaining and switching set, and abnormalities in selective attention.

The relationships between the cognitive impairments in PD and the motor symptoms are complex. Poor performance on cognitive tests cannot be purely related to motor abnormalities. For example, visuospatial deficits continue to be detectable using tasks that limit the role of eye movements (e.g., tachistoscope).

Psychiatric Abnormalities

Premorbid personality. In the 1940s, patients who appeared to suppress anger and be quite perfectionist were claimed to be more at risk for developing PD (Booth 1948; Sands 1942). Sands (1942) described the so-called masked personality in which the patient's outward appearance of calm belied the inner state of turmoil. More recent studies (Diller and Riklan 1956; Lishman 1978; Pollock and Hornabrook 1966) did not, however, show such strong relationships between premorbid personality and the development of PD. Although difficult to undertake, better designed studies with more modern personality inventories may help elucidate the relationships between premorbid psychological characteristics and psychiatric sequelae of neurodegenerative disease.

Affective disorder. Affective disorder is the most common psychiatric disturbance associated with PD, with estimates ranging from 20% to 90% (Mayeux et al. 1986a; Starkstein et al. 1989). Mayeux et al. (1986a) found that major depression and dysthymic disorder were the most frequent types. Some depression that occurs in PD, particularly early in the disorder, is believed to be reactive. However, relatively few associations between depression and disease factors such as duration of disease, degree of disability, and response to medications have been established. A higher frequency of depression has been found among patients with early-onset PD in which depression correlated with cognitive impairment and duration of disease. Mayeux et al. (1981) also found an association between depression and dementia. Based on their cerebrospinal fluid studies (Mayeux et al. 1984), Mayeux et al. (1988) used the precursor of serotonin 5-hydroxytryptophan to alleviate depression with some success. Atypical depressive disorders can also occur. Rubin et al. (1987) described a condition in which predominant anxiety occurs. Patients frequently develop phobias, such as the fear of falling, that often have some basis in reality.

Psychosis. Psychosis of a schizophrenic nature has been reported in PD in the absence of medication affects (Mjones 1949). However, most authors believe that the most common cause of psychosis in PD is medication. Celesia and Wanamaker (1972) observed psychotic episodes in 12% of their 153 patients. Most episodes were due to drugs and occurred in patients who were cognitively impaired. Anticholinergic drugs may be particularly likely to produce delirium with psychotic features, although they are also most effective in suppressing the tremor.

Treatment

Great strides have been made in treating the motor dysfunction in PD. L-Dopa or dopamine agonists combined with anticholinergic agents can effectively treat rigidity, bradykinesia, and tremor. Postural instability is resistant to beneficial effects of drugs. Complicated motor phenomenon, such as on-off fluctuations and freezing episodes, can occur, especially later in therapy, which can be very stressful to patient and caregiver. Treatment of the neuropsychiatric symptoms involves both behavioral and biological approaches.

Behavioral. Treatment must begin with a careful assessment that includes not only the medical aspects of the illness, but also the effects of the illness on the patient's life (e.g., functional disability as measured by ability to perform activities of daily living) and on the patient's family. Nursing and social work assessments can, therefore, play an important role in providing a baseline for following the course of the illness. Education about the disease process and referral to lay support organizations such as the Parkinson's Foundation are important. Frequent reassessments followed by modifications of care plans are necessary.

A variety of interventions are available for the individual patient, including individual psychotherapy, particularly to deal with reactive depressions early in the illness. For patients with dementia, some authors suggest that certain forms of cognitive training or rehabilitation may be helpful. (For a review, see Gilmore et al. 1989.) Particularly in the dementias associated with motor problems, physical and occupational therapy may be very helpful. Because these are disorders that affect the whole family, marriage therapy and family counseling may be appropriate in some circumstances. Careful attention should be paid to environmental modifications that may make the patient's life easier. For example, a safety check at home including the appropriate use of handrails, avoiding stairs if possible, and stowing away loose objects, such as rugs and electric cords is the most important intervention to prevent falls. As the illness progresses, particularly if there are associated neuropsychiatric symptoms, home care, day care, and eventually institutional care may be necessary. Early planning, both financial and legal, is helpful to minimize the difficulty of getting access to and financing for appropriate long-term care services. Discussions with the individual and family early in the disease, when the patient can participate in decision making and prepare advance directives (e.g., a living will), are probably desirable.

Biological. The most important role for the physician in caring for patients with dementia is to avoid so-called excess disability. In other words, intercurrent illnesses and psychological stress can increase the intensity of neuropsychiatric symptoms and need to be prevented as much as possible. Iatrogenic disease, usually caused by overuse of medication, needs to be monitored carefully, particularly if more than one physician is involved in care. The most effective biological interventions are probably those for the treatment of affective disorders and include the use of antidepressant medications, and, if necessary, ECT. Antidepressants or any drugs with profound anticholinergic side effects should be avoided.

Treatment of psychosis in these disorders is difficult because the medications used to treat the hallucinations and delusions can exacerbate some of the symptoms. The first step should be to identify drugs or other stressors that are contributing to the psychosis and eliminate them. If necessary, major tranquilizers can be used if monitored carefully for side effects on motor (especially worsening parkinsonism) and cognitive symptoms. In the future, drugs that appear to cause less extrapyramidal side effects than do currently available major tranquilizers, such as clozapine, may be useful in treating psychosis in these disorders. Sleep disturbances are common in patients with these disorders and primary focus should be placed on sleep hygiene (i.e., a regular pattern of sleep preparation behavior and avoidance of stimulants).

❑ OTHER DEGENERATIVE DEMENTIAS ASSOCIATED WITH MOTOR ABNORMALITIES

Progressive Supranuclear Palsy

Progressive supranuclear palsy (PSP) is a chronic progressive disorder (also known as the Steele-Richardson-Olszewski syndrome) associated with eye movement abnormalities, parkinsonism, and dementia. It may have onset with deficient downward gaze, which causes trouble walking downstairs. The prevalence of PSP has been estimated at 1.4/100,000 (Golbe et al. 1988). Median age at onset of symptoms is approximately 63 years with a median survival of 6–10 years (Golbe et al. 1988).

Clinical features. Dementia is often not severe in early cases of PSP. It may be characterized by forgetfulness, slowing of thought processes, emotional or personality changes, and impaired ability to manipulate knowledge in the relative absence of aphasia, apraxia, or agnosia (Albert et al. 1974). PSP patients are particularly impaired on tests of frontal lobe function. Not all patients with PSP have noticeable dementia (Maher et al. 1985). PSP patients may also have deficits in visual scanning and search as well as verbal fluency, digit span, verbal memory, and logical memory.

Diagnosis. The diagnosis of PSP is suggested by the presence of dementia with parkinsonism and eye movement abnormalities. There is usually extensive rigidity of the neck and spasticity of the face and extremities with bradykinesia and a parkinsonian gait. Restrictions on upward and downward gaze are present. This is most marked when tested to command (e.g., "Look up; look down"). When pursuit eye movements are tested (following a slowly moving object), the deficit in vertical gaze is also apparent. However, when tested with oculocephalic maneuvers (i.e., head turning), there is relative integrity in vertical eye movements. This has led to the distinction of the eye movement abnormality in PSP as being supranuclear, because the oculocephalic reflexes demonstrate the integrity of the lower motor neuron pathways for up and down gaze.

There is also axial dystonia and pseudobulbar palsy in the later stages. Bradyphrenia, perseveration, forced grasping, and utilization behaviors are also observed. The gait disturbance is associated with postural instability and a tendency toward retropulsion. Disturbance of gait, often with falling, is an early sign with disorders of articulation and behavior. Many patients are misdiagnosed as having PD, AD, or psychotic illness.

Neurobiology. X-ray computed tomography (CT) and magnetic resonance imaging (MRI) studies show early involvement of midbrain structures with later atrophy of the pons and frontotemporal regions. PET scanning has shown reduced spiperone binding in the basal ganglia. Fluorodeoxyglucose PET studies show marked frontal and temporal hypometabolism (Cambier et al. 1985; D'Antona et al. 1985; Maher et al. 1985). There is also decreased fluorodopa uptake in the striatum reflective of decreased striatal dopamine formation and storage (Leenders et al. 1988).

Neuropathological findings include neuronal loss associated with gliosis and neurofibrillary tangles, most marked in the substantia nigra, basal forebrain, subthalamic nucleus, pallidum, and superior colliculus. (The tangles in PSP are straight filaments, not twisted as in AD [Takahashi et al. 1989].) There is extensive disruption in fibrillar proteins in subcortical neurons, with antigenic similarities between PSP and AD neurofibrillary pathology (Galloway 1988; Probst et al. 1988). Additional areas involved to a lesser extent include the locus coeruleus, striatum, and a variety of upper brain stem and midbrain structures (Agid et al. 1987).

The neurochemistry of PSP is characterized by massive dopamine depletion in the striatum; reduced density of dopamine, subtype 2 (D_2), receptors in caudate and putamen (Pierot et al. 1988); widespread reduction in choline acetyltransferase levels in frontal cortex, basal forebrain, and basal ganglia (Whitehouse et al. 1988); diminished nicotonic receptors in the basal forebrain; diminished serotonin receptors in the temporal lobe (Maloteaux et al. 1988); and a variable reduction in GABAergic neurotransmitter systems in certain subcortical regions. The loss of striatal dopamine receptors, as demonstrated by PET scanning during life, may explain the poor therapeutic efficacy of dopamine agonist therapy in PSP. Available evidence concerning cortical and subcortical as well as multiple neurotransmitter system abnormalities demonstrates that PSP is not a pure subcortical or dopaminergic dementia (Cummings 1990).

Neuropsychiatric manifestations. PSP patients often have disturbances of sleep and depression, occasionally with schizophreniform psychoses (Aldrich et al. 1989). There is also memory loss, slowness of thought processes, changes in personality with apathy or depression, irritability, and forced inappropriate crying or laughing with outbursts of rage. PSP may also be associated with obsessive-compulsive behaviors (Destee et al. 1990). Patients with PSP are particularly impaired for tasks requiring sequential movements, shifting of concepts, monitoring the frequency of stimuli, or rapid retrieval of verbal information (Grafman et al. 1990). These are thought to be a reflection of frontal lobe impairment.

No treatment has been found to be effective in relieving the motor or cognitive deficiencies in PSP. L-Dopa treatment is generally not successful. A report of effective treatment of violent behavior in a PSP patient with trazodone has been published and may be explained by the serotonergic effects of the drug (Schneider et al. 1989).

Dementia With Degenerative Disorders of the Cerebellum

Classification of the diseases of the cerebellum associated with cognitive impairment is difficult. Disorders of the cerebellum may involve pure cerebellar dysfunction or combinations of abnormalities in the cerebellum and brain stem, cerebellum and basal ganglia, or cerebellum and spinal cord and brain stem. Involvement of the optic nerves (optic atrophy), retina (retinitis pigmentosa), or peripheral neuropathy may also be found.

Olivopontocerebellar atrophies. The olivopontocerebellar atrophies (OPCAs) are a heterogeneous group of disorders presenting with progressive ataxia and associated with cerebellar degeneration. Dementia may be found in types III and V (Gilman et al. 1981), using the classification of Konigsmark and Weiner (1970). The occurrence of dementia in type III OPCA is controversial. In type V OPCA, there is ataxia with parkinsonism, ophthalmoplegia, and dementia. OPCA may be associated with progressive autonomic failure and parkinsonism with striatonigral degeneration.

In a recent study of cognitive deficits in dominantly inherited OPCA of the Schut type, Kish et al. (1989) were able to demonstrate significant impairment in the functioning of the frontal lobes, as measured by delayed alternation tasks. How these test-specific cognitive abnormalities relate to the presence of any more global and pervasive syndrome of dementia remains to be determined. Kish et al. (1989) also reported reduction in brain choline acetyltransferase activity in dominantly inherited OPCA. Mean choline acetyltransferase activities in OPCA were reduced by 39%–72% in the cortex, thalamus, caudate, globus pallidus, basal forebrain, and media olfactory area. Atrophy of the cerebellum, pons, and middle cerebellar peduncles with areas of abnormal signal intensity is seen on MRI imaging (Savoiardo et al. 1989). Diminished glucose metabolism in the cerebellar vermis and hemispheres and brain stem is found in OPCA in PET studies (Rosenthal et al. 1988).

Friedreich's ataxia. Friedreich's ataxia (FA) presents with a slow onset of progressive ataxia and may be associated with dementia. Mental function changes are often seen but have not been well characterized. In some instances, a syndrome of "generalized intellectual deterioration" has been noted; in others, specific nonverbal intellectual impairments have been identified. In other cases, a variety of psychiatric disorders, including schizophrenia-like psychoses and depression, have been felt to be the primary cognitive behavioral abnormality. Changes in performance IQ, conceptual ability, and visual constructive tasks, as well as tasks of three-dimensional spatial functions have been found to be abnormal in FA. Cerebellar syndromes, including FA, are well reviewed by Gilman et al. (1981).

The mode of inheritance of FA is recessive. Mental deficiency may be present in approximately one-quarter of cases. Personality abnormalities may be marked and associated with juvenile delinquency and irritability. There may be excessive religiosity or mysticism. Psychotic states may also be detected including schizophrenia-like illnesses with paranoid delusions, agitated behavior, and nocturnal hallucinations.

The cerebellar ataxias may be either hereditary or sporadic. Abortive forms are common, sometimes showing little more than pes cavus or kyphoscoliosis. The cerebellar disorders are usually slowly progressive and associated with ataxia, ataxic gait, intention tremor, decreased rapid alternating movements, past pointing, loss of the ability to check rebound, and dysarthria. The ataxic disorders may not be accompanied by intellectual changes until late in the illness. In a study reported by Skre (1974), dementia was found in 36% of patients with autosomal dominant spinal cerebellar degeneration, 58% of those with autosomal recessive cerebellar disease, and 82% of those with autosomal recessive spinal cerebellar degeneration. Memory and attentional deficits are found with apathy and psychomotor retardation, occasionally with depression, and a schizophrenia-like psychosis.

Motor Neuron Disease With Dementia

Loss of strength with diminished muscle mass (amyotrophy) and dementia may be seen in motor neuron disease, such as amyotrophic lateral sclerosis (ALS) (Mitsuyama et al. 1985). Familial motor neuron disease may be associated with other neurodegenerative conditions including HD, Pick's disease, PD, and the spinal cerebellar degenerations (Rosenberg 1982). Approximately 5% of ALS patients may demonstrate dementia or parkinsonism (Tyler 1982). Whether patients with sporadic ALS but without dementia demonstrate a specific pattern of neuropsychological abnormalities (Gallassi 1985; Montgomery and Erickson 1987) remains to be elucidated.

The occurrence of dementia with ALS has been called "classical ALS with dementia" (Wikström et al. 1982), "dementia of motor neuron disease" (Horoupian et al. 1984), "progressive dementia with motor disease" (Mitsuyama et al. 1985), and "amyotrophy dementia complex" (Morita et al. 1987). The disease may begin with personality changes or with motor system degeneration. There may be early personality changes in association with frontotemporal atrophy on CT and a normal electroencephalogram (EEG). Spongy changes are found in 90% of cases with gliosis. Neurofibrillary tangles, Lewy bodies, or Pick's bodies are not found. Extensive neuronal loss with gliosis is found in the substantia nigra in some cases (Horoupian et al. 1984). There is a loss of neurons (particularly over 90 μm^2) in layers 2 and 3 of the cortical mantle, particularly in the frontal and temporal region. The syndrome of dementia with amyotrophy may also be found in Creutzfeldt-Jakob disease; however, in cases of Creutzfeldt-Jakob disease there is usually rapid onset with an interval from onset to death of less than 1 year. Personality changes and hallucinations may occur in patients with ALS, as well as impairments in judgment, memory, abstract thinking, and calculations and anomia.

In Western New Guinea, the Kii peninsula of Japan, and the island of Guam, a high incidence of ALS occurs, often associated with parkinsonism and dementia. On the island of Guam, 10% of adult deaths in the native Chomorro population result from ALS and 7% are attributed to the parkinsonism-dementia complex (Garruto, in press). In addition to bradykinesia and rigidity, mental slowing, apathy, and depression occur in the relative absence of aphasia, apraxia, or agnosia. Gross frontotemporal cortical atrophy is found at autopsy. Neurofibrillary tangles are present in great abundance with a relative absence of neuritic plaques in affected cortical regions, as well as in hippocampus, amygdala, and substantia nigra. Severe neuronal loss with depigmentation of the substantia nigra without Lewy body formation is seen. Pathological changes in the spinal cord include loss of anterior horn cells and neurofibrillary changes (Cummings and Benson 1988).

Other Conditions

Dementia may be associated with motor system impairment in a variety of other diseases of the nervous system (Table 25–1).

Thalamic degeneration may be found rarely in isolation or in association with multisystem atrophy. Abnormal movements of the limb and trunk are seen with tremor, choreoathetosis, and occasionally myoclonus. Alterations in sleep may be observed. Ataxia, paraparesis, blindness, spasticity, optic atrophy, nystagmus, and dysarthria may also be present. Aphasia, agnosia, and apraxia are usually absent. Depression may be prominent, and patients may be apathetic, with personality changes and hypersomnolence. Poor memory and calculations and occasionally incomprehensible spontaneous verbal output are also present. Judgment and calculations are impaired relatively early, and insight into the disease is limited. In the thalamus, there is severe gliosis and neuronal loss, with gliosis and neuronal loss also being found in limbic projection nuclei.

In Wilson's disease, the basal ganglia degenerate in association with abnormalities in liver function. Autosomal recessive inheritance of a deficiency in the copper-carrying protein, ceruloplasmin, leads to excessive copper disposition in the liver, cornea, and basal ganglia. Onset is usually in the second or third decade and is heralded by tremor, poor coordination, dystonia, rigidity, or changes in gait. There may also be dysarthria, dysphagia, or hypophonia. Chronic hepatitis or hemolytic anemia may be detected. Kayser-Fleischer rings are seen in nearly all patients and consist of brown or green discolorations near the limbus of the cornea. Ventricular enlargement and cortical atrophy on X-ray CT scanning and abnormalities in MRI signal in the basal ganglia with increased signal in the lenticular nuclei, caudate nuclei, thalamus, dentate nuclei, and brain stem occur. The diagnosis may be made on slit lamp exam of the cornea and laboratory studies demonstrating a serum ceruloplasmin level < 20 mg/dl, a 24-hour copper excretion > 100 mg, or liver biopsy demonstrating increased hepatic copper concentration.

Affective and behavioral changes are common in Wilson's disease and may include schizophrenia-like changes with depression or manic depressive states. Aggressive and self-destructive or antisocial acts may be noted, and schizoid hysterical or sociopathic personality traits have been reported. Intellectual deterioration in Wilson's disease is relatively mild. Pathologically, there is atrophy of the brain stem, dentate nucleus, and cerebellum with cavitary necrosis of the putamen. Wilson's disease is well treated with penicillamine and a copper-deficient diet. Neurological symptoms, including the dementia syndrome, improve with long-term therapy.

Fahr's disease (idiopathic basal ganglia calcification) is a rare inherited (autosomal dominant) disorder with idiopathic calcification of the basal ganglia. There are extrapyramidal movement abnormalities together with dementia and neuropsychiatric disturbances. X-ray CT scans demonstrate extensive calcification of the basal ganglia and periventricular white matter. Patients may present in early adulthood with a schizophrenia-like psychosis or mood disorder, or may present later in life with an extrapyramidal syndrome, dementia, and mood changes. Parkinsonism, choreoathetosis, cerebellar ataxia, dystonia, and paroxysmal chorea may also be seen. Apathy, poor judgment, and memory are usually prominent and language function is often spared.

Hallervorden-Spatz disease is a rare progressive autosomal recessive disease of childhood and adolescence characterized by stiffness of gait, distal wasting, dysarthria, and occasionally dementia. Pathologically, there is olive or golden brown discoloration of the medial segment of the globus pallidus. X-ray CT shows mild atrophy with flattening of the caudate nucleus. Granules of an iron-containing pigment similar to neuromelanin are found inside and outside of neurons and hyperplastic astrocytes. Increased amounts of iron and other metals (e.g., zinc, copper, and calcium) are found in the affected tissue.

Normal-pressure hydrocephalus (NPH) is a syndrome comprised of dementia, gait disturbance, and urinary incontinence. It may be associated with a history of meningitis, intracranial bleeding, or head injury (Friedland 1989). Idiopathic cases are also seen. Gait is characterized by a wide base with slow steps. No changes occur in motor strength or tone. It is thought that this disturbance results from an obstruction to the flow of cerebrospinal fluid around the convexities in the basal cisterns. Improvement can be seen after a cerebrospinal fluid shunting procedure, but it is difficult to predict those individuals who will respond to surgery. The best results are seen in cases in which the cognitive disturbances are relatively mild with early onset of urinary incontinence and gait disturbance.

❑ REFERENCES

Agid Y, Javoy-Agid F, Ruberg M, et al: Progressive supranuclear palsy: anatomoclinical and biochemical considerations. Adv Neurol 45:191–206, 1987

Albert ML, Feldman RG, Willis AL: The "subcortical dementia" of progressive supranuclear palsy. J Neurol Neurosurg Psychiatry 37:121–130, 1974

Aldrich MS, Foster NL, White RF, et al: Sleep abnormalities in progressive supranuclear palsy. Ann Neurol 25:577–581, 1989

Alexander GE, DeLong MR, Strick PL: Parallel organization of functionally segregated circuits linking basal ganglia and cortex. Ann Rev Neurosci 9:357–381, 1986

American Psychiatric Association: Diagnostic and Statistical Manual of Mental Disorders, 3rd Edition. Washington, DC, American Psychiatric Association, 1980

Arendt T, Bigl V, Arendt A, et al: Loss of neurons in the nucleus basalis of Meynert in Alzheimer's disease, paralysis agitans, and Korsakoff's disease. Acta Neuropathol (Berl) 61:101–108, 1983

Bamford K, Caine E, Kido D, et al: Clinical-pathologic correlation in Huntington's disease: a neuropsychological and computed tomography study. Neurology 39: 796–801, 1989

Bayles KA: Language and Parkinson's disease. Alzheimer Dis Assoc Disord 4(3):171–180, 1990

Boller F, Mizutani R, Roessmann U, et al: Parkinson's disease, dementia, and Alzheimer's disease: clinicopathologic correlations. Ann Neurol 7:329–335, 1980

Boller F, Passafiume D, Keefe NC, et al: Visuospatial impairment in Parkinson's disease. Arch Neurol 41:485–490, 1984

Booth G: Psychodynamics in parkinsonism. Psychosom Med 10:1–14, 1948

Brandt J, Butters N: The neuropsychology of Huntington's disease. Trends Neurosci 9:118–120, 1986

Brandt J, Strauss ME, Larus J, et al: Clinical correlates of dementia and disability in Huntington's disease. Journal of Clinical Neuropsychology 6:401–412, 1984

Brandt J, Folstein SE, Folstein MF: Differential cognitive impairment in Alzheimer's disease and Huntington's disease. Ann Neurol 23:555–561, 1988

Brandt J, Quaid SE, Folstein SE, et al: Presymptomatic diagnosis of delayed onset disease with linked DNA markers: the experience with Huntington's disease. JAMA 216:3108–3114, 1989

Brooks DJ, Ibanez V, Sawle GV, et al: Differing patterns of striatal 18F-Dopa uptake in Parkinson's disease, multiple system atrophy, and progressive supranuclear palsy. Ann Neurol 28:547–555, 1990

Brown RE, Marsden CD: Visuospatial function in Parkinson's disease. Brain 109:987–1002, 1986

Brown RE, Marsden CD: "Subcortical dementia": the neuropsychological evidence. Neuroscience 25:363–387, 1988

Butters N: The clinical aspects of memory disorders: contributions from experimental studies of amnesia and dementia. J Clin Exp Neuropsychol 6(1):17–36, 1984

Butters N: Alcoholic Korsakoff's syndrome: some unresolved issues concerning etiology, neuropathology and cognitive deficits. J Clin Exp Neuropsychol 7:179–208, 1985

Butters N, Tarlow S, Cermak LS, et al: A comparison of the information processing deficits of patients with Huntington's disease and Korsakoff's syndrome. Cortex 12:134–144, 1976

Butters N, Sax D, Montgomery K, et al: Comparison of the neuropsychological deficits associated with early and advanced Huntington's disease. Arch Neurol 35: 585–589, 1978

Butters N, Albert MS, Sax DS, et al: The effect of verbal mediators on the pictorial memory of brain-damaged patients. Neuropsychologia 21:307–323, 1983

Bylsma FW, Brandt J, Strauss ME: Aspects of procedural memory are differentially impaired in Huntington's disease. Archives of Clinical Neuropsychology 5:287–297, 1990

Caine ED, Shoulson I: Psychiatric symptoms in Huntington's disease. Am J Psychiatry 140(6):728–733, 1983

Caine ED, Ebert MHY, Eingartner H: An outline for the analysis of dementia: the memory disorder of Huntington's disease. Neurology 27:1087–1092, 1977

Caine ED, Hunt RD, Weingartner H, et al: Huntington's dementia: clinical and neuropsychological features. Arch Gen Psychiatry 35:377–384, 1978

Calne DB, Eisen A, McGeer E, et al: Alzheimer's disease, Parkinson's disease, and mononeurone disease: a biotropic interaction between aging and environment? Lancet II:1067–1070, 1986

Cambier J, Masson M, Viader F, et al: Le syndrome frontal de la maladie de Steele-Richardson-Olszewski. Rev Neurol 141:528–536, 1985

Celesia GG, Wanamaker WM: Psychiatric disturbances in Parkinson's disease. Diseases of the Nervous System 33:577–583, 1972

Chui HC, Mortimer JA, Slager U, et al: Pathologic correlates of dementia in Parkinson's disease. Arch Neurol 43:991–995, 1986

Cummings JL (ed): Subcortical Dementia. New York, Oxford University Press, 1990

Cummings JL, Benson DF: Psychological dysfunction accompanying subcortical dementias. Annu Rev Med 39: 53–61, 1988

Cummings JL, Darkins A, Mendez M, et al: Alzheimer's disease and Parkinson's disease: comparison of speech and language alterations. Neurology 38:680–684, 1988

D'Antona R, Baron JC, Samson Y, et al: Subcortical dementia: frontal cortex hypometabolism detected by positron tomography in patients with progressive supranuclear palsy. Brain 108:785–799, 1985

Destee A, Gray F, Parent M, et al: Obsessive-compulsive behavior and progressive supranuclear palsy. Rev Neurol 146(1):12–18, 1990

Diller L, Riklan M: Psychosocial factors in Parkinson's disease. J Am Geriatr Soc 4:1291–1300, 1956

Ebmeier KP, Calder SA, Crawford JR, et al: Clinical features predicting dementia in idiopathic Parkinson's disease: a follow-up study. Neurology 40:1222–1224, 1990

Epelbaum J, Ruberg M, Moyse E, et al: Somatostatin and dementia in Parkinson's disease. Brain Res 278:376–379, 1983

Farrer LA, Conneally PM: A genetic model for age at onset in Huntington's disease. Am J Hum Genet 37:350–357, 1985

Fedio P, Cox CS, Neophytides A, et al: Neuropsychological profiles in Huntington's disease: patients and those at risk, in Advances in Neurology, Vol 23: Huntington's disease. Edited by Chase TN, Wexler NS, Barbeau A. New York, Raven, 1979, pp 239–255

Folstein SE: Huntington's Disease: A Disorder of Families. Baltimore, MD, Johns Hopkins University Press, 1989

Folstein MF, Folstein SE, McHugh PR: Mini-Mental State: a practical method for grading the cognitive state of patients for the clinician. J Psychiatr Res 2:189–198, 1975

Folstein SE, Folstein MF, McHugh PR: Psychiatric syndromes in Huntington's disease. Adv Neurol 23:281–289, 1979

Folstein SE, Jensen B, Leigh RJ, et al: The measurement of abnormal movement: methods developed for Huntington's disease. Neurobehavioral Toxicology and Teratology 5:605–609, 1983a

Folstein SE, Abbott MH, Chase GA, et al: The association of affective disorder with Huntington's disease in a case series and in families. Psychol Med 13:537–542, 1983b

Folstein SE, Abbot MH, Franz ML, et al: Phenotypic heterogeneity in Huntington's disease. J Neurogenet 1: 175–184, 1984

Folstein SE, Chase GA, Wahl WE, et al: Huntington's disease in Maryland: clinical aspects of racial variation. Am J Hum Genet 41:168–179, 1987

Folstein SE, Brandt J, Folstein MF: Huntington's disease, in Subcortical Dementia. Edited by Cummings JL. New York, Oxford University Press, 1990, pp 87–107

Ford MF: Treatment of depression in Huntington's disease with monoamine oxidase inhibitors. Br J Psychiatry 149:654–656, 1986

Freedman M: Parkinson's disease, in Subcortical Dementia. Edited by Cummings JL. New York, Oxford University Press, 1990, pp 108–122

Friedland RP: 'Normal'-pressure hydrocephalus and the saga of the treatable dementias. JAMA 262:2577–2581, 1989

Gallassi P: Cognitive impairment in motor neuron disease. Acta Neurol Scand 71:480–484, 1985

Galloway PG: Antigenic characteristics of neurofibrillary tangles in progressive supranuclear palsy. Neurosci Lett 91(2):148–153, 1988

Garron DC: Huntington's chorea and schizophrenia. Adv Neurol 1:729–734, 1973

Garruto R: Pacific paradigms of environmentally induced neurological disorders. Neurotoxicology (in press)

Gilliam TC, Bucan M, MacDonald ME, et al: A DNA segment encoding two genes very tightly linked to Huntington's disease. Science 238:950–952, 1987

Gilman S, Bloedel JR, Lechtenberg R, et al (eds): Disorders of the Cerebellum. Philiadelphia, PA, FA Davis, 1981

Gilmore GC, Wykle M, Whitehouse PJ: Memory, Aging, and Dementia: Theory, Testing, and Treatment. New York, Springer-Verlag, 1989

Girotti F, Carella F, Scigliano G, et al: Effect of neuroleptic treatment on involuntary movements and motor performances in Huntington's disease. J Neurol Neurosurg Psychiatry 47:848–852, 1984

Girotti F, Soliveri P, Carella F, et al: Dementia and cognitive impairment in Parkinson's disease. J Neurol Neurosurg Psychiatry 51:1498–1502, 1988

Golbe LI, Davis PH, Schoenberg BS, et al: Prevalence and natural history of progressive supranuclear palsy. Neurology 38:1031–1034, 1988

Grafman J, Litvan I, Gomez C, et al: Frontal lobe function in progressive supranuclear palsy. Arch Neurol 47(5): 553–558, 1990

Gram L, Bentsen KD: Valproate: an updated review. Acta Neurol Scand 72:129–139, 1985

Growdon JH, Corkin S: Cognitive impairments in Parkinson's disease, in Advances in Neurology. Edited by Yahr MD, Bergmann KJ. New York, Raven, 1986, pp 383–392

Gusella J, Wexler NS, Conneally PM, et al: A polymorphic DNA marker genetically linked to Huntington's disease. Nature 306:234–238, 1983

Hakim AM, Mathieson G: Dementia in Parkinson's disease: a neuropathologic study. Neurology 29:1209–1214, 1979

Hayden MR, MacGregor JM, Beighton PH: The prevalence of Huntington's chorea in South Africa. South African Medical Journal 52:886–888, 1980

Hayden MR, MacGregor JM, Saffer DS, et al: The high frequency of juvenile Huntington's chorea in South Africa. J Med Genet 19:94–97, 1982

Hofman A, Schulte W, Tanja TA, et al: History of dementia and Parkinson's disease in 1st-degree relatives of patients with Alzheimer's disease. Neurology 39:1589–1592, 1989

Horoupian DS, Thal L, Katzman R, et al: Dementia and motor neuron disease: morphometric, biochemical, and Golgi studies. Ann Neurol 16:305–313, 1984

Huntington G: On chorea. Adv Neurol 1:33–35, 1872

Javoy-Agid F, Agid Y: Is the mesocortical dopaminergic system involved in Parkinson's disease? Neurology 30: 1326–1330, 1980

Jellinger K: Overview of morphological changes in Parkinson's disease, in Advances in Neurology, Vol 45: Parkinson's disease. Edited by Yahr MD, Bergmann KJ. New York, Raven, 1986, pp 1–18

Josiassen RC, Curry L, Roemer RA, et al: Patterns of intellectual deficit in Huntington's disease. Journal of Clinical Neuropsychology 4:173–183, 1982

Kessler H: Epidemiological studies of Parkinson's disease, III: a community based study. Am J Epidemiol 96:242–254, 1972

Kish SJ, Robitaille Y, el-Awar M, et al: Non-Alzheimer-type pattern of brain cholineacetyltransferase reduction in dominantly inherited olivopontocerebellar atrophy. Ann Neurol 26(3):362–367, 1989

Konigsmark BW, Weiner LP: The olivopontocerebellar atrophies: a review. Medicine (Baltimore) 49:227–241, 1970

Langston JW, Ballard P, Tetrud JW, et al: Chronic parkinsonism in humans due to a product of meperidine-analog synthesis. Science 219:979–980, 1983

Leenders KL, Palmer AJ, Quinn N, et al: Brain dopamine metabolism in patients with Parkinson's disease measured with positron emission tomography. J Neurol Neurosurg Psychiatry 49:853–860, 1986

Leenders KL, Frackowiak RS, Lees AJ: Steele-Richardson-Olszewski syndrome: brain energy metabolism, blood flow and fluorodopa uptake measured by positron emission tomography. Brain 111:615–630, 1988

Leigh RJ, Newman SA, Folstein SE, et al: Abnormal ocular motor control in Huntington's disease. Neurology 33: 1268–1275, 1983

Levin BE: Spatial cognition in Parkinson's disease. Alzheimer Dis Assoc Disord 4(3):161–170, 1990

Levin BE, Llabre MM, Weiner WJ: Cognitive impairments associated with early Parkinson's disease. Neurology 39:557–561, 1989

Levin BE, Llabre MM, Ansley J, et al: Do parkinsonians exhibit a visuospatial deficit? Adv Neurol 53:311–315, 1990

Lieberman A, Dziatolowski M, Coopersmith M, et al: Dementia in Parkinson's disease. Ann Neurol 6:355–359, 1979

Lishman WA: Organic Psychiatry: The Psychological Consequences of Cerebral Disorder. Oxford, England, Blackwell Scientific Publications, 1978

Lyle OE, Gottesman II: Subtle cognitive deficits as 15- to 20-year precursors of Huntington's disease. Adv Neurol 23:227–238, 1979

McHugh PR, Folstein ME: Psychiatric syndromes in Huntington's disease: a clinical and phenomenologic study, in Psychiatric Aspects of Neurologic Disease. Edited by Benson DF, Blumer D. New York, Grune & Stratton, 1975, pp 267–285

Maher ER, Smith EM, Lees AJ: Cognitive deficits in the Steele-Richardson-Olszewski syndrome (progressive supranuclear palsy). J Neurol Neurosurg Psychiatry 48:1234–1239, 1985

Maloteaux JM, Vanisberg MA, Laterre C, et al: [3H]GBR 12935 binding to dopamine uptake sites: subcellular localization and reduction in Parkinson's disease and progressive supranuclear palsy. Eur J Pharmacol 156 (3):331–340, 1988

Marder K, Flood P, Cote L, et al: A pilot study of risk factors for dementia in Parkinson's disease. Mov Disord 5:156–161, 1990

Martilla RJ, Rinne UK: Dementia in Parkinson's disease. Acta Neurol Scand 54:431–441, 1976

Martilla RJ, Rinne UK: Smoking and Parkinson's disease. Acta Neurol Scand 62:322–325, 1980

Martin JB, Gusella JF: Huntington's disease: pathogenesis and management. N Engl J Med 20:1267–1276, 1986

Martone M, Butters N, Payne M, et al: Dissociations between skill learning and verbal recognition in amnesia and dementia. Arch Neurol 41:965–970, 1984

Matison R, Mayeux R, Rosen J, et al: "Tip-of-the-tongue" phenomenon in Parkinson's disease. Neurology 32: 567–570, 1982

Mayeux R: Dementia in extrapyramidal disorders. Current Opinion in Neurology and Neurosurgery 3:98–102, 1990

Mayeux R, Stern Y, Rosen J, et al: Depression: intellectual impairment and Parkinson's disease. Neurology 31: 645–650, 1981

Mayeaux R, Stern Y, Rosen J, et al: Is "subcortical dementia" a recognizable clinical entity? Ann Neurol 14:278–283, 1983

Mayeux R, Stern Y, Cote L, et al: Altered serotonin metabolism in depressed patients with Parkinson's disease. Neurology 34:642–646, 1984

Mayeux R, Stern Y, Williams JBW, et al: Clinical and biochemical features of depression in Parkinson's disease. Am J Psychiatry 143:756–759, 1986a

Mayeux R, Stern Y, Herman A, et al: Correlates of early disability in Huntington's disease. Ann Neurol 20:727–731, 1986b

Mayeux R, Stern Y, Sano M, et al: The relationship of serotonin to depression in Parkinson's disease. Mov Disord 3:236–244, 1988

Mindham R, Steele C, Folstein MF, et al: A comparison of the frequency of major affective disorder in Huntington's disease and Alzheimer's disease. J Neurol Neurosurg Psychiatry 48:1172–1174, 1985

Mitsuyama Y, Kogo HH, Ata K: Progressive dementia with motor neuron disease: an additional case report and neuropathological review of 20 cases in Japan. Eur Arch Psychiatry Neurol Sci 235:1–8, 1985

Mjones H: Paralysis agitans: a clinical and genetic study. Acta Psychiatr Scand 54:1–195, 1949

Montgomery GK, Erickson LM: Neuropsychological perspectives in amyotrophic lateral sclerosis. Neurol Clin 5:61–81, 1987

Morita K, Kaiya H, Ikeda T, et al: Presenile dementia combined with amyotrophy: a review of 34 Japanese cases. Arch Gerontol Geriatr 6:263–277, 1987

Mortimer JA, Christensen KJ, Webster DD: Parkinsonian dementia, in Handbook of Clinical Neurology, Vol 2. Edited by Frederiks JAM. New York, Elsevier, 1985

Mortimer JA, Jun SP, Kuskowski MA, et al: Subtypes of Parkinson's disease defined by intellectual impairment. J Neurol Trans 24 (suppl):101–104, 1987

Moss MB, Albert MS, Butters N, et al: Differential patterns of memory loss among patients with Alzheimer's disease, Huntington's disease, and alcoholic Korsakoff's syndrome. Arch Neurol 43:239–246, 1986

Nahmias C, Garnett ES, Firnau G, et al: Striatal dopamine distribution in parkinsonian patients during life. J Neurol Sci 69:223–230, 1985

Nutt JG: Effects of cholinergic agents in Huntington's disease: a reappraisal. Neurology 33:932–935, 1983

Paulson GW: Diagnosis of Huntington's disease, in Advances in Neurology, Vol 23: Huntington's Disease. Edited by Chase TN, Wexler NS, Barbeau A. New York, Raven, 1979

Perry EK, Perry RH, Candy JM, et al: Cortical serotonin-S2 receptor binding abnormalities in patients with Alzheimer's disease: comparisons with Parkinson's disease. Neurosci Lett 51:353–357, 1984

Perry EK, Perry RH, Smith CJ, et al: Nicotinic receptor abnormalities in Alzheimer's and Parkinson's disease. J Neurol Neurosurg Psychiatry 50:806–809, 1987

Perry RH, Tomlinson BE, Candy JM, et al: Cortical cholinergic deficit in mentally impaired parkinsonian patients. Lancet 2:789–790, 1983

Pierot L, Desnos C, Blin J, et al: D1 and D2-type dopamine receptors in patients with Parkinson's disease and progressive supranuclear palsy. J Neurol Sci 86(2-3):291–306, 1988

Pirozzolo FJ, Hansch EC, Mortimer JA, et al: Dementia in Parkinson disease: a neuropsychological analysis. Brain Cogn 1:71–83, 1982

Pollock M, Hornabrook RW: The prevalence, natural history and dementia of Parkinson's disease. Brain 89: 429–448, 1966

Probst A, Langui D, Lautenschlager C, et al: Progressive supranuclear palsy: extensive neurophil threads in addition to neurofibrillary tangles: very similar antigenicity of subcortical neuronal pathology in progressive supranuclear palsy and Alzheimer's disease. Acta Neuropathol (Berl) 77(1):61–68, 1988

Rajput AH, Offord KP, Beard CM, et al: Epidemiology of parkinsonism: incidence, classification and mortality. Ann Neurol 16:278–282, 1984

Rinne JO, Rummukainen J, Paljarvi L, et al: Dementia in Parkinson's disease is related to neuronal loss in the medial substantia nigra. Ann Neurol 26:47–50, 1989

Rosenberg RN: Amyotrophy in multisystem genetic diseases, in Human Motor Neuron Diseases. Edited by Rowland LP. New York, Raven, 1982, pp 149–157

Rosenthal G, Gilman S, Koeppe RA: Motor dysfunction in olivopontocerebellar atrophy is related to cerebral metabolic rate studied with positron emission tomography. Ann Neurol 24:414–419, 1988

Ruberg M, Ploska A, Javoy-Agid F, et al: Muscarinic binding and choline acetyltransferase activity in parkinsonian subjects with reference to dementia. Brain Res 232:129–139, 1982

Rubin AJ, Kurlan R, Schiffer R, et al: Atypical depression and Parkinson's disease. Ann Neurol 20:150, 1987

Sands IR: The type of personality susceptible to Parkinson disease. Journal of the Mount Sinai Hospital 9:792–794, 1942

Savoiardo M, Strada L, Girotti F, et al: MR imaging in progressive supranuclear palsy and Shy-Drager syndrome. J Comput Assist Tomogr 13(4):555–560, 1989

Sax DS, O'Donnell B, Butters N, et al: Computer tomographic, neurologic, and neuropsychological correlates of Huntington's disease. Int J Neurosci 18:21–36, 1983

Schneider LS, Gleason RP, Chui HC: Progressive supranuclear palsy with agitation: response to trazodone but not to thiothixine or carbamazepine. J Geriatr Psychiatry Neurol 2(2):109–112, 1989

Shoulson I: Care of patients and families with Huntington's disease, in Movement Disorders. Edited by Marsden CD, Fahn S. London, Butterworths International Medical Reviews, 1982, pp 277–290

Shoulson I, Odoroff C, Oakes D, et al: A controlled clinical trial of baclofen as protective therapy in early Huntington's disease. Ann Neurol 25:252–259, 1989

Skre H: Spino-cerebellar ataxia in Western Norway. Clin Genet 6:265–288, 1974

Smith S, Butters N, White R, et al: Priming semantic relations in patients with Huntington's disease. Brain Lang 33:2740, 1988

Starkstein SE, Brandt J, Folstein S, et al: Neuropsychologic and neuropathologic correlates in Huntington's disease. J Neurol Neurosurg Psychiatry 51:1259–1263, 1988

Starkstein SE, Berthier ML, Bolduc PL, et al: Depression in patients with early versus late onset of Parkinson's disease. Neurology 39:1441–1445, 1989

Stewart JT, Mounts ML, Clark RL: Aggressive behavior in Huntington's disease: treatment with propranolol. J Clin Psychiatry 48(3):106–108, 1987

Strauss ME, Brandt J: Attempt at preclinical identification of Huntington's disease using the WAIS. J Clin Exp Neuropsychol 8:210–218, 1986

Strauss ME, Brandt J: Are there neuropsychologic manifestations of the gene for Huntington's disease in asymptomatic, at-risk individuals? Arch Neurol 47: 905–908, 1990

Sutcliffe RLG: Parkinson's disease in the district of Northhampton Health Authority, United Kingdom: a study of prevalence and disability. Acta Neurol Scand 72: 363–379, 1985

Tagliavini F, Pilleri G, Bouras C, et al: The basal nucleus of Meynert in idiopathic Parkinson's disease. Acta Neurol Scand 69:20–28, 1984

Takahashi H, Oyanagi K, Takeda S, et al: Occurrence of 15-nm-wide straight tubules in neocortical neurons in progressive supranuclear palsy. Acta Neuropathol (Berl) 79(3):233–239, 1989

Tedroff J, Aquilonious SM, Hartvig P, et al: Monoamine re-uptake sites in the human brain evaluated in vivo by means of 11C-nomifensine and positron emission tomography: the effects of age and Parkinson's disease. Acta Neurol Scand 77:192–201, 1988

Tyler HR: Nonfamilial amyotrophy with dementia or multisystem degeneration and other neurological disorders, in Human Motor Neuron Diseases. Edited by Rowland LP. New York, Raven, 1982, pp 173–179

Uhl GR, Hedreen JC, Price DL: Parkinson's disease: loss of neurons from the ventral tegmental area contralateral to therapeutic surgical lesions. Neurology 35:1215–1218, 1985

Villardita C, Smirni P, Le Pira F, et al: Mental deterioration, visuoperceptive disabilities and constructional apraxia in Parkinson's disease. Acta Neurol Scand 66: 112–120, 1982

von Hafften AH, Jensen CF: Paradoxical response to pindolol treatment for aggression in a patient with Huntington's disease. J Clin Psychiatry 50(6):230–231, 1989

Ward CD, Duvoisin RC, Ince SE, et al: Parkinson's disease in 65 pairs of twins and in a set of quadruplets. Neurology 33:815–824, 1983

Wasmuth JJ, Hewitt J, Smith B: A highly polymorphic locus very tightly linked to the Huntington's disease gene. Nature 332:734–736, 1988

Wechsler D: Wechsler Adult Intelligence Scale-Revised. San Antonio, TX, Psychological Corporation, 1981

Weingartner H, Caine ED, Ebert MH: Imagery encoding and retrieval of information from memory: some specific encoding-retrieval changes in Huntington's disease. J Abnorm Psychol 88:52–58, 1979

Wexler NS: Perceptual-motor, cognitive, and emotional characteristics of persons at-risk for Huntington's disease, in Advances in Neurology, Vol 23: Huntington's disease. Edited by Chase TN, Wexler NS, Barbeau A. New York, Raven, 1979, pp 257–271

Whitehouse PJ: The concept of subcortical and cortical dementia: another look. Ann Neurol 19:1–6, 1986

Whitehouse PJ, Hedreen JC, White CL, et al: Basal forebrain neurons in the dementia of Parkinson's disease. Ann Neurol 13:243–248, 1983

Whitehouse PJ, Vale WW, Zweig RM, et al: Reductions in corticotropin releasing factor-like immunoreactivity in cerebral cortex in Alzheimer's disease, Parkinson's disease, and progressive supranuclear palsy. Neurology 37:905–909, 1987

Whitehouse PJ, Martino AM, Marcus KA, et al: Reductions in acetylcholine and nicotine binding in several degenerative diseases. Arch Neurol 45:722–724, 1988

Wikström J, Paetau A, Palo J, et al: Classic amyotrophic lateral sclerosis with dementia. Arch Neurol 39:681–683, 1982

Chapter

26

Neuropsychiatric Aspects of Alzheimer's Disease and Other Dementing Illnesses

Jeffrey L. Cummings, M.D.

DEMENTING DISEASES ARE frequently accompanied by neuropsychiatric syndromes including personality alterations, mood changes, and psychosis. Behavioral disorders are often the principal determinants of residential placement of dementia patients and are currently the main target symptoms of pharmacotherapy in the dementias. In this chapter, I review the neuropsychiatric aspects of Alzheimer's disease (AD), frontal lobe degenerations, vascular dementias, and hydrocephalus, as well as discuss the evaluation and treatment of dementia syndromes and their neuropsychiatric aspects. Dementias associated with other brain diseases are discussed in earlier chapters of this volume addressing brain injury (Chapter 16), cerebral tumors (Chapter 20), acquired immunodeficiency syndrome (AIDS) and other infectious and inflammatory disorders (Chapter 21), endocrine disorders (Chapter 22), toxic disorders (Chapter 23), alcoholism and substance use disorders (Chapter 24), and non-Alzheimer, nonfrontal lobe degenerative diseases (Chapter 25).

This project was supported by the U.S. Department of Veterans Affairs.

❑ DEMOGRAPHY AND DEFINITIONS

Dementia is a syndrome of acquired persistent impairment of mental function involving at least three of the following five behavioral domains: memory, language, visuospatial skills, personality or mood, and cognition (including abstraction, judgment, calculation, and executive function) (Cummings and

Benson 1992). The requirement that the syndrome be *acquired* distinguishes dementia from mental retardation; the involvement of a minimum of three behavioral spheres differentiates dementia from monosymptomatic neuropsychological deficit syndromes such as aphasia and amnesia. Dementia is distinguished from the acute confusional state (delirium) by intact arousal, more preserved attention, and persistence of the intellectual changes. Dementia may be reversible (e.g., hypothyroid dementia), treatable without reversing existing intellectual deficits (e.g., prevention of further ischemic injury in patients with vascular dementia), or progressive (e.g., AD).

Dementia syndromes are age related, becoming more prevalent among the elderly. With increased longevity and a greater number of aged individuals in society, there is an expanding number of intellectually impaired patients, and dementia currently represents a major public health challenge. Estimates of the prevalence of dementia vary markedly, but most studies suggest that approximately 5% of persons over age 65 are severely demented and an additional 10% have mild to moderate intellectual compromise (Ineichen 1987; Jorm et al. 1987). The total financial impact of dementia on society in the United States has been estimated at approximately $30 billion annually (Hays and Ernst 1987).

❑ ALZHEIMER'S DISEASE

AD is a progressive degenerative disorder affecting primarily the neurons of the cerebral cortex. It is the single most common dementing illness of the elderly and afflicts between two million and four million United States citizens (Evans et al. 1989; Katzman 1986). AD usually begins after age 55, and its incidence and prevalence rise with age; men and women are approximately equally likely to have the disease. The course is inexorably progressive, and patients survive approximately a decade from diagnosis to death (Katzman et al. 1988). In some cases, AD is inherited as an autosomal dominant disorder, and there is an excess of Down's syndrome in the families of AD patients (Fitch et al. 1988; Heyman et al. 1983; Mohs et al. 1987).

Clinical Diagnosis

The diagnosis of AD is stratified as definite, probable, or possible according to the certainty of the available information (McKhann et al. 1984). A diagnosis of *definite AD* requires that the patient exhibit a characteristic clinical syndrome and that there be confirmatory histological evidence of AD pathology obtained from biopsy or autopsy.

The diagnosis of *probable AD* requires that the patient meet criteria for dementia based on a clinical examination, structured mental status questionnaire, and neuropsychological testing; there are deficits in at least two areas of intellectual function; there is progressive worsening of memory and other intellectual function; there is no disturbance of consciousness; the disease begins between ages 40 and 90; and there are no systemic or other brain disorders that could account for the deficits observed. Thus, accurate diagnosis depends on a combination of inclusionary clinical features as well as excluding other possible causes of dementia. AD should not be regarded as purely an exclusionary diagnosis.

Possible AD is diagnosed when there are variations in the onset, presentation, or course of a dementing illness that has no alternate explanation; there is a systemic illness or brain disease present that is considered not to be the cause of the dementia syndrome; or there is a single gradually progressive cognitive deficit in the absence of any other brain disorder. Focal neurological signs, sudden onset, or the early occurrence of a gait disorder or seizures make the diagnosis of AD unlikely. Neuropathological studies (Risse et al. 1990; Tierney et al. 1988) have demonstrated that between 65% and 90% of patients identified as having probable AD will have the diagnosis confirmed at autopsy.

The classic dementia syndrome of AD includes impairment of learning new information, poor recall of remote material, impaired naming and auditory comprehension, deterioration in constructional and visuospatial abilities, and poor calculation, abstraction, and judgment (Cummings and Benson 1986). Fluency of verbal output, repetition skills, and the ability to read aloud are retained until late in the disease. Motor and sensory functions are also spared throughout most of the course of the illness. In the final phases of the disease, there is near total abolition of intellectual function as well as progressive loss of ambulation and coordination, dysphagia, and incontinence. Aspiration pneumonia, urinary tract infection, sepsis associated with infected decubitus ulcers, or an independent age-related disease (e.g., heart disease or cancer) usually accounts for the patient's death.

Neuropsychiatric Aspects

Table 26–1 lists the principal neuropsychiatric syndromes occurring in AD (Cummings and Victoroff 1990). They include personality alterations, delusions, hallucinations, mood changes, anxiety, disturbances of psychomotor activity, and various miscellaneous behavioral changes including disturbances of sleep and appetite, altered sexual behavior, and Klüver-Bucy syndrome.

Personality changes are ubiquitous in AD, the most common being passivity or disengagement: patients exhibit diminished emotional responsiveness, decreased initiative, loss of enthusiasm, diminished energy, and decreased affection (Petry et al. 1988; Rubin et al. 1987). Self-centered, resistive, and disinhibited behaviors may also occur. Patients may be emotionally coarsened, labile, insensitive, rash, excitable, or unreasonable (Petry et al. 1988). Personality changes affect essentially all AD patients; they often occur early in the course and may predate intellectual abnormalities (Petry et al. 1989).

Delusions are also common in AD, affecting between 30% and 50% of patients (Cummings et al. 1987; Wragg and Jeste 1989). The most frequent delusions involve false beliefs of theft, infidelity of the spouse, abandonment, the house is not one's home, persecution, phantom boarder, and the Capgras phenomenon (Reisberg et al. 1987). There is no specific delusional content that distinguishes the psychosis of AD from other organic or idiopathic disorders with psychosis. Delusions are mos[illegible] in the middle phases of the illness, but th[illegible] occur early in the clinical course and they some[illegible] persist until late in the disease (Drevets and Ru[illegible] 1989). Delusions do not correlate with the severi[illegible] of dementia or with specific aspects of intellectual dysfunction. Delusional patients are more behaviorally disturbed and difficult to manage than those without delusions (Flynn et al. 1991), and AD patients with delusions exhibit more rapid intellectual decline than those without delusions (Drevets and Rubin 1989).

Hallucinations are not a common manifestation of AD; between 9% and 27% of patients have hallucinatory behavior. Visual hallucinations are most common, followed by auditory hallucinations or combined auditory and visual hallucinatory experiences. Typical visual hallucination content includes persons from the past (such as deceased parents), intruders, animals, complex scenes, or inanimate objects (Mendez et al. 1990). Auditory hallucinations are often persecutory and usually accompany delusions. Visual hallucinations may be indicative of a co-occurring delirium (Cummings et al. 1987).

A variety of mood changes have been observed in AD including depressive symptoms, elation, and lability. Few patients meet criteria of major depressive episodes, but elements of a depression syndrome are frequent, occurring in 20%–40% of AD patients (Cummings et al. 1987; Mendez et al. 1990). Tearfulness may be prominent, and thoughts of burden and worthlessness may be expressed. Suicide is rare in AD. Patients experiencing depression in the course of AD often have family histories of depressive disorders (Pearlson et al. 1990). Elation is reported in up to 20% of AD patients (Cummings and Victoroff 1990).

Anxiety has been reported in approximately 40% of patients with AD. The most common manifestation is excessive anticipatory concern regarding upcoming events (Mendez et al. 1990).

Psychomotor activity disturbances and troublesome behaviors are common in AD and become increasingly evident as the disease progresses. Wandering and pacing are pervasive behaviors in the middle and later stages of the illness, and providing safe contained spaces for wandering patients is a major challenge for residential facilities (Morishita 1990). Restlessness is reported in up to 60% of AD patients, angry outbursts in 50%, and assaultive behavior in 20% (Swearer et al. 1988; Teri et al. 1988).

TABLE 26–1. NEUROPSYCHIATRIC CHARACTERISTICS OF ALZHEIMER'S DISEASE

Personality alterations	**Anxiety**
Disengagement	**Psychomotor activity disturbances**
Disinhibition	Agitation or combativeness
Delusions	Wandering
Persecutory	Pacing
Theft	Purposeless activity
Infidelity	**Miscellaneous**
Capgras	Sexual activity changes
Hallucinations	Decreased sexual interest
Auditory	Increased sexual interest
Visual	Appetite changes
Mood changes	Sleep disturbances
Depressive symptoms	Klüver-Bucy syndrome
Elevated mood	
Catastrophic reactions	
Mood lability	

anges have also patients exhibit have transient reased sexual). Eating also ost patients sing weight as et al. 1989). Sleep dis- uent interruptions of nocturnal non, occurring in 45%–70% of patients am et al. 1988; Rabins et al. 1982; Swearer et al. 1988). The Klüver-Bucy syndrome is a complex behavioral disorder consisting of hyperorality, hypermetamorphosis, emotional placidity, agnosia, and altered sexual behavior. It may occur in fragmentary form in the late stages of AD (Lilly et al. 1983).

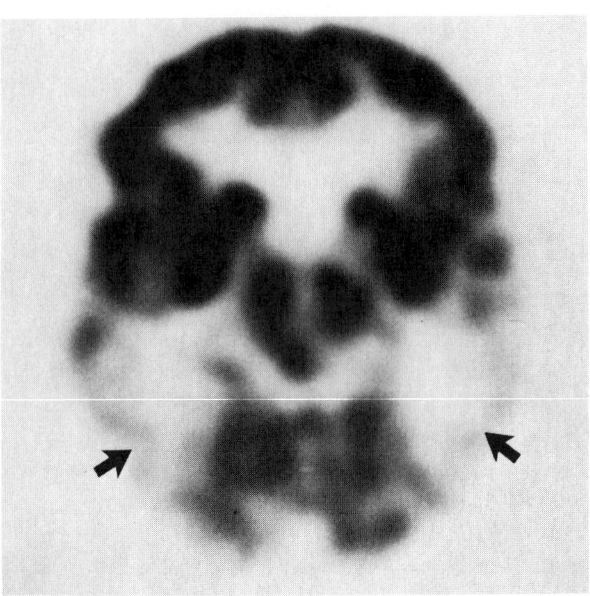

Figure 26–1. Transaxial positron-emission tomography (PET) scan revealing decreased glucose metabolism bilaterally in the parietal lobes (*arrows*) characteristic of Alzheimer's disease. (Image courtesy of M. Mahler and D. Sultzer.)

Laboratory Investigations

The results of most laboratory studies remain normal in AD. Routine assays of serum, urine, and cerebrospinal fluid (CSF) are unaffected. Computed tomography (CT) and magnetic resonance imaging (MRI) may reveal cerebral atrophy and help exclude intracranial processes that may imitate AD (e.g., neoplasms and subdural hematomas) but do not provide specific diagnostic information (Cummings and Benson 1992). Electroencephalography (EEG) usually reveals theta and delta slowing as the disease advances, and computed EEG studies with brain mapping demonstrate maximal abnormalities in the parietal regions of both hemispheres (Jordan et al. 1989).

Metabolic and perfusion studies offer substantial support for the diagnosis of AD. Positron-emission tomography (PET) using [^{18}F]fluorodeoxyglucose (FDG) reveals a characteristic pattern of hypometabolism (Figure 26–1). Early in the disease there is diminished glucose utilization in the parietal lobes, and the frontal lobes are affected as the disease progresses. Subcortical structures and primary motor and sensory cortices are spared (Foster et al. 1983; Jagust et al. 1988). Abnormalities in PET using FDG (FDG-PET) are demonstrable early in AD when memory is only mildly impaired and other cognitive functions are intact (Haxby et al. 1986).

Single photon emission computed tomography (SPECT) measures cerebral blood flow. Brain perfusion is determined by local cerebral metabolic activity, and the pattern of blood flow revealed by SPECT closely resembles the topography of cerebral glucose metabolism demonstrated by FDG-PET. SPECT reveals diminished cerebral perfusion, most marked in the parietal and posterior temporal lobes of both hemispheres, in the majority of AD patients (Figure 26–2) (Johnson et al. 1987; Miller et al. 1990).

Neuropathology

The major pathological alterations of AD include neuronal loss, cortical gliosis, intraneuronal cytoplasmic neurofibrillary tangles, neuritic plaques, granulovacuolar degeneration, and amyloid angiopathy of the cerebral vessels (Cummings and Benson 1992; Katzman 1986). The pathological burden of the disease is greatest in the medial temporal, posterior cingulate, and temporal-parietal junction regions. The frontal cortex is moderately involved, and the primary motor and sensory cortices have fewer pathological abnormalities (Brun and Gustafson 1976). Neurotransmitter alterations include marked reductions of choline acetyltransferase and somatostatin, as well as more modest and variable losses of serotonin, γ-aminobutyric acid (GABA), and norepinephrine (Cummings and Benson 1992; Procter et al. 1988).

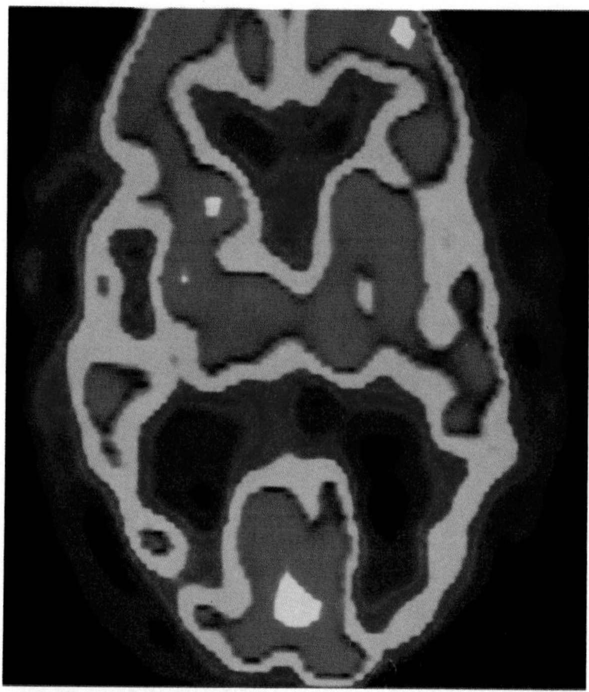

Figure 26–2. Transaxial single photon emission computed tomography (SPECT) scan of a patient with Alzheimer's disease revealing diminished cerebral perfusion in the temporoparietal regions bilaterally (red areas have normal blood flow; yellow regions have diminished perfusion). (Image courtesy of I. Mena.)

The pathological basis of the neuropsychiatric symptoms of AD remains to be determined. Temporal and parietal lobe changes may contribute to patients' indifference, and frontal lobe pathology may account for disinhibition, lability, and depressive symptoms. Delusions may reflect temporoparietal alterations and the cholinergic deficit of AD (Cummings and Victoroff 1990).

❑ FRONTAL LOBE DEGENERATIONS

Frontal lobe degenerations (FLD) are progressive idiopathic disorders that preferentially affect the frontal lobes. In some cases, distinctive histopathological changes such as Pick cells are noted at autopsy and a diagnosis of Pick's disease is supported; in others, no specific cellular changes are found (Brun 1987; Gustafson 1987). FLD can usually be distinguished from AD on the basis of clinical features, but there is insufficient information regarding differential characteristics to suggest that the different etiologies of FLD can be reliably identified clinically.

Pick's disease has been studied more thoroughly than other types of FLD and more demographic information is available regarding Pick-type dementia. Pick's disease typically begins in the sixth decade, although cases with onset as early as age 21 and as late as age 80 have been reported (Cummings and Benson 1992). Like AD, Pick's disease has a duration of approximately 10 years from diagnosis to death. Of patients with Pick's disease, 20%–50% inherit the disorder in an autosomal dominant fashion (Cummings and Benson 1992; Gustafson 1987); men and women are approximately equally likely to develop the disease (Heston et al. 1987). The prevalence of FLD is unknown, but in one large series Pick's disease accounted for 2.5% of pathologically studied dementias and non-Pick-type FLD accounted for 10% (Brun 1987).

Clinical and Neuropsychiatric Features

Neuropsychiatric features dominate the presentation of FLDs. Personality alterations are often florid, and depression or psychosis may be prominent. Patients may be apathetic or disinhibited (Miller et al. 1990). Apathetic individuals exhibit social and occupational withdrawal, loss of motivation, and interpersonal disengagement. Disinhibited patients are often boisterous, prone to make vulgar or socially inappropriate remarks, exhibit undue familiarity with strangers, have poor judgment, and may be unusually irritable. Mood changes may also be marked. Depression may occur early in the clinical course and is usually transient. Elation occurs in approximately one-third of the patients; delusions are evident in approximately one-fourth (Gustafson 1987; Miller et al. 1991). The Klüver-Bucy syndrome or fragments of the condition may be evident in the initial phases of the disease, and patients frequently gain weight as their eating habits become less discriminating (Cummings and Duchen 1981). Stereotyped behaviors with compulsive rituals and complex repetitive acts may also be observed in the course of FLD (Gustafson 1987).

Neuropsychological deficits are less marked in FLD than in AD. Memory, visuospatial skills, and mathematical abilities are relatively spared in the early and middle stages of FLD (Cummings and Benson 1992; Knopman et al. 1989). Patients have executive function deficits including difficulty with set shifting tasks (e.g., card sorting), word list generation (e.g., number of animals named in one minute), divided attention, and response inhibition (Miller et al. 1991). Language may be affected relatively early in the disease. Naming deficits, impairment of auditory comprehension, and increasingly sparse verbal output are common. Speech stereotypies, echolalia, and mutism may also occur (Cummings and Benson 1992; Graff-Radford et al. 1990; Gustafson 1987; Holland et al. 1985).

Laboratory Investigations

Results from routine studies of serum, urine, and CSF are normal in FLD. Neuroimaging with CT or MRI may provide supportive information if focal atrophy of the frontal or temporal lobes is revealed (Cummings and Benson 1992; Knopman et al. 1989; Wechsler et al. 1982). More definitive diagnostic information is provided by PET or SPECT scanning. FDG-PET reveals markedly diminished frontal lobe glucose utilization, particularly in the midfrontal convexity (Kamo et al. 1987). SPECT demonstrates severely diminished cerebral perfusion in the frontal lobes and, in some cases, in the anterior temporal lobes. Frontal hypoperfusion may be most marked in the frontal convexity or the orbitofrontal cortex (Figure 26–3) (Miller et al. 1991; Neary et al. 1988).

Neuropathology

The macroscopic pathology of Pick's disease includes marked atrophy of the frontal lobe anterior to the precentral sulcus and of the anterior temporal lobe (Cummings and Benson 1992). Neurons are atrophic, and there is gliosis of affected regions. Some of the remaining neurons contain intracytoplasmic argyrophilic Pick bodies, and examination of the dendrites reveals almost total absence of dendritic spines (Wechsler et al. 1982). Enlarged neurons with uniformly argyrophilic cytoplasm known as *ballooned cells* may occur in affected regions. Ultrastructurally, the Pick bodies are composed of straight filaments (Murayama et al. 1990). FLD patients without Pick's type pathology have nonspecific neuronal loss and gliosis in a lobar distribution (Brun 1987).

Neurochemical investigations have also been carried out in Pick's disease. Cortical choline acetyltransferase, L-glutamic acid decarboxylase, and dopamine are preserved (Yates et al. 1980). In the basal ganglia, dopamine, GABA, and substance P levels are reduced, and choline acetyltransferase levels are variably diminished (Kanazawa et al. 1988).

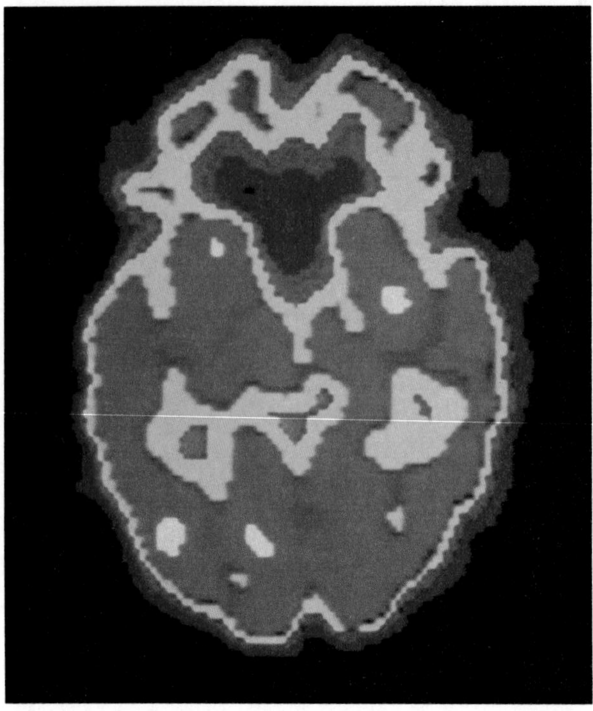

Figure 26–3. Transaxial single photon emission computed tomography (SPECT) scan of a patient with a frontal lobe degeneration demonstrating decreased cerebral blood flow in the frontal lobes (red areas have normal blood flow; yellow regions have diminished perfusion). (Image courtesy of I. Mena.)

Differential Diagnosis

FLD can usually be distinguished from AD on the basis of contrasting clinical characteristics. Although both are cortical diseases with gradually progressive courses and prominent language abnormalities, they differ in a number of other features. In AD, memory impairment, constructional disturbances, and acalculia appear early in the clinical course, whereas these deficits are delayed until the middle or late phases of FLD. Conspicuous personality changes and executive deficits herald the onset of FLD and are more modest and delayed in AD. CT and MRI reveal generalized atrophy in AD and frontal or temporal lobar atrophy in FLD. FDG-PET and SPECT demonstrate diminished posterior temporal and parietal function in AD and decreased frontotemporal function in FLD (Cummings and Benson 1992; Miller et al. 1991).

Several diseases can affect frontal lobe function in addition to FLD (Table 26–2). Amyotrophic lat-

TABLE 26–2. PRINCIPAL DEMENTIA SYNDROMES WITH PROMINENT FRONTAL LOBE INVOLVEMENT

Disorder	*Characteristic features*
Pick's disease	Cortical dementia with personality changes; language alterations; memory, constructional, and arithmetic deficits delayed; and intracytoplasmic neuronal Pick bodies
Frontal lobe degeneration—non-Alzheimer type	Clinical features similar to Pick's disease and nonspecific histologic alterations
Amyotrophic lateral sclerosis	Dementia with motor neuron syndrome
Neuronal intranuclear hyaline inclusion	Dementia with aggressive behavior; some patients have choreiform movements, ataxia, or tremor; and neuronal and disease glial inclusions
Progressive supranuclear palsy	Ophthalmoplegia, parkinsonism, and dysarthria
Progressive subcortical gliosis	Clinical features similar to Pick's disease and marked subcortical and white matter gliosis
Anterior cerebral artery occlusion	Apathy and paresis and sensory loss of lower limbs
Syphilis	Grandiosity and hypomania, positive serum serology, and abnormal cerebrospinal fluid protein, cell count, and Venereal Disease Research Laboratories test results
Hydrocephalus	Gait disturbance and incontinence, enlarged ventricles, and abnormal cisternography and pressure monitoring
Depression	Marked mood change and diminished glucose metabolism or perfusion of frontal lobes

eral sclerosis is sometimes accompanied by a frontal lobe type degenerative dementia (Figure 26–4) (Neary et al. 1990). This syndrome is identified by the characteristic motor neuron findings, although the dementia may antedate the motor findings by several months. Another rare degenerative disorder affecting the frontal lobes is neuronal intranuclear hyaline inclusion disease. This disease may have its onset in childhood or adult life and commonly includes an extrapyramidal syndrome with parkinsonism, tremor, chorea, or ataxia in addition to dementia. Aggressive belligerent behavior is common. Inclusions are found in glial cells, neurons of brain and digestive tract, and cells of the adrenal medulla (Munoz-Garcia and Ludwin 1986).

Progressive supranuclear palsy (PSP) is a degenerative disorder that produces a dementia syndrome in combination with parkinsonism, pseudobulbar palsy, and supranuclear gaze impairment (Grafman et al. 1990). FDG-PET and SPECT in PSP reveal markedly diminished frontal lobe activity (Foster et al. 1988). Progressive subcortical gliosis also affects frontal and temporal lobes. It is characterized by variable cortical involvement and marked subcortical and white matter gliosis (Verity and Wechsler 1987).

Nondegenerative diseases can also produce frontal lobe syndromes with dementia (Cummings 1985). Infarctions in the territories of the anterior cerebral arteries produce a syndrome of apathy and lack of initiative; there may be weakness and sensory loss in both lower extremities. Syphilitic brain infections preferentially affect the frontal lobes and may produce the grandiose hypomanic dementia syndrome of general paresis. White matter diseases that may disproportionately affect the frontal lobes include multiple sclerosis and Marchiafava-Bignami disease. Hydrocephalus (discussed below) may present with a frontal lobe syndrome. Depression is associated with reduced metabolism and perfusion of the frontal cortex, and the dementia syndrome of depression is characterized by frontal-lobe–type neuropsychological deficits (Baxter et al. 1989; Cummings and Benson 1992).

❑ VASCULAR DEMENTIA

Vascular dementia, also known as multi-infarct dementia (MID), is a dementing condition produced by cerebral ischemic injury. In its classic form, MID is characterized by an abrupt onset, stepwise deterioration, patchy pattern of intellectual deficits, focal neurological symptoms (transient ischemic attacks), focal neurological signs, a history of hypertension, and evidence of associated cardiovascular disease (American Psychiatric Association 1987; Hachinski et al. 1975). The majority of cases are produced by hypertensive cerebrovascular disease, but MID may also occur with multiple cerebral emboli, systemic hypotension, intracerebral hemorrhage, and inflammatory and infectious vascular disease (Cummings and Benson 1992; Meyer et al. 1988; Sulkava and Erkinjuntti 1987).

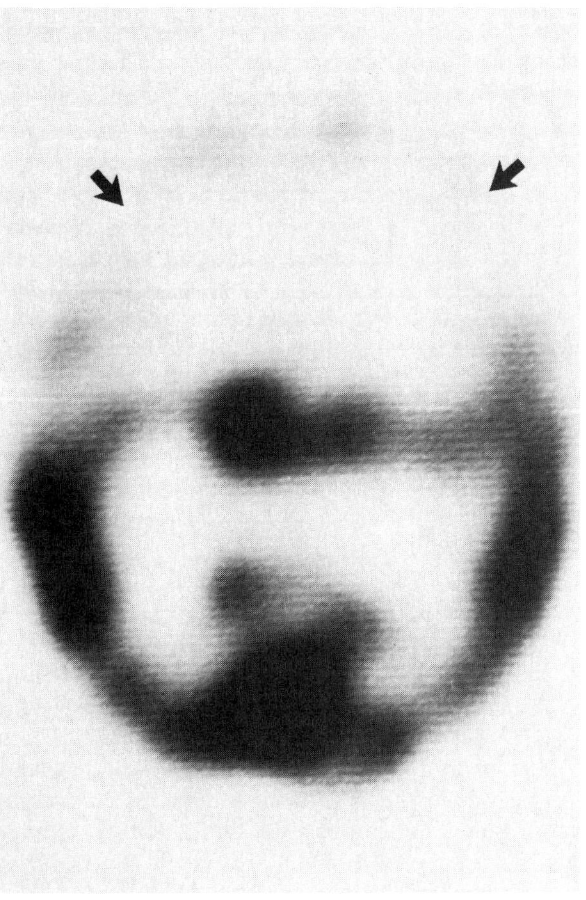

Figure 26–4. Transaxial single photon emission computed tomography (SPECT) scan of a patient with a frontal lobe syndrome in association with motor neuron disease. Note marked hypoperfusion of the frontal lobes (*arrows*).

Vascular dementia is the second most common cause of dementia in the elderly, accounting for 8%–35% of dementia syndromes (Cummings and Benson 1992). MID is most common after the age of 50 and affects men more often than women. Patients commonly survive for 6–8 years after onset, and death usually results from cardiovascular disease or stroke.

Clinical and Neuropsychiatric Features

Historically, MID is characterized by an abrupt onset in concert with the occurrence of a stroke and stepwise deterioration occurring synchronously with repeated cerebrovascular events. In some cases, however, neuropsychological abnormalities accumulate gradually, imitating the course of a degenerative dementia.

On examination, MID patients exhibit a combination of motor abnormalities, neuropsychological deficits, and neuropsychiatric symptoms. Motor findings may include weakness, spasticity, hyperreflexia, extensor plantar responses, bradykinesia, parkinsonism, and pseudobulbar palsy (Ishii et al. 1986). Gait abnormalities are common and may appear early in the course of the disorder.

The pattern of neuropsychological abnormalities in MID is characterized by "patchiness" with preservation of some abilities and mild to severe compromise of others. Thus the profile of deficits will vary among patients. In most cases, IQ testing and memory evaluations reveal diminished cognitive and memory abilities (Ladurner et al. 1982; Perez et al. 1975), and visuospatial abnormalities are also demonstrable in a majority of patients (Reichman et al., in press). Speech and language assessments reveal dysarthria with relative preservation of language functions (Hier et al. 1985; Powell et al. 1988). Slowing of cognitive function and impairment of executive function are common elements of the dementia syndrome.

Neuropsychiatric abnormalities are frequent in MID: personality changes, depression, lability of mood, and delusions occur regularly, but personality changes are the most common alterations. Apathy, abulia, and aspontaneity dominate the clinical syndrome; interpersonal relatedness and affect, however, are more preserved in MID than in AD (Dian et al. 1990; Ishii et al. 1986).

Major depressive disorders occur in 25%–50% of MID patients, and up to 60% of patients evidence symptoms of a depressive syndrome (Cummings 1988; Cummings et al. 1987; Erkinjuntti 1987). Sadness, anxiety, psychomotor retardation, and somatic complaints are the most common depressive symptoms reported. There is little relationship between the severity of depression and the degree of dementia, but very advanced patients lack depressive symptoms or have no recognizable means of expressing them (Cummings et al. 1987). Lability of mood and affect are also frequent in MID.

Psychosis with delusional ideation occurs in approximately 50% of MID patients. The delusional content is similar to that of AD and may include persecutory beliefs, fears of infidelity, phantom boarder syndrome, and the Capgras syndrome (Cummings et al. 1987; Flynn et al. 1991). Delusions most commonly occur with lesions involving the temporoparietal structures of either hemisphere.

Laboratory Investigations

Serum studies of MID patients should routinely include complete blood count, erythrocyte sedimentation rate, and serum cholesterol and triglyceride levels. In the absence of a history of hypertension or other stroke risk factors, more extensive laboratory studies should be pursued including antinuclear antibodies, antiphospholipid antibodies, and lupus anticoagulant levels (Briley et al. 1989; Cummings and Benson 1992; Young et al. 1989).

Neuroimaging studies provide support for the clinical diagnosis of MID. CT may reveal infarctions and evidence of periventricular ischemic changes (Aharon-Peretz et al. 1988; Erkinjuntti et al. 1987; Loeb and Gandolfo 1983). MRI is more revealing than CT and demonstrates small subcortical infarctions and ischemic white matter changes invisible on CT (Brown et al. 1988; Hershey et al. 1987). MRI is the technique of choice for identifying structural changes in MID (Figure 26–5). FDG-PET and SPECT show multiple irregular areas of hypometabolism or hypoperfusion consistent with focal regions of tissue infarction (Benson et al. 1983; Gemmell et al. 1987).

Classification and Neuropathology

Several subtypes of MID have been identified based on the size of vessel occluded and the area of tissue injured (Table 26–3) (Cummings and Benson 1992). Atherosclerosis may lead to occlusion of carotid arteries with large hemispheric infarctions; the most marked ischemic injury is in the borderzone regions between the three principal intracranial vessels. Occlusions of the anterior, middle, or posterior cerebral arteries produce hemisphere-specific deficit syndromes with neuropsychiatric complications (discussed in Chapter 19). Most MID is a product of sustained hypertension leading to fibrinoid necrosis of small arteries and arterioles. These vessels supply the deep gray matter nuclei including the striatum and thalamus, as well as the hemispheric white matter. Multiple small "lacunar" infarctions of the basal ganglia and thalamus produce the syndrome of lacunar state. Binswanger's disease is the syndrome characterized by extensive white matter ischemia.

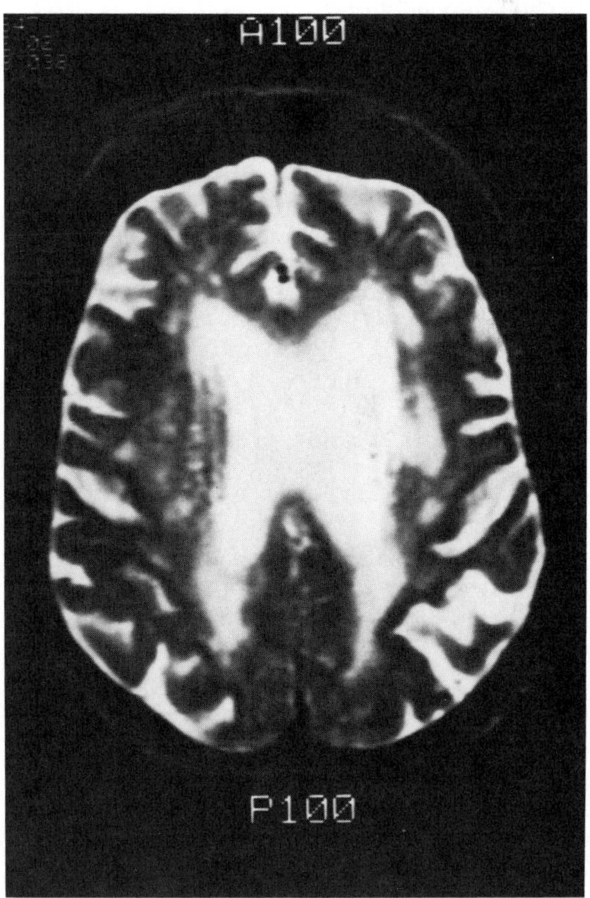

Figure 26–5. T2-weighted magnetic resonance imaging (MRI) scan of a patient with vascular dementia revealing irregular periventricular lesions and confluent high signal areas in the hemispheric white matter consistent with ischemic cerebral injury.

TABLE 26–3. SUBTYPES OF VASCULAR DEMENTIA

Syndrome	*Vessel size*	*Specific vessels*	*Common etiologies*
Multi-infarct dementia	Large	Carotid artery	Atherosclerosis and cardiac emboli
Multi-infarct dementia	Medium	Major intracranial branches	Atherosclerosis, hypertension, and cardiac emboli
Lacunar state	Small	Arterioles of deep gray nuclei	Hypertension
Binswanger's disease	Small	Arterioles of white matter	Hypertension
Angular gyrus syndrome	Medium	Middle cerebral artery branch	Cardiac emboli
Thalamic dementia	Small	Arterioles of thalamus	Hypertension

In most cases, lacunar state and Binswanger's disease coexist (Roman 1987).

The presence of dementia is not closely related to the total volume of infarcted tissue although large volumes of tissue injury are usually accompanied by intellectual impairment. Small lesions of the left angular gyrus or medial thalamic nuclei may disrupt multiple faculties and produce dementia syndromes.

Treatment

Treatment of MID consists of control of blood pressure in the upper-normal range and administration of aspirin for its platelet antiaggregant properties (Meyer et al. 1986, 1988). In rare circumstances, administration of anticoagulants or steroids may be warranted.

❑ HYDROCEPHALIC DEMENTIA

"Hydrocephalus" refers to enlargement of the cerebral ventricles with an increased amount of intraventricular CSF. Ventricular enlargement may be on an ex vacuo basis (from loss of cerebral tissue) or due to interruption of CSF flow (obstructive hydrocephalus). Hydrocephalus ex vacuo occurs in AD, MID, and other dementing illnesses and is not discussed further. There are two types of obstructive hydrocephalus: noncommunicating and communicating. Noncommunicating hydrocephalus arises from obstruction of CSF flow within the ventricular system or between the ventricles and the subarachnoid space. Communicating hydrocephalus occurs with obstruction of CSF flow within the subarachnoid space, preventing absorption of the CSF into the superior saggital sinus. Noncommunicating hydrocephalus is usually an acute process with headache, confusion, and ophthalmoplegia; intracranial pressure is typically elevated. Communicating hydrocephalus presents as a dementia syndrome and intracranial pressure is normal, hence the alternate name *normal-pressure hydrocephalus* (NPH). NPH accounts for approximately 5% of dementia syndromes in adults (Cummings and Benson 1992).

Clinical and Neuropsychiatric Features

The classic syndrome of NPH consists of dementia, gait disturbance, and incontinence. The dementia has prominent features of frontal-subcortical dysfunction including impaired attention and mental control, poor learning, visuospatial disturbances, and impaired abstraction and judgment (Cummings and Benson 1992; Gustafson and Hagberg 1978; Thomsen et al. 1986). Aphasia, apraxia, and agnosia are absent or mild. The gait abnormalities of NPH are variable but commonly include shortened stride length, diminished step height, and slow speed (Sudarsky and Simon 1987). Urinary incontinence is more common than loss of bowel control.

A variety of neuropsychiatric syndromes have been described in patients with NPH including personality alterations, anxiety, mood changes, and (rarely) psychosis. Apathy, inertia, and unconcern are the typical personality alterations; aggressive outbursts have also been reported (Crowell et al. 1973; Gustafson and Hagberg 1978). A wide range of mood disturbances has been described in NPH. Patients may manifest euphoria, mania, or depression (Gustafson and Hagberg 1978; Kwentus and Hart 1987).

Etiologies

NPH results from obstruction of CSF flow over the cerebral convexities with impaired absorption of fluid into the superior sagittal sinus (Table 26–4) (Cummings and Benson 1992). Classic NPH follows subarachnoid hemorrhage, head trauma, encephalitis, or meningitis. Less common causes include car-

TABLE 26–4. ETIOLOGIES OF NORMAL-PRESSURE HYDROCEPHALUS

Subarachnoid hemorrhage
Head trauma (especially with subarachnoid bleeding)
Meningitis
Encephalitis
Carcinomatous meningitis
Lymphomatous meningitis
Decompensation of congenital hydrocephalus
Aqueductal stenosis
Colloid cyst of third ventricle
Basilar impression
Ectatic basilar artery with intermittent third ventricular compression
Idiopathic

cinomatous meningitis and partial aqueductal obstruction. Many cases are idiopathic.

Diagnosis

The diagnosis of NPH depends on a combination of neuroimaging, CSF flow, and CSF pressure observations. CT studies reveal markedly enlarged ventricles and periventricular lucencies. The ventriculomegaly is most evident anteriorly with enlarged frontal and temporal horns. MRI demonstrates the same pattern of ventricular enlargement, increased periventricular signal on T2-weighted images, and an aqueductal flow void (Cummings and Benson 1992). Routine lumbar puncture reveals normal CSF pressure, and 24-hour pressure monitoring demonstrates increased B waves (Graff-Radford et al. 1989). Cisternography provides a means of assessing the pattern of CSF flow. After injection of radionuclide tracer into the lumbar subarachnoid space, there is reflux into the enlarged ventricular system and an absence of expected flow over the convexities to the superior sagittal sinus.

Treatment

Treatment for NPH is by ventriculoperitoneal shunting with diversion of CSF from the ventricles into the peritoneum. Lumboperitoneal shunts, diverting CSF from the lumbar subarachnoid space into the peritoneum, may also be used. Not all patients meeting diagnostic criteria for NPH improve following shunting. Increased B waves, shorter duration of dementia preceding surgery, known cause of the hydrocephalus, visible periventricular changes on CT or MRI, and onset of gait changes before dementia all predict a more favorable response to shunting (Graff-Radford et al. 1989; Thomsen et al. 1986). Patients who temporarily improve after removal of 50 ml of CSF are also likely to recover intellectual function after shunt placement (Wikkelso et al. 1982). Neuropsychiatric disturbances improve in concert with the cognitive impairment when shunting is successful.

❑ EVALUATION OF NEUROPSYCHIATRIC ALTERATIONS IN DEMENTIA

Evaluation of the dementia patient includes a careful history, mental status testing, and general physical and neurological examination. An assessment of past and current neuropsychiatric alterations (e.g., personality changes, anxiety, depression, mania, psychosis, and hallucinations) should be included. Appropriate laboratory studies include complete blood count, erythrocyte sedimentation rate, electrolytes, serum glucose, blood urea nitrogen, serum calcium and phosphorus levels, liver function tests, thyroid-stimulating hormone, vitamin B_{12} level, and serological test for syphilis (Cummings and Benson 1992). Additional tests such as human immunodeficiency virus (HIV) antibodies, antinuclear antibodies, antiphospholipid antibodies, lupus anticoagulant levels, heavy metal levels, serum drug levels, or other tests are obtained as dictated by specific clinical circumstances.

Neuroimaging procedures are an important part of the evaluation of the dementia patient (Martin et al. 1987). CT scanning is adequate for identifying intracranial tumors, hydrocephalus, larger strokes, abscesses, or subdural hematomas. Contrast enhancement may increase the detection of acute ischemic and demyelinating lesions. MRI is more sensitive to detection of ischemic injury and demyelination and capable of revealing more intracranial pathology than CT (Brown et al. 1988; Erkinjuntti et al. 1987). When available, MRI is the imaging procedure of choice in the evaluation of dementia.

PET and SPECT, imaging cerebral metabolism and perfusion, respectively, add another important dimension to the evaluation of dementia. In the degenerative disorders in which structural imaging techniques such as CT and MRI reveal only nonspecific atrophy, these tests reveal characteristic profiles of brain dysfunction helpful in differential diagnosis (Benson et al. 1983; Cummings and Benson 1992; Gemmell et al. 1987).

Electrophysiological studies, cisternography, CSF pressure monitoring, angiography, and other neurological investigations are used as indicated to explicate the diagnosis.

Treatment

There is no available therapy that ameliorates the course of AD or FLD; hydrocephalic patients have ventriculoperitoneal shunts placed; MID is currently managed with control of hypertension and administration of platelet antiaggregants (aspirin) (Meyer et al. 1986, 1989). Therapy of other diseases that can cause dementia is presented in Chapter 25.

Most treatment of dementia patients is directed at control of associated behavioral disturbances rather than the underlying dementing illness. Table 26–5 lists neuropsychiatric alterations that occur in

TABLE 26–5. NEUROPSYCHIATRIC ALTERATIONS OF DEMENTIA SYNDROMES AND THE PHARMACOLOGIC AGENTS COMMONLY USED IN THEIR TREATMENT

Symptom	*Available agents*	*Usual daily dose in mg po (range in mg)*
Psychosis	Haloperidol	1 (0.5–3)
	Fluphenazine	1 (1–5)
	Thiothixene	2 (1–10)
	Thioridazine	75 (30–150)
Agitation	Neuroleptics	
	Haloperidol	1 (0.5–3)
	Thiothixene	2 (1–10)
	Thioridazine	25 (10–75)
	Molindone	75 (5–125)
	Nonneuroleptics	
	Propranolol	120 (80–240)
	Trazodone	100 (100–400)
	Fluoxetine	40 (20–80)
	Buspirone	15 (15–30)
	Carbamazepine	1,000 (800–1,200)
	Lithium	900 (300–1,200)
	Lorazepam	1 (0.5–6)
Depression	Nortriptyline	50 (50–100)
	Desipramine	50 (50–150)
	Doxepin	50 (50–150)
	Trazodone	100 (100–400)
	Fluoxetine	40 (20–80)
Mania	Lithium	900 (300–1,200)
	Carbamazepine	1,000 (800–1,200)
	Clonazepam	4 (0.5–15)
	Valproic acid	1,500 (1,000–2,500)
Anxiety	Oxazepam	30 (20–60)
	Lorazepam	1 (0.5–6)
	Propranolol	120 (80–240)
Insomnia	Temazepam	15 (15–30)
	Lorazepam	1 (0.2–4)
	Nortriptyline	25 (20–75)
	Trazodone	100 (100–400)
	Thioridazine	25 (10–75)
Sexual aggression (in males)	Medroxyprogesterone	300 mg/week im

Source. Adapted from Cummings and Benson 1992.

dementia syndromes and the pharmacological agents most commonly used in their treatment.

In general, the drugs used in dementia are the same as those used for similar behaviors in patients without dementia, but dosages should be adjusted to reflect the fact that most dementias occur in aged individuals (Montamat et al. 1989; Thompson et al. 1983). Neuroleptics are the agents of choice for the control of delusions and agitation in dementia (Devanand et al. 1988; Helms 1985; Raskind and Risse 1986). Patients who are unresponsive or unable to tolerate these drugs may respond to treatment with trazodone, propranolol, carbamazepine, fluoxetine, lorazepam, buspirone, or lithium (Risse and Barnes 1986).

Depression is treated with nortriptyline, desipramine, doxepin, trazodone, or fluoxetine (Cummings and Benson 1992; Thompson et al. 1983). Agents used in the treatment of mania include lithium, carbamazepine, clonazepam, and valproic acid; anxiety may be managed with propranolol, oxazepam, or lorazepam. Sedating neuroleptics may be beneficial in the control of insomnia (Reynolds et al. 1988), but temazepam, lorazepam, nortriptyline, and trazodone may also afford relief. Males with sexually aggressive behavior may improve with administration of medroxyprogesterone (Cooper 1987).

Various nonpharmacological interventions may also be used with dementia patients in different phases of their illness including cognitive therapy, family therapy, supportive therapy, reminiscent therapy, and behavioral modification (Maletta 1988).

Care of dementia patients is delivered primarily by family members and the psychological, social, and legal needs of caregivers must be assessed. Depression is common among caregiving relatives (Cohen and Eisdorfer 1988), and individual or group therapy may be indicated. Families should be educated regarding social service resources such as home health aides, in-home respite care, day care programs, institutional respite care, and nursing home care. Legal consultation regarding durable power of attorney for health care and estate management is also warranted.

❑ REFERENCES

Aharon-Peretz J, Cummings JL, Hill MA: Vascular dementia and dementia of the Alzheimer type: cognition, ventricular size, and leuko-araiosis. Arch Neurol 45: 719–721, 1988

American Psychiatric Association: Diagnostic and Statistical Manual of Mental Disorders, 3rd Edition, Revised. Washington. DC, American Psychiatric Association, 1987

Baxter LR, Schwartz JM, Phelps ME, et al: Reduction of prefrontal cortex glucose metabolism common to three types of depression. Arch Gen Psychiatry 46:243–250, 1989

Benson DF, Kuhl DE, Hawkins RA, et al: The fluorodeoxyglucose 18-F scan in Alzheimer's disease and multi-infarct dementia. Arch Neurol 40:711–714, 1983

Briley DP, Coull BM, Goodnight SH Jr: Neurological disease associated with antiphospholipid antibodies. Ann Neurol 25:221–227, 1989

Brown JJ, Hesselink JR, Rothrock JF: MR and CT of lacunar infarcts. American Journal of Radiology 151:367–372, 1988

Brun A: Frontal lobe degeneration of non-Alzheimer type, I: neuropathology. Archives of Gerontology and Geriatrics 6:193–208, 1987

Brun A, Gustafson L: Distribution of cerebral degeneration in Alzheimer's disease. Archiv Psychiatrie Nervenkrankheiten 223:15–33, 1976

Cohen D, Eisdorfer C: Depression in family members caring for a relative with Alzheimer's disease. J Am Geriatr Soc 36:885–889, 1988

Cooper AJ: Medroxyprogesterone acetate (MPA) treatment of sexual acting out in men suffering from dementia. J Clin Psychiatry 48:368–370, 1987

Crowell RM, Tew JM Jr, Mark VH: Aggressive dementia associated with normal pressure hydrocephalus. Neurology 23:461–464, 1973

Cummings JL: Clinical Neuropsychiatry. New York: Grune & Stratton, 1985

Cummings JL: Depression in vascular dementia. Hillside J Clin Psychiatry 10:209–231, 1988

Cummings JL, Benson DF: Dementia of the Alzheimer type: an inventory of diagnostic clinical features. J Am Geriatr Soc 34:12–19, 1986

Cummings JL, Benson DF: Dementia: A Clinical Approach, 2nd Edition. Boston, MA, Butterworths, 1992

Cummings JL, Duchen LW: Kluver-Bucy syndrome in Pick disease: clinical and pathologic correlations. Neurology 31:1415–1422, 1981

Cummings JL, Victoroff JI: Noncognitive neuropsychiatric syndromes in Alzheimer's disease. Neuropsychiatry, Neuropsychology, and Behavioral Neurology 3:140–158, 1990

Cummings JL, Miller B, Hill MA, et al: Neuropsychiatric aspects of multi-infarct dementia and dementia of the Alzheimer type. Arch Neurol 44:389–393, 1987

Devanand DP, Sackeim HA, Mayeux R: Psychosis, behavioral disturbance, and the use of neuroleptics in dementia. Compr Psychiatry 29:387–401, 1988

Dian L, Cummings JL, Petry S, et al: Personality alterations in vascular dementia. Psychosomatics 31:415–419, 1990

Drevets WC, Rubin EH: Psychotic symptoms and the longitudinal course of senile dementia of the Alzheimer type. Biol Psychiatry 25:39–48, 1989

Erkinjuntti T: Types of multi-infarct dementia. Acta Neurol Scand 75:391–399, 1987

Erkinjuntti T, Ketonen L, Sulkava R, et al: CT in the differential diagnosis between Alzheimer's disease and vascular dementia. Acta Neurol Scand 75:262–270, 1987

Evans DA, Funkenstein H, Albert MS, et al: Prevalence of Alzheimer's disease in a community population of older persons: higher than previously reported. JAMA 262:2551–2556, 1989

Fitch N, Becker R, Heller A: The inheritance of Alzheimer's disease: a new interpretation. Ann Neurol 23:14–19, 1988

Flynn FG, Cummings JL, Gornbein J: Delusions in dementia syndromes: investigation of behavioral and neuropsychological correlates. Journal of Neuropsychiatry and Clinical Neurosciences 3:364–370, 1991

Foster NL, Chase TN, Fedio P, et al: Alzheimer's disease: focal cortical changes shown by positron emission tomography. Neurology 33:961–965, 1983

Foster NL, Gilman S, Berent S, et al: Cerebral hypometabolism in progressive supranuclear palsy studied with positron emission tomography. Ann Neurol 24:399–406, 1988

Gemmell HG, Sharp PF, Besson JAO, et al: Differential diagnosis in dementia using the cerebral blood flow agent 99mTc HM-PAO: a SPECT study. J Comput Assist Tomogr 11:398–402, 1987

Graff-Radford NR, Godersky JC, Jones MP: Variables predicting surgical outcome in symptomatic hydrocephalus in the elderly. Neurology 39:1601–1604, 1989

Graff-Radford NR, Damasio AR, Hyman BT, et al: Progressive aphasia in a patient with Pick's disease: a neuropsychological, radiologic, and anatomic study. Neurology 40:620–626, 1990

Grafman J, Litvan I, Gomez C, et al: Frontal lobe function in progressive supranuclear palsy. Arch Neurol 47: 553–558, 1990

Gustafson L: Frontal lobe degeneration of non-Alzheimer type, II: clinical picture and differential diagnosis. Archives of Gerontology and Geriatrics 6:209–223, 1987

Gustafson L, Hagberg B: Recovery of hydrocephalic dementia after shunt operation. J Neurol Neurosurg Psychiatry 41:940–947, 1978

Hachinski VC, Iliff LD, Zilhka E, et al: Cerebral blood flow in dementia. Arch Neurol 32:632–637, 1975

Haxby JV, Grady CL, Duara R, et al: Neocortical metabolic abnormalities precede nonmemory cognitive defects in early Alzheimer's-type dementia. Arch Neurol 43:882–885, 1986

Hays JW, Ernst RL: The economic costs of Alzheimer's disease. Am J Public Health 77:1169–1175, 1987

Helms PM: Efficacy of antipsychotics in the treatment of behavioral complications of dementia: a review of the literature. J Am Geriatr Soc 33:206–209, 1985

Hershey LA, Modic MT, Greenough G, et al: Magnetic resonance imaging in vascular dementia. Neurology 37:29–36, 1987

Heston LL, White JA, Mastri AR: Pick's disease: clinical genetics and natural history. Arch Gen Psychiatry 44: 409–411, 1987

Heyman A, Wilkinson WE, Hurwitz BJ, et al: Alzheimer's disease: genetic aspects and associated clinical disorders. Ann Neurol 14:507–515, 1983

Hier DB, Hagenlocker K, Shindler AG: Language disintegration in dementia: effects of etiology and severity. Brain Lang 25:117–133, 1985

Holland AL, McBurney DH, Moossy J, et al: The dissolution of language in Pick's disease with neurofibrillary tangles: a case study. Brain Lang 24:36–58, 1985

Ineichen B: Measuring the rising tide: how many dementia cases will there be in 2001? Br J Psychiatry 150:193–200, 1987

Ishii N, Nishihara Y, Imamura T: Why do frontal lobe symptoms predominate in vascular dementia with lacunes? Neurology 36:340–345, 1986

Jagust WJ, Friedland RP, Budinger TF, et al: Longitudinal studies of regional cerebral metabolism in Alzheimer's disease. Neurology 38:909–912, 1988

Johnson KA, Mueller ST, Walshe TM, et al: Cerebral perfusion imaging in Alzheimer's disease. Arch Neurol 44:165–168, 1987

Jordan SE, Nowacki R, Nuwer M: Computerized electroencephalography in the evaluation of early dementia. Brain Topography 1:271–274, 1989

Jorm AF, Korten AE, Henderson AS: The prevalence of dementia: a quantitative integration of the literature. Acta Psychiatr Scand 76:465–479, 1987

Kamo H, McGeer PL, Harrop R, et al: Positron emission tomography and histopathology in Pick's disease. Neurology 37:439–445, 1987

Kanazawa I, Kwak S, Sasaki H, et al: Studies on neurotransmitter markers of the basal ganglia in Pick's disease, with special reference to dopamine depletion. J Neurol Sci 83:63–74, 1988

Katzman R: Alzheimer's disease. N Engl J Med 314:964–973, 1986

Katzman R, Brown T, Thal LJ, et al: Comparison of rate of annual change of mental status score in four independent studies of patients with Alzheimer's disease. Ann Neurol 24:384–389, 1988

Knopman DS, Christensen KJ, Schut LJ, et al: The spectrum of imaging and neuropsychological findings in Pick's disease. Neurology 39:362–368, 1989

Kwentus JA, Hart RP: Normal pressure hydrocephalus presenting as mania. J Nerv Ment Dis 175:500–502, 1987

Ladurner G, Iliff LD, Lechner H: Clinical factors associated with dementia in ischaemic stroke. J Neurol Neurosurg Psychiatry 45:97–101, 1982

Lilly R, Cummings JL, Benson DF, et al: The human Kluver-Bucy syndrome. Neurology 33:1141–1145, 1983

Loeb C, Gandolfo C: Diagnostic evaluation of degenerative and vascular dementia. Stroke 14:399–401, 1983

McKhann G, Drachman D, Folstein M, et al: Clinical diagnosis of Alzheimer's disease: report of the NINCDS-ADRDA Work Group under the auspices of Department of Health and Human Services Task Force on Alzheimer's Disease. Neurology 34:939–944, 1984

Maletta GJ: Management of behavior problems in elderly patients with Alzheimer's disease and other dementias. Clin Geriatr Med 4:719–747, 1988

Martin DC, Miller J, Kapoor W, et al: Clinical prediction rules for computed tomographic scanning in senile dementia. Arch Intern Med 147:77–80, 1987

Mendez MF, Martin RJ, Smyth KA, et al: Psychiatric symptoms associated with Alzheimer's disease. Journal of Neuropsychiatry and Clinical Neuroscience 2: 28–33, 1990

Merriam AE, Aronson MK, Gaston P, et al: The psychiatric symptoms of Alzheimer's disease. J Am Geriatr Soc 36:7–12, 1988

Meyer JS, Judd BW, Tawakina T, et al: Improved cognition after control of risk factors for multi-infarct dementia. JAMA 256:2203–2209, 1986

Meyer JS, McClintic KL, Rogers RL, et al: Aetiological considerations and risk factors for multi-infarct dementia. J Neurol Neurosurg Psychiatry 51:1489–1497, 1988

Meyer JS, Rogers RL, McClintic K, et al: Randomized clinical trial of daily aspirin therapy in multi-infarct dementia. J Am Geriatr Soc 37:549–555, 1989

Miller BL, Mena I, Daly J, et al: Temporal-parietal hypoperfusion with single-photon emission computerized tomography in conditions other than Alzheimer's disease. Dementia 1:41–45, 1990

Miller BL, Cummings JL, Villanueva-Mayer J, et al: Frontal lobe degenerations: clinical, neuropsychological and SPECT characteristics. Neurology 41:1374–1382, 1991

Mohs RC, Breitner JCS, Silverman JM, et al: Alzheimer's disease: morbid risk among first-degree relatives approximates 50% by 90 years of age. Arch Gen Psychiatry 44:405–408, 1987

Montamat SC, Cusack BJ, Vestal RE: Management of drug therapy in the elderly. N Engl J Med 321:303–309, 1989

Morishita L: Wandering behavior, in Alzheimer's Disease: Treatment and Long-Term Mangement. Edited by Cummings JL, Miller BL. New York, Marcel Dekker, 1990, pp 157–176

Morris CH, Hope RA, Fairburn CG: Eating habits in dementia: a descriptive study. Br J Psychiatry 154:801–806, 1989

Munoz-Garcia D, Ludwin SK: Adult-onset neuronal intranuclear hyaline inclusion disease. Neurology 36: 785–790, 1986

Murayama S, Mori H, Ihara Y, et al: Immunocytochemical and ultrastructural studies of Pick's disease. Ann Neurol 27:394–405, 1990

Neary D, Snowden JS, Northen B, et al: Dementia of frontal lobe type. J Neurol Neurosurg Psychiatry 51:353–361, 1988

Neary D, Snowden JS, Mann DMA, et al: Frontal lobe dementia and motor neuron disease. J Neurol Neurosurg Psychiatry 53:23–32, 1990

Pearlson GD, Ross CA, Lohr WD, et al: Association between family history of affective disorder and the depressive syndrome of Alzheimer's disease. Am J Psychiatry 147:452–456, 1990

Perez FI, Rivera VM, Meyer JS, et al: Analysis of intellectual and cognitive performance in patients with multi-infarct dementia, vertebrobasilar insufficiency with dementia, and Alzheimer's disease. J Neurol Neurosurg Psychiatry 38:533–540, 1975

Petry S, Cummings JL, Hill MA, et al: Personality alterations in dementia of the Alzheimer type. Arch Neurol 45:1187–1190, 1988

Petry S, Cummings JL, Hill MA, et al: Personality alterations in dementia of the Alzheimer type: a three year follow-up study. J Geriatr Psychiatry Neurol 4:203–207, 1989

Powell AL, Cummings JL, Hill MA, et al: Speech and language alterations in multi-infarct dementia. Neurology 38:717–719, 1988

Procter A, Lowe SL, Palmer AM, et al: Topographical distribution of neurochemical changes in Alzheimer's disease. J Neurol Sci 84:125–140, 1988

Rabins PV, Mace NL, Lucas MJ: The impact of dementia on the family. JAMA 248:333–335, 1982

Raskind MA, Risse SC: Antipsychotic drugs and the elderly. J Clin Psychiatry 45 (suppl 5):17–22, 1986

Reichman WR, Cummings JL, Flynn F, et al: Visuospatial abnormalities in Alzheimer's disease and vascular dementia. Behavioral Neurology (in press)

Reisberg B, Borenstein J, Salob SP, et al: Behavioral symptoms in Alzheimer's disease: phenomenology and treatment. J Clin Psychiatry 48 (suppl 5):9–15, 1987

Reynolds CF III, Hoch CC, Stack J, et al: The nature and management of sleep/wake disturbance in Alzheimer's dementia. Psychopharmacol Bull 24:43–48, 1988

Risse SC, Barnes R: Pharmacologic treatment of agitation associated with dementia. J Am Geriatr Soc 34:368–376, 1986

Risse SC, Raskind MA, Nochlin D, et al: Neuropathological findings in patients with clinical diagnoses of probable Alzheimer's disease. Am J Psychiatry 147:168–172, 1990

Roman GC: Senile dementia of the Binswanger type. JAMA 258:1782–1788, 1987

Rubin EH, Morris JC, Storandt M, et al: Behavioral changes in patients with mild senile dementia of the Alzheimer's type. Psychiatry Res 21:55–62, 1987

Shapira J, Cummings JL: Alzheimer's disease: Changes in sexual behavior. Medical Aspects of Human Sexuality 23(6):32–35, 1989

Sudarsky L, Simon S: Gait disturbance in late-life hydrocephalus. Arch Neurol 44:263–267, 1987

Sulkava R, Erkinjuntti T: Vascular dementia due to cardiac arrhythmias and systemic hypotension. Acta Neurol Scand 76:123–128, 1987

Swearer JM, Drachman DA, O'Donnell BF, et al: Troublesome and disruptive behaviors in dementia. J Am Geriatr Soc 36:784–790, 1988

Teri L, Larson EB, Reifler BV. Behavioral disturbance in dementia of the Alzheimer's type. J Am Geriatr Soc 36:1–6, 1988

Thompson TL II, Moran MG, Nies AS: Psychotropic drug use in the elderly. N Engl J Med 308:134–138, 194–199, 1983

Thomsen AM, Borgesen SE, Bruhn P, et al: Prognosis of dementia in normal-pressure hydrocephalus after a shunt operation. Ann Neurol 20:304–310, 1986

Tierney MC, Fisher RH, Lewis AJ, et al: The NINCDS-

ADRDA Work Group criteria for the clinical diagnosis of probable Alzheimer's disease: a clinicopathological study of 57 cases. Neurology 38:359–364, 1988

Verity MA, Wechsler AF: Progressive subcortical gliosis of Neumann: A clinicopathological study of two cases with review. Archives of Gerontology and Geriatrics 6:245–261, 1987

Wechsler AF, Verity A, Rosenschein S, et al: Pick's disease: a clinical, computed tomographic, and histologic study with Golgi impregnation observations. Arch Neurol 39:287–290, 1982

Wikkelso C, Andersson H, Blomstrand C, et al: The clinical effect of lumbar puncture in normal pressure hydrocephalus. J Neurol Neurosurg Psychiatry 45:64–69, 1982

Wragg RE, Jeste DV: Overview of depression and psychosis in Alzheimer's disease. Am J Psychiatry 146:577–587, 1989

Yates CM, Simpson J, Maloney AFJ, et al: Neurochemical observations in a case of Pick's disease. J Neurol Sci 48:257–263, 1980

Young SM, Fisher M, Sigsbee A, et al: Cardiogenic brain embolism and lupus anticoagulant. Ann Neurol 26: 390–392, 1989

Chapter

27

The Neuropsychiatry of Schizophrenia

Henry A. Nasrallah, M.D.

SCHIZOPHRENIA IS ARGUABLY the most serious psychiatric disorder. The current "official" diagnosis of schizophrenia is determined by a set of inclusion and exclusion criteria, as per the guidelines published in the Diagnostic and Statistical Manual of Mental Disorders, Third Edition, Revised (DSM-III-R) (American Psychiatric Association 1987). Inclusion criteria include the presence of delusions and hallucinations, a marked decrement in functioning (work, social relations, or self-care), and continuous signs of the disturbance for at least 6 months. Exclusion criteria include the absence of a consistent mood disorder component such as schizoaffective disorder or mood disorder with psychotic features, as well as the lack of an organic factor that initiated and maintained the disorder. Schizophrenia is clinically subtyped into four types (catatonic, disorganized, undifferentiated, and residual), each characterized by the presence and absence of specific clinical features.

The syndrome of schizophrenia has become widely recognized as a brain disease (Henn and Nasrallah 1982; Nasrallah and Weinberger 1986). The evidence for the neurobiological basis of schizophrenia has been accumulating rapidly over the past two decades. The explosive advances in neuroscience research and the advent of computed brain imaging techniques have generated a windfall of new knowledge about brain structure and function in schizophrenia.

In this chapter, I present an overview of the neuropsychiatry of schizophrenia along two main themes: 1) brain lesions that produce a schizophrenia-like psychosis (also known as *symptomatic* or *secondary* schizophrenia) and 2) neurobiological findings in *primary* schizophrenia. Wherever possible I highlight the association of the clinical manifestations of the schizophrenic syndrome with regional brain pathology to underscore the pervasive involvement of many brain regions in schizophrenia.

❑ STRUCTURAL AND FUNCTIONAL BRAIN LESIONS ASSOCIATED WITH SCHIZOPHRENIA-LIKE PSYCHOTIC SYNDROMES

There are numerous medical conditions that are known to produce psychotic symptoms that resemble schizophrenia (Cummings 1985, 1988; Nasrallah 1986). Such clinical observations have generated many hypotheses regarding the brain "dysfunction" that may elucidate the neuropsychiatry of schizophrenia. The following is a description of disorders through the lifespan that may be associated with schizophrenia-like psychoses (Figure 27–1).

Genetic Abnormalities

There are several established genetic disorders that, in addition to producing physical anomalies, are also known to produce psychotic symptoms (e.g., delusions, hallucinations, and bizarre behavior) that strongly resemble schizophrenia (Propping and Friedl 1988). Table 27–1 lists genetic disorders that have been reported to present clinically with psychotic features. It is reasonable to predict that as the chemical mechanisms of these genetic disorders become known, considerable insights will accrue regarding the neurobiology of schizophrenia. Primary schizophrenia itself has been shown to have a strong genetic basis in family, twin, and adoption studies (Tsuang and Simpson 1988) as well as with molecular genetic methods (Gurling et al. 1989).

Congenital (Neurodevelopmental) Disorders

Several neurological congenital anomalies have been reported to be associated with psychotic symptoms, including corpus callosum agenesis (Swayze et al. 1990), aqueduct stenosis (Reveley and Reveley 1983), arachnoid cysts (Kuhnley et al. 1981), porencephaly (Owens et al. 1980), cerebral hamartoma (Taylor 1975), and cavum septum pellucidum (George et al. 1989). These reports lend support to the neurodevelopmental hypothesis of schizophrenia (Lewis and Murray 1987; Nasrallah 1990; Weinberger 1987), which postulates that schizophrenia is associated with disruption(s) of basic neurodevelopmental processes such as neuronal proliferation, migration, and elimination during fetal life, especially during the critical second trimester (Nowakowski 1987).

Perinatal Complications

A large literature extending over several decades suggests that neurological insults resulting from pregnancy and delivery complications (Table 27–2) are associated with schizophrenic psychoses in

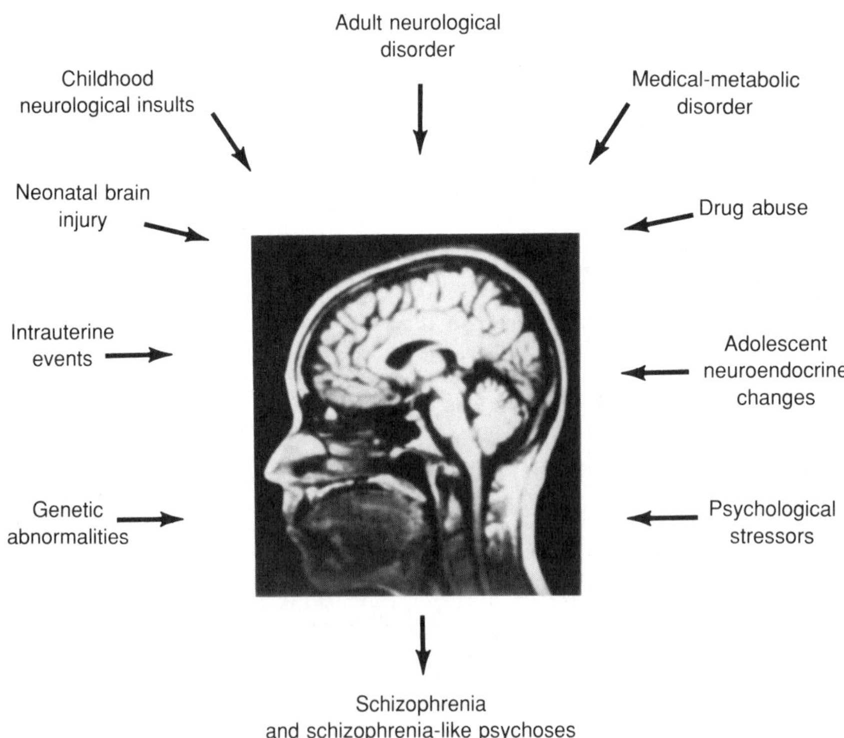

Figure 27–1. Various factors that may play a role in the production of schizophrenia or schizophrenia-like psychoses.

TABLE 27–1. GENETIC DISORDERS THAT MAY PRESENT WITH A SCHIZOPHRENIA-LIKE PSYCHOSIS

1. Albinism
2. Asperger's syndrome
3. Ataxia, dominant type
4. Congenital adrenal hyperplasia
5. Erythropoietic protoporphyria
6. Fabry's disease
7. Familial basal ganglia calcification
8. Glucose-6-phosphate dehydrogenase deficiency
9. Gaucher's disease
10. Hemochromatosis
11. Homocystinuria
12. Huntington's chorea
13. Hyperasparginemia
14. Ichthyosis vulgaris (autosomal dominant type)
15. Kartagener's syndrome
16. Klinefelter karyotype
17. Lawrence-Moon-Bardet-Biedl syndrome
18. Metachromatic leukodystrophy, adult type
19. Niemann-Pick's disease, late type
20. Phenylketonuria
21. Porphyria, acute intermittent type
22. Porphyria variegata
23. 18q or r (18) constitution
24. Turner's (or Noonan's) syndrome
25. Wilson's disease
26. XXX karyotype
27. XYY karyotype

Source. Adapted from Nasrallah 1986.

adulthood (Lyon et al. 1989; McNeil and Kaij 1978). It is postulated that perinatal complications may disrupt the brain structure and functions in a manner that facilitates the development of psychotic perceptions, thoughts, and behavior. One example of such disruption is interference with neuronal migration in the hippocampus (which is especially sensitive to hypoxia during the second trimester), resulting in gross hypoplasia of the hippocampal formation and aberrant histoarchitecture of pyramidal cells in parts of the hippocampus (Conrad and Scheibel 1987). More on the neuropathology of schizophrenia is presented later in this chapter.

Mednick et al. (1988) demonstrated that fetal exposure to influenza during the second trimester is associated with increased risk for the development of schizophrenia. However, it remains to be established whether perinatal brain injury alone (without a genetic predisposition to psychosis) is sufficient to produce schizophrenia in adulthood. Some studies (Lewis et al. 1987; Owen et al. 1989; Schwarzkopf et al. 1989a) have suggested that family history was less frequent among schizophrenic adults with a strong history of perinatal complications, but others (Parnas et al. 1982) have suggested that perinatal complications may be quite frequent

TABLE 27–2. OBSTETRIC AND PERINATAL COMPLICATIONS THAT MAY BE ASSOCIATED (WHEN IN EXCESS) WITH SCHIZOPHRENIA-LIKE PSYCHOSIS IN ADULTHOOD

Prenatal factors (during pregnancy)
- Maternal age above 39
- Nulliparous parity (first pregnancy is at higher risk)
- Viral infection
- Previous abortions
- Anemia
- Bleeding
- Physical injury
- Hypertension
- Albuminuria
- Generalized edema
- Medication intake other than vitamins
- Gestational diabetes or seizure disorders
- Venous thrombosis
- Psychiatric illness requiring medical attention
- Gestation under 36 weeks

Perinatal factors (during labor and delivery)
- Long labor
- Breech presentation
- Caesarean section
- Twins or multiple births
- General or epidural anesthesia
- Abruptio placentae
- Occult prolapse or neck-knot of cord
- Vacuum extraction
- Use of forceps
- Apgar score under 6
- Meconium in the amniotic fluid
- Meconium aspirated
- Physical trauma, (e.g., fractures to the newborn)
- Large placental infarcts
- Calcified placenta
- Birth weight under 2,500 g or above 4,000 g
- Postmaturity (more than 44 weeks)
- Hemolytic disease

Neonatal factors
- Respiratory distress
- Septicemia or meningitis
- Hyperbilirubinemia
- Anemia requiring transfusion
- Irritable or floppy infant
- Convulsions
- Difficulty regulating temperature
- Clinical dysmaturity
- Hypoxia
- Oxygen treatment

Source. Adapted from Nasrallah 1986.

in the offspring of schizophrenic mothers. It seems likely that perinatal brain injury may contribute to the heterogeneous spectrum of the schizophrenic syndrome and may help explain the discordance for schizophrenia in monozygotic twins (Suddath et al. 1990) or for variations in the age at onset (Wilcox and Nasrallah 1987a) or in deficit symptoms and course (Wilcox and Nasrallah 1987b).

Neurological Disorders in Childhood and Adulthood

Many neurological disorders have been reported to be occasionally associated with psychotic signs and symptoms. Davison and Bagley (1969) provided a comprehensive review of this literature, later condensed by Davison (1983). The following neurological disorders may present with psychosis:

1. *Epilepsy.* A higher frequency of psychosis is observed in patients with epilepsy than would be expected in the general population. This is especially true for left temporal lobe foci, an observation that led Flor-Henry (1969) to postulate a lateralized left dysfunction in schizophrenia. A recent study by Roberts et al. (1990) of temporal lobectomies demonstrated that even in chronic temporal lobe epilepsy, schizophrenia-like psychosis did not occur at random. Rather, psychosis a) was significantly associated with lesions that originated during fetal life (such as gangliomas), b) affected neurons in the medial temporal lobe (especially on the left), and c) produced first seizure at an early age (5–6 years). Such findings lend support to the neurodevelopmental model of schizophrenia and to the emerging importance of the medial temporal lobe in schizophrenia.
2. *Cerebral trauma.* Many studies of psychosis subsequent to cerebral trauma have been reported including large series of war casualties (Davison and Bagley 1969). Temporal and frontal lobe traumas appear to be more likely to produce psychotic features, with left temporal lobe injury producing positive symptoms and frontal lobe injury producing mainly negative symptoms.
3. *Cerebral tumors.* There are many reports of psychotic patients who died in long-term institutions and were found to have brain tumors at autopsy. Tumors in the temporal, hypophyseal, suprasellar, and supratentorial areas have been reported to be particularly likely to produce schizophrenia-like features. Tumors of the third ventricle strongly resemble catatonic schizophrenia in several reports. Hallucinations and delusions are more likely in temporal, frontal, and pituitary tumors. Psychotic symptoms have been reported to be associated with corpus callosum tumors, especially in the anterior part (genu) where frontal-temporal interhemispheric fibers are disrupted (Nasrallah and McChesney 1981).
4. *Cerebral infections.* Various types of encephalitides have been associated with psychotic symptoms, such as encephalitis lethargic epidemic sequelae in the 1920s (predominantly paranoid-hallucinatory features), postrheumatic Syndenham's chorea (Wilcox and Nasrallah 1988), and syphilis.
5. *Neurodegenerative disorders.* Psychotic symptoms are known to accompany or be a main feature of basal ganglia disorders (e.g., calcification, Huntington's chorea, Wilson's disease, and Parkinson's disease) as well as other neurodegenerative diseases (e.g., Alzheimer's disease, Pick's disease, and Leber's hereditary optic atrophy).
6. *Demyelinating disorders.* Up to 50% of patients with multiple sclerosis show psychiatric symptoms including psychosis. Also, several similarities between multiple sclerosis and schizophrenia prompted Stevens (1988) to suggest that these two disorders belong to the similar class of (possibly) viral etiology.
7. *Narcolepsy.* This sleep-wake cycle disorder of rapid-eye-movement (REM) sleep (Aldrich 1990) has frequently been reported to manifest hypnagogic sleep hallucinations, which used to be regarded as a psychotic symptom. However, some cases of narcolepsy are secondary to encephalitis, hypothalamic tumor, or Klein-Levin syndrome, and psychotic features may be a result of the primary disease. Because amphetamine-type central nervous system (CNS) stimulants are used in the treatment of narcolepsy, it has been suggested that some paranoid symptoms may be stimulant induced.
8. *Cerebrovascular disease.* Paranoid delusions and hallucinatory experiences have been reported in conjunction with subarachnoid hemorrhage, fat embolism, bilateral carotid artery occlusion, arteriovenous malformation, stroke, and subdural hematoma. In general, affective syndromes are

more likely than psychosis to be associated with cerebrovascular disease (Robinson and Forrester 1987).

Medical Diseases

Most systemic medical disorders influence brain function physiologically and/or metabolically and may produce psychotic symptoms. Physical illness has been reported to be very common at the onset of catatonic psychoses (Wilcox and Nasrallah 1986). The following medical disorders may produce psychotic manifestations:

1. *Infections.* As discussed in the previous section, infections that involve brain tissue may result in psychotic symptoms.
2. *Inflammatory disorders.* Likewise, inflammatory disorders, such as cerebritis associated with lupus erythematosus, may produce psychotic symptoms (Bluestein 1987).
3. *Endocrinopathies.* These include Addison's disease, hypothyroidism, hyperthyroidism, hypoparathyroidism, hyperparathyroidism, and hypopituitarism (Alarcon and Franceschini 1984; Leigh and Kramer 1984; Mikkelson and Reider 1979; O'Shanick et al. 1987; Reus 1986).
4. *Systemic medical diseases.* Such diseases include kidney failure and uremia, hepatic encephalopathy, hyponatremia, hypercalcemia, hypoglycemia (Stoudemire and Levenson 1990), and myasthenia gravis (Dorrell 1973).
5. *Nutritional deficiency states.* Deficiencies of thiamine (Wernicke-Korsakoff syndrome), vitamin B_{12} and folate (megaloblastic anemia) (McEvoy 1982), and niacin (Spivak and Jackson 1977) may also produce psychotic manifestations.

❑ DRUG-INDUCED PSYCHOTIC SYNDROMES

Numerous psychotic reactions seen in the clinical setting are now recognized to be associated with the use of both recreational and prescription drugs. Some of the drug-induced psychoses are almost indistinguishable from schizophrenia (such as amphetamine and phencyclidine [PCP] psychoses), whereas others may produce nonspecific or partial psychotic syndromes, sometimes with toxic-organic features. The following classes of drugs can produce psychotic syndromes:

1. *Stimulants.* The stimulants that can produce psychotic manifestations include amphetamine (Snyder 1973), cocaine (Gold and Giannini 1989), and methylphenidate (Janowsky et al. 1973). Their mechanism of action is believed to be via dopamine release or agonist effects.
2. *Hallucinogens.* Hallucinogens are drugs that usually produce visual hallucinations and bizarre behavior. Lysergic acid diethylamide (LSD), mescaline, psilocybin, and dimethyltryptamine are notable examples (Moreines 1989; Slaby 1989).
3. *Phencyclidine.* PCP can produce a mixture of positive and negative symptoms that can be indistinguishable from chronic schizophrenia (Giannini 1989).
4. *Catecholaminergic drugs.* These include drugs such as levodopa (L-dopa), amantadine, and ephedrine (Klawans 1978).
5. *Anticholinergics.* Numerous psychotropic drugs have anticholinergic activity including tricyclic antidepressants (TCAs) and antiparkinsonian agents (e.g., trihexyphenidyl and benztropine). In sufficiently high doses, anticholinergic drugs may produce a schizophrenia-like psychosis (Dysken et al. 1978)
6. *CNS depressants.* These include alcohol and benzodiazepine sedative-hypnotics (Roman 1978).
7. *Glucocorticoids.* Glucocorticoids can exaggerate preexisting psychosis or, in sufficient doses, may produce psychotic symptoms in a nonpsychotic person (Ling et al. 1981).
8. *Heavy metals.* The heavy metals that can produce psychotic syndromes include lead, mercury, manganese, arsenic, and thallium (Lishman 1987).
9. *Others.* Other drugs producing psychotic manifestations include digitalis (Gorelick et al. 1978), disulfiram (Nasrallah 1979), cimetidine (Adler et al. 1980), and bromide (Raskind et al. 1978).

To summarize the first part of this chapter, a variety of brain lesions or disturbances may manifest with psychotic signs and symptoms resembling those of schizophrenia. Although the sum total of the literature provides an extensive number of possible pathophysiological pathways to schizophrenia-like psychosis, the clues are too numerous to be reconciled into a coherent pathophysiological mechanism for schizophrenia. Perhaps the main relevant conclusion for the neuropsychiatry of schizophrenia that can be drawn from the literature is that many brain regions are probably involved in the production of schizophrenia phenomenology, but that certain regions (temporal, frontal, and limbic) appear to be of particular importance. A frequent clinical correlate of symptomatic schizophrenia is clouding of consciousness, which is not seen in true schizophrenia. In the second part of this chapter, I present neurobiological findings in primary schizophrenia. The conclusions to be drawn are quite similar to those of the first part, albeit the evidence is derived from different scientific perspectives and methods.

❑ NEUROBIOLOGICAL ABNORMALITIES ASSOCIATED WITH SCHIZOPHRENIA

Over the past 15 years, significant advances have been made in identifying replicable neurobiological abnormalities in schizophrenia. At least four developments may have contributed substantively to the timing of these advances:

1. The development of reliable operational diagnostic criteria that became widely used by researchers, initially the Research Diagnostic Criteria (RDC; Spitzer et al. 1978) and subsequently the DSM-III criteria (American Psychiatric Association 1980)
2. The computer "revolution" of the 1970s and 1980s that facilitated the development of high-tech research instrumentation
3. The development of brain-imaging biotechnology that enabled the in vivo investigation of brain structure and function
4. The quantum increase in neuroscience research activity and researchers

It is against this momentous backdrop that the neuropsychiatry of schizophrenia finally began to take shape. Many of the "psychiatric" signs and symptoms of schizophrenia are consistent with "neurological" abnormalities as well (Table 27–3).

In this section, I overview the current status of the neurobiological findings in schizophrenia and their etiopathophysiological and clinical significance. The implications for the neuropsychiatry of schizophrenia at the time of writing this chapter are presented. In addition, I highlight and discuss some of the major themes in this area.

TABLE 27–3. NEUROLOGICAL ABNORMALITIES REPORTED IN SCHIZOPHRENIA

"Higher" brain function
- Loss of insight re illness
- Loss of ambition and drive
- Loss of ability to plan
- Impaired judgment
- Lack of decision-making skill
- Failure to abstract
- Inability to initiate tasks
- Lack of social insight
- Gender identity confusion

Neurobehavioral
- Impaired attention
- Impaired recognition and perception of faces
- Impaired perception of prosody of speech
- Decreased ability to inflect own speech
- Flat affect
- Impaired memory, short-term
- Impaired memory, long-term

Motor function
- Abnormal smooth pursuit eye movement
- Tics
- Stereotypies
- Choreiform movements
- Grimacing
- Abnormal motor tone
- Increased blinking
- Apraxia
- Poor hopping
- Abnormal gait
- Abnormal finger tapping

Sensory integration
- Decreased pain sensation
- Decreased sense of smell
- Decreased temperature sensation
- Astereognosis
- Agraphesthesia
- Extinction
- Right-left confusion

Perceptual
- Hallucinations
- Auditory
- Visual
- Somatic
- Gustatory

In Vivo Regional Brain Abnormalities in Schizophrenia

The application of computed tomography (CT) and magnetic resonance imaging (MRI) to the in vivo study of the brain has resulted in the discovery of several regional structural abnormalities in schizophrenia. Similarly, the development and use of regional cerebral blood flow (rCBF), single photon emission computed tomography (SPECT), and positron-emission tomography (PET) have added significant new information about the functional disturbances in certain brain regions in schizophrenia. The following is a summary of the structural and/or functional pathology of various brain regions in schizophrenia.

The ventricular system. More than 75% of 60 CT studies since 1976, involving about 1,600 schizophrenic and 1,200 control subjects, have now demonstrated a significant pathological dilatation of the cerebral ventricular system in schizophrenia, particularly the lateral and third ventricles (Shelton and Weinberger 1986) (Figure 27–2).

This ventricular enlargement has been demonstrated by linear, area, and volumetric measurements on both CT and MRI scans. It has become one of the most established neurobiological findings in schizophrenia, implying the loss of brain tissue in periventricular regions in many but not all patients.

Clinically, ventriculomegaly is consistently shown to be unrelated to treatment(s) received or duration of illness (Nasrallah and Coffman 1985). Many studies have shown a correlation between ventriculomegaly and certain clinical variables including obstetric complications, poor premorbid adjustment, family history of psychosis, neuropsychological impairment, poor response to neuroleptic drugs, prominent negative symptoms, and presence of involuntary movements (Losonczy et al. 1986a). However, although Crow (1980) used ventricular enlargement to postulate the existence of two main subtypes of schizophrenia, other studies have failed to find correlations with many of those clinical variables (Nasrallah et al. 1983a) or failed to find evidence of a bimodal distribution of ventricular size (Farmer et al. 1987).

Several biological correlates of ventriculomegaly in schizophrenia have also been reported, including increased blood serotonin and cerebrospinal fluid (CSF) amino acids; decreased CSF 5-hydroxyindoleacetic acid (5-HIAA), homovanillic acid (HVA), dihydroxyphenylacetic acid (DOPAC), cyclic adenosine monophosphate (cAMP), and dopamine β-hydroxylase (DBH); defective smooth pursuit eye movements; neurological soft signs; decreased slow-wave sleep; temporal attenuation of the auditory P300 wave; and lack of inverse relationship of serum prolactin with psychosis ratings (Karson et al. 1988; Kleinman et al. 1984; Losonczy et al. 1986b; McCarley et al. 1989; Reveley et al. 1987; Smeraldi et al. 1987; van Kammen et al. 1988).

It should be noted that ventricular enlargement is not specific to schizophrenia and has been found in several other psychiatric disorders (Nasrallah and Coffman 1985; Nasrallah et al. 1989). However, this nonspecificity does not negate the specific significance that ventricular enlargement has within schizophrenia for pathogenesis and clinical course. Siblings of schizophrenic patients have larger ventricles than do control subjects, but only if they have a schizophrenia spectrum diagnosis (Olson et al. 1991). Affected siblings in monozygotic twins discordant for schizophrenia consistently have larger ventricles than do their nonaffected twins (Suddath et al. 1990).

More recently, the major thrust of research in this area has focused on whether ventriculomegaly in schizophrenia is static or progressive, an issue that has important pathophysiological implications. In the first follow-up study of ventricular size in schizophrenia, Nasrallah et al. (1986b) found no difference in mean ventricular size after 3 years, suggesting that ventricular dilatation is a static, thus probably a neurodevelopmental lesion rather than a degenerative lesion. This finding was supported by two subsequent follow-up studies (Illowsky et al. 1988; Vita et al. 1988), and by the presence of enlarged ventricles at the onset of the illness (Turner et al. 1986) and even before the appearance of the illness in the offspring of schizophrenic mothers (Schulsinger et al. 1984). However, some recent data from Kemali et al. (1989), Woods et al. (1990), and from my laboratory as well (Schwarzkopf et al. 1990) have demonstrated progressivity of ventricular size in at least a subgroup of schizophrenic patients. Thus the issue of static versus progressive ventricular enlargement in schizophrenia, with its important etiological (neurodevelopmental versus degenerative) implications, remains to be resolved.

Cerebrum and cranium. Schizophrenic patients have been shown to have smaller midsagittal craniums and cerebrums on MRI scans (Andreasen et al. 1986), a finding subsequently replicated by other MRI studies (DeMyer et al. 1988; Johnstone et al. 1989; Nasrallah et al. 1988; Schwarzkopf et al. 1989b) and CT studies (Pearlson et al. 1989). Smaller brain weight in schizophrenia (a decrease of 5%–8%) has also been reported in postmortem studies (Brown et al. 1986; Bruton et al. 1990; Pakkenberg 1987).

A

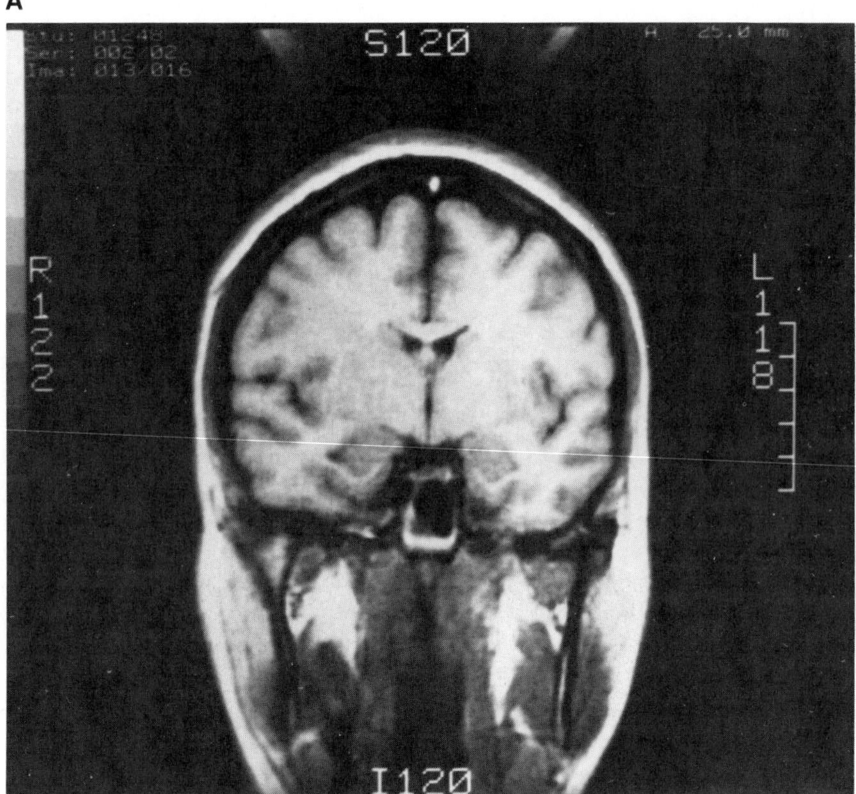

B

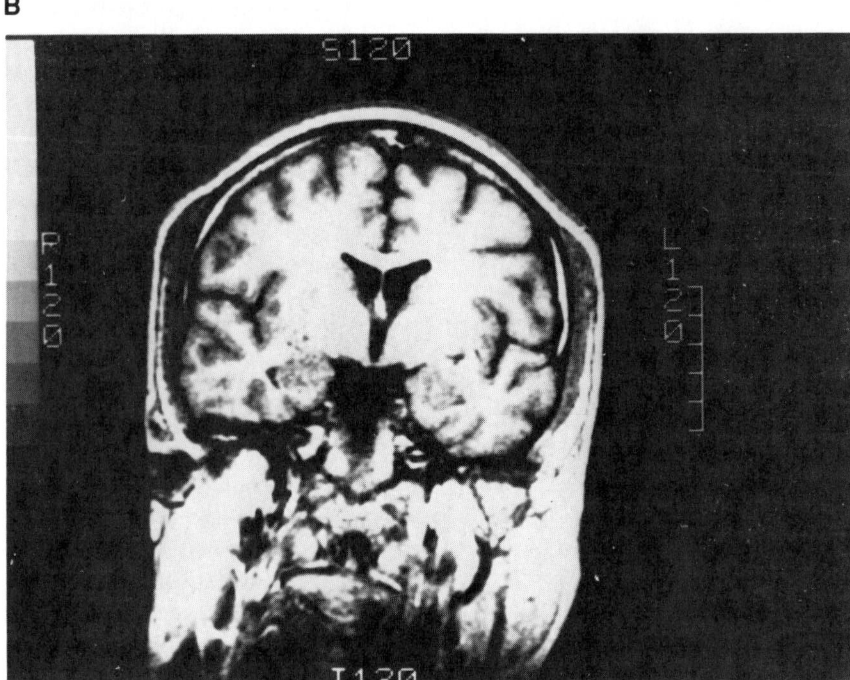

Figure 27–2. Coronal magnetic resonance imaging (MRI) scans showing normal lateral and third ventricles in a healthy control subject (*panel A*) and enlarged lateral and third ventricles in a schizophrenic patient (*panel B*) of the same age (28 years).

Results from my laboratory (Nasrallah et al. 1988; Schwarzkopf et al. 1991) suggest that the decrease in brain size in schizophrenia is particularly pronounced in patients with a family history of schizophrenia. Overall, the findings of smaller cerebrum and cranium in schizophrenia are consistent with a neurodevelopmental growth impairment, possibly under programmed genetic control rather than incidental environmental insult.

Sulcal widening. About 70% of 20 studies involving about 900 patients and 750 control subjects have confirmed the presence of enlarged cortical sulci and fissures in schizophrenia (Nasrallah et al. 1982; Pfefferbaum et al. 1988; Shelton and Weinberger 1986). There are no data yet as to whether this pathology is static or progressive, but there is support for a neurodevelopmental origin for widened sulci and fissures (Cannon et al. 1989). Clinical correlates of cortical sulcal widening include cognitive impairment (Yates et al. 1990), negative symptoms, and poor response to antipsychotic therapy (Nasrallah and Coffman 1985). In addition, prefrontal sulcal prominence was found to be inversely related to response to clozapine in chronic schizophrenia (Friedman et al. 1991).

Cerebellar vermis atrophy. About 90% of 13 CT studies on about 600 patients and 500 control subjects have reported a higher frequency of what appears to be "atrophy" of the cerebellum (widening of vermal sulci, enlargement of the fourth ventricle, and cerebellar cisterns) (Nasrallah et al. 1991; Shelton and Weinberger 1986). Overall, about 9% of schizophrenic patients compared to about 4% of controls show these cerebellar changes, which have also been reported to be associated with third ventricular enlargement (Nasrallah et al. 1985).

Reversed cerebral asymmetries. About a dozen CT studies examined the pattern of cerebral hemisphere asymmetry in schizophrenia (Shelton and Weinberger 1986). One-third of those studies reported abnormal structural cerebral asymmetries in schizophrenia compared with control subjects. There appears to have been a decline in interest in this area over the past few years. The significance of this abnormality remains unknown but may be explained by disruption of cerebral hemisphere growth and development in schizophrenia.

Frontal lobes. Frontal lobe dysfunction has been implicated in schizophrenia for decades, starting with Kraepelin and Bleuler (see Greden and Tandon 1991). Many of the manifestations of schizophrenia, such as negative symptoms, inability to plan, poor judgment, and impaired cognition, have been attributed to frontal lobe dysfunction (Levin 1984b) because of the strong similarity to the syndrome that follows damage to the frontal lobes (Mesulam 1986). However, although there is some evidence for structural abnormalities in the frontal lobe (smaller size) MRI scans in schizophrenia (Andreasen et al. 1986; Nasrallah et al. 1990), most of the evidence for frontal lobe impairment in schizophrenic patients is that of disrupted function.

Several cerebral blood flow (CBF) and PET studies have indicated a relative decrease in blood flow and glucose metabolism in the frontal lobe (Buchsbaum et al. 1984; Ingvar 1987; Weinberger and Berman 1988), but chronicity and neuroleptic use have been implicated in this "hypofrontality" (Figure 27–3). Weinberger et al. (1986) demonstrated with xenon-133 (^{133}Xe) inhalation that the rCBF in the dorsolateral prefrontal cortex (DLPFC) was significantly reduced in schizophrenic patients versus control subjects during the performance of the Wisconsin Card Sorting test (WCS; Heaton 1985), which presumably activates the DLPFC. Electroencephalographic (EEG) abnormalities in the frontal lobe indicate excessive EEG slow-wave activity (Morihisa et al. 1983; Shagass 1987).

The frontal lobes have also been linked to the smooth pursuit eye movement abnormalities that have been consistently found in schizophrenia (Iacono 1985; Levin 1984a) and to many of the neurological soft signs that are found in schizophrenic patients (Heinrich and Buchanan 1988).

The frontal lobes are quite important in the neuropsychiatry of schizophrenia. However, much more needs to be learned about their structure and function (Goldman-Rakic 1984) before their role in schizophrenia is defined. Because of the extensive projections between the frontal lobes and many other brain regions, it is not possible to conclude at this time whether the impairment of frontal lobe functions in schizophrenia is related to a primary or secondary lesion.

Temporal lobes. Evidence linking the temporal lobe with schizophrenia comes from many sources. As described above, there is an association between schizophrenia-like psychosis and lesions of the tem-

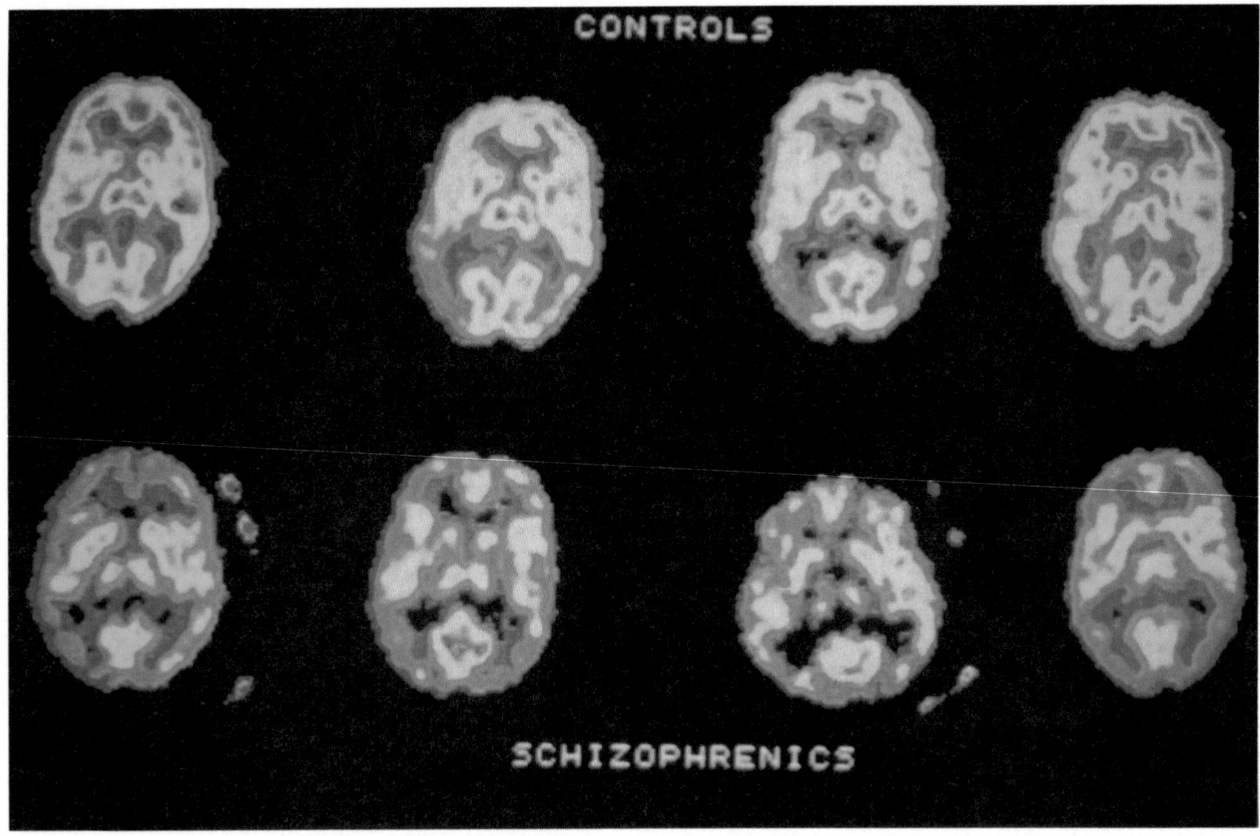

Figure 27–3. Positron-emission tomography (PET) scan in schizophrenic and healthy subjects (controls) showing the relatively reduced frontal metabolism (hypofrontality) in schizophrenia. (Courtesy of M. S. Buchsbaum, Director, PET Laboratory, University of California at Irvine.)

poral lobe (e.g., epilepsy, tumors, trauma, and infarcts). The evolving literature on the localization of psychotic symptoms suggests that Schneiderian delusions and hallucinations, commonly seen in schizophrenia, may reflect temporal lobe pathology, especially in temporolimbic areas (Trimble 1990). The medial temporal lobe is emerging as a key structure in the neurobiology of schizophrenia because of its important connections with higher cortical areas (Roberts 1990) and also because of the many neuropathological studies that have been published over the past few years (described below). Gross morphological abnormalities of the temporal lobes have been revealed on CT and MRI scans in schizophrenic patients, including reduced temporal gray matter (Suddath et al. 1989), left temporal lobe size (Rossi et al. 1990; Suddath et al. 1990), temporal horn enlargement (Crow et al. 1988), reduced limbic temporal volume (Bogerts et al. 1990), and focal temporal cortical atrophy (Yates et al. 1990). Figure 27–4 shows an example of hypoplasia of the medial temporal lobe structures (hippocampus-amygdala complex) on coronal MRI scans in a schizophrenic patient and a control subject.

Basal ganglia. For the past quarter century, the dopamine hypothesis of schizophrenia has continued to be a major pathophysiological model for this disorder (Carlsson 1988). Because the largest proportions of dopamine in the brain are found in the basal ganglia, it is logical to consider the basal ganglia as an important component of the neurobiology of schizophrenia. Further, basal ganglia disorders such as Huntington's chorea, which produces striatal degeneration, are known to be associated with schizophrenia-like psychosis. In addition to attributing motor abnormalities in schizophrenia to basal ganglia pathology (Manschreck 1986), other param-

A

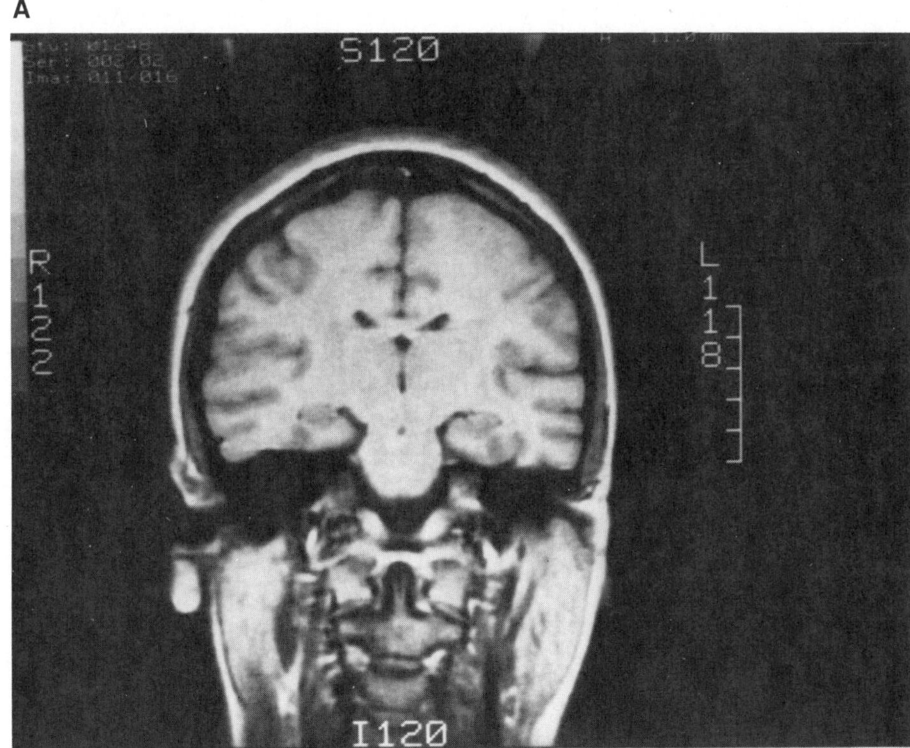

B

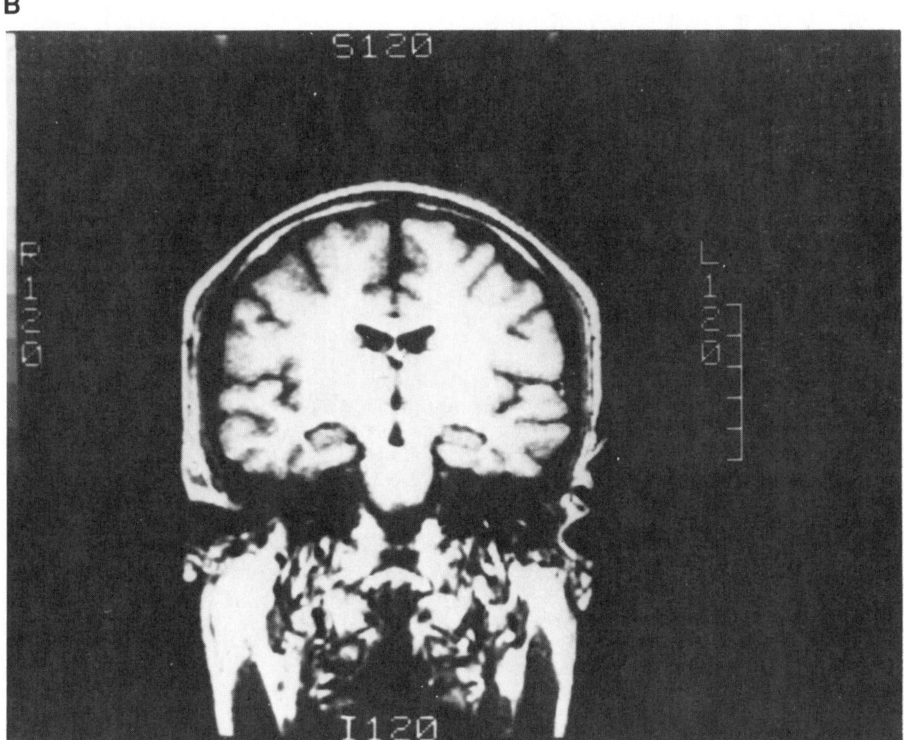

Figure 27–4. Coronal magnetic resonance imaging (MRI) scan showing normal (*panel A*) and hypoplastic (*panel* B) medial temporal lobe tissue (hippocampus-amygdala) in a control subject and schizophrenic patient, respectively.

eters such as reward, memory, attention, and higher cognitive functions have also been associated with the basal ganglia and their cortical projections (Lidsky et al. 1979). More recently, PET scan research has shown that the basal ganglia may be metabolically hyperactive in unmedicated schizophrenia (Early et al. 1987), and a possible relationship of this abnormality with thought disorder has been proposed (Early et al. 1989). Dopamine, subtype 2 (D_2), receptor imaging on PET scans was reported to show increased density in the basal ganglia (Wong et al. 1986), confirming postmortem findings (Seeman et al. 1984), but more recent studies did not demonstrate increased dopamine density in the basal ganglia (Farde et al. 1990). The use of different ligands may explain the different findings, but the role of the basal ganglia in schizophrenia remains a fertile area of neuropsychiatry research.

Parietal lobes. Although there has not been a substantial literature on the role of the parietal lobes in schizophrenia, there have been reports suggesting that the parietal lobes may be impaired in schizophrenia (Mesulam and Geschwind 1983). Particular reference is made to the role of the inferior parietal lobule in selective attention (Heilman et al. 1983). Further, some symptoms of schizophrenia, such as tactile discrimination and body image distortion (Erwin and Rosenbaum 1979), "physiognomization" of the environment and facial nonrecognition (Harrington et al. 1989), and even lack of insight into one's illness or need for treatment (David 1990), may be associated with parietal lobe dysfunction in schizophrenia.

Corpus callosum. Since the initial study of Rosenthal and Bigelow (1972) reporting a thicker corpus callosum in postmortem brains of schizophrenic patients, there have been several postmortem (Doty 1989; Nasrallah et al. 1983b) and in vivo MRI studies (Nasrallah et al. 1986a), some showing pathology and others not. A large literature about interhemispheric communications and integration was spawned by the possibility of an impaired callosal channel in schizophrenia (Nasrallah 1985). The possible relationship of neurodevelopmental factors to callosal morphology in schizophrenia has been suggested (Nasrallah 1989) but remains unconfirmed.

Neuropathological Findings in Schizophrenia

Postmortem histopathological studies of the brain in schizophrenia produced very few consistent findings up to the 1970s, leading Plum (1972) to pessimistically label schizophrenia "the graveyard of neuropathologists." However, in the 1980s, a remarkable consistency emerged in the neuropathological studies of schizophrenia by different investigators. Those studies almost unanimously suggest that schizophrenia is associated with a neurodevelopmental disruption, probably in the second trimester, as evidenced by changes in the usual histoarchitecture of brain tissue, and in failure of certain neuronal cells to migrate to their ultimate location. The following is a brief summary of the major published studies in this area:

1. A significant reduction (2%–40%) in the granule cell layer of the dentate gyrus in the hippocampus (McLardy 1974).
2. Pyramidal cell disarray in the left anterior and middle hippocampal regions, especially in the CA_1-prosubiculum and CA_1-CA_2 interfaces (Kovelman and Scheibel 1984; Scheibel and Kovelman 1981). These findings suggest faculty neuronal migration during the second trimester of fetal life. A partial replication of these findings was reported by Altshuler et al. (1987), but Christison et al. (1989) could not replicate them. More recently, Scheibel's laboratory reported another replication of their findings bilaterally (Conrad et al. 1991).
3. Reduced volume (20%–30%) of the limbic temporal lobe (amygdala, hippocampus, and parahippocampus) and a 20% decrease in the volume of the internal globus pallidus but no change in the external globus pallidus, caudate nucleus, putamen, or nucleus accumbens (Bogerts 1984; Bogerts et al. 1985).
4. A deficit in the neuronal density in layer VI of the prefrontal cortex, layer V of the cingulate gyrus, and layer III of the motor cortex, plus smaller and more sparse aggregates of neurons in the anterior cingulate gyrus (Benes 1987). The reduced number of glial cells per unit volume in the cingulate cortex of schizophrenia constituted a strong argument against a degenerative process and for a neurodevelopmental process such as excessive neuronal elimination or death.
5. Cytoarchitectonic deviation in the rostral entorhinal region of the parahippocampal gyrus, consisting of poorly developed upper layers with heterotrophic displacement of single pre-α cell groups (Jakob and Beckmann 1986). Again, no gliosis was observed, and the overall find-

ings are suggestive of a disruption of neuronal migration in the archipallium during development.

6. A reduction in the absolute number of neurons in the granular cell layer of the dentate gyrus by 10%–30%, without a difference in the number and density of glial cells (Bogerts 1986). The volume of the hippocampal segments CA_1-CA_2, CA_3, CA_4, and dentate gyrus was decreased.
7. Reduced white matter in the parahippocampal gyrus (Colter et al. 1987).
8. Significant reductions in the volume and neuron number without increased glial cell numbers in the entorhinal cortex (Falkai et al. 1988a).
9. Increased distance (20%–30%) between the pial surface of the entorhinal cortex and the center of the pre-α cell clusters in some patients, suggesting an impairment of pre-α cell migration from the inner to the outer layers of the entorhinal cortex during fetal brain development (Falkai et al. 1988b).
10. Significant shape distortion of the hippocampus and parahippocampal cortex, and a significantly smaller parahippocampal cortex (Altshuler et al. 1988).
11. Decreased volume and pyramidal cell density in all areas of the hippocampus, with the greatest difference observed in the left CA_4 (Jeste and Lohr 1989).

Although some neuropathological studies do report increased gliosis or cellular degeneration in schizophrenia (Stevens 1982), the majority of studies do not (Roberts and Bruton 1990). Because fetal brain tissue does not react to injury with a glial response until the third trimester, it could be postulated that the neuropathological lesions in schizophrenia occurred early in development (first and second trimester).

The above brief overview of recent findings regarding the gross and microscopic changes in the brains of schizophrenic patients points to the increasing evidence for a neurodevelopmental framework for the neurobiology and neuropsychiatry of schizophrenia. If the findings continue to be replicated, it will become more likely that the basis for the structural brain changes is mainly under genetic control (e.g., genes that program normal brain growth and development) with some modulation by "haphazard" perinatal and other environmental factors that contribute to the heterogeneity of the schizophrenic syndrome. It is quite possible that the neurodevelopmental lesion in schizophrenia is qualitatively the same in all patients, but quantitatively different across clinical subtypes. Research in the future should confirm or negate this postulate.

❑ CONCLUSIONS

It is impossible to review the neuropsychiatry of schizophrenia within the constraints of a chapter when the topic is broad enough to require an entire book. However, the literature and issues highlighted in this chapter are meant to bring the following conclusions into focus:

1. The exact neuropsychiatry of schizophrenia remains a mystery, but neurobiological clues are accumulating at a rapid pace and breakthroughs are probably within reach.
2. Lesions practically anywhere in the brain may be associated with schizophrenia-like psychoses, but lesions of the frontal, temporal, and limbic regions are more likely than others to produce psychotic features.
3. Several lines of evidence now point to the importance of neurodevelopmental factors in schizophrenia. Many of the neurobiological findings in schizophrenia can be explained within a neurodevelopmental model. Future research should focus on neurodevelopmental factors, including genetic and environmental, in the neurobiology of schizophrenia. A particularly promising brain region at present is the limbic temporal lobe and its projections.

❑ REFERENCES

Adler LE, Sadja L, Wilets G: Cimetidine toxicity manifested as paranoia and hallucinations. Am J Psychiatry 137:1112–1114, 1980

Alarcon RD, Franceschini JA: Hyper parathyroidism and paranoid psychosis: case report and review of the literature. Br J Psychiatry 145:477–512, 1984

Aldrich MS: Narcolepsy. N Engl J Med 323:389–394, 1990

Altshuler L, Conrad A, Kovelman JA, et al: Hippocampal pyramidal cell orientation in schizophrenia. Arch Gen Psychiatry 44:1094–1098, 1987

Altshuler L, Casanova ME, Goldberg T, et al: Shape and area measurements of hippocampus and parahippocampal gyrus in schizophrenics, suicide, and control brains. Neuroscience Abstracts 14:247, 1988

American Psychiatric Association: Diagnostic and Statistical Manual of Mental Disorders, 3rd Edition. Washington, DC, American Psychiatric Association, 1980

American Psychiatric Association: Diagnostic and Statistical Manual of Mental Disorders, 3rd Edition, Revised. Washington, DC, American Psychiatric Association, 1987

Andreasen NC, Nasrallah HA, Dunn V, et al: Structural abnormalities in the frontal system in schizophrenia: a magnetic resonance imaging study. Arch Gen Psychiatry 43:136–144, 1986

Benes FM: An analysis of the arrangement of neurons in the cingulate cortex of schizophrenic patients. Arch Gen Psychiatry 44:608–616, 1987

Bluestein HG: Neuropsychiatric manifestations of systemic lupus erythematosus. N Engl J Med 317:309–311, 1987

Bogerts B: Zur Neuropathologie der Schizophrenien. Fortschr Neurol Psychiatr 52:428–437, 1984

Bogerts B: Evidence for structural changes in the limbic system in schizophrenia, in Biological Psychiatry. Edited by Shagass C. Amsterdam, Elsevier, 1986, pp 1178–1180

Bogerts B, Meertz E, Schonfield-Bausch R: Basal ganglia and limbic system pathology in schizophrenia. Arch Gen Psychiatry 42:784–791, 1985

Bogerts B, Ashtari M, Degreef G, et al: Reduced temporal limbic structure volumes on magnetic resonance images in first episode schizophrenia. Psychiatry Research: Neuroimaging 35:1–13, 1990

Brown R, Colter N, Corsellis JAN, et al: Postmortem evidence of structural brain changes in schizophrenia: differences in brain weight, temporal horn area and parahippocampal gyrus compared with affective disorders. Arch Gen Psychiatry 43:36–42, 1986

Bruton CJ, Crow TJ, Frith CD, et al: Schizophrenia and the brain: a prospective clinicopathological study. Psychol Med 20:285–304, 1990

Buchsbaum MS, Delisi LE, Holcomb HH, et al: Anteroposterior gradients in cerebral glucose: glucose use in schizophrenia and affective disorders. Arch Gen Psychiatry 41:1159–1166, 1984

Cannon TD, Mednick SA, Parnas J: Genetic and perinatal determinants of structural brain deficits in schizophrenia. Arch Gen Psychiatry 46:883–889, 1989

Carlsson A: The current status of the dopamine hypothesis of schizophrenia. Neuropsychopharmacology 1:179–186, 1988

Christison GW, Casanova MF, Weinberger DR, et al: A quantitative investigation of hippocampal pyramidal cell size, shape, and variability of orientation in schizophrenia. Arch Gen Psychiatry 46:1027–1032, 1989

Colter N, Battal S, Crow TJ, et al: White matter reduction in the parahippo-campal gyrus of patients with schizophrenia. Arch Gen Psychiatry 44:1023, 1987

Conrad AJ, Scheibel AB: Schizophrenia and the hippocampus: the embryological hypothesis extended. Schizophr Bull 13:577–587, 1987

Conrad AJ, Abebe T, Austin R, et al: Hippocampal pyramidal cell disarray in schizophrenia as a bilateral phenomenon. Arch Gen Psychiatry 48:413–417, 1991

Crow TJ: Molecular pathology of schizophrenia: more than one disease process? Br Med J 280:66–69, 1980

Crow TJ, Colter N, Brown N, et al: Lateralized asymmetry of temporal horn enlargement in schizophrenia. Schizophrenia Research 1:155–156, 1988

Cummings JL: Organic delusions: phenomenology, anatomical correlations and review. Br J Psychiatry 146: 184–197, 1985

Cummings JL: Organic psychosis. Psychosomatics 29:16–26, 1988

David AS: Insight and psychosis. Br J Psychiatry 156:798–808, 1990

Davison K: Schizophrenia-like psychoses associated with organic cerebral disorders: a review. Psychiatr Dev 1:1–34, 1983

Davison K, Bagley CR: Schizophrenia-like psychoses associated with organic disorders of the CNS: a review of the literature, in Current Problems in Neuropsychiatry, Part II (British Journal of Psychiatry, Special Publication No 4). Edited by Herrington E. Ashford, Headley Bros, 1969, pp 113–184

DeMyer MK, Gilmor RL, Hendrie HC, et al: Magnetic resonance brain images in schizophrenic and normal subjects: influence of diagnosis and education. Schizophr Bull 14:21–37, 1988

Dorrell W: Myasthenia gravis and schizophrenia. Br J Psychiatry 123:249–252, 1973

Doty RW: Schizophrenia: a disease of interhemispheric processes at forebrain and brainstem levels? Behav Brain Res 34:1–33, 1989

Dysken MW, Merry W, Davis JM: Anticholinergic psychosis. Psychiatric Annals 8:30–35, 1978

Early TS, Reiman E, Raichle ME, et al: Globus pallidus abnormality in never-medicated patients with schizophrenia. Proc Natl Acad Sci U S A 84:561–563, 1987

Early TS, Posner MI, Reiman E, et al: Left striato-pallidal hyperactivity in schizophrenia, II: phenomenology and thought disorder. Psychiatr Dev 2:109–121, 1989

Erwin BJ, Rosenbaum G: Parietal lobe syndrome and schizophrenia: comparison of neuropsychological deficits. J Abnorm Psychol 88:234–242, 1979

Falkai P, Bogerts B, Rozumek M: Cell loss and volume reduction in the entorhinal cortex of schizophrenics. Biol Psychiatry 24:515–521, 1988a

Falkai P, Bogerts B, Roberts GW, et al: Measurement of the alpha cell migration in the entorhinal region: a marker for developmental disturbances in schizophrenia? Schizophrenia Research 1:157–158, 1988b

Farde L, Wiesel FA, Stone-Elander S, et al: D2 dopamine receptors in neuroleptic-naive schizophrenic patients: a positron emission tomography study with [^{11}C] raclopride. Arch Gen Psychiatry 47:213–219, 1990

Farmer A, Jackson R, McGuffin P, et al: Cerebral ventricular enlargement in chronic schizophrenia: consistencies and contradictions. Br J Psychiatry 150:324–330, 1987

Flor-Henry P: Psychosis and temporal lobe epilepsy: a controlled investigation. Epilepsia 10:363–395, 1969

Friedman L, Knutson L, Shurell M, et al: Prefrontal sulcal prominence is inversely related to response to clozapine in schizophrenia. Biol Psychiatry 29:865–877, 1991

George MS, Scott T, Kellner CH, et al: Abnormalities of the septum pellucidum in schizophrenia. Journal of Neuropsychiatry and Clinical Neurosciences 1:385–390, 1989

Giannini AJ: Phencyclidine, in Drugs of Abuse. Edited by Giannini AJ, Slaby AE. Oradell, NJ, Medical Economics, 1989, pp 145–159

Gold MS, Giannini AJ: Cocaine and cocaine addiction, in Drugs of Abuse. Edited by Giannini AJ, Slaby AE. Oradell, NJ, Medical Economics, 1989, pp 83–96

Goldman-Rakic PS: The frontal lobes: uncharted provinces of the brain. Trends Neurosci 7:425–429, 1984

Gorelick DA, Kussin SZ, Kahn I: Paranoid delusions and auditory hallucinations associated with dioxin intoxication. J Nerv Ment Dis 166:817–820, 1978

Greden JF, Tandon R (eds): Negative Schizophrenic Symptoms: Pathophysiology and Clinical Implications. Washington, DC, American Psychiatric Press, 1991

Gurling HMD, Sherrington RP, Brynjolfsson J, et al: Recent and future molecular genetic research into schizophrenia. Schizophr Bull 15:373–382, 1989

Harrington A, Oepin G, Spitzer M: Disordered recognition and perception of human faces in acute schizophrenia and experimental psychosis. Compr Psychiatry 30:376–384, 1989

Heaton R: Wisconsin Card Sorting Test. Odessa, TX, Psychological Assessment Resources, 1985

Heilman KM, Watson RT, Valenstein E, et al: Localization of lesions in neglect, in Localization in Neuropsychology. Edited by Keretz A. New York, Academic, 1983, pp 471–492

Heinrich DW, Buchanan RW: The significance and meaning of neurological signs in schizophrenia. Am J Psychiatry 145:11–18, 1988

Henn FA, Nasrallah HA (eds): Schizophrenia as a Brain Disease. New York, Oxford University Press, 1982

Iacono WG: Psychophysiologic markers of psychopathology: a review. Can J Psychol 26:96–112, 1985

Illowsky BP, Juliano DM, Bigelow LB, et al: Stability of CT scan findings in schizophrenia: results of an 8-year follow-up study. J Neurol Neurosurg Psychiatry 51: 209–213, 1988

Ingvar DH: Evidence for frontal/pre-frontal cortical dysfunction in chronic schizophrenia: the phenomenon of hypofrontality reconsidered, in Biological Perspectives of Schizophrenia. Edited by Helmchen H, Henn FA. New York, John Wiley, 1987, pp 201–211

Jakob J, Beckmann H: Prenatal developmental disturbance in the limbic allocortex in schizophrenics. J Neural Transm 65:303–326, 1986

Janowsky MS, El-Yousef MK, Davis JM, et al: Provocation of schizophrenic symptoms by intravenous administration of methylphenidate. Arch Gen Psychiatry 28: 185–191, 1973

Jeste DV, Lohr JB: Hippocampal pathologic findings in schizophrenia: a morphometric study. Arch Gen Psychiatry 46:1019–1024, 1989

Johnstone EC, Owens DGC, Bydder GM, et al: The spectrum of structural brain changes in schizophrenia: age of onset as a predictor of cognitive and clinical impairments and their cerebral correlates. Psychol Med 19:91–103, 1989

Karson CN, Coppola R, Daniel DG, et al: Alpha frequency in schizophrenia: an association with enlarged cerebral ventricles. Am J Psychiatry 145:861–864, 1988

Kemali D, Maj M, Galderisi S, et al: Ventricle-to-brain ratio in schizophrenia: a controlled follow-up study. Biol Psychiatry 26:756–759, 1989

Klawans HL: Levodopa-induced psychosis. Psychiatric Annals 8:19–22, 1978

Kleinman JE, Karson CN, Weinberger DR, et al: Eye-blinking and cerebral ventricular size in chronic schizophrenic patients. Am J Psychiatry 141:1430–1432, 1984

Kovelman JA, Scheibel AB: A neurohistological correlate of schizophrenia. Biol Psychiatry 19:1601–1621, 1984

Kuhnley EJ, White DH, Granoffal R: Psychiatric presentation of arachnoid cyst. J Clin Psychiatry 42:167–169, 1981

Leigh H, Kramer SI: The psychiatric manifestations of endocrine disease, in Advances In Internal Medicine, Vol 29. Edited by Stollerman GH. Chicago, Year Book Medical, 1984, pp 413–445

Levin S: Frontal lobe dysfunctions in schizophrenia, I: eye movement impairments. J Psychiatr Res 18:27–55, 1984a

Levin S: Frontal lobe dysfunctions in schizophrenia, II: impairments of psychological and brain functions. J Psychiatr Res 18:57–72, 1984b

Lewis SW, Murray RM: Obstetric complications, neurodevelopmental deviance and risk for schizophrenia. J Psychiatr Res 21:413–421, 1987

Lewis SW, Reveley AM, Reveley MA, et al: The familial/sporadic distinction as a strategy in schizophrenia research. Br J Psychiatry 151:306–313, 1987

Lidsky TI, Weinhold PM, Levin FM: Implications of basal ganglionic dysfunction for schizophrenia. Biol Psychiatry 14:3–12, 1979

Ling MH, Perry PJ, Tsuang MT: Side effects of corticosteroid therapy: psychiatric aspects. Arch Gen Psychiatry 38:471–474, 1981

Lishman AL: Organic Psychiatry: The Psychological Consequences of Cerebral Disorder. London, Blackwell Scientific, 1987, pp 537–544

Losonczy MF, Song IS, Mohs RC, et al: Correlates of lateral ventricular size in chronic schizophrenia, I: behavioral and treatment response measures. Am J Psychiatry 143:976–981, 1986a

Losonczy MF, Song IS, Mohs RC, et al: Correlates of lateral ventricular size in chronic schizophrenia, II: biological measures. Am J Psychiatry 143:1113–1118, 1986b

Lyon M, Barr CE, Cannon TD, et al: Fetal neural development and schizophrenia. Schizophr Bull 15:149–161, 1989

McCarley RW, Faux SF, Shenton M, et al: CT abnormalities in schizophrenia: a preliminary study of their correlation with P300/P200 electrophysiological features and positive/negative symptoms. Arch Gen Psychiatry 46:698–708, 1989

McEvoy JP: The chronic neuropsychiatric disorders associated with alcoholism, in Encyclopedic Handbook of Alcoholism. Edited by Pattison EM, Kaufman E. New York, Gardner, 1982, pp 167–179

McLardy T: Hippocampal zinc and structural deficit in brains from chronic alcoholics and some schizophrenics. Journal of Orthomolecular Psychiatry 4:32–36, 1974

McNeil TF, Kaij L: Obstetric factors in the development of schizophrenia: complications in the birth of preschizophrenic patients, in The Nature of Schizophrenia. Edited by Wynne LC, Cromwell RL, Matthysse S. New York, John Wiley, 1978, pp 401–429

Manschreck TC: Motor abnormalities in schizophrenic disorders, in Handbook of Schizophrenia, Vol 1: The Neurology of Schizophrenia. Edited by Nasrallah HA, Weinberger DR. Amsterdam, Elsevier, 1986, pp 65–96

Mednick SA, Machon RA, Huttunen MO, et al: Adult schizophrenia following prenatal exposure to an influenza epidemic. Arch Gen Psychiatry 45:189–192, 1988

Mesulam MM: Frontal cortex and behavior. Ann Neurol 15:320–325, 1986

Mesulam MM, Geschwind N: On the possible role of neocortex and its limbic connections in the process of attention and schizophrenia. J Psychiatr Res 14:249–261, 1983

Mikkelson EJ, Reider HA: Post-parathyroidectomy psychosis: clinical and research implications. J Clin Psychiatry 40:352–355, 1979

Moreines R: The psychedelics, in Drugs of Abuse. Edited by Giannini AJ, Slaby AE. Oradell, NJ, Medical Economics, 1989, pp 207–242

Morihisa JM, Duffy FH, Wyatt RJ, et al: Brain electrical activity mapping in schizophrenic patients. Arch Gen Psychiatry 40:719–728, 1983

Nasrallah HA: Vulnerability to disulfiram psychosis. West J Med 130:575–577, 1979

Nasrallah HA: The unintegrated right cerebral hemisphere as alien intruder: a possible mechanism for Schneiderian delusions in schizophrenia. Compr Psychiatry 26:273–282, 1985

Nasrallah HA: The differential diagnosis of schizophrenia: genetic, perinatal, neurological, pharmacological and psychiatric factors, in Handbook of Schizophrenia, Vol 1: The Neurology of Schizophrenia. Edited by Nasrallah HA, Weinberger DR. Amsterdam, Elsevier, 1986, pp 49–63

Nasrallah HA: Right hemispheric speech, callosal size, perinatal brain insult and schizophrenia. Ann Neurol 26:290–291, 1989

Nasrallah HA: Brain structure and function in schizophrenia: evidence for fetal neurodevelopmental impairment. Current Opinion in Psychiatry 3:75–78, 1990

Nasrallah HA, Coffman JA: Computerized tomography in psychiatry. Psychiatric Annals 15:239–249, 1985

Nasrallah HA, McChesney CM: Psychopathology of corpus callosum tumors. Biol Psychiatry 16:663–669, 1981

Nasrallah HA, Weinberger DR (eds): Handbook of Schizophrenia, Vol 1: The Neurology of Schizophrenia. Amsterdam, Elsevier, 1986

Nasrallah HA, McCalley-Whitters M, Jacoby CG: Cortical atrophy in schizophrenia and mania: a comparative CT study. J Clin Psychiatry 43:439–441, 1982

Nasrallah HA, Kuperman S, Hamra B, et al: Schizophrenia patients with and without large cerebral ventricles: a controlled clinical comparison. J Clin Psychiatry 44: 407–409, 1983a

Nasrallah HA, McCalley-Whitters M, Rauscher FP, et al: A histological study of the corpus callosum in subtypes of chronic schizophrenia. Psychiatry Res 8:151–160, 1983b

Nasrallah HA, Jacoby CG, Chapman S, et al: Third ventricular enlargement on CT scans: association with cerebellar atrophy. Biol Psychiatry 20:443–450, 1985

Nasrallah HA, Andreasen NC, Coffman JA, et al: A controlled magnetic resonance imaging study of corpus callosum thickness in schizophrenia. Biol Psychiatry 21:274–282, 1986a

Nasrallah HA, Olson SC, McCalley-Whitters M, et al: Cerebral ventricular enlargement in schizophrenia: a preliminary follow-up study. Arch Gen Psychiatry 43:157–159, 1986b

Nasrallah HA, Olson SC, Coffman JA, et al: Magnetic resonance brain imaging, perinatal injury, and negative symptoms in schizophrenia. Schizophrenia Research 1:171–172, 1988

Nasrallah HA, Coffman JA, Olson SC: Structural brain-imaging findings in affective disorders: an overview. Journal of Neuropsychiatry and Clinical Neurosciences 1:21–26, 1989

Nasrallah HA, Schwarzkopf SB, Olson SC, et al: Gender differences in schizophrenia on MRI scans. Schizophr Bull 16:205–210, 1990

Nasrallah HA, Schwarzkopf SB, Olson SC, et al: Perinatal brain injury and cerebellar vermal lobules I-X in schizophrenia. Biol Psychiatry 29:567–574, 1991

Nowakowski RS: Basic concepts of CNS development. Child Dev 58:568–595, 1987

Olson SC, Nasrallah HA, Lynn MB: Lateral and third ventricular volumes in schizophrenics and their siblings: effect of spectrum diagnosis. Schizophrenia Research 4:407–408, 1991

O'Shanick GJ, Gardner DF, Kornstein SG: Endocrine disorders, in Principles of Medical Psychiatry. Edited by Stoudemire A, Fogel BS. Orlando, FL, Grune & Stratton, 1987, pp 641–657

Owen MJ, Lewis SW, Murray RM: Family history and cerebral ventricular enlargement in schizophrenia: a case control study. Br J Psychiatry 154:629–634, 1989

Owens DGC, Johnstone EC, Bydder GM, et al: Unsuspected organic disease in chronic schizophrenia demonstrated by computed tomography. J Neurol Neurosurg Psychiatry 43:1065–1069, 1980

Pakkenberg B: Post-mortem study of chronic schizophrenic brains. Br J Psychiatry 151:744–752, 1987

Parnas J, Schulsinger F, Teasdale T, et al: Perinatal complications and clinical outcome with the schizophrenia spectrum. Br J Psychiatry 140:416–420, 1982

Pearlson GD, Kim WS, Kubos KL, et al: Ventricle-brain ratio, computed tomographic density and brain area in 50 schizophrenics. Arch Gen Psychiatry 46:690–697, 1989

Pfefferbaum A, Zipursky RB, Lim KO, et al: Computerized tomographic evidence for generalized sulcal and ventricular enlargement in schizophrenia. Arch Gen Psychiatry 45:633–640, 1988

Plum F: Prospects for research on schizophrenia, 3: neurophysiology, neuropathological findings. Neurosciences Program Bulletin 10:384–388, 1972

Propping P, Friedl W: Genetic studies of biochemical, pathophysiological, and pharmacological factors in schizophrenia, in Handbook of Schizophrenia, Vol III: Nosology, Epidemiology, and Genetics of Schizophrenia. Edited by Tsuang MT, Simpson JC. Amsterdam, Elsevier, 1988, pp 579–608

Raskind MA, Kitchell M, Alvarez C: Bromide intoxication in the elderly. J Am Geriatr Soc 26:222–224, 1978

Reus VI: Behavioral disturbances associated with endocrine disorders. Annu Rev Med 37:205–214, 1986

Reveley AM, Reveley MA: Aqueduct stenosis and schizophrenia. J Neurol Neurosurg Psychiatry 46:18–22, 1983

Reveley MA, DeBelleroche J, Recordati A, et al: Increased CSF amino acids and ventricular enlargement in schizophrenia: a preliminary study. Biol Psychiatry 22: 413–420, 1987

Roberts GW: Schizophrenia: the cellular biology of a functional psychosis. Trends Neurosci 13:207–211, 1990

Roberts GW, Bruton CJ: Notes from the graveyard: neuropathology and schizophrenia. Neuropathol Appl Neurobiol 16:3–16, 1990

Roberts GW, Done DJ, Bruton C, et al: A "mock-up" of schizophrenia: temporal lobe epilepsy and schizophrenia-like psychosis. Biol Psychiatry 28:127–143, 1990

Robinson RG, Forrester AW: Neuropsychiatric aspects of cerebrovascular disease, in Textbook of Neuropsychiatry. Edited by Hales RE, Yudofsky SC. Washington, DC, American Psychiatric Press, 1987, pp 191–208

Roman D: Schizophrenia-like psychosis following mandrax overdose. Br J Psychiatry 121:619–621, 1978

Rosenthal RLB, Bigelow LB: Quantitative brain measurements in chronic schizophrenia. Br J Psychiatry 121: 259–264, 1972

Rossi A, Stratta P, Casacchia M, et al: Reduced temporal lobe areas in schizophrenia: preliminary evidences from a controlled multiplanar magnetic resonance imaging study. Biol Psychiatry 27:61–68, 1990

Scheibel AB, Kovelman JA: Disorientation of the hippocampal pyramidal cell and its processes in the schizophrenic patient. Biol Psychiatry 16:101–102, 1981

Schulsinger F, Parnas J, Petersen ET, et al: Cerebral ventricular size in the offspring of schizophrenic mothers: a preliminary study. Arch Gen Psychiatry 41:602–606, 1984

Schwarzkopf SB, Nasrallah HA, Olson SC, et al: Perinatal complications and genetic loading in schizophrenia: preliminary findings. Psychiatry Res 27:233–239, 1989a

Schwarzkopf SB, Nasrallah HA, Olson SC, et al: Smaller MRI brain measures in familial vs sporadic schizophrenics: a replication. Schizophrenia Research 2:128, 1989b

Schwarzkopf SB, Olson SC, Nasrallah HA: Third and lateral ventricular volumes in schizophrenia: support for progressive enlargement of both structures. Psychopharmacol Bull 26:385–391, 1990

Schwarzkopf SB, Nasrallah HA, Olson SC, et al: Family history and brain morphology in schizophrenia: an MRI study. Psychiatry Research: Neuroimaging 40:49–60, 1991

Seeman P, Ulpian C, Bergeron C, et al: Bimodal distribution of dopamine receptor densities in brains of schizophrenics. Science 225:728–730, 1984

Shagass C: Deviant cerebral functional topography as revealed by electrophysiology, in Biological Perspectives of Schizophrenia. Edited by Helmchen H, Henn FA. New York, John Wiley, 1987, pp 201–211

Shelton RC, Weinberger DR: X-ray computerized tomography studies in schizophrenia: a review and synthesis, in Handbook of Schizophrenia, Vol 1: The Neurology of Schizophrenia. Edited by Nasrallah HA, Weinberger DR. Amsterdam, Elsevier, 1986, pp 207–250

Slaby AE: Psychotropic and psychedelic emergencies, in Drugs of Abuse. Edited by Giannini AJ, Slaby AE. Oradell, NJ, Medical Economics, 1989, pp 161–206

Smeraldi E, Gamabini O, Bellodi L, et al: Combined measure of smooth pursuit eye movements and ventricle-brain ratio in schizophrenic disorders. Psychiatry Res 21:293–301, 1987

Snyder SH: Amphetamine psychosis: a "model" schizophrenia mediated by catecholamines. Am J Psychiatry 130:61–68, 1973

Spitzer RL, Endicott J, Robins E: Research Diagnostic Criteria, 3rd Edition. New York, New York State Psychiatric Institute. Biometrics Research Division, 1978

Spivak JL, Jackson DL: Pellagra: an analysis of 18 patients and a review of the literature. Johns Hopkins Med J 140:295–302, 1977

Stevens JR: Neuropathology of schizophrenia. Arch Gen Psychiatry 39:1131–1139, 1982

Stevens JR: Schizophrenia and multiple sclerosis. Schizophr Bull 14:231–241, 1988

Stoudemire GA, Levenson JL: Psychiatric consultation to internal medicine, in American Psychiatric Press Review of Psychiatry, Vol 9. Edited by Tasman A, Goldfinger SM, Kaufmann CA. Washington, DC, American Psychiatric Press, 1990, pp 466–490

Suddath RL, Casanova MF, Goldberg TE, et al: Temporal lobe pathology in schizophrenia: a quantitative magnetic resonance imaging study. Am J Psychiatry 146: 464–472, 1989

Suddath RL, Christison GW, Torrey EF, et al: Anatomical abnormalities in the brains of monozygotic twins discordant for schizophrenia. N Engl J Med 322:789–794, 1990

Swayze VW, Andreasen NC, Ehrhardt JC, et al: Developmental abnormalities of the corpus callosum in schizophrenia. Arch Neurol 47:805–808, 1990

Taylor DC: Factors influencing the occurrence of schizophrenia-like psychosis with TLE. Psychol Med 5:249–257, 1975

Trimble MR: First-rank symptoms of Schneider: a new perspective? Br J Psychiatry 156:195–200, 1990

Tsuang MT, Simpson JC (eds): Handbook of Schizophrenia, Vol III: Nosology, Epidemiology, and Genetics of Schizophrenia. Amsterdam, Elsevier, 1988

Turner SW, Toone BK, Brett-Jones JR, et al: Computerized tomographic scan changes in early schizophrenia: preliminary findings. Psychol Med 16:219–225, 1986

van Kammen DP, van Kammen WB, Peters J, et al: Decreased slow-wave sleep and enlarged lateral ventricles in schizophrenia. Neuropsychopharmacology 1: 265–271, 1988

Vita A, Sacchetti E, Valvassori G, et al: Brain morphology in schizophrenia: a 2- to 5-year CT scan follow-up study. Acta Psychiatr Scand 78:618–621, 1988

Weinberger DR: Implications of normal brain development for the pathogenesis of schizophrenia. Arch Gen Psychiatry 44:660–669, 1987

Weinberger DR, Berman KF: Speculation on the meaning

of cerebral metabolic hypofrontality in schizophrenia. Schizophr Bull 14:157–168, 1988

Weinberger DR, Berman KF, Zec RF: Physiological dysfunction of dorsolateral prefrontal cortex in schizophrenia, I: regional cerebral blood flow (CBF) evidence. Arch Gen Psychiatry 43:114–125, 1986

Wilcox JA, Nasrallah HA: Organic factors in catatonia. Br J Psychiatry 149:782–784, 1986

Wilcox JA, Nasrallah HA: Perinatal insult as a risk factor in paranoid and nonparanoid schizophrenia. Psychopathology 20:285–287, 1987a

Wilcox JA, Nasrallah HA: Perinatal distress and prognosis of psychotic illness. Neuropsychobiology 17:173–175, 1987b

Wilcox JA, Nasrallah HA: Sydenham's chorea and psychopathology. Neuropsychobiology 19:6–8, 1988

Wong DF, Wagner HN, Tune LE, et al: Positron emission tomography reveals elevated D2 dopamine receptors in drug-naive schizophrenics. Science 234:1558–1563, 1986

Woods BT, Yurgelun-Todd D, Benes FM, et al: Progressive ventricular enlargement in schizophrenia: comparison to bipolar affective disorder and correlation with clinical course. Biol Psychiatry 27:341–352, 1990

Yates WR, Swayze VW, Andreasen NC: Neuropsychological effect of global and focal cerebral atrophy in schizophrenia. Neuropsychiatry, Neuropsychology and Behavioral Neurology 3:98–106, 1990

Chapter

28

Neuropsychiatric Disorders of Childhood and Adolescence

Edwin H. Cook, Jr., M.D.
Bennett L. Leventhal, M.D.

NEUROPSYCHIATRIC DISORDERS commonly have their onset in childhood and adolescence. From 5% to 8% of children and adolescents have one of the neuropsychiatric disorders described in this chapter. In addition, although children and adolescents not infrequently experience traumatic brain injury (TBI), many of those sustaining TBI in adulthood may have been at higher risk because of attentional, cognitive, visuospatial, or other neuropsychological impairment present since childhood.

Two factors increase the morbidity associated with neuropsychiatric disorders in childhood and adolescence. One is that children with a neuropsychiatric disorder substantially affect their parents and siblings. Second, children with these disorders often have long lives with disability. Even when compared with early dementia of the Alzheimer type beginning at age 50, a child with a pervasive developmental disorder (PDD) will have a disorder for an additional 47–50 years. Although with Alzheimer's disease or adult cerebrovascular disease there is a consequent loss of productivity at the height of a career, it is unknown what potential benefits to society are lost to neuropsychiatric disorders of childhood onset, and these benefits are often replaced with large economic burdens and human suffering.

❑ DEVELOPMENTAL ISSUES

Overview

Developmental factors must be considered to understand the neuropsychiatric disorders of childhood and adolescence. A distinguishing feature of such disorders is that they occur most commonly as a result of disordered neurological development rather than of damaged or degenerated structures that developed normally. As a result, focal neurological signs are less commonly present. This led to a theory that the outcome of neurological deficits would be better if sustained earlier in childhood when the greater plasticity of the central nervous system (CNS) would allow greater adaptation to lesions (Lenneberg 1967).

Reasoning backward from adult neuropsychology, the absence of specific aphasias, such as those seen as a result of cerebrovascular disease in adulthood, was believed to be evidence of this greater plasticity. However, two factors must be considered. First, even cerebrovascular disorders have a different pathology in childhood (e.g., atherosclerotic changes are rarely associated with childhood-onset neuropsychiatric disorders). With compromise of the vascular supply, children much more commonly experience "watershed" infarcts, which are less well understood than are thrombotic events. Second, most childhood-onset neuropsychiatric disorders occur because the normal processes of brain maturation do not occur in a sufficiently organized manner. Thus there is little or no period of normal brain functioning. Indeed, it has recently been shown that patients with congenital unilateral hemiplegia show declines in IQ throughout childhood (Banich et al. 1990). Moreover, although children with hemiplegia acquired after birth do not show similar declines in IQ with advancing age, they also do not show any evidence of IQ improvement consistent with general plasticity in the development of cognition (Banich et al. 1990). Even though there does appear to be some age-related plasticity in the development of language, there does not appear to be such plasticity in the development of visuospatial skills (Levine et al. 1987).

The Developing Brain

Recent developments in the related field of developmental neurobiology must be mentioned more to stimulate the reader to read further in these areas than to suggest a completed understanding of neural development. Our understanding of developmental neurobiology is increasing rapidly (see Chapter 1). For example, it took 30 years to identify, purify, and sequence nerve growth factor (NGF), but 3 months to identify the third member of the NGF family, neurotrophin-3. Therefore, a brief summary of events in the developing nervous system follows, but readers are directed not only to monographs that include more comprehensive reviews of these topics (Arenander and de Vellis 1989; Purves and Lichtman 1985), but also to current journals.

The development of the nervous system comprises the most complex events in human biological development. After the formation of the blastula, each cell is not only influenced by its genotype, but its phenotype as well. For example, the ectoderm induces formation of the mesoderm during gastrulation, and further induction of nervous tissue proceeds only with macromolecular signals from the underlying mesoderm. After neural induction, proliferation of the neural ectoderm proceeds. Neural stem cells divide into more differentiated cells according to a genomically specified, but microenvironmentally determined sequence. After a specified number of divisions, cells migrate away from the ventricular regions. Although neurons have been a proper focus of study, less scientific attention has been devoted to the glia, which not only have important metabolic roles in the sustenance of the nervous system, but also signal and provide a matrix for proper cellular migration. Abnormalities in neuronal migration have been identified in relationship to mental retardation and developmental disorders associated with epilepsy (Falconer et al. 1990).

After the brain has assumed a relatively mature gross morphology at birth, it continues to undergo dramatic changes in microscopic anatomy. One well-studied change is the myelination of axons, which begins prenatally and continues in some areas throughout childhood and adolescence. A striking temporal correlation between neuropsychological development and myelination of related structures has been highlighted (Meyersburg and Post 1979). In contrast, the number of synapses appears to peak at 18 months and to decline thereafter, at a time when the infant's symbolic capacities (especially language) are increasing rapidly (Huttenlocher 1982). In addition to the changing numbers of synapses, the continuing rearrangement of synapses adds to the complexity of developmental events.

Each of the single steps described above is among the most complex in biology. Each requires proper regulation between genomically triggered epigenetic events and regulation of transcription (largely receptor-mediated transcriptional regulation) by the microenvironment. Whether the disruption is primarily genomic (e.g., Down's syndrome) or environmental (e.g., fetal alcohol syndrome [FAS]), the pathophysiological event involves an interaction between these two processes. The best example of a macroenvironmental therapeutic intervention for a primary genomic disorder is dietary manipulation in phenylketonuria (PKU), in which a deficiency of phenylalanine hydroxylase is treated by a low-phenylalanine diet. In FAS, the presence of alcohol or metabolites during development leads to differences in the phenotypic expression of the genome of at least some of the nervous system.

During development, it appears that the nervous system regulates itself by overproduction of axonal and dendritic processes with subsequent retraction of some processes and synapse elimination. At least two disorders, tuberous sclerosis and neurofibromatosis, involve the failure of control of cell differentiation and/or proliferation within the nervous system as documented by diagnostically characteristic gross morphological changes. It may also be that many of the other neuropsychiatric disorders with more subtle neurological abnormalities, such as obsessive-compulsive disorder (OCD), Tourette's disorder, and attention-deficit hyperactivity disorder (ADHD), involve more subtle abnormalities in regulation of plasticity within the developing nervous system.

In addition to chemical-environmental effects from outside of the developing fetus such as alcohol and cocaine, perceptions of the larger environment by the child may also affect the regulation between genome and microenvironment in determination of the phenotype. A classic set of experiments showing morphological changes after visual deprivation in the developing cat (Wiesel et al. 1974) is now being elaborated in studies of the neurobehavioral response of primates to different rearing environments (Insel et al. 1988).

An interesting relationship between developmental neurobiology and neurodegenerative disorders is developing. The clinical parallel is the presence of plaques and tangles in both Down's syndrome and Alzheimer's disease caused by amyloid deposition (Rumble et al. 1989). However, the possibility of a more general connection due to the role of neurotrophic factors in both the development and maintenance of the CNS must be considered (Knusel et al. 1991; Maisonpierre et al. 1990).

❑ DEVELOPMENTAL DISORDERS

Because developmental neurobiology forms the foundation for normal development, it follows that the most common neuropsychiatric disorders in childhood are developmental disorders. In patients with mental retardation, cognitive, language, and motor development are significantly delayed relative to chronological norms. In specific developmental disorders, aspects of cognitive, language, or motor development are affected. It is relatively unusual for a developmental disorder to have a single area of dysfunction because any perturbation of neurological development is likely to affect the development of different regions of the brain. In addition, the learning of many academic skills such as arithmetic is dependent on other functions such as reading. As developmental neuropsychology matures as an independent discipline rather than solely as an extension of adult neuropsychology, the natural patterns of relatively specific developmental disorders will be better described and may then be better understood in the context of developmental neurobiology. Autistic disorder is important in this context, because it is one of the first developmental disorders to be studied more from the perspective of normal and abnormal child neuropsychological development than as a downward extension of an adult disorder. In autistic disorder, specific patterns of social and language abnormalities not seen in mental retardation or specific developmental disorders are present.

Mental Retardation

Overview. Mental retardation is one of the most common neuropsychiatric disorders, occurring in 2%–3% of school-age children. Mental retardation has received much less neuropsychiatric study than less prevalent and less severe disorders. This is partly due to the exclusion of patients with mental retardation from both clinical and research efforts. However, because of increasing integration of mentally retarded individuals into communities, such exclusion has been reduced; the neuropsychiatric care of mentally retarded patients continues to be substandard relative to the care provided patients without mental retardation, except for a few centers with expertise in this area.

Characteristic features. Mental retardation is defined by a reduced rate of mental development relative to chronologically and culturally based norms (Table 28–1). A combination of a measured IQ below 70 (2 standard deviations below the mean) and functional deficits in social, occupational, or academic functioning is required for diagnosis. Although IQ is determined by comparing the performance of in-

TABLE 28–1. DSM-III-R AXIS II DIAGNOSIS OF DEVELOPMENTAL DISORDERS[a]

Mental retardation[b] (IQ)	
Mild	(50–55 to 70)
Moderate	(35–40 to 50–55)
Severe	(20–25 to 35–40)
Profound	(Below 20–25)
Unspecified mental retardation	
Pervasive developmental disorders	
Autistic disorder	
Pervasive developmental disorder not otherwise specified (NOS)	
Specific developmental disorders	
Academic skills disorders	
Developmental arithmetic disorder	
Developmental expressive writing disorder	
Developmental reading disorder	
Language and speech disorders	
Developmental articulation disorder	
Developmental expressive language disorder	
Developmental receptive language disorder	
Motor skills disorder	
Coordination disorder	
Others	
Specific developmental disorder NOS	
(Single specific developmental disorder)	
Developmental disorders NOS	
(More than one specific developmental disorder)	

[a]Patients with developmental disorders are at higher risk for Axis I disorders.
[b]Mental retardation is most often not comorbid with pervasive developmental disorders, but pervasive developmental disorders are most often associated with mental retardation.
Source. Adapted from American Psychiatric Association 1987. Used with permission.

dividuals on an intelligence test such as the Wechsler Intelligence Scale for Children-Revised (WISC-R; Wechsler 1974) and determining the position of the individual on a theoretically normal distribution, it is also useful to have a "bedside" measure of development that allows a practical appreciation of a mentally retarded individual's functional impairment. The Developmental Quotient (DQ) is an informal tool for this purpose (Figure 28–1).

The DQ is determined by using as much information as possible to determine the highest age level of acquired skills in several areas, including gross motor development, fine motor development, personal-social skills, language development, and academic development, and comparing these with milestones of normally developing children. Mental age divided by chronological age (if greater than 16 years, divide by 16) gives the DQ expressed as a percentage (Figure 28–1). For example, a 5-year-old child who has just begun speaking in two word sentences (mental age 2 years), would have a DQ of 40. An adult who recently learned to ride a bicycle and is reading at a first-grade level would have an estimated mental age of 6 years and a DQ of 37.

$$\text{Developmental Quotient (DQ)} = \frac{\text{Mental age (MA)}}{\text{Chronological age (CA)}}$$

Note. If chronological age is more than 16 years, enter 16 as CA.

Figure 28–1. Developmental Quotient.

The DQ becomes more informative as more information is included. It is also a useful exercise to realize that the DQ may vary greatly across functional domains within individuals. An example of the use of the DQ is in an emergency room assessment in which formal testing is usually not available to assist in determining the mental capacities of an individual but the family is still able to provide a history of the skills that could be performed before any recent change in condition. In addition, if the IQ is widely discrepant with the DQ, it may be a clue to a deterioration in function since the last IQ testing, or it may be a clue to factors compromising the validity of the IQ testing. This process is roughly analogous to the process of reconciling the clinical neurological examination with laboratory findings.

Eighty-five percent of children, adolescents, and adults with mental retardation have mild mental retardation (IQ 50–55 to 70). Most individuals with mild mental retardation do not have dysmorphic features. One can see by application of the DQ that an adult with mild mental retardation will have a mental age ranging from roughly 8 to 11, which corresponds to the usual grade school intellectual level of most adults with mental retardation. At this level of function, most patients with mild mental retardation are able to live in the community and hold jobs, but require support from both their families and communities to maintain such community integration, particularly in managing changes in relationships, jobs, or other life circumstances. In caring for individuals with mental retardation it is helpful to think of social and coping skills as among the most complex cognitive functions necessary for successful adaptation.

Moderate mental retardation is the next most common form, occurring in about 0.2%–0.3% of the population. With an IQ range between 35–40 and 50–55, the mental age ranges from roughly 5 to 8.

Assessment of individuals at this level and below often requires administration of IQ tests such as the Stanford-Binet Intelligence Scale (Thorndike et al. 1986), because tests such as the WISC-R often are not valid for individuals with IQs below 40. For children over 31 months, for whom a basal level on the Stanford-Binet cannot be achieved, a DQ obtained by administration of the Mental Scale of the Bayley Scales of Infant Development (Bayley 1969) is predictive of IQ determined by the Stanford-Binet scale at a later age (Goldstein and Sheaffer 1988). Individuals with moderate mental retardation usually learn to communicate at the level of a preschool or early grade school child, although expressive language is often more impaired than other skills at this level and below. The extent of expressive language impairment relative to general intelligence often is associated with an increased risk of psychiatric disorder, particularly involving aggression directed toward the self and/or others.

Severe mental retardation (IQ 20–25 to 35–40) is characterized by a mental age between approximately 3 and 5 years. Individuals with increasingly severe levels of mental retardation have increasing frequencies of seizure disorders, "hard" neurological signs such as spasticity, and identified etiologies such as chromosomal and metabolic disorders (discussed below). In addition, self-injurious behavior (SIB) and stereotypic behavior, such as hand flapping, increase to a frequency of 50% in patients with profound mental retardation (IQ below 20–25).

Although individuals with profound mental retardation have mental ages as low as the first year of life, the mismatch between chronological age and mental age should not be allowed to obscure the observation that they have as many or more capacities and psychological and physical needs as infants without mental retardation.

Neuropsychiatric features. Children with mental retardation often have nonspecific abnormalities on electroencephalograms (EEGs) or neuroimaging scans. Specific etiologies include toxic, metabolic, and genetic disorders (discussed in more detail below). A full discussion of the range of etiology of mental retardation is beyond the scope of this chapter, and readers are directed to other sources (Menkes 1990b).

Treatment. Most cases of mental retardation or other developmental disorders do not have an identifiable etiology. However, numerous metabolic, genetic, and endocrinologic etiologies have been suggested. When a child is diagnosed with a developmental disorder, evaluation of identifiable etiologies or associated neurological conditions should be completed. Such a workup should include, but not be limited to, a detailed history and physical examination with particular attention to dysmorphology, an EEG, serum chemistry panel, thyroid function testing, and quantitative urinary amino and organic acids testing. Each of these investigations may reveal partially treatable forms of developmental disorder. To assist in determining etiology, a structural imaging scan of the brain may be performed. However, if sedation is required, the minimal risk of sedation must be weighed against the currently infinitesimal benefit of structural scans in developmental disorders, especially in the absence of recent loss of functional skills, other recent mental status changes, or traumatic injury. Computed tomography (CT) may be more helpful than magnetic resonance imaging (MRI) in the diagnosis of some disorders, including tuberous sclerosis, because of the improved contrast of certain abnormal tissue, although MRI more commonly identifies neuropathology. Chromosomal testing is useful to diagnose syndromes such as Down's syndrome and fragile X syndrome. Although most useful for genetic counselling, such information may also directly affect management, such as prevention of paralysis by screening Down's syndrome patients for atlantoaxial instability with cervical spine films in flexion and hyperextension (Cullen et al. 1989). Atlantoaxial instability may lead to spinal cord injuries during physical exercise (particularly tumbling exercises) because of severe subluxation between the C_1 and C_2 vertebrae.

Neuropsychiatric treatment of children, adolescents, and adults consists primarily of habilitation and treatment of associated psychiatric disorders in the majority of cases. Individuals with mental retardation and other developmental disorders are at risk for psychiatric illness (Lund 1985). Factors accounting for this increased risk include not only CNS dysfunction but peer rejection and decreased coping strategies (Reiss and Benson 1984). Concomitant psychiatric disorder often accounts for discrepancies between DQ and IQ or current levels of functioning and previous levels of functioning. Patients with mental retardation may have any associated DSM-III-R Axis I or Axis II diagnosis (American Psychiatric Association 1987), although cognitive and language limitations may make diagnosis more difficult. If an Axis I diagnosis or Axis II diagnosis is made, treatment for someone with mental retardation is similar to that for someone without it.

Many patients with relatively severe disorders of behavior or social and emotional functioning do not fit into categories established for patients without mental retardation. Aggression toward self (i.e., SIB) or others is often a presenting problem leading to restriction of the patient from community integration. If an Axis I diagnosis is not present to guide treatment, the first intervention should be to assess the living situation of the patient. All children should have individualized educational programs, and all adults should have individualized habilitative programs that provide them with a sense of accomplishment and personal growth. Possible physical or sexual abuse should be considered in patients with regression, although most cases of regression are caused by an extreme response to milder stressors or onset or recurrence of Axis I disorders.

In addition to improving positive programming, operant behavioral interventions are often helpful in reducing aggressive behaviors. Patients with mild mental retardation often respond well to token economies, whereas patients with lower levels of functioning often benefit from more intensive operant behavioral paradigms (LaVigna and Donnellan 1986). A particularly useful intervention that avoids aversive interventions is differential reinforcement of other behavior in which reinforcement is provided after a specified period of no undesired responding (e.g., reinforcement after each 15 minute period of no aggression) (LaVigna 1987).

If there are no Axis I disorders identified and nonpharmacological interventions have been optimized, pharmacological management may be considered. The first step is to assess possible negative psychotropic effects of current medications. This includes sedative effects from phenobarbital and phenytoin, as well as from neuroleptics. Adjustment of the current regimen may include changing to a less sedating anticonvulsant or to an anticonvulsant with possibly positive psychotropic effects (e.g., substitution of carbamazepine where appropriate for patients with cycling periods of irritability and/or activity). Adjustment of neuroleptic may include the addition of amantadine or anticholinergic agents to reduce akathisia. Some patients with mental retardation may require more gradual tapering of neuroleptics than others because of decreased cognitive-based coping skills necessary for adaptation to the subjective experience of neuroleptic withdrawal.

If the patient is not currently being treated with medication, empirical treatment is sometimes warranted to reduce the distress of the patient and allow improved self-regulation. Assessment is enhanced by baseline and periodic use of the Aberrant Behavior Checklist (Aman et al. 1985). Five subscales (irritability, withdrawal and lethargy, stereotypy, hyperactivity, and inappropriate speech) are relatively sensitive indicators of pharmacological response. For patients with behavioral problems associated with repetitive stereotypic behavior including SIB or ritualized pacing, a trial of potent serotonin (5-hydroxytryptamine [5-HT]) reuptake inhibitors used in the treatment of OCD may be started empirically with close follow-up (see discussion on OCD below). If aggressive behavior is part of an overall presentation of inattention, hyperactivity, and impulsivity, stimulant therapy may be of benefit, particularly for patients with moderate or mild mental retardation (see discussion on ADHD below). If aggressive behavior is impulsive but behavior is not pervasively hyperactive and inattentive, a trial of a β-blocker such as propranolol may be warranted. Alternatively, buspirone may be of benefit for nonspecific treatment of irritability at a low dosage (5 mg tid). Clonidine is particularly effective in short-term reduction of aggression and irritability, but tolerance is common after a few weeks to a few months (see discussion on Tourette's disorder below). Some mentally retarded patients with SIB have responded to naltrexone.

Autistic Disorder and Pervasive Developmental Disorder

Overview. Although the full syndrome of autistic disorder is relatively uncommon (with a prevalence of 2–4 per 10,000), it is one of the most severe neuropsychiatric disorders. Although the original description of autistic disorder (Kanner 1943) did not describe its common association with mental retardation, autistic disorder is associated with mental retardation in 7 out of 10 cases. However, autistic disorder represents a qualitative abnormality in development (gaze aversion seen in autistic disorder is not a behavior seen in normal development), as opposed to mental retardation which is defined as a quantitative (slower rate of maturation) abnormality of development.

Characteristic features. The paradigmatic PDD is autistic disorder. It affects social, communicative, and imaginative development. Abnormal development of social reciprocity is one of the most striking features of autistic disorder, although the social, communicative, imaginative, and cognitive elements of the disorder are inextricably linked.

The natural developmental history of autistic disorder is relatively consistent. Children often have impaired reciprocal social interactions with their caretakers identifiable within the first 6 months, including impaired early anticipation of being held or social smiling (Rutter 1985). Joint attention with mothers, which normally develops within the first year, does not develop normally in most cases (Mundy and Sigman 1989). However, more than 30% of autistic children have a regression or arrest in development, most notably affecting maternal-infant social interaction, after initial normal development (Dahl et al. 1986). Some of the more easily identifiable abnormalities, such as gaze aversion and stereotypies, often peak between 3 and 5 years, whereas more subtle problems in social reciprocity, language usage and speech delivery, and understanding and expression of emotions persist into adulthood (Rutter 1985). Diagnostic confusion commonly occurs because of failure to consider the developmental course of the disorder.

The restriction of imaginative interests is most dramatically demonstrated by atypical behaviors, such as stereotypic complex hand and body movements; but the absence of imaginative activity is most characteristic of the disorder. The distress and anxiety associated with interruption of routines, such as going to the store in exactly the same way each time or ordering of the environment, are similar to some of the symptoms of OCD; these symptoms respond partially to serotonin (5-HT) reuptake inhibitors such as fluoxetine (Cook et al. 1990) and clomipramine (Gordon et al. 1991). Although about 70% of individuals with autistic disorder also have mental retardation (Lord and Schopler 1988; Rutter et al. 1967), differential diagnosis of the presence of autistic disorder is important because autistic patients have different learning characteristics and may respond adversely if their preoccupations or frequent distress at normally reinforcing social interactions are not considered. Although intrusive preoccupations and rituals may respond to behavioral interventions similar to those used in the treatment of OCD, behavioral contingency programs that are improperly generalized from treatment of children with disruptive behavior disorders such as ADHD often increase aggressive behaviors in patients with autistic disorder. Programs developed for individuals with autistic disorder should be developed with these issues in mind.

Twenty-five percent or more of autistic children develop epilepsy, with many having the relatively rare age at onset during adolescence (Deykin and Macmahon 1979; Volkmar and Nelson 1990). In addition, the syndrome is often associated with attentional impairment, affective lability, and aggressive and impulsive behavior. The clinical features of autistic disorder are often similar to those of patients who have sustained TBI.

Standardized assessments are available for the diagnosis of autistic disorder in children, adolescents, and adults. These tests include a parent interview, the Autism Diagnostic Interview (ADI; Le Couteur et al. 1989), and two observation schedules, the Childhood Autism Rating Scale (CARS; Mesibov et al. 1989) and Autism Diagnostic Observation Schedule (ADOS; Lord et al. 1989). The ADI is a semistructured interview in which the interviewer asks specified probes about social, communicative, and imaginative development and follows up with further questions until specific examples of language and behavior are given by the parent. The ADOS consists of an interview with the child or adult who may have autistic disorder, during which a set of tasks designed to "press" the patient for social and conversational interaction is presented. A limitation of the current version of the ADOS is that a mental age of 3 years is required. The CARS is a less structured assessment of the child or adult who may have autistic disorder, but may be given to children and adults with a mental age less than 3 years.

There are many children and adolescents who have abnormalities in social, communicative, and imaginative development, but do not meet criteria for the diagnosis of autistic disorder. Although some of these patients may be similar to children with avoidant disorder of childhood and adolescence or OCD, they are considered to also have PDD, with a subclassification of PDD not otherwise specified (PDD NOS) (Table 28–1). Currently, PDD is subclassified into autistic disorder and PDD NOS, but the classification system is likely to become more differentiated to include more clinically or etiologically defined subgroups. One example is Asperger's syndrome, in which motor clumsiness and preoccupation with restricted interests but relatively preserved language and cognitive function are present (Wing 1981). Recently, social communication spectrum disorder has been proposed to include children who have social communication deficits, but are not diagnosed within the current nosology (Tanguay 1990).

Neuropsychiatric features. No case of autistic disorder has been described in which a sufficient connection has been made between the disorder and a neuropathological finding. However, several neurological disorders have been associated with autistic disorder in a minority of cases, including chromosomal disorders (e.g., fragile X syndrome), neurocutaneous disorders (e.g., tuberous sclerosis), metabolic disorders (e.g., PKU), congenital viral infections (e.g., rubella), and various others occurring in a total of about 10% of cases (Ritvo et al. 1990). There is evidence of a genetic component of the disorder in at least a subgroup of cases (Folstein and Rutter 1988).

Treatment. Assessment and treatment of autistic disorder are similar to those described for mental retardation above. However, autistic children almost invariably require an emphasis in educational and habilitative plans on improving functional communication and social skills and reducing repetitive or ritualistic behaviors that interfere with adaptive functioning.

❑ ATTENTION-DEFICIT HYPERACTIVITY DISORDER

Overview. Child and adolescent neuropsychiatry was heavily influenced when a link was established between adults who had sequelae from the encephalitis lethargica epidemic in 1917 involving inattention and children who had symptoms of hyperactivity, inattention, and impulsivity. This link was strengthened by the therapeutic effects of dextroamphetamine for both conditions. This led to the term *minimal brain dysfunction* used to describe what is now termed *attention-deficit hyperactivity disorder*. Although many children with ADHD have evidence of neuropsychiatric dysfunction, the etiology of this dysfunction has not been established, and head injury is at most a rare cause (Rutter et al. 1983). Neurological "soft signs" were initially described as evidence in support of an association between ADHD and specific "brain damage," but soft signs at age 7 have been demonstrated to be related to anxiety, withdrawal, and depression rather than to ADHD (Shaffer et al. 1985).

ADHD continues to be an important neuropsychiatric disorder of childhood because of its prevalence in about 3%–5% of school-age children and because of the psychosocial problems with which it is associated. In addition, several outcome studies have demonstrated that ADHD frequently persists into adulthood and is a strong risk factor for incarceration and substance abuse in adulthood (Gittelman et al. 1985).

Characteristic features. Similar to other child and adolescent neuropsychiatric disorders, ADHD is an etiologically heterogenous syndrome. However, the developmental course is relatively consistent. Hyperactivity is the most common initial symptom, occasionally with even prenatal symptoms (increased kicking in utero) frequently described retrospectively. Hyperactivity continues to be the most commonly identified and interfering symptom until the children are about 10 years old, when activity level often becomes less prominent and attentional dysfunction becomes more important, partly in relationship to increased expectations in school. Attentional dysfunction often continues to be a problem into adulthood, although its actual impact depends on academic and career demands. Impulsivity becomes the major problem during adolescence. At this time social demands require that aggressive and appetitive (sexual and substance-related) impulses be under much more effective self-control. Lack of such control is common in affected adolescents and young adults with ADHD. Table 28–2 lists the DSM-III-R criteria of ADHD.

Because ADHD is common, it is not surprising that other disorders are frequently comorbid. The most common of these is conduct disorder, which appears to increase the risk of antisocial behavior in adolescence and adulthood. Table 28–3 lists the DSM-III-R criteria for conduct disorder. Comorbidity with mood and anxiety disorders has also been described. Such comorbidity increases the risk of impulsive suicidal acts.

Treatment. Practice parameters for the assessment and treatment of ADHD have been established by the American Academy of Child and Adolescent Psychiatry (American Academy of Child and Ado-

TABLE 28–2. DSM-III-R DIAGNOSTIC CRITERIA FOR ATTENTION-DEFICIT HYPERACTIVITY DISORDER

Note: Consider a criterion met only if the behavior is considerably more frequent than that of most people of same mental age.

A. A disturbance of at least 6 months during which at least eight of the following are present:
   1. Often fidgets with hands or feet or squirms in seat (in adolescents may be limited to subjective feelings of restlessness)
   2. Has difficulty remaining seated when required to do so
   3. Is easily distracted by extraneous stimuli
   4. Has difficulty awaiting turn in games or group situations
   5. Often blurts out answers to questions before they have been completed
   6. Has difficulty following through on instructions from others (not due to oppositional behavior or a failure of comprehension), e.g., fails to finish chores
   7. Has difficulty sustaining attention in tasks or play activities
   8. Often shifts from one uncompleted activity to another
   9. Has difficulty playing quietly
   10. Often talks excessively
   11. Often interrupts or intrudes on others, e.g., butts into other children's games
   12. Often does not seem to listen to what is being said to him or her
   13. Often loses things necessary for tasks or activities school or at home (e.g., toys, pencils, books, assignments)
   14. Often engages in physically dangerous activities without considering possible consequences (not for the purpose of thrill-seeking), e.g., runs into street without looking

Note: The above items are listed in descending order of discriminating power based on data from a national field trial of the DSM-III-R criteria for disruptive behavior disorders.

B. Onset before the age of 7

C. Does not meet the criteria for a pervasive developmental disorder

Criteria for severity of attention-deficit hyperactivity disorder:
Mild: Few, if any, symptoms in excess of those required for diagnosis **and** only minimal or no impairment in school and social functioning
Moderate: Symptoms of functional impairment intermediate between "mild" and "severe"
Severe: Many symptoms in excess of those needed to make the diagnosis **and** significant and pervasive impairment in functioning at home and school and with peers

Source. Reprinted from American Psychiatric Association: Diagnostic and Statistical Manual of Mental Disorders, 3rd Edition, Revised. Washington, DC, 1987, pp 52–53. Used with permission.

lescent Psychiatry 1991), and readers are advised to consult these parameters as well as other sources devoted to this topic (Barkley 1983; Donnelly and Rapoport 1985).

Assessment of children with ADHD, as of other children and adolescents with developmental neuropsychiatric syndromes, consists of obtaining history from the parents (including family history), school information (including grades, behavioral and emotional functioning, peer relationships, and achievement testing), a diagnostic interview of the child, and completion of standard parent rating scales such as the Abbreviated Parent Questionnaire (Conners 1970) and ADD-H: Comprehensive Teacher's Rating Scale (ACTeRs; Ullmann et al. 1984). Psychological evaluation, psychoeducational evaluation, speech and language evaluation, and other assessments may be necessary because of the frequent association of ADHD and specific developmental disorders ranging from speech and language disorders to developmental arithmetic disorders.

Multimodal treatment begins with education of the parents, children, and teachers about the disorder. This is particularly important so that symptoms of hyperactivity and inattention can be differentiated from oppositional behaviors. A trial of a stimulant medication, such as methylphenidate or dextroamphetamine, is often indicated. Methylphenidate is usually the drug of choice because of less potent cardiovascular effects (increased pulse and blood pressure) than dextroamphetamine.

TABLE 28–3. DSM-III-R DIAGNOSTIC CRITERIA FOR CONDUCT DISORDER

A. A disturbance of conduct lasting at least 6 months, during which at least three of the following have been present:
   1. Has stolen without confrontation of a victim on more than one occasion (including forgery)
   2. Has run away from home overnight at least twice while living in parental or parental surrogate home (or once without returning)
   3. Often lies (other than to avoid physical or sexual abuse)
   4. Has deliberately engaged in fire-setting
   5. Is often truant from school (for older person, absent from work)
   6. Has broken into someone else's house, building, or car
   7. Has deliberately destroyed others' property (other than by fire-setting)
   8. Has been physically cruel to animals
   9. Has forced someone into sexual activity with him or her
   10. Has used a weapon in more than one fight
   11. Often initiates physical fights
   12. Has stolen with confrontation of a victim (e.g., mugging, purse-snatching, extortion, armed robbery)
   13. Has been physically cruel to people

Note: The above items are listed in descending order of discriminating power based on data from a national field trial of the DSM-III-R criteria for disruptive behavior disorders.

B. If 18 or older, does not meet criteria for antisocial personality disorder

Criteria for severity of conduct disorder:
Mild: Few if any conduct problems in excess of those required to make the diagnosis, **and** conduct problems cause only minor harm to others
Moderate: Number of conduct problems and effect on others intermediate between "mild" and "severe"
Severe: Many conduct problems in excess of those required for diagnosis, **or** conduct problems cause considerable harm to others, e.g., serious physical injury to victims, extensive vandalism or theft, prolonged absence from home

Source. Reprinted from American Psychiatric Association: Diagnostic and Statistical Manual of Mental Disorders, 3rd Edition, Revised. Washington, DC, 1987, p 55. Used with permission.

The starting dosage for children over age 5 is usually 5 mg at 8 A.M. and noon to control symptoms during school hours. If children have ADHD symptoms that cause significant problems at home, the medication may be given at 4 P.M. and on weekends. The dosage may be tapered up to 20 mg tid depending on clinical response. Pulse, blood pressure, height, and weight should be monitored. In addition, teacher and parent behavior rating scales should be completed and scored before and after each dosage change to assist in assessment of drug response. Patients should also be monitored for possible development of tics. A relative contraindication for stimulant treatment is the presence of tics, although the benefit of stimulant therapy for many patients with tics outweighs the risk of tic exacerbation. Patients who have limiting side effects on methylphenidate can be treated with imipramine or desipramine with baseline and periodic electrocardiograph (ECG) monitoring. The dosage of desipramine or imipramine necessary to treat ADHD is often in the range of 10–20 mg at bedtime, rather than usual antidepressant dosage. In addition, response of ADHD symptoms occurs within days, in contrast to antidepressant response, which occurs within weeks.

In addition to pharmacological treatment, parent training (Forehand and Atkeson 1977) and educational intervention for ADHD and frequently associated specific developmental disorders including language disorders are also important in the treatment of children and adolescents with ADHD. For older children, cognitive-behavioral therapy may assist the child in developing strategies to minimize impulsive behavior (Kendall and Braswell 1985).

❑ OBSESSIVE-COMPULSIVE DISORDER

Overview. OCD has recently increased in importance as a childhood neuropsychiatric disorder for several reasons. A careful epidemiological study (Flament et al. 1989) revealed a lifetime prevalence for OCD of at least 0.4% for high school students. In addition, the efficacy of clomipramine in reducing the obsessions and compulsions of OCD has added it to the list of neuropsychiatric disorders in which knowledge of specific diagnosis indicates specific treatment (Leonard et al. 1989).

Characteristic features. Diagnosis of OCD requires the presence of either obsessions, (recurrent and persistent ideas, thoughts, or images), or compulsions (repetitive, purposeful, and intentional behaviors that are performed according to certain rules or in a stereotyped manner). In addition, the obsessions and/or compulsions must cause marked distress and significantly interfere with a person's school or occupational functioning, usual social activities, or relationships. Table 28–4 lists the DSM-III-R diagnostic criteria for OCD.

OCD can start as early as age 2 years, although there appears to be an increased incidence at age 7 and in late adolescence. About 20% of children and adolescents with OCD have affected first-degree relatives. Ego-dystonicity (subjective experience that the obsessions or compulsions have intruded into the person's usual thoughts and actions), which is often present in patients with OCD of adolescent and adult onset, is frequently absent in those with childhood onset of the disorder (Swedo and Rapoport 1989).

Neuropsychiatric features. OCD has been reported in association with encephalitis lethargica (Schilder 1938), TBI (McKeon et al. 1984), and Sydenham's chorea (Swedo et al. 1989a). Patients with OCD have been shown to have an increased incidence of tics and other neurological soft signs (Denckla 1989; Hollander et al. 1990). Soft signs include neurodevelopmental deficits in balance, postural control, gait, and timed repetitive and alternating movements. The revised Physical and Neurological Examination for Soft Signs (PANESS; Denckla 1985) is a preferred assessment instrument of neurological soft signs. A quantitative CT scan study (Luxenberg et al. 1988) revealed decreased size of the caudate nuclei in adult male patients with primary OCD. Through examination with positron-emission to-

TABLE 28–4. DSM-III-R DIAGNOSTIC CRITERIA FOR OBSESSIVE-COMPULSIVE DISORDER

A. Either obsessions or compulsions:

Obsessions: 1, 2, 3, and 4:

1. Recurrent and persistent ideas, thoughts, impulses, or images that are experienced, at least initially, as intrusive and senseless, e.g., a parent's having repeated impulses to kill a loved child, a religious person's having recurrent blasphemous thoughts
2. The person attempts to ignore or suppress such thoughts or impulses or to neutralize them with some other thought or action
3. The person recognizes that the obsessions are the product of his or her own mind, not imposed from without (as in thought insertion)
4. If another Axis I disorder is present, the content of the obsession is unrelated to it, e.g., the ideas, thoughts, or images are not about food in the presence of an eating disorder, about drugs in the presence of a psychoactive substance use disorder, or guilty thoughts in the presence of a major depression

Compulsions: 1, 2, and 3:

1. Repetitive, purposeful, and intentional behaviors that are performed in response to an obsession, or according to certain rules or in a stereotyped fashion
2. The behavior is designed to neutralize or to prevent discomfort or some dreaded event or situation: however, either the activity is not connected in a realistic way with what it is designed to neutralize or prevent, or it is clearly excessive
3. The person recognizes that his or her behavior is excessive or unreasonable (this may not be true for young children; it may no longer be true for people whose obsessions have evolved into overvalued ideas)

B. The obsessions or compulsions cause marked distress, are time-consuming (take more than an hour a day), or significantly interfere with the person's normal routine, occupational functioning, or usual social activities or relationships with others

Source. Reprinted from American Psychiatric Association: Diagnostic and Statistical Manual of Mental Disorders, 3rd Edition, Revised. Washington, DC, 1987, p 247. Used with permission.

mography (PET), cerebral metabolic rate has appeared to be increased in bilateral prefrontal, left orbital frontal, left premotor, right sensorimotor, and anterior cingulate regions in patients with OCD of childhood onset (Swedo et al. 1989b). However, none of the neurological or neuroimaging findings has been confirmed to be specific for obsessive-compulsive disorder or to identify a homogeneous subgroup.

Treatment. Treatment of OCD includes psychopharmacological treatment with potent serotonin (5-HT) reuptake inhibitors, including clomipramine, fluvoxamine, sertraline, fluoxetine, and paroxetine. Currently, only clomipramine has been approved for the specific indication of OCD in the United States. After baseline history, physical examination, and ECG, clomipramine is started at a dosage of 25 mg/day and gradually increased, as tolerated, to a dosage of 100 mg or 3 mg/kg body weight (whichever is smaller) over the first 2 weeks. Clomipramine should be given in divided doses with meals to decrease gastrointestinal side effects. Over the next several weeks, the dosage should be increased to the lesser of 3 mg/kg body weight or 200 mg for children and adolescents between ages 10 and 17 years, or to 250 mg for adults. A second ECG should be performed if there are cardiac symptoms or if a dosage of 3 mg/kg body weight is reached. After titration, the total daily dosage can be given at bedtime as tolerated.

As an alternative, cognitive-behavioral treatment focusing on sufficient exposure to a precipitating stimulus with prevention of obsessions or compulsions appears to be as efficacious as psychopharmacological treatment (Berg et al. 1989). Cognitive-behavioral therapy has the advantage of not having the physical side effects of pharmacological management, but many patients are unable to comply because of psychological discomfort with the procedure or limitations in cognitive and language skills. Dynamically based psychotherapy and family therapy are often useful adjuncts to treat the effects of OCD on interpersonal and family relationships, but have not been shown to be useful in the treatment of the core symptoms of obsessions or compulsions in OCD.

❑ TOURETTE'S DISORDER

Characteristic features. Tourette's disorder is characterized by the presence of multifocal motor and phonic tics. Tics are sudden, repetitive, stereotyped motor movements that may be visualized directly or heard (in the case of phonic tics). Motor tics vary in complexity from eye blinking and arm jerking to copropraxia (obscene gestures). Phonic tics vary in complexity from throat clearing and coughing to immediate echolalia (immediate repetition) and coprolalia. Tics vary in intensity and frequency throughout the day and wax and wane over periods of days to months. Tics can usually be suppressed to some extent. In addition, they are often exacerbated by stress or fatigue and often ameliorated in novel or highly structured environments. Table 28–5 lists the DSM-III-R diagnostic criteria for Tourette's disorder.

The natural developmental progression of Tourette's disorder includes motoric hyperactivity, inattention, and impulsivity, which frequently precede the development of tics in as many as 50% of patients. In addition, associated specific developmental disorders often are evident relatively early in the course of the disorder. Tics are often first manifest when children are between the ages of 5 and 8 years. They frequently start with transient

TABLE 28–5. DSM-III-R DIAGNOSTIC CRITERIA FOR TOURETTE'S DISORDER

A. Both multiple motor and one or more vocal tics have been present at some time during the illness, although not necessarily concurrently.
B. Tics occur many times a day (usually in bouts), nearly every day or intermittently throughout a period of more than 1 year.
C. The anatomic location, number, frequency, complexity, and severity of the tics change over time.
D. Onset before age 21.
E. Occurrence not exclusively during psychoactive substance intoxication or known central nervous system disease, such as Huntington's chorea and postviral encephalitis.

Source. Reprinted from American Psychiatric Association: Diagnostic and Statistical Manual of Mental Disorders, 3rd Edition, Revised. Washington, DC, 1987, p 80. Used with permission.

blinking or other tics involving facial or neck muscles. A rostral-caudal progression of the development of tics is common as is the diminution of one tic followed by the emergence of another. Complex tics become more common with increasing age. Tics frequently diminish during adolescence and early adulthood (Leckman and Cohen 1988).

Neuropsychiatric features. Obsessions and compulsions frequently develop during late childhood and adolescence (mean onset 9.5 years) in 10%–40% of patients with Tourette's syndrome (Jagger et al. 1982). A single study of tics and obsessions and compulsions (Pauls and Leckman 1986) was consistent with autosomal dominant transmission of a gene with variable expression; in some family members, particularly females, OCD rather than Tourette's syndrome or chronic motor tics was expressed in a manner consistent with autosomal dominant transmission. Neurochemical findings include decreased cerebrospinal fluid (CSF) 5-hydroxyindoleacetic acid (5-HIAA) after probenecid loading compared with that of other children and adolescent patients with serious developmental disorders, medical illnesses, and cognitive processing disturbances (Cohen et al. 1978). Nonspecific developmental, nonepileptiform EEG abnormalities have been documented in 45% of cases, although this finding is similar to that of the other child and adolescent neuropsychiatric disorders described above (Waldo et al. 1978).

Treatment. Pharmacological treatment of Tourette's syndrome includes treatment with clonidine, which has been documented in controlled trials to be effective in reducing tics in Tourette's syndrome (Cohen et al. 1980). After history, physical examination, ECG, and fasting glucose testing, clonidine may be initiated at a dose of 0.05 mg/day (one-half tablet). It may be increased by 0.05 mg every third day until doses in the range of 0.15–0.30 mg/day are achieved (3–5 μg/kg body weight per day). Clonidine should be administered tid or qid, although it is impractical to give less than 0.05 mg at any given time because of the small size of the tablet. Main side effects are drowsiness, dry mouth, and hypotension. Patients should be cautioned not to abruptly discontinue clonidine therapy, even though clinically significant rebound hypertension in nonhypertensive patients has not been reported.

Neuroleptics at relatively low dose, including haloperidol (Bruun et al. 1976) and pimozide (Shapiro and Shapiro 1984), have been shown to be effective. Haloperidol doses of 5 mg or less per day are generally adequate to control tics in as many as 80% of patients. Pimozide is often preferable because it has less of a sedative effect. After baseline history, physical examination, and ECG (Q-T interval > 0.47 seconds is a contraindication), pimozide may be initiated at a dose of 1 or 2 mg/day in divided doses. The dose may be increased every third day to a maximum of 0.2 mg/kg body weight per day or 10 mg/day. Periodic ECGs should be obtained during titration and the Q-T interval should not exceed 0.47 seconds or 25% above baseline. The risk of tardive dyskinesia with neuroleptics is compounded by the early age at onset of the disorder, and the dosage of pimozide or haloperidol should be maintained at the lowest level possible (Riddle et al. 1987).

Behavioral treatment, family counselling and therapy, individual therapy, academic interventions, and occupational and social adaptations are other components of treatment, with priorities for therapies (including pharmacotherapy) dependent to a large extent on associated learning disabilities, ADHD, OCD, and psychosocial consequences of Tourette's syndrome (Towbin et al. 1988).

❑ SEIZURE DISORDERS

Seizure disorders in childhood are commonly associated with developmental disorders. The prevalence rates for epilepsy increase with decreasing IQ. When intractable epilepsy occurs in the setting of an IQ less than 80, the prognosis for spontaneous remission of seizures appears to be decreased (Huttenlocher and Hapke 1990; Lindsay et al. 1979a). In contrast, the presence of focal atrophic brain abnormalities does not affect the prognosis of intractable seizures (Huttenlocher and Hapke 1990). Another relationship between developmental disorders and epilepsy is that although the onset of epilepsy during adolescence is relatively rare, it is more common in adolescent patients with autistic disorder (Deykin and Macmahon 1979). It is interesting that long-term potentiation and associated *N*-methyl-D-aspartate (NMDA) receptors in the hippocampus (see Chapter 1) have been linked to animal models of both learning and epilepsy, but application of these models awaits a fuller understanding of the processes and the availability of NMDA-receptor–related drugs for clinical trials.

Psychiatric morbidity related to seizure disorders is determined by several factors including underlying neuropathology, neural effects of ictal and interictal states, psychological effects of loss of consciousness or altered consciousness, family reaction to epilepsy, and psychotropic effects of anticonvulsant treatment. Several of these issues have been addressed in detail in Chapter 17. An interesting finding in children has been that as many as 85% of children with temporal lobe epilepsy had psychiatric disorders including mental retardation (25%) and disruptive behavior disorders (including "hyperkinetic syndrome" and catastrophic rage), but only 30% had psychiatric disorders when followed up in adulthood (Lindsay et al. 1979b).

Anticonvulsant therapy is an obvious mainstay in the treatment of children and adolescents with nonfebrile seizure disorders. However, phenobarbital and phenytoin should generally be avoided because sedation associated with both medications is not optimal for academic performance. Phenobarbital is of particular concern because of an apparent association with hyperactivity in children (Vining et al. 1987) and depression and suicidality in adolescents (Brent et al. 1987). Although carbamazepine has been reported to have therapeutic psychotropic effects (Ballenger and Post 1980), adverse psychotropic effects in some children and adolescents have also been reported (Pleak et al. 1988). All of these drugs, alone or in combination, are in common clinical use. Blood levels of the drugs are available and should be used in the regular monitoring of treatment.

Surgical treatment of intractable epilepsy in children has been receiving more attention recently. Although some authors have proposed that such treatment is important in reducing the risk of cognitive sequelae of seizure disorders, there is no evidence that in the absence of the hypoxic complications of status epilepticus that seizure disorders affect cognitive outcome (Ellenberg et al. 1986). It is worth emphasizing that seizure disorders and mental retardation may be signs and symptoms of underlying common neuropathology. Therefore, the justification for surgical treatment does not include reduction of risk for cognitive sequelae unless medical management has not been able to prevent status epilepticus. Surgical treatment of epilepsy should be considered only when seizures are refractory to medical treatment to the point that there is definitive compromise in function because of seizure frequency or duration. Although there have been claims of behavioral improvement after surgical treatment (Gillingham 1988), these have been anecdotal and must be weighed with extreme caution until controlled trials document that the benefit outweighs the considerable risk of loss of cognitive or language function.

The loss of control associated with epilepsy presents a challenge to normal development. Although many children easily master this challenge, some children react by becoming either overly passive or rebellious. However, this is often complicated by ictal or interictal effects on cognition or impulse regulation. Family responses to epilepsy often include overcontrol (Voeller and Rothenberg 1973) or decreased expectations (Long and Moore 1979), which contribute to the individual child's attempts to master a frequently chronic illness and perform academically.

❑ TERATOGENIC EXPOSURE

The most common toxic exposures associated with neuropsychiatric disorders in children are prenatal and postnatal exposure to alcohol and lead. Exposure to teratogenic substances leads to obvious congenital malformations such as FAS and to less severe congenital anomalies. However, some patients with minimal congenital anomalies may have more severe behavioral or cognitive sequelae.

Organic Toxins

Alcohol. The classical expression of FAS includes mild to moderate mental retardation, microcephaly, irritability, intrauterine and postnatal growth retardation, short palpebral fissures, midfacial hypoplasia, and prognathism. This level of expression of FAS is seen in 1–2 live births per 1,000. However, partial expression has been estimated at as high as 5 live births per 1,000 and has been termed *fetal alcohol effect* (FAE) (Clarren and Smith 1978; Hoyseth and Jones 1989).

Although some patients have severe facial dysmorphology, others have attenuated dysmorphic features. Although mental retardation has been reported in as many as 85% of cases, some bias toward severely affected cases was probably present. However, 15 of 87 children without mental retardation at a learning disorders clinic had mothers who had a history of alcoholism during pregnancy (Shaywitz et al. 1980).

ling involved in the development of the nervous system.

Cognitive deficits in affected males typically consist of moderate to severe mental retardation, although affected males without mental retardation have been identified. IQ during development has been shown to decrease from a mean of 54 between ages 5 and 10 years to 38 between ages 15 and 20. This appears to be due to a "plateau" effect rather than a loss of acquired skills (Dykens et al. 1989). Cognitive skills are not evenly deficient across developmental domains. Fragile X males have the most severe impairments in visual spatial skills and sequential processing skills. Hyperactivity and attentional deficits are common. Language abnormalities include rapid speech rhythm, perseverative speech, echolalia, and poor communicative intent. Qualitative social impairment includes social avoidance, poor peer relations, and gaze aversion. Auditory hypersensitivity, abnormal sensory interests (such as smelling), and self-injury are common.

The similarity of the fragile X neuropsychiatric phenotype to the syndrome of autistic disorder overlaps so considerably that 10 of 17 patients with fragile X syndrome were diagnosed as having autistic disorder or PDD NOS (Reiss and Freund 1990). Although the frequency of fragile X syndrome patients in studies of autistic children may not be greater than that expected based on level of mental retardation, the high frequency of qualitative impairments in social, communicative, and regulation of activities and interests in patients with fragile X syndrome suggests that there may be common developmental neurobiological processes involved. The recent findings of cerebellar vermal hypoplasia in both autistic disorder (Courchesne et al. 1988) and fragile X syndrome (Reiss et al. 1991) provide preliminary evidence of such an association. Diagnosis of fragile X syndrome currently only reliably leads to increased knowledge for parents about etiology and genetic risk; less is known about treatment implications. Although fragile X patients in one study (Hagerman et al. 1988) responded to stimulants for treatment of attentional dysfunction and hyperactivity as much as children with ADHD, side effects may be seen more commonly at doses above 0.3 mg/kg body weight. Further studies may reveal a differential response to psychotropic agents. Fragile X syndrome may be one of the next syndromes in which a molecular understanding of pathogenesis may contribute directly to the development of therapeutic strategies.

❑ TRAUMATIC BRAIN INJURY IN CHILDHOOD AND ADOLESCENCE

Most severe TBI during childhood and adolescence occurs during motor vehicle accidents. Milder TBI is sustained in the home for preschool children and during falls for children between ages 6 and 12 years. However, child abuse accounts for a significant minority of cases of severe head injuries during infancy. Prevention of head injuries is a major public health issue that is best addressed through efforts to modify parental behavior and supervision (e.g., increasing use of infant and child car seats and decreasing substance use during driving). However, these interventions alone cannot prevent all injury. Many parental behaviors that put children at risk for TBI also interact through genetic and environmental effects. Although accidents occur with an element of randomness, children with impaired impulse regulation (i.e., with ADHD or developmental disorders) are at much higher risk for "accidents." The sex-related prevalence of these disorders may account for the 3:1 incidence of TBI in boys compared with girls.

More than 90% of TBI is caused by closed head injury. The acute course of mild TBI includes brief unconsciousness followed by confusion, somnolence, and listlessness. Vomiting, pallor, and irritability often follow. Although as many as 40% of patients with mild TBI have linear skull fractures, this finding does not predict neuropsychiatric morbidity. Treatment of mild TBI includes neurological examination and CT scan depending on clinical judgment. Observation for epidural and subdural hematomas is essential. It also appears best to counsel children and parents that the sequelae of mild TBI are usually transient and that active reintroduction of normal activities is recommended. Because post-TBI changes in parental behavior such as overprotection appear to adversely affect the child's adjustment, this needs to be avoided. However, if a child has a premorbid disruptive behavior disorder such as ADHD, this should be appropriately treated (Rutter et al. 1983). The failure to consider premorbid functioning can lead to an overestimate of the long-term sequelae of mild TBI.

Severe TBI ranges from closed head injuries with posttraumatic amnesia lasting more than 7 days but no neurological signs to prolonged coma or death. Intensive supportive care has decreased mortality from severe TBI considerably. In addition to maintenance of adequate ventilation and circulation, repeated neurological examination (especially after extended stupor or coma) will identify changes in status such as those caused by mass lesions such as epidural or subdural hematomas. Children more commonly have increased intracranial pressure, which often requires aggressive management including induced hypothermia, if necessary.

After the emergence from coma, stupor is followed by impairment in regulation of consciousness indicated by delirium with fluctuating levels of consciousness. Patients in this phase need much the same care as other patients with delirium (see Chapter 12). Memory deficits are prominent and include both pretraumatic and posttraumatic amnesia. The duration of posttraumatic amnesia is considered the strongest predictor of cognitive or behavioral sequelae. In a study of patients with severe TBI (Chadwick et al. 1981), only patients with posttraumatic amnesia lasting more than 14 days had evidence of persistent intellectual impairment 1 year after TBI. Of the 17 patients in this subgroup, only 8 had persistent intellectual impairment. However, the first few weeks and months were characterized by intellectual deficit with the mean WISC-R Performance IQ being 77 when measured after posttraumatic amnesia had ended.

Psychiatric consequences of severe head injury include new onset of psychiatric disorders at a rate higher than that for control subjects only in patients with posttraumatic amnesia lasting more than 7 days. Transient or persistent intellectual impairment increases the risk of new-onset psychiatric disorder, although severe TBI is a risk factor for psychiatric disorder without intellectual impairment. In addition, preinjury behavioral characteristics and psychosocial adversity contribute to psychiatric morbidity after head injury. Although it was proposed that ADHD symptoms would be characteristic sequelae of TBI (and transient difficulties with attentional function characteristic of delirium are common during the acute [6–9 months] recovery phase), only social disinhibition was found to be a relatively specific sequela of severe TBI (Brown et al. 1981).

❑ REFERENCES

Aman MG, Singh NN, Stewart AW, et al: The Aberrant Behavior Checklist: a behavior rating scale for the assessement of treatment effects. American Journal of Mental Deficiency 39:485–491, 1985

American Academy of Child and Adolescent Psychiatry: Practice parameters for the assessment and treatment of attention-deficit hyperactivity disorder. J Am Acad Child Adolesc Psychiatry 30:I–III, 1991

American Psychiatric Association: Diagnostic and Statistical Manual of Mental Disorders, 3rd Edition, Revised. Washington, DC, American Psychiatric Association, 1987

Arenander AT, de Vellis J: Development of the nervous system, in Basic Neurochemistry, 4th Edition. New York, Raven, 1989, pp 479–506

Ballenger JC, Post RM: Carbamazepine in manic-depressive illness: a new treatment. Am J Psychiatry 137:782–790, 1980

Banich MT, Levine SC, Kim H, et al: The effects of developmental factors on IQ in hemiplegic children. Neuropsychologia 28:35–47, 1990

Barkley RA: Hyperactive Children. New York, Guilford Press, 1983

Bayley N: Bayley Scales of Infant Development. New York, Psychological Corporation, 1969

Bellinger D, Leviton A, Waternaux C, et al: Longitudinal analyses of prenatal and postnatal lead exposure and early cognitive development. N Engl J Med 316:1037–1043, 1987

Berg CZ, Rapoport JL, Wolff RP: Behavioral treatment for obsessive-compulsive disorder in childhood, in Obsessive-Compulsive Disorder in Children and Adolescents. Edited by Rapoport JL. Washington, DC, American Psychiatric Press, 1989, pp 169–188

Brazelton TB: Neonatal Behavioral Assessment Scale. Philadelphia, PA, JB Lippincott, 1973

Brent DA, Crumrine PK, Varma RR, et al: Phenobarbital treatment and major depressive disorder in children with epilepsy. Pediatrics 80:909–917, 1987

Brown G, Chadwick O, Shaffer D, et al: A prospective study of children with head injuries, III: psychiatric sequelae. Psychol Med 11:63–78, 1981

Bruun RD, Shapiro AK, Shapiro E, et al: A follow-up of 78 patients with Gilles de la Tourette's syndrome. Am J Psychiatry 133:944–947, 1976

Chadwick O, Rutter M, Brown G, et al: A prospective study of children with head injuries, II: cognitive sequelae. Psychol Med 11:49–61, 1981

Chasnoff IJ, Griffith DR, MacGregor S, et al: Temporal patterns of cocaine use in pregnancy: perinatal outcome. JAMA 261:1741–1744, 1989

Clarren SK, Smith DW: The fetal alcohol syndrome. N Engl J Med 298:1063–1067, 1978

Cohen DJ, Shaywitz BA, Caparulo B, et al: Chronic, multiple tics of Gilles de la Tourette's disease: CSF acid monoamine metabolites after probenecid administration. Arch Gen Psychiatry 35:245–250, 1978

Cohen DJ, Detlor J, Young JG, et al: Clonidine ameliorates Gilles de la Tourette Syndrome. Arch Gen Psychiatry 37:1350–1357, 1980

Conners CK: Symptom patterns in hyperkinetic, neurotic, and normal children. Child Dev 41:667–682, 1970

Cook EH, Terry EJ, Heller W, et al: Fluoxetine treatment of borderline mentally retarded adults with obsessive-compulsive disorder. J Clin Psychopharmacol 10:228–229, 1990

Cook EH, Rowlett R, Jaselskis C, et al: Fluoxetine treatment of patients with autism and mental retardation. J Am Acad Child Adolesc Psychiatry (in press)

Courchesne E, Yeung CR, Press GA, et al: Hypoplasia of cerebellar vermal lobules VI and VII in autism. N Engl J Med 318:1349–1354, 1988

Cullen S, O'Connell E, Blake NS, et al: Atlantoaxial instability in Down's syndrome: clinical and radiological screening. Ir Med J 82:64–65, 1989

Dahl EK, Cohen DJ, Provence S: Clinical and multivariate approaches to the nosology of pervasive developmental disorders. J Am Acad Child Psychiatry 25:170–180, 1986

Dekaban AS: Abnormalities in children exposed to x-radiation during various stages of gestation: tentative timetable of radiation injury to the human fetus, part I. J Nucl Med 9:471–477, 1968

Denckla MB: Revised neurological examination for subtle signs (1985). Psychopharmacol Bull 21:773–789, 1985

Denckla MB: Neurological examination, in Obsessive-Compulsive Disorder in Children and Adolescents. Edited by Rapoport JL. Washington, DC, American Psychiatric Press, 1989, pp 107–115

Deykin EY, Macmahon B: The incidence of seizures among children with autistic symptoms. Am J Psychiatry 136:1310–1312, 1979

Donnelly M, Rapoport JL: Attention deficit disorders, in Diagnosis and Psychopharmacology of Childhood and Adolescent Disorders. Edited by Wiener JM. New York, John Wiley, 1985, pp 179–197

Dykens EM, Hodapp RM, Ort S, et al: The trajectory of cognitive development in males with fragile X syndrome. J Am Acad Child Adolesc Psychiatry 28:422–426, 1989

Ellenberg JH, Hirtz DG, Nelson KB: Do seizures in children cause intellectual deterioration? N Engl J Med 314:1085–1088, 1986

Falconer J, Wada JA, Martin W, et al: PET, CT, and MRI imaging of neuronal migration abnormalities in epileptic patients. Can J Neurol Sci 17:35–39, 1990

Fergusson DM, Fergusson JE, Horwood LJ, et al: A longitudinal study of dentine lead levels, intelligence, school performance and behavior, part III: dentine lead levels and attention/activity. J Child Psychol Psychiatry 29:811–824, 1988

Flament M, Whitaker A, Rapoport JL, et al: An epidemiological study of obsessive-compulsive disorder in adolescence, in Obsessive-Compulsive Disorder in Children and Adolescents. Edited by Rapoport JL. Washington, DC, American Psychiatric Press, 1989, pp 253–267

Folstein SE, Rutter ML: Autism: familial aggregation and genetic implications. J Autism Dev Disord 18:3–30, 1988

Forehand R, Atkeson BM: Generality of treatment effects with parents as therapists: a review of assessment and implementation procedures. Behavior Therapy 8:575–593, 1977

Gillingham FJ: Surgical treatment of epilepsy: restoration of personality? Acta Neurochir 44S:102–105, 1988

Gittelman R, Mannuzza S, Shenker R, et al: Hyperactive boys almost grown up, I: psychiatric status. Arch Gen Psychiatry 42:937–947, 1985

Goldstein DJ, Sheaffer CI: Ratio developmental quotients from the Bayley are comparable to later IQs from the Stanford-Binet. Am J Ment Retard 92:379–380, 1988

Gordon C, Rapoport J, Hamburger S, et al: Differential response of autistic disorder to clomipramine. J Am Acad Child Adolesc Psychiatry 30:164, 1991

Hagerman RJ, Murphy MA, Wittenberger MD: A controlled trial of stimulant medication in children with the fragile X syndrome. Am J Med Genet 30:377–392, 1988

Hans SL: Developmental consequences of prenatal exposure to methadone. Ann NY Acad Sci 562:195–207, 1989

Hollander E, Schiffman E, Cohen B, et al: Signs of central nervous system dysfunction in obsessive-compulsive disorder. Arch Gen Psychiatry 47:27–32, 1990

Hoyseth KS, Jones PJH: Ethanol induced teratogenesis: characterization, mechanisms and diagnostic approaches. Life Sci 44:643–649, 1989

Huret JL, Delabar JM, Marlhens F, et al: Down syndrome with duplication of a region of chromosome 21 containing the CuZn superoxide dismutase gene without detectable karyotypic abnormality. Hum Genet 75:251–257, 1987

Huttenlocher PR: Synaptogenesis in the human visual cortex: evidence for synapse elimination during normal development. Neurosci Lett 33:247–252, 1982

Huttenlocher PR, Hapke RJ: A follow-up study of intractable seizures in childhood. Ann Neurol 28:699–705, 1990

Insel TR, Scanlan J, Champoux M, et al: Rearing paradigm in a nonhuman primate affects response to beta-CCE challenge. Psychopharmacology 96:81–86, 1988

Jagger J, Prusoff BA, Cohen DJ, et al: The epidemiology of Tourette's syndrome: a pilot study. Schizophr Bull 8:267–278, 1982

Jankovic J, Caskey TC, Stout JT, et al: Lesch-Nyhan syndrome: a study of motor behavior and cerebrospinal fluid neurotransmitters. Ann Neurol 23:466–469, 1988

Kanner L: Autistic disturbances of affective contact. Nervous Child 2:217–250, 1943

Kendall PC, Braswell L: Cognitive-Behavioral Therapy for Impulsive Children. New York, Guilford, 1985

Knusel B, Winslow JW, Rosenthal A, et al: Promotion of central cholinergic and dopaminergic neuron differentiation by brain-derived neurotrophic factor but not neurotrophin 3. Proc Natl Acad Sci U S A 88:961–965, 1991

Kremer EJ, Pritchard M, Lynch M, et al: Mapping of DNA instability at the fragile X to a trinucleotide repeat sequence p(CCG)n. Science 252:1711–1714, 1991

Kun LE, Mulhern RK, Crisco JJ: Quality of life in children treated for brain tumors: intellectual, emotional, and academic function. J Neurosurg 58:1–6, 1983

LaVigna GW: Nonaversive strategies for managing behavior problems, in Handbook of Autism and Pervasive Developmental Disorders. Edited by Cohen DJ, Donnellan AM. New York, John Wiley, 1987, pp 418–429

LaVigna GW, Donnellan A: Alternatives to Punishment:

Solving Behavior Problems With Non-Aversive Strategies. New York, Irvington, 1986

Leckman JF, Cohen DJ: Descriptive and diagnostic classification of tic disorders, in Tourette's Syndrome and Tic Disorders: Clinical Understanding and Treatment. Edited by Cohen DJ, Bruun RD, Leckman JF. New York, John Wiley, 1988, pp 3–20

Le Couteur A, Rutter M, Lord C, et al: Autism Diagnostic Interview: a standardized investigator-based instrument. J Autism Dev Disord 19:363–388, 1989

Lenke RR, Levy HL: Maternal phenylketonuria and hyperphenylalaninemia: an international survey of the outcome of untreated and treated pregnancies. N Engl J Med 303:1202–1208, 1980

Lenneberg E: Biological Foundations of Language. New York, John Wiley, 1967

Leonard HL, Swedo SE, Rapoport JL, et al: Treatment of obsessive-compulsive disorder with clomipramine and desipramine in children and adolescents: a double-blind crossover comparison. Arch Gen Psychiatry 46: 1088–1092, 1989

Levine S, Huttenlocher P, Banich M, et al: Factors affecting cognitive functioning of hemiplegic children. Dev Med Child Neurol 29:27–35, 1987

Lindsay J, Ounsted C, Richards P: Long-term outcome in children with temporal lobe seizures, I: social outcome and childhood factors. Dev Med Child Neurol 21:285–298, 1979a

Lindsay J, Ounsted C, Richards P: Long-term outcome in children with temporal lobe seizures, III: psychiatric aspects in childhood and adult life. Dev Med Child Neurol 21:630–636, 1979b

Long CG, Moore JR: Parental expectations for their epileptic children. J Child Psychol Psychiatry 20:299–312, 1979

Lord C, Schopler E: Intellectual and developmental assessment of autistic children from preschool to schoolage: clinical implications of two follow-up studies, in Diagnosis and Assessment in Autism. Edited by Schopler E, Mesibov G. New York, Plenum, 1988, pp 167–181

Lord C, Rutter M, Goode S, et al: Autism Diagnostic Observation Schedule: a standardized observation of communicative and social behavior. J Autism Dev Disord 19:185–212, 1989

Lund J: The prevalence of psychiatric morbidity in mentally retarded adults. Acta Psychiatr Scand 72:563–570, 1985

Luxenberg JS, Swedo SE, Flament MF, et al: Neuroanatomical abnormalities in obsessive-compulsive disorder detected with quantitative X-ray computed tomography. Am J Psychiatry 145:1089–1093, 1988

McKeon J, McGuffin P, Robinson P: Obsessive-compulsive neurosis following head injury: a report of 4 cases. Br J Psychiatry 144:190–192, 1984

McMichael AJ, Baghurst PA, Wigg NR, et al: Port Pirie cohort study: environmental exposure to lead and children's abilities at the age of four years. N Engl J Med 319:468–475, 1988

Mahaffey KR, Annest JL, Roberts J, et al: National estimates of blood lead levels: United States, 1976–1980: association with selected demographic and socioeconomic factors. N Engl J Med 307:573–579, 1982

Maisonpierre PC, Belluscio L, Squinto S, et al: Neurotrophin-3: a neurotrophic factor related to NGF and BDNF. Science 247:1446–1451, 1990

Menkes JH: Metabolic diseases of the nervous system, in Textbook of Child Neurology. Edited by Menkes JH. Philadelphia, PA, Lea & Febiger, 1990a, pp 28–138

Menkes JH: Textbook of Pediatric Neurology. Philadelphia, PA, Lea & Febiger, 1990b

Menkes JH: Toxic and metabolic disorders, in Textbook of Child Neurology. Edited by Menkes JH. Philadelphia, PA, Lea & Febiger, 1990c, pp 497–525

Mesibov GB, Schopler E, Schaffer B, et al: Use of the Childhood Autism Rating Scale with autistic adolescents and adults. J Am Acad Child Adolesc Psychiatry 28:538–541, 1989

Meyersburg HA, Post RM: An holistic developmental view of neural and psychological processes: a neurobiologic-psychoanalytic integration. Br J Psychiatry 135:139–155, 1979

Miller RW: Delayed effects in atomic-bomb survivors: major observations by the Atomic Bomb Casualty Commission are evaluated. Science 166:569–574, 1969

Mundy P, Sigman M: The theoretical implications of joint-attention deficits in autism. Development and Psychopathology 1:173–183, 1989

New England Congenital Hypothyroidism Collaborative: Elementary school performance of children with congenital hypothyroidism. J Pediatr 116:27–32, 1990

Nyhan WL: Behavior in the Lesch-Nyhan syndrome. Journal of Autism and Childhood Schizophrenia 6:235–252, 1976

Oberlé I, Rousseau F, Heitz D, et al: Instability of a 550-base pair DNA segment and abnormal methylation in fragile X syndrome. Science 252:1097–1102, 1991

Okano Y, Eisensmith RC, Güttler F, et al: Molecular basis of phenotypic heterogeneity in phenylketonuria. N Engl J Med 324:1232–1238, 1991

Park JP, Wurster-Hill DH, Andrews PA, et al: Free proximal trisomy 21 without the Down syndrome. Clin Genet 32:342–348, 1987

Pauls DL, Leckman JF: The inheritance of Gilles de la Tourette's syndrome and associated behaviors. N Engl J Med 315:993–997, 1986

Pleak RR, Birmaher B, Gavrilescu A, et al: Mania and neuropsychiatric excitation following carbamazepine. J Am Acad Child Adolesc Psychiatry 4:500–503, 1988

Purves D, Lichtman JW: Principles of Neural Development. Sunderland, MA, Sinauer, 1985

Rakic P: Defects of neuronal migration and the pathogenesis of cortical malformations, in Progress in Brain Research. Edited by Boer GJ, Feenstra MGP, Mirmiran M, et al. New York, Elsevier, 1988, pp 15–37

Realmuto GM, Garfinkel BD, Tuchman M, et al: Psychiatric diagnosis and behavioral characteristics of phenylketonuric children. J Nerv Ment Dis 174:536–540, 1986

Reiss AL, Freund L: Fragile X syndrome. Biol Psychiatry 27:223–240, 1990

Reiss AL, Aylward E, Freund LS, et al: Neuroanatomy of

the fragile X syndrome: the posterior fossa. Ann Neurol 29:26–32, 1991

Reiss S, Benson BA: Awareness of negative social conditions among mentally retarded, emotionally disturbed outpatients. Am J Psychiatry 141:88–90, 1984

Riddle MA, Hardin MT, Towbin KE, et al: Tardive dyskinesia following haloperidol treatment in Tourette's syndrome. Arch Gen Psychiatry 44:98–99, 1987

Ritvo ER, Mason-Brothers A, Freeman BJ, et al: The UCLA-University of Utah epidemiological survey of autism: the etiologic role of rare diseases. Am J Psychiatry 147:1614–1621, 1990

Rovet J, Ehrlich R, Sorbara D: Intellectual outcome in children with fetal hypothyroidism. J Pediatr 110:700–704, 1987

Rumble B, Retallack R, Hilbich C, et al: Amyloid A4 protein and its precursor in Down's syndrome and Alzheimer's disease. N Engl J Med 320:1446–1452, 1989

Rutter M: Infantile autism, in The Clinical Guide to Child Psychiatry. Edited by Shaffer D, Ehrhardt AA, Greenhill LL. New York, Free Press, 1985, pp 48–78

Rutter M, Greenfield D, Lockyer L: A five to fifteen year follow-up study of infantile psychosis, II: social and behavioural outcome. Br J Psychiatry 113:1183–1199, 1967

Rutter M, Chadwick O, Shaffer D: Head injury, in Developmental Neuropsychiatry. Edited by Rutter M. New York, Guilford, 1983, pp 83–111

Schilder P: The organic background of obsessions and compulsions. Am J Psychiatry 94:1397–1416, 1938

Shaffer D, Schonfeld I, O'Connor PA, et al: Neurological soft signs. Arch Gen Psychiatry 42:342–351, 1985

Shapiro AK, Shapiro E: Controlled study of pimozide vs. placebo in Tourette's syndrome. J Am Acad Child Psychiatry 23:161–173, 1984

Shaywitz SE, Cohen DJ, Shaywitz BA: Behavior and learning difficulties in children of normal intelligence born to alcoholic mothers. J Pediatr 96:978–982, 1980

Swedo SE, Rapoport JL: Phenomenology and differential diagnosis of obsessive-compulsive disorder in children and adolescents, in Obsessive-Compulsive Disorder in Children and Adolescents. Edited by Rapoport JL. Washington, DC, American Psychiatric Press, 1989, pp 13–32

Swedo SE, Rapoport JL, Cheslow DL, et al: High prevalence of obsessive-compulsive symptoms in patients with Sydenham's chorea. Am J Psychiatry 146:246–249, 1989a

Swedo SE, Schapiro MB, Grady CL, et al: Cerebral glucose metabolism in childhood-onset obsessive-compulsive disorder. Arch Gen Psychiatry 46:518–523, 1989b

Tanguay PE: Infantile autism and social communication spectrum disorder. J Am Acad Child Adolesc Psychiatry 29:854, 1990

Thorndike R, Hagen E, Sattler J: Standford-Binet Intelligence Scale 4th Edition. Chicago, Il, Riverside, 1986

Towbin KE, Riddle MA, Leckman JF, et al: The clinical care of individuals with Tourette's syndrome, in Tourette's Syndrome and Tic Disorders: Clinical Understanding and Treatment. Edited by Cohen DJ, Bruun RD, Leckman JF. New York, John Wiley, 1988, pp 329–352

Ullmann RK, Sleator EK, Sprague RL: A new rating scale for diagnosis and monitoring of ADD children. Psychopharmacol Bull 20:160–164, 1984

Verkerk AJMH, Pieretti M, Sutcliffe JS, et al: Identification of a gene (FMR-1) containing a CGG repeat coincident with a breakpoint cluster region exhibiting length variation in fragile X syndrome. Cell 65:905–914, 1991

Vining EPG, Mellits D, Dorsen MM, et al: Psychologic and behavioral effects of antiepileptic drugs in children: a double-blind comparison between phenobarbital and valproic acid. Pediatrics 80:165–174, 1987

Voeller KKS, Rothenberg MB: Psychosocial aspects of the management of seizures in children. Pediatrics 51: 1072–1082, 1973

Volkmar FR, Nelson DS: Seizure disorders in autism. J Am Acad Child Adolesc Psychiatry 29:127–129, 1990

Waldo MC, Cohen DJ, Caparulo BS, et al: EEG profiles of neuropsychiatrically disturbed children. J Am Acad Child Psychiatry 17:656–670, 1978

Watts RW, Spellacy E, Gibbs DA, et al: Clinical, postmortem, biochemical and therapeutic observations on the Lesch-Nyhan syndrome with particular reference to the neurological manifestations. Q J Med 51:43–78, 1982

Wechsler D: Manual for the Wechsler Intelligence Scale for Children. Revised. New York, Psychological Corporation, 1974

Wiesel TN, Hubel DH, Lam DM-K: Autoradiographic demonstration of ocular-dominance columns in the monkey striate cortex by means of transneuronal transport. Brain Res 79:273–279, 1974

Wing L: Asperger's syndrome: a clinical account. Psychol Med 11:115–129, 1981

Yarbro MT, Anderson JA: L-Tryptophan metabolism in phenylketonuria. J Pediatr 68:895–904, 1966

Zimmer DB, Van Eldik LJ: Levels and distribution of the calcium-modulated proteins S100 and calmodulin in rat C6 glioma cells. J Neurochem 50:572–579, 1988

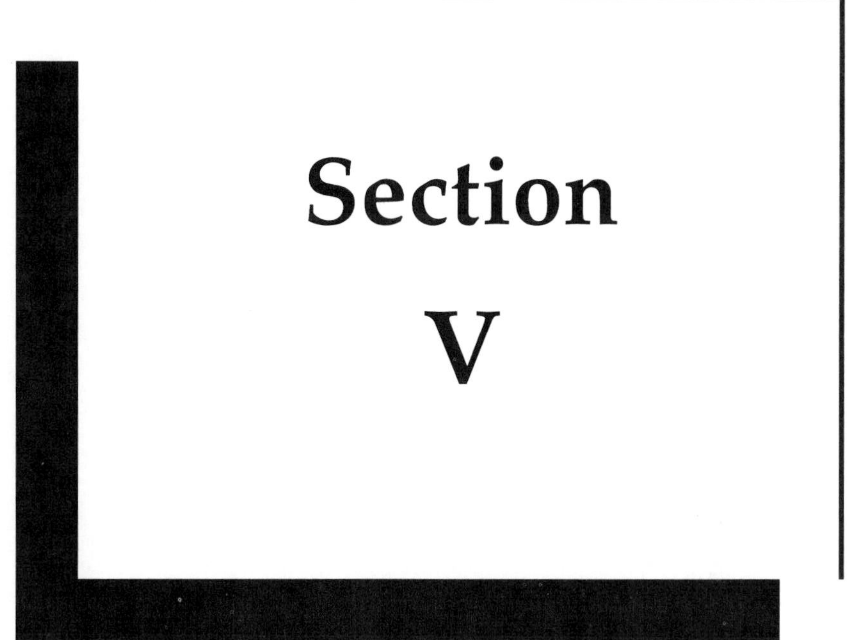

Section V

Neuropsychiatric Treatments

Chapter

29

Psychopharmacological Treatment in Neuropsychiatry

Steven L. Dubovsky, M.D.

PSYCHOTROPIC MEDICATIONS are used extensively in patients with neurological illnesses. This chapter addresses the major classes of physical intervention used in psychiatry, with special attention to the neurological setting. Introductory discussions are followed by summaries of the major side effects of psychiatric and neurological uses and the important interactions. Each section is more or less self-contained to permit easy access by the clinician to information about each topic.

Because the focus of this chapter is on psychopharmalogical applications in the neuropsychiatric setting, the reader is referred to more general texts and to the review articles cited as recommended reading for discussions of broader issues in biological therapies in psychiatry.

❑ HETEROCYCLIC ANTIDEPRESSANTS

First reported to be effective in depression in 1957 after imipramine was synthesized in a search for a structural analogue to chlorpromazine, heterocyclic antidepressants (HCAs) have become the first line of drug therapy for depression. All HCAs are of approximately equal efficacy; their side-effect profiles, however, permit considerable flexibility in treating patients with neurological illnesses. Antidepressants currently available in the United States are summarized in Table 29–1.

Antidepressants referred to as *heterocyclics* have a number of different structures, all of which include rings containing carbon, nitrogen, and/or oxygen atoms (Figure 29–1). The tricyclic antide-

TABLE 29–1. HETEROCYCLIC ANTIDEPRESSANTS CURRENTLY AVAILABLE IN THE UNITED STATES

Drug	*Trade name*	*Structure*	*Usual daily dose (mg)*	*Upper daily limit (mg)*	*Usual daily dose in elderly (mg)*
Amitriptyline	Elavil	Tertiary amine[a]	150–300	300	50–100
Nortriptyline	Pamelor; Aventyl	Secondary amine[a]	75–125[b]	150[b]	25–50
Protriptyline	Vivactil	Secondary amine[a]	30–40	60	15–20
Imipramine	Tofranil	Tertiary amine[a]	150–200[b]	300	25–100
Desipramine	Norpramin; Pertofrane	Secondary amine[a]	150–250[b]	300	25–100
Trimipramine	Surmontil	Tertiary amine[a]	150–200	300	50–100
Clomipramine	Anafranil	Tertiary amine[a]	150–250	300	75–150
Doxepin	Sinequan	Tertiary amine[a]	150–250	300	25–50
Amoxapine	Asendin	Dibenzoxazepine	150–300	600	75–300
Maprotiline	Ludiomil	Tetracyclic	150–200	300	50–75
Trazodone	Desyrel	Triazolopyridine	150–400[c]	600	50–150
Fluoxetine	Prozac	Propylamine	5–40	100	5–20
Bupropion	Wellbutrin	Aminoketone	300–450[c]	450	150–300

[a]Tricyclic.
[b]Dosage should be adjusted according to blood level.
[c]Dose may have to be divided because of short half-life.

pressants (TCAs) are structurally related to the phenothiazines. The tertiary (i.e., three methyl groups) amines imipramine and amitriptyline differ from each other only in the presence of a nitrogen versus a carbon atom in position 5 of the middle ring. Desipramine and nortriptyline, the secondary amine congeners of these TCAs, have one less methyl group. Newer antidepressants provide variations on the tricyclic structure or novel arrangements such as tetracyclic or bicyclic formulas.

Because HCAs are extensively metabolized by the liver after oral administration, conditions that affect microsomal enzyme activity can significantly alter antidepressant levels. Alcohol, anticonvulsants, barbiturates, oral contraceptives, and antidepressants themselves may stimulate liver enzymes, decreasing blood levels of the antidepressant and leading to unexpected treatment failures or relapses in compliant patients. Some substances (e.g., phenothiazines and methylphenidate) compete with HCAs for metabolizing enzymes, slowing the rate of breakdown of both the antidepressant and the other drug. This may be one basis for the synergistic action of neuroleptics and stimulants with antidepressants (Baldessarini 1985).

The long half-life of most HCAs (from 10–20 hours for imipramine to 80 hours for protriptyline [Baldessarini 1985; Lydiard 1985]) makes once-daily dosing possible for all preparations except trazodone and bupropion. Inherited patterns of metabolism of HCAs probably account for two clinical phenomena. First, a patient with a blood relative who has responded to a particular medication is more likely to respond to that drug as well. Second, there is wide interindividual variation in blood levels produced by the same dose of a given drug. The clinical significance of the latter observation is complicated because response to antidepressants has been shown to be clearly correlated with blood levels only for nortriptyline, imipramine, desipramine, and possibly amitriptyline (American Psychiatric Association 1985; Lydiard 1985), and questions have even arisen about these correlations (Lydiard 1985).

Nortriptyline usually has a therapeutic window of 50–150 ng/ml, but some individuals only respond at levels of 100–150 mg/ml (Rubin et al. 1985). The likelihood of clinical response increases as blood levels of imipramine (plus desipramine) approach 200–225 ng/ml; higher levels may lead to more side effects without a better clinical effect. Desipramine is more predictably effective at concentrations greater than 125 ng/ml, and some patients exhibit decreased effectiveness at levels greater than 250 ng/ml. Although the relationship between blood levels and effectiveness of other antidepressants remains to be clarified, preliminary observations suggest that a range of 125–300 ng/ml of parent compound plus demethylated metabolite of tricyclics may be satisfactory for most patients (Baldessarini 1985; Lydiard 1985).

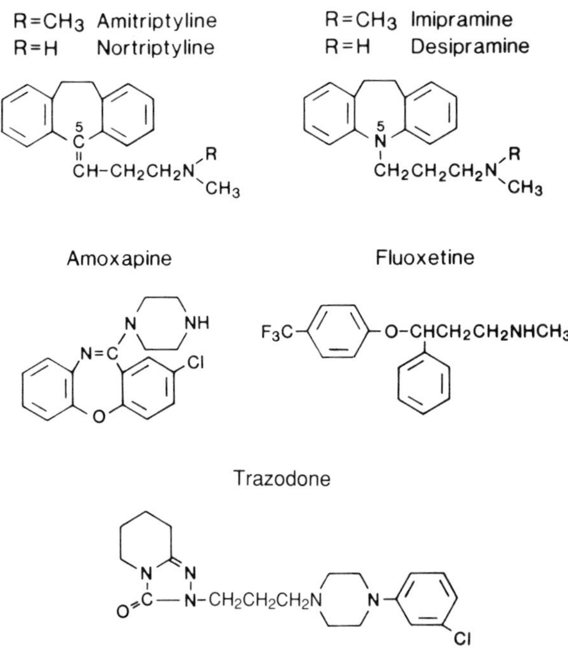

Figure 29–1. Structures of some heterocyclic antidepressants.

Antidepressant blood levels are most appropriately used to adjust the dose of nortriptyline, desipramine, and imipramine; to investigate the reason for failure to respond to an adequate dose of other antidepressants; to evaluate slow metabolism as a cause of toxicity at low doses; and possibly to determine the correct dose of an antidepressant under urgent circumstances (American Psychiatric Association 1985). Blood levels should be measured in adults about 1 week after each dose adjustment (90% of the steady-state concentration is achieved in 3.3 half-lives). Up to 2 weeks should elapse after a dosage change in elderly and medically ill patients before blood levels of antidepressants are measured (Baldessarini 1985; Lydiard 1985).

Recommendations about dosage limitations for several HCAs are beginning to emerge. In the treatment of depression, doses of fluoxetine greater than 40 mg may produce no more improvement but more side effects (Wernicke et al. 1988). The long half-life of this drug, which lengthens the time to achieve a steady state, may explain why up to 8 weeks are necessary for some patients to achieve a therapeutic response to a given dosage of fluoxetine (Schweitzer et al. 1990). On the other hand, doses up to 100 mg/day of fluoxetine may be necessary to treat obsessive-compulsive disorder (OCD), bulimia, and obesity (Ayd 1990a). Higher doses of chlorimipramine may also be necessary for OCD (Greist et al. 1990). Doses greater than 225 mg of maprotiline and 450 mg of bupropion should not be exceeded because of an increased risk of seizures.

Mechanisms of Action

For many years the effectiveness of antidepressants was attributed to blockade of uptake into the presynaptic neuron of brain monoamine transmitters, especially norepinephrine, serotonin, and (to a lesser extent) dopamine (Richelson 1984). Although it is still thought that the beneficial effect of some antidepressants could, in part, be related to increased functional availability of serotonin (Charney et al. 1984), recent research has suggested that some of the chronic actions of HCAs on receptor mechanisms may actually decrease net noradrenergic activity (Siever and Davis 1985; Sugrue 1983). β-Adrenergic receptor down-regulation may be one antidepressant effect associated with its therapeutic action. This change might be primary or could be a homeostatic response to increased amounts of neurotransmitter resulting from reuptake blockade.

On the other hand, most antidepressants do seem to enhance serotonergic transmission and some (e.g., bupropion) increase dopaminergic transmission. As they have begun to look beyond single transmitter systems, investigators have become interested in the effects of antidepressants on dysregulated interactions between multiple transmitter systems (Goodman and Charney 1985; Siever and Davis 1985) and on cell membrane, G proteins, or intracellular second messengers that might explain how multiple transmitter systems are affected (Dubovsky and Franks 1983). These and other hypotheses remain more or less inferential, and any observed effect of antidepressants on a particular biologic system may be incidental to the action that actually produces therapeutic benefit. In addition, some transmitter changes (e.g., acutely enhanced noradrenergic tone) may explain side effects (e.g., jitteriness) rather than a primary action.

Psychiatric Uses of HCAs in the Presence of Neurological Disease

HCAs have been found to be useful in the treatment of depression, panic anxiety, generalized anxiety, bulimia, posttraumatic stress disorder, OCD, and probably some symptoms associated with borderline personality disorder (Goodman and Charney 1985). Using antidepressants for psychiatric indications in neurological patients requires great skill when the psychiatric disorder is caused, obscured, or complicated by disease of the brain and when side effects of the medications can aggravate the neurological illness.

Depression and Organic Brain Disease

A number of drugs and illnesses can produce depression, which may or may not be accompanied by signs of delirium or dementia. About 40% of stroke patients develop depression; the risk is greater with left-hemisphere strokes, especially in the frontal lobe (Robinson et al. 1990). Human immunodeficiency virus (HIV) infection commonly is associated with mental changes that include depression and mania, which may occur in an apparently clear sensorium. Anticonvulsants, tranquilizers, antineoplastic agents, and adrenal steroids are common causes of depression in neurological patients. Of patients taking prednisone, 1% of those taking 40 mg/day, 5% of those taking 40–80 mg/day, and 18% of those taking 80 mg/day develop depression, mania, delirium, or psychosis, especially if the dose is increased or decreased rapidly (Rogers 1985). Psychiatric symptoms usually begin within 10 days of beginning steroids and remit shortly after the drug is discontinued, but the onset of symptoms may be delayed and they may continue after withdrawal of the medication (Rogers 1985).

The most appropriate approach to organically induced depression is to treat the underlying disorder or withdraw the offending drug. However, if the illness cannot be reversed immediately or if it would be unsafe to reduce the dose of medication, an antidepressant may ameliorate the depressive symptoms. Precautions discussed below for administering antidepressants to patients with compromised brain reserves should be observed.

Antidepressants may also be useful for patients in whom depression mimics or is accompanied by organic brain disease, even when an obvious irreversible cause of dementia is present. For example, depression may further slow thinking, increase confusion, or make the patient less inclined to marshal whatever intellectual resources remain, resulting in an apparent cognitive deficit that is out of proportion to the actual degree of organic impairment. Depression probably also produces primary cognitive deficits, particularly those attributable to right-hemisphere dysfunction. A course of antidepressant therapy may be reasonable for newly diagnosed dementia patients without reversible causes on the grounds that there may be a component of depressive pseudodementia.

A different problem occurs when organic disturbances that affect the right hemisphere or the balance between the hemispheres impair the ability to express emotion normally. Instead of being obvious, depressive affect, thinking, and behavior in these instances may be expressed as distorted derivatives such as failure to recover from the neurological illness, emotional lability, negativism, paranoia, hostility, confusion, mutism, catatonia, assaultiveness, noncompliance, and expression of a wish to die (Ross and Rush 1981). Only a course of antidepressants or electroconvulsive therapy (ECT) may resolve the behavioral disorder, which may persist after the underlying neurological disorder has been successfully treated (Dubovsky 1986b; Ross and Rush 1981).

Because they can further impair cortical function or depress the reticular activating system, strongly anticholinergic and sedating antidepressants can be problematic for patients with organic brain syndromes. Appropriate HCAs for demented patients include desipramine, maprotiline, trazodone, or fluoxetine.

Antidepressants in the Elderly

Because organic brain syndromes and other neurological syndromes frequently occur in elderly patients, it is important to know about the differences between patients in this age group and younger patients that influence dosage and choice of antidepressants (Salzman 1985). First, there is slower demethylation of tertiary amines (which tend to produce more anticholinergic, sedative, and hypotensive side effects) to the less toxic secondary amines. The clearance of all antidepressants is slowed in the elderly, and this leads to higher blood levels and prolonged activity of all compounds. At the same time, the central nervous system (CNS) of elderly individuals is more sensitive to the toxic as well as therapeutic effect of antidepressants. For these reasons, secondary compounds are often less troublesome than tertiary preparations, as are methylphenidate and newer antidepressants with less anticholinergic and sedating potential.

For elderly patients, the dose of all antidepressants should be increased slowly, and the final dose should usually be lower than that for younger patients (Table 29–1). Using an antidepressant for which blood level can meaningfully be measured is a useful strategy when the clinician is unsure of the appropriate dose of these drugs. Nortriptyline has been shown to be low in hypotensive potential in the elderly, and this is probably also true of desipramine. TCAs have antiarrhythmic properties that may make it possible to discontinue or reduce the dose of other type I antiarrhythmics such as procainamide, quinidine, and disopyramide.

Antidepressants in Patients With Seizure Disorders

Particularly at higher doses, many antidepressants lower the seizure threshold in epileptic patients, and spontaneous seizures have occasionally been reported in patients without a history of epilepsy who were taking these drugs (Fiori 1977). Maprotiline in doses greater than 225 mg/day and bupropion in doses greater than 450 mg/day are the worst offenders (Pinder et al. 1977), but in lower doses the risk of seizures associated with them is not necessarily higher than that for all HCAs (about 0.5% [Davidson 1989]). The risk of seizures with bupropion is highest in patients with organic brain disease, electroencephalogram (EEG) abnormalities, brain tumors, bulimia, concomitant medications that lower seizure threshold, and high blood levels of bupropion (Davidson 1989). Because amoxapine frequently causes seizures when taken in overdose, it should probably also be avoided in epileptic patients (Litovitz and Troutman 1983). Doxepin and monoamine oxidase inhibitors (MAOIs) may be relatively safe for patients with epilepsy, and secondary amines may be preferable to tertiary amines.

Antidepressants and Movement Disorders

The incidence of depression is high in Parkinson's disease, and levodopa (L-dopa) may increase or produce depression in susceptible patients. From a theoretical standpoint, at least, the more anticholinergic antidepressants such as amitriptyline, protriptyline, doxepin, trimipramine, and imipramine could benefit parkinsonian patients. However, because many of these patients are elderly and are already taking anticholinergic drugs, the same side effect can prove troublesome. The dopaminergic properties of bupropion may prove useful for some parkinsonian patients. Bromocriptine, an ergot alkaloid with established antiparkinsonian properties, may also have antidepressant effects by itself and may augment antidepressants (Sitland-Marslen et al. 1990).

Because it can produce extrapyramidal syndromes (EPS), amoxapine is contraindicated in parkinsonian patients. This drug might be useful, however, for depressed patients with Tourette's syndrome. Its structural relationship to loxapine, a neuroleptic, may also make amoxapine useful in depression associated with bizarre or psychotic symptoms, which are sometimes expressed as atypical physical and neurological complaints. Fluoxetine, which may cause EPS as well as aggravate EPS caused by neuroleptics (Ciraulo and Shader 1990), should be avoided in parkinsonian patients and those taking neuroleptics.

Antidepressants and Urologic Syndromes

Some urologic complications of neurological disease require careful adjustment of antidepressant regimens. Because anticholinergic side effects can be particularly risky for uncatheterized patients with neurogenic bladder, drugs with low anticholinergic potency such as fluoxetine, trazodone, bupropion, and desipramine are preferable. Methylphenidate is even safer when urinary retention is a major concern. Desipramine, amoxapine, maprotiline, and methylphenidate seem less likely to cause erectile and orgasmic dysfunction, which can be a problem with other antidepressants, particularly highly serotonergic drugs such as fluoxetine, clomipramine, and MAOIs. This problem may or may not respond to the antiserotonin drug cyproheptadine or to yohimbine or bethanechol, or it may remit spontaneously. Trazodone causes priapism in 1 in 6,000 cases, usually within 3 days to 18 months of starting doses of 50–400 mg/day (Thompson et al. 1990). Patients with a past history of prolonged erections in association with medication appear to be at greatest risk. A few cases of clitoral enlargement have also been reported (Thompson et al. 1990).

Antidepressant Withdrawal

Antidepressants are usually discontinued slowly (e.g., 25 mg/month of imipramine) to monitor for return of depression. More rapid discontinuation (25 mg every 3–5 days) is possible, but abrupt withdrawal of HCAs may result in abstinence symptoms (probably related to cholinergic rebound) that appear within 12–48 hours after the last dose and last up to 2 weeks after stopping the drug (Dilsaver and Greden 1984; Lawrence 1985). Withdrawal phenomena, which have been estimated to occur in 3%–100% (average 20%–50%) of cases of abrupt discontinuation of HCAs, include gastrointestinal symptoms such as nausea, vomiting, and diarrhea; influenza-like syndromes; anxiety; agitation; insomnia; early-onset nightmares; parkinsonism; and hypomania. Withdrawal symptoms can be attenuated by more gradual discontinuation or, if the antidepressant must be stopped quickly, by adding 0.8 mg of atropine every 3–4 hours (Dilsaver and Greden 1984).

Neurological Uses of Antidepressants

Antidepressants have a number of actions that can be beneficial in some neurological syndromes even if depression is not present. Amitriptyline, imipramine, and doxepin appear to have analgesic effects in chronic pain in doses lower than the usual antidepressant dose (e.g., amitriptyline 75 mg/day) (Rosenblatt et al. 1984). Amitriptyline, imipramine, and trazodone in both low (e.g., imipramine 100 mg/day) and usual antidepressant doses have reduced pain caused by diabetic neuropathy in a few patients (Hoogiverf 1985). Depression is common in patients with chronic pain, and chronically depressed patients frequently complain of pain. However, the antinociceptive action of antidepressants may be unrelated to their effect on depression because the doses for the two disorders are different and one condition may improve while the other remains unchanged. Severe intractable pain of terminal cancer may be controlled by the combination of intravenous haloperidol, lorazepam, and hydromorphone (Adams 1988).

Tinnitus associated with depression is improved but not eradicated by nortriptyline (Sullivan et al. 1989). Fluvoxamine has improved memory in alcohol amnestic disorder but not alcohol dementia (Martin et al. 1989). Amitriptyline has been found to ameliorate pathological laughing and crying (pseudobulbar affect) associated with organic brain disease (Schiffer et al. 1985), and protriptyline may be helpful to some patients with sleep apnea.

In usual doses, amitriptyline has been widely used as a prophylactic agent for migraine headaches (Mathew 1981). Other antidepressants have not been studied systematically in this context, although there is no reason to believe that amitriptyline should be the only effective drug. However, propranolol and other standard antimigraine drugs produce the same or better migraine prophylaxis (Goodman and Charney 1985), and highly serotonergic antidepressants such as fluoxetine may make migraines worse. Histamine, subtype 2 (H_2), receptor blockade may explain the beneficial effects of trimipramine (25–50 mg/day) and doxepin (50–150 mg/day) in peptic ulcer disease (Richelson 1985b). These drugs are as effective as cimetidine, but cheaper, easier to monitor, and less toxic. Their anticholinergic effects, however, are additive with other anticholinergic drugs taken by ulcer patients.

Neurological Side Effects of HCAs

HCAs have a number of side effects that require consideration in neurological practice. Important syndromes and drugs that commonly cause these side effects are listed in Table 29–2 (Baldessarini 1985; Baldessarini and Marsh 1990; Demuth et al. 1985; Fiori 1977; Herman et al. 1990; Teicher et al. 1990).

Interactions of HCAs With Neurological Drugs

Cyclic antidepressants interact with many medications that are used in neurological and psychiatric practice. Some important interactions include the following (Baldessarini 1985; Bernstein 1983; Graham et al. 1974; Lydiard 1985; Pearson 1990; Salzman 1985):

1. Additive anticholinergic effects with antiparkinsonian drugs, antihistamines, and neuroleptics.
2. Increase of antidepressant levels by neuroleptics, methylphenidate, amphetamine, and disulfiram.
3. Increase of neuroleptic and stimulant levels by antidepressants.
4. Decrease of antidepressant levels by alcohol, anticonvulsants (such as phenytoin), carbamazepine and barbiturates, oral contraceptives, cigarette smoking, and chloral hydrate. (Benzodiazepines [BZDs] do not have a significant effect on antidepressant metabolism.)
5. Increased antidepressant levels due to displacement of binding of antidepressants to albumin

TABLE 29–2. SOME SIDE EFFECTS OF HETEROCYCLICS

Side effect	*Manifestations*	*Drugs*
Anticholinergic	Delirium with tachycardia, warm dry skin, and mydriasis	Amitriptyline, trimipramine, protriptyline, and doxepin (especially when combined with other anticholinergic drugs)
Postural hypotension (α-adrenergic blockade)	Dizziness, unsteadiness, light-headedness, and stumbling on standing up	Tertiary amines, protriptyline, trazodone, and maprotiline
Cardiovascular	Sinus tachycardia	Especially anticholinergic compounds
	Suppression of ventricular arrhythmias	
	Worsening of conduction defects	All but trazodone and fluoxetine
	Cardiac depression	
	Sinus bradycardia	
	Worsening of ventricular arrhythmias	Trazodone
Sedation	Oversedation, impaired cognition, and worsening of organic brain syndrome	Amitriptyline, trimipramine, trazodone, doxepin, and maprotiline
Psychomotor impairment	Impaired driving during first few weeks	Amitriptyline, imipramine, and doxepin; not fluoxetine
Auditory	Tinnitus	Imipramine, probably other TCAs
Urologic	Priapism leading to impotence	Trazodone
	Sexual dysfunction	All antidepressants, especially MAOIs, fluoxetine, and clomipramine
Decreased seizure threshold	Spontaneous seizures or exacerbation of epilepsy	Amoxapine, maprotiline, and tertiary amines
Neuromuscular	Fine tremor and myoclonic jerks	Most tricyclics, maprotiline, trazodone, and fluoxetine
	Peripheral neuropathy	Amitriptyline
	Proximal myopathy	Imipramine
	Phospholipid accumulation in nerve tissue	Imipramine
Extrapyramidal	Parkinsonism and rabbit syndrome	Amoxapine, fluoxetine, imipramine, and amitriptyline in high doses
	Tremor and akathisia	Fluoxetine and amoxapine
	Tardive dyskinesia	Amoxapine
Sleep changes	Increased REM latency, decreased total REM, increased stage 4, and nightmares occasionally when entire dose taken at night	Most heterocyclics
	Insomnia	Fluoxetine and MAOIs
EEG changes	Suppressed alpha	Amitriptyline
	Increased synchronization at low doses	Especially tertiary amines
	Arousal in high doses	
Dermatologic	Skin rash, eosinophilia, and photosensitivity	Tricyclics and maprotiline
Psychiatric	Mania and rapid cycling	Any antidepressant
	Mania in nonbipolar patients	Fluoxetine
	Anxiety, insomnia, and hypervigilance	Noradrenergic HCAs and fluoxetine
	Suicidal or angry obsessions	Fluoxetine
	Aggressive, assaultive, and suicidal behavior	Amitriptyline, imipramine

Note. TCAs = tricyclic antidepressants; MAOIs = monoamine oxidase inhibitors; REM = rapid eye movement; EEG = electroencephalogram; HCAs = heterocyclic antidepressants.

produced by aspirin, phenothiazines, phenylbutazone, aminopyrine, and scopolamine.
6. Potentiation by antidepressants of norepinephrine and amphetamine.
7. Blockade by antidepressants of substances, such as guanethidine, bethanidine, debrisoquin, and tyramine, that must actively be taken up into presynaptic nerve terminals.
8. Blockade of the central antihypertensive effect of clonidine.
9. Increased levels of TCAs, carbamazepine, and possibly neuroleptics by fluoxetine.

Alternatives to Antidepressants

When HCAs are ineffective or produce intolerable side effects in neurological patients, stimulants may ameliorate depression. Doses of 10–90 (usually 15–60) mg/day of methylphenidate or 10–60 (usually 10–45) mg/day of dextroamphetamine have been found useful in treating depression associated with a variety of neurological illnesses. Cognitive deterioration as well as depression may improve in patients with HIV encephalopathy treated with stimulants (Holmes et al. 1989). Addiction and tolerance have not been problems in medically ill patients taking this drug, which can often be discontinued after a month or two without a return of depression (Kaufman et al. 1984). Appetite and sleep often increase as depression begins to remit.

Buspirone may have antidepressant properties in doses of 40–90 mg/day (Rickels et al. 1991; Robinson et al. 1989) and does not aggravate organic mental syndromes. Buspirone may also improve agitation in mentally retarded individuals and those with dementia. Some unipolar and more bipolar depressed patients who cannot tolerate or do not respond to antidepressants may respond to lithium or carbamazepine, with rapid cyclers perhaps responding better to carbamazepine (Ballenger 1988). ECT (discussed below) is an option in more severe cases, even if dementia is present.

When medications for depression cannot be tolerated and ECT is not feasible or appropriate, artificial bright light may be helpful. Bright light therapy is most effective for treatment and prophylaxis of clear-cut seasonal affective disorder but may also be helpful alone or as an adjunct to an antidepressant for the large number of depressed patients with worsening mood in the winter and some without any obvious seasonal variation (Rosenthal et al. 1985). Bright light may also be used to reset sleep phase syndromes such as those associated with work shift change or jet lag. A response usually occurs within a week, and relapse often occurs within 2–3 days of stopping the therapy.

Exposure to 2,500 lux of light for at least 2 hours/day appears necessary with the patient placed within 1 meter of the light; the duration of exposure can sometimes be reduced after the patient responds. Very bright light (e.g., 10,000 lux) may require a briefer exposure, but this has not been proven. Controversy remains about the importance of the timing of the light (e.g., in the morning for patients with a phase delay of the sleep-wake cycle). Patients should experiment with different timing if one schedule does not work, but they should be aware that exposure to light in the evening may cause insomnia. Like any antidepressant treatment, bright light may precipitate hypomania, although this is more likely to remit quickly after withdrawal of the treatment than is HCA-induced mania. Finally, light therapy has not yet been found to be harmful to the eyes.

❑ MONOAMINE OXIDASE INHIBITORS

After the discovery that iproniazid, a monoamine oxidase inhibitor (MAOI) antituberculous drug, could produce euphoria and hyperactivity, there was great enthusiasm for this class of drug as a potential antidepressant. Later, the risk of hepatotoxicity with iproniazid, the need for dietary restrictions, and studies (probably using inadequate doses) suggesting that MAOIs were not effective antidepressants led to an equally rapid decline in their use, at least in the United States. More recent research has solidified the place of MAOIs in the psychiatric armamentarium, especially for the treatment of depression associated with anxiety, mood reactivity, sensitivity to rejection, leaden paralysis, and reverse vegetative symptoms; chronic depression; depression resistant to other therapies; phobic-anxiety states; panic anxiety; agoraphobia; bulimia; OCD; and posttraumatic stress disorder (Baldessarini 1985; Bernstein 1983; Klein et al. 1980; Pare 1985; Quitkin et al. 1979).

Five MAOIs are now in common psychiatric use in the United States (Table 29–3). Nonhydrazines are theoretically safer for patients with liver disease; the risk of hepatic damage is greatest with isocarboxazid. Tranylcypromine inhibits monoamine oxidase (MAO) faster than other MAOIs and may have

TABLE 29–3. MONOAMINE OXIDASE INHIBITORS (MAOIs) AVAILABLE IN THE UNITED STATES

Class	*Drug*	*Trade name*	*Usual daily dose (mg)*	*Acceptable dose limit (mg)*[a]
Hydrazine	Phenelzine	Nardil	45–60	90
	Isocarboxazid	Marplan	20–30	40
Nonhydrazine	Tranylcypromine	Parnate	20–40	80
	Pargyline	Eutonyl	10–25	100
Phenylethylamine	L-Deprenyl (selegiline)	Eldepryl	10–40[b]	60

[a]Higher doses necessary for rapid metabolizers.
[b]Antiparkinsonian dose = 5–10 mg/day.

amphetamine-like properties related to release and blockade of reuptake of norepinephrine. L-Deprenyl (selegiline), a new MAOI used to treat Parkinson's disease, is an effective antidepressant at higher doses.

MAOIs are usually given in divided doses. With the possible exception of pargyline, the last dose of an MAOI should not be taken too late in the day, or activation produced by the drug may result in insomnia. One principal route of metabolism for MAOIs other than phenelzine appears to be by acetylation in the liver (Klein et al. 1980; Pare 1985). About half of the physically healthy Caucasian population are "slow acetylators," which makes them more sensitive to MAOIs because of higher levels with the same dose. "Rapid acetylators," on the other hand, may not achieve therapeutic concentrations easily and may need doses that exceed the recommended range.

Serum concentrations of MAOIs generally are not measured in clinical practice. Inhibition of platelet MAO may be a more valid measure of activity of drugs that affect this enzyme, 80% inhibition being necessary for the effect to become clinically apparent. Because there is often a good correlation between dose administered and response, the test is usually unnecessary in addition to being impractical. However, platelet MAO inhibition may be helpful in deciding whether to increase the dose beyond the usual range in compliant but unresponsive patients who may be rapid metabolizers. Brain MAO inhibition lags 2–3 weeks beyond the rather immediate inhibition of platelet MAO by MAOIs (Klein et al. 1980).

Located on mitochondria, MAO is a ubiquitous enzyme whose function is to inactivate biogenic amines such as norepinephrine, serotonin, dopamine, and tyramine. The enzyme exists in two forms. MAO-A exhibits a preference for serotonin, dopamine, and tyramine and is the principal form of MAO in the lungs, intestine, and placenta. MAO-B preferentially breaks down phenylethylamine and is the principal isoenzyme in platelets and kidney. The brain and liver contain both MAO-A and MAO-B (Baldessarini 1985), although the brain may contain more MAO-B (Tabakoff et al. 1985).

MAOIs irreversibly destroy both forms of MAO, which take up to 2 weeks to regenerate themselves after the drug is stopped. For this reason, dietary restrictions should be observed for 2 weeks after drug discontinuation. Because MAO-A metabolizes tyramine in the gut and limits the amount that is absorbed, inhibition of this enzyme allows increased amounts of tyramine to enter the bloodstream. The inherent pressor effects of tyramine are augmented because more is absorbed while its inactivation by MAOI is slowed throughout the body and in sympathetic nerve terminals.

Two strategies have been investigated to limit adverse reactions related to increased tyramine absorption produced by MAOIs. The first is to develop MAOIs that are selective for one or the other isoenzyme. For example, clorgyline inhibits only MAO-A, whereas L-deprenyl is selective for MAO-B. Because L-deprenyl does not affect the intestinal form of MAO (i.e., MAO-A), the rate of tyramine breakdown in the gut is not decreased, tyramine absorption is not increased, and hypertensive reactions to ingestion of tyramine-containing foods are supposed to be less likely to occur. However, although L-deprenyl is effective for Parkinson's disease at doses at which it inhibits only MAO-B (5–10 mg), it loses its selectivity at doses greater than 10 mg/day, which are necessary for an antidepressant effect. Until claims that deprenyl does not increase sensitivity to tyramine even at nonselective doses (Mann et al. 1989) are confirmed, dietary restrictions should probably be observed at antidepressant doses of L-deprenyl (up to 30–60 mg/day).

Still in its early stages of development, the second approach to reducing the adverse effects of alteration of tyramine metabolism has been to explore "reversible" MAOIs. Theoretically, tyramine could compete with such drugs everywhere in the body for MAO, which would then be temporarily inhibited but not destroyed by the MAOI. If too much tyramine were ingested, the increased amounts would displace the MAOI from the enzyme and would then be metabolized normally.

Mechanisms of Action

It would be tempting to attribute the clinical effectiveness of MAOIs to increased availability of monoamines secondary to reduced degradation; however, this is only one of their actions. Moreover, there may be more than one action that is responsible for the clinical effect, or a combination of mechanisms may be important. For example, inhibition of MAO leads to accumulation not only of neurotransmitters but of substances (e.g., octopamine) that are normally present only in trace amounts. Octopamine, and possibly other compounds, may function as false noradrenergic transmitters that alter functional activity in systems that use those transmitters. Any acute effects on neurotransmitter availability may also be balanced by more enduring changes in receptor functioning. For example, like other antidepressants, MAOIs enhance serotonergic transmission. Further research into possible mechanisms of action of the MAOIs will undoubtedly be stimulated by the recent resurgence of clinical interest in this class of drugs.

Psychiatric Uses of MAOIs in the Presence of Neurological Disease

MAOIs may be very useful in the treatment of depressed neurological patients who are not taking medications (discussed below) that might interact with the antidepressant. Anticholinergic MAOIs, like phenelzine, can exacerbate confusion and memory loss in patients with dementia, and tranylcypromine may be less troublesome than the more sedating and anticholinergic of the HCAs. The principal risk in cognitively impaired patients is that they will forget to adhere to the dietary restrictions.

Pargyline, an MAOI marketed as an antihypertensive, probably has antidepressant properties (Bernstein 1983). To a lesser extent, phenelzine can also ameliorate high blood pressure and may therefore be useful in hypertensive depressed patients. The potential hypotensive effects of MAOIs warrant slow and cautious increases in dosage in patients with marginal cerebrovascular reserve who cannot tolerate a decrease in blood pressure. Depressed patients with Parkinson's disease may be most appropriately treated with L-deprenyl; however, interactions with L-dopa could occur at higher doses of deprenyl.

Because MAOIs may have advantages in treatment of depression with prominent anxiety as well as primary anxiety states (Klein et al. 1980; Sheehan et al. 1980), they should probably be considered more frequently in neurological patients whose symptoms are caused or exaggerated by anxiety, especially when mixed with depression. Patients with light-headedness, dizziness, numbness, paresthesias, and other symptoms of hyperventilation, who may be misdiagnosed as having labyrinthitis, vestibular neuronitis, multiple sclerosis, or hypoglycemia, may be particularly good candidates, especially if HCAs have been ineffective or difficult to tolerate. Tolerance to antipanic and antidepressant effects may occur more frequently with MAOIs than with other antidepressants.

MAOIs in the Elderly

Lower doses and slower increments in dosage are necessary when MAOIs are prescribed for elderly patients. For example, treatment with phenelzine should be initiated at a dose of 7.5 mg, with increases of 7.5–15 mg every 3–6 days to a therapeutic range of 15–60 mg/day. The starting dose of tranylcypromine in the elderly should be 5 mg, with 2.5- to 5-mg increments daily to a total dose of 5–15 mg (Salzman 1985).

Elderly patients are particularly vulnerable to the effects of hypertensive reactions that can result from adverse MAOI interactions (described below). However, hypertensive crises do not occur more frequently in older individuals than in anyone else (Jenike 1984). Some older patients, and some younger ones, become paradoxically sedated from MAOIs, but tolerance tends to develop to this side effect. Many elderly patients tolerate phenelzine without significant hypotension.

MAOIs in Patients With Other Neurological Syndromes

MAOIs are generally safe for use in patients with epilepsy; however, seizures have occurred in some nonepileptic patients following overdose. Interactions with antiparkinsonian drugs can complicate the use of the anticholinergic MAOIs such as phenelzine; L-deprenyl in antiparkinsonian doses does not interact with other antiparkinsonian drugs. Patients with carcinoid and pheochromocytoma should not receive MAOIs.

Neurological Uses of MAOIs

As already mentioned, L-deprenyl is an antiparkinsonian drug. Because they strongly suppress rapid-eye-movement (REM) sleep, MAOIs have been used to treat narcolepsy. Furazolidone, an MAOI antibiotic, may prove useful as a treatment for peptic ulcer and gastritis (Huai-Yu et al. 1985).

Neurological Side Effects of MAOIs

A serious but infrequent adverse effect of the hydrazine-type MAOIs is hepatocellular damage, which, in rare cases, can be fatal. Hydrazines can also cause reversible peripheral neuropathy, which may be a result of direct neural toxicity or of interference with pyridoxine metabolism; treatment with pyridoxine may be helpful in the latter instances. Other MAOI side effects that are important in a neurological setting are summarized in Table 29–4 (Bernstein 1983; Lieberman et al. 1985; Meyler and Herxheimer 1968; Pare 1985).

Interactions of MAOIs With Neurological Drugs

The most dangerous interaction of an MAOI is the hypertensive reaction that can occur when the MAOI is combined with certain tyramine-containing foods and various medications, some of which are listed in Table 29–5. A recent study of the tyramine content of traditionally prescribed foods found that for many of these, unlikely quantities (e.g., 15–20 bottles of beer or 50 glasses of wine) would have to be ingested to induce a hypertensive reaction (Shulman et al. 1989), suggesting that many substances end up on the proscribed list because of one or two case reports of headache or mild hypertension not proven to be due to an MAOI interaction. Shulman et al. (1989) recommend that a briefer and possibly more realistic list would include all aged cheeses, concentrated yeast extracts (e.g., Marmite), sauerkraut, broad bean pods (e.g., fava beans), aged meats, salami, air-dried sausage, old chicken liver, protein extracts, spoiled protein-containing foods, and all Chinese food and soups. They suggest that such a list might decrease the incidence of adverse interactions by increasing compliance. Proscribed foods should not be eaten for 2 weeks after stopping MAOIs.

Headache, fever, agitation, vomiting, and chest pain signal a hypertensive crisis; these may progress to intracerebral bleeding or heart failure. Some authorities recommend that patients have available one or two 50-mg chlorpromazine tablets to take for the α-blocking effect if they accidentally violate the dietary restrictions and develop symptoms of a hypertensive crisis (Baldessarini 1985). Others are concerned that hypotension from the chlorpromazine might be more dangerous than mild hypertension

TABLE 29–4. ADVERSE EFFECTS OF MONOAMINE OXIDASE INHIBITORS (MAOIs)

System	*Manifestation*
Autonomic nervous system	Orthostatic hypotension, dry mouth, constipation, and delay in micturition
Central nervous system	Toxic psychosis, insomnia, irritability, headache, and ataxia
Neuromuscular	Muscle twitching, myoclonus, motor tension, tremor, muscle and joint pain, peripheral neuropathy, carpal tunnel syndrome, and hyperreflexia
Liver	Jaundice, hepatocellular damage, and elevated liver enzymes
Genitourinary	Impotence and anorgasmia (in men and women; may respond to cyproheptadine)
Miscellaneous	Edema, skin rash, blood dyscrasia (rare), aggravation of asthma, fever, and constipation

TABLE 29–5. COMMON SUBSTANCES THAT MAY INTERACT WITH MONOAMINE OXIDASE INHIBITORS (MAOIs)

Foods
- Aged cheese (cottage cheese and cream cheese are OK)
- Pickled herring
- Sauerkraut
- Dry sausage (including Genoa salami, hard salami, pepperoni, and Lebanon bologna)
- Soy sauce
- Chinese food
- Chicken liver
- Broad bean pods (fava bean)
- Fermented beer
- Yeast extract
- Any spoiled, aged, pickled, fermented, or smoked protein-containing food
- Sour cream
- Avocados
- Overripe bananas or banana peel
- Raisins

Drugs and over-the-counter medications
- Dextromethorphan
- Cold preparations
- Any nasal decongestant
- Hay-fever medications
- Sinus medications
- Asthma inhalants
- Antiappetite drugs
- Amphetamines or cocaine
- Weight loss pills
- Pep pills
- Demerol
- Tricyclic antidepressants
- Robitussin-PE
- Cotylenol
- Alka-Seltzer Plus

Cold and allergy preparations that will *not* interact
- Aspirin
- Diphenhydramine (Benadryl)
- Acetaminophen (Tylenol)
- Cēpacol
- Chloraseptic
- Sucrets
- Plain Alka-Seltzer
- Chlor-Trimeton
- Plain Robitussin

resulting from most "cheese reactions" (Bernstein 1983). A 10-mg tablet of nifedipine chewed and placed under the tongue for sublingual absorption can ameliorate hypertensive reactions with fewer side effects (Clary and Schweizer 1987). The definitive treatment of a severe hypertensive crisis is 2–5 mg of intravenous phentolamine.

Although hypertension, rigidity, tremor, fever, convulsions, and coma can occur when MAOIs are combined with HCAs, these two classes of drugs are frequently administered together without adverse consequences. In fact, by blocking uptake of tyramine into nerve terminals, HCAs (except those mentioned below) may protect to some degree against hypertensive reactions related to ingestion of tyramine (Pare 1985). Trazodone in doses of 50–75 mg can be used safely to treat MAOI-induced insomnia (Jacobsen 1990).

Imipramine, clomipramine, fluoxetine, and meperidine can interact with MAOIs to produce hypotension, hypothermia, seizures, coma, and fatal cardiac arrhythmias, probably due to serotonin syndrome. Because of the long elimination half-life of fluoxetine, MAOIs should not be administered within at least 6 weeks of this drug's use. The possibility of serotonin syndrome also warrants great caution combining buspirone and MAOIs. Because hydrazine and nonhydrazine MAOIs may interact severely with each other, it is advisable to wait 2 weeks before switching from one class of MAOI to another.

Because it takes 2 weeks for MAO to recover after it has been inhibited by MAOIs, most clinicians wait this length of time after completely discontinuing MAOIs before allowing the patient to take a food or medication that might lead to a hypertensive reaction if MAO were still inhibited. Decline in blood level of the drug and increase in MAO activity after abrupt discontinuation of MAOIs are gradual, but discontinuation syndromes have occurred when MAOIs were withdrawn too rapidly. Withdrawal syndromes have included psychosis, mania, insomnia, headache, tremors, nightmares, weakness, paresthesias, and delirium (Lawrence 1985). MAOIs should therefore gradually be discontinued by decreasing the dose by one pill every few days. In addition to hypertensive reactions and serotonin syndrome, the following potentially dangerous interactions have been reported with MAOIs (Baldessarini 1985; Lieberman et al. 1985; Meyler and Herxheimer 1968; Pare 1985):

1. Ataxia, hyperreflexia, ankle clonus, myoclonus, nystagmus, dysarthria, paresthesias, and more severe signs of serotonin syndrome when L-tryptophan is added.

2. Potentiation of general anesthetics, sedatives, antihistamines, and narcotic analgesics. Concern about such interactions makes some physicians recommend that anesthesia for surgery or ECT be delayed until MAOIs can be discontinued; however, anesthesia has been administered safely to patients who are still taking MAOIs.
3. Potentiation of the pressor effects of amphetamine and tyramine, but not norepinephrine and epinephrine.
4. Additive anticholinergic effects with neuroleptics and antiparkinsonian drugs.
5. Potentiation of the sedative effects with neuroleptics and antiparkinsonian drugs.
6. Severe hyperpyrexia and coma with dextromethorphan.
7. Increased hypoglycemic effect of insulin.
8. Excitation with reserpine and tetrabenazine.

❑ LITHIUM

Lithium was introduced in 1859 as a treatment for gout, and it could be found in patent medicines during the late 1800s and early 1900s (Bernstein 1983). The modern use of this ion began in 1949 when Cade, an Australian psychiatrist who believed that urate might be an endotoxin in mania, injected lithium urate into guinea pigs and found that it tranquilized them. Theorizing that lithium was the active agent, he found that it did indeed calm a small group of manic patients.

At the same time that Cade reported on its effectiveness in mania, lithium chloride was in wide use as a salt substitute. Unfortunately, the combination of strict sodium restriction, which increased lithium resorption by the kidney, and liberal use of the substitute resulted in fatal lithium intoxication in a number of hypertensive patients. Fears of lithium that arose from these catastrophes delayed its approval in the United States as a psychiatric drug until 1970.

Lithium carbonate, which is less irritating to the gastrointestinal tract than other lithium salts (Baldessarini 1985), is available in 300-mg capsules and tablets. Lithium citrate comes in liquid form. There is no parenteral preparation.

Lithium is eliminated primarily by direct excretion by the kidney. Equilibrium between ingestion and excretion takes about 5–6 days, and the half-life of lithium in chronic administration is about 24 hours. Even during long-term therapy, a peak in blood level that is 2–3 times the steady-state concentration is reached 1–2 hours after each oral dose. It had been thought that because there is only a two- to threefold difference between therapeutic and toxic concentrations, lithium should usually be administered in divided doses to avoid peaks that might be high enough to be problematic. However, recent work suggests that administration of the entire dose every night or 150% of the daily dose every other night reduces side effects and improves compliance without decreasing effectiveness (Jensen et al. 1990). It has been postulated that brief peaks in blood levels during sleep are not harmful, whereas the deeper troughs associated with this method may reduce the risk of short- and long-term adverse effects (Mellerup and Plenge 1990). Sustained release preparations are absorbed relatively slowly and are associated with less abrupt increases in serum levels without decreasing effectiveness (Jensen et al. 1990).

The dose of lithium is always adjusted according to blood level, which is measured 10–12 hours after the last dose to ensure an accurate estimate of the steady-state concentration. Acutely manic patients usually require 0.8–1.5 mEq/L, which is generally achieved at a dose of 1,200–2,400 mg/day (Bernstein 1983; Klein et al. 1980). Levels greater than 1.2 mEq/L rarely are necessary in adults, although some adolescents may respond only to higher concentrations. Levels greater than 1.5 mEq/L in adults almost always result in more side effects than therapeutic benefit. Maintenance blood levels usually range from 0.5 to 1.0 mEq/L (from 900 to 1,500 mg/day). Recent research suggests that relapse rates are lower but side effects more frequent at lithium levels of 0.8–1.0 mEq/L, whereas relapse rates are higher but side effects less common at levels of 0.4–0.6 mEq/L (Gelenberg et al. 1989).

Mechanisms of Action

Lithium inhibits the release of norepinephrine from brain synaptosomes and enhances serotonergic transmission. Lithium substitutes incompletely for sodium, calcium, and magnesium in many biologic systems, inhibiting their action (Singer and Rotenberg 1973).

Lithium may also reduce hyperactive intracellular signalling through the phosphatidylinositol (PI) and calcium ion (Ca^{2+}) signals. Lithium inhibits reconstitution of the PI parent compound at a number of points in its metabolic cycle, an effect that may be more marked in hyperactive cells (Berridge 1984). In view of evidence of hyperactive intracellular Ca^{2+} signalling in bipolar patients and its reduction by lithium, it is possible that the diverse changes in transmitter and physiological systems in bipolar illness are related to an underlying change in the PI/Ca^{2+} systems that is modified by lithium (Dubovsky et al. 1991). It has also been suggested that lithium acts on the cell membrane or a G protein to reduce hyperactive signalling by both the PI and cyclic adenosine monophosphate (cAMP) systems (Schreiber et al. 1991).

Psychiatric Uses of Lithium in the Presence of Neurological Disease

Lithium is the drug of choice for prophylaxis of recurrent mania. It is also effective in the treatment of acute mania. Because the clinical effect is not completely manifest for 1 to several weeks after lithium is initiated, neuroleptics frequently are also required during acute treatment if the patient is agitated or psychotic.

There seems little doubt about lithium's ability to prevent or attenuate antidepressant-induced mania and recurrent bipolar depression. It may be an antidepressant in cases of acute bipolar depression or affective psychoses. Whether lithium is a useful treatment or prophylaxis of acute or recurrent unipolar depression is controversial. Many clinicians have found that lithium can augment the antidepressant effect of HCAs, especially in bipolar depression and to a lesser extent in unipolar depression (Jefferson 1990; Roy and Pickar 1985). Lithium may also increase response rates in manic patients treated with carbamazepine and valproate, schizophrenic patients treated with neuroleptics, and OCD patients treated with clomipramine and fluoxetine (Jefferson 1990; Jenike 1990). Lithium may control impulsive, aggressive, and self-destructive behavior in some emotionally labile patients with brain damage and personality disorders.

Lithium and Organic Brain Disease

When a patient being treated with lithium becomes delirious, the first consideration is lithium intoxication, which may occur at therapeutic levels. Lithium should therefore be withheld until the cause of an acute organic brain syndrome is determined and the illness is treated. Hypothyroidism, which may be induced by lithium treatment itself, can aggravate lithium toxicity. Even at therapeutic levels, lithium may aggravate preexisting organic brain syndromes. However, some agitated dementia patients tolerate lithium well.

Alternatives to Lithium

Patients with dementia who require treatment for a bipolar disorder and who become more confused on lithium may benefit from one of the alternative treatments listed in Table 29–6. Of these experimental alternatives, carbamazepine, valproate, and ECT have been studied most thoroughly.

Roughly 60%–70% of manic patients are moderately to markedly responsive to carbamazepine for the first year, but up to one-half of these patients, particularly those with an accelerating frequency of episodes, may become tolerant to carbamazepine prophylaxis (Post et al. 1990). Some lithium-resistant patients may respond better to carbamazepine. Valproate, which may be most effective when given with another antimanic drug, seems especially useful for manic patients with abnormal EEGs and possibly for patients with rapid cycling and mixed states (Chou 1991). Verapamil has been given to a small number of manic patients with dementia without adverse effects (Dubovsky et al. 1986). Because nimodipine, a calcium channel blocker used to treat cerebrovascular disease, may retard deterioration in some forms of dementia, it is another possible alternative, although there are no published studies of its effectiveness as an antimanic drug. Propranolol might theoretically be useful in manic patients with brain damage.

Clonazepam in doses of 2–16 mg/day has been found useful in reducing agitation and other acute manic symptoms, and other BZDs such as lorazepam may also be effective (Dubin 1988). Potential adverse effects in patients with organic brain disease include sedation, cerebellar signs, and paradoxical

TABLE 29–6. EXPERIMENTAL ALTERNATIVES TO LITHIUM

Bromocriptine
Carbamazepine
Clonazepam
Electroconvulsive therapy (ECT)
Lorazepam
Valproic acid
Verapamil

excitement or increased confusion unless lorazepam's anticonvulsant properties predominate in patients with seizure disorders. Lorazepam may also reduce agitation in acute mania. None of these drugs has been studied systematically as a mood stabilizer in patients with brain damage. ECT, on the other hand, has been found to be effective for mania.

Lithium in Patients With Other Neurological Disorders

Because lithium lowers the seizure threshold and occasionally induces seizures in nonepileptic patients (Massey and Folger 1984), increased doses of anticonvulsants may be necessary when patients with epilepsy take lithium. On the other hand, in at least one report (Shukla et al. 1988) lithium did not increase seizure frequency or anticonvulsant requirement in a small group of bipolar epileptic patients taking doses sufficient to control the mood disorder. The antiepileptic drugs carbamazepine, valproic acid, and clonazepam (Table 29–6) are logical alternatives to lithium when seizure control is difficult.

Chronic lithium therapy occasionally produces EPS (Klein et al. 1980), which can be a problem for parkinsonian patients. Sodium depletion leads to increased renal conservation of lithium; hypokalemia increases the risk of neurological and cardiovascular side effects of lithium, even at therapeutic lithium concentrations (Jefferson and Greist 1977).

Lithium and the Elderly

Even if renal clearance is normal, a general decrease in organ reserve makes the elderly more vulnerable to confusion and other toxic effects of lithium (Table 29–7). The dose of lithium should therefore be increased more slowly in the elderly, and the final dose should be lower (e.g., maintenance serum concentration from 0.4 to 0.7 mEq/L) than in younger patients. Because lithium suppresses automaticity of the sinoatrial (SA) node and conduction through the atrioventricular (AV) node, patients with cardiovascular disease require very close monitoring. Alternate treatment should be considered if electrocardiographic (ECG) changes occur or if adverse effects on the heart develop.

Neurological Uses of Lithium

In anecdotal reports and uncontrolled studies, lithium has been said to ameliorate cluster headaches, Huntington's disease, and spasmodic torticollis; it has also been subjected to preliminary trials in tardive dyskinesia (TD) (Baldessarini 1985). The leukocytosis induced by lithium makes it a useful therapy for leukopenia induced by chemotherapeutic agents. Lithium-induced diabetes insipidus may counteract the syndrome of inappropriate secretion of antidiuretic hormone, which can be a primary disorder or a complication of some tumors and infections of the brain and lung.

Neurological Side Effects of Lithium

Lithium produces two types of side effects: those at therapeutic levels (Table 29–7) and those that are due to toxicity. Impairment of memory and concentration may be bothersome to students. Prolonged memory loss and other neurological sequelae have been reported after episodes of lithium toxicity (Saxena and Maltikarjuna 1988). All lithium side effects are less frequent at blood levels less than 0.6 mEq/L, but the prophylactic effect may be less reliable (Gelenberg et al. 1989; Vestergaard et al. 1988). Toxic reactions are common when blood levels are greater than 1.5–2.0 mEq/L, but they may occur at therapeutic levels in some patients, especially if the patient is dehydrated or taking a neuroleptic, carbamazepine, or calcium channel blocker.

The onset of toxicity is heralded by a coarse tremor, ataxia, vertigo, dysarthria, disorientation, nausea, and vomiting. These signs and symptoms may progress to muscle fasciculation, gross confusion, delirium, hyperreflexia, arrhythmias, seizures, coma, irreversible brain damage, and death. Treatment of lithium intoxication involves stopping all drugs, hydration, diuresis, maintenance of electrolyte balance, and dialysis if toxicity is extreme. Lithium has been reported to cause increased intracranial pressure (Saul 1985).

Interactions of Lithium With Neurological Drugs

Lithium levels are increased by sodium-wasting diuretics, angiotensin-converting enzyme (ACE) inhibitors, and nonsteroidal anti-inflammatory drugs, but not aspirin or sulindac (Jefferson 1990; Ragheb 1990). Potassium-wasting diuretics can increase the risk of toxicity even at therapeutic levels (Bernstein

TABLE 29–7. COMMON LITHIUM SIDE EFFECTS UNRELATED TO TOXICITY

Side effect	*Manifestations*	*Comments*
Tremor	Irregular, fine resting of fingers and hands most likely to appear after rapid increase in dose; myoclonic jerking may also occur.	May respond to decreasing the dose, adding propranolol or amantadine, switching to lithium carbonate in slow-release tablets, or bedtime doses.
Mental symptoms	Difficulty concentrating, dazed feeling, impaired memory, confusion, dizziness, and flat affect.	Can appear in normal subjects as well as affective patients. May respond to decreasing the dose.
Polyuria and polydipsia	May be due to nephrogenic diabetes insipidus (metabolic effect) or tubular damage (structural effect).	Lithium-induced kidney disease is probably mild and clinically is insignificant. Nevertheless, renal function should be monitored regularly, and the lowest possible dose should be prescribed. Patients should be advised to avoid dehydration. Thiazide diuretics or amiloride may decrease polyuria.
Thyroid function	Hypothyroidism or enlarged thyroid with normal thyroxine but increased thyroid-stimulating hormone; decreased thyroid function may initiate rapid cycling in some bipolar patients.	Treatment with thyroxine or discontinuation of lithium usually restores normal thyroid function.
Cardiac changes	Decreased automaticity of SA node; delayed conduction through AV node.	Arrhythmias and conduction disturbances are much more common at toxic levels. A baseline ECG should be obtained if there is any suspicion of preexisting cardiac disease to compare suspected postlithium changes. Observe caution when combining with propranolol or verapamil.
EEG changes	REM suppression, high-voltage slow waves, superimposed beta, epileptiform discharges, and disorganization of background rhythm.	Seizures may occur in nonepileptic patients at therapeutic levels.
Gastrointestinal, dermatologic, metabolic, and endocrine effects	Diarrhea, indigestion, skin rash, acne, hair, loss, weight gain, altered glucose hypertolerance, and parathyroidism.	Weight gain is probably due to fluid retention plus altered carbohydrate metabolism. Insulin requirement may be changed. Cataracts, depression, or renal disease on lithium should prompt serum calcium studies.
Irreversible neurological damage	Memory deficits and cerebellar symptoms.	Occasionally reported after an episode of severe toxicity.

Note. ECG = electrocardiogram; REM = rapid eye movement; EEG = electroencephalogram; SA = sinoatrial; AV = atrioventricular.

1983). A number of antibiotics, especially tetracyclines, spectinomycin, and metronidazole, may increase lithium levels, although this association has not been established definitively. Theophylline and possibly caffeine occasionally lower serum lithium concentrations (Perry et al. 1984).

Since the report by Cohen and Cohen (1974) of irreversible neurotoxicity in patients treated with lithium plus haloperidol, there has been considerable debate about the risks of combining lithium and neuroleptics, particularly with haloperidol and thioridazine, and with carbamazepine. Even though some experts feel that these combinations present no increased risk of neurotoxicity (Baldessarini 1985; Bernstein 1983), reports still emerge of irreversible neurological syndromes, often following lithium intoxication (Izzo and Brody 1985). In a recent study (Miller and Menninger 1987), 17% of patients treated with lithium-neuroleptic combinations developed reversible neurotoxicity consisting mainly of EPS and delirium. Neurotoxicity was found to be more likely to occur with higher neuroleptic doses and possibly with higher lithium levels. Neurotoxicity has also been reported when lithium is combined with clonazepam (Koczerinski et al. 1989), neuroleptics, carbamazepine, and calcium channel blockers (Chou 1991).

Many of these drugs, particularly neuroleptics, are often coadministered with lithium to control agitation while waiting for lithium's antimanic effect to appear. However, it is not clear that such combinations are superior in the short run to neuroleptics alone. Some authors therefore recommend using neuroleptics with or without BZDs, or carbamazepine, until the patient's behavior is controlled, at which point lithium is begun and the neuroleptic is withdrawn (Chou 1991).

❑ INTERACTIONS OF ALTERNATIVES TO LITHIUM WITH NEUROLOGICAL DRUGS

Interactions of ECT, clonazepam, and lorazepam are considered in the sections describing them. Carbamazepine induces its own metabolism and metabolism of other anticonvulsants, alprazolam, coumadin, neuroleptics, and oral contraceptives. Calcium channel blockers, erythromycin, and isoniazid increase carbamazepine levels, leading to toxicity. Combining carbamazepine with lithium or neuroleptics can cause neurotoxicity. Verapamil and diltiazem have produced neurotoxicity when combined with lithium or carbamazepine.

❑ ELECTROCONVULSIVE THERAPY

Convulsive therapies were initially developed as a treatment for schizophrenia because it was thought that schizophrenia and epilepsy rarely occurred together. The original convulsants were gases and liquids, but in 1938 an electrical stimulus was shown to be easier to administer and control. Epilepsy was eventually shown not to protect against schizophrenia, and ECT turned out to be truly useful in schizophrenia in only 15% of cases (mainly those with associated affective symptoms). However, double-blind studies comparing real to sham ECT provided strong evidence that ECT was a highly effective treatment for depression (Brandon et al. 1984).

ECT is usually administered under barbiturate anesthesia with succinylcholine or similar muscle relaxants to spare the patient the peripheral manifestations of major motor seizures. An anticholinergic drug such as atropine or glycopyrrolate (which does not cross the blood-brain barrier) may be administered to dry secretions and prevent bradycardia caused by central stimulation of the vagus nerve. Many psychiatrists begin ECT with unilateral nondominant electrode placement, which may minimize memory loss, and proceed to bilateral treatment if satisfactory seizures cannot be obtained or if the patient does not improve. The usual course is 6–12 treatments or 200–600 seizure seconds (Fink 1979). However, some patients require more treatment and suprathreshold stimulation, and seizure time may not be correlated with treatment response.

Mechanisms of Action

ECT induces changes in several transmitter-receptor systems, particularly acetylcholine, norepinephrine, dopamine, and serotonin (Fink 1974, 1990); down-regulates β-adrenergic receptors; and may decrease cerebrospinal fluid calcium levels (Carman and Wyatt 1977). It is also conceivable that, analogous to cardioversion, an electrical stimulus to the brain could suppress reentrant or hyperactive circuits that were provoked by recurrent stimulation (kindling) (Dubovsky 1986b; Fink 1990). Another possibility is that the process by which the artificially induced seizure is terminated, and not the seizure itself, is therapeutic.

An interesting but unproven hypothesis is that ECT increases brain levels of one or more neuropeptides that stabilize mood and vegetative physiology (Fink 1990). It has also been postulated that ECT restores interhemispheric balance by enhancing right-brain function and dampening left-brain function (Small et al. 1988). There are as yet insufficient data to support any of these ideas, but it is clear that the effect of the electrical current on the brain, and not peripheral manifestations of the seizure, memory loss, adjunctive medications, or the psychological meaning of the treatment, is the source of its beneficial action.

Psychiatric Uses of ECT in Patients With Neurological Disease

ECT is usually reserved for severely depressed patients who have not responded to medication or who are too ill to wait for antidepressants to take effect. It may also be effective in mania, catatonia, and some cases of schizophrenia (Bernstein 1983; Black et al. 1987). To prevent relapse, patients who respond to ECT should be maintained on antidepressants. Patients who cannot tolerate or do not respond to maintenance medication may benefit from maintenance ECT (Thienhaus et al. 1990), although this is not a proven prophylactic treatment (Thornton et al. 1990).

Space-occupying lesions in the brain (or any condition with increased intracranial pressure) have traditionally been considered to be a contraindication to ECT (Bernstein 1983; Fink 1974). However, ECT has been administered to patients with brain tumors and with elevated intracranial pressure without ill effects (Dubovsky 1986b). Obviously, the potential benefits would have to outweigh the considerable risks to justify the use of ECT in such patients, and the treatment is probably safer in patients with small tumors, no lateralizing signs, and normal intracranial pressure. A few reports of irreversible brain damage suggest that ECT should not be used within several months of carbon monoxide poisoning (Dubovsky 1986b).

There have been reports that ECT has improved physical as well as psychiatric status in some patients with neurological illnesses including epilepsy, Parkinson's disease, multiple sclerosis, pituitary insufficiency, anterior cerebral artery occlusion, hypertensive retinal hemorrhage, neurodermatitis, and diabetes mellitus (Dubovsky 1986b). These anecdotal studies do not prove that ECT is helpful or even benign in most patients with neurological disease, but they do suggest that ECT does not necessarily have to be withheld under these circumstances. There is no convincing evidence that ECT permanently worsens dementia or causes brain damage (Weiner 1984).

Neurological Uses of ECT

According to the 1978 American Psychiatric Association (APA) Task Force Report on Electroconvulsive Therapy, most American psychiatrists "would find it strange" to use a treatment that can produce an acute organic brain syndrome in delirious patients (Dubovsky 1986b). Over the years, however, a number of studies of single and small groups of patients have reported that ECT induced rapid clearing of delirious states associated with intoxication and withdrawal from numerous drugs, delirium tremens, cerebritis, meningitis, encephalitis, syphilis, uremia, pneumonia, and delirium superimposed on dementia (Dubovsky 1986b). One to four treatments have usually been sufficient, even when the underlying pathological process has not yet been corrected. There are no controlled studies of this application of ECT, but it remains a potential therapy for life-threatening delirium. The most recent APA Task Force therefore considers ECT appropriate for some delirious patients (American Psychiatric Association Task Force 1990).

Because repeated seizures raise the threshold for further convulsions, ECT has been used as a treatment for intractable epilepsy and as a means of clearing prolonged postictal clouding of consciousness (Dubovsky 1986b). Several reports exist of improvement of Parkinson's disease and enhanced response to antiparkinsonian therapy generally lasting for weeks after ECT, even if depression was not improved (Anderson et al. 1987). In one study (Fink 1988), a small number of depressed parkinsonian patients experienced improvement for 4–8 years after a course of ECT.

Neurological Side Effects of ECT

Confusion and memory loss are major neurological side effects of ECT. These may be proportional to the degree to which the stimulus exceeds the seizure threshold and the use of bilateral versus unilateral treatment, although the latter approach may be less effective (Sackheim et al. 1987). A small number of patients continue to complain that their memories or personalities have been permanently damaged after ECT, but objective studies have not yet provided evidence of memory loss persisting more than 6 months after treatment (Weiner 1984). It is not clear whether such problems do not really occur or whether they just cannot be measured. Some of these patients have preexisting brain lesions that are not aggravated but not improved by ECT. Despite the frequent occurrence of an acute confusional state, ECT improves right-hemisphere function in association with improvement of depression (Rossi et al. 1990).

With modern anesthetic management, serious complications or death develop in fewer than 1 in 8,000 patients, making ECT one of the safest interventions that use general anesthesia (Fink 1974). Any morbidity or mortality that does occur is usually secondary to cardiovascular complications such as arrhythmia, myocardial infarction, or hypertension. The major risks are those associated with brief general anesthesia.

Interactions of ECT

Concerns that HCAs might predispose to cardiac complications and that MAOIs could potentiate pressor agents and anesthetics or could cause severe hypotension lead many clinicians to discontinue these drugs 2 weeks before beginning ECT. Although this is the safest course, research has suggested that ECT can be safe even when these antidepressants are still being taken (Azar and Lear 1984; El-Gazour et al. 1985). In addition, patients taking antidepressants during ECT may be less likely to relapse, although this has been disputed (American Psychiatric Association Task Force 1990).

Lithium may increase the severity of post-ECT confusion, memory loss, delirium, and prolonged seizures (El-Mallakh 1988; Penney et al. 1990), necessitating a longer hospital stay (Penney et al. 1990). To avoid these problems, it has been suggested that lithium be discontinued a week before ECT and that it be withheld for several days after ECT is completed (Small and Milstein 1990). Lithium enhances the action of neuromuscular blocking agents (Bernstein 1983; Packman et al. 1978; Small and Milstein 1990), although this is usually not clinically significant (El-Mallakh 1988). Anticonvulsants and BZDs may make it more difficult to initiate a seizure during ECT.

❑ ANTIPSYCHOTIC DRUGS

Chlorpromazine, the first of the modern antipsychotic drugs, was synthesized in France in 1950 in an attempt to find a new agent that would potentiate general anesthesia. Because it seemed to have marked sedative properties, it was given to manic and then to schizophrenic patients. This resulted in the discovery of its antipsychotic potential. Six classes of antipsychotic agents are now available in the United States: phenothiazines, thioxanthenes, butyrophenones, indolones, dibenzoxazepines, and dibenzodiazepines (Figure 29–2).

Antipsychotic drugs act on psychosis of any cause, not just schizophrenia. No antipsychotic is inherently more effective than any other, although some differences (described below) exist in activity against negative versus positive symptoms and against treatment-resistant cases.

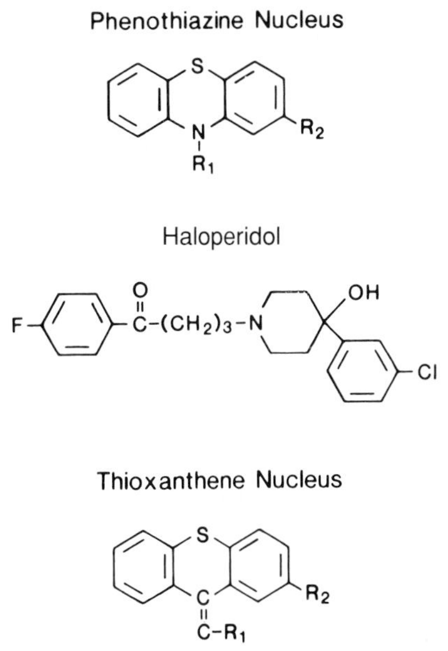

Phenothiazine Nucleus

Haloperidol

Thioxanthene Nucleus

Figure 29–2. Structures of some antipsychotics.

Neuroleptics (derived from the Greek for "to clasp the neuron") are antipsychotic drugs that control symptoms of psychosis and produce neurological side effects. All currently available antipsychotic drugs except clozapine are neuroleptics. Available antipsychotic drugs differ primarily in their anticholinergic properties, potency (i.e., effectiveness at a given dose), and tendency to produce sedation and hypotension. The oral and intramuscular doses of these drugs are summarized in Table 29–8.

Although high doses are sometimes necessary for severely psychotic patients, doses greater than 1,000 mg/day of chlorpromazine or its equivalent are probably no more effective in controlling psychotic symptoms than doses of 300–600 mg/day, even for acutely psychotic patients (Baldessarini et al. 1988; Davis and Andriukaitis 1986). Higher doses produce more side effects, including akinesia, that can be mistaken for negative symptoms. In addition, patients treated with higher doses may be more noncompliant (Baldessarini et al. 1988). One exception may be psychotically depressed patients who require higher neuroleptic doses (e.g., up to 60–90 mg/day perphenazine). The optimal dose of neuroleptic for acute mania is not known but may be

TABLE 29–8. ANTIPSYCHOTIC DRUGS AVAILABLE IN THE UNITED STATES

Drug by class	*Trade name*	*Usual daily oral dose (mg)*	*Usual single im dose (mg)*	*Sedative properties*	*Anticholinergic properties*	*Hypotensive effects*
Phenothiazines						
Chlorpromazine	Thorazine	300–800	25–50	Very high	High	Moderate-high
Triflupromazine	Vesprin	100–150	20–60	Moderate	Moderate	Moderate
Thioridazine	Mellaril	200–700[a]	—	High	Very high	Moderate-high
Mesoridazine	Serentil	75–300	25	High	Moderate-high	Moderate
Acetophenazine	Tindal	60–120	—	Moderate	Moderate	Low
Perphenazine	Trilafon	8–40	5–10	Moderate	Moderate-low	Low-moderate
Trifluoperazine	Stelazine	6–20	1–2	Low	Low	Low
Fluphenazine	Prolixin	1–20	12.5–50	Low	Low	Low
Thioxanthenes						
Chlorprothixene	Taractan	50–400	25–50	High	High	Moderate
Thiothixene	Navane	6–30	2–4	Low-moderate	Low	Moderate
Butyrophenones						
Haloperidol	Haldol	6–20	2–5[b]	Low	Very low	Very low
Diphenylbutyl-piperidines						
Pimozide	Orap	1–10[c]	—	Moderate-high	Moderate-low	Low
Dibenzoxazepines						
Loxapine	Loxitane	60–100	12.5–50	Low-moderate	Moderate	Low
Dihydroindolones						
Molindone	Moban	50–100	—	Low-moderate	Moderate	Very low
Dibenzodiazepines						
Clozapine	Clozaril	300–450[d]	—	Very high	Moderate	Moderate-high

[a]Maximum 800 mg.
[b]Intravenous doses may be higher.
[c]Second line drug because of cardiotoxicity.
[d]Maximum 900 mg.

lower than commonly used doses (Chou 1991). Fluphenazine decanoate, 12.5 mg (0.5 ml), is usually administered intramuscularly every 2–3 weeks for every 10 mg of fluphenazine hydrochloride given daily; 10–15 mg of haloperidol decanoate should probably be administered intramuscularly every 4 weeks for every 1 mg of oral haloperidol given daily (Kane 1986).

There are different metabolic pathways in the intestine and the liver for antipsychotic drugs (Ko et al. 1985). Chlorpromazine and thioridazine have many active metabolites, whereas butyrophenones and thioxanthenes may be metabolized only to inactive compounds. Parenteral administration avoids hepatic first-pass metabolism that occurs after oral dosage, increasing availability of the neuroleptic four to ten times (Baldessarini 1985). Some low-potency neuroleptics such as chlorpromazine and thioridazine may induce their own metabolism, resulting in decreased drug levels after a few weeks of treatment (Baldessarini 1985).

Blood levels vary widely in different patients given the same dose of a neuroleptic. Because there is no established correlation between serum concentration and clinical response (with the possible exception of haloperidol), blood levels are used only to determine if levels are very low in nonresponding patients and not as a standard approach to adjusting the dose (Ko et al. 1985). However, some neuroleptics may have a therapeutic window, with diminished responsiveness at higher doses (Baldessarini et al. 1988). The half-life of all antipsychotics is long (20–40 hours), and metabolites may be detected in the urine months after the drug is discontinued. This may explain why recurrence of psychosis may be delayed when medication is stopped.

Mechanisms of Action

The potency of neuroleptics appears to parallel their ability to block dopamine, subtype 2 (D_2), receptors, suggesting that dopamine blockade or depolarization inactivation may be important in their antipsychotic action (Creese et al. 1976; Kane 1986). However, the usual cautions apply before assuming that an observed action of a drug, and not some as yet unsuspected mechanism or combination of actions, explains why the drug is effective in a particular disorder. For example, neuroleptics also block muscarinic, histamine, α-adrenergic, Σ-dopaminergic, and serotonin receptors (Richelson 1985a). In addition, clozapine exhibits weak binding to dopamine, subtype 1 (D_1), and D_2 receptors while it blocks serotonin-2 (5-HT_2), H_2, muscarinic, and α-adrenergic receptors (Ereshefsky et al. 1989; Kane et al. 1988; Marder and Van Putten 1988). An action on the brain stem reticular formation may account for the attenuating effect of antipsychotic drugs on schizophrenic individuals' tendency to become overwhelmed by sensory input (Richelson 1985a).

Psychiatric Uses of Antipsychotic Drugs in the Presence of Neurological Disease

Antipsychotic drugs are used to treat psychotic and agitated states. Their widest application has been in the treatment of schizophrenia, mania, and depression. Most neuroleptics ameliorate positive symptoms such as delusions, hallucinations, and agitation better than negative symptoms such as indifference, withdrawal, blunted affect, and anergia (Schooler 1986). Family therapy enhances the beneficial effects of neuroleptics in schizophrenia (Schooler 1986).

Clozapine is a new antipsychotic drug that appears to be more effective than traditional neuroleptics for negative schizophrenic symptoms (Ereshefsky et al. 1989). About one-third of severely ill schizophrenic patients resistant to neuroleptics demonstrate meaningful improvement with clozapine (Marder and Van Putten 1988). Clozapine is less likely to cause EPS, TD, or neuroleptic malignant syndrome (NMS), although these adverse effects may occur (Kane et al. 1988). Clozapine has a 1%–2% incidence of agranulocytosis, which is probably an immune phenomenon that is reversible if the medication is discontinued rapidly. Weekly blood counts are therefore mandatory. Clozapine is indicated for treatment-resistant schizophrenia, schizophrenia with prominent negative symptoms, and psychotic patients with severe TD or EPS (Marder and Van Putten 1988). It is usually evident within 6 weeks whether a response will occur (Kane et al. 1988).

Combined data from formal studies of over 3,500 patients demonstrate with great certainty ($P < 10^{-100}$) that neuroleptics reduce relapse rates in schizophrenia (Davis and Andriukaitis 1986). After initially responding, however, 20%–30% of schizophrenic patients relapse during the first 1–2 years of continuation treatment (Kane et al. 1988). Relapse rates are higher among less stable schizophrenic patients than among more stable ones (40% versus 10%–15%) (Schooler 1986).

In patients with chronic schizophrenia, psychotic symptoms return an average of 4.5 months after neuroleptics are discontinued. The risk of relapse appears to be the same no matter how long patients have been taking the neuroleptic. Each month after a group of schizophrenic patients discontinues antipsychotic drugs, a relatively constant percentage of additional patients will relapse (Davis and Andriukaitis 1986).

Some impulsive borderline patients with transient psychotic symptoms benefit from the short-term use of low doses of nonsedating neuroleptics such as haloperidol. The use of neuroleptics in the treatment of organic brain syndromes is considered below. The risk of TD makes neuroleptics poor choices in nonpsychotic anxiety and most types of insomnia. Neuroleptics are necessary adjuncts in the treatment of psychotic depression and possible adjuncts to serotonergic antidepressants in treatment-resistant OCD (Jenike 1990).

Because neuroleptics produce EPS, they are usually contraindicated for patients with Parkinson's disease. Clozapine, however, appears to be well tolerated (Friedman and Lammon 1989). Theoretically, at least, another choice would be an antipsychotic drug with strong anticholinergic properties, such as thioridazine or one of the alternatives to neuroleptics described below.

Many antipsychotic drugs lower the seizure threshold, especially clozapine, loxapine, and low-potency neuroleptics such as chlorpromazine and thioridazine. This appears to be a dose-related effect, especially for clozapine, which has a low incidence of seizures at doses less than 300 mg/day, a 1%–2% incidence of seizures at doses of 30–60 mg/day, and a 5% incidence at doses of 600–900 mg/day (Ereshefsky et al. 1989; Miller 1991). Haloperidol and molindone seem safest in seizure-prone individuals (Baldessarini 1985; Fenwick 1989). The dopamine blockade produced by neuroleptics increases prolactin secretion, which is a definite problem for patients with prolactin-secreting pituitary tumors and a possible concern for patients with breast cancer. Bromocriptine may reduce neuroleptic-induced galactorrhea related to hyperprolactinemia.

As with many drugs, lower doses of neuroleptics are required in the elderly; the initial dose should be about one-third of the usual adult starting dose (Raskin 1985). Higher-potency drugs with lower anticholinergic and hypotensive potential such as haloperidol, molindone, loxapine, fluphenazine, trifluoperazine, and perphenazine are safer in older patients with heart disease (Baldessarini 1985). Thioridazine, which has been reported to cause cardiotoxicity, and chlorpromazine, which has quinidine-like myocardial depressant properties, should generally not be the first-line treatments for cardiac patients.

Alternatives to Antipsychotic Drugs in the Treatment of Psychosis

When acutely psychotic patients are in urgent need of treatment but cannot tolerate neuroleptics, several alternative strategies may be considered. If the patient has mania, one of the experimental alternatives listed in Table 29–6 may be useful. ECT may be effective in extreme situations, especially if the psychosis is depressive, manic, schizophreniform, or schizoaffective, and it may reduce psychotic symptoms in some schizophrenic patients (Van Valkenberg and Clayton 1983). Clonidine, clonazepam, diazepam, alprazolam, and lorazepam may augment the action of neuroleptics in ameliorating acute psychotic symptoms, thereby reducing the amount of neuroleptic needed (Bodkin 1990; Salzman et al. 1986).

Lorazepam has been used most widely as an adjunct or alternative to neuroleptics. The usual dose is 1–2 mg every 2–4 hours in cases not requiring intravenous haloperidol-lorazepam (Bodkin 1990). Lorazepam and other BZDs may be rapidly effective treatments for catatonia, as may amobarbital and ECT (Bodkin 1990; Fricchione 1989). Reserpine, baclofen, droperidol, and L-tryptophan have also been used as antipsychotic agents (Richelson 1985a). Alprazolam may occasionally augment the action of neuroleptics against negative symptoms, perhaps when panic disorder is also present, but it may induce mania or increase agitation in bipolar patients (Bodkin 1990).

Short-acting barbiturates such as amobarbital (see below) may be used for emergency tranquilization and treatment of catatonia if a contraindication to their use does not exist (Bodkin 1990; Salzman et al. 1986). Intravenous doses of 5–45 mg of droperidol may rapidly control agitation and assaultive behavior; intramuscular absorption may be almost as rapid as the intravenous route (Dubin et al. 1986).

Neurological Uses of Antipsychotic Drugs

Although it has never been directly compared to intramuscular dosing, intravenous haloperidol is thought to be a more effective treatment for severe agitation and psychosis caused by delirium than oral or intramuscular dosing because rapid onset and multiple high doses are often necessary (Fernandez et al. 1988). Single intravenous doses of haloperidol as high as 75 mg and total 24-hour doses greater than 500 mg have been administered without any ill effects (Fernandez et al. 1988; Tesar et al. 1985). Control of agitations is achieved within 20–90 minutes in many cases (Adams et al. 1986), and the patient is often alert and oriented within 24–36 hours (Fernandez et al. 1988). According to Ayd (1984b), haloperidol is safe even for delirious cardiac patients because it "has virtually no effects on cardiac, pulmonary, renal, hepatic or hematopoietic functions and no absolute contraindications to its use" (p. 33). Extrapyramidal reactions are also rare with high intravenous doses of haloperidol (Fernandez et al. 1988). Intramuscular or intravenous droperidol is preferred by some clinicians.

Intravenous haloperidol therapy is begun with a 1- to 5-mg dose. Cassem's group (Tesar et al. 1985) has recommended escalating the dose rapidly to 30- to 75-mg boluses administered as frequently as necessary to control agitation and psychosis in delirious patients. Adams (1988; Adams et al. 1986) and Fernandez et al. (1988), who have studied this drug in patients with metastatic brain cancer, recommend starting with 5 mg of intravenous haloperidol followed by 0.5 mg of intravenous lorazepam. If no improvement occurs within 20 minutes, further doses of 10 mg of haloperidol and 0.5–10 mg of lorazepam are administered every 30 minutes until the patient is sedated (total daily dose up to 100–240 mg/day of each medication). When severe pain is felt to contribute to delirium, 0.5–4.0 mg of hydromorphone is added to each dose. Once the patient is sedated, lorazepam is withdrawn and the dose of haloperidol is reduced. Maintenance therapy includes 5–10 mg of haloperidol and 0.5 mg of lorazepam intravenously or orally.

In extreme cases in which repeated dosing is ineffective, an intravenous haloperidol drip (e.g., 15–25 mg/hour) may be effective (Fernandez et al. 1988). Other BZDs, and possibly intramuscular lorazepam, may also be adjuncts or substitute for neuroleptics (Dubin 1988). Intravenous or oral haloperidol may be useful in reducing ictal and interictal violence associated with epilepsy (Fenwick 1989), and addition of lorazepam or any BZD would be expected to antagonize any associated reduction or seizure threshold. On the other hand, administering frequent intramuscular doses in an attempt to control psychosis rather than agitation (rapid neuroleptization) is no more effective in acute schizophrenia than are standard approaches, although it is more likely to cause EPS (Dubin 1988; Escobar et al. 1983; Modestin et al. 1983).

For many years, low doses of high-potency neuroleptics (e.g., haloperidol 0.5–2.0 mg 1–4 times a day) have been used to control recurrent agitation in patients with dementia when nonpharmacological measures such as keeping the patient oriented failed and when it was clear that intercurrent delirium was not present. Ideally, the drug should be administered intermittently to coincide with anticipated episodes of agitation. Even with this schedule, however, the risk of TD is significant in this group of patients. In addition, the primary mechanism by which neuroleptics reduce agitation in these patients may be sedation. As tolerance develops to the sedative effect, it may be necessary to escalate the dose, further increasing the risk of neurological side effects.

Propranolol is a safe and effective alternative to neuroleptics for controlling violent outbursts in patients with brain damage. In an initial dose of 20 mg tid gradually increased to a maximum of 640–1,000 mg/day and titrated according to heart rate, this drug has been found to ameliorate unpredictable attacks of rage and assaultiveness in adults and children with a variety of organic brain syndromes (Silver and Yudofsky 1985; Yudofsky et al. 1983). Some patients respond immediately; others take up to 1 month to improve. Carbamazepine, fluoxetine, trazodone, and buspirone may also be useful treatments for intermittent agitation associated with organic brain disease (Silver and Yudofsky 1985; Stewart et al. 1990).

Propranolol, nadolol, carbamazepine, and lithium have shown promise in the treatment of episodic dyscontrol in adults, adolescents, and children with brain damage (Campbell and Spencer 1988; Stewart et al. 1990), and lithium may reduce aggression in mentally retarded children and adults (Campbell and Spencer 1988). Naltrexone has been used to control self-destructive behavior in severely mentally retarded patients (Kars et al. 1990). Stimulants may be used for aggression associated with attention-deficit hyperactivity disorder (Stewart et al. 1990). Carbamazepine is useful for the rare instances of interictal aggression associated with partial complex seizures (Stewart et al. 1990).

Most neuroleptics (except thioridazine) have antiemetic properties that make them useful treatments in low doses for nausea and vomiting induced by chemotherapy, vestibular syndromes, dysautonomia, and related physical factors (Baldessarini 1985; Richelson 1985a). For unknown reasons, chlorpromazine in low doses orally, intramuscularly, or as a suppository can ameliorate intractable hiccups. The phenothiazine trimeprazine (Temaril), which does not have antipsychotic properties, is an antipruritic agent at a dose of 10 mg/day. A well-known use of the potent neuroleptics, especially haloperidol and pimozide, is for control of chorea and agitation in Huntington's disease and of involuntary movements and obscene vocalizations in Tourette's disorder. However, a 25% incidence of ECG changes and a risk of sudden death make pimozide a second-line drug (Teicher and Glod 1990).

Neurological Side Effects of Antipsychotic Drugs

Seizures associated with clozapine are considered above. Neuroleptics have many side effects that mimic or exacerbate neurological disease, the most familiar of which is EPS. Parkinsonism consists of a resting tremor, shuffling gait, bradykinesia, stooped posture, excess salivation, and a mask-like face. Some of these signs can be mistaken for schizophrenic mannerisms and withdrawal, leading the clinician to increase the dose of medication inappropriately. Akathisia, a feeling of intense inner restlessness and need to keep moving, may sometimes be confused with psychotic agitation, whereas dystonia and oculogyric crises may be interpreted as psychotic posturing. Recognizing these syndromes is important because they usually call for a decrease rather than an increase in dosage. Most EPS (with the exception of akathisia) are uncommon with clozapine.

Acute EPS usually appear shortly after neuroleptic therapy is instituted. They often resolve within 3 months, making it possible in some cases to discontinue medications used to treat the side effect. Many experts prefer to wait to see if extrapyramidal side effects appear before prescribing an antiparkinsonian agent to avoid administering medications that may not be necessary and that have adverse effects of their own (see below). In addition, the concerns have been raised that patients may abuse anticholinergics (Ayd 1990b).

Prophylactic antiparkinsonian therapy may be indicated for patients at risk of acute dystonic reactions, such as individuals with a past history or family history of acute dystonia with neuroleptics and adolescents and young adult males receiving high-potency neuroleptics (Ayd 1986). These patients may not require the antiparkinsonian drug for more than a week (Ayd 1990b). Because the duration of action of neuroleptics is much longer than that of agents used to treat EPS, these side effects may reemerge when antiparkinsonian and antipsychotic drugs are discontinued at the same time (Baldessarini 1985). Lithium can aggravate neuroleptic-induced EPS.

A great deal of concern exists about TD (Table 29–9) a syndrome of involuntary movements of the tongue, lips, extremities, and trunk that usually, but not always, appears after long-term neuroleptic therapy. The risk of TD may be proportional to the total amount of neuroleptic that has been taken (Ko et al. 1985). Other risk factors include being older, female, and not schizophrenic and having brain damage (Kane et al. 1985). Another possible risk factor is intermittent use of high doses (Chou 1991). A study of 668 patients taking neuroleptics for an average of 8 years found that 40% had TD, which persisted for more than 6 months in 22% of the entire sample (Kane et al. 1985). Other estimates vary from 15% to 20% of younger patients and up to 70% of the elderly (Ereshefsky et al. 1989). Patients with a history of severe acute extrapyramidal reactions may be more likely to develop TD later, but it is not known whether aggressive treatment of these early side effects will decrease the risk of the later syndrome. Anticholinergic drugs may unmask TD, which can be temporarily suppressed but not cured by an increase in the dose of neuroleptic.

Antiparkinsonian drugs, which were once thought to reduce the risk of TD, may actually increase the risk (Dickey and Morrow 1990; Teicher and Glod 1990). Discontinuing the neuroleptic improves TD in some patients, sometimes after a delay of several years, but no specific treatment is known. The calcium channel blockers have shown some promise in animal models and a few series of patients. Clozapine is a potential treatment, but it is not known whether its capacity to suppress TD is enduring.

The most dreaded complication of neuroleptic treatment is neuroleptic malignant syndrome (NMS). This potentially lethal condition occurs in 0.5%–1.0% of patients taking neuroleptics (Guze and Baxter 1985). Mortality has decreased from original reports of 20%–30% thanks to earlier recognition and treatment (Dickey and Morrow 1990). NMS is more likely to occur with intramuscular administration of antipsychotic drugs and may be more common with high-potency preparations, especially haloperidol, thiothixene, fluphenazine, and trifluoperazine (Mueller 1985); however, it has also been reported in patients taking chlorpromazine, promethazine, thioridazine, metoclopramide, carbidopa-levodopa, and various other drugs; in patients taking clozapine plus lithium; and after withdrawal of amantadine and carbidopa-levodopa (Mueller 1985; Pelonero et al. 1985). Patients are more vulnerable to develop NMS if they are less than 40 years old, male, unresponsive to the usual doses of neuroleptics, and debilitated or have brain damage, nonschizophrenic disorders, and neurological illnesses (Mueller 1985). Concurrent use of lithium may increase the risk of NMS (Sakkas et al. 1989).

NMS may appear soon after the offending medication is begun, or its onset may be delayed for months. The major manifestations affect tempera-

TABLE 29–9. NEUROLOGICAL SIDE EFFECTS OF NEUROLEPTIC DRUGS AND THEIR TREATMENT

Syndrome	*Manifestations*	*Treatment or prevention*
Akathisia	Motor restlessness and feeling of inability to remain still; may be persistent or tardive.	Propranolol, clonazepam, lorazepam, diazepam, clonidine, amantadine, or antiparkinsonian drug (e.g., benztropine).
Acute dystonia	Spasm of muscles of neck, tongue, face, eyes, or trunk.	Decrease dose of neuroleptic; diphenhydramine or antiparkinsonian drug.
Parkinsonism	Stiffness, tremor, bradykinesia, shuffling gait, and salivation.	Oral antiparkinsonian drug for 4 weeks to 3 months; decrease dose of the antipsychotic drug.
Perioral (rabbit) tremor	Perioral tremor usually appearing after long-term therapy.	Decrease dose or change to a medication in another class.
Tardive dyskinesia	Dyskinesias of tongue and face, choreoathetoid movements of neck and trunk usually, but not always, appearing after years of treatment following a reduction in dose; incidence higher in the elderly, brain damaged, nonschizophrenic patients, children and adolescents.	Risk may be reduced by prescribing the least amount of drug possible for as little time as is clinically feasible, and using long drug-free holidays for patients who need to continue taking the drug.
	Symptoms are worsened by antiparkinsonian drugs and masked, but not cured, by higher dose of neuroleptic.	Calcium channel blockers, clonazepam, and clozapine reduce signs of tardive dyskinesia; reserpine temporarily ameliorates tardive dyskinesia but may also cause it.
Anticholinergic delirium (acute organic brain syndrome)	Psychotic symptoms, dry skin, hyperpyrexia, mydriasis, and tachycardia.	Discontinue drug; iv physostigmine for severe agitation or fever.
Neuroleptic malignant syndrome	More commonly caused by high-potency drugs; appears days to months after beginning treatment; elevated creatine phosphokinase, white blood count, and urinary myoglobin; hyperthermia, muscle rigidity, autonomic instability; parkinsonian symptoms, catatonia stupor, neurological signs; 10%–30% fatality.	Obtain serum creatine phosphokinase if altered neurological status, fever, and muscle rigidity appear; if creatine phosphokinase and urine myoglobin levels are elevated, discontinue neuroleptic and give iv dantrolene plus po bromocriptine. Ensure hydration and cooling.
Seizures	Especially with clozapine, low potency, neuroleptics, and loxapine.	Use lower doses or coadminister anticonvulsants.
α-Adrenergic blockade	Orthostatic hypotension, more common with low-potency drugs; inhibition of ejaculation (may also be related to calcium channel blockade).	Advise patient to stand up slowly; treat acute hypotension with norepinephrine, not epinephrine; avoid β–adrenergic stimulation; change to another medication.
	Priapism, especially with chlorpromazine and thioridazine; may occur at any dose at any time.	Do not administer to patients with a history of prolonged erections with medication.

continued on next page

TABLE 29–9. (Continued)

Syndrome	*Manifestations*	*Treatment or prevention*
Heat stroke	Decreased sweating; thirst and possible hypothalamic dysfunction cause fever, decreased sweating, and collapse.	Discontinue drug; hydrate and cool.
Behavioral toxicity	Confusion, disorganization, increased aggression, especially in children and adolescents.	Use alternative treatment for aggression.
Sedation	More common with lower-potency neuroleptics and clozapine.	Start with low dose and increase dose slowly.
Leukopenia and agranulocytosis	Sudden appearance within the first 2 months of treatment with high doses of low-potency neuroleptics; 1%–2% incidence with clozapine, usually within the first 6–18 weeks.	Advise patient to call immediately for sore throat, fever, etc., and obtain immediate blood count; discontinue drug; regular complete blood counts will usually identify clozapine-induced agranulocytosis before it becomes irreversible.
Temperature dysregulation	Transient mild hyperthermia common with clozapine.	Rule out fever secondary to infection and give antipyretics; does not progress to neuroleptic malignant syndrome.
Pigmentary retinopathy	Reported with doses of thioridazine equal to or greater than 800 mg/day.	Prescribe less than 800 mg/day of thioridazine.
Impaired psychomotor performance	May be independent of sedation.	Advise patient of risk of impaired driving.
Photosensitivity	Easy sunburning.	Advise patient to avoid strong sunlight and to use sunscreens.
Jaundice	Rare complications of low-potency phenothiazine use.	Switch to a low dose of a low-potency agent in a different class.
Hypersalivation	May be very severe with clozapine, where it is not due to extrapyramidal syndrome.	Decrease dose or add anticholinergic drug.

ture regulation, muscle tone, autonomic regulation, the extrapyramidal system, and mental status. Severe hyperthermia can lead to heat stroke and brain damage. Muscular rigidity may progress to rhabdomyolysis, myoglobinuria, and renal failure. Other disturbances include dyspnea, dysphagia, autonomic instability with hypertension, diaphoresis, tachycardia, parkinsonian symptoms, delirium, catatonia, and psychosis. NMS is associated with elevations of white blood count, serum creatine phosphokinase, and urinary myoglobin. NMS requires intensive medical treatment that usually involves cooling, hydration, and, when supportive measures are not completely effective, amantadine, bromocriptine, or intravenous dantrolene (Mueller 1985).

Patients who recover from NMS frequently still require treatment for the underlying psychiatric disorder. Although there are no proven guidelines for managing this situation, several suggestions have been offered (Guze and Baxter 1985; Mueller 1985; Pelonero et al. 1985; Rosebush and Stewart 1989). The most appealing option is to use one of the alternative treatments described earlier in this chapter. If a neuroleptic is necessary, it has been recommended that a low-potency compound of a different class from that of the drug that caused the NMS be tried. Supplementation with BZDs may make it easier to use the lowest possible dose. The patient's temperature, blood pressure, pulse, and mental status should be monitored closely, and the neuroleptic should be discontinued if early signs of NMS reappear. Waiting at least 2 weeks before readministering neuroleptics seems to decrease the risk of a recurrence of NMS substantially (Rosebush and Stewart 1989).

Descriptions of parkinsonian syndromes, TD, and NMS, as well as other important neurological side effects of neuroleptics, are provided in Table 29–9.

Interactions of Neuroleptics With Neurological Drugs

Sedating neuroleptics potentiate other CNS depressants, whereas anticholinergic effects are additive with other anticholinergic drugs. Neuroleptics are sometimes used to increase the analgesic effect of narcotics, but respiratory depression may be potentiated as well. Like HCAs, chlorpromazine and other neuroleptics can interfere with the action of antihypertensive agents like guanethidine. Anticonvulsants that induce microsomal enzyme systems (e.g., phenytoin and carbamazepine) enhance metabolism of neuroleptics, sometimes decreasing blood levels and clinical effectiveness substantially (Kahn et al. 1990; Miller 1991), whereas neuroleptics may reduce anticonvulsant effectiveness by lowering the seizure threshold (Teicher and Glod 1990). Neuroleptics raise blood levels of TCAs by as much as 500%; TCAs also raise neuroleptic levels, but the effect is not clinically significant. By interfering with gastrointestinal absorption, antiparkinsonian drugs, cimetidine, lithium, and some antacids also lower neuroleptic levels and may decrease the therapeutic efficacy of the antipsychotic drug (Ayd 1986). The combination of clozapine and BZDs may occasionally cause collapse (Sassim and Grohmann 1988), and clozapine is not prescribed with carbamazepine because of the risk of additive bone marrow suppression, which may have occurred in one fatality reported by the manufacturer.

❑ ANTIANXIETY DRUGS

Bromides, the first sedatives, were introduced in the mid-1800s; barbiturates followed 50 years later. Bromides proved to be toxic, and the risks of dependence and death with overdose when barbiturates were used to treat anxiety became evident by the early 1950s. Propanediol carbamates such as meprobamate were developed at about this time, but they also proved to be addicting and dangerous in overdose. Since the introduction of chlordiazepoxide in 1961, the BZDs have proved to be both effective and safer than other drugs in the treatment of anxiety and insomnia. These medications, too, can produce tolerance and excessive sedation, problems that may be reduced with newer non-BZD anxiolytics such as buspirone.

Technically, the term *benzodiazepine* refers to the fusion of a benzene ring and a 7-atom diazepine ring. Most BZDs in clinical use also have a 5-aryl substituent ring. Alprazolam and triazolam have, in addition, a triazolo ring fused to positions 3 and 4 (Figure 29–3). Properties and doses of some BZDs and other relatively safe antianxiety drugs are described in Table 29–10. Because barbiturates and related drugs are generally no longer recommended for anxiety and insomnia, they are not discussed for these indications in this chapter.

BZDs are well absorbed orally, but (with the exception of lorazepam) they have unpredictable availability after intramuscular use. Most BZDs are

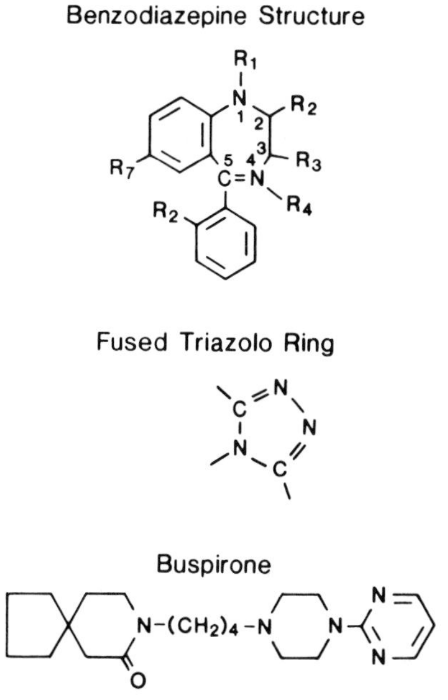

Benzodiazepine Structure

Fused Triazolo Ring

Buspirone

Figure 29–3. Structures of some anxiolytics.

TABLE 29–10. COMMONLY USED ANTIANXIETY DRUGS

Class and medication	*Trade name*	*Usual daily antianxiety dose (mg)*	*Onset of effect*
Short half-life benzodiazepines[a]			
Alprazolam	Xanax	1.5–6.0	Intermediate
Halazepam	Paxipam	20–120	Intermediate
Lorazepam	Ativan	1.5–6.0	Intermediate
Midazolam	Versed	7.5–45	Intermediate (oral); fast (iv)
Oxazepam	Serax	45–100	Slow
Quazepam[b]	Doral	7.5–15	Fast
Temazepam	Restoril	15–30	Intermediate-slow
Triazolam	Halcion	0.125–0.25	Fast
Long half-life benzodiazepines[c]			
Chlordiazepoxide	Librium	10–100	Slow
Clonazepam	Klonopin	0.5–4.0	Intermediate-slow
Clorazepate	Tranxene	7.5–60	Fast
Diazepam	Valium	2–30	Fast
Flurazepam	Dalmane	7.5–30	Fast
Azaspirone			
Buspirone	BuSpar	15–60	Slow
Antihistamines			
Hydroxyzine	Atarax	50–200	Slow
Diphenhydramine	Benadryl	50–200	Slow
β-Adrenergic blockers			
Propranolol	Inderal	40–120	Slow

[a]Half-life 5–20 hours.
[b]Major metabolite has half-life of 50–160 hours.
[c]Half-life 20–200 hours.

metabolized in the liver by complex enzyme systems. Unlike the barbiturates and many other psychoactive drugs, BZDs do not induce their own metabolism or the breakdown of other medications. With a few exceptions (e.g., lorazepam), the inactivation of BZDs is inhibited by cimetidine and oral contraceptives.

Onset of action following a single dose of a BZD is to a large extent a function of lipid solubility, which determines the speed with which the drug is absorbed into the bloodstream and then diffuses into the brain; rapid diffusion out of the brain leads to more rapid termination of action of more lipid-soluble drugs. This is why a single dose of diazepam has a faster onset and shorter duration of action than lorazepam, which has a shorter half-life but is less lipid soluble.

Elimination half-life contributes to duration of action during chronic dosing. BZDs with extremely short half-lives such as triazolam and midazolam do not accumulate but may be associated with discontinuation syndromes after a single dose. Drugs with intermediate (5–24 hour) half-lives accumulate somewhat and are associated with discontinuation syndromes that are intense and rapid in onset. BZDs with longer (> 24 hour) half-lives exhibit the greatest accumulation and may be more likely to cause falls in the elderly. Discontinuation syndromes are more gradual in onset and less severe in this group, but they last longer.

Variable patterns of metabolism of BZDs to active or inactive metabolites result in a broad range of half-lives (Table 29–10). Because blood level peaks can produce undue sedation, BZDs are often given 2–4 times a day for daytime anxiety despite half-lives of 2 days or more (Baldessarini 1985).

Mechanisms of Action

Much has been learned about the potentiation by BZDs of γ-aminobutyric acid (GABA), the transmitter that inhibits activation of monoamine-containing neurons (e.g., in the locus coeruleus) that mediate arousal and anxiety-related behaviors (Harvey 1985). Receptors for BZDs are linked to GABA receptors, which in turn facilitate opening of chloride ion channels. As chloride influx increases, so does the net negative internal charge, which hyperpolarizes the neuron. BZDs enhance affinity of the GABA receptor for GABA, thereby increasing its inhibitory action. BZD inverse agonists (e.g., the β-carbolines) decrease facilitation of GABA receptor affinity by BZD receptors and make it easier to depolarize the neuron.

BZDs and related anxiolytics appear to relieve anxiety through actions on BZD receptors in affective and arousal centers. Side effects such as sedation, elevated seizure threshold, and muscle relaxation are related to actions on BZD receptors in other regions of the nervous system such as the cortex, pyramidal cells, and spinal neurons. One approach to reducing adverse effects has been to develop compounds like alpidem and zolpidem with selective affinity for limbic but not cortical or spinal BZD receptors (Bartholini 1988). Quazepam, a recently marketed BZD-hypnotic, is supposed to have selective affinity for limbic receptors. However, its major metabolite, desalkylflurazepam, which has a long half-life, is more nonselective than the parent compound is selective (Shader and Greenblatt 1990).

Another approach to reducing side effects is with the azaspirones: buspirone, gepirone, and ipsapirone (the latter two have not yet been released). These drugs, which reduce anxiety without producing sedation, muscle relaxation, or elevated seizure threshold, have been thought not to have a primary effect on the BZD-GABA receptor complex but to have a more prominent action in stabilizing serotonergic transmission (Eison et al. 1986). However, buspirone may also enhance BZD receptor binding (Ayd 1984a).

Psychiatric Uses of Antianxiety Drugs in the Presence of Neurological Disease

Antianxiety drugs are most appropriately used to treat time-limited anxiety or insomnia that represents response to an identifiable stress or change in sleep phase. Because generalized anxiety disorder is often episodic, intermittent treatment of this condition is often appropriate.

When chronic anxiolytic therapy is necessary, buspirone may be better tolerated by patients with organic mental syndromes; however, its delayed onset of action makes it ineffective when taken as needed. TCAs are as effective as BZDs for generalized anxiety disorder in some patients (Hoehn-Saric et al. 1988), and the sedating TCAs are often useful as hypnotics.

Alprazolam may have antidepressant properties in patients with panic disorder, but the therapeutic index of this drug is too low for use as a primary antidepressant for most patients (Borison et al. 1989). Other BZDs may also reduce depression in mixed anxiety-depression, and these may be appropriate adjuncts when secondary anxiety does not respond to an antidepressant, particularly in epileptic patients.

Azaspirones administered in higher doses (e.g., 60–90 mg/day of buspirone) may have antidepressant properties that could make them useful as adjuncts to antidepressants or as a primary treatment for depression complicated by anxiety when the patient cannot tolerate effective doses of an antidepressant. Buspirone may also augment the antiobsessional effect of the serotonergic antidepressants.

Alprazolam and clonazepam are the only BZDs that have been studied for panic anxiety, but in equivalently high doses other BZDs may also be useful. A single dose of propranolol has been helpful to patients with stage fright, and atenolol may decrease social phobia (Gorman et al. 1985). Because buspirone can produce dysphoria at higher doses (Dommisse and DeVane 1985), it is not addicting.

Discontinuation Syndromes

Three syndromes may develop after abrupt discontinuation of BZDs (Busto et al. 1986; Noyes et al. 1988). Relapse, or return of the original anxiety disorder, occurs in 60%–80% of anxious patients, often after weeks to months. Rebound, which appears after hours to days in 25%–75% of patients, is intensification of the original symptoms that usually lasts several days. Withdrawal, which may be mild to severe in 40%–100% of cases, includes autonomic and CNS symptoms that are different from those of the original disorder.

The risk of withdrawal is greatest in patients who take 40–60 mg/day of diazepam or its equivalent for more than 1 month or who take lower doses for more than 8 months (Dubovsky and Weissberg 1986; Harvey 1985). Even one dose of a BZD-hypnotic can produce some rebound insomnia (Harvey 1985).

Withdrawal from BZDs is phenomenologically similar to withdrawal from other CNS depressants (Table 29–11). The real cause may not be apparent when acute psychosis, agitation, delirium, or a generalized seizure are secondary to BZD withdrawal, especially when the patient conceals the extent of drug use. These symptoms may not appear for some time after the patient has been admitted to the hospital if a long-acting BZD is being used or if the patient continues to take the medication after admission. Family members may provide important information about drug intake, but the patient's history is frequently unreliable. Toxicology screens may reveal additional unsuspected substances, but BZD blood levels are usually zero during an abstinence syndrome.

Because CNS depressants cross-react with each other, withdrawal from any combination of them may be diagnosed by administering phenobarbital or pentobarbital. Once signs and symptoms of withdrawal appear, 200 mg of pentobarbital or 60–100 mg of phenobarbital are administered orally on an empty stomach. If pentobarbital is used, the amount necessary to suppress abstinence is estimated from the amount of intoxication that is observed 1 hour after administration of the test dose. Intoxication is judged by the degree of signs such as sedation, nystagmus, dysarthria, postural hypotension, and ataxia. It is important to record the level of these findings both before and after the test dose is given because all but nystagmus may be seen in both intoxication and withdrawal.

TABLE 29–11. SYMPTOMS OF WITHDRAWAL FROM CENTRAL NERVOUS SYSTEM DEPRESSANTS

Dysphoria, irritability, and depression
Anxiety,[a] anorexia, agitation, panic, and restlessness
Increased sensitivity to light and sound
Headache, sweating, faintness, and dizziness
Myalgia, tremor, and muscle twitching
Rebound insomnia and bad dreams
Delirium, paranoia, and psychosis
Seizures

[a]Daytime anxiety may be a symptom of recurrent withdrawal when short-acting benzodiazepines are taken chronically at night for sleep.

Multiple significant signs of intoxication using this method indicate that there is no tolerance and that no further treatment is needed. Moderate intoxication suggests that 400–800 mg/day of pentobarbital is needed to suppress withdrawal. Nystagmus in the absence of other intoxication symptoms suggests that 800–1,000 mg/day of pentobarbital is necessary. No intoxication after the test dose suggests that more than 1,200 mg/day of pentobarbital is needed to prevent the abstinence syndrome; further requirements can be estimated with additional doses of pentobarbital (Dubin et al. 1986). These doses, or an equivalent amount of phenobarbital, are then administered in divided dose for 1–2 days, after which the barbiturate is withdrawn at a rate of 10% every day.

If phenobarbital is the initial medication, 60- to 100-mg doses are administered every 2–6 hours until the patient is intoxicated; the maximum daily phenobarbital dose is 500 mg (Smith and Wesson 1970). The total amount is given the next day in divided doses every 6 hours and then withdrawn initially at the same rate as for pentobarbital. More rapid withdrawal may be necessary after 4–7 days because the long half-life (24–120 hours) may result in drug accumulation when a steady state is reached. Nevertheless, this drug is preferable to pentobarbital because seizures are less likely to occur if dosage reduction is too rapid and because phenobarbital is available in injectable form if the patient refuses treatment. Within the guidelines listed above, each dose of pentobarbital or phenobarbital should be adjusted according to the patient's clinical status. A flow sheet indicating signs of withdrawal or intoxication before and after each dose makes it easier to judge the patient's overall response and the amount of the next dose.

❑ ORGANIC BRAIN SYNDROMES AND ANXIOLYTICS

When anxiety is a symptom of organic brain disease, steps should be taken to compensate for the underlying disturbance of concentration, attention, and memory while the medical or neurological disorder is being diagnosed and treated. This is accomplished by measures such as frequent orienting, keeping a light on at night, and avoiding unnecessary changes in the patient's surroundings. Although they may be useful in some forms of agitation, oral BZDs and barbiturates are often ineffective anxiolytics in patients with delirium and dementia because these medications further depress cortical and reticular activating system function, which clouds the patients' sensorium even more. Buspirone does not cloud consciousness and is a more appropriate anxiolytic for patients with dementia. Buspirone may also reduce episodic and chronic agitation in patients with dementia, as may trazodone.

Antihistamines (e.g., hydroxyzine 50–100 mg po or im) are sometimes used to sedate patients with organic brain disease who require an EEG, because these drugs have minimal effects on the EEG. Antihistamines have also been used as sleeping pills for the elderly and patients with dementia, but their anticholinergic properties may be problematic and their antianxiety effect is unpredictable. Low doses of sedating antidepressants such as amitriptyline, doxepin, or trazodone may be useful hypnotics for dementia patients as well as for patients with insomnia induced by fluoxetine or MAOIs. Care should be taken to assess the suicide potential of such patients because antidepressants are more dangerous than BZDs when taken in overdose.

Even after special tests, it is occasionally not clear whether complex symptoms such as memory loss, confusion, agitation, or psychosis are due to a psychiatric or a neurological disorder. If the patient does not have a space-occupying lesion, increased intracranial pressure, porphyria, or allergy to the drug, amobarbital 100–400 mg iv administered very slowly can sometimes distinguish between the two. With a little sedation, the patient may become more cooperative with mental status testing. Dramatic transient improvement when the patient is tranquilized suggests a functional etiology. Worsening of symptoms during the amobarbital interview, which is usually due to intensification of the underlying disorder of consciousness by the CNS depressant, suggests an organic cause.

The amobarbital interview may also help to distinguish between neurologically based and functional paralysis, blindness, deafness, aphonia, and sensory loss. The latter disorders may disappear briefly under amobarbital, whereas the former only improve slightly or are unchanged. Failure of symptoms to remit during the interview does not exclude a psychogenic syndrome.

Antianxiety Drugs in the Elderly

As with other centrally acting drugs, lower doses and smaller increments in dosage are necessary for older patients. Shorter-acting BZDs such as triazolam are preferable as sleeping pills to longer-acting ones such as flurazepam. BZDs with simpler metabolic pathways such as lorazepam or oxazepam may be safer than medications with multiple active metabolites, and buspirone is probably safest. Elderly patients who complain of insomnia should not take a hypnotic unless it is clear that difficulty sleeping is not a symptom of another major disorder such as dementia, depression, gastroesophageal reflux, sleep apnea, or restless legs syndrome. Dementia and sleep apnea in particular may be aggravated by nighttime sedation.

Neurological Uses of BZDs and Related Drugs

Phenobarbital is familiar to most clinicians as a first-line anticonvulsant. Clonazepam is a BZD anticonvulsant with a half-life ranging from 20 to 40 hours that is used to treat generalized, myoclonic, and absence epilepsy (Chouinard and Penry 1985). Clonazepam may be helpful in some cases of trigeminal neuralgia and pain syndromes elsewhere in the body that are associated with paroxysmal dysesthesias, pain on stimulation or normal tissue, burning sensations, and hyperesthesia (Bouckonis and Litman 1985). Clonazepam has utility in paroxysmal choreoathetosis that might predict effectiveness in the treatment of TD (Chouinard and Penry 1985). A dose of 1.5–4.0 mg/day has been used for neuralgia, whereas the purported antimanic dose is 4–16 mg/day (Chouinard and Penry 1985).

Neurological Side Effects of Antianxiety Drugs

The most important adverse effects of BZD use are tolerance, abstinence syndromes, sedation, and impaired psychomotor performance. Tolerance to sedation often develops within a week or so, but tolerance to psychomotor impairment takes longer and in some cases may not develop at all (Moskowitz and Smiley 1985). Patients taking BZDs often are not aware of impaired driving, but the risk of a serious accident may be increased fivefold over that for nonusers of BZDs, and even more if the patient also drinks (Dubovsky 1990). Not only may BZDs produce additive psychomotor impairment with alcohol, they may also increase the risk of relapse of alcoholism. The risk of addiction to BZDs is low in patients without a history of substance abuse; anxious patients with such a history should be treated with buspirone or antidepressants (Dubovsky 1990).

TABLE 29–12. PSYCHIATRIC SIDE EFFECTS OF NEUROLOGICAL DRUGS

Symptom	*Medications*	*Comments*
Depression	Amantadine	Common at usual doses
	Anticonvulsants	Usually at higher blood levels
	Corticosteroids, ACTH	More common with high doses; may occur on withdrawal
	Benzodiazepines	Depression may also decrease in anxious, depressed patients
	Barbiturates	Common side effect
	Narcotics	
	L-Dopa	Greater risk with prolonged use
	Antihypertensives	Has been reported with many preparations
	Propranolol	Can occur at usual doses
	Vinblastine	Rare
	Asparaginase	Common side effect with higher doses
	Cimetidine	
	Oral contraceptives	In as much as 15% of all cases
	Ibuprofen	Rare
	Metoclopramide	Usual doses
Mania	Baclofen	Usually appears after sudden withdrawal
	Bromocriptine	Symptoms may continue after drug is withdrawn
	Captopril	Symptoms may continue after drug is withdrawn
	Corticosteroids, ACTH	Usually at higher doses
	Dextromethorphan	
	L-Dopa	More frequent in elderly; risk increases with prolonged use
	Antidepressants	In bipolar and some chronically depressed patients
	Digitalis	In bipolar patients with higher doses
	Cyclobenzaprine	Reported in one patient
Hallucinations	Amantadine	Rare; more common in elderly
	Anticonvulsants	Visual and auditory
	Antihistamines	Especially with higher doses
	Anticholinergics	Usually with delirium
	Corticosteroids, ACTH	See above[a]
	Digitalis	Usually at higher blood levels
	Indomethacin	Especially in elderly
	Methysergide	Occasional
	Propranolol	At usual or increased doses
	Methylphenidate	More likely in children
	L-Dopa	See above[a]
	Ketamine	Common
	Cimetidine	Usually in higher doses and in elderly
Nightmares	Antidepressants	When entire dose is taken at night
	Amantadine	Especially in elderly
	Baclofen	Usually after sudden withdrawal
	Ketamine	Also produces hallucinations, crying, changes in body image, and delirium
	L-Dopa	Often after dosage increase
	Pentazocine	During treatment
	Propranolol	See above[a]
	Digitalis	See above[a]
Paranoia	Asparaginase	May be common
	Bromocriptine	Not dose related
	Corticosteroids, ACTH	See above[a]
	Amphetamines	Even at low doses
	Indomethacin	Especially in elderly
	Propranolol	At any dose
	Sulindac	Reported in a few patients

TABLE 29–12. (Continued)

Symptom	*Medications*	*Comments*
Aggression	Bromocriptine	Not dose related; may persist
	Tranquilizers and hypnotics	A release phenomenon
	L-Dopa	See above[a]
	Phenelzine	May be separate from mania
	Digitalis	See above[a]
	Carbamazepine	In children and adolescents

Note. ACTH = adrenocorticotropic hormone.
[a]Same comments apply as for previous reactions on this drug.

Paradoxical reactions to BZDs such as anxiety, irritability, aggression, agitation, and insomnia are common in children, the elderly, and patients with brain damage. Behavioral toxicity may occur in psychotic patients treated with BZDs, whereas alprazolam may induce mania (Bodkin 1990). Because characteristically hypervigilant patients may become panic stricken, suspicious, or belligerent when their faculties are dulled by sedating effects of tranquilizers, antianxiety drugs should be either avoided or used in very low doses when they are absolutely necessary; buspirone may be better tolerated. BZDs are rarely fatal when ingested in overdose unless they are accompanied by other CNS depressants (Baldessarini 1985), and the LD50 (median lethal dose) of buspirone is as much as 100 times the therapeutic dose.

Like the barbiturates, low doses of BZDs decrease alpha activity on the EEG and increase low-voltage fast activity (Harvey 1985). In contrast with the barbiturates, EEG changes with BZDs are more obvious in the frontal regions and are less likely to spread through the brain. Most BZDs increase stage 2 non-REM sleep and decrease stage 4 sleep, making them useful in treating some but not all nightmares (Harvey 1985). Low doses of flurazepam, temazepam, and possibly other BZDs do not shorten the total time in REM sleep; even when time in each REM period is decreased, the number of REM cycles is increased. Patients with depression who have increased REM density may spend even more time in REM sleep when they take BZDs, resulting in unpleasant or vivid dreams.

Buspirone can cause nausea, dizziness, headache, or excitement. Concerns have been raised about the possibility that this drug could cause EPS and TD, but because it binds to presynaptic autoreceptors rather than postsynaptic D_2 receptors, does not induce postsynaptic dopamine receptor supersensitivity, is devoid of clinical neuroleptic activity, and does not aggravate Parkinson's disease, these concerns do not appear to be justified (Dubovsky 1990; Neppe 1989; Sussman 1987).

Interactions of Antianxiety Drugs With Neurological Drugs

Barbiturates induce hepatic microsomal systems that metabolize many other drugs, including a number of anticonvulsants. This is not true of BZDs, but ethanol and phenytoin decrease BZD breakdown slightly (Harvey 1985). A more significant problem is the additive CNS depressant effect of most anxiolytics with other depressant drugs, including anticonvulsants. BZDs can augment respiratory depression induced by opioids other than meperidine. Buspirone has not yet been found to have any clinically significant interactions with the exception of possible serotonin syndrome with MAOIs (Ayd 1984a).

❑ PSYCHIATRIC SIDE EFFECTS OF NEUROLOGICAL DRUGS

Most drugs that affect the CNS can produce changes in thinking, emotion, and behavior that mimic primary psychiatric syndromes. The psychiatric symptoms may appear in a clear sensorium, or they may be accompanied by signs and symptoms of delirium. Antiparkinsonian drugs (e.g., trihexyphenidyl and benztropine) and some neuroleptics and antidepressants can produce anticholinergic delirium characterized by agitation, psychosis, hallucinations, tachycardia, mydriasis, fever, and warm dry skin. Common disturbances and their causes are summarized in Table 29–12 (Dubovsky and Weissberg 1986; Medical Letter 1985).

Psychiatric Uses of Neurological Drugs

As the boundary between neurology and psychiatry continues to be explored, a number of drugs used routinely in neurological practice are proving useful for psychiatric syndromes. Some of the better studied applications, doses, and side effects are reviewed in Table 29–13 (Altamura et al. 1987; Chouinard 1988; Dickey and Morrow 1990; Dubin et al. 1986; Jefferson 1990; Larsen et al. 1985; McElroy et

TABLE 29–13. PSYCHIATRIC APPLICATIONS OF SOME NEUROLOGICAL DRUGS

Medication (usual dose in psychiatry mg/day)	*Psychiatric uses*	*Side effects*
Carbamazepine (400–2,000; blood level 8–12 µg/ml)	Mania, especially when resistant to lithium Rapid cycling Antidepressant augmentation Posttraumatic stress syndrome Adjunct to neuroleptics in schizophrenia and schizoaffective disorder Restless legs syndrome Chronic pain with dysesthesias Trigeminal neuralgia	Rash (10%–15%) Bone marrow suppression (1:40,000 to 1:125,000) Hepatotoxicity Dizziness Ataxia Sedation Diplopia Dysarthria Inappropriate antidiuretic hormone secretion Mania and aggressiveness in children Loses effectiveness when stored in humid conditions
Valproic acid 1,000–3,000; blood level 50–120 µg/ml)	Mania, especially when resistant to lithium and carbamazepine Ultra rapid cycling Usually combined with another antimanic drug	Tremor Gastrointestinal distress Weight gain Hepatotoxicity
Clonazepam (2–10)	Mania, especially as sedative or hypnotic Panic disorder Psychosis associated with epilepsy Augmentation of neuroleptics in schizophrenia Akathisia Chronic pain Tic disorders Possibly obsessive-compulsive disorder	Sedation Impaired performance Tolerance to anticonvulsant and psychotropic effects
Bromocriptine (5–200)	Neuroleptic malignant syndrome Neuroleptic-induced galactorrhea and amenorrhea Extrapyramidal syndrome Refractory depression Cocaine craving and withdrawal Restless legs syndrome	Nausea and vomiting Abdominal cramps Headaches Dizziness Delirium Psychosis Nonrecurrent syncope after first dose
Calcium channel blockers (e.g., verapamil 240–480)	Mania Adjunct in panic disorder Tourette's syndrome Tardive dyskinesia MAOI-induced hypertensive reaction	Headache Constipation Postural hypotension Increased carbamazepine and valproate levels Increased lithium toxicity Increased carbamazepine toxicity

Note. MAOI = monoamine oxidase inhibitor.

al. 1988; Okuma et al. 1989; Post et al. 1987; Stewart et al. 1990). These drugs are also discussed in the appropriate sections earlier in this chapter.

❑ REFERENCES

*Suggested reading

*Adams F: Emergency intravenous sedation of the delirious medically ill patient. J Clin Psychiatry 49(suppl): 22–26, 1988

Adams F, Fernandez F, Andersson BE: Emergency pharmacotherapy of delirium in the critically ill cancer patient. Psychosomatics 27(suppl):33–37, 1986

Altamura AC, Mauri MC, Mautero M, et al: Clonazepam/haloperidol combination therapy in schizophrenia: a double-blind study. Acta Psychiatr Scand 76:702–706, 1987

*American Psychiatric Association: Tricyclic antidepressants: blood level measurements and clinical outcome: a report of the Task Force on the Use of Laboratory Tests in Psychiatry. Am J Psychiatry 142:155–162, 1985

American Psychiatric Association Task Force on Electroconvulsive Therapy: The Practice of Electroconvulsive Therapy: Recommendations for Treatment, Training, and Privileging. Washington, DC, American Psychiatric Association, 1990

*Anderson K, Baldwin J, Gottfries CG, et al: A double-blind evaluation of electroconvulsive therapy in Parkinson's disease with "on-off" phenomenon. Acta Neurol Scand 76:191–199, 1987

Ayd F: Buspirone: a review. International Drug Therapy Newsletter 19:37–42, 1984a

Ayd F: Intravenous haloperidol-lorazepam therapy of delirium. International Drug Therapy Newsletter 19:33–35, 1984b

*Ayd F: Prophylactic antiparkinsonian drug therapy: pros and cons. International Drug Therapy Newsletter 21:5–6, 1986

Ayd FJ: Fluoxetine: less seems to be more in depression? International Drug Therapy Newsletter 25:27, 1990a

*Ayd FJ: The World Health Organization's position on prophylactic anticholinergics. International Drug Therapy Newsletter 25:31–32, 1990b

Azar I, Lear E: Cardiovascular effects of electroconvulsive therapy in patients taking tricyclic antidepressants. Anesth Analg 63:1140, 1984

Baldessarini RJ: Drugs and the treatment of psychiatric disorders, in The Pharmacological Basis of Therapeutics. Edited by Gilman AG, Goodman LS, Rall TW, et al. New York, Macmillan, 1985, pp 387–445

*Baldessarini RS, Marsh E: Fluoxetine and side effects. Arch Gen Psychiatry 47:191–192, 1990

*Baldessarini RJ, Cohen BM, Teicher MH: Significance of neuroleptic dose and plasma level in the pharmacological treatment of psychosis. Arch Gen Psychiatry 45:79–91, 1988

Ballenger JC: The clinical use of carbamazepine in affective disorders. J Clin Psychiatry 49 (suppl):13–19, 1988

Bartholini G: Concluding remarks. Pharmacol Biochem Behav 29:833–834, 1988

Bernstein JG: Handbook of Drug Therapy in Psychiatry. Boston, MA, John Wright-PSG, 1983

Berridge MJ: Inositol triphosphatase and diacylglycerol as second messengers. Biochem J 220:345–360, 1984

Black DW, Winokur G, Nasrallah A: Treatment of mania: a naturalistic study of electroconvulsive therapy vs lithium in 438 pts. J Clin Psychiatry 48:132–139, 1987

Bodkin JA: Emerging uses for high-potency benzodiazepines in psychotic disorders. J Clin Psychiatry 51 (suppl):41–46, 1990

Borison RL, Siriha P, Albrecht JW, et al: Double-blind comparison of 3 and 6 mg fixed doses of alprazolam vs placebo in outpatients with major depression. Psychopharmacol Bull 25:186–189, 1989

Bouckonis AJ, Litman RE: Clonazepam in the treatment of neuralgic pain syndromes. Psychosomatics 26:933–936, 1985

Brandon S, Crowley P, MacDold C, et al: Electroconvulsive therapy: results in depressive illness from the Leicestershire trial. Br Med J 288:22–25, 1984

Busto V, Sellers EM, Naranjo C, et al: Withdrawal reaction after long-term therapeutic use of benzodiazepines. N Engl J Med 315:854–859, 1986

*Campbell M, Spencer EIK: Psychopharmacology in child and adolescent psychiatry: a review of the past five years. J Am Acad Child Adolesc Psychiatry 27:269–279, 1988

Carman JS, Wyatt RJ: Alterations in cerebrospinal fluid and serum total calcium with changes in psychiatric state, in Neuroregulators and Psychiatric Disorders. Edited by Usdin E, Hamburg DA, Barchas JD. New York, Oxford University Press, 1977, pp 488–494

Charney DS, Heninger GR, Sternberg DE: Serotonin function and mechanisms of action of antidepressant treatment. Arch Gen Psychiatry 41:359–365, 1984

*Chou JCY: Recent advances in treatment of acute mania. J Clin Psychopharmacol 11:3–21, 1991

Chouinard G: The use of benzodiazepines in the treatment of manic-depressive illness. J Clin Psychiatry 49:15–20, 1988

Chouinard G, Penry JK: Neurologic and psychiatric aspects of clonazepam: an update: proceedings of a symposium. Psychosomatics 26 (suppl):1–37, 1985

Ciraulo DA, Shader RI: Fluoxetine drug-drug interactions, I: antidepressants and antipsychotics. J Clin Psychopharmacol 10:48–50, 1990

Clary C, Schweizer E: Treatment of MAOI hypertensive crisis with sublingual nifedipine. J Clin Psychiatry 48: 249–250, 1987

Cohen WJ, Cohen NH: Lithium carbonate, haloperidol and irreversible brain damage. JAMA 230:1283–1287, 1974

Creese I, Burt DR, Snyder SH: Dopamine receptor binding predicts clinical and pharmacologic potencies of antischizophrenic drugs. Science 192:481–483, 1976

Davidson J: Seizures and buspirone: a review. J Clin Psychiatry 50:256–261, 1989

*Davis JM, Andriukaitis S: The natural course of schizophrenia and effective maintenance drug treatment. J Clin Psychopharmacol 6 (suppl 1):2S–10S, 1986

Demuth GW, Breslov RE, Drescher J: The elicitation of a movement disorder by trazodone: case report. J Clin Psychiatry 46:535–536, 1985
Dickey W, Morrow JI: Drug-induced neurological disorders. Prog Neurobiol 34:331–342, 1990
Dilsaver SC, Greden JF: Antidepressant withdrawal phenomena. Biol Psychiatry 19:237–253, 1984
Dommisse CS, DeVane CL: Buspirone: a new type of anxiolytic. Drug Intelligence and Clinical Pharmacy 19: 624–628, 1985
*Dubin WR: Rapid tranquilization: antipsychotics or benzodiazepines? J Clin Psychiatry 49 (suppl):5–11, 1988
Dubin WR, Weiss KJ, Dorn JM: Pharmacotherapy of psychiatric emergencies. J Clin Psychopharmacol 6:210–222, 1986
Dubovsky SL: Calcium antagonists: new class of psychiatric drugs? Psychiatric Annals 16:724–728 1986a
*Dubovsky SL: Using electroconvulsive therapy for patients with neurological disease. Hosp Community Psychiatry 37:819–825, 1986b
*Dubovsky SL: Generalized anxiety disorder: new concepts and psychopharmacologic therapies. J Clin Psychiatry 51 (suppl):3–10, 1990
Dubovsky SL, Franks RD: Intracellular calcium ions in affective disorders: a review and an hypothesis. Biol Psychiatry 18:781–797, 1983
Dubovsky SL, Weissberg MP: Clinical Psychiatry in Primary Care, 3rd Edition. Baltimore, MD, Williams & Wilkins, 1986
Dubovsky SL, Franks RD, Allen S, et al: Calcium antagonists in mania. Psychiatry Res 18:309–320, 1986
Dubovsky SL, Lee C, Christiano J, et al: Lithium lowers platelet intracellular calcium ion concentration in bipolar patients. Lithium 2:167–174, 1991
Eison AS, Eison MS, Stanley M, et al: Serotonergic mechanisms in behavioral effects of buspirone and gepirone. Pharmacol Biochem Behav 24:710–717, 1986
El-Gazour AR, Ivankovich AD, Braverman B, et al: Monoamine oxidase inhibitors: should they be discontinued preoperatively? Anesth Analg 64:592–596, 1985
El-Mallakh RS: Complications of concurrent lithium and electroconvulsive therapy: a review of clinical material and theoretical considerations. Biol Psychiatry 23:595–601, 1988
*Ereshefsky L, Watanabe MD, Tran-Johnson TK: Clozapine: an atypical antipsychotic agent. Clin Pharm 8: 691–709, 1989
Escobar JI, Barron A, Kiriakos R: A controlled study of "neuroleptization" with fluphenazine hydrochloride injections. J Clin Psychopharmacol 3:359–363, 1983
*Fenwick P: The nature and management of aggression in epilepsy. Journal of Neuropsychiatry and Clinical Neurosciences 1:418–425, 1989
Fernandez F, Holmes VF, Adams F, et al: Treatment of severe refractory agitation with a haloperidol drip. J Clin Psychiatry 49:239–241, 1988
Fink M: Induced seizures and human behavior, in Psychobiology of Convulsive Therapy. Edited by Fink M, Kety S, McGaugh J, et al. Washington, DC, VH Winston, 1974, pp 1–20
Fink M: Convulsive Therapy: Theory and Practice. New York, Raven, 1979
*Fink M: ECT for Parkinson's disease? Convulsive Therapy 4:189–191, 1988
Fink M: How does convulsive therapy work? Neuropsychopharmacology 3:73–82, 1990
Fiori MG: Tricyclic antidepressants: a review of their toxicology. Current Developments in Psychopharmacology 4:72–94, 1977
Fricchione G: Catasonia: a new indication for benzodiazepines? Biol Psychiatry 26:761–765, 1989
Friedman JH, Lammon MC: Clozapine in treatment of psychosis in Parkinson's disease. Neurology 39:1219–1221, 1989
*Gelenberg AJ, Kane JM, Keller MB, et al: Comparison of standard and low serum levels of lithium for maintenance treatment of bipolar disorder. N Engl J Med 321: 1489–1493, 1989
Goodman WK, Charney DS: Therapeutic applications and mechanisms of action of monoamine oxidase and heterocyclic antidepressant drugs. J Clin Psychiatry 46:6–22, 1985
Gorman JM, Leibowitz MR, Fyer AJ, et al: Treatment of social phobia and atenolol. J Clin Psychopharmacol 5: 298–301, 1985
Graham LF, Fredrickson-Overo K, Kirk L: Influences of neuroleptics and benzodiazepines on metabolism of tricyclic antidepressants in man. Am J Psychiatry 131: 863–866, 1974
*Greist JH, Jefferson JW, Rosenfeld R, et al: Clomipramine and obsessive compulsive disorder: a placebo-controlled double-blind study of 32 patients. J Clin Psychiatry 51:292–297, 1990
Guze BH, Baxter LR: Neuroleptic malignant syndrome. N Engl J Med 313:163–166, 1985
Harvey SC: Hypnotics and sedatives, in the Pharmacological Basis of Therapeutics, 7th Edition. Edited by Gilman AG, Goodman LS, Rall TW, et al. New York, Macmillan, 1985, pp 339–371
Herman JB, Brotman AW, Pollack MH, et al: Fluoxetine-induced sexual dysfunction. J Clin Psychiatry 51:27–29, 1990
Hoehn-Saric R, McLeod DR, Zimmerl WD: Differential effects of alprazolam and imipramine in generalized anxiety disorder. J Clin Psychiatry 49:293–301, 1988
*Holmes VF, Fernandez F, Levy JK: Psychostimulant response in AIDS-related complex patients. J Clin Psychiatry 50:5–8, 1989
Hoogiverf B: Amitriptyline treatment of painful diabetic neuropathy: an inadvertent single-patient clinical trial. Diabetes Care 8:526–527, 1985
Huai-Yu, Guszhen L, Jundong G, et al: Furazalidone in peptic ulcer. Lancet 2:276–277, 1985
Izzo KL, Brody R: Rehabilitation in lithium toxicity. Arch Phys Med Rehabil 66:779–782, 1985
*Jacobsen FM: Low-dose trazodone as a hypnotic when treated with MAOIs and other psychotropics. J Clin Psychiatry 51:298–302, 1990
Jefferson JW: Lithium: the present and the future. J Clin Psychiatry 51 (suppl):4–8, 1990
Jefferson JW, Greist JH: Primer of Lithium Therapy. Baltimore, MD, Williams & Wilkins, 1977

Jenike MA: The use of monomine oxidase inhibitors in the treatment of elderly patients. J Am Geriatr Soc 32: 571–575, 1984

Jenike MA: Approaches to the patients with treatment-refractory obsessive-compulsive disorder. J Clin Psychiatry 51 (suppl):15–21, 1990

*Jensen HV, Olafsson K, Bille A, et al: Lithium every second day: a new treatment regimen? Lithium 1:55–58, 1990

Kahn EM, Schulz C, Perel JM, et al: Change in haloperidol level due to carbamazepine: a complexatory factor in combined medication for schizophrenia. J Clin Psychopharmacol 10:54–57, 1990

Kane JM: Dosage strategies with long-acting injectable neuroleptics, including haloperidol decanoate. J Clin Psychopharmacol 6:205–235, 1986

Kane JM, Woerner M, Borenstein M, et al: Integrating incidence and prevalence of tardive dyskinesia. Paper presented at the Fourth World Congress of Biological Psychiatry, Philadelphia, PA, September 1985

*Kane JM, Honigfeld G, Singer J, et al: Clozapine for the treatment-resistant schizophrenia. Arch Gen Psychiatry 45:789–796, 1988

Kars H, Broekenia W, Glaudenmans-Gelderen I, et al: Naltrexone attenuates self-injurious behavior in mentally retarded patients. Biol Psychiatry 27:741–746, 1990

Kaufman MW, Cassem N, Murray G, et al: The use of methylphenidate in depressed patients after cardiac surgery. J Clin Psychiatry 45:82–84, 1984

Klein DF, Gittelman R, Quitkin F, et al: Diagnosis and Drug Treatment of Psychiatric Disorders: Adults and Children, 2nd Edition. Baltimore, MD, Williams & Wilkins, 1980

Ko GN, Korpi ER, Linnoila M: On the clinical relevance and methods of quantification of plasma concentrations of neuroleptics. J Clin Psychopharmacol 5:253–262, 1985

Koczerinski D, Kennedy SH, Swinson RP: Clonazepam and lithium: a toxic combination in the treatment of mania? Int Clin Psychopharmacol 4:195–199, 1989

Larsen S, Telstad W, Sorensen O, et al: Carbamazepine therapy in restless legs: discrimination between responders and nonresponders. Acta Medica Scandinavia 218:223–227, 1985

Lawrence JM: Reactions to withdrawal of antidepressants, antiparkinsonian drugs, and lithium. Psychosomatics 11:869–877, 1985

Lieberman JA, Kane JM, Reife R: Neuromuscular effects of monamine oxidase inhibitors. J Clin Psychopharmacol 5:217–220, 1985

Litovitz TL, Troutman WG: Amoxapine overdose: seizures and fatalities. JAMA 250:1069–1071, 1983

Lydiard RB: Tricyclic-resistant depression: treatment resistance or inadequate treatment. J Clin Psychiatry 46: 412–417, 1985

*McElroy SL, Keck PE, Pope HJ, et al: Valproate in the treatment of rapid-cycling bipolar disorder. J Clin Psychopharmacol 8:275–279, 1988

Mann JJ, Aarons SF, Wilner PJ, et al: A controlled study of the antidepressant efficacy and side effects of (-)-deprenyl. Arch Gen Psychiatry 46:45–50, 1989

*Marder SR, Van Putten T: Who should receive clozapine? Arch Gen Psychiatry 45:865–867, 1988

Martin PR, Adinoff DB, Eckardt MJ, et al: Effective pharmacotherapy of alcoholic amnestic disorder with fluvoxamine: preliminary findings. Arch Gen Psychiatry 46:617–621, 1989

Massey EW, Folger WN: Seizures activated by therapeutic levels of lithium carbonate. South Med J 77:1173–1175, 1984

Mathew NT: Prophylaxis of migraine and mixed headache: a randomized controlled study. Headache 21: 105–109, 1981

*Medical Letter: Drugs that cause psychiatric symptoms. Med Lett Drugs Ther 26:75–78, 1985

Mellerup ET, Plenge P: The side effects of lithium. Biol Psychiatry 28:464–465, 1990

Meyler L, Herxheimer A: Side Effects of Drugs. Baltimore, MD, Williams & Wilkins, 1968

Miller DD: Effect of phenytoin on plasma clozapine concentration in two patients. J Clin Psychiatry 52:23–25, 1991

Miller F, Menninger J: Correlation of neuroleptic dose and neurotoxicity in patients given lithium and a neuroleptic. Hosp Community Psychiatry 38:1219–1221, 1987

Modestin J, Toffler G, Pia M: Haloperidol in acute schizophrenic inpatients: a double-blind comparison of two dosage regimens. Pharmacopsychiatry 16:121–126, 1983

Moskowitz H, Smiley A: Effects of chronically administered buspirone and diazepam in driving-related skills performance. J Clin Psychopharmacol 5:45–55, 1985

Mueller PS: Neuroleptic malignant syndrome. Psychosomatics 26:654–662, 1985

Neppe VM: Innovative Psychopharmacotherapy. New York, Raven, 1989, pp 35–57

*Noyes R, Garvey MJ, Cook BL, et al: Benzodiazepine withdrawal: a review of the evidence. J Clin Psychiatry 49:382–389, 1988

Okuma T, Yamashita I, Takahashi R, et al: Clinical efficacy of carbamazepine in affective, schizoaffective, and schizophrenic disorders. Pharmacopsychiatry 2:47–53, 1989

Packman AM, Meyer DA, Verdun RM: Hazards of succinylcholine administration during electrotherapy. Arch Gen Psychiatry 35:1137–1141, 1978

Pare CMB: The present status of monoamine oxidase inhibitors. Br J Psychiatry 146:576–584, 1985

Pearson HJ: Interaction of fluoxetine with carbamazepine (letter). J Clin Psychiatry 51:126, 1990

Pelonero AL, Levenson JL, Silverman JL: Neuroleptic therapy following neuroleptic malignant syndrome. Psychosomatics 26:946–947, 1985

Penney JF, Dinwiddie SH, Zorunuski CF, et al: Concurrent close temporal administration of lithium and ECT. Convulsive Therapy 6:139–145, 1990

Perry PJ, Calloway RA, Cook BL, et al: Theophyllus-precipitated alterations of lithium clearance. Acta Psychiatr Scand 69:528–539, 1984

Pinder RM, Brogden RN, Speight TM, et al: Maprotiline: a review of its pharmacological properties and therapeutic efficacy in mental states. Drugs 13:321–352, 1977

Post RM, Uhde TW, Roy-Byrne PP, et al: Correlates of

antimanic responses to carbamazepine. Psychiatry Res 21:71–83, 1987

*Post RM, Leverich GS, Rosoff AS, et al: Carbamazepine prophylaxis in refractory affective disorders: a focus on long-term follow-up. J Clin Psychopharmacol 10: 318–327, 1990

Quitkin F, Rifkin A, Klein DF: Monoamine oxidase inhibitors: review of effectiveness. Arch Gen Psychiatry 36: 749–760, 1979

Ragheb M: The clinical significance of lithium-nonsteroidal antiinflammatory drug interactions. J Clin Psychopharmacol 10:350–354, 1990

Raskin DE: Antipsychotic medication and the elderly. J Clin Psychiatry 46:36–40, 1985

Richelson E: The newer antidepressants: structures, pharmacokinetics, pharmacodynamics, and proposed mechanisms of action. Psychopharmacol Bull 20:213–223, 1984

Richelson E: Pharmacology of neuroleptics in use in the United States. J Clin Psychiatry 46:8–14, 1985a

Richelson E: Treatment of peptic ulcer disease with tricyclic antidepressants. International Drug Therapy Newsletter 20:21–23, 1985b

*Rickels K, Schweizer E, Csanalosi I, et al: Long-term treatment of anxiety and risk of withdrawal. Arch Gen Psychiatry 45:444–450, 1988

Rickels K, Amsterdam JD, Clary C, et al: Buspirone in major depression: a controlled study. J Clin Psychiatry 52:34–38, 1991

Robinson DS, Alms DR, Shrotriya RC, et al: Serotonergic anxiolytics and treatment of depression. Psychotherapy 22 (suppl):27–36, 1989

Robinson RG, Lipsey JR, Price TP: Diagnosis and clinical management of post-stroke depression. Psychosomatics 26:769–778, 1985

Robinson RG, Morris PLP, Fedoroff JP: Depression and cerebrovascular disease. J Clin Psychiatry 51 (suppl):26–31, 1990

Rogers MP: Rheumatoid arthritis: psychiatric aspects and use in psychotropics. Psychosomatics 26:915–925, 1985

*Rosebush P, Stewart T: Neuroleptic malignant syndrome. Am J Psychiatry 146:717–725, 1989

Rosenblatt RM, Reich J, Dehrung D: Tricyclic antidepressants in treatment of depression and chronic pain: analysis of the supporting evidence. Anesth Analg 63:1025–1032, 1984

*Rosenthal NE, Sack DA, Carpenter CJ, et al: Antidepressant effects of light in seasonal affective disorder. Am J Psychiatry 142:163–170, 1985

*Ross ED, Rush AJ: Diagnosis and neuroanatomical correlates of depression in brain damaged patients. Arch Gen Psychiatry 38:1344–1354, 1981

Rossi A, Stratta P, Nistico R, et al: Visuospatial impairment in depression: a controlled ECT study. Acta Psychiatr Scand 81:245–249, 1990

*Roy A, Pickar D: Lithium potentiation of imipramine in treatment-resistant depression. Br J Psychiatry 148: 528–583, 1985

Rubin EH, Biggs JT, Preskorn SH: Nortriptyline pharmacokinetics and plasma levels: implications for clinical practice. J Clin Psychiatry 46:418–424, 1985

Sackheim HA, Decina P, Portnoy S, et al: Studies of dosage seizure threshold and seizure duration in ECT. Biol Psychiatry 22:249–268, 1987

Sakkas P, Davis JM, Jin H: Vulnerability and presentation of NMS. Paper presented at the annual meeting of the American Psychiatric Association, San Francisco, CA, May 1989

Salzman C: Geriatric psychopharmacology. Annu Rev Med 36:217–228, 1985

Salzman C, Green A, Rodriguez-Villa F, et al: Benzodiazepines combined with neuroleptics for management of severe disruptive behavior. Psychosomatics 27 (suppl):17–21, 1986

Sassim N, Grohmann R: Adverse drug reactions with clozapine and simultaneous application of benzodiazepines. Pharmacopsychiatry 21:306–307, 1988

Saul RF: Pseudotumor cerebri secondary to lithium carbonate. JAMA 253:2869–2871, 1985

Saxena S, Maltikarjuna P: Severe memory impairment with acute overdose lithium toxicity. Br J Psychiatry 152:853–854, 1988

Schiffer RB, Herndon RM, Rudide RA: Treatment of pathological laughing and weeping with amitriptyline. N Engl J Med 312:1480–1482, 1985

Schooler NR: The efficacy of antipsychotic drugs and family therapy in the maintenance treatment of schizophrenia. J Clin Psychopharmacol 6:115–195, 1986

Schreiber G, Avissar S, Danon A, et al: Hyperfunctional G proteins in mononuclear leukocytes of patients with mania. Biol Psychiatry 29:273–280, 1991

*Schweitzer E, Rickels K, Amsterdam JD, et al: What constitutes an adequate antidepressant trial for fluoxetine? J Clin Psychiatry 51:8–11, 1990

Shader RI, Greenblatt DJ: Newly-marketed medications: ABCs of mind your Qs. J Clin Psychopharmacol 10:81–82, 1990

Sheehan DV, Ballenger J, Jacobson G: Treatment of endogenous anxiety with phobic, hysterical and hypochondriacal symptoms. Arch Gen Psychiatry 37:51–59, 1980

Shukla S, Mukherjee S, Decina P: Lithium in the treatment of bipolar disorders associated with epilepsy: an open study. J Clin Psychopharmacol 8:201–204, 1988

*Shulman KI, Walker SE, Mackenzie S, et al: Dietary restriction, tyramine, and the use of monoamine oxidase inhibitors. J Clin Psychopharmacol 9:397–402, 1989

*Siever LJ, Davis KL: Overview: toward a dysregulation hypothesis of depression. Am J Psychiatry 142:1017–1031, 1985

Silver JM, Yudofsky S: Propranolol for aggression: literature review and clinical guidelines. International Drug Therapy Newsletter 20:9–12, 1985

Singer I, Rotenberg D: Mechanisms of lithium action. N Engl J Med 289:254–260, 1973

Sitland-Marslen PA, Wells BG, Froemming JH, et al: Psychiatric applications of bromocriptine therapy. J Clin Psychiatry 51:68–82, 1990

Small JG, Milstein V: Lithium and electroconvulsive therapy. J Clin Psychopharmacol 10:346–350, 1990

Small JG, Milstein V, Miller MJ, et al: Neurophysiological effects of ECT. Psychopharmacol Bull 24:391–395, 1988

Smith DE, Wesson DR: A new method for treatment of barbiturate dependence. JAMA 213:294–295, 1970

Stewart JT, Myers WC, Burkett RC, et al: A review of pharmacotherapy of aggression in children and adolescents. J Am Acad Child Adolesc Psychiatry 29:269–277, 1990

Sugrue MF: Do antidepressants possess a common mechanism of action? Biochem Pharmacol 32:1811–1817, 1983

Sullivan MD, Sakai CS, Dobie RA, et al: Treatment of depressed tinnitus patients with nortriptyline. Ann Otol Rhinol Laryngol 98:867–872, 1989

*Sussman N: Treatment of anxiety with buspirone. Psychiatric Annals 17:144–150, 1987

Tabakoff B, Lee JM, De Leon-Jones L, et al: Ethanol inhibits the activity of the B form of monoamine oxidase in human platelet and brain tissue. Psychopharmacology 87:152–156, 1985

*Teicher MH, Glod CA: Neuroleptic drugs: indications and guidelines for their rational use in children and adolescents. Journal of Child and Adolescent Psychopharmacology 1:33–56, 1990

Teicher MH, Glod C, Cole JO: Emergency of intense suicidal preoccupation during fluoxetine treatment. Am J Psychiatry 147:207–210, 1990

Tesar GE, Murray GB, Cassem VH: Use of high-dose intravenous haloperidol in the treatment of agitated cardiac patients. J Clin Psychopharmacol 5:344–347, 1985

*Thienhaus OJ, Margletta S, Bennett JA: A study of the clinical efficacy of maintenance ECT. J Clin Psychiatry 51:141–144, 1990

Thompson JW, Ware MR, Blashfield RK: Psychotropic medication and priapism: a comprehensive review. J Clin Psychiatry 51:430–433, 1990

Thornton JE, Mulsant BH, Dealy R, et al: A retrospective study of maintenance electroconvulsive therapy in a university-based psychiatric practice. Convulsive Therapy 6:121–129, 1990

Van Valkenberg C, Clayton PJ: Electroconvulsive therapy and schizophrenia. Biol Psychiatry 20:699–700, 1983

Vestergaard P, Poulstrup I, Schou M, et al: Prospective studies in a lithium cohort. Acta Psychiatr Scand 78: 434–441, 1988

Weiner RD: Does ECT cause brain damage? Behav Brain Res 7:1–53, 1984

Wernicke JF, Dunlop SR, Dornseif BE, et al: Low-dose fluoxetine for depression. Psychopharmacol Bull 24: 183–188, 1988

*Yudofsky S, Williams D, Gorman J: Propranolol in the treatment of rage and violent behavior in patients with chronic brain syndrome. Am J Psychiatry 138:218–220, 1983

Chapter

30

Psychotherapy of Patients With Neuropsychiatric Disorders

David V. Forrest, M.D.

CONSIDERING PSYCHOTHERAPY in neuropsychiatry in a separate chapter does not imply that it ought to be separated in the minds of psychiatrists from the neurological and pharmacotherapeutic aspects of care. Indeed, psychiatrists will frequently rely on their medical background to help the patient interpret the real meaning of a neuropsychiatric disorder, to translate diagnostic jargon into emotionally relevant human meaning, and to help fine-tune complex treatment regimens that may include pharmacotherapy or other somatotherapy. All psychiatrists would do well to spend some time in attendance at neurological clinics or rounds to refresh their knowledge of the burgeoning pharmacopoeia in use there. Just as contact with patients with gross neurological impairment helps us assess neurological abnormalities in our psychiatric patients, so too can familiarity with the needs of more impaired psychiatric patients—especially those with schizophrenia, organic mental disorders, and substance use disorders—help us frame a psychotherapeutic approach that is tailored to the cognitive and affective needs of neurological patients.

Many of the same mechanisms overlap in neurological and psychiatric conditions. Woods and Short (1985) found that 50% of 270 newly admitted patients with major psychiatric disorders at McLean Hospital had neurological abnormalities, and Schiffer (1983) established psychiatric diagnoses in 41.9% of 241 inpatients and outpatients on a neurology service in Rochester. In formulating an approach to neuropsychiatry, the psychiatrist cannot be content with offering vague homilies about the necessity of support and outreach or the importance of acting as a liaison with other disciplines regarding consciousness-raising about patients' feelings. Psychiatrists are now expected to interact effectively with other professionals who speak in terms of the structure and function of the nervous system. Nor are personal warmth, kindness, and being well analyzed sufficient personal characteristics in themselves, although empathy remains the best motivation for learning about the brain functions involved. Empathic medical psychotherapy techniques must be adapted to the specific neurological features of the patient.

❑ PSYCHODYNAMIC ASPECTS OF THE MENTAL EXAMINATION

Not only neuropsychiatrists but also general psychiatrists who practice at the state of the art now find it valuable to expand a patient's mental status examination to include components of the neurological exam. A good outline helps. Although brief ones such as the Mini-Mental State Exam (MMSE; Folstein et al. 1975) may suffice as a routine ritual, from time to time one will wish to employ a more extensively elaborated paradigm such as those of Strub and Black (1985) or Taylor (1981). But structured examinations and formal neuropsychological testing, even those as extensive as the Halstead-Reitan battery and computerized neuropsychological tasks, do not bring out the information necessary to formulate a comprehensive treatment plan and only crudely hint at the difficulties that will be encountered as the psychiatrist adjusts the treatment to individuals. The checklists must be set aside, and a shift must be made to a psychodynamically oriented interview with ample open-ended questions that will enable the psychiatrist to appreciate the unique personality and affective qualities of each patient. Such an interview should provide an understanding of the hereditofamilial, constitutional, developmental, experiential, and interpersonal contributions to the formation of personality structure and the major traumata and conflicts the patient encountered along the way. The impact of the illness is assessed similarly and placed in the context of the person's longitudinal history, in the tradition that Adolph Meyer brought to 20th-century American psychiatry. The psychiatrist goes beyond assessing the elements of function, as in physical medicine, and is interested in the operational aspects of how the patient will fare at home and at work, as in rehabilitation medicine.

Employment of any structured mental examination, whether systematic and of great length or limited to a few tests of attention (such as serial 7s) and supraspan memory (such as recall of a specific street, tree, and flower after 5 minutes), marks a shift away from a psychotherapeutic relatedness to the patient toward an evaluative mode that always has a distancing effect and sometimes is experienced as threatening or even outrageous by the patient. The analogy with the physical exam is not complete because the patient's very ability to make sense of the proceedings is being questioned. This is a time for great compensatory warmth and reassurance on the part of the examiner, which pays the scientific dividend of eliciting the patient's best performance. The patient may experience emotions as strong as self-loathing and humiliation, depending on the deficits involved and the degree of investment in the integrity of those functions.

The examining psychiatrist must ensure that a methodical approach is not mistaken by the patient for scorn or that a smug supplying of the correct answers (which are of little interest to the patient) is not taken for an air of superiority. Seemingly "playing to the crowd" at the patient's expense, whether before assembled family or in front of residents and medical students, is to be scrupulously avoided. Sympathetic recognition of all deficits should be directed first to the patient. For instance, the psychiatrist may comment, "Exercises such as this seem to exaggerate the difficulty. I wonder if you've noticed any trouble keeping your attention on the task." Even complex concepts such as the operationally crucial faculty of constructional ability, which involves so much of the brain and is often worth testing through copied diagrams such as of a house and a smoking pipe, can often be evaluated empathetically. For example, the psychiatrist may ask, "Has it been difficult lately to plan your day or to grasp the overall picture in complicated situations? Have you noticed difficulty in getting things together to do something? Have things seemed different on TV or in the newspaper?"

Contact in Neuropsychiatric Patients

On first entering the patient's room, the psychiatrist should be aware that impairments in the patient's hierarchy of capacities are likely to impede any beneficial encounter between patient and physician in specific ways that require adaptations and compensations in psychotherapeutic technique. Each capacity in Table 30–1 is dependent on the integrity of those that precede it.

The psychiatrist makes a sequence of judgments about the patient's ability to engage in therapeutic contact that begins with rudimentary neurological functions, proceeds through higher cortical functions, and ends with the subtler capacities for relatedness and self-perspective by which patients are evaluated for insight-oriented psychotherapy. *Consciousness* is the most basic function, and it is not uncommon that a psychiatrist will be called to the bedside of a patient who is moving in and out of coma. Although reports of recall of things said in the patient's presence under coma or anesthesia may arouse skepticism (and no one has ever been able to learn anything while asleep because of a lack of activation and attention), it is best not to say things that would disturb the patient if he or she was awake because the level of the coma may be uncertain or variable or the patient may become aware of his or her surrounding while still poorly able to respond. The most important element of the physician's communication in the presence of a patient with diminished consciousness is his or her own affect, which may be primitively grasped even when the words do not come through. A reassuring manner, especially with the family and special duty nurses who will stay with the patient after the physician leaves, creates a protective ambience that may inhibit emerging agitation. It is important to avoid overstimulating or overloading the patient with diminished consciousness (soft radio or TV can reassure such a patient, but not at the same time a psychiatrist is talking) and to talk about familiar and unthreatening matters, limiting the time of contact and assessing the patient's tolerance for interventions.

Attention is a faculty of a slightly higher order than consciousness, and *retention* cannot occur when attention cannot be sustained until the objects of attention can be absorbed. Anxiety and agitation may be based on the inability to attend to the outside world long enough to process it. *Orientation* is a process of remembering and integrating a sufficient sampling of perceptions in a short enough time. An information model of brain function is helpful. To give a trivial example, a contact lens may increase the acuity of vision, but the wearer will see more poorly if forced to blink constantly so that the active process of gathering information by looking is diminished. Confusing overload, poor lighting, field cuts, or poor attention, memory, and cortical reception and integration of the visual modality all diminish the information available. Simplification and repetition of communication and instructions are helpful, as are allowing familiarization with the doctor and giving the patient enough time to collect himself or herself when agitated or flustered.

Recognition might be seen as a first step in each of the component processes of making sense of the world of space and time and form in which we have evolved and to which we are adapted. The natural intelligence of the brain in computer jargon consists of an astonishing number of parallel processors that can be specifically impaired. For example, banks of neurons exist with the incredible specialization of recognizing lines at each of many different angles to the upright that separate forms in the perceived world. Close experience with even a *single* case of agnosia demonstrates that the state of the art of neurological description, as well presented by Cummings (1985) and Heilman and Valenstein (1984), remains an extremely rudimentary and insufficient basis for psychotherapeutic and rehabilitative interventions. This means that custom tailoring to the individual patient and a willingness to discover a myriad of complexities of impairment from a primer level of geometric perceptions to the level of the components of interpersonal and social relevance are therefore required.

Construction is the putting together of the parts or elements of the mental contents, whether perceptions or recognitions, to build meaningful wholes, especially spatial and temporal connection and fit. The patient with problems of construction cannot assemble anything, even a copied drawing, and fails to see how actions will fit into time slots of the day. *Drives* are a basic level of motivational push, often betrayed by evidences of anxiety, aggressiveness, or assertive confidence that underlie the faculty of a concerted will or *conation. Affect* consists of emotional colorings that could be summarized under headings—joy, fear, anger, shame, guilt, and sadness—for which group norms in response to videotaped stimuli can be reliably measured (Forrest 1982). Drives, conation, and affect, although often primarily disturbed in schizophrenic patients and complexly forced, labile, or deranged in those with pseudobulbar palsy or other language-preserving subcortical disease such as supranuclear palsy, are recruited to make communicative sense in patients with cortical disease such as aphasia. An example would be the previously soft-spoken and propitious

TABLE 30–1. HIERARCHY OF CAPACITIES FOR PSYCHOTHERAPEUTIC CONTACT THAT MAY BE IMPAIRED IN NEUROPSYCHIATRIC PATIENTS

Capacity	*Adaptations in psychiatric technique*
Consciousness	Adopt a reassuring manner. Avoid agitation by avoiding overstimulation. Limit time of visit. Assess changing tolerance for interventions. Keep affect positive even if patient is apparently unconscious or not fully conscious.
Attention	Eliminate distractions. Keep contacts one on one. Speak clearly and simplify language. Use brief syntax. Make sure your presence is registered. Note perceptual impairments such as field cuts or hearing deficits and position self helpfully.
Retention	Repeat from time to time. Simplify. Break down communications into simple steps. Reinforce with other channels and modalities (e.g., writing and diagrams). Practice mnemonics with patient. Identify self each visit and keep your appearance constant.
Orientation	Remind patient (as needed) of time, place, and person. Keep calendar and clock in view. Visit at the same time daily.
Recognition	Tailor approach to compensate for specific impairments of any of the many parallel brain processors, from trouble with simple geometric perceptions through facial recognition to more complex perceptual components of relationship. Adapt communication to assist and circumvent dysphasic channels (e.g., reassure with affects when verbal reception is poor).
Construction	Assist in putting together cause and effect, as well as spatial and temporal connection. Help to see how necessary activities or outing will fit into time slots of the day. Offer structures.
Emotion	Assess underlying drives of anxiety, aggressiveness, and sexuality. Do not stress patient's having difficulty with control. Identify and read out to the patient degrees of joy, fear, anger, shame, guilt, or sadness being felt by the patient. Name more specific emotions under these main headings to reduce resistance and increase the feeling of being understood.
Conation	Help patient build on fragile will and find his or her own direction in confusion. Do not be overbearing as your very presence may be commanding to the point of causing automatic obedience or opposition, echopraxia, echolalia, or cataplexy. Respect elements of prosocial intentionality in actions.
Motivation	Facilitate positive incentives by behavioral manipulation and removal of negative influences. Help patient identify latent longings for improved adaptation. Guard against helplessness.
Proposition	Accept that the first stage of proposition during recovery is usually opposition, as with a child in the "terrible twos." Respect the inherent positive energy, but set limits. Encourage half-baked initiatives and help structure only after they get going. Don't discourage the patient or complicate things.
Delineation	Help patient see origins of affects in self or from others and help him or her work on impairment in self, not project it onto world. Use projections onto the psychiatrist or onto paralyzed body parts as clues to self-concepts. Excessive blame taking may often best be handled as a failure of delineation from family anger or disappointment about the patient's not being sufficiently restored to normal.
Relation	Note quality of and changes in relations with significant others. The patient's caring about the needs of others is an extremely good sign that social function will recover and psychotherapy will be helpful. Balance looking out for the patient's needs against validating reasonable perceptions and needs of spouse and family, on whom the patient is dependent.

person who displays emotion-laden obscenity while recovering language after a stroke.

Motivation, which is akin to the motor action of getting moving or being moved to action (and caring to be), is a reminder of the overlap in neurotransmitter distribution between the emotional and motor systems. Motivation gets the patient to take practical action—to get going and keep moving—and reflects the concept of "working through" what is learned in psychoanalytic psychotherapy, which can be considered motorically as a moving through or acting through. *Proposition* is a quality of active outflow from the neuraxis that involves initiation, construction, and execution of one's own meaningful entities of language and action. Often in neurological recovery, as in the development of the young child, the first stages may be oppositional (e.g., spitting out pills or contradicting or disbelieving everything said). The patient should in part be encouraged in this rudimentary attempt at exerting the will, or at least understood, much as a "terrible twos" child is tolerated to some degree. The negativism can be appreciated as evidence of energy and possibly growth, even as limits must be set on it when the individual paints himself or herself into a corner (e.g., refusing to get dressed or undressed).

Delineation of boundaries between self and other and between inner and outer reality is a function frequently disturbed in brain illness, resulting in a host of projections onto other people, the environment, and the parts of the body whose functions are impaired. Projections onto the psychiatrist may impair therapy but are valuable clues and must be worked with. Usually these projections are highly critical mirror images of the great disrepute in which the patient holds himself or herself. Negative attributes of the self may also be projected by the patient and allocated to various other persons who are perceived in shallow cardboard stereotypes; this process is called *splitting*. Sometimes the patient is too depressed to project and is introjective to an unrealistic degree, assuming blame for all the woe in the world. This is also a failure of delineation. Projection with splitting and fusion are probably not regressions to a normal infantile state, but rather pathological formations to be understood as part of the repertory of defenses available to the injured brain. These defenses may be more accessible if previously used by a pathological premorbid personality, but sufficiently severe brain impairment can elicit them in anyone.

Relation completes the list of ingredients for psychotherapeutic participation and is also the domain psychotherapy seeks to improve. Requiring contributions from all the previously described capacities, relatedness as studied by modern psychodynamic psychiatry is both an intrapsychic and interpersonal idea based on a patient's coming to terms with the inner representations of other people and with the actual feedback of social reality. The "quality of object relations" is one of the most important prognostic criteria for psychotherapy. Impairment of the ability to relate may arise from diseases of the brain as well as from other so-called functional disorders. The preservation of the ability to care about the needs of a person other than the self is an extremely good sign for the recovery of social function and for psychotherapy to help the recovery on its way. It is important to distinguish between true caring and a more primitive, merely pragmatic concern that the other person may not function as a supplier of needs. This lesser level of relatedness, in a neurological patient who was premorbidly capable of mature love and appreciation of other persons, is comparable to the stunted relatedness of many patients (such as those with sociopathic personality disorders or who are alcoholic or bulimic) who tend to see others, including the physician, as vending machines of care or mere providers, to borrow the language of third-party payment. The psychiatrist should guard against anger elicited by such atavistic relatedness and, while maintaining the greatest empathy for the family members, should avoid siding against the patient.

Defenses: The Neuropsychodynamic Continuum

The psychiatrist who is well trained in psychodynamic psychotherapy brings to the study of defense mechanisms in neuropsychiatry a relevant but incomplete description. Defenses are psychodynamic mechanisms employed by a person in interaction with the surprises and dangers of the world and with drives and emotions from within. Traditionally, defenses have been classified on a dimension from the most mature to the most immature. The most mature defenses are viewed as the healthiest ones (such as sublimation, suppression, and laughter). Less mature defenses (such as reaction formation, rationalization, displacement, and isolation) are thought to be characteristic of a neurotic level of function. The most immature defenses (such as denial, splitting, merging, projection, and projective identification) are considered the sickest, typifying psychotic functioning. But "healthy" people in sufficiently desperate or emotional circumstances may also employ the "immature" or "sick" defenses (Forrest 1980). Stern (1985) has questioned whether the "immature" defenses, such as merging, are ever characteristic of normal infants. Although psychodynamic theory originally recognized a somatic contribution to the mental defenses (Freud 1895), it did not specify which mental defenses are associated with organic impairment or how the defenses are related to organic processes. Indeed, it may be incorrect to assume that "sicker" or "more primitive" defenses are consistently associated with worse organic disease, and the "healthier" defenses with milder impairment. Much depends on the level of distress.

In approaching defenses in neuropsychiatry, parallels might be sought between the mental mechanisms of defense and defensive brain (or cortical) reactions. Despite Freud's contributions (1891) to aphasiology and the fact that psychiatrists have been aware of mental defenses and cortical reactions for 90 years, the two domains have not been meaningfully interrelated. Too often, case discussions shift from the mental to the cortical realm and back with no carryover. Such interrelating could become the basis for useful adaptations of psychotherapeutic technique as well as correlations of premorbid coping styles with postmorbid reactions. At the very least, the confused patient and baffled family could be helped to see which defensive reactions are exacerbations of characterological armor (under varying degrees of voluntary control and amenable to interpretation) and which are more primitive, automatic defenses of an injured brain that may be compensated for by tolerant understanding and environmental manipulation. Between these two extremes lie defensive formations that are rooted in both psyche and brain. Finally, one must not assume that a learning process is absent in cortical defenses, so that improvement occurs only with spontaneous recovery, or that the mental defenses have a plasticity that is completely reeducable by psychotherapy.

Certain analogical comparisons on the basis of operational principles may be made among cortical defenses, mental defenses, and a bridging area of what might be termed *neuropsychic defenses*. In Table 30–2, parallels are drawn among similar defensive structures of similar shape that are 1) mental defenses of the psyche, 2) somatopsychic or neuromental defenses clearly influenced by the neurological state, and 3) cortical neurological reactions. Potential continua among these three types of defensive structures are implied.

❑ TECHNIQUES FROM PSYCHOTHERAPY OF SCHIZOPHRENIA

Schizophrenia is a symptom formation that is more complex than an organic deficit, but its treatment may serve as a model for psychiatric work with less familiar neurological conditions. All of the dysfunctional features previously catalogued for schizophrenia (Forrest 1983) may be variably present in the neurological patient with a brain injury (especially those with mesolimbic involvement) and require sensitive adjustments of technique by the neuropsychiatrist similar to those I have described for schizophrenia (Forrest 1983).

The mechanisms that occur both in schizophrenia and in neurological patients with disordered brain function include undifferentiated "catastrophic" reactions to stresses when the patient becomes overwhelmed, originally described in patients with brain injuries (Goldstein 1942, 1952); involuntary concreteness or metonymy (taking a part of a concept for the entire concept); incapability of moving among levels of abstraction, especially regarding interpersonal relations (Searles 1965); fear of novel situations (neophobia); segmentalization and deautomatization of previously automatic sequences of emotional response (like shaking hands on meeting a person); slow habituation and extinction of reactions to stimuli; and probabilistic incapacity (poor ability to evaluate the likely outcome of actions and events).

Frequently there is an additional feature of language disturbance not present in schizophrenia. Although the schizophrenic person almost always exhibits an impairment of language in a larger sense (i.e., in its consensual or interpersonal use, and in the attachment of affects to language and thought), other patients with impaired brain function usually have some difficulty *accessing* language. This problem is typically absent in schizophrenia (Benson 1975), despite what seem at times paraphasic substitutions of uncommon phrases that are reminiscent of fluent posterior or jargon aphasias. Having sufficient contact with the schizophrenic person will usually dispel the impression of impediment and

TABLE 30–2. NEUROPSYCHIATRIC DEFENSE CONTINUUM

Continuum	*Mental defenses*	*Neuromental defenses*	*Cortical reactions*
Nonrecognition	Denial of damage, avoidance, disavowal; or conscious caring for paralyzed limb	Neglect of body part or side, with preservation of the concept of a damaged limb (Weinstein and Friedland 1977)	Hemi-inattention because of diminished cortical representation
Misdirection	Circumstantiality, tangentiality	Overinclusion, ellipsis	Inattention, distractibility
Nondenotation	Metaphor, metonymy, symptom and symbol formation, circumlocution, poetic language and logic	Rhyming, clang associations, neologism, substitution	Aphasic paraphasias, jargon, dysnomia
Nonrecall (or nongrasp)	Obsessive ordering, hysterical evasion, paranoid reductiveness, schizoid invention, sociopathic approximate answers (Ganser syndrome) (Enoch and Trethowan 1979)	Confabulation, structure by constant talking, compensatory grandiloquence (poststroke, to prove smart), ignore what one can't structure, repeating and quoting self	Amnestic or state-dependent lapses, failure of processing with information overload
Referential loss	Delusions of reference and influence and of dementia in depression (pseudo-dementia)	Delusions of loss or impoverishment; metaphorical substitution of time, feces, money, or other measurable things for unacceptable and incomprehensible loss of brain function	Diminished capacity for construction, proposition, and planning
Affect application	Helplessness, hopelessness; compensation; or plaintive self-denigration with realization of deficit; schizophrenic substitutions of (sociopolitical or religiophilosophical) abstractions for interpersonal focus on emotions	Beneficence toward or degradation of self or object world without realization or recognition of deficit; parapathic substitutions of schizophrenic language for affects	Apathy, emotionalism, organic mania; flat affect in schizophrenia
Regression	Ontogenic regression to less mature states of mind, with diminished object constancy, tantrums, or catastrophic reactions to stress (Goldstein 1942)	Stereotypy and other complex innate primitive patterns such as mechanical repetition in stimulant abuse, touching the face in Huntington's disease, and regression to silly humor or puns (*Witzelsucht*)	Phylogenetic regression to neural reactions characteristic of lower mammalian and vertebrate predecessors (e.g., grasp and snout)
Kindling or temporolimbic hyperconnection (interictal)	Hypermoralism, intensified religiosity, and proselytizing; sense of urgency and mission; anger and remorse; and graphomania	Viscosity, emotional deepening, sensations of immanence, transcendence, and divine presence; thought insertion	Organic sensations of otherness or bodily intrusion; hyposexuality

(continued)

TABLE 30–2. (Continued)

Continuum	*Mental defenses*	*Neuromental defenses*	*Cortical reactions*
Impaired worldview	"My relationship to the world has changed."	"The world is bigger, harder to deal with, more confusing," or (in schizophrenia) more aesthetically awesome	"The world has been changed, reduplicated, substituted" in patients with brain injury
Impaired view of others	Transference reactions: "It's I who changed, my perceptions differ because I'm injured;" degrees of insight; interpersonal shallowness and manipulativeness	Misidentification: "People have changed, are different, are to blame, have been replaced by impostors"; splitting and projective identification; "underlying defect" in borderline syndrome of failure of delineation	Prosopagnosia: state-dependent change in cognition of people or their relation to self
Sex object shift	Avoidance of parental object to preserve ties to family	Failure to integrate affects and sexuality	Failure to differentiate sexual object (Klüver-Bucy syndrome of bilateral hippocampal damage) or own gender
Impaired ego boundary	Creativity and regression in the service of the ego	Disturbing nightmares, other vulnerability to internal and external processes, and schizophrenia (Hartmann 1984)	Diminished stimulus barrier (Hartmann 1984)
Impairment of conation or will	Identification with the aggressor, and introjection and incorporation in health, neurosis, and depression	Made cognition, made volition, and command hallucinations in schizophrenia	Echolalia, echopraxia, and involuntary reflex activity in brain injury
Impaired movement or spatial play	Disorientation, agoraphobia, diminished sense of mastery and mobility and of bodily feedback and control, and lowered confidence in actions	Vestibular defensiveness, fear of moving, fear of falling or of whirling (twirling a soft sign in children), incoordination, and clumsiness	Vertigo, motor or proprioceptive impairment incoordination, poor eye tracking, ataxia, and tremor

reveal instead *increased* access to elements of thought and language that are improperly freighted with affect. The crucial practical difference for psychotherapy is that emotions in most neurological patients are recruited to overcome cognitive and linguistic problems and to make interpersonal sense, whereas in schizophrenia cognitive and linguistic elements—often exaggerated and fanciful—are recruited to compensate for poor command of affects, and the result frustrates interpersonal sense.

As any psychiatrist must do, in order to function effectively the neuropsychiatrist must be crucially attuned to nuances of a patient's affect. One's own perception of affect can be calibrated against the highly reliable means of affect scoring of short videotaped interview segments by professional audiences (Forrest 1982). The six affects—joy, fear, anger, shame, guilt, and sadness—can each be rated on a scale of 0 to 4+ like any other medical measurement. Under the general affect rubrics, cognitive shadings of emotions can be specified. The most common error in treating patients with impaired brain function is not adjusting one's own projection of emotional tone to the patient's needs. For example, patients with hyperemotionalism may require us to throttle down our emotions (see Table 30–3). House et al. (1989) found that 29% of 89 stroke patients in their study had emotionalism and that it was responsive to emotional experiences. The greater challenge for most neuropsychiatrists is to increase the benevolent emotion they project toward certain patients who for various reasons are receiving signals poorly (Table 30–4). Psychotherapy in neuropsychiatry should be eclectic, adapting elements that are helpful from various modalities (Table 30–5).

In the next section, I discuss interventions that are specific for neuropsychiatric conditions.

❑ TRAUMATIC BRAIN INJURY

Childs (1985) has stated that the most difficult sequelae of head injury to treat are the psychosocial disabilities; impaired cognition is next in degree of difficulty, and impaired physical abilities are the least difficult. Also, perhaps contrary to common assumption, the patient's family suffers most severely from the disruption of emotions and object relations, next most from the intellectual impairments, and least from the physical impairments (Oddy et al. 1978). This is why psychotherapy can play a crucial role in individual and family recovery after head injury.

The emotional climate is worsened by the typical emergence of bad temper in the patient 3 or more months after the injury. The family's optimism that full recovery will occur, based on successes in physical rehabilitation, turns to disappointment when the patient's impulse control worsens. The doctors often bear the transferred brunt of family anger, which may result in family members splitting the staff into good and bad. Interventions should aim at legitimizing family disappointment and avoiding comments that abet the splitting. Unconscious or unacknowledged family anger at the patient for being injured contributes to the patient's internalized anger within the family system and must be addressed to head off severe self-loathing and possible suicidal trends as the protection of denial wears off.

Regression in the patient's mental processes may parallel neurological regression, and both mental and neuromental defenses (discussed above) par-

TABLE 30–3. THERAPEUTIC ADAPTATIONS TO NEUROPSYCHIATRIC PATIENTS: TUNING AFFECTIVE PROJECTIONS DOWN

Tune affective projections down for patients with emotional sensitization, including

1. Patients with temporal lobe and other epileptic personalities with hyperemotionalism and viscosity.
2. Patients with Alzheimer's disease and other dementias (when marked by hyperemotionalism and anger).
3. Patients with explosive rage syndromes.
4. Pseudobulbar palsy patients with emotional lability.
5. Patients whose character armor is paranoid or obsessive.
6. Patients with irritable euphoric or manic syndromes (as may appear with the diffuse cerebral involvements of human immunodeficiency virus [HIV]-positive patients, multiple sclerosis patients, or other patients with euphoric dementias).
7. Schizophreniform patients with flatness (such patients may require a throttled down affect to prevent their extreme ego weakness from becoming overwhelmed by intrusive Schneiderian effects of another ego).
8. Stroke patients with emotionalism associated with a more general mood disturbance (especially in patients with left frontal and temporal regions [House et al. 1989]).

Hints for tuning down affective intensity

1. Avoid countertransference of clinging to patient, aggravating viscosity, or mutual dependency.
2. End sessions on time.
3. Limit calls and be able to hang up the phone gracefully.
4. Avoid being too warm and loving with aggressive patients.
5. Preserve boundaries and formality of relationship.
6. Avoid too much eye contact.
7. Mitigate overly intense habits of gaze.
8. Avoid identifying too much with patient's aggressiveness or hyperemotionalism, a mechanism of identification with the aggressor, or Stockholm syndrome in the captive audience of the treating doctor.

TABLE 30–4. THERAPEUTIC ADAPTATIONS TO NEUROPSYCHIATRIC PATIENTS: TUNING AFFECTIVE PROJECTIONS UP

Tune affective productions up for patients with emotional blunting (the majority of neuropsychiatric patients), including

1. Confused patients.
2. Patients who, for varying reasons, are receiving signals more poorly.
3. Patients who are hearing and visually impaired.
4. Patients who have become isolated or paranoid because of poor perception or reception.
5. Stroke syndrome patients with receptive dysphasia.
6. Patients disoriented to person, place, or time.
7. Parkinsonian patients with flattened affect, whose facial display is flatter than they inwardly feel.
8. Depressed, affectively impoverished, or apathetic patients.
9. Patients with histrionic or childlike personalities (including children) who relate and communicate disproportionately through affective channels.

Hints for tuning up affective intensity

1. Increase affective output by emoting more strongly.
2. Become a beacon for, that is, become easier to pay attention to, the brain-injured, disoriented, or confused patient trying to track events and stay in reality.
3. Project yourself in the way of an actor or stage announcer.
4. Avoid merely increasing the volume of your voice in flat or tinny tones as obsessive professionals are wont to do.
5. Project admiration for the patient's courage.
6. Project consolation for the patient's emotional pain.
7. Project caring for the patient's subjective experience of journeying toward greater understanding and meaning.
8. Bathe the patient in warmth and helpfulness.
9. Avoid being sappily affectionate.
10. Avoid confusing seductive or sexual messages of courtship.
11. Avoid projecting blame.
12. Keep eye contact attentive with relaxed momentary breaks, highly interested but never intruding, peering, leering, or cute.
13. Make voice larger, clearer in enunciation, with more breath and amplitude, but not necessarily louder.
14. Keep word choice simplified and direct, as when one speaks with persons new to English or with children.
15. Abbreviate syntax for patients with poorer concentration and short-term memory.
16. Convey the message in a few words and delete the extra qualifying words that obsessive professionals love (e.g., "essentially,," "not unlike,," "some degree of") and jargon words.
17. Repeat important statements without varying them or inverting subject and predicate.
18. Avoid extra clauses and relations of conjunction between clauses, conditional tenses, and all but simple present, past, and future words.
19. Coordinate gestures with words and use emotional expressions as markers of syntax the way announcers do, capitalizing on parallel channels of human communication.

allel pathological brain reactions. Often, borderline or other organic personality disorders result that comprise an array roughly paralleling functional personality syndromes (Childs 1985). It is important to interview family and friends to determine the premorbid personality of the patient in calculating effects of injury, which may be easier to change. Highly resistant to change, but worth the early prescription of a diet to help stave off weight gain, is the omnivoracious syndrome of organic bulimia from hypothalamic damage. Sexual and emotional inappropriateness, especially from frontal injury, may express regressive needs for clinging contact and responds to structured schedules of nonsexual human contact.

Psychotherapeutic interventions optimally begin soon after the patient is hospitalized, and management of the emotional climate is crucial to recovery. Childs (1985) has recommended placing a priority on the reestablishment of object constancy in cognitively impaired patients by staff members who are carefully selected for their lack of personal tension or anger and work one-on-one all day with each patient. This familiar and consistent other person enacts an early stage in cognitive retraining of a regressively lost relational skill. This is accom-

TABLE 30–5. MODALITIES OF PSYCHOTHERAPY IN NEUROPSYCHIATRY

Helpful aspects of the psychoanalytic approach for neuropsychiatry:
1. Respect for the patient's autonomy and self-determination.
2. Theoretic concept of defense organization.
3. Most sufficient map of mental, cognitive, and emotional function.
4. Model based on conflict among mental structures.

Inappropriate aspects of the psychoanalytic approach for neuropsychiatry:
1. Too passive a receptiveness rather than making affective contact.
2. Too much reliance upon free association and dreams.
3. Searching for remote causes and relationships.
4. Attribution of treatment events to abstract forces and entities in talking to the patients.
5. Overemphasis on transference versus reality issues.
6. Intentional lack of frames and structures.
7. Interpersonal relations considered as inner object relations.
8. Avoidance of direct answers or being a "blank screen" rather than being a beacon to security.

Other modalities of psychotherapy in neuropsychiatry
1. Behaviorist approaches to the patient's learning system as a black box may be helpful in structuring relearning, but they are "brainless" in their theoretical avoidance of capacities, defenses, conflicts, recruitment of affect to aid cognition, and other neuromental dynamics that are helpful in explanation.
2. Interpersonal and family approaches are surprisingly helpful communication systems despite the clear nidus of difficulty in a neuropathologically "designated patient," because of the impact on relatives and their involvement in the care of the disabilities. As there is both direct influence and imitation and a hereditary factor in neurotic, characterological, and major psychiatric disorders, the families of patients with acquired neuropsychiatric disorders may themselves be less disordered and more of a help in the treatment.

plished with a soothing voice and touch, with limitation of talk to familiar subjects and to the patient only, and the restriction of stimulation to a single channel (no conflicting conversations or television in the background). Later, active exercises based on Luria's prescription include practice in following directions requiring progressively more sequential steps (one step first, then increase up to five, in sequence) (Luria 1973), problem solving, and movement from the concrete to the abstract, retracing Piaget's developmental steps and hoping for generalization of learning (Piaget 1954; Piaget and Inhelder 1971). Newcombe (1983) reviewed such developing techniques as the use of imagery in mnemonics for the patient with left-hemisphere damage, constant structures of temporal framework and other memory aids (e.g., cooking buzzers, electronic diaries, and alarm clock-calendars), attention practice with single-digit chains and electronic or computer games, maps and drawing exercises for nonverbal visuospatial and constructional defects, and time-out rooms with talking books.

Other measures that the psychiatrist should consider include the following adapted from Berry (1984) (Table 30–6):

1. Identify the affective quality of the grieving stage the family is undergoing (denial, anger, and grief resolution). Prepare them for fluctuations of improvement and regression, and expect incomplete resolution of grief when the condition is chronic in nature.
2. Structure events each day for internalization by the cognitively impaired. Once automatized again, the structure can be withdrawn. Circadian rhythms should be reestablished as soon as possible and held inviolate. This means helping the patient experience bodily cycles (endogenous insulin and steroid secretion cycles, sleep, and exercise) at the same time each day by a routine schedule that can be continued after discharge.
3. Establish positive rewards such as increased privileges and independence to reinforce responsible behavior. Structure behavioral feedback with a point-scoring system for each daily activity. For example, a patient who completes a program of hygiene, rather than omitting some items on an individualized checklist, wins more points that can then be "spent" on a favorite snack or activity.

TABLE 30–6. MEASURES TO ASSIST RECOVERY OF PATIENTS WITH BRAIN INJURY

1. Relate interventions to family grieving stage (denial, anger, grief resolution).
2. Structure daily events to assist patient's internalizing of routine and reestablishing circadian rhythms.
3. Establish positive rewards to reinforce responsible behavior; individualize rewards to what patient likes.
4. Approach disabilities with expectancy they will be overcome cheerfully, never as excuse for misbehavior.
5. Individualize treatment goals to patient's specific problems; for example, reward withdrawn frontal patients for conversation and aggressive patients for not reacting.
6. Break maladaptive habits by vigilance and restraint, because motivation to become involved in positive change follows elimination of irresponsible behavior.
7. Orient family extensively to structure needed before discharge to home so gains are maintained.

Note. Adapted from Berry 1984.

4. Treat disabilities as difficulties to overcome, never as excuses for misbehavior. A high level of expectance is maintained that the patient will seek help with problems such as clumsiness, anxiety, irritability, inattention, and expressive dysphasias and give his or her best effort cheerfully, modeled on the patience and good-natured approach of the staff, rather than fly off the handle, break something, or become intoxicated.
5. Individualize treatment goals to reflect the patient's specific problems out of the myriad of possible ones. For example, withdrawn patients earn rewards for initiation of conversation, which is most difficult for those with frontal damage, and aggressive patients earn rewards by not reacting in situations of interpersonal stress. Individualize rewards to what the patient likes.
6. Regard irresponsible behaviors as maladaptive habits that are to be broken by vigilance and restraint as necessary. Motivation often follows rather than precedes the elimination of irresponsible behavior so that the patient internalizes the role of self-therapist.
7. Orient the family extensively to the current level of inpatient structure that is necessary before attempting home placement so that gains can be maintained.

Self-Expectations, Language, and Other Psychotherapeutic Correlates

Tyerman and Humphrey (1984) studied expectations about recovery in 25 patients with severe head injuries. Typically, the patients expected to return from their present concept of a self with a head injury to a past (premorbid) self within a year. The authors concluded that although unrealistic expectations may emotionally protect and motivate the profoundly disabled individual at first, eventually these expectations can work against rehabilitation and adjustment. Consequently, it helps if the psychiatrist, from the first contact with the patient, grasps the probable limitations of the prognosis without becoming discouraged about the real possibilities of contributing to the patient's progress. Follow-up at 2 years after severe head injury (Tyerman and Humphrey 1984), as compared with follow-up at 7 years (Oddy et al. 1985) or at 10–15 years (Thomsen 1984), found the same cognitive and physical defects, although long-term improvement continued in social and work function. Data such as these suggest two things to the psychiatrist: that at some point the patient must have come to terms with and mourned the loss of the premorbid intact state of functioning, and that there is more to a person's recovery for the psychiatrist to address than these measurable cognitive deficits.

Van Zomeren and van den Burg (1985) found that the severity of posttraumatic amnesia and difficulty resuming previous work were related at 2-year follow-up to "impairment complaints" of forgetfulness, slowness, poor concentration, and inability to divide attention over two simultaneous activities. Other complaints, such as anxiety or intolerances of noise, glaring light, or bustle, were not related to posttraumatic amnesia or resumption of previous work. In their study, "very severe" closed head injury was defined by the Russell classification (Russell 1971) as having a posttraumatic amnesia of 1 week or more. Not just neurophysical status and memory loss but personality changes affect work capacity, and these changes are especially important at 2-year follow-up in the loss of preaccident friendships (Weddell et al. 1980).

Verbal impairment to some degree is found in all patients with closed head injuries who had been referred to a rehabilitation medicine center. In a study of 56 cases by Sarno (1980), 32% had classic aphasia, 38% had motor dysarthria, and 30% had no discernible aphasic deficit in spontaneous speech but clear evidence of verbal deficit on testing. Dysarthric patients without exception showed subclinical linguistic effects. Because psychotherapy depends on the use of language with an emotional dimension, the psychiatrist should be alert to subtle evidence of dysarthria, identify any linguistic problems, and consciously adapt the psychotherapeutic technique to the deficit in the particular patient.

Sexual Disturbances After Brain Injury

Sexual disturbances may follow brain injury, especially damage to the limbic system (e.g., following rupture of aneurysms of the circle of Willis at the base of the brain). Weinstein (1974) suggested several useful generalizations about these organic sexual problems. First and foremost, he stated, "In man, sex is not only a drive or emotion but a vital component of identity, a means of social relatedness and a form of communication. . . . Changes in sexual behavior observed in brain-damaged patients are often abnormal by reason of the [inappropriate] circumstances in which they occur, rather than their intrinsic nature" (pp. 10, 16) or by their being different from the person's habitual conduct. It is often helpful to make it clear to the family that the patient with a brain injury has not become oversexed or a "sex maniac" (when the patient's drives have indeed not become amplified, as they may in certain patients with Klüver-Bucy syndrome or mania) and that the patient is just enacting a normal sexuality in the wrong context because of a more general disorder of judgment.

Another principle to remember with these patients is that sexual behavior in individuals with brain damage is usually marked by a loss of specificity as to objects or forms of excitation, rather than a new focus. Although specific behavior such as fetishism has been linked to temporal lobe seizure activity (as well as hyper- and hyposexuality), intermediary personality factors and learning are more probably the cause than postulated so-called sexual centers, as has recently been suggested for heterosexual pursuit.

Stoller (1991) found that sadomasochistic sex practices have great specificity of erotic stimulus choice. This is reminiscent of the specificity of brain perceptual pathways, but could reflect learning at vulnerable times. The interstitial nucleus 3 of the anterior hypothalamus (INAH 3) was found by LeVay (1991) to be twice as large in heterosexual men as in either homosexual men or women and is associated with male-typical sexual pursuit in animals. Again, how much is acquired is at issue in humans.

Verbal seductiveness frequently occurs in a situation of stress, such as when a patient is asked about his or her illness or is being tested, and thus may have a defensive, avoidant quality. Another stress-related phenomenon is ludic play, which Piaget (1952) described in young children, and which in patients with brain damage appears as punning or joking about illness, caricaturing disabilities, or imitating or mimicking the examiner's behavior. Often patients classify their disabilities in sexual terms, or sex enters into the content of their confabulations and delusions in the acute state, which Weinstein (1974) declared are useful signs that sexual behavior will be acted out later in a real-life situation. Some patients seek relatedness through physical contact that may "put off" visitors or staff, all the more so when the dementia is secondary to a contagious disease. I have seen 2 cases of Creutzfeldt-Jakob presenile dementia, one in a young woman and one in a man, in which the touch of the doctor's hand was sexualized in a sad and clearly readable attempt to cling to human contact. Interestingly, patients with brain injuries are often described in positive terms as emotional, sensitive, and sympathetic as well as excitable and dramatic.

Another feature of patients with brain injury noted by Weinstein is the interesting phenomenon of an unusually strong, stereotypical male-female dichotomy, in which character traits are allocated in black-and-white fashion to men and women or father and mother. Weinstein (1974) noted that this stereotypic sexism (which might be described as symbolically splitting goodness into one parent and badness into the other) is common in patients whose behavior includes sexual self-exposure and sexual actions directed toward children. A general tendency in patients with brain injuries toward stereotyping or forming judgments of other people on the basis of superficial criteria is characteristic and may lead to projective splitting of the ward staff into individuals labeled "good" and "bad." Weinstein (1974) also noted that the content of confabulations and delusions in the acute state of brain damage may predict later sexual and marital disturbances, especially in male patients whose confabulations employ themes of women and children.

A study of the psychosexual consequences of brain injury in 21 male patients by Kreutzer and Zasler (1989) showed most patients reported a lessening of sexual drive, erectile function, and frequency of intercourse; reduced self-esteem and self-perceived sex appeal; and no relationship between the level of affect and sexual behavior. Despite the changes, the quality of the patients' marital relationships appeared preserved.

❑ STROKE

As in patients with head injury, the psychiatrist should be aware of prognostic parameters in stroke patients when communicating with patient and family. These include psychosocial factors. Kotila et al. (1984) studied 154 survivors from a group of 255 stroke patients and found no difference in outcome between subarachnoid hemorrhage patients and infarction patients when matched for age (the younger subarachnoid patients fare better as a group). Major negative influences on outcome were old age, acute-stage hemiparesis, impairment of intelligence and memory, visuoperceptual deficits, nonadequate emotional reactions, and living alone. Clear improvement could be expected from the acute stage to 3 months, continuing to a lesser degree to 12 months. At 12 months, 78% of these patients were living at home and 58% were independent in activities of daily living. Of those patients who were gainfully employed before having a stroke, 55% had returned to work after 12 months. The authors emphasized that emotional reactions as well as neurological deficits influence outcome and should be considered in assessing prognosis.

Stevens et al. (1984) found that the type A behavior pattern was more common (71%) than type B (29%) in patients who had carotid artery atherosclerosis on Doppler ultrasonography. Nondiseased individuals were almost equally divided between type A (53%) and type B (47%) behavior. This premorbid personality classification suggests that type A personality factors, such as an intolerance of disability and recuperation requirements, may be frequent in stroke patients and may benefit from psychiatric intervention. A stroke is unwelcome at any age, but Goodstein (1983) noted that for the older patient, a stroke activates preexisting fears of losing control or sanity, dying, and becoming disfigured or impaired physically or sexually. The elderly are also more insecure about sudden recurrences, long stays away from home, and running out of retirement funds. Goodstein recommended that therapeutic endeavors be individually tailored to address the poor patient motivation based on subtle mental syndromes that are often associated with cerebrovascular accidents.

Management of Defenses After Mild Stroke: The "Old Guy"

A case of a minor cerebrovascular event that tipped the balance into neuropsychiatric dysfunction is illustrative of the management problems for these patients.

Case 1

Mr. A, a right-handed 73-year-old retired businessman, had survived a full episode of delirium tremens 5 years previously, including a coma, with no apparent residual. Recently, he sustained an episode of hemiparesis lasting only 5 minutes and leaving no motor residual. Neurological workup including computed tomography (CT) scan was negative, and he soon returned home. Yet it was clear Mr. A was very changed. He became preoccupied with the amount of his bowel movements and anal cleanliness, greatly reduced his food intake, and lost 20 pounds. He greatly resisted each stage of daily living, from getting up and dressed to going out. He repeated that he was an "old guy," that he would die soon, and that there was little hope for him. Cleared by his neurologist, he was referred for neuropsychiatric treatment by his family internist. On examination he showed intact comprehension and production of language. He could read and assess newspaper articles (although he thought that the events had not happened) and was physically robust. Furthermore, his affective display was not persistently depressed nor was it flat. He was often cheerful and could joke in a nettling way. He was not consistently angry but at times was quite verbally abusive of his family and doctors for bothering with such a hopeless case. He claimed also to be "uninterested" in the doctors. The main problems were his repetitious, almost reflexive naysaying and a need to make *image tarnishing* statements, to borrow a term from complex partial epilepsy.

Underlying these problems was not mere depression or pseudodementia but Mr. A's profound inability to construe his own reduced position in the world. One could infer this from his negative statements and neurological defenses. This deficiency was betrayed by his conviction that any given time interval would be insufficient to accomplish a given goal in daily living, whether it was getting to the barber or obtaining clothes for the next winter.

Money and electricity were handled in the same conserving way as calories and feces. He tore up checks his wife tried to write, was convinced he was poor, refused to carry his billfold for fear it would be stolen, and went about turning off lights. Attempts by his family to contradict such statements resulted in stubborn resistance. The behaviors, which were regressive and symbolically anal retentive, were not discussed as such but rather as expressions of his legitimate fear that he had lost some mental capacity to deal with the world.

Mr. A's family was advised to praise the strength of his harmless stubborn behavior as evidence of the preservation of his willpower. They were told his opposition was a stage of recovery of independence, as in children, that would likely be followed by an improved stage of proposition and initiation of positive actions. Judiciously small amounts of neuroleptic drugs were prescribed for anxiety. Admiration was expressed for the patient's preserved concern for his wife's medical problems. This promising sign went beyond a merely selfish interest in her being there to help him; it was believed to be evidence of a preserved capacity for loving object relations, implying an ability to maintain an inner representation of significant others.

If the capability for empathic, loving relatedness is lost, as it frequently is late in a variety of organic and degenerative brain states such as Parkinson's disease, the patient may not be able to invest an inner representation of the spouse with emotion. The tragic result late in the course of the disease may be a lack of appreciation of the spouse's loving care. A patient in an advanced stage of the disease may not even miss the caregiving spouse on his or her death if the patient's practical needs are satisfied. This can alienate or demoralize the most important caregiver. Often the psychiatrist must sensitively weigh a couple's unequal relationship—one that meets the needs of the spouse who is the patient and constructively employs the spouse who is not the patient against that spouse's potential need to recognize a discouraging lack of emotional mutuality and real relatedness received in exchange.

Postdischarge Planning

A number of studies have underscored the importance of social support in the patient's adjustment to physical deficits from a stroke. Evans and Northwood (1983) related the wide variation in individual differences in adjustment to expressed interpersonal needs for social support. Labi et al. (1980) studied long-term stroke survivors and found a significant proportion manifested social disability, despite complete physical restoration. The parameters of social function in the study were socialization inside and outside the home, hobbies, and interests; much of the subjects' disability could not be accounted for by age, physical impairment, or specific neurological deficits. The distribution of documented functional disabilities suggested that, in addition to organic deficits, psychosocial factors were major determinants. Many times the psychiatrist will be laboring at the border of a patient's neurological and reactive-interpersonal problems and be required to keep a balance between the two. But passive resignation is appropriate neither to neurological deficits in the light of the new views of neuroplasticity nor, of course, to interpersonal disability—although the latter, including rigidities of character, may be harder to change.

Davidson and Young (1985), considering outpatient management from the nursing standpoint after completion of a formal rehabilitation program, remarked that so much of the patient's energy is consumed with activities of daily living that "complex planning and timing were necessary to continue a few pleasurable activities" (p. 123). Also discussing the contribution of nursing, Smith-Brady (1982) noted that, because most of the spontaneous improvement occurs before discharge, inpatient rehabilitation programs should take advantage of this and aim at increasing postdischarge compliance, which is related to the patient's comprehension of the disease, his or her physical condition, and the prescribed therapy. In addition to educating the patient, Smith-Brady recommended getting the patient to agree to "interpersonal contracts." For recalcitrant patients who are noncompliant, Jain (1982) recommended operant conditioning techniques. Good performances in activities of daily living are rewarded with small privileges, increased eating with extra physical therapy, and attendance and good performance in therapies with tokens worth weekend passes.

The psychiatrist should be aware, as Wilson and Smith (1983) determined, that poststroke patients will often attempt to drive. However, these patients may have special difficulty in entering and leaving highways and handling traffic at traffic circles, are relatively unaware of other vehicles, and have difficulty reversing and parking their cars accurately on the right or doing two things at once in an emergency. Many of these problems are predictable from the clinical examination, and the patient should be warned. In addition to these deficits, problems with diminished vision, personality change, the prominence of denial and projection as mental defenses, and alcoholism are likely to increase the risks of driving for these patients. The justifiably decreased tolerance of society for impaired drivers should make psychiatrists cautious in encouraging post-stroke patients to assume the liability of taking the wheel once more. Even if driving is a major source of self-esteem and independence, ego-building substitutes often should be found.

Defenses and Object Relations in Hemiplegia

Critchley's discussion (1979) of patients' reactions to hemiplegia, which he calls "misoplegia, or hatred of hemiplegia" (pp. 115–120), contains observations of a variety of defensive maneuvers that epitomize the possibilities of "neurologizing" the dynamic defenses of psychiatry. In the loss of the sensation and control of parts of the body, the most remarkable changes occur in relatedness to those parts that Critchley calls "personification of the paralyzed limbs." This develops after an initial period of anosognosia and may be an overcompensation. The patient becomes a detached onlooker and the limb a foreign body outside the self. A patient may refer to the paralyzed limb as if it were an object such as a pet or a plaything, a person of another gender (often with a nickname), a "poor little withered hand" that the patient would kiss, or, in the case of a weak hand, as a "little monkey" the patient would like to feed. Sometimes personality traits are attributed to the paralyzed limb, as in "the curse," "lazy bones," "old useless," "the delinquent," or "the dummy." In one case, the paralyzed limb was called "Schumann," whom the patient disliked, whereas the unimpaired hand was called "Chopin." Illusions about the appearance of the limb ("like the hand of a mummy"), averting one's gaze from it, striking it, or screaming abuse at it are what Critchley calls "misoplegia in the highest degree."

Critchley summarized the four hypotheses put forth to explain the misoplegia:

1. That it is a specific focal neurological manifestation of involvement of the parietal lobe on the nondominant side of the brain
2. That it is an organic repression or denial syndrome (Weinstein and Friedland 1977; Weinstein and Kahn 1955) present in varying degrees in every victim of brain damage and in damage of nonparietal areas
3. That the lack or presence of insight into the effects of a cerebral lesion depends almost entirely on the nature of the premorbid personality or, in Hughlings-Jackson's terms, "the kind of brain that was in existence prior to the appearance of the lesion" (quoted in Critchley 1979)
4. That it is an iatrogenic product of the interpersonal relationship between the doctor and a suggestible patient

Critchley's discussion is limited to listing these possibilities that go beyond the limited scope of neurology. This invites the neuropsychiatrist to go much further in helping to comprehend the contributions from the last three hypotheses. When we evaluate the patients' communications in the light of our familiarity with such psychodynamic defenses as splitting and projective identification, and with transference phenomena, we see these mechanisms are very apparent in and affected by neurological impairments. Splitting and lateralization into good and bad sides of the body, which ordinarily require a psychotic personality to be manifested in the absence of neurological disease, become accessible, readily used defenses against the changed representation of the impaired body part, in brain and mind. Beneath the level of denotative meaning and concrete representation that neurology comprehends, metaphors appear that speak to psychiatrists in fuller connotations about the state of the personality in relation to the diseased limb.

Approach to Patients Who Are Unstable on Their Feet

The fearful, usually elderly patient who feels unstable on his or her feet is a common neuropsychiatric problem. An educational therapeutic approach is often helpful and may serve as a model of that approach within the context of an ongoing therapeutic relationship. The patient is taught that there are at least six components of balance, any and all of which, once improved, will contribute to them all. This immediately begins to dispel the sense of helplessness and maps a multipronged offensive effort that the patient can marshal. Table 30–7 suggests the possible multiple foci of attention to the problem.

The neuromental dimension is often the most important. The patient often expresses the feeling

TABLE 30–7. ASSISTING PATIENTS WITH UNSTEADY GAIT

1. Prescribe physical exercise; coach in morale, need for practice before going out, "training for octogenarian marathon"; get physical medicine or rheumatology consultations as needed.
2. Improve patient's footing and feedback from feet; attend to shoes or cane if needed (prevail over vanity); curtail patient's ethanol, pill taking; test Romberg and cobalamin levels.
3. Consider treatable inner ear problem (vertigo occurs in bed; ear, nose, and throat specialist referral and nylidrin may be tried) versus postural hypotension (on rising); for aging inner ear, advise patient to avoid rapid head movements and to keep head level in elevators.
4. Improve patient's visual security; teach patient to wait for eyes to adapt before moving in dark (e.g., in a theater); examine patient's eyes; consider cataract, motor problems with blinking, Meige dystonic eye closing, and gaze palsies, any of which can reduce visual input.
5. Avoid perfusion problems; rise slowly from chair or bed and wait before stepping away; do not crane neck to shave or look out for cars; "imitate Ed Sullivan," turning head and neck together; allow for postprandial shunting and micturition syncope; suggest diet, exercise, and internist visit for healthy heart.
6. Approach interpersonal world (unsteadiness can symbolize isolation and lack of support by emphasis on gait problems); avoid insulting by saying the unsteadiness is not real or hysterical; plan and map outings with graded difficulty with rest points (practicing recruiting of strangers' help) and use of public toilets; use hired cars to get to doctor or to mall to meet friends.

of a lack of support in symbolic somatic language of unsteadiness and a fear of falling. Frequently the patient has become isolated through the deaths of relatives and friends, and therapy must deal with a resistance to affiliate that usually expresses the sentiment that the loved ones cannot be replaced. This sentiment must be given its due, as it is a form of loving memorial. But progress is rapid once the patient sees associating with others as compatible with loving memories. Even the acquisition of a pet that stays in the home can improve the sense of security. Physical immobility diminishes the patient's sense of participation in life. While not working on the gait in the ways described above, patients are encouraged to correspond with distant friends, authors whose books and articles they have enjoyed, and new contacts through clubs and interests that encourage correspondence.

One such patient, an 82-year-old intellectual woman still active on a freelance basis, found her gait was unstable only en route to my office and not on the way home. As she would rise to the occasion of the session, actively voicing her problems, it became clear that the increased activation, attention, and focus of her mental state enhanced balance. She was encouraged not only to rehearse the trip beforehand physically at home in the hallway, but to pay close attention to television or vehemently read aloud favorite passages from books, priming herself cognitively before embarking from home. Central to her therapy was helping her to relax her scorn of new acquaintances and her tendency to take any excuse to give up on them, while memorializing her departed husband.

❑ SPINAL CORD INJURY

A quarter of a million Americans live permanently paralyzed from spinal cord injuries, with 10,000 new cases each year (most often young persons), with devastating career impact and emotional cost for the patients and their families (National Advisory Neurological Disorders and Stroke Council 1990).

Premorbid personality traits may also be relevant to the prevention and postinjury care of patients with spinal cord injuries, but the issue is controversial. In a study of 56 patients 16 to 50 years old, 50 of whom were males, Ditunno et al. (1985) found no correlations between a scale designed to measure sensation-seeking behavior and the dimension of prudence-imprudence in the incidents causing spinal cord injuries. Sensation-seeking scores were no higher for the patients with spinal cord injury than for a comparable normal population.

These patients, insofar as they are brain intact, may exhibit emotional reactions that are similar to those of mourning in the death of a loved one or other situations of severe loss (Bracken and Shepard 1980). Consequently, it is not surprising that premorbid personality and the influence of significant others play a central role in coping with injury.

Bodenhamer et al. (1983) added a "positive outlook" scale to scales that measured anxiety, depression, and social discomfort, and they found that patients with spinal cord injuries reported less depression and more anxiety and optimism than their caregivers predicted. The authors concluded, "Traditional theoretical models of adjustment to disability have provided very limited predictive utility for professionals in understanding individual responses to spinal cord injury" (p. 192). Bodenhamer et al. (1983) also pointed out that traditional stage theories of what is said to be a mourning-like adjustment must be individualized.

Manifest depression is not an inevitable psychological sequel to spinal cord injury. Howell et al. (1981) found diagnosable depression in only 5 of 22 patients with spinal cord injuries of less than 6 months' duration. Palmer (1985), reviewing depressions and adrenocortical function following spinal cord injury, noted that whereas depression is frequent (presumably amenable to psychotherapy), endogenous depression (presumably amenable to pharmacotherapy) is infrequent, and the dexamethasone suppression test is of questionable validity because of spinal cord injury-related changes in adrenocortical regulation. Malec and Neimeyer (1983) found that measures of distress and depression (e.g., the Beck Depression Inventory [BDI; Beck 1978], Derogatis Symptom Checklist [SCL-90; Derogatis 1977], and the Minnesota Multiphasic Personality Inventory [MMPI; Hathaway and McKinley 1970]) administered at admission predicted both duration of inpatient rehabilitation and achievement of critical bladder care and skin care behaviors after discharge.

But the best predictor of future self-care by these patients was past self-care behavior, augmented by knowledge of personality tendencies. Green et al. (1984), studying persons who had had spinal cord injuries at least 4 years previously, administered the Tennessee Self-Concept Scale (Fitts 1965) and found, in comparison with scale norms, that the respondents had significantly *higher* personal self, moral-ethical self, and social self scores, although they had significantly lower physical self scores. The higher-than-normal self-concept scores were related to perceived independence, provision of one's own transportation, assistance needed, and living arrangements. These findings suggest the possibility of *enhanced* self-concepts through mastery of handicaps and that the psychiatrist often need not settle for limitations in the patient's mental health. Wool et al. (1980) studied the learned helplessness theory, which takes the hypothesis that experiences of failure breed feelings of helplessness and depression, whereas experiences of self-controlled success produce competence and feelings of industriousness. Results from studying 24 patients with recent spinal cord injuries using standard learned helplessness tasks suggested that the psychiatrist might "immunize" these patients "against debilitating emotional reactions to paralysis with a success-oriented rehabilitation regimen during the initial stages of recovery" (p. 324).

Bracken et al. (1981) considered the coping and adaptation of 190 patients with spinal cord injuries in an acute care hospital. Affective reactions that persisted to discharge were correlated with severity of motor disability and, to a lesser degree, with sensory disability. Affective reactions were also associated with negative coping reactions that could interfere with rehabilitation therapy. This indicated the need for intensive psychotherapeutic intervention prior to discharge.

In a longitudinal study, Rosenstiel and Roth (1981) found that their best adjusted patients with spinal cord injuries predominantly employed the defenses of rationalization and denial, in keeping with an earlier point that the psychiatrist ought to respect the so-called more primitive defenses, if they work. Other traits that favored adjustment were avoidance of catastrophizing and of worrying what their life would be like, thinking about goals to be achieved after leaving the rehabilitation center, and employment of internal forms of mental rehearsal in anticipation of going home. This is reminiscent of Hamburg's sequence of cognitive defenses against a threat, which includes 11 elements: 1) regulate the timing and dosage of the threat; 2) deal with stresses one at a time; 3) seek information from multiple sources; 4) formulate expectations; 5) delineate manageable goals; 6) rehearse coping strategies and practice in safe situations; 7) test coping strategies in situations of moderate risk; 8) appraise feedback from those situations; 9) try more than one approach, keeping several options open; 10) commit to one approach; and 11) develop buffers against disappointment and develop contingency plans (Hamburg 1985).

But consider how the person stressed with brain damage is deprived of these optimal mental and psychosocial mechanisms of mastery. The stress arises from within and cannot be eliminated by avoidance or flight. The organic disease cannot be viewed at a distance from the self because it is in the very organ's self-perception. On the other hand, the cognitively distorted perceptions of a paralyzed limb involve highly metaphorical removals from the self and illustrate the difficulty one has in grasping an illness of one's own brain. The virtual impossibility of clearly grasping the disease of the perceiving organ itself renders the regulation of the timing, dosage, and sequence of multiple threats as formidable problems for psychotherapy. Formulation of expectations and delineation of goals are frequently impossible when the requisite cognitive skills are absent. "Safe" and "moderate risk" situations are lacking for the patient haunted by a global sense of impairment that intrudes into every pleasurable aspect of life, especially the seemingly simple pastimes that, when we analyze them neuropsychiatrically, are brain tests of one sort or another. For instance, think of the faculties required for reading novels, playing cards, crocheting, taking a drive, model building, tennis, golf, billiards, or appreciation of ballet. Even the taste of food is frequently altered; network television, despite its simplicity, may seem confusing. Finally, the choice of multiple options, the use of feedback from situations, and the possibility of contingency plans are all techniques that may be quite unreachable for the patient with brain damage.

The task of psychotherapy with the patient with brain damage is to assess his or her capability for each step of the cognitive sequence of defenses, to help break down difficult steps into subroutines, and to assist in bridging gaps with the psychiatrist's own analytic functions.

On a phenomenological level of prediction, DeJong et al. (1984) found that the best predictors of independent living outcome (i.e., ability to live in a less restrictive environment and to be productive in employment and other contributions to family and community life) were marital status, education, transportation barriers, economic disincentives, and severity of disability. Table 30–8 summarizes management issues for patients with spinal cord injuries.

TABLE 30–8. MANAGING PATIENTS WITH SPINAL INJURY

1. Recognize injured patients are not generally greater risk-takers.
2. Expect mourning reactions to loss of use of body.
3. Evaluate premorbid personality to understand coping techniques.
4. Consider anxiety and optimism as well as depression.
5. Individualize traditional stage theories of mourning.
6. Avoid giving priority to medication over psychotherapy.
7. Gauge self-care ability based on past self-care.
8. Expect enhanced self-concepts with experience of mastery.
9. Avoid learned helplessness with early rehabilitation.
10. Treat interfering affective reactions before discharge.
11. Respect "primitive" rationalization and denial if they work.
12. Help avoid catastrophizing and worrying.
13. Encourage mental rehearsal for goals after discharge.
14. Consider spouse and socioeconomic and educational level in plans.

Sexual Therapy for Patients With Spinal Cord Injury

Sexual therapy for the patient with a spinal cord injury, like sexual counseling for other patients, requires that the psychiatrist be comfortable and specially trained in such work (Table 30–9). Schuler (1982) culled the techniques from five programs. The myth that patients with spinal cord injuries are asexual should be dispelled, and these patients should be helped to derive satisfaction from their sexual relations. The psychiatrist should emphasize resolving the high rate of marital discord. This includes not provoking guilt in the spouses with homilies about mutual responsibility, but instead giving close attention to the spouse's role in the vital area of sexuality. It is important to educate the couple about how the level of the lesion affects whether reflexive, psychogenic, or no orgasms can be expected, and to encourage female patients to learn about phantom orgasms. Ovulation still occurs in women, and testicular atrophy is avoided in many men who receive excellent care. Pregnancy is possible with artificial insemination. Attitudes toward sexuality may be changed with the exploration of neglected erogenous zones in each partner, and sexuality should be redefined as any activity that is mutually stimulating.

A person with spinal cord injuries can be taught to prepare a new partner by explaining the physical condition and improving communication. New techniques that use mechanical devices for stimulation and the expanded use of fantasy may be intro-

TABLE 30–9. MANAGING SEXUALITY IN PATIENTS WITH SPINAL CORD INJURY

1. Avoid thinking of patients as asexual.
2. Place priority on resolving marital conflict.
3. Avoid provoking guilt in spouses.
4. Educate about potential mechanisms of orgasm.
5. Inform that pregnancy is still possible.
6. Help explore substitute erogenous zones.
7. Redefine sexuality as any mutually stimulating activity.
8. Help prepare explanations for a new partner.
9. Discuss use of mechanical devices and fantasy.
10. Be sensitive to potential for embarrassment.
11. Take a psychosexual history to gauge shyness.
12. Help overcome rigid stereotypes about passivity.
13. Suggest bladder emptying before sex to avoid spasms.
14. Introduce colloquial language if comfortable.
15. Employ coed groups for viewpoints of both sexes.

TABLE 30–10. FAMILY ISSUES IN SPINAL CORD INJURY

1. Prepare children for first contact with parent's disability.
2. Support noncorporeal basis of parental authority.
3. Explore children's fear of lack of parental control.
4. Inquire about ideas of family badness or divine punishment.
5. Suggest family religious counseling if appropriate.
6. Help family preserve long-term goals.
7. Meet sufficiently with patient and family to involve them with rehabilitation.

duced. The psychiatrist should be sensitive to a patient's embarrassment and should be willing to spend sufficient time to discuss the topics. A psychosexual history may be used to obtain information that initially may be controversial (e.g., prosthetic devices, oral sex, and masturbation). Disabled male patients and their spouses must be helped to overcome any rigid sex-role stereotypes of male domination and female passivity. Romano and Lassiter (1972) have provided specific information pertinent to sexual activity of patients with spinal cord injuries, such as the necessity of foreplay, the use of certain positions, and the importance of emptying the bladder beforehand to prevent spasms. Communication is improved and made more specific by introducing colloquial language while conducting the counseling (Romano 1973). Support groups that include both men and women are strongly recommended.

The Family Model in Spinal Cord Injury

Whereas family attitudes about the injured person's entitlements are pervasive, all members of the family are affected differently according to their roles (Table 30–10). Children must be specially prepared for their first confrontation with their parent's disability (Romano 1976), especially in dealing with fantasies of divine punishment. Children and other family members who construe human relationships in overly corporeal terms may also fear that with paralysis, the disabled parent has lost all effectiveness as an authority to admire or control them. Questions about the meaning of suffering almost always arise in persons with strong religious beliefs; often persons whose religiousness is less than mature have fantasies that they or their entire families are being punished for their intrinsic badness. Steinglass et al. (1982) considered the suddenness of the impact of spinal cord injury on families and how an overemphasis on short-term stability of family life may lead patients to sacrifice family needs for growth and development. A 1-day group meeting for patient and family improves family involvement with the rehabilitation process and decreases feelings of anxiety, helplessness, and isolation (Rohrer et al. 1980).

❑ EPILEPSY

General Therapeutic Principles

Twenty million Americans will have at least one seizure during their lives, and 2 million will have spontaneously recurrent seizures. These seizures are termed *epilepsy*, 70% of which is under control (National Advisory Neurological Disorders and Stroke Council 1990). Most epilepsy is well compensated. In a community-based sample of 125 adult nonretarded adults who had epilepsy in 1980, Trostle et al. (1989) found even those still having seizures or taking anticonvulsants were relatively well-adjusted. In a study of 57 consecutive patients with epilepsy, Roberts and Guberman (1989) found 33% had been treated for mental disorder.

In formulating psychotherapy, the neuropsychiatrist may consider the functional context (Sands 1982) in which epilepsy occurs. Differing age-related needs and tasks may be delayed or arrested at each stage of life by seizures, which usually have a regressive, exhibitionistic, and shame-producing impact. In the preschooler, it is important to consider the impact on the affective climate of the family and whether the family reaction manifests enlightenment or neurotic enmeshment. In the school-age child, the psychiatrist should consider the effects of peer acceptance or scapegoating on medication compliance; in the adolescent, issues related to epilepsy and driving, dating, sexuality, employability, and substance abuse should be explored. It is also important to determine if there is any linkage of seizure occurrence to menstruation and, if so, what the teenage girl's ideas about this relationship may be. The visibility of medication side effects may be mortifying for an adolescent. For a young adult, the psychiatrist should help the patient consider the degree of autonomy as opposed to inhibition of independence. Travel becomes relevant for such a patient, as well as issues regarding the pursuit of a career and the acceptance of seizures by employers, prospective mates, or the patient's own family. In the older adult, the psychiatrist needs to help the patient accept any necessary limitations on living alone or to face issues such as forced retirement or placement in a nursing home.

The following case illustrates how a psychiatrist may constructively interpret for a patient the functional context of epilepsy:

Case 2

A 35-year-old government official who was recently diagnosed as having idiopathic epilepsy also was experiencing mild to moderate depression about work advancement and marital difficulties. He omitted his medication on two occasions and experienced grand mal seizures at work, about which he seemed surprisingly indifferent. Gains from this behavior were considered in therapy, from the primary gain of an electroconvulsive therapy-like effect of the seizures on his depression to such secondary gains as the dramatic expression of repressed anger and self-punishment derived from career frustrations. The psychiatrist was able to help the patient achieve greater self-understanding and compliance through interpretations and discussion of these issues.

Further specific principles of neuropsychiatric management in epilepsy are given in Table 30–11.

Management of Interictal Behavior and Personality Changes

For most of the traits of the Bear-Fedio Inventory (Bear and Fedio 1977) for temporal lobe behavioral syndrome, Sørensen et al. (1989) found that a group of patients with psoriasis scored intermediate between the epileptic group and control subjects, suggesting "the mere presence of a chronic disorder with potential social stigmatization influences personality" (p. 620).

From Blumer (1982), we may adapt hints for the management of the behavior and personality changes that he associated with the interictal states of temporal lobe epilepsy (complex partial seizure state) and that may occur in other seizure states:

TABLE 30–11. PSYCHOTHERAPEUTIC APPROACH TO EPILEPSY

1. Educate the patient and family based on social background, dispelling myths.
2. Have patient and family keep a log of seizure activity and triggering factors, especially emotions; maintain expectancy that behavioral shaping based on close observation will be helpful.
3. Avoid provoking situations or rewarding seizures; treat seizure in a child like a tantrum, avoiding display of attention afterward.
4. Be pragmatic, for example, limit fluids away from home and consider other contributions to incontinence, rather than focus on earliest sources of shame, if symptom relief is goal.
5. Formulate case specifically for patient's personality, avoiding "wastebasket" concepts such as "the epileptic personality."
6. Avoid encouraging dependency because epilepsy already fosters dependency; recruit patients' active role in improving the handling of seizures, as many feel they have some conscious control over seizures.
7. Adapt treatment to enmeshment with others when present, employing marital or family approaches; for shame and shyness, consider therapy in groups including nonepileptic patients.

1. Viscosity, or stickiness, to a subject in conversation (or to the interviewer) by a laborious, detailed, and emphatic conversation and delay at the door on the way out, may be worked with, if the psychiatrist is neither rejecting nor overly passive. Self-critical patients with left temporal foci accept this better than patients with right temporal foci, who tend to deny.
2. Deepened emotionality is associated with conflict around a hyperreligious overpreoccupation with righteousness and a Dostoevskian concern with crime and punishment. Roberts and Guberman (1989) found that 51% of 57 consecutive patients with epilepsy had undergone religious conversion in the past. In these patients, cheerful hypermoralism alternates with briefer episodes of explosive verbalized anger and threatened violence, followed by remorse or denial. A patient may lack insight but will benefit from the psychiatrist's explaining how others learn to avoid the patient because of this deepened emotionality. These patients may also be coached to drop the proselytizing mode and to switch mental sets, removing themselves physically from entanglements. This works best when the patient is at a less intense emotional point.
3. Hyposexuality is seldom complained of, but further isolates patients with temporal lobe epilepsy, especially males. Rarely, there may be inappropriate sexual arousal postictally. Although the hyposexuality may be drug responsive, the psychiatrist should address the isolation and the needs of the spouse and encourage closeness. Toone et al. (1989) demonstrated hyposexuality, low sex hormone levels, and increased anterior pituitary hormones in 60 male epileptic patients.
4. Mood swings, especially those that build up over several days to a seizure, may be difficult for relatives, who try to avoid outbursts.
5. Schizophrenia-like psychosis may occur after many years in the presence of a personality more like that of the patient with temporal lobe epilepsy than that of the schizoid patient. The psychiatrist should adapt the treatment approach to specific features, as with patients who are schizophrenic. Psychosis may diminish when anticonvulsants are discontinued for a few days. Continuous aura and temporal lobe status are rare.
6. Memory disorders, related in severity to seizure severity and bitemporality, occur retrograde and anterograde during postictal confusion. Having the patient write memos at the first sign of an aura may help. Psychomotor automatisms also are a postictal phenomenon to be identified and explained.

❑ ALZHEIMER'S DISEASE

The neuropsychiatrist should approach the impact of Alzheimer's disease on the patient and his or her family in a way that is comprehensive yet sensitive to the stage of the disease. As is often the case, in this condition in which "nothing can be done," there is much that the psychiatrist can do. The following suggestions are adapted and amplified from Aronson (1984), Jenicke (1985), and Rabins et al. (1982):

Because attention and memory are impaired in patients with Alzheimer's disease, a dyadic psychotherapeutic learning process is usually impossible. But in speaking with the patient and the family together, the psychiatrist should convey by affects directed toward the patient that the patient is valued by the psychiatrist. This provides for attitudinal modeling by the family that is more crucial than any words that might be said and helps prevent retaliatory behavior by the patient against the family. The patient faces the potential of the most dehumanizing possible losses in status and valuation by the family and needs comforting in coming to terms with the beginnings of these changes while he or she is still aware of them. Genuine feelings of appreciation of the Alzheimer's patient may be difficult for physicians and other professionals to have because we are selected and trained to overvalue intellect and memory in ourselves.

The single overriding principle for treatment of the family unit of the Alzheimer's patient is the maintenance of family homeostasis and equilibrium despite the great changes in roles that result. Both patient and family benefit most if the family life can preserve its function as a holding environment for all its members and a social entity in which the members can feel loved and loving.

Sleep is the first consideration in home care. The family cannot care for the patient and will resent the patient more if family members are suffering from sleep deficits caused by the patient's reversed sleep cycle. A strict diurnal schedule is prescribed as with any insomnia, with sufficient daily activity and exercise so that the characteristically physically vigorous patient does not have an unusual amount of leftover energy during the night.

Quality-of-life considerations for the family should be immediately addressed by the psychiatrist. Discussions should counter the family's irrational feelings of guilt, family shame, punitive self-denial, and taking responsibility for the disease, all of which may lead to resentment and the potential for abuse of the patient. The physician must *prescribe* family fun with and without the patient.

Financial planning based on clinical reality should be addressed as soon as possible after diagnosis. Early consultation with a social worker to access available care resources and legal advice about the shifting of financial responsibility can help avoid bankrupting the family. The psychiatrist neither shuns relevant financial concerns nor takes sides in financial disputes. Aspects of the patient's clinical condition may enter into court proceedings, and the psychiatrist should, as always, keep clinical notes grounded in specific observations, quotes, and evaluations. The family should be encouraged to keep a log of evidence of the patient's incapacity to accomplish tasks in case it is necessary to demonstrate this. It is imperative to have colleagues determine competency to preserve the treatment relationship. Care of the patient, a new dependent, will require help from the whole family, but children and other immature members may find it especially taxing and might be less than helpful because of their own unanswered needs for support and their inability to tolerate a family situation that does not conform with ideal expectations. This is especially difficult when the Alzheimer's patient is a role model for a teenager. Exhibition of sexual inappropriateness, incontinence, or abusive hitting will humiliate an adolescent thoroughly. Encouragement of substitute role models for these family members is vital.

Certain practical measures are directly applicable to the patient's condition and thereby indirectly helpful to the family. The psychiatrist should assist the family in avoiding situations that are stressful to the patient's diminished processing ability. Just as a person with cardiac failure should not be physically overtaxed, a person with brain failure should not be pressed to evaluate multiple inputs or negotiate complex interpersonal situations, compensate for changes in plans or schedules that were attuned to bodily cycles, or even weather a physical illness without special help. Catastrophic reactions may be prevented or minimized by directing the patient's attention away from stressful tasks, thereby capitalizing on distractibility and poor memory.

The family can prevent the patient from making errors and straying by eliminating dangerous choices. Just as one childproofs a house, so too one Alzheimer-proofs. Weapons, dangerous tools, or substances that could erroneously be ingested by the patient must be locked away and outside door locks installed that cannot be opened at night. Keys to the car can be made unavailable, thus avoiding driving and confrontation about it; knobs can be removed from stoves, and matches hidden. The patient should not be left alone with minors who would be vulnerable to molestation. Comforting, favorite radio or TV shows can be set by a timer in the patient's room. Secondary systems of memory enhancement may be employed, such as posted signs, arrows, daily schedules, and identifying labels on objects or clothes. Household clutter should be avoided. Simple syntax should be used in all conversations so that the patient's memory and attention are not taxed.

Frank fear in the patient should be investigated as a possible index of victimization by the family. As Rathbone-McCuan and Goodstein (1985) have pointed out, "A disoriented aged person generally exhibits serenity in a familiar setting unless there is a sense of threat" (p. 337). "Granny-bashing" may require social support for the abusers in much the same way that child abuse does.

The psychiatrist should employ knowledge of the 15 predictable functional assessment stages in the progression both of normal aging and of Alzheimer's disease as described by Reisberg (1985) to weigh the presence of other, treatable factors. For example, incontinence should only occur late in Alzheimer's disease; if the patient experiences this sooner, there may be a treatable infection. Loss of the ability to dress properly never precedes loss of the ability to choose clothing properly, and could mean the patient is misbehaving. However, skills that the patient had yesterday may be gone today, and the family should be helped to accept the deterioration. As the sad saying goes, first it's forgetting names; then forgetting to zip up; then forgetting to zip down.

A welcome approach that combines psychodynamic and familial interpersonal principles is the study by Pruchno and Resch (1989) of defenses and coping strategies in the mental health of the spouses who care for Alzheimer's patients. Problem-focused instrumental strategies best preserved the caregivers' positive affect, and wishfulness, acceptance, and intrapsychic adaptations prevented other symptom formation.

It is an emotional reality that families may premourn the loss of the personality of Alzheimer's patients before the death of these patients and may thereby devalue what is left of the person. Often the patient is protected by the disease from awareness of this emotional abandonment, but at times when sensibility lingers the caring doctor remains the last real representative of "other people." Table 30–12 summarizes management issues for Alzheimer's patients.

TABLE 30–12. MANAGEMENT ISSUES FOR PATIENTS WITH ALZHEIMER'S DISEASE

1. Convey valuation of patient for attitudinal modeling.
2. Maintain equilibrium of family when roles must shift.
3. Prescribe sleep and exercise schedule so patient sleeps at night.
4. Discuss family guilt and shame about affected member.
5. Prescribe family fun with and without patient.
6. Refer to social worker to access care resources.
7. Suggest legal help with financial responsibility.
8. Avoid taking sides in family financial disputes.
9. Encourage log of incapacities in advanced patient.
10. Note effect of newly dependent patient on dependent family members.
11. Attend to age-specific needs of children, teenagers.
12. Encourage substitute role models for children.
13. Discuss wounded pride about loss of ideal family image.
14. Assist family in avoiding situations that tax brain failure.
15. Coach family in avoiding changes in plans and schedules.
16. Give added help at times of stress like physical illness.
17. Capitalize on poor memory to distract patient from stress.
18. Lock up weapons, poisons, money, and car keys.
19. Remove matches, lighters, and knobs from stove.
20. Do not leave patient alone with minors vulnerable to molesting.
21. Set timers for comforting radio and TV programs in patient's room.
22. Post signs, labels, and arrows as memory reinforcers.
23. Avoid household clutter and distracting background sounds.
24. Speak in short clauses and simple syntax to patient.
25. Investigate frank fear in patient for possible abuse.
26. Check emerging problems against known stages to see if avoidable.
27. Help patient find appropriate substitute activities with friends.
28. Attend closely to mental health needs of spouse.
29. Note overconcern about care, concealing feeling of family that patient would be "better off dead."
30. Recognize family may premourn physical death of patient.

Further Opportunities for Psychotherapy in Dementia

At initial evaluations, after the family has been called in, Miller (1989) has suggested that psychiatrists pay close attention to the way the family responds when the patient with dementia turns to them at moments of forgetting. If family members "wince, grunt, show surprise, coach, attempt to correct, or otherwise intervene," this provides firsthand evidence of their attitudes toward the patient. The family should be interviewed alone to permit them to ask questions about their being at risk for developing dementia, the speed of the patient's deterioration, and possible guilt about not seeking treatment for the patient earlier.

Often, family members can be helped with overall planning of the management of the major logistical problems posed by a family member with dementia, rather than persisting in previous arrangements that no longer work; to grieve for the "lost" but still living loved one; and to accept the patient's placement out of the home when desperately indicated. But nursing home placement may often be delayed by appropriate psychiatric management of a patient's noncognitive behavioral and mood disturbances (Steele et al. 1990). Day care, senior citizen centers, visiting nurses and other home health care, and geriatric transportation may also help. Family members who are the most capable and helpful are also often the most guilt-ridden. Some become martyrs, ignoring their own health and needs (and requiring psychotherapy). Miller (1989) has suggested open discussion among family members of the common feeling that the patient with dementia would be better off dead—a feeling often concealed in going to any lengths to promote care of the patient.

In considering psychotherapy for patients with dementia themselves, Miller (1989) would treat those who can still realize their cognitive disability.

These patients can be helped to adjust to increments of irreversible cognitive decline and the dependency that follows, to avoid self-blame, to retain self-esteem, and to modulate any accentuation of paranoid, obsessive, or avoidant personality traits that occurs. Those patients with more severe dementia who have lost their self-awareness (the "third eye" or observing ego) also often lose the painful feelings of frustration, embarrassment, depression, and hostility of earlier stages of the disease.

Specific interventions by the psychiatrist can address patient concerns. The card-playing patient who fears losing friends as she loses memory can be given suggestions of other ways to relate to them, and the friends' guilt can be dispelled by explaining the disease is not caused by the patient's lack of effort. A patient's worries about becoming a burden can be helped by focusing on capabilities and choices for the future, such as of a nursing home, and by establishing external systems of memory aid.

Parkinson's Disease

In describing the "shaking palsy" as a purely motor rather than mental degeneration, Parkinson (1817) himself referred to depression and terminal delirium. Reflecting the more recent recognition of concomitant mental involvement, Mayeux and Stern (1983) described some of the specific mental processes that are impaired. Building on such observations, the psychiatrist may make a more educated psychotherapeutic approach to the patient with this syndrome.

Because the degree of intellectual impairment tends to increase as the severity of motoric symptoms increases (Mayeux and Stern 1983), the psychiatrist should also assume that the patient will have greater impairment in the ability to make therapeutic contact if motor ability is more impaired. Furthermore, the psychiatrist should not conclude that all psychopathology is reactive to impairment, or that the constriction of the patient's life is due solely to motoric limitations. Beatty et al. (1989) found the MMSE useful in assessing the cognitive impairments of Parkinson's disease, and they also found that tests of frontal lobe function such as the Wisconsin Card Sorting Test (Heaton 1985) did not indicate that the cognitive impairments these patients experienced arose principally from typical frontal lobe dysfunction. Instead, such tests suggested that cerebral dysfunction extended beyond subcortical-frontal circuits.

Mayeux and Stern (1983) found that bradykinesia and rigidity, but not tremor, gait disturbance, or posture, predicted overall intellectual performance for a patient taking the MMSE. The neuropsychiatrist should not hesitate to examine the patient neurologically to gauge potential areas of mental difficulty. Although this would appear to be a roundabout approach compared with doing a mental status, it is often less threatening and efficiently yields a preliminary clinical impression.

The types of motor impairments tell us much about the patient's quality of thought, insight, and ability to relate to the therapist. Mayeux and Stern (1983) and Hallet (1979) have noted that the activities that are impaired require directed attention to the task, sequencing of cognitive processes, and often additional motor interaction. In more psychiatric terms, these activities involve an inherent motoric or spatial mental action.

Other disturbances characteristic of patients with Parkinson's disease are impaired perceptual motor or visuospatial functions, especially the inability to perform sequential or predictive voluntary movements (Stern et al. 1984). This results in impaired internal spatial representation (from which may arise the initiation of independent thought and mental action) and articulatory difficulty without impaired language reception or production. In fact, Parkinson's disease is distinct from other neuropsychiatric disorders because of the paucity of language impairment, a significant boon to the psychiatrist trying to do psychotherapeutic work.

Memory in these patients is often slowed without being impaired. Trouble with word finding, which worsens with increased motoric symptoms in some parkinsonian patients, was considered a form of the "tip of the tongue" phenomenon similar to anomia in aphasic patients with frontal lesions. Mayeux (1984) summarized a review of the literature on Parkinson's disease and Huntington's disease by stating that "nearly every patient with a movement disorder has some type of behavioral dysfunction, whether it is personality change or intellectual impairment" (p. 537). Such work specifying the cognitive correlations of motor disorders opens the way for greater interest by psychiatrists in motor phenomena. Psychotherapeutic work may be coordinated with data from employment or physical and occupational therapy sessions, which the psychiatrist may profitably attend to observe and evaluate the mood, cognition, organization, and willpower that emerge during the patient's physical action. The close linkage of motor and mental action may be turned to advantage by using a number of behavioral techniques. (Many of those which follow are mentioned by Duvoisin [1984].)

Patients should be encouraged to keep fit by regular moderate exercise, especially if their occupations are sedentary. Fitness does not stop the progression of Parkinson's disease but helps patients cope with symptoms. Free moving calisthenics and sports such as swimming are best, but safety, especially with patients who freeze motorically, must be considered.

It is important to employ sensory, rhythmic, and other cues and reminders to keep the bradykinetic patient moving. A patient can put taplike nails in the shoes to provide an auditory cue to keep the rhythm of walking constant and prevent festination. A small piece of raw carrot in the mouth may remind the patient to swallow and prevent drooling. Many techniques helpful to movement and mental state seem mechanical: wearing slippery rather than rubber soles to permit shuffling without falling, dispensing with canes and walkers when there is retropulsion, raising the back legs of chairs and toilet seats 2 inches to facilitate rising, and removing doorsills to prevent a patient from freezing in a doorway. An L-shaped extension at the tip of a cane can be stepped over so that the patient can keep moving.

Other measures are more cognitive, such as teaching a patient how to initiate rising from a chair by placing hands on the arms of the chair, or by taking someone's hand (often without having to be pulled at all) and having the patient move his or her own head forward. Similarly, patients can be taught ways to initiate sexual intercourse when rolling over in bed is difficult. If a patient who is attempting to walk through a door focuses beyond the doorjamb or wears eyeglasses with sideblinds, this may avoid inhibition of passing through by the frame effect. An earphone radio or tape recorder (such as a Walkman) can be rigged with a mercury switch attached to the eyeglasses that keep a favorite station or music going only when the patient stands up straight. A simple device to quantify tremor (Forrest 1990) reassures patients of preserved control of intentional movements.

These and other measures to help parkinsonian patients show that outpatient physical therapy and outpatient psychiatric treatment can be of great help in keeping the patient at home rather than in a nursing home.

Parkinson's disease is a disorder of knife-edge tolerances and balances. The response to levodopa (L-dopa) is so dramatic that the patient and family are exquisitely conscious of the central role of drug effects. Indeed, patients become such believers in their medication that it is difficult to pry them beyond a mechanistic view of their movement disorder and beyond their demanding dependence on the neurologist to monitor their prescriptions. Because of this fervent pharmacologism, the psychiatrist must deal not only with the patient's pathology but with the symbiotic relationship between patient and drug that includes not only motor and mental improvement but an array of side effects.

Patient and family, building on this medication response, may try to convey the idea that the psychiatrist is dealing with a cumbersome apparatus—a thing rather than a person. The psychiatrist should avoid becoming so totally immersed in the intricacies of compelling medicomotor phenomena such as on-off reactions and sudden transient freezing that the emotional issues are neglected.

A previous strategy of being reluctant to make the diagnosis or treat it in the earliest stages may be changing as deprenyl and antioxidant therapy may now be used to slow the course and keep the patient employed (National Advisory Neurological Disorders and Stroke Council 1990). The early parkinsonian patient should be watched closely for symptoms of depression. The psychiatrist should seriously consider the increased suicide risk, especially in males who overvalue physical mobility and power and are extremely anxious about their continued performance in competitive and exacting sports such as tennis and golf. Activities less aggravating for the mild parkinsonian patient may be chosen. More confusion than meets the eye (because of the preservation of language) contributes to the consternation that these patients feel over adaptation to the new challenge of disability. Further, the early pharmacotherapy of the disorder often employs anticholinergic agents with their additional potential for confusion.

Cantello et al. (1989) showed that parkinsonian patients with major depression, compared with nondepressed parkinsonian patients, nonparkinsonian depressed individuals, and control subjects, lack sensitivity to the euphoriant effects of methylphenidate that are dopamine dependent. Degeneration of the dopamine system may predispose patients with Parkinson's disease to major depression.

Starkstein et al. (1990) studied 105 outpatients with Parkinson's disease and found that 40% had major or minor depression and that depression was associated with left-hemisphere involvement in patients with unilateral symptoms. Thus depression in the early stages of Parkinson's disease may be generally related to left-hemisphere dysfunction. Another peak of depression late in the course of the disease correlated with impairment of activities of daily living and of cognitive function. This may indicate different sources of depression early and late in the course, or that depression has an adverse impact on the course of the disease. Such understanding can better legitimize a psychotherapeutic effort to deal with the more reactive components of depression.

The psychiatrist should explore the patient's image of the disease process. Although it does not present the hereditary family models of advanced disease as does Huntington's chorea, Parkinson's disease is sufficiently common to be a vivid caricature on the minds of some patients, who fear they will become an exaggeration of the motor tendencies of the aged that are assumed by stage actors and comics who portray shuffling old duffers. Fear of humiliation because of such an image may be allayed by emphasizing the medical manageability of the condition, its usual slow progression, and intense research efforts including transplantation that are based on our knowledge of the pathophysiology of the disease.

Often, antiparkinsonian drugs lose their efficacy with time. This can result in severe disillusionment to parkinsonian patients and their families, or increasing the doses can aggravate side effects.

Emotional sequelae of L-dopa treatment may include domineering behavior, increased libido, manic hyperactivity or depression, confused irrational behavior, and activation of latent psychosis or of vivid nightmares that may disturb sleep and visual hallucinations ("dopa madness"). Psychiatrists may be called on to help with these effects. Attention to the requirements for a patient's orientation (e.g., night-lights and familiar schedules), decreasing the stimulus level to diminish irritability, encouraging the beleaguered spouse to set limits, informing the spouse that the libidinal changes seldom persist, and most of all, assuring compliance with the times of dosing may all be helpful.

Later symptoms of emotional flattening, apathy, and impoverishment of the ability to relate to loved ones can be especially painful for the spouse on whom the patient may greatly rely without much gratitude or recognition. These feelings often are not articulated by the spouse unless he or she is encouraged by the psychiatrist when not in the patient's presence, but without siding against the patient.

Dopamine and Personality in Parkinson's Disease

Personality is not only a learned and habitual phenomenon simply to be unlearned in the psychotherapeutic analysis of character defenses. Evidence is growing that neurotransmitters have specific influences on personality. Dopamine has been associated with novelty seeking (analogous to exploratory behavior in animals), serotonin with harm avoidance, and norepinephrine with reward dependence. Menza et al. (1990), viewing Parkinson's disease with its low dopamine levels as a natural experiment, have shown by rating scales completed by patients and their families that there is significantly less novelty-seeking behavior in Parkinson's patients both currently and premorbidly as compared with control subjects from rheumatology and orthopedics, and no differences in the serotonin- and norepinephrine-mediated behaviors. The psychotherapeutic approach to the "reflective, rigid, stoic, slow-tempered, frugal, and orderly behaviors," as Menza et al. (1990, p. 286) characterized them, can include admiration of these traits as virtues. Often patients and their families react with amusement and pleasure to the enumeration of these traits, finding them acceptable to their "American Gothic" self-image. Table 30–13 summarizes management issues for patients with Parkinson's disease.

❑ HUNTINGTON'S DISEASE

In a large kindred of Huntington's disease families living along the shores of Lake Maracaibo in Venezuela, in whom in 1983 the G8 DNA marker was localized to chromosome 4, all descendants were said to "inherit" the disease and only those who were affected by it were said to "have" it (see Gusella et al. 1983). Wexler (1985) pointed out that although this distorts genetic truth, it expresses the experience of being at risk as a distinct state of mind. Because this state is stressful and conflict-ridden, the psychiatrist may be consulted on various issues.

Ambiguity about whether one will be affected, as with any later-onset autosomal dominant disease, may dominate the mental life of people at risk. Ad-

TABLE 30–13. MANAGEMENT ISSUES FOR PATIENTS WITH PARKINSON'S DISEASE

1. Estimate problems of therapeutic contact by motor impairment.
2. Estimate cognitive impairment by bradykinesia and rigidity.
3. Employ neurological exam readily as less threatening than cognitive exam.
4. Capitalize on language preservation without underestimating impairment of spatial planning.
5. Coordinate psychotherapy with occupational and physical therapy sessions.
6. Encourage exercise and fitness to help cope with symptoms.
7. Employ sensory, mechanical, and cognitive aids to movement.
8. Anticipate symbiotic relationship with pharmacotherapy process.
9. Avoid neglecting emotional issues amidst dosing schedule.
10. Observe early in course for depression and suicide risk.
11. Choose activities and sports appropriate to abilities.
12. Distinguish early neuropsychiatric depression from later reaction to impairment.
13. Explore patient's embarrassment about image of appearance.
14. Emphasize manageability and slow progression of illness.
15. Anticipate disillusionment as drugs lose efficacy in time.
16. Anticipate side effects of levodopa treatment.
17. Aid orientation with night-lights and schedules.
18. Decrease stimulus level to decrease irritability.
19. Anticipate spouse's pain confronted by affective flattening.
20. Praise reflective, stoic, frugal, and orderly premorbid personality.

ministration of the genetic test for persons at risk requires much sensitivity to the emotional dimensions of determining whether an individual possesses the gene, and the test should always be administered as part of a personal physician-patient relationship. Even if it is ascertained that the marker mentioned previously is found to be a universal one and the presymptomatic diagnostic test based on it becomes widely available, a 5% error can arise by recombination, and the half of those at risk who will not be exempted will face ambiguity about when the disabling symptoms will begin. The peak onset of Huntington's disease is in the third and fourth decades of life, and patients who do not know their genetic state can be comforted by a lower probability of inheriting the illness as they pass these decades symptom free. Only a tiny percentage of those at risk have taken the test, for a variety of reasons including cost and fears of discrimination, especially by insurers (Mechcatie 1990).

As Shoulson (1978) pointed out, most individuals translate the 50/50 risk into a 100% certainty they will or will not develop the disease and should be told they have a 50% risk of *not* doing so. Lack of control over one's destiny may lead to feelings of helplessness or to the development of an overcontrolling personality—effects that test results will not suddenly change. The overlap of initial symptoms of Huntington's disease and everyday experience, such as incidences of clumsiness, irritability, nocturnal myoclonus, emotional instability, or infrequent lapses of memory or judgment, can lead to hypochondriacal worries, converting each new experience into a self-test or the attribution of inadequacies to a fantasied version of the disease. Symptom seeking can lead to the loss of years of healthy productivity when a premature decision is made by an individual that the disease has begun. Conversely, symptom denial may prevent acceptance of the symptomatic help that is needed or may cause the person to suddenly collapse into depression or suicidal behavior. The psychiatrist may help the patient by taking over the responsibility of the symptom search, distinguishing between those symptoms that overlap with normality and the disease, or by teaching the patient to delegate this function to the neurologist.

Stigmatization for being part of a Huntington's disease family may affect employment and, even in the absence of evidence that the person is affected, lead to job discrimination. Most people feel some irrational guilt about a problem with their genetic inheritance for which they had no responsibility, and, unless specifically helped, these individuals may accept discrimination against them as rightful.

Patients at risk may have difficulty getting married unless the testing has shown them to be not at risk. With prenatal prediction, *even affected persons* will have the option of bearing children free of the gene for Huntington's disease, but they may not be willing to do so for fear the disease may render their parenting abnormal and deficient. In most cases, persons at risk have seen one of their own parents deteriorate before reaching their own childbearing age. Survival guilt arises in the unaffected family members who consciously or unconsciously wished the disease on other family members "in exchange" for their own health. The psychiatrist should explore such feelings with these individuals and remind them that genetic probabilities—not fantasies—determine the outcome. The allocation of genes remains 50/50 per individual, whether or not other siblings are affected. Salutary effects in being at risk are not to be ignored. Many persons at risk, fearing the healthy time of their lives may be limited, are superproductive, feel heroic as well as damaged, develop an internal locus of control to a high degree as a compensation, and have warm relations with their healthy parents and others. Table 30–14 summarizes management issues for persons at risk for Huntington's disease.

Approach to Affected Patients

Knowing one has Huntington's disease and knowing which parent is affected often leads to an unreasonable conscious or unconscious blaming of the gene-donating parent. This can disrupt vital processes of internalization of character from that present during development. Psychotherapy can help patients deal with their longings for a healthy parental model and control primitive, envious rage against unaffected siblings. Positive aspects of the affected parent as a model should be sought. Psychotherapy can help with fantasies that the disease is a punishment, that anyone is to blame, and that alternative behaviors could have prevented it, while recognizing such thoughts are defenses against helplessness and lack of control. There are also instances when knowledge of the risk of the disorder has been denied by persons at risk, and even their professional caregivers, with the result of needless transmission of the gene to another generation (Table 30–15).

The disease itself adds the further incapacitation of a movement disorder to a progressive unremitting dementia affecting higher intellectual skills and judgment. Frequently, speech is impaired. Patients with Huntington's disease remain oriented to their surroundings, are able to recognize family and caregivers, and are able to convey their likes and dislikes somewhat better than patients with Alzheimer's disease and other dementias. In keeping with this, they have more depression and less psychosis. Burns et al. (1990) found in cognitively matched Alzheimer's disease and Huntington's disease patients that the patients with Huntington's disease were both more aggressive and more apathetic than those with Alzheimer's disease and that irritability was related to the premorbid trait of bad temper in Huntington's disease but not Alzheimer's disease. Choreic movements eventually may increase a patient's caloric needs to 6,000 calories/day at the same time the

TABLE 30–14. MANAGEMENT ISSUES FOR HUNTINGTON'S DISEASE: PERSONS AT RISK

1. State probability as a 50% risk of *not* developing the disease.
2. Anticipate hypochondriasis and symptom seeking in persons at risk.
3. Expect also possible denial of symptoms and avoidance of help.
4. Take over symptom search for patient.
5. Help family with guilt and shame and to resist destigmatization.
6. Advise regarding risk childbearing and childrearing will be affected.
7. Interpret negative wishes toward relatives.
8. Advise that genes, not wishes, determine outcome.
9. Note any salutary effects on personality of being at risk.
10. Recognize many will eschew testing, sometimes for practical reasons related to stigma.

TABLE 30–15. MANAGEMENT ISSUES FOR HUNTINGTON'S DISEASE: AFFECTED PATIENTS

1. Interpret blaming of gene-donating parent.
2. Help patient internalize healthy heritage from affected patient.
3. Ventilate wishes for healthy parental model.
4. Work with envy and rage against unaffected siblings.
5. Discuss fantasies that disease is a punishment.
6. Recognize ideas of blame and prevention are strategies for control.
7. Do not participate in denial of transmissibility.
8. Recognize movement disorder adds disability to dementia.
9. Note preservation of recognition may lead to depression.
10. See family has aid of physiatrists and nutritionists.
11. Improvise mechanical assistances to movement function.
12. Discuss family ambivalence about preserving life in downhill course.
13. Help family take pride in giving nutrition and learning Heimlich maneuver for choking.
14. Encourage caregivers to pace themselves and take recreation.

coordination required to eat and swallow the food is impaired. The psychiatrist should help the patient and family to accept the expert assistance of physiatrists and nutritionists. Improvisations for mechanical assistance may also be drawn from the ingenuity of the family.

Family and staff ambivalence may arise around the sad irony of the daily struggle to keep the patient adequately nourished, in view of the disease's progressive downhill course and the likelihood that the patient will one day die of choking. But there is comfort for the family and staff in treating the patient properly, managing nutrition in an efficient way, and knowing the Heimlich maneuver. Care of patients with Huntington's disease is a great burden, and those who do it need to monitor and pace themselves to avoid undue discouragement while deriving the satisfaction of having been compassionate and useful.

Symptomatic prescription of neuroleptic drugs as antichoreics and of antidepressants should be weighed against the paucity of effectiveness data. As with any dementia, moderation in the use of confusing or obtunding psychotropic medication can minimize the difficulties a patient experiences in adjusting to new environments. As much as possible, psychotherapeutic measures can be relied on to aid orientation, as discussed above in the section on Alzheimer's disease.

❑ MULTIPLE SCLEROSIS

Whitlock (1984) reviewed the variety of affective conditions in multiple sclerosis (MS) and concluded that it is difficult to separate the reactive from the organic (frontal and limbic) sources. The influential view of Cottrell and Wilson (1926) that 63% of the patients were unusually euphoric has been supplanted by numerous studies, beginning with that of Braceland and Giffin (1950), which showed more depression among these patients.

Minden and Schiffer (1990), in reviewing affect disorders in MS, stated that the euphoria is usually described as a mental serenity, a cheerful feeling of physical well-being found more frequently later in the course, an affect disassociated from the cognitive awareness of the disability. This is not a fluctuating, reversible affect but a persistent change of personality. It is poorly documented because of sample variability and the lack of a rating scale for positive emotions, but, according to Minden and Schiffer, neurologists concur that if it exists, it is produced by demyelination and not a mental reaction.

Berrios and Quemada (1990) have discussed the scientific aspects of the relation of depressive illness to the disorder and have found the linear correlations of current approaches wanting. Careful attention to pattern recognition may help decide whether the depression is genuine or only a behavioral phenocopy. Psychiatrists may question the assumption of a unicausal direct explanation. Although a positive affect is unlikely to stir a clamor for psychotherapeutic change, it is advisable to have a close look to address the patient's possible pain beneath the euphoria in view of the frequent depressive symptoms that do respond to psychotherapy, and to consider the presence of hypomania. Minden and Schiffer (1990) have noted the higher rate of bipolar disorder found in MS patients, and the fact that mania and hypomania may occur with steroid treatment, especially if the patient has a family history of depression or alcoholism. Emotional instability of a labile nature responds so well to antidepressants that psychotherapy alone should not be considered.

Ron and Logsdail (1989) found no evidence that psychiatric symptoms in isolation were the first manifestation of MS in a series of 116 patients and that whereas elation correlated with widespread magnetic resonance imaging (MRI) abnormalities, flattening of affect, delusions, and thought disorder correlated with temporoparietal pathology on MRI. The elation in MS patients (as with the frequently seen indifference or insouciance in the similarly diffuse cortical involvement of human immunodeficiency virus [HIV]-positive patients) does not generally require pharmacotherapeutic management, in my experience.

Grant et al. (1989) found that 77% of new MS patients, as compared to only 35% of control subjects, experienced marked life stress in the year before onset of symptoms, perhaps explaining the timing of symptom exacerbation for some patients by a psychosomatic process of further destabilizing an already unstable neuroimmunological system.

Certain specific interventions, adapted here from Simons (1984), LaRocca et al. (1983), and Michele Madonna and others of the New York City Chapter of the National Multiple Sclerosis Society (personal communication, December 1985), may be considered by the psychiatrist attempting to address the nature of symptoms in MS.

Psychiatrists should help the patient focus on the lack of certainty in prognosis in a positive sense, rather than on the myriad of possible symptoms. It is important to point out that the absence of sure knowledge by the physician reflects the general uncertainty of life, including variability of the disease over time. The ability to accurately diagnose MS is improving, and although there are "uncertain" cases that meet the Poser criteria (Poser et al. 1983) for clinical probable or lab-supported probable cases the label "possible" MS to describe a wider group should be avoided. The psychiatrist should emphasize the presence of medical support and treatment rather than the lack of cure. One must be aware that the mysterious nature of the disease encourages magical theories of self-blame and of taking the illness as an ominous metaphor.

The psychiatrist should not reinforce the sick role for these patients; rather, it is necessary to reiterate the concept that, although suffering from a disease, the MS patient is not ill in the traditional sense. These patients may "have disabilities," but they are not "disabled." Thus encouraging the realistic, but temporary and selective, omission of activities that are onerous for the patient becomes important, while simultaneously working this out with the family. But family fun needs to be preserved as well.

Psychiatrists should recognize differences in patients' expectations about self-reliance and involvement in their own care, versus passivity toward medical authority, in this illness, which has a great capacity to stimulate dependence upon doctors.

If direct questioning reveals that the MS patient has sexual difficulties, the psychiatrist should distinguish between degrees of organic and psychogenic sexual dysfunction in males by nocturnal penile tumescence monitoring. A crude way to test dysfunction that is cheaper than a sleep lab is to have the patient paste a circle of postage stamps around his flaccid penis for 3 consecutive nights; if the stamps are torn apart, the patient sees that the erection mechanism works. If indicated, the psychiatrist can instruct the patient about techniques of cooperative intromission despite the patient's lack of erection, as discussed by Barrett (1982). A urological referral is indicated to discuss local treatment options of injections and prosthetic implants to aid erectile capability (J. Flax, personal communication, August 1990). Altered sexual response can precede severe disability and does not imply loss of libido or love in either sex. This area should be approached cautiously, and the spouse should be involved in sexual counseling eventually. It is important to remember that many people have erectile difficulties and inorgasmia unrelated to MS. A spouse's resistance to the labeling of a partner as "disabled" may indicate a lesser likelihood of marital breakdown than immediate acceptance.

In assessing the potential of MS for creating disappointment with the self, the psychiatrist needs to recognize that MS is a disease of young adults (women:men=1.7:1) that occurs in the prime of their lives (age 20–50), when they may have the highest performance expectations of themselves.

Because extensive frontal lobe involvement of MS greatly impairs analytic ability, planning and organizing, flexibility, and emotional lability and limits the value of psychotherapy, it is important not to reach beyond reasonable therapeutic goals or to attempt sweeping revision of defenses when neuropsychiatric assessment suggests such involvement of the frontal lobe.

Psychiatrists should help these patients to manage fatigue and other limitations by assisting them in selecting and planning participation in activities, rather than seeing the patients withdraw or regress as a result of frustration at attempting too much. It is imperative to focus on what the patient is able to do, not what he or she is unable to do. This means that the psychiatrist should advise the patient to avoid undue stress, which temporarily worsens symptoms, and reassure the patient that these flare-ups do not permanently advance the disease.

The MS patient's greatest fears are of becoming wheelchair bound, blind, and incontinent. Newly diagnosed patients should be kept from attending support groups with very advanced patients. The psychiatrist should apprise them of the likelihood of remission or successful management of their symptoms. Table 30–16 summarizes management issues for MS patients.

The following case is illustrative of many of the needs that are expressed directly and indirectly by patients with MS:

Case 3

A 44-year-old married woman whose MS was associated with sensory symptoms and neurogenic bladder lay curled in a fetal position on her hospital bed trying to rest despite her concern about the noise of activities outside her door. During the interview, she revealed (in a plaintive voice) a preoccupation with toxic and nutritional theories of MS and resentment toward her parents for having ex-

TABLE 30–16. MANAGEMENT ISSUES FOR PATIENTS WITH MULTIPLE SCLEROSIS

1. Expect more depression than euphoria, especially early.
2. Look past euphoria for coexistent depressive symptoms.
3. Consider possible bipolar disease or steroid effects during psychotherapy.
4. Avoid relying on psychotherapy alone for emotional instability.
5. Avoid unnecessarily medicating euphoria.
6. Note likely presence of life stress before episode.
7. Suggest psychotherapy, especially after diagnosis.
8. Disclose diagnosis to significant others, not to all.
9. Assist those who are dating with disclosure after rapport with partner.
10. Help patient see uncertainty of prognosis in a positive sense of possibility.
11. Plan for the possibility of disability, as in choosing a new home, but hope for the best.
12. Anticipate magical theories of self-blame in view of mysterious nature of the disease's etiology and fluctuations.
13. Avoid reinforcing sick or disabled role.
14. Select activities to substitute for those posing difficulties.
15. Accept differences in patients' relying on self versus doctors.
16. Inquire directly about sexual difficulties.
17. Approach sexual area cautiously and involve spouse eventually.
18. Consider urological treatment options for male patients.
19. Adapt therapeutic goals and discourse in impaired planning ability.
20. Help to manage fatigue by selection and planning.
21. Focus on capacities, not disabilities.
22. Advise avoidance of stresses that worsen symptoms.
23. Reassure that flare-ups do not permanently advance the disease.
24. Keep newly diagnosed patients from support groups for wheelchair bound, blind, or incontinent cases.

Source. Items 7–9 and 11 were adapted from Scheinberg 1983.

pected her to work long hours at a family business that exposed her to benzene fumes. Her physician was receptive to her complaint that the hospital was serving the improper diet but added that there was no evidence that fatigue or toxins caused MS to be worse. The patient was encouraged to find that she enjoyed nontiring activities on the ward, and she was advised by her physician not to try to experience all her sorrow at one sitting. Further psychotherapeutic exploration focused on her guilt about having MS and disappointing her parents, which was implicit in her self-justifying listing of all the things she had done for her children, and her complaints about her hospital care.

❑ BRAIN TUMOR

Because of the variety of sites and resulting deficits, the neuropsychiatric approach to neoplastic disease is difficult to generalize and arises from the needs of each particular case. Nevertheless, neurologists agree that the brain tumors most likely to produce behavioral difficulties in patients for which a psychiatrist might be consulted are those of the temporal lobe, and the tumors do so by becoming an irritative focus for temporal lobe epilepsy. Blumer and Benson (1975) noted the difficulties for psychotherapy that are caused by the viscous type of verbal expression in patients with temporal lobe epilepsy, including a deepening of emotional response that is not reversed by anticonvulsant therapy, as are the changes in sexuality and episodic aggressivity. These authors argue in favor of nondrug psychiatric management of temporal lobe emotional features.

Hochberg and Slotnick (1980) used neuropsychological tests of higher cortical functions to examine 13 survivors of primary astrocytomas who failed to return to premorbid educational or vocational levels. In the absence of tumor regrowth, all had trouble solving problems or coping with novel situations, although previously acquired abilities, overlearned material, and psychometric intelligence appeared unchanged from the premorbid level. The difficulties these patients experienced were diffuse, not related to tumor type or location, and not explained by focal deficits, psychotic or depressive thought disorders, metabolic difficulties, or hydrocephalus.

Blumer and Benson (1975) stated that the "pseudodepressed" change in personality caused by lesions of the convexity of the frontal lobes warrants early and ongoing rehabilitative efforts and mobilization; that is, patients should not be allowed to sit around. Patients with the "pseudopsychopathic" alteration of personality, more attributed to lesions of the orbital surface, have misbehavior that tries the patience of family members, who may benefit by psychiatric support. In patients with recurrent or intractable central nervous system (CNS) tumors, more diffuse signs of increased intracranial pressure sometimes supplant the specific personality changes already mentioned. Communication of underlying fear should always be expected, as when a patient with brain tumor denied all distress but lay with his arms crossed over his chest, as in a coffin (J. Jaffe, personal communication, April 1986).

Jaffe (personal communication, August 1990) found that psychiatric consultation in several hundred neurosurgical brain tumor and arteriovenous malformation cases led to an appreciation of how much warm understanding and explanation by a consistent figure can minimize the distress before and after surgery. Certain communications are frequently useful. For example, the CNS anatomic basis of puzzling peripheral symptoms can be explained, because patients are not so familiar with brain symptoms as they are with cardiac symptoms. With arteriovenous malformations, questions are raised regarding the permissibility of exertion, emotion, and sexuality, and there is a frequent confusion of the fact that the malformation is growing with the idea of malignancy. Psychiatric support may head off withdrawal of permission to continue the long arteriovenous malformation procedures, which are performed without general anesthesia to ascertain the preservation of function.

Brain tumor patients may need to be informed that malignancy admits of degrees and is not a black-and-white issue. When patients are allowed to discuss the issues without ridicule or withdrawal of support, the frequently occurring transient psychotic symptoms they experience while undergoing high-dose steroid treatment can be reported and described by these patients with much relief. In intractable cases that face a terminal course, reassurance may be given to these patients about competency, with assistance in arranging for their wishes to be respected. The patient who has fears of a painful and frightening death can be told death will likely come after lapsing into a coma and (with the exception of certain headache patients) will bring little or controllable pain. Table 30–17 summarizes management issues for patients with brain tumors.

TABLE 30–17. MANAGEMENT ISSUES FOR PATIENTS WITH BRAIN TUMORS

1. Correlate observations of specific impairments with tumor location, as in the case of temporal lobe involvement.
2. Also expect diffuse difficulties and trouble with novel situations.
3. Mobilize patients with frontal "pseudodepressed" changes.
4. Watch for communication of fears, sometimes nonverbally.
5. Provide warmth, understanding, and explanation as a consistent figure before and after surgery.
6. Explain puzzling anatomic symptoms, such as contralateral effects.
7. Discuss permissibility of exertion and sex in arteriovenous malformations.
8. Distinguish between growth and malignancy of tumor.
9. Explain that malignancy may differ in degree and is not black and white.
10. Invite reporting of psychotic symptoms on high-dose steroids.
11. Reassure about competency and arrange for wishes to be respected in terminal patients.
12. Reassure that death will come after a coma and that there will be little or controllable pain.

❑ PROGNOSIS AND THE ATTITUDES OF PROFESSIONALS

Neuropsychiatry has been thought to involve poor prognoses; but when the statistics are in the patient's favor, they may aid the psychiatrist's supportive role. For example, in Thorngren et al.'s study (1990) of stroke patients discharged from the hospital to independent living, 1 year later 90% were still in their own homes, 99% could walk independently, 92%–95% could climb a staircase, and 90% could manage their daily hygiene. Six percent had died, and 25% had had a rehospitalization.

When the statistics are not so favorable, the psychiatrist's objective and relativistic viewpoint may be tested. Frequently, psychiatrists and other physicians have such high demands for their own performance that they must guard against identifying too easily with suicidal impulses in patients who might later be grateful for aggressive intervention against depression and suicide. Lessons that can be learned from this include the need for a relativistic viewpoint that can adopt the patients' differing standards for acceptable living. It is also imperative to recognize that emotional exhaustion and burnout may sometimes affect young professionals with high standards more than most people, who have more relaxed standards of performance and may be better able to contemplate enduring life with prolonged morbidity and a chronic downhill course. In general, patients with neurological deficits affecting their performance may be better able to accept them than some of their physicians, and it is up to us to help them make the most of living.

❑ REFERENCES

Aronson MK: Alzheimers and other dementias (Carrier Letter #102). Belle Meade, NJ, Carrier Foundation, November 1984

Barrett M: Sexuality and MS. New York, National Multiple Sclerosis Society, 1982

Bear DM, Fedio P: Quantitative analysis of interictal behavior in temporal lobe epilepsy. Arch Neurol 34:454–467, 1977

Beatty WW, Staton RD, Weir WS, et al: Cognitive disturbances in Parkinson's disease. J Geriatr Psychiatry Neurol 2:22–33, 1989

Beck AT: Depression Inventory. Philadelphia, PA, Philadephia Center for Cognitive Therapy, 1978

Benson DF: Disorders of verbal expression, in Psychiatric Aspects of Neurological Disease. Edited by Benson DF, Blumer D. New York, Grune & Stratton, 1975, pp 121–135

Berrios GE, Quemada JI: Depressive illness in multiple sclerosis. Clinical and theoretical aspects of the association. Br J Psychiatry 156:10–16, 1990

Berry V: Partners/Families and Professionals Together: A Model of Posttraumatic Rehabilitation. Austin, TX, Ranch Treatment Center, 1984

Blumer D: Specific psychiatric complications in certain forms of epilepsy and their treatment, in Epilepsy: A Handbook for the Mental Health Professional. Edited by Sands H. New York, Brunner/Mazel, 1982, pp 97–111

Blumer D, Benson DF: Personality changes with frontal and temporal lobe lesions, in Psychiatric Aspects of Neurologic Disease, Vol 1. Edited by Benson DF, Blumer D. New York, Grune & Stratton, 1975, pp 151–170

Bodenhamer E, Achterberg-Lawlis J, Kevorkian G, et al: Staff and patient perceptions of the psychosocial concerns of spinal cord injured persons. Am J Phys Med 62(4):182–193, 1983

Braceland FJ, Giffin ME: The mental changes associated with MS (an interim report; ARNMD 28:450–455). Baltimore, MD, Williams & Wilkins, 1950

Bracken MB, Shepard MJ: Coping and adaptation following acute spinal cord injury: a theoretical analysis. Paraplegia 18(2):74–85, 1980

Bracken MB, Shepard MJ, Webb SB Jr: Psychological response to acute spinal cord injury: an epidemiological study. Paraplegia 19(5):271–283, 1981

Burns A, Folstein S, Brandt J, et al: Clinical assessment of irritability, aggression, and apathy in Huntington and Alzheimer disease. J Nerv Ment Dis 178:20–26, 1990

Cantello R, Aguggia M, Gilli M, et al: Major depression in Parkinson's disease and the mood response to intravenous methylphenidate: possible role of the "hedonic" dopamine synapse. J Neurol Neurosurg Psychiatry 52:724–731, 1989

Childs AH: Brain injury: "now what shall we do?": problems in treating brain injuries. Psychiatric Times, April 1985, pp 15–17

Cottrell SS, Wilson SAK: The affective symptomatology of disseminated sclerosis. Journal of Neurology and Psychopathology 7:1, 1926

Critchley M: The Divine Banquet of the Brain and Other Essays. New York, Raven, 1979

Cummings JL: Clinical Neuropsychiatry. New York, Grune & Stratton, 1985

Davidson AW, Young C: Repatterning of stroke rehabilitation clients following return to life in the community. Journal of Neurosurgical Nursing 17(2):123–128, 1985

DeJong G, Branch LG, Corcoran PJ: Independent living outcomes in spinal cord injury: multivariate analyses. Arch Phys Med Rehabil 65(2):66–73, 1984

Derogatis LR: SCL-90-R: Manual–I. Baltimore, MD, Johns Hopkins University School of Medicine, 1977

Ditunno PL, McCawley C, Marquette C: Sensation-seeking behavior and the incidence of spinal cord injury. Arch Phys Med Rehabil 66(3):152–155, 1985

Duvoisin RC: Parkinson's Disease: A Guide for Patient and Family, 2nd Edition. New York, Raven, 1984

Enoch MD, Trethowan WH: Uncommon Psychiatric Syndromes, 2nd Edition. Chicago, IL, Year Book Medical, 1979, pp 50–62

Evans RL, Northwood LK: Social support needs in adjustment to stroke. Arch Phys Med Rehabil 64(2):61–64, 1983

Fitts WH: Manual for Tennessee Self-Concept Scale. Nashville, TN, Counselor Recordings and Tests, 1965

Folstein MF, Folstein SE, McHugh PR: "Mini-Mental State": a practical method of grading the cognitive state of patients for the clinician. J Psychiatr Res 12:189–198, 1975

Forrest DV: E. E. Cummings and the thoughts that lie too deep for tears: of defenses in poetry. Psychiatry 43:13–42, 1980

Forrest DV: Selected American Expressions for the Foreign-Born Psychiatrist and Other Professionals. New York, Educational Research, 1982

Forrest DV: Therapeutic adaptations to the cognitive features of schizophrenia, and Therapeutic adaptations to the affective features of schizophrenia, in Treating Schizophrenic Patients. Edited by Stone MH, Albert HD, Forrest DV, et al. New York, McGraw-Hill, 1983

Forrest DV: The tremometer: a convenient device to measure postural tremor from lithium and other causes. Journal of Neuropsychiatry and Clinical Neurosciences 2:391–394, 1990

Freud S: On Aphasia: A Critical Study (1891) (authorized translation). New York, International Universities Press, 1953

Freud S: Project for a scientific psychology (1895), in The Standard Edition of the Complete Psychological Works of Sigmund Freud, Vol 1. Translated and edited by Strachey J. London, Hogarth Press, 1966, pp 283–397

Goldstein K: Aftereffects of Brain Injuries in War. New York, Grune & Stratton, 1942

Goldstein K: The effect of brain damage on the personality. Psychiatry 15:245–260, 1952

Goodstein RK: Overview: cerebrovascular accident and the hospitalized elderly: a multidimensional clinical problem. Am J Psychiatry 140:141–147, 1983

Grant I, Brown GW, Harris T, et al: Severely threatening events and marked life difficulties preceding onset or exacerbation of multiple sclerosis. J Neurol Neurosurg Psychiatry 52:8–13, 1989

Green BC, Pratt CC, Grigsby TE: Self-concept among persons with long term spinal cord injury. Arch Phys Med Rehabil 65(12):751–754, 1984

Gusella JF, Wexler NS, Coneally PM, et al: A polymorphic DNA marker genetically linked to Huntington's disease. Nature 306:234–238, 1983

Hallet M: Physiology and pathophysiology of voluntary movement. Current Neurology 2:351–376, 1979

Hamburg D: Brain, behavior and health (VanGieson Award Address). Presented at the New York State Psychiatric Institute, New York, November 1985

Hartmann H: The Nightmare. New York, Basic Books, 1984

Hathaway SR, McKinley JC: Minnesota Multiphasic Personality Inventory, Revised. Minneapolis, MN, University of Minnesota, 1970

Heaton R: Wisconsin Card Sorting Test. Odessa, TX, Psychological Assessment Resources, 1985

Heilman KM, Valenstein E: Clinical Neuropsychology, 2nd Edition. Oxford, Oxford University Press, 1984

Hochberg FH, Slotnick B: Neuropsychologic impairment in astrocytoma survivors. Neurology (NY) 30(2):172–177, 1980

House A, Dennis M, Molyneux A, et al: Emotionalism after stroke. BMJ 298:991–994, 1989

Howell T, Fullerton DT, Harvey RF, et al: Depression in spinal cord injured patients. Paraplegia 19(5):284–288, 1981

Incagnoli T, Goldstein G, Golden CJ (eds): Clinical Application of Neuropsychological Test Batteries. New York, Plenum, 1986

Jain S: Operant conditioning for management of a noncompliant rehabilitation case after stroke. Arch Phys Med Rehabil 63(8):374–376, 1982

Jenicke MA: Alzheimer's Disease: Diagnosis, Treatment and Management. Philadelphia, PA, Clinical Perspectives on Aging, Wyeth Labs Div American Home Products Corp, 1985

Kotila M, Waltimo O, Niemi ML, et al: The profile of recovery from stroke and factors influencing outcome. Stroke 15:1039–1044, 1984

Kreutzer JS, Zasler ND: Psychosexual consequences of traumatic brain injury: methodology and preliminary findings. Brain Inj 3:177–186, 1989

Labi MJ, Phillips TF, Greshman GE: Psychosocial disability in physically restored long-term stroke survivors. Arch Phys Med Rehabil 61:561–565, 1980

LaRocca N, Kalb R, Kaplan SR: Psychological changes, in Multiple Sclerosis: A Guide for Patients and Their Families. Edited by Scheinberg LC. New York, Raven, 1983, pp 175–194

LeVay S: A difference in hypothalamic structure between heterosexual and homosexual men. Science 253:1034–1037, 1991

Luria AR: The Working Brain: An Introduction to Neuropsychology. New York, Basic Books, 1973

Malec J, Neimeyer R: Psychologic prediction of duration of spinal cord injury rehabilitation and performance of self care. Arch Phys Med Rehabil 64(8):359–363, 1983

Mayeux R: Behavior manifestations of movement disorders: Parkinson's and Huntington's disease. Neurol Clin 2:527–540, 1984

Mayeux R, Stern Y: Intellectual dysfunction and dementia in Parkinson disease, in The Dementias. Edited by Mayeux R, Rosen WG. New York, Raven, 1983

Mechcatie E: Guidelines for Huntington's genetic testing, follow up. Clinical Psychiatry News 18(2):2, 22, 1990

Menza MA, Forman NE, Goldstein HS, et al: Parkinson's disease, personality and dopamine. Journal of Neuropsychiatry 2:282–287, 1990

Miller MD: Opportunities for psychotherapy in the management of dementia. J Geriatr Psychiatry Neurol 2:11–17, 1989

Minden SL, Schiffer RB: Affective disorders in multiple sclerosis: review and recommendations for clinical research. Arch Neurol 47:98–104, 1990

National Advisory Neurological Disorders and Stroke Council: Implementation Plan: Decade of the Brain. Washington, DC, National Institute of Neurological Disorders and Stroke, 1990

Newcombe F: The psychological consequences of closed head injury: assessment and rehabilitation. Injury 14: 11–136, 1983

Oddy M, Humphrey M, Uttley D: Subjective impairment and social recovery after closed head injury. J Neurol Neurosurg Psychiatry 41:611–616, 1978

Oddy M, Coughlan T, Tyerman A, et al: Social adjustment after closed head injury: a further follow-up seven years after injury. J Neurol Neurosurg Psychiatry 48: 564–568, 1985

Palmer JB: Depression and adrenocortical function in spinal cord injury patients: a review. Arch Phys Med Rehabil 66(4):253–256, 1985

Parkinson J: An Essay on the Shaking Palsy. London, Sherwood, Neely and Jones, 1817

Piaget J: Play, Dreams and Imitation in Childhood. London, Routledge & Kegan Paul, 1952

Piaget J: The Construction of Reality in the Child. Translated by Cook M. New York, Basic Books, 1954

Piaget J, Inhelder B: Mental Imagery in the Child. Translated by Chilton PA. New York, Basic Books, 1971

Poser CM, Paty DW, Scheinberg L, et al: New diagnostic criteria for multiple sclerosis: guidelines for research protocols. Ann Neurol 13:227–231, 1983

Pruchno RA, Resch NL: Mental health of caregiving spouses: coping as mediator, moderator, or main effect? Psychol Aging 4:454–463, 1989

Rabins PV, Mace NL, Lucas MJ: The impact of dementia on the family. JAMA 248:333–335, 1982

Rathbone-McCuan E, Goodstein RK: Elder abuse: clinical considerations. Psychiatric Annals 15:331–339, 1985

Reisberg B: Alzheimer's disease update. Psychiatric Annals 15:319–322, 1985

Roberts JK, Guberman A: Religion and epilepsy. Psychiatr J Univ Ottawa 14:282–286, 1989

Rohrer K, Adelman B, Puckett J, et al: Rehabilitation in spinal cord injury: use of a patient-family group. Arch Phys Med Rehabil 61(5):225–229, 1980

Romano MD: Sexual counseling in groups. Journal of Sex Research 9:69–78, 1973

Romano MD: Preparing children for parental disability. Soc Work Health Care 1:309–315, 1976

Romano MD, Lassiter RE: Sexual counseling with the spinal cord injured. Arch Phys Med Rehabil 53:568–573, 1972

Ron MA, Logsdail SJ: Psychiatric morbidity in multiple sclerosis: a clinical and MRI study. Psychol Med 19: 887–895, 1989

Rosenstiel AK, Roth S: Relationship between cognitive activity and adjustment in four spinal cord-injured individuals: a longitudinal investigation. Journal of Human Stress 7:35–43, 1981

Russell WR: The Traumatic Amnesias. Oxford, Oxford University Press, 1971

Sands H: Psychodynamic management of epilepsy, in Epilepsy: A Handbook for the Mental Health Professional. Edited by Sands H. New York, Brunner/Mazel, 1982, pp 135–157

Sarno MT: The nature of verbal impairment after closed head injury. J Nerv Ment Dis 168:685–692, 1980

Scheinberg LC: Multiple Sclerosis: A Guide for Patients and Their Families. New York, Raven, 1983

Schiffer RB: Psychiatric aspects of clinical neurology. Am J Psychiatry 140:205–211, 1983

Schuler M: Sexual counseling for the spinal cord injured: a review of 5 programs. J Sex Marital Ther 8:241–252, 1982

Searles H: The differentiation between concrete and metaphorical thinking in the recovering schizophrenic patient, in Selected Papers in Schizophrenia and Related Subjects. New York, International Universities Press, 1965, pp 560–583

Shoulson I: Clinical Care of the Patient and Family With Huntington's Disease. New York, Committee to Combat Huntington's Disease, 1978

Simons AF: Problems of providing support for people with M.S. and their families, in Multiple Sclerosis: Psychological and Social Aspects. Edited by Simons AF. London, Heinemann Medical Books, 1984, pp 1–20

Smith-Brady R: Assessing adherence in stroke regimens. Nurs Clin North Am 17:499–512, 1982

Sørensen AS, Hansen H, Andersen R, et al: Personality characteristics and epilepsy. Acta Psychiatr Scand 80: 620–631, 1989

Starkstein SE, Preziosi TJ, Bolduc PL, et al: Depression in Parkinson's disease. J Nerv Ment Dis 178:27–31, 1990

Steele C, Rovner B, Chase GA, et al: Psychiatric symptoms and nursing home placement of patients with Alzheimer's disease. Am J Psychiatry 147:1049–1051, 1990

Steinglass P, Temple S, Lisman SA, et al: Coping with spinal cord injury: the family perspective. Gen Hosp Psychiatry 4:259–264, 1982

Stern DN: The Interpersonal World of the Infant: A View From Psychoanalysis and Developmental Biology. New York, Basic Books, 1985

Stern Y, Mayeux R, Rosen J: Contribution of perceptual motor dysfunction to construction and tracing disturbances in Parkinson's disease. J Neurol Neurosurg Psychiatry 47:987–989, 1984

Stevens JH, Turner CW, Rhodewalt F, et al: The type A behavior pattern and carotid artery atherosclerosis. Psychosom Med 46:105–113, 1984

Stoller RJ: Pain and Passion: A Psychoanalyst Explores the World of S & M. New York, Plenum, 1991

Strub RL, Black FW: The Mental Status Examination in Neurology, 2nd Edition, With a Foreword by Norman Geschwind. Philadelphia, PA, FA Davis, 1985

Taylor MA: The Neuropsychiatric Mental Status Exam. New York, SP Medical & Scientific, 1981

Thomsen IV: Late outcome of very severe blunt head trauma: a 10–15 year second follow-up. J Neurol Neurosurg Psychiatry 47:260–268, 1984

Thorngren M, Westling B, Norrving B: Outcome after stroke in patients discharged to independent living. Stroke 21:236–240, 1990

Toone BK, Edeh J, Nanjee MN, et al: Hyposexuality and epilepsy: a community survey of hormonal and behavioral changes in male epileptics. Psychol Med 19:937–943, 1989

Trostle JA, Hauser WA, Sharbrough FW: Psychological and social adjustment to epilepsy in Rochester, Minnesota. Neurology 39:633–637, 1989

Tyerman A, Humphrey M: Changes in self concept following severe head injury. Int J Rehabil Res 7:11–23, 1984

van Zomeren AH, van den Burg W: Residual complaints of patients two years after severe head injury. J Neurol Neurosurg Psychiatry 48:21–28, 1985

Weddell R, Oddy M, Jenkins D: Social adjustment after rehabilitation: a 2-year follow-up of patients with severe head injury. Psychol Med 10:257–263, 1980

Weinstein EA: Sexual disturbances after brain injury. Medical Aspects of Human Sexuality 8(10):10–31, 1974

Weinstein EA, Friedland RP: Behavioral disorders associated with hemi-inattention, in Advances in Neurology, Vol 18. Edited by Weinstein EA, Friedland RP. New York, Raven, 1977, pp 51–62

Weinstein EA, Kahn RL: Denial of Illness: Symbolic and Physiological Aspects. Springfield, IL, Charles C Thomas, 1955

Wexler NS: Genetic jeopardy and the new clairvoyance, in Progress in Medical Genetics, Vol 6. New York, Praeger, 1985

Whitlock A: Emotional disorder in multiple sclerosis, in Multiple Sclerosis: Psychological and Social Aspects. Edited by Simons AF. London, William Heinemann Medical Books, 1984, pp 72–81

Wilson T, Smith T: Driving after stroke. International Rehabilitation Medicine 5(4):170–177, 1983

Woods BT, Short MP: Neurological dimensions of psychiatry. Biol Psychiatry 20:192–198, 1985

Wool RN, Siegel D, Fine PR: Task performance in spinal cord injury: effect of helplessness training. Arch Phys Med Rehabil 61(7):321–325, 1980

❑ ANNOTATED REFERENCES

Aronson MK: Alzheimers and other dementias (Carrier Letter #102). Belle Meade, NJ, Carrier Foundation, November 1984

Available from Carrier Foundation, Belle Meade, NJ 08502

Barrett M: Sexuality and MS. New York, National Multiple Sclerosis Society, 1982

Available from National Multiple Sclerosis Society, 205 E. 42nd Street, New York, NY 10017

Berry V: Partners/Families and Professionals Together: A Model of Posttraumatic Rehabilitation. Austin, TX, Ranch Treatment Center, 1984

Available from Ranch Treatment Center, Head Injury Articles, P.O. Box 4008, Austin, TX 78765

Forrest DV: Selected American Expressions for the Foreign-Born Psychiatrist and Other Professionals. New York, Educational Research, 1982

Available from Educational Research Lab, New York State Psychiatric Institute, 722 W. 168th Street, New York, NY 10032

National Advisory Neurological Disorders and Stroke Council: Implementation Plan: Decade of the Brain. National Institute of Neurological Disorders and Stroke, June 8, 1990

Available from National Coalition for Research in Neurological Disorders, 3050 K Street N.W., Suite 310, Washington, DC 20007

Shoulson I: Clinical Care of the Patient and Family With Huntington's Disease. New York, Committee to Combat Huntington's Disease, 1978

Available from the Committee to Combat Huntington's Disease, Inc., 250 West 57th Street, New York, NY 10107

Chapter

31

Cognitive Rehabilitation and Behavior Therapy of Neuropsychiatric Disorders

Mark R. Lovell, Ph.D.
Christopher Starratt, Ph.D.

As psychiatry's role in the assessment and treatment of individuals with neurological impairment has expanded dramatically over the last decade, so has the need for a broad-based understanding of methods of promoting recovery from brain injury and disease. The role of the psychiatrist in the diagnosis and treatment of the sequelae of central nervous system (CNS) dysfunction has become a crucial one and promises to become even more central with the continued development of sophisticated neuropharmacological treatments for both cognitive and psychosocial components of brain impairment (Gualtieri 1988). In addition to these exciting new developments, an understanding of nonpharmacological, behavioral methods of assessment and treatment can greatly enhance the patient's recovery from cognitive deficits as well as provide a useful adjunct treatment for behavioral deficits and excesses that are commonly associated with CNS dysfunction. In this chapter, we review the role of psychological treatments for the neuropsychological (cognitive) and behavioral consequences of CNS dysfunction.

In response to the increase in the number of patients requiring treatment for CNS dysfunction, there has been a proliferation of treatment agencies structured to provide rehabilitation services, as well as an accompanying increase in research efforts designed to assess the efficacy of these treatment programs. There has been a particularly intense focus over the last few years on the development of rehabilitation programs designed specifically to treat the neuropsychological and psychosocial sequelae of neuropsychiatric disorders. Before turning to a discussion of specific treatment modalities, that may be useful with neuropsychiatric patients, we briefly review neuroanatomical influences on the recovery process.

❑ NEUROANATOMICAL AND NEUROPHYSIOLOGICAL DETERMINATES OF RECOVERY

Recovery from brain injury or disease can be conceptualized as involving a number of separate, but interacting processes. Although a complete discussion of existing research concerning neuroanatomical and neurophysiological aspects of the recovery process is beyond the scope of this chapter, we provide here a brief review. (For a more complete review of current theories of recovery from brain injury, see Gouvier et al. 1986.)

After an acute brain injury, such as a stroke or head injury, there is likely to be some degree of improvement due to a lessening of the temporary or treatable consequences of the injury. Factors such as degree of cerebral edema and extent of increased intracranial pressure are well known to temporarily affect brain function after a closed head injury or stroke (Lezak 1976). Cellular waste material that is released after injury to the cell has also been shown to affect neural functioning. In addition, the regrowth of neural tissue to compensate for an injured area has been shown to occur to some minimal extent in animal studies on both the anatomical (Kolata 1983) and physiological levels (Wall and Egger 1971) and may have some limited relevance for humans. With many acute brain injuries, there is an improvement in functioning as these temporary effects subside. However, with degenerative illnesses, such as Alzheimer's disease and Huntington's disease, the condition actually worsens over time.

The differences in prognosis between various neurological disorders obviously affects the structuring of the rehabilitation program. For example, the expectations and goals of a rehabilitation program structured to improve memory function in patients with head injury are likely to be much different from the goals set for a patient with Alzheimer's disease. The program designed for the patient with head injury is likely to focus on teaching the patient alternative strategies for remembering new information, whereas a program designed for an Alzheimer patient would probably focus on improving the patient's functioning with regard to activities of daily living.

❑ COGNITIVE REHABILITATION OF NEUROPSYCHIATRIC DISORDERS

The terms *cognitive rehabilitation* and *cognitive retraining* have been variously used to describe treatments designed to maximize recovery of the individual's abilities in the areas of intellectual functioning, visual processing, language, and, particularly, memory.

It is important to note that techniques used to improve cognitive functioning after a neurological event represent an extremely heterogeneous group of procedures that vary widely in their focus depending on the nature of the patient's cognitive difficulties, the specific skills and training of the staff members, and the medium through which the information is presented (i.e., computer versus individual therapy versus group therapy). Under ideal conditions, a cognitive rehabilitation program should be tailored to the individual patient's particular needs and based on a thorough, individualized neuropsychological assessment of the patient's psychometric deficits, as well as an estimation of how these deficits are likely to affect the patient in his or her daily life. Because patients with different neurological or neuropsychiatric syndromes often have different cognitive deficits, the focus of the treatment is likely to vary a great deal. For example, a treatment program designed primarily to treat patients with head injury is likely to be focused on the amelioration of attentional and memory deficits, whereas a rehabilitation program designed for stroke patients is likely to focus on a more specific deficit such as language disorders or other disorders that tend to occur after lateralized brain damage, with less emphasis on co-occurring attentional and memory deficits.

It must be emphasized that, despite the recent surge in interest in psychiatric problems in patients with neurological impairment, there has been little systematic research concerning the effectiveness of cognitive and behavioral treatment strategies in this group. Most of our information comes from experience with patients in pure rehabilitation settings. The following brief review of cognitive rehabilitation strategies is designed to treat specific cognitive deficits that may be associated with neuropsychiatric disorders.

Attentional Processes

Disorders of attention are common sequelae of a number of neurological disorders and are particularly common after traumatic brain injury. Recognition and treatment of attentional disorders are extremely important because an inability to focus and sustain attention may directly limit the patient's ability to actively participate in the rehabilitation program and may, therefore, affect progress in other areas of cognitive functioning. It must be stressed that attention is not a unitary process. A number of components have been identified, including alertness and the ability to selectively attend to incoming information, as well as the capacity to focus and maintain attention or vigilance (Posner and Rafal 1987).

Rehabilitation programs designed to improve attentional processes usually attempt to address all of these processes. One such program is the Orientation Remedial (OR) module developed by Ben-Yishay and associates (Ben-Yishay and Diller 1981) at New York University. The OR program consists of five separate tasks that are presented by microcomputer and vary in degree of difficulty. These tasks involve 1) training the patient to attend and react to environmental "signals," 2) training the patient to time his or her responses in relation to changing environmental cues, 3) training the patient to be actively vigilant, 4) training in time estimation, and 5) training the patient to synchronize responding with complex rhythms. Progress on these tasks is a prerequisite for further training on "higher-level" tasks.

Memory

Within the field of cognitive rehabilitation, much of the emphasis has been placed on the development of treatment approaches to improve memory. This is not surprising given the pervasiveness of memory disorders in many different neurologically impaired populations. In general, rehabilitation strategies for improving memory can be divided into three primary categories depending on whether the technique involves 1) the use of mnemonic strategies, 2) the use of repetitive practice and drills, or 3) approaches that rely on external devices or procedures to improve memory.

Mnemonic strategies. Mnemonic strategies are approaches to memory rehabilitation that are specifically designed to promote the encoding and remembering of a specific type of information depending on the patient's particular memory impairment. There are currently a number of different types of mnemonic strategies that may be of use in neuropsychiatric settings. *Visual imagery* is one of the most well known and commonly used mnemonic strategies (Glisky and Schacter 1986) and involves the use of visual images to assist in the learning and retention of verbal information. Probably the oldest and best known visual imagery strategy is the "method of Loci," which involves the association of to-be-remembered verbal information with locations that are familiar to the patient (i.e., the room in a house, location on a street, and so on). When recall of the information is required, the patient visualizes each room and the item(s) that are to be remembered in each location (Moffat 1984). Initial research has suggested that this method may be particularly useful for elderly patients (Robertson-Tchabo et al. 1976).

A related method of learning and remembering new information is generally referred to as *peg mnemonics* and requires the patient to learn a list of peg words and to associate these words with a given visual image, such as one-bun, two-shoe, and so on. After the learned association of the numbers with the visual image, sequential information can be remembered in order by association with the visual image (Gouvier et al. 1986). Although this strategy has been widely used by professional mnemonists and did show some early promise in use with brain injury patients (Patten 1972), more recent research has suggested that this approach may not be highly effective because of an inability of patients with brain injury to generate visual images (Crovitz et al. 1979) and because of difficulty maintaining this information over time.

Another type of visual imagery procedure that has been widely used in clinical settings and studied extensively is *face-name association*. As the name implies, this procedure has been used with brain injury patients to promote the remembering of peoples' names based on visual cues and involves association of components of the name with a distinctive visual image. For example, the name *Angela Harper* might be encoded by the patient visualizing an angel playing a harp. Obviously, the ease with which this method can be used with brain injury patients depends on their ability to form internal visual images, as well as the ease with which the name can be transferred into a distinct visual image. Whereas a name such as *Angela Harper* may be relatively easy to find visual associations for, a name such as *Jane Johnson* may be much more difficult to encode in this manner. Overall, visual imagery strategies may be useful for specific patient groups (i.e., patients with impairment in verbal memory who need to use nonverbal cues to assist them in recall) and in patient groups whose impairments are mild enough to allow them to recall the series of steps necessary to spontaneously use these strategies once they return to their natural environments.

In addition to the extensive use of visual imagery strategies for improving memory in patients with brain injury, the use of verbally based mnemonic strategies has also become quite popular, particularly with patients who have difficulty employing visual imagery. One such procedure, *semantic elaboration*, involves constructing a story out of new to-be-remembered information. This type of procedure may be particularly useful in cases where the patient may be unable to use imagery strategies because of a reduced ability to generate internal visual images.

Rhyming strategies involve remembering verbal information by incorporating the information into a rhyme. This procedure was originally demonstrated by Gardner (1977) with a globally amnestic patient who was able to recall pertinent personal information by the learning and subsequent singing of the following rhyme:

> Henry's my name; Memory's my game; I'm in the V.A. in Jamaica Plain; My bed's on 7D; The year is '73; Every day I make a little gain.

For patients who have difficulty learning and remembering written information, Glasgow et al. (1977) used a structured procedure for approaching the information called *PQRST*. This strategy involves application of five steps: 1) *P*review the information, 2) form *Q*uestions about the information, 3) *R*ead the information, 4) *S*tate the questions, and 5) *T*est for retention by answering the questions after the material has been read.

Repetitive practice. Cognitive rehabilitation strategies that emphasize repetitive practice of the to-be-remembered information have become extremely popular in rehabilitation settings despite little experimental evidence that these procedures produce lasting improvement in memory. Repetitive practice strategies rely heavily on the use of drills and appear to be based on a "mental muscle" conceptualization of memory (Harris and Sunderlund 1981), which infers that memory can be improved merely by repeated exposure to the information that is to be learned. Although it is generally accepted that patients with brain injury can learn specific pieces of information through repeated exposure, studies designed to demonstrate generalization of this training to new settings or tasks has not been encouraging. (For a review, see Schacter and Glisky 1986.)

In view of the lack of evidence that repeated practice strategies are effective in producing improvement in memory in patients with brain damage, Glitsky and Schacter (1986) suggested that attempts to remedy memory disorders should be focused on the acquisition of "domain-specific knowledge" that is likely to be specifically relevant to the patient's ability to function in everyday life. This approach differs from the use of traditional cognitive remediation strategies in that 1) the goal of this treatment is not to improve memory functioning "in general," but rather to deal with specific problems associated with memory impairment; 2) the information acquired through this treatment has practical value to the individual; and 3) the information learned through training exercises is chosen on the basis of its having some practical value in the patient's natural environment. Initial research has established that even patients with severe brain injury are indeed capable of acquiring discrete pieces of information important to their ability to function on a daily basis (Glasgow et al. 1977; Wilson 1982).

External memory aids. External aids to memory can take various forms, but generally they fall into two categories: 1) memory-storage devices and 2) memory-cuing strategies (Harris 1984). Probably the most basic memory-storage devices take the form of written lists and memory books. Lists and memory books are widely used with brain injury patients and often include the patient recording information vital to his or her daily function (e.g., the daily schedule of activities and chores to be performed) and then consulting this information at a given time.

These strategies are not designed to provide a general improvement in the patient's ability to learn and retain new information but are used as memory-support devices.

With recent advances in the field of microelectronics, hand-held electronic storage devices have become increasingly popular in rehabilitation settings. Although these devices allow for the storage of large amounts of information, their oftentimes complicated operations requirements may obviate their use in all but the mildest cases of brain injury or disease. Another problem inherent to external storage devices is the requirement that the device be consulted at the appropriate time to be useful. This may be a difficult task for the patient with brain injury and often involves the use of cuing strategies that remind the patient to engage in a behavior at a given time.

The application of cuing involves the use of prompts designed to remind the patient to engage in a specific behavioral sequence at a given time. To be maximally effective, the cue should be given as close to the time that the behavior is required, must be active rather than passive (i.e., such as an alarm clock), and should provide a reminder of the specific behavior that is desired (Harris 1984). One particularly useful cuing device that is currently in use is the alarm wristwatch. This device can be set to sound an alarm at a given time. Although this does not provide specific information concerning the desired response, it can serve as a useful cue to prompt the patient to check a list or other storage device for further instructions. Thus a patient with brain injury can be cued to engage in some behavior on a regular basis.

Visual-Perceptual Disorders

In addition to memory impairment, individuals with brain injury may have difficulties with visual perception. Deficits in visual perception most commonly occur in patients who have suffered right-hemisphere cerebral vascular accidents (Gouvier et al. 1986). Given the importance of visual perceptual processing to many occupational tasks and to the safe operation of an automobile (Sivak et al. 1985), the rehabilitation of deficits in this area could have important implications for the recovery of the neuropsychiatric patient.

One deficit that is particularly common in stroke patients is the hemispatial neglect syndrome. This deficit is characterized by an inability to recognize stimuli in the contralateral visual field. One strategy that has been used extensively to treat hemispatial neglect is visual scanning training. This procedure, which has been designed to promote scanning to the neglected hemifield, has been extensively used at the Rusk Institute of Rehabilitation, New York Medical Center (Diller and Weinberg 1977) and by others (Gianutsos et al. 1983). The New York Medical Center program uses a light board with 20 colored lights and a target that can be moved around the board at different speeds. The patient can be systematically trained to attend to the neglected visual field. This procedure, with the addition of other tasks (e.g., a size estimation and body awareness task) was found to improve visuoperceptual functioning in a group of brain injury patients compared with a group of similar patients who received standard occupational therapy (Gordon et al. 1985). Other researchers have produced similar therapeutic gains in scanning and other aspects of visuoperceptual functioning through rehabilitation strategies. (For a more complete review of this area, see Gianutsos and Matheson 1987; Gordon et al. 1985.)

Intellectual and Executive Functions

Patients who have sustained a brain injury often suffer a breakdown in their ability to reason, form concepts, solve problems, execute and terminate behavioral sequences, and engage in other complex cognitive activities (Goldstein and Levin 1987). Deficits in these areas are among the most debilitating to the neuropsychiatric patient because they often underlie changes in the patient's basic abilities to function interpersonally, socially, and vocationally. Despite a general recognition of the impact that disorders of intellectual and executive processes have on the individual, relatively little effort has been dedicated to the systematic development of rehabilitation programs to ameliorate these disorders. This may be due, at least in part, to the complex and multifaceted nature of intellectual and executive functions.

It is important to emphasize that intellectual and executive functioning cannot be conceptualized as unitary constructs, but rather involve a number of processes that include motivation, abstract thinking, and concept formation, as well as the ability to plan, reason, and execute and terminate behaviors. Therefore, breakdowns in intellectual and executive functioning can occur for a number of different reasons depending on the underlying core deficit(s) and can vary based on the area of the brain that is injured. For example, injury to the parieto-occipital brain area is likely to result in a problem-solving deficit secondary to difficulty with comprehension of logico-grammatical structure, whereas a frontal lobe injury may impede problem solving by disrupting the individual's ability to plan and to carry out the series of steps that are necessary to process the grammatical material (Luria and Tsvetkova 1990).

An apparent breakdown in the patient's ability to function intellectually can also occur secondary to deficits in other related areas of neuropsychological functioning such as attention, memory, and language. The type of rehabilitation strategy chosen depends on the underlying core deficit that needs to be addressed. The goal of rehabilitation with a patient with a left parieto-occipital lesion might be to help the patient develop the skill to correctly analyze the grammatical structure of the problem. Rehabilitation efforts with a frontal lobe patient might emphasize impulse control and execution of the appropriate behavioral sequence to solve the problem.

Because of the multitude of factors that can result in intellectual and executive functioning difficulties in patients with brain injury, programs designed to rehabilitate these deficits have necessarily involved attempts to address them in a hierarchical manner, as originally proposed by Luria (1963). One such program was developed at New York University by Ben-Yishay and associates (Ben-Yishay and Diller 1983). Ben-Yishay developed a two-tiered approach that defines five basic deficit areas (arousal and attention, memory, impairment in underlying skill structure, language and thought, and feeling tone) and two domains of higher-level problem solving. This model proposes that deficits in the higher-level skills are often produced by core deficits and that the patient's behavior is likely to depend on an interaction between the two domains (Goldstein and Levin 1987).

Speech and Language

Disorders of speech and language are common sequelae of neurological damage, particularly when the dominant (usually left) hemisphere is injured. As the ability to communicate is often central to the patient's personal, social, and vocational readjustment after brain injury or disease, rehabilitation efforts in this area are extremely important. In most rehabilitation settings, speech and language therapies have traditionally been the province of speech pathologists. Therapy has often involved a wide variety of treatments depending on the training, interest, and theoretical orientation of the therapist. The goal of therapy has variously been the improvement of comprehension (receptive language) and expression (expressive language), and it has been demonstrated that patients who receive speech therapy after a stroke improve more than patients who do not (Basso et al. 1979).

❑ USE OF COMPUTERS IN COGNITIVE REHABILITATION

The use of the microcomputer in cognitive rehabilitation has increased dramatically over the last decade, just as its use has increased in many other facets of everyday life. The microcomputer has a great deal of potential for use in rehabilitation settings and may offer several advantages over more conventional, therapist-based treatments (Grimm and Bleiberg 1986). Microcomputers may have the advantage of being potentially self-instructional and self-paced, of requiring less direct staff time, and of accurately providing direct feedback to the patient regarding his or her performance. Microcomputers also facilitate research by accurately and consistently recording the large amounts of potentially useful data that are generated during the rehabilitation process.

Notwithstanding the above mentioned advantages, several cautions must be mentioned concerning the use of microcomputers in the rehabilitation process. First, it must be emphasized that the microcomputer is merely a tool (albeit a highly sophisticated one) whose usefulness is limited by the availability of software that meets the needs of the individual patient and the skill of the therapist in implementing the program or programs. As noted by Harris (1984), the danger exists that cognitive rehabilitation will become centered around the software that is available through a given treatment program rather than being based on the individual needs of the patient. Second, microcomputers are not capable of simulating human social interaction and should not be used in lieu of human therapeutic contact.

❑ BEHAVIORAL DYSFUNCTION AFTER BRAIN INJURY

At the beginning of this section it is important to stress that our understanding of the full range of behavioral dysfunction in individuals with brain injury or disease remains far from complete. Unfortunately, there have been relatively few follow-up studies to date that have systematically investigated the efficacy of neuropsychiatric treatment programs. In addition, as is the case with the cognitive rehabilitation literature, much of what we know comes from studies conducted in rehabilitation settings rather than in hospitals specifically designed to treat patients with neuropsychiatric disorders. Most recent studies in this area have focused on patients with traumatic brain injury.

Behavioral disruption associated with other neurological disorders, such as cerebrovascular accidents and progressive dementing disorders, has also received considerable attention but has not been the subject of a great deal of research to evaluate treatment procedures that are likely to be effective. Despite the relatively sparse literature on treatment outcome in this area, the studies that have been reported have been useful in guiding the development of practical strategies for dealing with the behavioral-psychiatric consequences of brain injury. In particular, behaviorally based treatments have been heavily used.

Behavioral dysfunction after brain injury can have a marked impact on the recovery process itself, as well as on the more general aspects of psychosocial adjustment. It is indeed a tragedy that the patients most needing cognitive rehabilitation services are often kept out of many treatment facilities because of their disruptive behavior. In fact, research studies (Levin et al. 1982; Lishman 1978; Weddell et al. 1980) have shown that behavioral dysfunction is often associated with reduced ability to comply with rehabilitation programs, return to work, engage in recreational and leisure activities, and sustain positive interpersonal relationships. Levin and Grossman (1978) reported behavioral problems 1 month after traumatic brain injury in areas such as emotional withdrawal, conceptual disorganization, motor slowing, unusual thought content, blunt affect, excitement, and disorientation. At 6 months after injury, those patients who had poor social and occupational recovery continued to manifest significant cognitive and behavioral disruption. Complaints of tangential thinking, fragmented speech, slowness of thought and action, depressed mood, increased anxiety, and marital and/or family conflict were also frequently noted (Levin et al. 1979).

Other behavioral changes reported to have the potential to cause psychosocial disruption include increased irritability (Rosenthal 1983), social inappropriateness (Lewis et al. 1988), aggression (Mungas 1988), expansiveness, helplessness, suspiciousness, and anxiety (Grant and Alves 1987).

Behavioral dysfunction is not limited to individuals with traumatic brain injury. Patients with lesions in specific brain regions secondary to various pathological conditions can exhibit characteristic patterns of dysfunctional behavior as well. For example, frontal lobe dysfunction secondary to stroke, tumor, or other disease processes is often associated with a cluster of symptoms including social disinhibition, reduced attention and distractibility, impaired judgment, affective lability, and more pervasive mood disorder (Bond 1984; Stuss and Benson 1984). In contrast, Prigatano (1987) noted that individuals who have temporal lobe dysfunction can display heightened interpersonal sensitivity, which can evolve into frank paranoid ideation.

In addition to differences between patients with different types of brain injury or disease, there is remarkable variability with regard to the severity and extent of behavioral disruption after injury within each patient group. Eames and Wood (1985), for example, vividly described the variability in severity of impairment of a group of patients who were treated on a special unit for behaviorally disordered patients with head injury. Verbal and physical aggression, inappropriate social and sexual behavior, self-injury, irritability, and markedly altered levels of drive and motivation represent the kinds of behaviors that their patients exhibited. The magnitude of their dysfunction precluded many of them from participation in traditional rehabilitation programs. They were unable to be managed at home, in extended care facilities, or even in general inpatient psychiatric settings.

Perhaps, not too surprisingly, individuals with mild head injuries are less prone to debilitating behavioral changes but still can experience physical, cognitive, and affective changes of sufficient magnitude to affect their ability to return to preaccident activities (Dikman et al. 1986; Levin et al. 1987).

It seems clear that adjustment (and failure to adjust) after brain injury appears to be related to a multitude of neurological and nonneurological factors, each requiring consideration when deciding on an appropriate course of intervention for any observed behavioral dysfunction. In addition to the extent and severity of the neurological injury itself, some of the other factors that can contribute to the presence and type of behavioral dysfunction include time since injury, premorbid psychiatric and psychosocial adjustment, financial resources, social supports, and personal awareness of (and reaction to) acquired deficits (Eames 1988; Goldstein and Ruthven 1983; Gross and Schutz 1986; Meier et al. 1987).

Given the large number of factors that are known to influence recovery from brain injury, a multidimensional approach to the behavioral treatment of patients with brain injury is likely to result in an optimal recovery. This approach should take into consideration the patient's premorbid level of functioning (both in terms of psychological adjustment and neuropsychological functioning), as well as his or her current psychological and neuropsychological resources. Individuals with more severe types of cognitive impairments are more likely to profit from highly structured behavioral programs; whereas individuals who are more intact neuropsychologically may be able to profit from interventions that have a more active cognitive component that requires them to use abstract thought, as well as to use self-evaluative and self-corrective processes. Not surprisingly, therapeutic approaches that fall under the general heading of "behavior therapy" represent an intervention approach that is gaining increasing interest as a component of the overall treatment plan for neuropsychiatrically impaired patients.

❑ BEHAVIORAL THERAPY WITH BRAIN-IMPAIRED PATIENTS

The domain of behavioral therapies has undergone considerable expansion over the past 20 years. Although it is not our primary purpose in this chapter to review the history of behaviorally based therapies, it is useful to keep in mind that behavioral assessment and treatment have extended far beyond their early roots in classical and operant conditioning and have been adapted for use with numerous special populations, most recently including the persons with brain injury. (For more comprehensive and critical presentations of the recent status and direction of behavior therapies, see Haynes 1984; Hersen and Bellack 1985; Kazdin 1979. For excellent compendiums describing both assessment and treatment approaches in clinically useful terms, see Bellack and Hersen 1985b; Hersen and Bellack 1988.)

Despite a broadening scope that has included the treatment of neurologically impaired patients, behavioral approaches remain committed to the original principles derived from experimental and social psychology. They also emphasize the empirical and objective implementation and evaluation of treatment (Bellack and Hersen 1985a).

The general assumptions about the nature of behavioral disorders that form the basis of behavioral approaches include the following (Haynes 1984):

1. Disordered behavior can be expressed through overt actions, thoughts, verbalizations, and physiological reactions.
2. These reactions are not necessarily going to vary in the same way for different individuals or for different behavioral disorders.
3. Changing one specific behavior may result in changes in other, related behaviors.
4. Environmental conditions play an important role in the initiation, maintenance, and alteration of behavior.

These assumptions lead to approaches that emphasize the objective evaluation of "observable" aspects of the individual and his or her interaction with the environment. The range of observable events is bounded only by the clinician's ability to establish a reliable, valid quantification of the target behavior or environmental condition. As previously noted, this could range from a specific physiological reaction, such as heart rate, to a self-report of the number of obsessive thoughts occurring during a 24-hour period.

Intervention focuses on the active interaction between the individual and environment. The goal of treatment is to alter those aspects of the environment that have become associated with the initiation or maintenance of maladaptive behaviors or to alter the patient's response to those aspects of the environment in some way.

The application of a behavioral intervention with a neuropsychiatric patient requires careful consideration of both the neuropsychological and environmental aspects of the presenting problem. Although this may seem obvious, it is important to remember that the attempted synthesis of these two separate disciplines is still in the early stages of development. Few clinicians have the training, time, or energy to become and remain equally competent in both neuropsychology and behavioral psychology. There is, however, a growing effort to explore areas of commonality between these two specialties. Professional interest groups among behavioral psychologists are attempting to define more precisely the domain of "behavioral neuropsychology" (Horton and Barrett 1988).

At present, the accumulated body of evidence remains limited regarding the specific types of behavioral interventions that are most effective in treating the various dysfunctional behaviors observed in individuals with different kinds of brain injuries. Despite this, there is optimism, based on the current literature, that behavior therapy can be effectively used with brain injury patients (Horton and Miller 1985). Indeed, there are an increasing number of books, primarily on the rehabilitation of patients with brain injury, that describe the potential applications of behavioral approaches with neurologically impaired persons (Edelstein and Couture 1984; Goldstein and Ruthven 1983; Seron 1987; Wood 1984). Such sources provide an excellent introduction to the basic models, methods, and limitations of behavioral treatments of the brain injured.

Behavioral approaches can be broadly classified into at least three general models (Calhoun and Turner 1981): 1) a traditional behavioral approach, 2) a social learning approach, and 3) a cognitive-behavioral approach. The degree to which the client or patient is required to participate actively in the identification and alteration of the environmental conditions assumed to be supporting the maladaptive behavior varies across these models.

Traditional Behavioral Approach

This approach emphasizes the effects of environmental events that occur after (consequences), as well as before (antecedents), a particular behavior of interest. We address these two aspects of environmental influence separately.

Interventions aimed at the consequences of behavior. Any *consequence* that increases the probability of a specific behavior occurring again under similar circumstances is termed a *reinforcer*. Consequences can have the effect of either increasing or decreasing the likelihood of a particular behavior occurring again.

When a behavior is followed by an environmental consequence that increases the likelihood that the behavior will occur again, this event is called a *positive reinforcer*. When a behavior is followed by the *removal* of a negative or aversive environmental condition it is called a *negative reinforcer*. When a behavior is followed by an aversive environmental event, that condition is termed a *punisher*. The effect of punishers is to reduce the probability that the behavior will occur under similar conditions. There has often been confusion concerning the difference between negative reinforcers and punishers. It is useful to remember that reinforcers (positive or negative) always increase the likelihood of the behavior occurring again, whereas punishers decrease the likelihood of a behavior occurring again. When the reliable relationship between a specific behavior and an environmental consequence is removed, the behavioral effect is to reduce the target behavior to a near zero level of occurrence. This process is called *extinction*.

Interventions aimed at the antecedents of behavior. Behavior is controlled or affected not only by the consequences that follow a behavior but also by events that precede the behavior. These events are called *antecedents*. For example, an aggressive patient may only have outbursts in the presence of the nursing staff but never in the presence of the physician. In this case, failure to search for potential antecedents that may be eliciting (e.g., female gender or physical size) may leave half of the behavioral assessment undone and may result in difficulty decreasing the aggressive behavior. This type of approach may be particularly useful in patients for whom the behavior is disruptive enough that approaches aimed at manipulation of consequences hold some danger for staff and family (e.g., in the case of the patient with explosive or violent outbursts). In this situation, treatment is structured to decrease the likelihood of an outburst by restructuring the events that lead to violent behavior. Some patients are able to learn to anticipate these antecedents themselves, whereas for others it becomes the task of the treating staff to identify and modify antecedents that lead to unwanted behavior. For example, if the stress of verbal communication leads to aggressive behavior in an aphasic patient, the patient may be initially trained to use an alternative form of communication such as writing or sign language (Franzen and Lovell 1987).

Social Learning Approach

With this approach, cognitive processes that mediate between environmental conditions and behavioral response are included in explanations of the learning process. Social learning approaches take advantage of learning through "modeling" by systematically arranging opportunities for patients to observe socially adaptive examples of social interaction. Practice of the components of social skills in role-playing situations where the patient can receive corrective feedback is also stressed. Intervention that focuses on "social skills training" is one example of a treatment that is often useful with brain injury patients who have lost the ability to effectively monitor their behavior and respond appropriately in a given situation. Socially skilled behavior is generally divided into three components: social perception, social problem solving, and social expression. Training can occur at any one of these levels. For the patient who has lost the ability to interact appropriately with regard to conversational skills, this appropriate behavior may be "modeled" by staff members. (For a comprehensive review, see Bandura 1977.)

Cognitive-Behavioral Approach

The term *cognitive-behavioral approach* represents a heterogeneous group of procedures that emphasize the individual's cognitive mediation (self-messages) in explaining behavioral responses within environmental contexts. The thoughts, beliefs, and predictions about one's own actions and potential environmental consequences are emphasized. Treatment focuses on changing maladaptive beliefs and increasing the amount of self-control an individual has within the current social environment by changing maladaptive thoughts or beliefs. This approach is particularly useful when used with patients who have relatively intact language and self-evaluative abilities.

❑ CASE EXAMPLES OF BEHAVIORAL INTERVENTION

In this section we present two case examples of how behavioral interventions can be applied within the context of the comprehensive care provided in an acute neuropsychiatric inpatient setting. Although the focus of the cases is on the behavioral treatment, patients are followed by an interdisciplinary treatment team representing neuropsychiatry, neuropsychology, psychiatric nursing, occupational therapy, recreational therapy, speech-language pathology, and physical therapy. The emphasis here is on the application of behavioral procedures, not on the attribution of outcome. The cases selected represent typical behavior complaints within this type of setting.

Case 1: Poor Impulse Control With Verbal and Physical Aggression

Ms. A was a 21-year-old, single white woman who suffered from meningitis at the age of 6 months. She apparently had a second episode at age 10 years, with a resultant left frontal subdural hematoma that was evacuated. She was diagnosed as moderately mentally retarded and attended special education classes until age 20. She lived at home until admission, although her parents were seriously considering placement in a group home, largely to provide Ms. A with greater psychosocial and vocational opportunities than they were able to provide at home. They were also advancing in age and were concerned about how much longer their own physical health would allow them to care for their daughter. It was unclear how much awareness the patient had of these plans.

Ms. A was admitted to the neuropsychiatric hospital with a presenting complaint of verbal and physical aggression, verbal threats of violence, and self-destructive threats. Medically, she had a poorly controlled seizure disorder, which was being treated with primidone, carbamazepine, and diazepam. A neurodiagnostic evaluation was conducted. A computed tomography (CT) scan noted an old left temporal craniotomy. Her electroencephalogram (EEG) was interpreted as abnormal with excessive background slowing and persistent asymmetry, left slower than right. A single photon emission computed tomography (SPECT) scan was also interpreted as abnormal with bifrontal perfusion deficits, left greater than right, and increased perfusion of the basal ganglia.

Intellectually, Ms. A obtained an IQ score of 35, placing her in the severe range of mental retardation. Problem solving and reasoning with low verbal demands were at even lower levels than her IQ estimate. Her neuropsychological impairments were sufficiently severe to preclude the use of all but very elementary mnemonic strategies (i.e., reminders from staff to practice more appropriate behavior on the unit and at home). She demonstrated marked graphomotor and verbal perseveration. Her voice volume was very loud with limited capacity to self-modulate, even when prompted. Speech was mildly pressured but prosodic. Behaviorally, she was demanding and verbally and physically threatening to both staff and patients, and she often refused to comply with unit rules.

The staff's formulation of the patient's difficulties included the possibility that consequences for disruptive behavior had not been consistently applied at home. In addition, it seemed likely that Ms. A had some awareness that she may be leaving home soon and did not possess the cognitive capacity or social skills to deal with this stressor in an adaptive way. Three behavioral interventions were introduced simultaneously: 1) positive reinforcement for displays of socially appropriate behavior, 2) training in simple de-escalation procedures, and 3) social skills training in a group context.

Specific behaviors targeted for modification included inappropriate touching, loud voice, and noncompliance with staff direction. A signature card was carried by the patient to all her therapies (e.g., physical therapy, occupational therapy, and recreation). She was reminded at the beginning of each therapy session what was expected of her (e.g, keep hands to self, use "inside" voice, and follow directions). At the end of each session, behavior was reviewed by the patient and therapist. The therapist would initial boxes on her card associated with target behavior compliance. On return to the unit, Ms. A would present her card to her primary nurse. If she had obtained two of three signatures, she could select a "treat" (6 oz of soft drink or 15 minutes of extra individual staff time). In addition, while on the unit, Ms. A was given specific feedback hourly regarding her behavior. Social praise was provided for compliance. Gradually, she was encouraged to take a more active role in these hourly reviews to increase her own selfmonitoring.

De-escalation training was used to help Ms. A begin developing alternative strategies for dealing with anger. A series of interventions was reviewed with her twice per day. If she began to threaten, she was directed to a diversional activity she had previously identified as relaxing (looking at magazines) to help her feel "calmer." If she was still "upset," the diversional activity was followed by time-out in her room. If this was not successful, increasing external control was imposed, including oral medication, opened-door seclusion, intramuscular medication, and locked seclusion. These latter procedures were obviously restricted to those situations in which Ms. A represented a clear danger to herself or others on the unit and followed standard hospital policy regarding the use of prn medication and seclusion.

Finally, social skills training was used to allow Ms. A to learn and practice more appropriate ways of relating to other people. Modeling (demonstrations of appropriate behavior by staff), rehearsal, and feedback were used. Because she was probably going to live away from home for the first time, emphasis was placed on the skills needed to make and maintain new friendships.

Assessment of the effectiveness of the treatment included direct measurement of the target behaviors. Nursing rated the occurrence of verbal or physical threats, rated voice volume, and recorded the number of times Ms. A complied with a request during 5 minute rating periods twice a day. An indirect measure of effectiveness included monitoring the number of prn medications administered, amount of time in seclusion, and number of timeouts in room per day. Reduction in need for more intensive, externally imposed intervention was interpreted as a demonstration of increased self-control.

Ms. A showed a good response to treatment. Within 3 weeks, she demonstrated little verbally or physically threatening behavior and no inappropriate touching, and she was following all directions. Her failures to comply with treatment diminished from an average of 10 refusals a day for the first 3 days of treatment to zero by the seventh day of treatment. Similarly, time spent in "time-out" in her room and in seclusion also diminished almost completely. Her voice volume remained loud, but she was making a more active effort at controlling it. As discharge approached, an expected reemergence of these behaviors was noted, but with less severity.

Case 2: Poststroke Depression With Fear of Falling

Ms. B was a 76-year-old married white woman who was referred for inpatient neuropsychiatric hospitalization with complaints of increased depression, especially over the 4 months preceding the hospitalization. She had apparently fallen while alone at home during this time. Although her daughter arrived soon after the fall occurred, the patient had been unable to get up from the floor and was quite afraid that assistance would not arrive. Since the fall, she had become increasingly isolative and withdrawn, somatically preoccupied, and much less mobile.

Neuropsychological evaluation demonstrated multiple areas of cognitive deficits. Ms. B had particular difficulty with new learning and memory as well as with visuospatial and visuoconstructional ability. In contrast, her language skills were intact. Neurodiagnostic evaluation was completed. Magnetic resonance imaging (MRI) was interpreted as showing multiple lacunar infarcts as well as a focal right occipital infarct. EEG was interpreted as abnormal with transient background slowing, right greater than left. SPECT was interpreted as essentially normal.

Ms. B's primary problems were depression and anxiety, particularly associated with ambulation. Considering its impact on her social functioning, this fear of ambulation appeared to be of phobic proportions. Medical complications associated with decreased ambulation and poor vascular circulation were also of concern. The occurrence of a stroke at the time of the fall was considered likely, but not definite.

Ms. B was included in both individual and group treatment focusing primarily on three areas: 1) reduction of anxiety associated with ambulation, which was reducing her willingness to walk; 2) improvement in depressed mood with a reduction in her preoccupation over negative, self-defeating thoughts; and 3) promotion of a limited, realistic awareness of her cognitive or physical strengths and limitations.

Interventions included in vivo desensitization for anxiety associated with ambulation (she was slowly but systematically exposed to conditions surrounding ambulation). Ms. B demonstrated the ability to learn the general concept of deep breathing. Because of cognitive limitations, she had more difficulty with systematic progressive muscle relaxation, but clearly understood the concept of deep breathing and attempted to relax her muscles when she felt increased anxiety associated with attempts at ambulation. This approach was generalized to her physical therapy sessions as well as to her "ambulation homework" with nursing on the unit three times a day. Verbal praise was systematically provided for both successful execution as well as for effort.

A simplified cognitive-behavioral approach was used to address the catastrophic thoughts that were associated with ambulation. Despite difficulty with memory, Ms. B had good verbal skills and could understand alternative concrete self-statements. She would usually tell herself that she needed to be extremely careful when she walked; that she would be too weak to continue and that she might fall and no one would be there to help her. Practice focused on challenging these beliefs and having her make positive statements, initially while seated and then during ambulation.

Ms. B also believed that she was a "failure" because she was no longer able to engage in her previous responsibilities at home, such as cooking and cleaning. Her verbal skills were highlighted for her and she was encouraged to redefine or reframe her role in the home as one of "companion" to her husband and grandchildren.

Depressive thoughts were particularly problematic, from a cognitive-behavioral standpoint, because of her reduced memory. She had difficulty remembering all the successes and accomplishments she was experiencing. This perpetuated her misbelief that she "would never get better." To increase her ability to monitor her own course and progression, a chart was used that targeted specific activities such as preparing her belongings for evening care, walking on the unit, and extending compliments to other people on the unit. This was reviewed with nursing every evening.

At discharge, Ms. B described feeling less hopeless. Her Geriatric Depression Scale (Yesavage et al. 1983) scores improved from the "severely depressed" to the "moderately depressed" range. It is important to note however, that Ms. B's self-report of depression was significantly different from staff observations of her behavior and her self-report most likely represented an underestimate of her improvement. Because of her memory impairment, she remained preoccupied with her physical deficits and was unable to remember improvements in her functioning during hospitalization. This underscores the need for multiple levels of assessment when working with neuropsychiatric patients. She stated that she believed both she and her family had a more realistic idea of what she was capable of doing. She reported feeling less angry, sad, and resentful. She was able to ambulate with a walker with minimal anxiety. She continued to have somewhat unrealistic expectations about her capacity to continue routine household chores, although her family had a clearer idea of her limits and planned on continuing to emphasize her role as a companion.

❑ CONCLUSIONS

Neuropsychological and behavioral dysfunction associated with brain injury is varied and complex. Effective intervention requires an integrated interdisciplinary approach that focuses on the individual patient and his or her specific needs. Behaviorally based formulations can provide a valuable framework from which to understand the interaction between an individual with compromised physical, neuropsychological, and emotional functioning, and the psychosocial environment in which he or she is trying to adjust. Much work remains to define the most effective cognitive and behaviorally based treatments for various neuropsychiatric disorders. The evidence to date suggests that this area is indeed an area worthy of continued pursuit.

❑ REFERENCES

Bandura A: Social Learning Theory. Englewood Cliffs, NJ, Prentice-Hall, 1977

Basso A, Capotani E, Vignolo L: Influence of rehabilitation on language skills in aphasic patients. Arch Neurol 36:190–196, 1979

Bellack AS, Hersen M: General considerations, in Handbook of Clinical Behavior Therapy With Adults. Edited by Hersen M, Bellack AS. New York, Plenum, 1985a, pp 3–19

Bellack AS, Hersen M: Dictionary of Behavior Therapy Techniques. New York, Pergamon, 1985b

Ben-Yishay Y, Diller L: Rehabilitation of cognitive and perceptual deficits in people with traumatic brain damage. Int J Rehabil Res 4:208–210, 1981

Ben-Yishay Y, Diller L: Cognitive deficits, in Rehabilitation of the head-injured adult. Edited by Griffith, EA, Bond, M, Miller, J. Philadelphia, Davis, 1983

Bond M: The psychiatry of closed head injury, in Closed Head Injury: Psychosocial, Social and Family Consequences. Oxford, England, Oxford University Press, 1984

Calhoun KS, Turner SM: Historical perspectives and current issues in behavior therapy, in Handbook of Clinical Behavior Therapy. Edited by Turner SM, Calhoun KS, Adams HE. New York, Wiley, 1981, pp 1–11

Crovitz H, Harvey M, Horn R: Problems in the acquisition of imagery mnemonics: three brain damaged cases. Cortex 15:225–234, 1979

Dikmen S, McLean A, Temkin N: Neuropsychological and psychosocial consequences of minor head injury. J Neurol Neurosurg Psychiatry 49:1227–1232, 1986

Diller L, Weinberg J: Hemi-inattention in rehabilitation: the evolution of a rational remediation program. Adv Neurol 18:63–82, 1977

Eames P: Behavior disorders after severe head injury: their nature, causes and strategies for management. Journal of Head Trauma Rehabilitation 3:1–6, 1988

Eames P, Wood R: Rehabilitation after severe brain injury: a follow-up study of a behavior modification approach. J Neurol Neurosurg Psychiatry 48:613–619, 1985

Edelstein BA, Couture ET: Behavioral Assessment and Rehabilitation of the Traumatically Brain-Damaged. New York, Plenum, 1984

Franzen MD, Lovell MR: Behavioral treatments of aggressive sequelae of brain injury. Psychiatric Annals 17: 389–396, 1987

Gardner H: The Shattered Mind: The Person After Brain Damage. London, Routledge & Kegan, 1977

Gualtieri CT: Pharmacotherapy and the neurobehavioral sequelae of traumatic brain iniury. Brain Inj 2:101–109, 1988

Gianutsos R, Matheson P: The rehabilitation of visual perceptual disorders attributable to brain injury, in Neuropsychological Rehabilitation. Edited by Meier MJ, Benton AL, Diller L. New York, Guilford, 1987, pp 202–241

Gianutsos R, Glosser D, Elbaum J, et al: Visual imperception in brain injured adults:multifacted measures. Arch Phys Med Rehabil 64:456–461, 1983

Glasgow RE, Zeiss RA, Barrera M, et al: Case studies on remediating memory deficits in brain damaged individuals. J Clin Psychol 33:1049–1054, 1977

Glisky EL, Schacter DL: Remediation of organic memory disorders: current status and future prospects. Journal of Head Trauma Rehabilitation 4:54–63, 1986

Goldstein FC, Levin HS: Disorders of reasoning and problem solving ability, in Neuropsychological Rehabilitation. Edited by Meier MJ, Benton AL, Diller L. New York, Guilford, 1987, pp 327–354

Goldstein G, Ruthven L: Rehabilitation of The Brain-Damaged Adult. New York, Plenum, 1983

Gordon W, Hibbard M, Egelko S, et al: Perceptual remediation in patients with right brain damage: a comprehensive program. Arch Phys Med Rehabil 66:353–359, 1985

Gouvier WD, Webster JS, Blanton PD: Cognitive retraining with brain damaged patients, in The Neuropsychology Handbook: Behavioral and Clinical Perspectives. Edited by Wedding D, Horton AM, Webster J. New York, Springer, 1986, pp 278–324

Grant I, Alves W: Psychiatric and psychosocial disturbances in head injury, in Neurobehavioral Recovery From Head Injury. Edited by Levin HS, Grafman J, Eisenberg HM. New York, Oxford University Press, 1987, pp 222–246

Grimm BH, Bleiberg J: Psychological rehabilitation in traumatic brain injury, in Handbook of Clinical Neuropsychology, Vol 2. Edited by Filskov SB, Boll TJ. New York, Wiley, 1986, pp 495–560

Gross Y, Schutz LF: Intervention models in neuropsychology, in Clinical Neuropsychology of Intervention. Edited by Uzzell BP, Gross Y. Boston, MA, Martinus Highoff, 1986, pp 179–204

Harris JE: Methods of improving memory, in Clinical Management of Memory Problems. Edited by Wilson BA, Moffat N. Rockville, MD, Aspen, 1984, pp 46–62

Harris JE, Sunderland A: A brief survey of the management of memory disorders in rehabilitation units in

Britain. International Rehabilitation Medicine 3:206–209, 1981

Haynes SN: Behavioral assessment of adults, in Handbook of Psychological Assessment. Edited by Goldstein G, Hersen M. New York, Pergamon, 1984, pp 369–401

Hersen M, Bellack AS: Handbook of Clinical Behavior Therapy With Adults. New York, Plenum, 1985

Hersen M, Bellack AS: Dictionary of Behavioral Assessment Techniques. New York, Pergamon, 1988

Horton AM, Barrett D: Neuropsychological assessment and behavior therapy: new directions in head trauma rehabilitation. Journal of Head Trauma Rehabilitation 3:57–64, 1988

Horton AM, Miller WA: Neuropsychology and behavior therapy, in Progress in Behavior Modifications. Edited by Hersen M, Eisler R, Miller PM. New York, Academic, 1985, pp 1–55

Kazdin AE: Fictions, factions, and functions of behavior therapy. Behavior Therapy 10:629–654, 1979

Kolata G: Brain-grafting work shows promise (letter). Science 4617:1277, 1983

Levin HS, Grossman RG: Behavioral sequelae of closed head injury: a quantitative study. Arch Neurol 35:720–727, 1978

Levin HS, Grossman RG, Ross JE, et al: Long-term neuropsychological outcome of closed head injury. J Neurosurg 50:412–422, 1979

Levin HS, Benton AL, Grossman RG: Neurobehavioral Consequences of Closed Head Injury. New York, Oxford University Press, 1982

Levin HS, Mattis S, Ruff R, et al: Neurobehavioral outcome following minor head injury: a three center study. J Neurosurg 66:234–243, 1987

Lewis FD, Nelson J, Nelson C, et al: Effects of three feedback contingencies on the socially inappropriate talk of a brain-injured adult. Behavior Therapy 19:203–211, 1988

Lezak MD: Neuropsychological Assessment. New York, Oxford University Press, 1976

Lishman WA: Organic Psychiatry. St. Louis, MO, Blackman Scientific, 1978

Luria AR: Restoration of Function After Brain Injury. New York, Macmillian, 1963

Luria AR: The Working Brain. New York, Basic Books, 1973

Luria AR, Tsvetkova LS: The Neuropsychological Analysis of Problem Solving. Orlando, FL, Paul Deutsch, 1990

Meier MJ, Strauman S, Thompson WG: Individual differences in neuropsychological recovery: an overview, in Neuropsychological Rehabilitation. Edited by Meier MJ, Benton AL, Diller L. New York, Guilford, 1987, pp 71–110

Moffat N: Strategies of memory therapy, in Clinical Management of Memory Problems. Edited by Wilson BA, Moffat N. Rockville, MD, Aspen, 1984, pp 63–88

Mungas D: Psychometric correlates of episodic violent behavior: a multidimensional neuropsychological approach. Br J Psychiatry 152:180–187, 1988

Patten BM: The ancient art of memory. Arch Neurology 26:25–31, 1972

Posner HI, Rafal RD: Cognitive theories of attention and the rehabilitation of attentional deficits, in Neuropsychological Rehabilitation. Edited by Meier MJ, Benton AL, Diller L. New York, Guilford, 1987, pp 182–201

Prigatano GP: Personality and psychosocial consequences after brain injury, in Neuropsychological Rehabilitation. Edited by Meier MJ, Benton AL, Diller L. New York, Guilford, 1987, pp 355–378

Robertson-Tchabo EA, Hausman CP, Arenberg D: A classical mnemonic for older learners: a trip that works. Educational Gerontologist 1:215–216, 1976

Rosenthal M: Behavioral sequelae, in Rehabilitation of the Head Injured Adult. Edited by Rosenthal M, Griffith ER, Bond MR, et al. Philadelphia, PA, FA Davis, 1983, pp 297–308

Schacter DL, Glisky EL: Memory rehabilitation: restoration, alleviation, and the acquisition of domain specific knowledge, in Clinical Neuropsychology of Intervention. Edited by Uzzell B, Gross Y. Boston, MA, Martinus Nijhof, 1986, pp 257–287

Seron X: Operant procedures and neuropsychological rehabilitation, in Neuropsychological Rehabilitation. Edited by Meier MJ, Benton AL, Diller L. New York, Guilford, 1987, pp 132–161

Sivak M, Hill C, Henson D, et al: Improved driving performance following perceptual training of persons with brain damage. Arch Phys Med Rehabil 65:163–167, 1985

Stuss DT, Benson DF: Neuropsychological studies of the frontal lobes. Psychol Bull 95:3–28, 1984

Wall P, Egger M: Mechanisms of plasticity of new connection following brain damage in adult mammalian nervous systems, in Recovery of Function: Theoretical Considerations for Brain Injury Rehabilitation. Edited by Bach-y-Rita. Baltimore, MD, Park, 1971

Weddell R, Oddy M, Jenkins D: Social adjustment after rehabilitation: a two year follow up of patients with severe head injury. Psychol Med 10:257–263, 1980

Wilson B: Success and failure in memory training following a cerebral vascular accident. Cortex 18:581–594, 1982

Wood RL: Behavior disorders following severe brain injury: their presentation and psychological management, in Closed Head Injury: Psychological, Social and Family Consequences. Edited by Brooks N. New York, Oxford University Press, 1984, pp 195–219

Yesavage JA, Brink TL, Rose TL, et al: Development and validation of a geriatric depression screening scale: a preliminary report. J Psychiatric Res 17:37–49, 1983

Chapter

32

Family Caregivers of Persons With Neuropsychiatric Illness: A Stress and Coping Perspective

Frederick E. Miller, Ph.D., M.D.
William Borden, Ph.D.

FAMILY CAREGIVERS OF persons with neuropsychiatric illness have emerged as an important group in social-psychological research efforts over the last decade, and investigators have documented a range of problems in living associated with the strain of the caregiving experience in such disparate conditions as Alzheimer's disease, stroke, traumatic brain injury, mental retardation, and acquired immunodeficiency syndrome (AIDS).

From the perspective of stress and coping theory, neuropsychiatric disorders may be viewed as adverse life events that tax adaptive resources and threaten the well-being of the family caregivers, placing them at risk for stress-related dysfunction and psychopathology. Consistent with this line of theorizing, one group of findings (Rabins et al. 1982) showed that some family members develop discrete signs of physical or mental distress (notably depression, anxiety, demoralization, depletion, and psychosomatic symptoms) after onset and progression of illness and disability. Other investigations (e.g., Cohler et al. 1989), however, have suggested that many family members appear to manage the demands of the illness experience without overt signs of dysfunction. A third area of work (Borden 1991a, 1991b) indicated that some [illegible] members report personal growth and enduring positive changes as a consequence of the illness experience. Increasingly, researchers and clinicians have recognized the significance of individual differences among family caregivers in determining levels of functioning and well-being and, in turn, have realized the need to develop multivariate models of caregiver adaptation.

The importance of family support in community-based care of chronically ill patients, particularly the frail elderly, has been documented in a series of investigations over the last decade (Cohler et al. 1989). Contrary to the social myth that older persons are alienated from their families, study of intergenerational relations has shown that older adults maintain close, interdependent relationships with other family members (Shanas 1979). Although family life involves regular exchanges of resources and services between parents and adult children, research indicates that caregiving responsibilities typically fall on elderly spouses or parents who are themselves in senescent phases of the life cycle and therefore vulnerable to losses associated with aging (Borden 1988; Walsh 1987).

Studies have also shown that when the family is unable to manage problems associated with chronic conditions, members attempt to link the ill person with formal or professional service systems (Aronson and Lipkowitz 1981; Brody 1978, 1985; Brody et al. 1978; Streib and Beck 1981; Sussman 1976; Troll 1971). In the absence of such formal support to the family caregiver, however, members experience increasing difficulty in maintaining the ill person in the home setting. Nevertheless, institutionalization may be delayed at considerable psychological and physical expense to the caregiving family (Eisdorfer and Cohen 1981).

As numerous accounts in the mass media have demonstrated, family members often are deeply involved with the patient and instrumental in providing daily care. By way of example, one series of books, *A Child Called Noah* (Greenfeld 1972), *A Client Called Noah* (Greenfeld 1986), and *A Place for Noah* (Greenfeld 1978) documents a family's struggle to care for a child with developmental and emotional disabilities. An increasing number of works chronicle families in their efforts to care for older adults with organic brain syndromes (Borden 1988). Such accounts have served to increase awareness of the difficulty inherent in the caregiving experience and foster a sense of empathy for families with chronically ill members.

Despite growing recognition of the demands imposed by the caregiving role, the psychiatric profession appears to have lagged in its efforts to address the needs of family members and provide services to caregivers at risk for stress-related dysfunction and psychopathology. Overall, there has been relatively little consideration of family caregiver issues or attention to clinical intervention with this population in the general psychiatric literature. In an effort to provide a base for the development of comprehensive psychiatric care in this area, in this chapter we 1) provide an overview of work to date in the study of neuropsychiatric illness and family caregivers, with an emphasis on emergent research issues; 2) describe a model of stress, coping, and adaptation that provides an organizing frame of reference for identification of core tasks in psychiatric intervention; and 3) consider the implications of research to date for psychosocial intervention with family caregivers. In doing so, we include general criteria for assessment, treatment, and management decisions in this underserved population.

As the subsequent discussions emphasize, the caregiving experience is influenced by a range of biological, psychological, and social factors, and assessment of adaptational outcomes must consider individual differences in perceptions of stressors, coping strategies, social relationships, and support resources. Further, although caregiving is generally characterized as a stressful, taxing experience, emerging lines of research suggest that many family members also perceive beneficial outcomes over the course of caretaking and experience considerable fulfillment and meaning in assuming such roles (Borden 1991b). Accordingly, it is important to consider negative as well as positive outcomes of the caretaking experience in development of further research, theory, and practice.

❑ STRESS RESEARCH

The general body of research on stress and illness provides a context for clinical and theoretical interest in neuropsychiatric illness and family caregivers. The early work of Cannon (1932), Selye (1950), and Meyer (1951) led to an interest in life events as potential stressors in development of physical and mental illness. Over the last quarter century studies have focused on responses to crisis events, such as divorce, financial hardship, and job loss, as well as on reactions to such developmental events as parenthood, the empty nest, retirement, and widowhood. By extension, medical and psychiatric conditions have been studied as events in themselves requiring adjustment and adaptation. Over the years a growing number of reports, informed by findings in the stress and illness literature, have suggested that family members of persons with chronic neuropsychiatric illness commonly experience symptoms of depression, anxiety, and depletion, as well as feelings of helplessness and hopelessness (Rabins et al. 1982). In addition, various physical conditions, such as hypertension, peptic ulcer, migraine, and colitis, as well as exacerbation of chronic illness, such as diabetes mellitus, coronary artery disease, and rheumatoid arthritis, have been associated with the stress of caring for a chronically ill member (Borden 1991a). In the light of such discussion, researchers have focused their investigations on aspects of the illness experience believed to precipitate stress-related dysfunction in family caregivers. The central question integrating such studies is what set of characteristics best predicts development of physical or mental symptoms in family members.

Basic Lines of Study

Basic lines of research have examined variables in five areas: 1) severity of illness, as determined by extent of physical and mental impairment; 2) social support; 3) family characteristics; 4) gender and social roles; and 5) developmental stages of the illness experience. A review of representative studies in each of these areas will focus our understanding of basic research issues at present and provide a rationale for development of clinical intervention strategies.

Severity of illness. The earliest line of research, based largely on conceptual models of life events study, set out to explore the relationship between characteristics of chronic illness and burden in family caregivers. Studies relied largely on objective measures of patient functional status and focused generally on two aspects of neuropsychiatric illness: behavioral symptoms (e.g., wandering, insomnia, delusions, and inability to recognize family members), and physical impairment (e.g., incontinence and inability to feed self, dress, or bathe). A series of British studies, among the first in this area of investigation, compared the effects of dementing conditions and functional psychiatric disorders on family members. Hoenig and Hamilton (1966) reported significant degrees of burden in 80% of the families of elderly patients with functional psychiatric or cognitive impairment. They noted that dementing conditions caused more problems than any other disorders, both in terms of subjective complaints by family members and observable negative effects on the household in areas such as physical health and income. Severity of symptomatology, inferred by global measures of behavioral disturbance and functional status, was associated with greater degrees of burden in dementing illness.

In a study of family members that provided home care for patients with functional psychiatric disorders and dementing illnesses, Grad and Sainsbury (1968) identified a series of patient behaviors that appeared to predict degree of burden. Aggressive behaviors, delusions, hallucinations, confusion, and inability to provide self-care were correlated with family stress. Family members specified frequent somatic complaints, threats of self-harm or harm of others, and excessive demands for attention as the most provocative behaviors. As in previous studies, severity of dementia, as inferred by objective assessment of symptomatology, was identified as a potential determinant of family burden.

In a related study, Sainsbury and Grad (1970) found that the care of geriatric patients produced significant difficulties for more than 75% of the families in their sample, with the burden rated as "severe" in 40%. Negative changes in mental health were reported by 63% of the family members; 58% noted changes in physical health. Half of them described interruption of social and leisure activities, and 19% reported financial hardship. Patients with dementing illnesses caused difficulties in the aforementioned areas for 84% of the families.

Subsequent studies, focused on severity and manifestation of neuropsychiatric illness, have emphasized behavioral disturbance rather than physical impairment in discussions of caregiver strain. In a study of 50 geriatric cases by Sanford (1975), family caregivers reported the following patient behaviors as most stressful: sleep disturbance, immobility, wandering, and aggressive or dangerous behaviors. Physical violence and hitting, memory disturbance, catastrophic reactions, and suspiciousness were patient behaviors most frequently listed as causing serious problems for caregivers in the study by Rabins et al. (1982).

Greene et al. (1982) found that the highest levels of caregiver distress were significantly associated with apathetic or withdrawn patient behavior. Caregivers of dementia patients with depression reported experiencing the most negative feelings about the patients. Wilder et al. (1983) reported that noxious behaviors associated with dementia, such as expressions of anger and aggression as well as excessive demands for attention, appeared to correlate with family stress. Further, the study indicated that such behaviors often precipitated institutionalization of the patient. Patient demands for attention and emotional management were associated with caregiver strain, anxiety, and depression in studies by Gelleard and Boyd-Watts (1982), Johnson and Johnson (1983), and Poulshock and Deimling (1984).

In summary, research in this area has attempted to document the relationship between clinical features of neuropsychiatric illness and stress on the assumption that behavioral symptoms and physical impairment are salient predictors of burden and dysfunction in family members. No significant relationship between objective measures of physical impairment and caregiver distress has been found, although patient behavioral disturbance has been associated with caregiver distress. We must interpret findings cautiously, however, in view of conceptual and methodological limitations that emerge in review of the work. Major difficulties include the lack of clarity in definitions of basic concepts such as stress, burden, and caregiving; gross measurement of variables and inconsistent levels of analysis; failure to consider individual caregiver characteristics; and reliance on small, opportunity samples.

Social support. A second line of study examines the functions of social support in family efforts to mediate stressors associated with chronic illness. Work in this area is based on the assumption that social support buffers potentially harmful effects of stressor events and strengthens coping capacity and adaptive ability (Cobb 1976; Johnson 1985; Kaplan et al. 1977; Sarason 1985). Although evidence for the mediating effect of social support is equivocal (Cohen and Syme 1985; Henderson 1981), reviews have suggested that support variables exert a direct effect on a number of mental health measures (Lin et al. 1985).

In a global study of psychosocial stressors and dementia, Zarit et al. (1980) found that the only variable significantly related to perceived caregiver burden was the number of visits from children, grandchildren, or siblings. Similarly, Johnson (1983) found that caregiving spouses who reported frequent contact with their adult children experienced less depression than those with irregular or minimal interaction, presumably because of varying degrees of social support.

Zarit et al. (1985) suggested that lack of social support is more predictive of family stress than specific symptoms or impairment associated with the dementing process. They reported that family members tended to become isolated over the course of the illness, initiating social contact less frequently and receiving fewer visits from persons outside the household. Their clinical studies supported earlier findings that family members who continued to receive emotional support, as inferred by phone calls and visits from other family members and friends, experienced less strain than those who reported diminished social contact.

Although few studies have focused specifically on social support and caregiving in clearly specified types of neuropsychiatric illness, the foregoing findings are consistent with the outcomes of numerous studies that investigated the relationship between social support, family stress, and chronic illness. Fengler and Goodrich (1979) reported isolation from friends and limitation of activities in the wives of elderly men disabled by severe chronic illness (including organic brain syndromes) and hypothesized that deficits in social support may lead to stress-related difficulties in caregivers. In general, accounts have indicated that family caregivers tend to withdraw from social contact and activity over the course of chronic illness, experiencing feelings of loneliness, helplessness, and alienation (Cantor 1983; McCubbin et al. 1982; Robinson and Thurnher 1979).

Findings in this area have provided a rationale for the development of family support groups, self-help groups, and formal support services such as day care and respite programs (Groves et al. 1984). Some studies have indicated that formal support services help to relieve stress in family members (Frankfather 1977; Kahn and Tobin 1981), whereas other reports did not show significant relationships between burden and support services (Noelker and Poulshock 1982). Groves (1988) suggested that support from family and friends exerts a greater influence on caregiver distress than support from formal service programs.

In summary, research in the area of social support suggests that the progression of a chronic dementing condition may erode sources of social support and stability. Diminished availability of emotional and instrumental support is identified as a potential direct or indirect determinant of stress-related dysfunction in family members. Although few studies have focused specifically on social support and caregivers of persons with clearly specified neuropsychiatric illness, work to date points toward a significant relationship between support variables and caregiver adaptation (Bankoff 1983).

In interpreting findings, however, we must take into account a series of methodological difficulties that emerge in definition and assessment of social support. Measures have tended to rely on global demographic indicators of support, such as marital status, family size, and living arrangements. Such methods of assessment are based on the questionable notion that degree of support may be inferred from size or type of social network. Few studies have considered individual differences in caregiver perception of support needs and resources. Furthermore, there has been little consideration of the ways certain types of support (e.g., family or peer) may differentially relate to coping and adaptation. Finally, theoretical speculation as to how support neutralizes maladaptive physical, psychological, or social responses to stressors is absent in most accounts.

Family characteristics. A third focus of investigation examines the influence of family characteristics on stress and adaptation in members. Instrumental and affective problem-solving processes, communication processes, affective responsiveness, and behavior control are important issues in this area of study (Borden 1988). Although most reports have been based on single case studies or preliminary empirical research, reviews of the literature have suggested that the increased dependency of the person with neuropsychiatric impairment leads to shifts in the power or authority structure of the family, thereby necessitating major role changes (Lansky 1984; Niederehe and Fruge 1985).

Tasks and responsibilities must be reassigned as the illness progresses, and the process of reorganizing power within the family system may precipitate tension, conflict, and disequilibrium. For example, differences may emerge between the primary caregiver and other family members about the most effective way to care for the patient or about the veracity of the caregiver's perception of patient deficits and needs (Blazer 1978; Koopman-Boyden and Wells 1979; Rabins et al. 1982).

Neuropsychiatric illness in a parent or sibling may inhibit other members' efforts to separate from the family, particularly in enmeshed systems, and members may find it difficult to maintain a sense of separateness in their caregiving activities. Families showing evidence of rigid role assignments, maladaptive communication patterns, chronic marital conflict, and reliance on defenses such as repression and denial appear to be especially vulnerable to breakdown and dysfunction (Lansky 1984; Niederehe and Fruge 1985). The structure and function of the family, accordingly, are hypothesized to serve as important mediating variables in the process of adaptation (Bruhn 1977).

Some accounts have suggested that the preexisting quality of family relationships, especially the marital relationship, is a major determinant of the spouse's ability to tolerate the stress of caregiving (Borden 1988; Niederehe and Fruge 1985; Zarit et al. 1985). The hypothesis is that greater degrees of satisfaction in the relationship buffer illness-related stressors. This line of thinking is supported by findings that showed a significant relationship between quality of affective relations and caregiver strain (Cantor 1983; Cicirelli 1983; Robinson 1983; Zarit et al. 1985).

Finally, some authors have hypothesized that the strain of the illness intensifies preexisting intrapsychic conflict in family members, thereby leading to development of stress-related dysfunction. Groves et al. (1984), for example, observed that unconscious conflict related to loss, such as the death of a parent, may be unmasked by losses inherent in the disease process or in senescence. They suggested that family members with unresolved issues are at greatest risk of developing stress-related difficulties.

In summary, the influence of family structure and interaction on caregiver functioning has received little attention in empirical work to date. Spouses, children, siblings, and other relatives have been treated categorically as family caregivers in a number of studies, making it difficult to determine variance associated with relationship status, family structure, or caregiving patterns. Further, there has been little consideration of the impact of differences in family cohesion and adaptability, problem-solving and communication processes, and role traditionality on caregiver well-being. Specific issues have been identified in clinical accounts, however, and preliminary study has documented the importance of this area in further study of caregiver distress.

Gender and social roles. A fourth group of reports, focused largely on the caregiving process, considers the influence of gender and social roles on stress and adaptation in family members. As commentators have observed, families are expected to care for the impaired elderly with little or no support from the community or government (Blumenthal 1979; Cohler et al. 1989; Eisdorfer 1985). Social norms endorse family self-sufficiency in community-based care of the older adult, and most families expect to manage caregiving tasks within the family unit. Research has indicated that women most frequently assume responsibility for caregiving, as spouses or daughters (Brody 1981, 1985; Johnson and Catalano 1981). Shifts in the employment status of women over the last decade have reduced their availability for such activities, however, and commentators have suggested that women may experience increased stress as a result of conflict between the traditional familial role of caring for an ill member, marital and parenting tasks, and development of career goals (Hudson 1986).

The differential effects of gender on coping and adaptation in family caregivers have received little attention to date. However, there is some evidence that women tend to report higher levels of psychological distress than do men (Borden 1991 a; Borden and Berlin 1990; Cantor 1983; Johnson 1983; Noelker and Poulshock 1982). Fitting et al. (1986) reported that husband and wife caregivers experienced similar degrees of burden but found that wives exhibited more symptoms of depression and demoralization. Interestingly, 25% of husbands reported an improved relationship with their spouse since assuming the caregiver role, whereas about a third of the wives reported a deterioration in the marital relationship. The authors cast potential explanations for such a finding in terms of developmental role changes associated with gender (Neugarten and Gutmann 1968), husbands' repayment of support and nurturance received through the marriage, and guilt associated with the recognition of sacrifices wives had made.

In a longitudinal study of subjective burden in husbands and wives caring for spouses with chronic dementing disorders, Zarit et al. (1985) found that women initially reported more distress than men, although no differences were found at the end of a 2-year follow-up period. They hypothesized that wives may have emphasized distress at the outset but assumed a stoic attitude over time or adopted more effective coping strategies.

The influence of social norms on caregiving is implicit in discussions of role conflict. Brody (1985) described a norm, which holds that offspring should provide their aging parents with care of comparable quality and quantity as that which they received from their parents during childhood. Adherence to such a norm, she suggested, leads to disappointment and guilt because the expectation is an unattainable ideal. George (1986) proposed two contradictory norms as potential sources of stress in family members caring for a demented parent: reciprocity, which holds that members should experience equitable levels of gain and loss; and solidarity, which holds that members should be given as much help as they need on an unconditional basis. Provision of ongoing care in a dementing illness inevitably violates such expectations, she hypothesized, thereby exacerbating stress and conflict in family members. In a study of 510 family caregivers (George 1986), she found that such norms appeared to contribute to feelings of distress and diminished self-esteem in adult children, although spouses appeared to experience relatively little normative conflict in assuming the role of primary caregiver. We may speculate that features of the marital relationship neutralize feelings of inequity or resentment in spousal caregivers. George noted, however, that 52% of the spouse sample expressed a desire for more assistance from children and other relatives, suggesting that normative conflicts may emerge in the parent-child relationship rather than in the spousal subsystem.

In summary, the developmental literature leads us to expect gender-related differences in caregiver characteristics and outcomes (Barnett et al. 1987; Gilligan 1982). Although some reports have suggested that women are more inclined to report symptoms of depression and demoralization than are men, other studies failed to show gender-related differences in the experience of caregiver burden. Researchers have emphasized the need for prospective studies, using multiple indicators of caregiver functioning, in efforts to understand the effects of gender on adaptation.

Developmental stages of the illness experience. A fifth line of study examines developmental aspects of the illness experience in neuropsychiatric conditions. Clinicians have described phases of family adjustment and adaptation, seeking to understand stress responses in the context of developmental issues associated with various disorders. The work of Teusink and Mahler (1984) is representative. They developed a stage model of family adjustment in dementing illness consisting of five phases: 1) initial denial of difficulty associated with dementing condition; 2) overinvolvement with the patient in an effort to compensate for symptoms of the illness; 3) anger, when compensatory efforts fail; 4) guilt, in response to feelings of anger; and 5) acceptance of the illness. Such stages parallel phases of adaptation in the demented patient as described by Cohen et al. (1984).

Several investigators have considered specific aspects of the adjustment process. In studies of traumatic brain injury and degenerative neurological disorders, Romano (1974) and Falek (1979) noted that families often denied the nature or extent of cognitive impairment at the outset, moving toward acceptance of the condition in stages resembling those hypothesized for the acceptance of terminal illness. Borden (1988) considered the implications of the diagnostic process and noted that family members may alter or cease normal patterns of interaction with the patient once they learn that a condition is irreversible. At the same time, diagnosis of the condition may help to account for seemingly inexplicable behaviors and thereby reduce anxiety in members, particularly in early stages of the illness.

In the context of such models, stress-related symptoms in family members are seen as normative reactions in efforts to adjust to progressive losses associated with the illness. Developmental processes, rather than specific stressor variables, are viewed as primary determinants of stress and adaptation. Although stage models have been criticized on the grounds that they oversimplify adaptive processes, prospective study is needed to document shifts in caregiver perceptions, needs, resources, and coping strategies over the course of the illness experience.

Tables 32–1, 32–2, 32–3, and 32–4 provide a means of organizing areas of study within the

TABLE 32–1. DETERMINANTS OF CAREGIVER FUNCTIONING—PATIENT

Characteristics	*Related research (chronological order)*
Health status	
Dementia	Hoenig and Hamilton 1966; Grad and Sainsbury 1968; Sainsbury and Grad 1970; Sanford 1975; Ross and Kedward 1977; Godber 1977; Blazer 1978; Koopman-Boyden and Wells 1979; Rabins et al. 1982; Gelleard and Boyd-Watts 1982; Johnson and Johnson 1983; Wilder et al. 1983; Poulshock and Deimling 1984
Time since diagnosis	
Global severity of disorder	
Cognitive deficits	
Physical impairment	
Behavioral disturbance	
Caregiving needs	
Physical care needs	
Mental care needs	
Health problems unrelated to dementia	
Psychological	
Premorbid personality features	Anecdotal clinical accounts; not yet systematically investigated in empirical study
Perception of illness	
Perception of spousal and familial relationships	
Perception of social support	
Coping strategies	
Social	
Age	Fengler and Goodrich 1979; Hirschfield 1983; Cantor 1983; Poulshock and Deimling 1984
Sex	
Race	
Ethnicity	
Religion	
Occupation before disability or retirement	
Income level	

TABLE 32–2. DETERMINANTS OF CAREGIVER FUNCTIONING—CAREGIVER

Characteristics	*Related research (chronological order)*
Health status	
Mental conditions	Blumenthal and Morycz 1980; Zarit et al. 1980
Physical conditions	
Psychological	
Personality features	Niederhe and Fruge 1982; Groves et al. 1984; Lansky 1984; Zarit et al. 1985; Fitting et al. 1986; Hudson 1986
Perception of illness	
Perception of patient response to illness	
Perception of caregiver tasks	
Physical tasks	
Mental tasks	
Social norms and roles	
Perception of spousal and familial relationships	
Perception of social support	
Coping strategies	
Social	
Age	Fengler and Goodrich 1979; Hirschfield 1983; Cantor 1983; Poulshock and Deimling 1984
Sex	
Race	
Ethnicity	
Religion	
Occupation	
Income	

person-environment construct. These tables specify classes of patient, caregiver, family, and social-environmental characteristics identified as potential determinants of caregiver functioning in theoretical, empirical, and clinical reports to date.

Overview

As we have seen, work to date provides important data about potential sources and signs of stress-related dysfunction in family caregivers. Before we consider the importance of stress and coping perspectives in identifying tasks and strategies in clinical intervention, however, it will be useful to review the implications of the studies as a whole.

First, discussions of caregiver functioning have emphasized consequences of patient impairment or behaviors associated with neuropsychiatric conditions that call for a response or intervention from the caretaker. The implicit assumption, consistent with biological models of stress, has been that caregiver stress is determined by objective, external demands. Although objective measures of physical health status have failed to document a relationship between severity of illness and caregiver distress, there is modest evidence of an association between behavioral disturbance and caregiver strain in some studies.

Second, it is increasingly clear that individual differences in caregiver perceptions of the illness experience and coping behaviors play a central role in distress and adaptation. Highly demanding patients are not necessarily perceived as burdensome by caregivers. Accordingly, patient characteristics must be considered in the context of caregiver characteristics such as perception of events and coping strategies used in dealing with taxing conditions.

Third, there is evidence of a modest relationship between social support and caregiver strain in the illness experience. The assumption is that greater degrees of support buffer the effects of stressors and result in lower levels of strain. To date, however, studies have relied on relatively gross measures of support variables. Outcome differences related to caregiver perception of social networks and resources have been examined only in preliminary ways, and it is reasonable to expect that assessment of perceived support will yield more meaningful findings.

TABLE 32–3. DETERMINANTS OF CAREGIVER FUNCTIONING—FAMILY

Characteristics	*Related research (chronological order)*
Family constellation	
Family functioning[a]	
Problem solving	Bruhn 1977; Blazer 1978; Koopman-Boyden and Wells 1979; Groves et al. 1984; Lansky 1984; Niederehe and Fruge 1985
Instrumental	
Affective	
Communication	
Roles	
Affective responsiveness	
Behavioral control	
Adaptability	
Cohesion	
Family response to illness	
Perception of disorder	
Perception of caregiver needs	
Degree of involvement in caregiving tasks	
Family life stage (developmental issues)	
Family life events	

[a]Selection of such characteristics have been based on models of family functioning described by Epstein et al. (1982)—McMaster model. See Walsh (1987) for comprehensive review of family issues in later life.

Fourth, clinical narratives and descriptive studies have suggested that perceived quality of the caregiver's relationship with the ill person before onset of symptoms may influence levels of strain. One assumption has been that caregivers who appraise relationships in positive terms experience less burden because the recalled sense of fulfillment helps to neutralize the demands of the caregiving experience (Borden 1991a).

Finally, findings increasingly point to the importance of gender in consideration of adaptational outcomes. Although earlier accounts suggested that men and women experience comparable levels of strain in the caregiving role, a growing number of investigations have documented significant differences in outcomes, with women reporting lower levels of psychological well-being (Borden and Berlin 1990).

TABLE 32–4. DETERMINANTS OF CAREGIVER FUNCTIONING—SOCIAL-ENVIRONMENTAL

Characteristics	*Related research (chronological order)*
Living arrangements	
Physical setting	Sanford 1975
Home	
Institution	
Caregiving constellation	
Geographical factors	
Caregiving context	
Informal social structure (family and friends)	Fengler and Goodrich 1979; Zarit et al. 1980; Kahn and Tobin 1981; Johnson 1983; Cantor 1983
Formal social structure (health and supportive services)	

❑ STRESS AND COPING

Given the increasing importance placed on individual differences in analysis of findings, two constructs, coping and psychological well-being, emerge as central concepts in the development of further study and clinical intervention. A brief review of work in each of these areas will help provide a rationale for discussion of clinical intervention strategies described below.

Coping

Although the issue of caregiver stress is increasingly linked with the concept of coping in theoretical discussion, there has been remarkably little consideration of coping processes in study of neuropsychiatric illness and family caregivers. The construct of coping emerges as a central focus in further research in the light of theoretical work and empirical study in the behavioral sciences. The concept is implied by the notion of stress, and theoretical perspectives as well as research findings indicate that adaptational outcomes are determined by perceptions of events as well as by the thoughts, feelings, and actions used in efforts to mediate taxing situations (Lazarus and Folkman 1984; Lazarus and Launier 1978; Moos and Tsu 1977).

In critical reviews of the literature, Moos and Billings (1982) and Lazarus and Folkman (1984) distinguished two approaches in work on the concept of coping. The earliest line of thinking, based on animal models of stress, focused on the notion of arousal and defined coping as acts that control aversive situations and reduce drive or activation. Avoidance and escape behaviors were emphasized. Critics noted that such approaches failed to address cognitive and affective processes that figure in human coping efforts.

The second line of development, drawing on concepts of ego psychology, was concerned with thoughts, feelings, and actions that persons used to mediate difficulties in relationships and situations. Hierarchies of coping strategies, ranging from immature to mature mechanisms, were conceptualized by numerous theoreticians and clinicians over the last quarter century (Vaillant 1977). Such models emphasized traits or styles that presumably predisposed persons to cope in particular ways over the life course. Empirical work has suggested, however, that ego psychological formulations underestimated the complexity and the variability of coping processes. Further difficulties emerged from the equation of coping with positive adaptational outcomes; less successful efforts to manage stressors were seen as defensive or primitive in character.

Coping should not be equated with mastery over the environment, according to social-psychological views, because many sources of stress cannot be mastered. Commentators have suggested that denial, minimization, or acceptance of stressful situations may be adaptive in some instances. The implication of such arguments is that no strategy can be considered inherently better or worse than any other. Judgments concerning the adaptiveness of a strategy must be made in the context of the person-situation configuration.

In an effort to extend traditional formulations of coping processes, Lazarus and Folkman (1984) conceptualized coping as ongoing cognitive and behavioral efforts to manage specific internal and external demands that are perceived as taxing or exceeding the adaptive resources of the person. By way of overview, they distinguished three types of cognitive appraisal: 1) primary appraisal, or judgment that an experience is a) stressful (i.e., involving loss, harm, threat, or challenge), b) irrelevant, or c) benign-positive; 2) secondary appraisal, or judgment concerning what potential and actual options are available to mediate the stressor and the consequences of each alternative; and (3) reappraisal, or modified judgment based on new information from the person or environment. The appraised meaning of the situation is a primary determinant of coping experience, in their view.

As Lazarus's and Folkman's use of the word *effort* suggests (1984), coping may include anything the person thinks or does in an attempt to deal with a stressful experience, independent of outcome. Use of the word *manage* is intended to avoid the equation of coping with mastery. Managing may mean minimization, avoidance, tolerance, or acceptance of stressful conditions as well as attempts to master the environment.

The functions of coping are described as 1) modification or management of a stressful problem (problem-focused coping) and 2) regulation of emotional responses to the problem (emotion-focused coping). Problem-focused coping efforts attempt to eliminate sources of stress or deal with the tangible consequences of a problem. Strategies in this category include seeking information, advice, or concrete sources of assistance and initiation of problem-solving actions, such as development of plans or skills in efforts to resolve difficulties.

Emotion-focused coping efforts, on the other hand, involve attempts to neutralize emotion aroused by the problem and thereby maintain affective equilibrium. Strategies in this category include direct attempts to control emotion, such as detachment, wishful thinking, emphasizing positive aspects of a situation, acceptance, and efforts to discharge emotions, such as letting off steam, crying, or exercise (Lazarus and Folkman 1984; Moos and Billings 1982). Support for such functions has come from theoretical work as well as empirical study of coping experience (Lazarus and Launier 1978).

Although there has been little consideration of coping processes in study of neuropsychiatric illness and family caregivers, several investigators have examined features of coping experience in global study of organic brain syndrome and psychosocial stressors. Johnson (1983) found that family caregivers frequently attempted to deal with the strain of dementing illness either by psychological distancing from the patient or by extreme involvement with the patient, often marked by withdrawal from other relationships. Clinicians have pointed out that excessive involvement with the patient may preclude engagement of informal and formal sources of social support that potentially help to reduce the burden.

Levine et al. (1983) reported that family members best able to cope with caregiving demands attempted to develop specific strategies for solving illness-related problems, such as wandering and activities of daily living. Use of prayer was also associated with positive outcomes in their study. Similarly, reliance on problem-solving strategies and emotion-focused strategies that emphasize positive elements of the caregiving situation emerged as salient predictors of psychological well-being in a study by Borden (1991a). Capacity to see beyond the illness, or futurity, was associated with reduced role strain in dementia caregivers. On the basis of theoretical work and exploratory study, we can assume that family caregivers rely on a range of thoughts, feelings, and actions in problem-focused and emotion-focused efforts to deal with the vicissitudes of the illness experience.

Psychological Well-Being

Researchers have increasingly assumed that stress and coping are important determinants of health status. By extension, workers have attempted to assess the consequences of specific coping behaviors in terms of physical and mental phenomena. The implicit assumption has been that greater degrees of stress, unmediated by effective coping strategies, are manifested in physical or mental signs of illness.

In limiting evaluation of adaptational outcomes to assessment of distinct pathological signs, however, investigators have failed to consider psychological and social indicators of functional status beyond the boundary of discrete symptom configurations or illness states. There has been little distinction between the absence of illness and relative degrees of health. Absence of physical or mental symptoms does not necessarily speak to how "well" one is feeling. As clinical experience has shown (Borden 1988), persons may report feeling distressed or "ill" when symptomatology is minimal. At the same time, clinical accounts indicate that many family caregivers experience varying types and degrees of physical difficulty (e.g., hypertension, arthritis, back pain, and cardiac problems) but report minimal feelings of strain. Older adults, in particular, may experience negative changes in health status without reporting feelings of distress (Lieberman and Tobin 1983). It is increasingly clear that study of adaptational outcomes requires knowledge of positive indicators of health status, as well as understanding of dysfunction and pathology. (The limitations of pathology-based approaches in stress and coping research are described in a critical review by Lazarus and Folkman [1984]).

The construct of psychological well-being emerges as an important concept in multidimensional assessment of adaptational outcome. Psychological well-being has been defined in a variety of ways, including lack of illness, the balance between positive and negative affect, quality of life, and positive indicators of adaptational outcome. Increasingly, well-being is understood as a cognitive appraisal of functional status and outcome along multiple dimensions, including emotional states, morale, life satisfaction, and perceptions of relationships.

Psychological well-being would appear to be an important indicator of adaptational outcome in research on neuropsychiatric illness and caregiver functioning for three reasons. First, the concept addresses multidimensional aspects of functioning that pathology-based perspectives generally fail to consider, including emotional states, morale, social functioning, and life satisfaction. There has been little systematic study of such factors in work to date. Second, assessment of the characteristic relies on subjective perception of life experience as opposed to objective assessment of reactions to specific life events. As such it reflects the increasing importance placed on subjective experience in the study of caregiver functioning. Third, the construct examines affective reactions to life experience along a continuum; accordingly, the full range of affective experience, positive as well as negative, is considered in assessment of adaptational outcomes. Such a range allows workers to examine degrees of well-being, thereby shifting the emphasis from stress and pathology to adjustment and adaptation.

We know little about what it means to cope adaptively in the context of the illness experience at present, given the emphasis on pathology and dysfunction in caregiver studies to date. Researchers have inferred "health" or "well-being" in the absence of distinct symptom configurations or illness states. However, such assessments have failed to distinguish absence of illness from perceptions of relative health status (e.g., from feeling "so-so" to feeling "good enough" to feeling "wonderful"). Spouses may experience diminished states of well-being without developing signs of mental or physical illness, as suggested in numerous clinical accounts (Borden, in press), just as they may show symptoms of diagnosable conditions without experiencing distressing degrees of strain. In order to achieve a more complete understanding of coping and adaptation in the illness experience, we must include negative as well as positive indicators of health, or well-being, in evaluation of adaptational outcome.

❑ TRANSACTIONAL MODEL OF STRESS AND COPING

Although investigators have generally failed to describe theoretical models of stress implicit in research hypotheses and designs, it would appear that much of the work on impairment associated with neuropsychiatric illness and caregiver functioning has been based on relatively simple antecedent-consequent or stimulus-response models. That is, researchers have attempted to identify global antecedent variables (e.g., neuropsychiatric symptoms) as causes of unitary outcomes (e.g., ill-effects), without examining specific aspects of such characteristics or mediating processes. Characteristics are thereby treated as if they are unitary, static, and directly linear in relationship (i.e., certain objective stimuli produce certain stress responses). Such designs fail to reflect the interactive configuration of person and environment and, in doing so, overlook specific processes such as perception and coping that would appear to be central mediators of stress and adaptation.

The Lazarus-Folkman model (Lazarus and Folkman 1984), developed in an effort to extend traditional antecedent-consequent frameworks, shifts the focus from stress and pathology to coping and adaptation. Stress is understood as a particular relationship between the person and the environment that is appraised by the individual as taxing or exceeding adaptive resources and endangering well-being. In this model, coping, as noted earlier, is defined as ongoing cognitive and behavioral efforts to mediate internal and external demands that are appraised as taxing or exceeding the adaptive resources of the person. Given the emphasis on perceptual and coping processes, the model is especially useful in conceptualizing areas of research and intervention with family caregivers in neuropsychiatric illness.

The schema in Figure 32–1, based on the Lazarus-Folkman model, conceptualizes the interactive pattern of patient, caregiver, family, and environmental characteristics in terms of antecedent factors and mediating processes. As the schema shows, caregiver outcome is mediated by 1) caregiver perception and appraisal of physical, psychological, and social characteristics, specified as antecedent conditions, and 2) caregiver coping strategies. Physical, mental, and social outcomes in caregiver functioning, in turn, are believed to influence caregiver perception of conditions and coping strategies over time.

Such a framework provides an integrative schema in conceptualization of research questions and hypotheses. Whereas the traditional antecedent-consequent models imply that an environmental stimulus generates stressful responses in a unicausal fashion (Lazarus and Folkman 1984), this schema provides a means of conceptualizing multiple characteristics as mediators of caregiver outcome: person and environmental characteristics are cast as interactive determinants in the stress and coping configuration. As such the model provides a more comprehensive and complex means of analysis than that found in traditional antecedent-consequent frameworks. Units of intervention may involve the

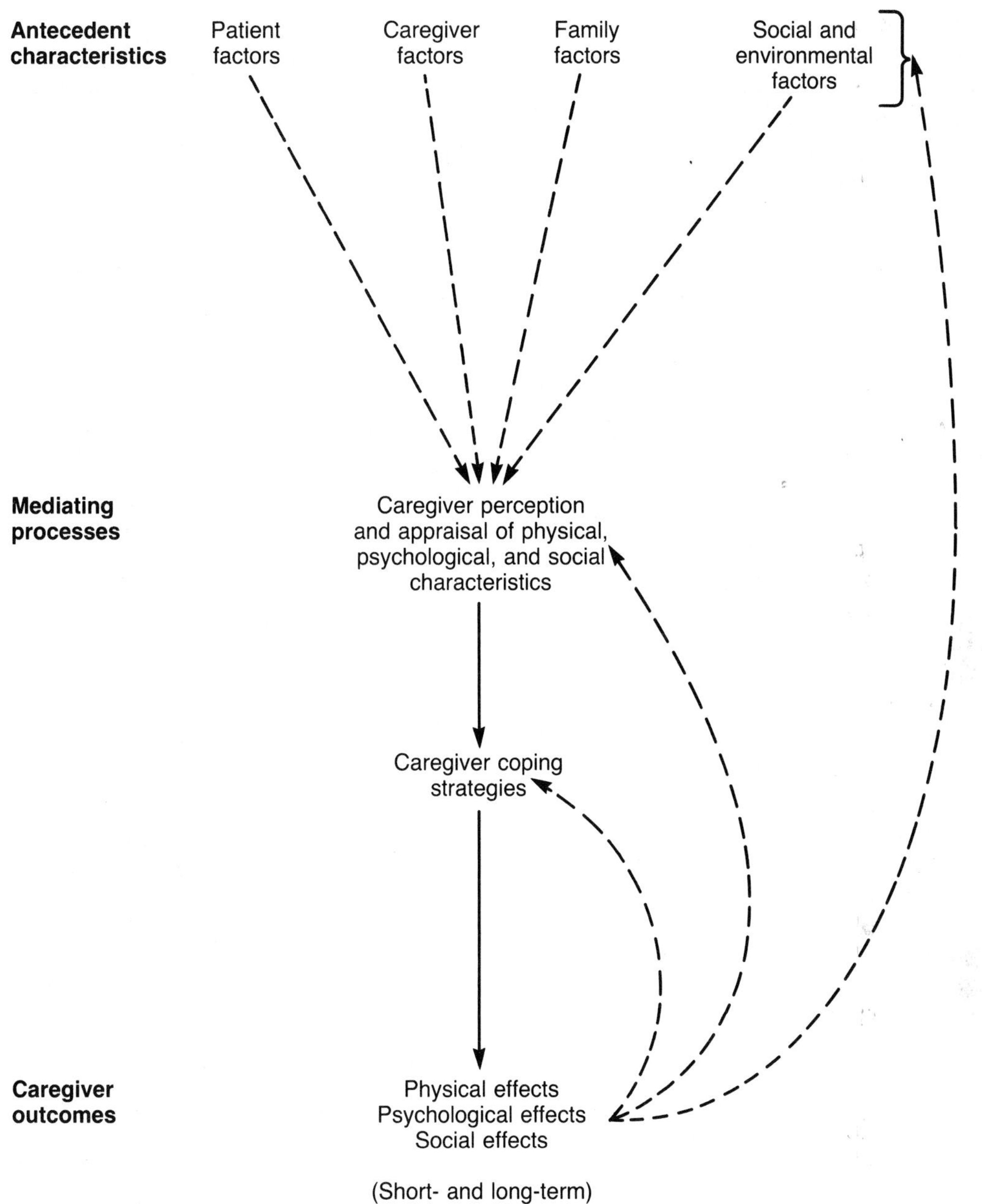

Figure 32–1. Multivariate model of caregiver functioning.

caregiver, the caregiver-patient dyad, the family, or the social-environmental field.

❑ CLINICAL INTERVENTION

Clinicians must recognize the range of biological, psychological, and social factors that influence the character of the caregiving experience, just as they must distinguish individual needs and identify optimal forms of intervention at various stages of neuropsychiatric illness. As work to date has made clear, caregiving is a heterogeneous process, and there is considerable variation in the ways family members deal with the demands of the role over the course of the illness experience. Although varying degrees of strain appear to be inevitable, research and clinical practice suggest that development of coping skills and mobilization of social support work to buffer the negative impact of caregiving demands.

Assessment

Caregivers vary widely in their abilities to deal with the demands of the illness experience, and individual differences in appraisal of illness characteristics, social relationships, and coping strategies are important factors in determining levels of well-being (Borden 1991a). Accordingly, assessment strategies must focus not only on objective phenomena, but also on subjective perceptions and meanings of illness characteristics, appraisals of family and peer relationships, and use of coping strategies. Assessment should specify the conditions under which the caregiver experiences strain and determine whether the difficulty is located primarily in the appraisal process (e.g., a person inappropriately views symptoms as intentional, hostile acts or views problems as uncontrollable), or the coping process (e.g., a person has inadequate problem-solving skills, relies on maladaptive strategies, or lacks relevant information).

Intervention

In the context of psychotherapeutic treatment, three tasks emerge from review of work to date. First, intervention should specifically seek to reduce distress in appraisal of illness characteristics. Treatment efforts should help caregivers manage reactions to illness phenomena and reframe maladaptive attributions about the conditions. Second, intervention should facilitate development of coping skills that help caregivers solve specific problems and alter stressful circumstances in the context of the illness experience. Third, intervention efforts should promote use of social networks in efforts to mobilize sources of emotional and instrumental support. Self-help groups and social casework, as well as family and group psychotherapy, may be effective in helping caregivers develop sources of support. Natural helping networks also emerge as important factors in planning interventions.

Overall, work to date points to the importance of educational, psychotherapeutic, and supportive modes of intervention in the development of comprehensive service programs. Education of family members about the nature and course of neuropsychiatric conditions would appear to provide the basis for management of illness-related problems. Instructing caregivers in specific problem-solving techniques, such as behavioral and cognitive procedures, may help them reduce behavioral problems associated with neuropsychiatric conditions such as dementia, stroke, and traumatic brain injury. Further, education in stress management and other self-care procedures may provide varying degrees of relief from caregiving burdens.

In summary, the results of work to date show that development of intervention programs must be based on a broad understanding of the psychological and social needs of family caregivers and acknowledge differences in members' capabilities to provide care. Planners must realize that the demands and burdens of caregiving vary not only among individuals but change over time.

Intervention Approaches

Clinicians have developed a series of intervention approaches in their efforts to help family caregivers of persons with neuropsychiatric illness, ranging from provision of respite care, education, and social support to skills training and formal psychotherapy. Presently, however, there is no consistent evidence to suggest the superiority of any one approach (Montgomery and Borgatta 1985). Although we emphasize the value of interventions from the perspective of caregiver burden, it is important to note that any reduction in caregiver distress may also be expected to have a positive effect on patient psychiatric symptoms as well.

Self-help organizations such as the Alzheimer's Disease and Related Disorders Association (ADRDA) and the National Alliance for the Mentally Ill (NAMI) have emerged as major forces, paving the way for legislation and public funding favorable to care for neuropsychiatrically ill patients. Some groups have mounted advocacy programs through public education and letter writing campaigns. Many offer support groups facilitated by members. Although there are no studies documenting the social and psychological effects of these grass-roots organizations, at present, it would appear that such efforts increase the social support networks of family caregivers. The relationship between social isolation and caregiver distress has been documented in a number of studies, and it is reasonable to assume that participation in such groups fosters development of supportive relationships. Furthermore, membership in such organizations may provide a sense of belonging and affiliation.

Reports have also suggested that most family caregivers do not request formal assistance for themselves, and caregivers often appear reluctant to make use of family support services (Montgomery and Borgatta 1985). Such reluctance may stem from past negative experiences with the psychiatric profession as well as from states of depletion in which caregivers feel they have expended their energy in caring for the member and cannot generate additional resources to seek help for themselves. Anderson et al. (1986) described the empathic stance that should guide clinicians in engaging family caregivers in the treatment process. Clinicians must demonstrate an understanding of the hardships caregivers face and be willing to bear the brunt of the family's frustrations in initial contacts. It is our impression that there are critical periods of receptiveness to involvement in support programs, often distinguished by crisis, and that specific populations, notably mothers, spouses, and aging caretakers, are most likely to seek help.

Most support programs involve some form of education. Systematic programs include didactic presentations on the diagnosis, course, and treatment of conditions and specific coping and management strategies. Studies have documented the effectiveness of such programs in reducing the frequency of psychiatric hospitalizations and in increasing the community tenure of patients who will eventually be hospitalized (Eisdorfer and Cohen 1981). Some studies have suggested that family educational programs facilitate engagement of persons in rehabilitation programs and, in doing so, promote recovery after stroke and traumatic brain injury (Chiverton and Caine 1989). Educational programs also appear to be effective in reducing family strain and increasing coping skills in caregivers. Even short-term educational programs appear useful in promoting feelings of mastery, competence, and the ability to function independently (Chiverton and Caine 1989).

Respite services seek to lessen the burden of daily care by temporarily relieving family members from caregiving responsibilities. Although there may be a high degree of satisfaction with such programs from the perspective of the family, formal studies of the impact of family respite on patient community tenure and caregiver burden are equivocal (Montgomery and Borgatta 1985). Further investigation is needed before any conclusions about the benefits of respite care can be drawn.

A number of intervention programs have employed family caregivers in cognitive and physical rehabilitation of their ill relative. Giving family caregivers explicit rehabilitative tasks to perform may help prevent them from placing unrealistic demands on the patient and thereby reduce frustration and aggressive behavior. Quayhagen and Quayhagen (1989) documented the effectiveness of a program in which family caregivers received training in communication, memory, and problem-solving skills. Subjects showed diminished burden and higher levels of psychological well-being. Other studies have demonstrated ways in which family members may usefully maintain behaviorally based treatment programs initiated during hospitalization and promote adjustment and adaptation (Pinkston and Linsk 1984).

There has been relatively little study of the effectiveness of individual psychotherapy and family therapy in relieving stress and burden in family caregivers. Clinical accounts have suggested, however, that preexisting psychiatric conditions are often exacerbated by the stress of caregiving and that traditional psychotherapy and other forms of therapeutic intervention may be of great value.

In summary, comprehensive support services for family caregivers of neuropsychiatrically ill patients should include educational, support, and respite programs as well as means of engaging the family in ongoing rehabilitation of the patient. Additional consideration should include therapeutic interventions that help family members deal with grief following the losses imposed by the illness experience. Miller et al. (1990) described the mourning that families often experience in schizophrenia and bipolar illness and suggested that similar processes occur in adjustment to neuropsychiatric illness.

❑ SUMMARY

Commentators have acknowledged the potential conflict between "research" and "service" objectives in discussion of chronic illness and caregiver burden (Borden 1988), and writers have questioned the costs and benefits of extended empirical study in the face of what would appear to be self-evident problems and solutions. Little progress will be made, however, until we achieve a better understanding of caregiving experience as seen in specific types of illness. Researchers must continue to move beyond global descriptions of persons, problems, and outcomes and consider the effects of biological, psychological, and social characteristics on caregiver functioning in the context of multidimensional models of stress and coping. In doing so, we will advance our understanding of adaptive processes and continue to establish criteria for effective assessment, treatment, and management decisions in intervention with this vulnerable and underserved population.

❑ REFERENCES

Anderson C, Reiss D, Hogarty G: Schizophrenia and the Family. New York, Guilford, 1986

Aronson MK, Lipkowitz R: Senile dementia, Alzheimer's type: the family and the health care delivery system. J Am Geriatr Soc 29:568–571, 1981

Bankoff E: Social support and adaptation to widowhood. Journal of Marriage and the Family 45:827–839, 1983

Barnett R, Biener L, Baruch G: Gender and Stress. New York, Free Press, 1987

Blazer D: Working with the elderly patient's family. Geriatrics 33:176–183, 1978

Blumenthal MD: Psychosocial factors in reversible and irreversible brain failure. Journal of Clinical and Experimental Gerontology 1:39–50, 1979

Blumenthal MD, Morycz RK: Late-life brain disease and family burden. Unpublished manuscript. University of Pittsburgh, School of Medicine, Department of Psychiatry, Pittsburgh, PA, 1980

Borden W: Stress, appraisal, and coping in spouses of demented elderly: Predictors of psychological well-being. Doctoral dissertation, University of Chicago, Chicago, IL, 1988

Borden W: Stress, coping, and adaptation in spouses of older adults with chronic dementia: predictors of psychological well being. Social Work Research and Abstracts 27:14–22, 1991a

Borden W: Beneficial outcomes in adjustment to HIV seropositivity. Social Service Review September 3:601–603, 1991b

Borden W: Psychosocial intervention following adverse life events: a narrative perspective. Social Work (in press)

Borden W, Berlin S: Gender, coping, and psychological well being in spouses of older adults with chronic dementia. Am J Orthopsychiatry 60:605–610, 1990

Brody EM: The aging of the family. Annals of the American Academy of Political and Social Science 438:13–27, 1978

Brody EM: Women in the middle and family help to older people. Gerontologist 21:471–480, 1981

Brody EM: Parent care as a normative family stress. Gerontologist 25:19–29, 1985

Brody SJ, Poulshock SW, Masciocchi CF: The family caring unit. Gerontologist 18:556–561, 1978

Bruhn JG: Effects of chronic illness on the family. J Fam Pract 4:1057–1060, 1977

Cannon W: The Wisdom of the Body. New York, Norton, 1932

Cantor M: Strain among caregivers: a study of the experience in the United States. Gerontologist 23:597–604, 1983

Chiverton P, Caine ED: Education to assist spouses in coping with Alzheimer's Disease. J Am Geriatr Soc 37:593–598, 1989

Cicirelli V: Adult children's attachment and helping behavior to elderly parents: a path model. Journal of Marriage and the Family 45:815–825, 1983

Cobb S: Social support as a moderator of life stress. Psychosom Med 3:300–314, 1976

Cohen D, Kennedy G, Eisdorfer C: Phases of change in the patient with Alzheimer's dementia: a conceptual dimension for defining health care management. J Am Geriatr Soc 32:11–15, 1984

Cohen S, Syme SL: Social Support and Health. Orlando, FL, Academic, 1985

Cohler B, Borden W, Groves L, et al: Caring for family members with Alzheimer's Disease, in Alzheimer's Disease Treatment and Family Stress. Edited by Lebowitz B, Light E. Washington, DC, U.S. Government Printing Office, 1989

Eisdorfer C: Health care policy and long term care. Rehabilitation Psychology 30(2):121–128, 1985

Eisdorfer C, Cohen D: Management of the patient and family coping with dementing illness. J Fam Pract 12: 831–837, 1981

Epstein NB, Bishop DS, Baldwin L: McMaster model of family functioning, in Normal Family Processes. Edited by Walsh F. New York, Guilford, 1982, pp 115–141

Falek A: Observations on patient and family coping with Huntington's Disease. Omega 10:35–42, 1979

Fengler AP, Goodrich N: Wives of elderly disabled men: the hidden patients. Gerontologist 19:175–183, 1979

Fitting M, Rabins P, Lucas M, et al: Caregivers for demented patients: a comparison of husbands and wives. Gerontologist 26:248–252, 1986

Frankfather D: The Aged in the Community: Managing Senility and Deviance. New York, Praeger, 1977

Gelleard CJ, Boyd-Watts WD: Problems in caring for the elderly mentally infirm at home. Archives of Gerontology and Geriatrics 1:151–158, 1982

George LK: Caregiver burden: conflict between norms of reciprocity and solidarity, in Elder Abuse: Conflict in the Family. Edited by Pillemer K, Wolf R. Dover, MA, Auburn House, 1986

Gilligan C: In a Different Voice. Cambridge, MA, Harvard University Press, 1982

Godber C: Planning services for the elderly demented patient. Age Ageing 6:100–105, 1977

Grad J, Sainsbury P: The effects that patients have on their families in a community care and a control psychiatric service: a two-year followup. Br J Psychiatry 114:265–278, 1968

Greene JG, Smith R, Gardiner M, et al: Measuring behavioural disturbance of elderly demented patients in the community and its effects on relatives: a factor analytic study. Age Ageing 11:121–126, 1982

Greenfeld J: A Child Called Noah: A Family Journey. New York, Hartcourt Brace Jovanovich, 1972

Greenfeld J: A Place for Noah. New York, Harcourt Brace Jovanovich, 1978

Greenfeld J: A Client Called Noah: A Family Journey Continued. New York, Harcourt Brace Jovanovich, 1986

Groves L: Psychological distress of caregivers in Alzheimer's Disease. Unpublished doctoral dissertation, Northwestern University, Chicago, IL, 1988

Groves L, Lazarus LW, Newton N, et al: Brief psychotherapy with families of patients with Alzheimer's disease, in Clinical Approaches to Psychotherapy with the Elderly. Edited by Lazarus LW. Washington, DC, American Psychiatric Press, 1984, pp 37–53

Henderson S: Social relationships, adversity, and neurosis. Br J Psychiatry 138:391–398, 1981

Hirschfield MJ: Home care versus institutionalization: family caregiving and senile brain disease. Int J Nurs Stud 20:23–32, 1983

Hoenig J, Hamilton MW: Elderly psychiatric patients and the burden on the household. Psychiatria Neurologia [Basel] 154:281–293, 1966

Hudson MF: Elder mistreatment: current research, in Elder Abuse: Conflict in the Family. Edited by Pillemer K, Wolf RS. Dover, MA, Auburn House, 1986, pp 178–196

Johnson CL: Dyadic family relations and social support. Gerontologist 23:377–383, 1983

Johnson C, Catalano D: Childless elderly and their family support. Gerontologist 21:610–618, 1981

Johnson CL, Johnson FA: A microanalysis of senility: the responses of the family and health professionals. Cult Med Psychiatry 7:77–96, 1983

Johnson M: Interweaving of informal and formal care: a challenge to some of the myths. Paper presented at the International Congress of Gerontology, New York, July 12, 1985

Kahn RL, Tobin S: Community treatment for aged persons with altered brain function, in Clinical Aspects of Alzheimer's Disease and Senile Dementia. Edited by Miller N, Cohen G. New York, Raven, 1981

Kaplan BH, Cassel J, Gore S: Social support and health. Med Care 15:47–58, 1977

Koopman-Boyden P, Wells L: The problems arising from supporting the elderly at home. N Z Med J 89:265–269, 1979

Lansky J: Family psychotherapy of the patient with chronic organic brain syndrome. Psychiatric Annals 14:2–17, 1984

Lazarus R, Folkman S: Stress, Appraisal, and Coping. New York, Springer, 1984

Lazarus R, Launier R: Stress-related transactions between person and environment, in Perspectives in Interactional Psychology. Edited by Pervin LA, Lewis M. New York, Plenum, 1978

Levine N, Dastorr D, Gendron C: Coping with dementia: a pilot study. J Am Geriatr Soc 31:12–18, 1983

Lieberman MA, Tobin S: The Experience of Old Age: Stress, Coping, and Survival. New York, Basic Books, 1983

Lin N, Woelfel MW, Light SC: The buffering effect of social support subsequent to an important life event. J Health Soc Behav 26:247–263, 1985

McCubbin HI, Cauble AE, Patterson JM (eds): Family Stress, Coping, and Social Support. Springfield, IL, Charles C Thomas, 1982

Meyer A: The life chart and the obligation of specifying positive data in psychopathological diagnosis, in The Collected Papers of Adolph Meyer, Vol III: Medical Teaching. Edited by Winters EE. Baltimore, MD, Johns Hopkins University Press, 1951

Miller F, Dworkin J, Ward M, et al: Unresolved grief in families of the seriously mentally ill. Hosp Community Psychiatry 41:1321–1325, 1990

Montgomery RJ, Borgatta EF: Family support project: final report, Administration on Aging. Seattle, WA, University of Washington Press, 1985

Moos R, Billings AG: Conceptualizing and measuring coping resources and processes, in Handbook of Stress. Edited by Goldberger L, Breznitz S. New York, Macmillan, 1982, pp 212–230

Moos RH, Tsu VD: The crisis of physical illness: an overview, in Coping with Physical Illness. Edited by Moos RH. New York, Plenum, 1977, pp 3–22

Neugarten B, Gutmann D: Age-sex roles and personality in middle age: a thematic apperception study, in Middle Age and Ageing. Edited by Neugarten B. Chicago, IL, University of Chicago Press, 1968, pp 54–73

Niederehe G, Fruge E: Dementia and family dynamics. J Geriatr Psychiatry 17:21–56, 1985

Noelker LS, Poulshock SW: The Effects on Families of Caring for Impaired Elderly in Residence (Final Report, Administration on Aging Grant 90-AR-2112). Cleveland, OH, Benjamin Rose Institute, 1982

Pinkston E, Linsk N: Behavioral family intervention with the impaired elderly. Gerontologist 24:576–583, 1984

Poulshock SW, Deimling GT: Families caring for elders in residence: issues in measurement of burden. J Gerontol 39:230–239, 1984

Quayhagen MP, Quayhagen M: Differential effects of family-based strategies in Alzheimer's Disease. Journal of the Geriatric Society of America 29:150–155, 1989

Rabins P, Mace NL, Lucas MJ: The impact of dementia on the family. JAMA 248:333–335, 1982

Robinson BC: Validation of a caregiver strain index. J Gerontol 38:344–348, 1983

Robinson B, Thurnher M: Taking care of aged parents. Gerontologist 19:586, 1979

Romano M: Family response to traumatic head injury. Scand J Rehabil Med 6:1–4, 1974

Ross HE, Kedward HB: Psychogeriatric hospital admissions from the community and institutions. J Gerontol 32:420–427, 1977

Sainsbury P, Grad J: The psychiatrist and the geriatric patient: The effects of community care on the family of the geriatric patient. J Geriatr Psychiatry 4:23–41, 1970

Sanford JR: Tolerance of debility in elderly dependents by supporters at home: Its significance for hospital practice. BMJ 3:471–473, 1975

Sarason IG: Social support: conceptual and methodological issues. Paper presented at the 93rd conference of the American Psychological Association, Los Angeles, CA, August 1985

Selye H: The physiology and pathology of exposure to stress. Acta Montreal 1950

Shanas E: Social myth as hypothesis: the case of the family relations of old people. Gerontologist 19:3–9, 1979

Streib G, Beck R: Older families: a decade review. Journal of Marriage and the Family 42:937–956, 1981

Sussman MB: Family life of older people, in Handbook of Aging and the Social Sciences. Edited by Binstock R, Shanas E. New York, Van Nostrand Reinhold, 1976, pp 415–449

Teusink JP, Mahler S: Helping families cope with Alzheimer's Disease. Hosp Community Psychiatry 35:152–156, 1984

Troll LE: The family of later life: A decade review. Journal of Marriage and the Family 33:263–290, 1971

Vaillant G: Adaptation to Life. Boston, MA, Little, Brown, 1977

Walsh F: The family in later life, in The Family Life Cycle, Revised Ed. Edited by Carter E, McGoldrick M. New York. Gardiner Press, 1987, pp 105–136

Wilder D, Teresi J, Bennett R: Family burden and dementia, in The Dementias. Edited by Mayeur P, Rosen H. New York, Raven, 1983, pp 87–101

Zarit SH, Reever KE, Bach-Peterson J: Relatives of the impaired elderly: Correlates of feelings of burden. Gerontologist 20:649–655, 1980

Zarit SH, Orr NK, Zarit JM: Families Under Stress: The Hidden Victims of Alzheimer's Disease. New York, New York University Press, 1985

Chapter

33

Ethical and Legal Issues in Neuropsychiatry

Robert I. Simon, M.D.

TODAY, THE PRACTICE OF psychiatry requires a working knowledge of neurobiological procedures, treatments, and research. Few psychiatrists continue to provide only psychological treatment for all their patients, nor do clinicians view most patients as suffering solely from "pure" psychological disorders. Even patients with so-called problems in living frequently require psychotropic medications. Under the salutary influence of the medical model, mind and body are again merging together in psychiatric practice. The broad definition of a neuropsychiatrist used in this chapter reflects this merging of mind and body. The term *neuropsychiatrist* refers to a psychiatrist who diagnoses patients with organic and other mental disorders and treats them with somatic therapies. The term *neuropsychiatric patient* refers to a patient with organic mental disorder or a patient primarily requiring somatic therapy.

The body of law applied to the practice of psychiatry does not differ for the treatment of functional or organic mental disorders. The diagnosis, treatment, and management of patients with organic mental disorders, however, presents not only unique clinical and ethical concerns, but legal considerations as well. For example, an assessment of competency may be required to determine a neuropsychiatric patient's capacity to make health care decisions or ability to manage his or her personal affairs.

This is particularly true for patients suffering from Alzheimer's disease or acquired immunodeficiency syndrome (AIDS)-related dementia. Accordingly, the ethical and legal issues such as informed consent, the right to refuse treatment, alternative care providers, and advance directives are likely to be confronted in treating neuropsychiatric patients.

Individuals who have been criminally charged must be legally competent to stand trial. Defendants with neuropsychiatric impairments may not meet that standard. Therefore, these defendants are likely candidates for pretrial evaluations of their mental status and cognitive capability for understanding the charges against them and their ability to assist in their legal defense. Moreover, depending on the nature and duration of a neuropsychiatric disorder, a criminal defendant may seek acquittal or have the charges reduced based on the argument that the defendant was legally insane at the time the offense occurred.

Vulnerability to psychiatric malpractice suits may be increased in certain areas of neuropsychiatric practice. For example, the use of various somatic therapies, the assessment and prediction of violence, involuntary hospitalization, and discharging potentially dangerous patients all represent potential areas of liability for the neuropsychiatric practitioner.

Lastly, lawsuits involving head injuries have increased annually and have become a major source of personal injury litigation. Because of the complexities often associated with establishing the extent and cause of a plaintiff's damages, forensic expertise in neuropsychiatry is frequently needed to address the common psychiatric sequelae that may be caused by head injuries.

This chapter presents a brief review of some of the salient clinical, ethical, and legal issues that link neuropsychiatry to criminal law and civil personal injury litigation. Readers interested in a more comprehensive summary of the medical and psycholegal aspects of general psychiatry, which would incorporate neuropsychiatry, are encouraged to read additional contemporary texts (1–7).

❑ ETHICAL CONSIDERATIONS

During the first half of this century, the principle of patient autonomy was clearly recognized in the medical malpractice case *Schloendorf v. Society of New York Hospital* (8). Justice Cardozo firmly enunciated the principle of patient self-determination by stating that "every human being of adult years and sound mind has a right to determine what shall be done with his own body, and a surgeon who performs an operation without his patient's consent commits an assault, for which he is liable in damages" (p. 126).

Since the late 1950s and early 1960s, the medical profession has moved away from an authoritarian, physician-oriented stance toward a more collaborative relationship with patients concerning their health care decisions. This is especially reflected in contemporary ethical principles (9). Thus on ethical grounds, psychiatry endorses granting competent patients the legal right to autonomy in determining their medical care. Quite apart from any legal compulsion, most psychiatrists disclose truthful and pertinent medical information to their patients as a way of enhancing the therapeutic alliance (10,11).

The ethical principles of beneficence, nonmaleficence, and the respect for the dignity and autonomy of the patient provide the moral-ethical foundation for the doctor-patient relationship. Accordingly, patients with dementia or other brain disorders that significantly interfere with the capacity to make decisions require more active intervention by the psychiatrist. For example, the psychiatrist has a legal and ethical duty to obtain consent from substitute decision makers when a patient is incapable of making an informed decision. The rights of all patients are the same—only how these rights are exercised is different (12).

The ethics of social justice call for the fair allocation of medical resources in accord with medical need (13). Although seemingly a new development, the ethical concerns about equitable health care distribution are found in the *Hippocratic Oath* and in the tradition of medicine and psychiatry (14). Thus neuropsychiatric patients are ethically entitled to have access to the same medical resources available to other patients. For example, it would be unethical to discriminate against patients with AIDS-related dementia by not providing adequate treatment and management resources.

Ethical issues arise daily for psychiatrists who become involved in the critical care of neuropsychiatric patients. Medical decision making, informed consent, resuscitation, "brain death," organ transplantation, the withholding and withdrawing of life support, and the allocation of medical resources all give rise to complex ethical and legal problems (15). Moreover, that which is considered ethical in clinical practice today may become a legal requirement tomorrow.

Specific ethical issues are also addressed in connection with the various clinical and legal topics discussed throughout this chapter.

❑ LEGAL ISSUES

Health Care Decision Making

The following case example illustrates thorny clinical-legal issues surrounding a patient's capacity to make informed health care decisions.

Case 1

A 72-year-old woman is progressively exhibiting deficits in recent and past memory, concentration, orientation and social and self-care functioning. These symptoms greatly impair her ability to effectively manage a restaurant that she owns. She is hospitalized on a general medical service for evaluation of vague complaints of pain and "disorientation." A psychiatric consultant makes a presumptive clinical diagnosis of primary degenerative dementia of the Alzheimer type, senile onset. The psychiatrist concludes that the patient is unable to handle her business affairs. Because she appears questionably competent to make health care decisions (i.e., to give a competent consent to start antidepressant medication), the physician obtains permission for treatment from the family. Meanwhile, the family seeks an adjudication of incompetency. After reviewing the psychiatrist's evaluation, the court declares the patient incompetent for managing her finances, but not for health care decisions. A limited guardianship is created.

Nearly every area of human endeavor is affected by the law and, as a fundamental condition, requires one to be mentally competent (Table 33–1). Essentially, *competent* is defined as "having sufficient capacity, ability [or] possessing the requisite physical, mental, natural, or legal qualifications" (16). This definition is deliberately vague and ambiguous because the term *competent* is a broad concept encompassing many different legal issues and contexts. As a result, its definition, requirements, and application can vary widely depending on the circumstances in which it is being measured (e.g., health care decisions, executing a will, or confessing to a crime).

In general, competency refers to some *minimal* mental, cognitive, or behavioral ability, trait, or capability required to perform a particular legally recognized act or to assume some legal role. The term *capacity*, which is often interchanged with the word *competency*, refers to an individual's actual ability to understand or to form an intention with regard to some act. In patients with traumatic brain injuries, fluctuation in mental capacity is common, particularly in the days or even months following injury. Generally, patients with brain disorders of diverse etiologies often manifest considerable variability in mental functioning from day to day.

As a distinction, the term *incompetent* is applied to an individual who fails one of the tests of capacity and is therefore considered by law not mentally capable of performing a particular act or assuming a particular role. The adjudication of incompetence is subject or issue specific. In other words, the fact that a neuropsychiatric patient is adjudicated incompetent to execute a will does not automatically render that patient incompetent to do other things, such as consent to treatment, testify as a witness, marry, drive, or make a legally binding contract. In case 1 above, the court created a limited guardianship for financial matters only.

Generally, the law will recognize only those decisions or choices that have been made by a competent individual. The law seeks to protect incompetent individuals from the harmful effects of their acts. Persons over the age of majority, which is now 18 (17), are presumed to be competent (18). This presumption is rebuttable, however, by evidence of

TABLE 33–1. SOME AREAS OF LAW IN WHICH COMPETENCY IS AN ISSUE

Civil law
Act in public or professional capacity
Authorize disclosure of medical records
Consent to treatment
Contract
Guardianship—care for one's self and property[a]
Make a will
Obtain a driver's license
Receive benefits (e.g., Social Security)
Retain private counsel
Sue or be sued
Testify in court
Vote
Criminal law
Assume responsibility for a criminal act
Be executed
Consent to sexual intercourse
Entertain premeditation or "specific intent" of a crime
Make a confession
Make a plea
Provide testimony in court
Stand trial
Be sentenced
Waive the insanity defense
Waive the right to counsel
Family law
Adopt
Divorce
Marry
Terminate parental relations with a child

[a]See, for example, In re Guardianship of Pamela, 519 NE2d 1335 (Mass Sup Jud Ct 1988).

Source. Adapted from Bisbing SB: Competency and capacity, in Legal Medicine: Legal Dynamics of Medical Encounters. St. Louis, MO, Mosby Year Book, 1991, p 136.

not necessarily mean the defendant lacks the requisite cognitive ability to aid in his own defense at trial. The ultimate determination of incompetency is solely for the court to decide (78). Moreover, the impairment must be considered in the context of the particular case or proceeding. Mental impairment may render an individual incompetent to stand trial in a complicated tax fraud case, but not incompetent for a misdemeanor trial.

Psychiatrists and psychologists that testify as expert witnesses regarding the effect of neuropsychiatric problems on a defendant's competency to stand trial will be most effective if their findings are framed according to the degree to which the defendant is cognitively capable of meeting the standards enunciated in *Dusky*. Use of instruments like the CSTI to pragmatically illustrate actual functional conformity to competency standards is especially useful.

Insanity defense. In American jurisprudence, one of the most controversial issues is the insanity defense. Defendants with mental or neuropsychiatric disabilities who are found competent to stand trial may seek acquittal on the basis that they were not criminally responsible for their actions due to insanity at the time the offense was committed.

The vast majority of criminals choose to commit crimes for a number of reasons, but the law presumes all of them to do so rationally and of their own free will. As a result, the law concludes that they are deserving of some form of punishment. Some offenders, however, are so mentally disturbed in their thinking and behavior that they are thought to be incapable of acting rationally. Under these circumstances, civilized societies have deemed it unjust to punish a "crazy" or insane person (79). This is in part due to fundamental principles of fairness and morality. Additionally, the punishment of a person who cannot rationally appreciate the consequences of his or her actions thwarts the two major tenets of punishment: retribution and deterrence.

There is more than one insanity defense standard in the United States—depending on which state or jurisdiction has control over the defendant raising the defense. For example, in the Superior Court of the District of Columbia the standard states:

> A person is not responsible for [his] criminal conduct at the time of such conduct as a result of a mental disease or defect [80] if he lacked substantial capacity either to recognize the wrongfulness of his conduct or to conform his conduct to the requirements of the law. (81)

By contrast, defendants tried in a federal court are governed by the standard enunciated in the Comprehensive Crime Control Act (CCCA) of 1984 (82). The CCCA provides that it is an affirmative defense to all federal crimes that, at the time of the offense, "the defendant, as a result of a severe mental disease or defect, was unable to appreciate the nature and quality or the wrongfulness of his acts. Mental disease or defect does not otherwise constitute a defense" (83). This codification eliminates the volitional or irresistible impulse portion of the insanity defense. That is, it does not allow an insanity defense based on a defendant's inability to conform his or her conduct to the requirements of the law. The defense is now limited to only those defendants who are unable to appreciate the wrongfulness of their acts (i.e., the *cognitive portion* of the defense).

The threshold issue in making an insanity determination is not the existence of a mental disease or defect, per se, but the lack of substantial mental capacity because of it. Therefore, lack of capacity due to causes other than mental illness may be sufficient. For instance, mental retardation may represent an adequate basis for the insanity defense under certain circumstances. There are less commonly considered disorders that may be related to central nervous dysfunction that could potentially render a defendant legally incapable of conforming his or her behavior to the dictates of the law. These disorders include metabolic conditions (e.g., functional hypoglycemia) (84), premenstrual syndrome (PMS) (85), and episodic dyscontrol syndrome (86,87a).

Depending on the severity of the condition and its actual impact on an offender's cognitive and affective processes, a defense of insanity might be warranted. At the very least, however, these conditions (see Table 33–4) should be investigated as mitigating factors that may have caused the offender to suffer from *diminished capacity*.

Diminished capacity. It is possible for a person to have the required *mens rea* and yet still be declared legally insane. For example, a defendant's actions may be considered so "crazy" as to convince a jury that he or she was criminally insane and therefore not legally responsible, yet his or her knowledge of what they were doing (e.g., committing a murder) was relatively intact. From this distinction, the law

TABLE 33–4. PERSONALITY AND COGNITIVE CHANGES ASSOCIATED WITH FRONTAL CORTEX DAMAGE

Social and Behavioral Changes
Impulsivity and distractibility
Apathy, general lack of concern for consequences of behavior
Exacerbation of preexisting behavioral traits such as anxiousness, suspiciousness, disorderliness
Uncharacteristic lewdness with loss of social restraint, inattention to personal hygiene and appearance
Increased risk taking, unrestrained consumption of alcohol and food to the point of gluttony
Intrusiveness, uncharacteristic profanity, boisterousness
Affect Changes
Apathy, shallowness, indifference
Lability of affect, manic states, irritability
Lack of control of rage and violent behavior
Intellectual Changes
Reduced ability to use language, symbols and logic
Impaired ability to focus, concentrate, and determine time and place orientation
Impaired ability to calculate, process abstract information, reason, and conduct arithmetic processing

Source. Adapted from MacKinnin RA, Yudofsky SC: Psychiatric Evaluation in Clinical Practice. Philadelphia, PA, JB Lippincott, 1986.

recognized that there are "shades" of mental impairment that obviously can affect *mens rea* but not necessarily to the extent of completely nullifying it. In recognition of this fact, the concept of diminished capacity was developed (87b).

Broadly viewed, diminished capacity permits the accused to introduce medical and psychological evidence that relates directly to the *mens rea* for the crime charged, without having to assert a defense of insanity (87b). For example, for the crime of assault with the intent to kill, psychiatric testimony would be permitted to address whether the offender acted with the purpose of committing homicide at the time of the assault. When a defendant's *mens rea* for the crime charged is nullified by clinical evidence, the defendant is acquitted only of that charge. Patients suffering from neuropsychiatric disorders who commit criminal acts may be eligible for a diminished capacity defense.

There are several other exculpatory and mitigating defenses that, although lesser known and statistically limited in success, bear mentioning because of their potential connection to neuropsychiatric conditions or causes.

The *automatism* (or unconscious) defense recognizes that some criminal acts may be committed involuntarily (87b). Automatism is defined as "having performed in a state of mental unconsciousness or dissociation without full awareness" and is applied to actions or conduct occurring "without will, purpose, or reasoned intention" (88).

The classic, although rare, example is the person who commits an offense while sleepwalking. Courts have held that such an individual does not have conscious control of his or her physical actions and therefore acts involuntarily (89). Other situations relevant to neuropsychiatry in which the automatism defense might be used arise when a crime is committed during a state of unconsciousness caused by a concussion following a head injury, involuntary ingestion of drugs or alcohol, metabolic disorders such as anoxia or hypoglycemia, or epileptic seizures (90).

There are, however, limitations to the automatism defense. Most notably some courts hold that if the person asserting the automatism defense was aware of the condition before the offense and failed to take reasonable steps to prevent the criminal occurrence, then the defense is not available. For example, if a defendant with a known history of uncontrolled epileptic seizures loses control of a car during a seizure and kills someone, that defendant will not be permitted to assert the defense of automatism.

Ordinarily, *intoxication* is not a defense to a criminal charge. Because intoxication, unlike mental illness, mental retardation, and most neuropsychiatric conditions, is usually the product of a person's own actions, the law is naturally cautious about viewing it as a complete defense or a mitigating factor. Most states view voluntary alcoholism as relevant to the issue of whether the defendant possessed the *mens rea* necessary to commit a specific intent crime or whether there was premeditation in a crime of murder. Generally, however, the mere fact that the defendant was voluntarily intoxicated will not justify a finding of automatism or insanity. A distinct difference does arise when, because of chronic, heavy use of alcohol, the defendant is suffering from an alcohol-induced organic mental disorder, such as alcohol hallucinosis, withdrawal delirium, amnestic disorder, or dementia associated with alcoholism. If competent neuropsychiatric evidence is presented that an alcohol-related neuropsychiatric disorder caused significant cognitive or volitional impairment, a defense of insanity or diminished capacity could be upheld.

Another "mental state" defense occasionally raised by defendants regarding assault-related crimes is that the assaultive behavior was involuntarily precipitated by abnormal electrical patterns in their brain. This condition is frequently diagnosed as *temporal lobe epilepsy* (91). Recently, episodic dyscontrol syndrome (92) has also been advanced as a neuropsychiatric condition causing involuntary aggression. Studies have hypothesized that there are "centers of aggression" in the temporal lobe or limbic system—primarily the amygdala. This hypothesis has promoted the idea that sustained aggressive behavior by these persons may be primarily the product of an uncontrollable, randomly occurring, abnormal brain dysrhythmia. Hence, the legal argument is raised that these individuals should not be held accountable for their actions. Despite its simplicity and occasional success in the courts, there are few empirically significant data to support this theory at this time (93).

Defenses based on *metabolic disorders* have also been tried. The so-called Twinkie defense was used as part of a successful strategy to defend Dan White in the murders of San Francisco Mayor George Moscone and Supervisor Harvey Milk. This defense was based on the theory that the ingestion of large amounts of sugar contributed to a state of temporary insanity (94). The forensic psychiatric report stated that the defendant had been "filling himself up with Twinkies and Coca-Cola" (95; p. 16). After specifying a number of factors that contributed to the murders, the forensic examiner concluded with his opinion concerning Dan White's ingestion of certain food:

> Finally, there is much evidence to suggest recently recognized physiological aberrations consequent to consumption of noxious edibles by susceptibles. There are cases in the literature challenged with large quantities of refined sugar. Furthermore, there are studies of cerebral allergic reactions to the chemicals in highly processed foods; some studies have documented a marked reduction in violent and antisocial behavior in "career criminals" upon the elimination of these substances from their diet, as well as the production of rage reactions in susceptible individuals when challenged by the offending food substances. For these reasons, I would suggest a repeat electroencephalogram preceded by a glucose-tolerance test, as well as a clinical challenge of Mr. White's mental functions with known food antigens, in a controlled setting. (95; pp. 21–22)

Hypoglycemic states also may be associated with significant psychiatric impairment (96). The brain is dependent on a steady supply of glucose through the blood stream. When the glucose level drops significantly, the brain has no backup energy source to compensate. When this occurs, metabolism naturally slows down and cerebral function is impaired. Because the cerebral cortex and parts of the cerebellum metabolize glucose at the highest rate, they are the first to suffer when there is an energy depletion (97). When a substantial glucose depletion occurs, a wide variety of responses may occur including episodic and repetitive dyscontrol, temporary amnesia, depression, and hostility with spontaneous recovery (quick recovery following the consumption of appropriate nutrients). The degree of mental abnormality associated with hypoglycemic states varies from mild to severe according to blood glucose level. It is the degree of disturbance, not the mere presence of an etiological metabolic component, that is determinative in a mental state defense. This principle also applies to mental dysfunctions produced by metabolic disorders originating in the hepatic, renal, adrenal, and endocrine systems.

❑ NEUROPSYCHIATRIC MALPRACTICE

Neuropsychiatric malpractice is medical malpractice. Malpractice is the provision of substandard professional care that causes a compensable injury to a person with whom a professional relationship existed. Although this concept may seem relatively clear and simple, it has its share of conditions and caveats. For example, the essential issue is not the existence of substandard care, per se, but whether there is actual compensable liability. For a physician to be found liable to a patient for malpractice, several fundamental concepts must be established.

Medical malpractice is a tort or civil wrong (i.e., a noncriminal or noncontract-related wrong) committed as a result of negligence by physicians or other health care professionals that causes injury to a patient in their care. *Negligence*, the fundamental concept underlying a malpractice lawsuit, is simply described as doing something that a person with a duty of care (to the patient) should not have done or failing to do something that a person with a duty of care should have done. The fact that a psychiatrist commits an act of negligence does not automatically make him or her liable to the patient bringing the lawsuit. Liability for malpractice is based on the plaintiff's (e.g., patient's) establishing by a preponderance of the evidence that 1) there was a duty of care owed by the defendant (duty), 2) that duty of care was breached (deviation), 3) the plaintiff suffered actual damages (damages), and 4) the deviation was the direct cause of the damages (direct causation). These elements are sometimes referred to as the four Ds of malpractice.

Each of these elements must be met or there can be no finding of liability, regardless of any finding of negligence. In other words, a physician can actually have been negligent but still not be found liable. For example, if the plaintiff suffered no real injuries because of the negligence or if there was an injury but it was not directly due to the doctor's negligence, then a claim of malpractice will be defeated.

Critical to the establishment of a claim of professional negligence is the requirement that the defendant's conduct was substandard or was a deviation in the standard of care owed to the plaintiff. The law presumes and holds all physicians (psychiatrists) to a standard of ordinary care, which is measured by its reasonableness according to the clinical circumstances in which it is provided.

Somatic Therapies

Generally speaking, psychiatric intervention with neuropsychiatric patients, especially those exhibiting serious affective, delusional, or aggressive disorders, is essentially composed of drug therapy and electroconvulsive therapy (ECT). A brief review of the standard of care of these procedures is instructive in understanding the basis for any lawsuits involving neuropsychiatric treatment procedures.

The therapeutic use of a somatic therapy, including ECT, is evaluated no differently from any other medical or psychiatric procedure with respect to its application and potential liability. The same general standard of ordinary and reasonable care will, therefore, govern the assessment of whether a psychiatrist's use or failure to use a somatic intervention is actionable (98).

It is generally acknowledged within the psychiatric profession that there is no absolute standard protocol for the administration of psychotropic medication or ECT. The existence of certain guidelines, procedures, and authoritative resources regularly accepted or used by a significant percentage of psychiatrists, however, should alert clinicians to consider them as a reference and counsel. For example, APA published comprehensive findings in the form of task force reports on ECT (99) and tardive dyskinesia (100). The task force report on ECT was recently updated by APA and should be considered the leading resource with regard to ECT treatment. The revised task force report on tardive dyskinesia is due soon.

It is important to note that "on their own," these or any other publications, do not, per se, establish the standard of care by which a court might evaluate a psychiatrist's treatment. They do represent, however, a credible source of information with which a reasonable psychiatrist should at least be familiar and have considered (101). It is the failure to consider these and other sources (e.g., current reviews of the clinical literature) that the courts will most likely look to in establishing contemporary psychiatric practices and determining the standard of care.

There is some evidence that there is less professional autonomy and flexibility associated with the use of ECT. Normally, the "reasonable care" standard that is applied to psychiatric treatment is construed in a fairly broad manner because psychiatry is currently considered inexact. Some psychiatric treatments such as ECT, however, appear to be more rigidly regulated than others. For example, the Joint Commission on Accreditation of Healthcare Organizations (JCAHO) considers ECT a special treatment procedure, requiring hospitals to have written, informed consent policies concerning its use (102). These standards, coupled with any specific regulations a facility might have promulgated regarding ECT, could serve as establishing the basis for liability if violated. Nevertheless, no official guidelines should be interpreted as a substitute for sound clinical judgment.

The "standard" for judging the use and administration of medication, on the other hand, appears to be consistent with the more flexible and general "reasonable care" requirement. The third reference source that bears highlighting is the use of the *Physicians' Desk Reference (PDR)* to establish or dispute a psychiatrist's pharmacotherapy procedures. The *PDR* is a commercially distributed, privately published reference regarding medication products used in the United States. The Food and Drug Administration (FDA) requires that drug manufacturers have their official package inserts reported in *PDR* (103). Accordingly, to keep abreast of new medication treatments and provide patients with current and accurate medication information, psychiatrists should periodically consult publications like *PDR*. **However**, although numerous courts have cited *PDR* as a credible source of medication-related information in the medical profession (104), it does not by itself, establish *the* standard of care. Instead, the *PDR* may be used as one piece of evidence to establish the standard of care in a particular situation (105). The *PDR* or any other reference, however, cannot serve as a substitute for a clinician's judgment.

Fortunately, courts recognize the importance of professional judgment and will give psychiatrists and other medical specialists some latitude in explaining any special diagnostic or treatment considerations that guided their decision making. For example, the research data regarding pharmacologic treatment of aggression in neurologically impaired patients indicate that there is a variety of potentially useful drug therapies—some that are considered experimental or on the cutting edge (106). Yet no drug is presently approved by the FDA for the treatment of aggression (107).

Accordingly, the courts will consider the fact that no one treatment of choice exists and that treatment applications are still being developed. Moreover, evidence that a treatment procedure is accepted by at least a respectable minority of professionals in the field could establish that the modality is a reasonable professional practice. For example, reliance on the "12-Step Guide to the Clinical Use of Propranolol" (108) for the treatment of patients with organic personality disorder, explosive type, might be considered reasonable care in a lawsuit against a psychiatrist for the negligent treatment of a violent patient who injures the plaintiff. The determining factor would be whether these "guidelines" could be established as representing reasonable clinical practice.

Notwithstanding these special concerns, the standard of care associated with the use of a somatic therapy to treat a neuropsychiatric patient should, at a minimum, include some variation of the following considerations and measures:

- Pretreatment
  - Complete clinical history (e.g., medical and psychological) (109)
  - Complete physical examination, if needed
  - Administration of necessary laboratory tests and review of all past test results (110)
  - Disclosure of sufficient information to obtain informed consent, including information regarding the consequences of *not* receiving treatment
  - Thorough documentation of all decisions, informed consent information, patient responses, and any other relevant treatment data
- Posttreatment
  - Careful monitoring of the patient's response to treatment, including frequent patient interviews and appropriate laboratory testing (111)
  - Prompt adjustments in treatment, as needed
  - Obtaining a renewed informed consent when appreciably altering treatment or initiating new treatment

Different treatment approaches will require different preparations and precautions. Moreover, the final word regarding pre- and posttreatment measures depends on the clinician and not the law. However, the above considerations should be viewed as general guidelines that are commonly associated with reasonable care when somatic therapies are implemented.

Theories of Liability in Neuropsychiatry

The term *psychiatric malpractice* is a misnomer because the same basic legal principles will be applied to any lawsuit alleging malpractice by a patient, regardless of medical subspecialty. Adjectives such as *psychiatric* or *neuropsychiatric* reflect the general recognition that the theories of liability to be discussed represent the most common areas of malpractice associated with that subspecialty. The following is a limited review of the most common litigation areas in treating neuropsychiatric patients.

Medication. The potential for negligence by a psychiatrist would appear greatest in clinical situations involving the use of psychotropic medications. Although no reliable compilation of malpractice claims data has been published, anecdotal information suggests that medication-related lawsuits constitute a significant share of the litigation filed against psychiatrists. For example, insurance data collected by the Medical Protective Company revealed that medication-related injuries constituted 20% of the total claims against psychiatrists between 1980 and 1985 (112) (Table 33–5). Similar figures are reported by APA's insurance committee and other commentators studying the incidence of psychiatric malpractice claims (113).

TABLE 33–5. PSYCHIATRY CLAIMS CLOSED, 1980–1985

Claims	Percent of total
Incarceration/suicide attempts	21%
Drugs (overdose or addiction)	20%
Miscellaneous (failure to diagnose physical condition, breach of contract, and other claims)	18%
Psychotherapy/depression	14%
Failure to treat psychosis	14%
Restraints (paralysis or fracture)	7%
Sexual misconduct	6%
Dollars	
Incarceration/suicide attempts	42%
Sexual misconduct	16%
Restraints (paralysis or fracture)	16%
Drugs (overdose or addiction)	10%
Miscellaneous	8%
Failure to treat psychosis	5%
Psychotherapy/depression	3%

Source. Cited from *Psychiatric News.*

A review of the relevant case law indicates that a variety of mistakes, omissions, and poor pharmacological treatment practices commonly result in malpractice actions brought against a psychiatrist or other physician. The following list, although not intended to be exhaustive, provides a workable framework for identifying problem areas associated with medication treatment:

1. *Failure to properly evaluate.* Sound clinical practice requires that the patient be properly examined before any form of somatic treatment is initiated. The nature and extent of an examination is largely dictated by the type of treatment being contemplated. At the very minimum, physical examination, clinical history, and mental status examination should be conducted. A recent physical examination may suffice or the patient may be referred by psychiatrists who do not perform physical examinations. Moreover, the duty to ensure that proper informed consent is obtained can also be fulfilled at this time.

   A number of lawsuits have resulted from the failure to properly evaluate a patient before administering psychotropic medication (114). As a result of this omission, the patient's condition is misdiagnosed and remains untreated. Additionally, the patient is exposed (without giving informed consent) to unnecessary side effects and risks.
2. *Failure to monitor or supervise.* Probably the most common act of negligence associated with pharmacotherapy is the failure to supervise the patient's progress on the medication, including monitoring the patient for adverse side effects.

   Once psychotropic medication has been prescribed, it is the physician's duty to monitor or supervise the patient. This monitoring may require the use of laboratory testing; physical examination and medical referral, if necessary; and, of course, direct interviewing of the patient and other reliable parties. Serum drug levels are now obtainable for a number of psychotropic medications. The primary indications for these laboratory tests include assessing therapeutic and toxic levels of medication and patient compliance with treatment. The use of carbamazepine, valproic acid, and clozapine requires close monitoring of the hematopoietic system and liver. A failure to properly supervise patients on psychotropic medication can unnecessarily subject them to harmful side effects and can delay a change to more effective treatment. If a patient is harmed from these omissions, a malpractice action might result (115).
3. *Negligent prescription practices.* The selection of a medication, initial dosage, form of administration, and other related procedures are all decisions left to the sound discretion of the treating

psychiatrist. The law recognizes that the physician is in the best position to "know the patient" and to determine what course of treatment is best under the circumstances. Accordingly, the standard by which a psychiatrist's prescription practices will be evaluated is whether they are reasonable. In administering psychotropic medication, psychiatrists need only conform their procedures and decision making to those that are ordinarily practiced by other psychiatrists under similar circumstances.

Negligent prescription procedures usually involve several common practices representing fairly serious deviations from generally accepted treatment practice. These include exceeding recommended dosages and then failing to adjust the medication level to therapeutic levels, negligent mixing of drugs (or polypharmacy), prescribing medication for unapproved uses, prescribing "unapproved" medications, and failing to disclose medication effects.

As stated above, any physician who prescribes medication has a duty to explain the purpose, action, and risks of the drug within reason and as circumstances permit. Obtaining competent informed consent may be complicated by the fact that a significant number of neuropsychiatric patients have diminished cognitive capacity due to mental illness, physical trauma, or chronic organic impairment.

Each time a medication is changed and a new drug is introduced, informed consent should be obtained. A failure to properly inform a patient of the risks and consequences of ingesting a medication is ample grounds for a malpractice action, if the patient is injured as a result (116).

4. *Other.* Areas of negligence involving medication that have also resulted in legal action include failure to treat side effects once they have been recognized or should have been recognized, failure to monitor a patient's compliance with prescription limits, failure to prescribe medication or appropriate levels of medication according to the treatment needs of the patient, failure to refer a patient for consultation or treatment by a specialist, and negligent withdrawal from medication.

Tardive dyskinesia. The following case example illustrates the potential for legal liability when a patient taking neuroleptics is not monitored carefully.

Case 5

A 56-year-old woman with a 30-year history of mild mental retardation and schizophrenia is seen for medication appointment every 6–9 months. She has been taking major tranquilizers for nearly 30 years. The patient lives in a rural area, making it difficult to see her psychiatrist more often. During a 9-month interval between appointments, she develops oral-lingual dyskinesia. On discontinuation of the neuroleptic, her dyskinetic symptoms spread and become more severe. The patient is unable to work and maintain herself. Her family brings a lawsuit against the psychiatrist for negligence in failing to monitor the patient and her medications.

The development of neuroleptic medications in the mid-1950s created a considerable stir in the psychiatric community with regard to the improvement of patient management and treatment. Shortly after the introduction of neuroleptic medications as therapeutic agents, however, researchers and clinicians observed unusual muscle movements (later referred to as tardive dyskinesia [TD]) in certain patients treated with these drugs. Numerically, the number of psychiatric patients being treated with neuroleptics is quite high (117), and it is estimated that at least 10%–20% (96) and perhaps as many as 50% of all patients (118) exposed to neuroleptic drugs for more than 1 year exhibit some degree of probable TD. These projections are even higher for elderly patients (119). Given these data, the potential for TD litigation appears obvious. Despite the possibility of numerous TD-related suits, however, relatively few psychiatrists have been sued under this cause of action. In addition, patients who develop TD may not have the physical and psychological staying power required to pursue litigation.

Cases involving allegations of negligence after a patient developed TD are based on the same legal elements as any other malpractice action. Moreover, the bases for negligence mirror those that have been previously identified with general medication cases including (but not limited to) failure to properly evaluate a patient, failure to obtain informed consent, and negligent diagnosis of a patient's condition.

For example, in *Hyde v. University of Michigan Board of Regents* (120), a woman was awarded $1,000,000 from a medical center that misdiagnosed her condition—TD—as Huntington's chorea. This verdict was later reversed on the basis of a subsequent case that expanded the state's sovereign immunity coverage (121).

In *Dovido v. Vasquez* (122), a net award of $700,000 went to a 42-year-old plaintiff who suffered from TD as a result of the defendant psychiatrist's negligent prescription of extremely high doses of fluphenazine.

In *Clites v. State* (123), the plaintiff was a mentally retarded man who had been institutionalized since age 11 and treated with major tranquilizers from ages 18 to 23. TD was diagnosed at age 23, and the plaintiff subsequently sued. The family claimed that the defendants had negligently prescribed medication, had not informed the family of the possibility of developing TD, and failed to monitor and subsequently treat the patient's resulting side effects. The jury returned a verdict for the plaintiff and awarded damages in the amount of $760,165. This award was affirmed on appeal. The court ruled that the defendants were negligent because they deviated from the standards of the "industry." Specifically, the court cited various omissions in common psychiatric practice that, they concluded, reasonable psychiatrists would have provided. Among the "deviations" they noted were a failure to conduct regular physical examinations and laboratory tests, failure to intervene at the first sign of TD, the inappropriate use of multiple medications at the same time, the use of drugs for convenience (e.g., "behavior management") rather than therapy, and the failure to obtain the plaintiff's informed consent.

As case 5 demonstrates, patients receiving neuroleptic medication need to be monitored frequently. For example, seeing such patients every 6 months (or even less frequently) may lead to legal claims of failure to properly monitor the patient.

The defenses and preventive measures applicable to TD-related malpractice claims are consistent with those used in any case alleging negligent drug treatment. Generally speaking, the application of sound clinical practice that is appropriately communicated to the patient and documented in the treatment chart will serve as an effective foil to any allegation of negligence should TD develop (124).

Moreover, for the psychiatrist who is treating chronic aggression with antipsychotic drugs, it is instructive to consider the observations of one commentator who noted

> The use of antipsychotic medication in treating chronic aggression involves a substantial risk of the emergence of tardive dyskinesia, because the prevalence of tardive dyskinesia among patients on long-term neuroleptic treatment is about 25% . . . .
>
> While antipsychotic agents are the treatment of choice for aggression due to psychosis and also may be helpful in the acute short-term management of violence through sedative action, we do not recommend their use in the long-term management of aggression, especially that which is secondary to organic brain syndrome. (125; pp. 397, 400)

ECT. Although a significant proportion of psychiatrists believe ECT is a viable treatment for certain mental disorders (126), it has been estimated that no more that 3%–5% of all psychiatric inpatients in the United States receive this form of treatment (127). As can be expected from these figures, the potential number of legal actions alleging negligence associated with ECT is likely to be low. Commentators who have reported on the incidence of ECT-related malpractice suits have corroborated this suspicion (128).

Despite this low potential, lawsuits involving ECT are occasionally brought. Cases involving ECT-related injuries have represented a variety of circumstances in which negligence has occurred. These cases can be categorized into three groups: pretreatment, treatment, and posttreatment.

Although there is some variation in pre-ECT evaluations, generally five procedures—recommended by the APA Task Force on ECT (99)—should be observed: 1) a psychiatric history and examination to evaluate the indications for ECT, 2) a medical examination to determine risk factors, 3) an anesthesia evaluation, 4) informed consent (written), and 5) an evaluation by a physician privileged to administer ECT.

Although the APA Task Force on ECT Recommendations do not define in any absolute sense the standard of care for ECT, the task force report may be proffered as evidence of the standard of care by attorneys in malpractice suits involving ECT. Official treatment guidelines, however, should never be a substitute for the psychiatrist's sound clinical judgment. Nevertheless, failure to adequately conduct one of these *pretreatment* procedures could endanger the welfare of the patient and ultimately result in a lawsuit for negligence.

It is well established that a psychiatrist will not be held liable for a mere mistake in judgment, nor will a psychiatrist be held to a standard of 100% accuracy or perfect performance (129). Therefore, a bad result does not automatically establish a claim for malpractice (130). Instead, a patient must prove, by a preponderance of the evidence, that the physician deviated from the standard of care and that deviation proximately caused the patient some injury or damage. The procedure for evaluating the care and treatment afforded a patient when ECT is used is no different. Cases involving ECT-related injuries in which the negligence has centered around the actual *treatment* process include 1) failure to use a muscle relaxant to reduce the chance of a bone fracture, 2) negligent administration of the procedure, and 3) failure to conduct an evaluation of an injured patient, including the failure to obtain X rays, before continuing treatment.

It is not uncommon for patients being treated with ECT to experience certain side effects such as temporary confusion, disorientation, and memory loss following its administration (22,126). Due to this temporary debilitating effect, sound clinical practice requires that the psychiatrists provide reasonable *posttreatment* care and safeguards. Courts have held that the failure to properly attend to a patient for a period of time following the administration of ECT can result in malpractice liability. Posttreatment circumstances in which legal liability may occur include 1) failure to evaluate complaints of pain or discomfort following treatment, 2) failure to evaluate a patient's condition before resuming ECT treatments, 3) failure to properly monitor a patient to prevent falls, and 4) failure to properly supervise a patient who had been injured as a result of ECT.

As a source of civil liability, ECT-related law suits today are quite rare and are not likely to represent a significant problem area for psychiatrists. But, as Perlin cautioned, "recent developments in right-to-refuse treatment law and statutory regulation of intrusive therapy are likely to ensure that any future ECT litigation will still be considered carefully" (131; pp. 47–48).

The violent patient. The following case example illustrates the legal liability associated with the treatment and management of the violent patient.

Case 6

A 16-year-old male suffers extensive frontal lobe damage after an automobile accident. The patient's main difficulties are low frustration tolerance, impulsiveness, and violent outbursts. He threatens to kill a student at his high school who has been teasing him. The patient is consistently noncompliant with neuroleptic treatment. His private psychiatrist persuades him to enter a psychiatric hospital and asks a consultant to perform a neuropsychiatric evaluation. A regimen of various pharmacological agents is recommended. In addition, the psychiatrist and other staff employ behavior modification and biofeedback.

One month after admission, the patient is assessed to be "psychiatrically stable" and is released. Three days after his discharge, he fatally shoots the high-school student that he had earlier identified as tormenting him. The deceased student's parents file suit against the hospital, treating psychiatrist, and the consulting psychiatrist for negligent treatment and negligent discharge of the patient. They also allege the failure to warn them and their son of the threats made by the patient.

Aggressive and violent behaviors are common among patients exhibiting neuropsychiatric disorders. Aggressive and threatening behavior often precipitates admissions to psychiatric hospitals. In one survey it was found that 10% of patients at a state psychiatric facility had had assaultive behavior in the 2 weeks before admission (132). In addition, it is not uncommon for neuropsychiatric patients to exhibit aggression after hospitalization (133). Besides the clinical challenges that these patients represent, they also create certain legal concerns.

For psychiatrists who treat violent or potentially violent patients, probably the greatest risk of a lawsuit involves *failure to control aggressive outpatients* and *the discharge of violent inpatients*.

Psychiatrists can be sued for failing to protect society from the violent acts of their patients if it was reasonable for the psychiatrist to have known about the patient's dangerous proclivities and if he or she was in a position to do something that may have safeguarded the public. Since the landmark case *Tarasoff v. Regents of the University of California* (134), in which the California Supreme Court held that mental health professionals had a duty to protect third parties from imminent threats of serious harm made by patients in their care, courts and state legislatures have increasingly held psychiatrists to a fictional standard of having to predict the future behavior (dangerousness) of potentially violent patients that they are treating.

Psychiatrists who treat violent, aggressive, or potentially dangerous outpatients must be cognizant of their responsibility not only to the patient but also to any person or persons that might be a foreseeable victim of the patient's aggression. Accordingly, psychiatrists must adequately assess the patient's risk of violence to self or others as part of the general psychiatric examination. Furthermore, the mental capacity of patients at risk for violence must also be evaluated. This is particularly critical for neuropsychiatric patients manifesting cognitive deficits and diminished impulse control. Serious depression may be a consequence of compromised brain functioning that may go undetected. Patients with brain disorders may lack the capacity to properly inform the psychiatrist of violent intentions. Generally, the psychiatrist must exercise close supervision of patients lacking full mental capacity, both cognitively and affectively.

If a patient threatens harm to a third party, a majority of states require that the psychiatrist perform some act that might prevent the harm from occurring. In states with duty-to-warn statutes, the responses available to psychiatrists and psychotherapists are defined by law. In states offering no such guidance, health care providers are required to use clinical judgment appropriate to the situation that will accomplish the objective of safeguarding the object of the patient's threat. Typically, a variety of options are clinically and legally available including voluntary hospitalization, involuntary hospitalization (if civil commitment requirements are met), warning the intended victim of the threat, notifying the police, adjusting medication, and seeing the patient more frequently (135).

The following case example illustrates discharge or release considerations involved in working with violent or potentially violent patients.

Case 7

A 37-year-old epileptic man is discharged from a psychiatric hospital after treatment for alcohol intoxication and random violence. The patient has had numerous, similar psychiatric hospital admissions before. The violent acts occur only when alcohol intoxication is combined with the discontinuance of his anticonvulsant medication. The psychiatrist works closely with the patient to ensure follow-up treatment within the first week of discharge. The patient seems motivated to stop drinking, promising to continue attending Alcoholic Anonymous meetings begun in the hospital. The psychiatrist call the patient's outpatient therapist to be sure the first appointment is kept.

Violent or potentially violent patients in an inpatient setting represent a unique and challenging situation for treating psychiatrists. In a hospital there is more control over the patient than is available in an outpatient setting. Courts strictly evaluate decisions made by psychiatrists who treat inpatients that might adversely affect the patient or a third party.

The psychiatric-legal issues surrounding seclusion and restraint of violent inpatients are complicated and discussed fully elsewhere (136). Seclusion and restraint as clinical management modalities have both indications and contraindications (Tables 33–6 and 33–7). The legal regulation of seclusion and restraint has become increasingly more stringent over the past decade.

Lawsuits stemming from the release of a foreseeably dangerous patient who subsequently injures or kills himself or someone else are a source of considerable litigation. Such litigation is much more common than outpatient duty-to-warn lawsuits. Case 7 illustrates some of the clinical issues surrounding discharge of the potentially violent patient. Psychiatrists should not discharge patients and then forget about them. The patient's willingness to cooperate with the psychiatrist, however, is critical to maintaining follow-up treatment. The psychiatrist's obligation focuses on structuring the follow-up visits in a fashion that encourages compliance. A study of Veteran's Administration (VA) outpatient referrals showed that of 24% of inpatients referred to the VA mental health clinic, approximately 50% failed to keep their first appointments (137). Limitations do exist, however, on the extent of the psychiatrist's ability to ensure follow-up care. This must be acknowledged by both the psychiatric and legal communities (138).

In either the outpatient or inpatient situation, psychiatrists will comply with this responsibility if they reasonably assess a patient's potential risk for violence and act in a clinically appropriate manner based on their findings. Professional standards do

TABLE 33–6. INDICATIONS FOR SECLUSION AND RESTRAINT

1. Prevent clear, imminent harm to the patient or others
2. Prevent significant disruption to treatment program or physical surroundings
3. Assist in treatment as part of ongoing behavior therapy
4. Decrease sensory overstimulation[a]
5. At patient's voluntary reasonable request

[a]Seclusion only.

Source. Reprinted from Simon RI: Concise Guide to Clinical Psychiatry and the Law. American Psychiatric Press, Washington, DC, 1988. Used with permission.

TABLE 33–7. CONTRAINDICATIONS TO SECLUSION AND RESTRAINT

1. Extremely unstable medical and psychiatric conditions[a]
2. Delirious or demented patients unable to tolerate decreased stimulation[a]
3. Overtly suicidal patients[a]
4. Patients with severe drug reactions, overdoses, or requiring close monitoring of drug dosages[a]
5. For punishment or convenience of staff

[a]Unless close supervision and direct observation provided.
Source. Reprinted from Simon RI: Concise Guide to Clinical Psychiatry and the Law. American Psychiatric Press, Washington, DC, 1988. Used with permission.

exist for the assessment of the risk factors for violence (139). No standard of care exists, however, for the prediction of violent behavior. The clinician should assess the risk of violence frequently, updating the risk assessment at significant clinical junctures (e.g., room and ward changes, passes, and discharge). A risk-benefit assessment should be conducted and recorded before issuing a pass or discharge.

Involuntary hospitalization. The following case example illustrates a common clinical indication for initiating a medical certification for involuntary hospitalization.

Case 8

A 72-year-old woman, living by herself, ceases to be able to care for herself due to a progressive dementia, but she refuses to allow anyone to enter her home. One night, she is heard screaming. The police are called; they forcibly enter the home and take her to an emergency room. The patient is profoundly confused, disoriented, and dehydrated. The emergency room physician signs medical certification papers indicating that she is gravely disabled by severe dementia and is a danger to herself. The patient is detained on a 7-day hold for psychiatric examination before her commitment hearing. At the hearing, the judge hears psychiatric evidence that the patient is severely demented. The court orders involuntary hospitalization for a period of 30 days.

A person may be involuntarily hospitalized only if certain statutorily mandated criteria are met. Three main substantive criteria serve as the foundation to all statutory commitment requirements: the individual must be 1) mentally ill, 2) dangerous to self or others, and/or 3) unable to provide for his or her basic needs. Generally, each state spells out which criteria are required and what each means. Terms such as *mentally ill* are often loosely described, thus displacing the responsibility for proper definition onto the clinical judgment of the petitioner.

In addition to individuals with mental illness, certain states have enacted legislation that permits the involuntary hospitalization of three other distinct groups: developmentally disabled (mentally retarded) persons, persons addicted to substances (alcohol and drugs), and mentally disabled minors. Special commitment provisions may exist governing requirements for the admission and discharge of mentally disabled minors as well as numerous due process rights afforded these individuals.

Involuntary hospitalization of neuropsychiatric patients usually arises when violent behavior threatens to erupt and when patients become unable to care for themselves. These patients frequently manifest mental disorders and conditions that readily meet the substantive criteria for involuntary hospitalization. In case 8, the patient suffers from severe dementia and is unable to care for herself. Thus she clearly meets the substantive criteria of mental illness and grave disability (inability to provide for her basic needs).

Clinicians must remember that they do not commit the patient. This is done solely under the jurisdiction of the court. The psychiatrist merely initiates a medical certification that brings the patient before the court, usually after a brief period of evaluation. Clinicians should not attempt to second-guess the court's ultimate decision concerning involuntary hospitalization. The psychiatrist must be guided by the treatment needs of the patient in seeking medical certification.

The most common type of lawsuit involving involuntary hospitalization usually relates to a physician's or psychiatrist's failure to adhere to the statutory requirements in good faith, which results in a wrongful commitment. Oftentimes, these lawsuits are brought under the theory of false imprisonment. Other areas of liability that may arise from wrongful commitment include assault and battery, malicious prosecution, abuse of authority, and intentional infliction of emotional distress.

In many states, psychiatrists are granted immunity from liability as long as they use reasonable professional judgment and act in good faith when petitioning for commitment (56). However, evidence of willful, blatant, or gross failure to adhere to statutorily defined commitment procedures will not likely immunize a psychiatrist from a lawsuit.

National Practitioner Data Bank. On September 1, 1990, the National Practitioner Data Bank established by the Health Care Quality Improvement Act of 1986 (42 U.S.C. Section 11101 [Supp V 1987]) went into effect. The data bank will track disciplinary actions and malpractice judgments and settlements against physicians, dentists, and other health care professionals (140).

Hospitals, health maintenance organizations (HMOs), professional societies, state medical boards, and other health care organizations are required to report any disciplinary action taken against providers lasting more than 30 days. Disciplinary actions include limitation, suspension, or revocation of privileges or professional society membership. Under the Health Care Quality Improvement Act, immunity from liability is granted for health care entities and providers making peer review reports in good faith (141).

Hospitals are required to request from the data bank information concerning all physicians applying for staff privileges. Every 2 years, a query of the data bank will be required concerning each physician or other practitioner on the hospital staff. Hospitals that do not comply face loss of immunity for professional peer review activities.

Personal Injury Litigation

This final case example illustrates the double agent role of a therapist who becomes an expert witness for the patient.

Case 9

A 42-year-old woman has been treated by insight psychotherapy for moderate anxiety and depression for 3 years. When her car is struck from behind by a truck while she is waiting at a traffic light, she suffers a moderate concussion. Severe symptoms of a postconcussion syndrome persist for 10 months after the accident. The treating psychiatrist agrees to act as the patient's expert witness. At the trial, the psychiatrist is closely questioned about psychiatric problems that preexisted the accident. Highly personal, embarrassing details of the patient's life are brought out by opposing counsel's cross examination of the psychiatrist. The jury awards the patient nominal monetary damages. The patient never returns to therapy.

Head injuries. Traumatic head injury is an enormous medical, social, and economic problem. It is estimated that the annual incidence of serious head injury is over 500,000 new cases (142). The National Head Injury Foundation estimated that at least 50,000 of these patients suffer chronic disability each year (143).

Patients with compromised brain function may manifest difficulties in judgment, mood regulation, memory, orientation, insight, impulse control, and the maintenance of a clear sensorium. In addition, they are likely to suffer from a plethora of psychiatric symptoms. The plaintiff's (person bringing suit) organic and psychiatric injuries are likely to produce large economic losses due to unemployment, which may be permanent. In combination with current and future medical expenses, it is easy to see that compensable damages from head trauma can be substantial.

To establish in court the nature and extent of any psychiatric and neurological problems and to determine their relationship to the event causing the head trauma, expert testimony will be needed. One of the most important experts in this type of litigation is the psychiatrist.

Neuropsychiatric expert. The ensuing civil litigation in head injury cases generally requires the evaluation and testimony of a psychiatrist, as well as neurologist, neuropsychologist, and other mental health professionals. These professionals can become involved in litigation as witnesses in two ways: as *treating physicians* or as *forensic experts.*

Psychiatrists who venture into the legal arena must be aware of the fundamentally different roles between a treating psychiatrist and the forensic psychiatric expert. For the treating psychiatrist, treatment and expert roles do not mix. Unlike the orthopedist who possess objective, concrete information, such as the X ray of a broken limb to demonstrate orthopedic damages in court, the treating psychiatrist must rely heavily on the subjective reporting of the patient. In a clinical context, psychiatrists are interested primarily in the patient's perception of difficulties, not necessarily objective reality. As a consequence, many psychiatrists do not speak to third parties to gain information about a patient or corroborate their statements. The law, however, is only interested in what can reasonably be established as fact. Uncorroborated, subjective patient data are frequently attacked in court as being speculative, self-serving, and unreliable. The treating psychiatrist usually is not well equipped to counter these charges.

Credibility issues also abound. The treating psychiatrist is, and must be, a total ally of the patient. This bias toward the patient is a proper treatment stance that fosters the therapeutic alliance. Furthermore, to effectively treat psychiatric patients, the patient must be "liked" by the psychiatrist. No therapist can effectively treat a patient for very long who is fundamentally disliked (by the therapist). Moreover, the therapist looks for psychiatric disorders. This again is an appropriate bias for the treating psychiatrist.

In court, credibility is a critical virtue to possess when testifying. Opposing counsel will take every opportunity to portray the treating psychiatrist as a subjective mouthpiece for the plaintiff, which may or may not be true. Also, as case 9 demonstrates, court testimony by the treating psychiatrist may compel the disclosure of information that may not be legally privileged but is nonetheless seen as private and confidential by the patient. This disclosure by the trusted therapist is bound to cause psychological damage to the therapeutic relationship (144). In addition, psychiatrists must be careful to inform patients about the consequences of releasing treatment information, particularly in legal matters. Section 4, Annotation 2 of the Principles of Medical Ethics with Annotations Especially Applicable to Psychiatry (1989) states:

> The continuing duty of the psychiatrist to protect the patient includes fully apprising him/her of the connotations of waiving the privilege of privacy. This may become an issue when the patient is being investigated by a government agency, is applying for a position, or is involved in legal action. (145, p. 6)

Finally, when the treating psychiatrist testifies concerning the need for further treatment, a conflict of interest is readily apparent. In making such treatment prognostications, the therapist stands to benefit economically from further treatment. Although this may not be the psychiatrist's intention whatsoever, opposing counsel is sure to point out that the psychiatrist has a financial interest in the case.

Although opposing counsel may attempt to depict the forensic expert as a "hired gun," he or she is usually free of these encumbrances. No doctor-patient relationship is created during forensic evaluation with its treatment biases toward the patient. The expert can review various records and speak to numerous people who know the litigant. Furthermore, the forensic expert is not as easily distracted from considering exaggeration or malingering because of a clear appreciation of the litigation context and the absence of treatment bias. Finally, the forensic psychiatrist is not placed in a conflict-of-interest position of recommending treatment from which the treating psychiatrist would necessarily benefit.

The treating psychiatrist should attempt to remain solely in a treatment role. The Ethical Guidelines of the American Academy of Psychiatry and the Law state: "A treating psychiatrist should generally avoid agreeing to be an expert witness or to perform an evaluation of his patient for legal purposes because a forensic evaluation usually requires that other people be interviewed and testimony may adversely affect the therapeutic relationship" (146). If it becomes necessary to testify on behalf of the patient, the psychiatrist should testify as a fact witness rather than as an expert witness. As a fact witness, the psychiatrist will be asked to describe the number and length of visits and the diagnosis and treatment. No opinion evidence will be requested concerning causation of the injury or extent of damages. In some jurisdictions, however, the court may convert a fact witness into an expert at the time of trial.

Particularly in the area of neuropsychiatry, both the treating psychiatrist and the expert psychiatric witness need to coordinate their efforts with other medical and nonmedical professionals. Obtaining additional information from others who are also assisting the patient makes for both good treatment as well as credible testimony. Psychiatrists, however, must remain ever mindful of the many double agent or conflicting roles that can develop when mixing psychiatry and litigation (147).

❑ CONCLUSIONS

The neuropsychiatrist today must be informed concerning the legal regulation of psychiatric practice. Without a working knowledge of the law, the neuropsychiatrist's ability to provide good clinical care will be significantly impaired by fear and uncertainty. Neuropsychiatrists who are forensically knowledgeable are in a much better position to practice relatively unencumbered within the requirements of the law while also minimizing the potential adverse clinical impacts of burgeoning legal regulation.

❑ NOTES

1. Simon RI: Clinical Psychiatry and the Law. Washington, DC, American Psychiatric Press, 1987
2. Rozovsky FA: Consent to Treatment: A Practical Guide. Boston, MA, Little, Brown, 1984, pp 87–122
3. Perlin ML: Mental Disability Law: Civil and Criminal v. I–III. Charlottesville, VA, Michie, 1989
4. Brakal S, Parry J, Weiner BA: Mental Disability and the Law. Chicago, ABA Foundation, 1986
5. Curran WJ, McGarry AL, Petty CS: Modern Legal Medicine: Psychiatry and Forensic Science. Philadelphia, PA, FA Davis, 1985
6. Curran WJ, McGarry AL, Shah SA: Forensic Psychiatry and Psychology. Philadelphia, PA, FA Davis, 1986
7. Shuman DW: Psychiatric and Psychological Evidence. Colorado Springs, CO, Shephard's McGraw-Hill, 1986
8. Schloendorff v Society of New York Hospital, 211 NY 125, 126, 105 NE 92, 93 (1914), overruled, Bing v Thunig, 2 NY2d 656, 143 NE2d 3, 163 NYS2d 3 (1957)
9. American Psychiatric Association: Opinions of the Ethics Committee on the Principles of Medical Ethics with Annotations Especially Applicable to Psychiatry. Washington, DC, American Psychiatric Press, 1989
10. Simon RI: Clinical Psychiatry and the Law. Washington, DC, American Psychiatric Press, 1987, p 113
11. Simon RI: Beyond the doctrine of informed consent: a clinician's perspective. The Journal for the Expert Witness, The Trial Attorney, The Trial Judge 4 (Fall): 23–25, 1989
12. Parry JW, Beck JC: Revisiting the civil commitment/involuntary treatment stalemate using limited guardianship, substituted judgment and different due process considerations: a work in progress. Medical and Physical Disability Law Reporter 14:102–114, 1990
13. Ruchs VR: The "rationing" of medical care. N Engl J Med 311:1572–1573, 1984
14. Dyer AR: Ethics and Psychiatry: Toward Professional Definition. Washington, DC, American Psychiatric Press, 1988, p 34
15. Luce JM: Ethical principles in critical care. JAMA 263:696–700, 1990
16. Black HC: Black's Law Dictionary, 6th Edition. St Paul, MN, West, 1990, p 284
17. The Legal Status of Adolescents 1980. US Department of Health and Human Services, 41 (1981)
18. Meek v City of Loveland, 85 Colo 346, 276 P 30 (1929)
19. Scaria v St Paul Fire & Marine Ins Co, 68 Wis2d 1, 227 NW2d 647 (1975)
20. Smith JT: Medical Malpractice: Psychiatric Care. Colorado Springs, CO, Shephards McGraw-Hill, 1986
21. See, e.g., Gulf SIR Co v Sullivan, 155 Miss 1, 119 So 501 (1928)
22. See, e.g., Planned Parenthood v Danforth, 428 US 52, 74 (1976) (abortion); Ill Ann Stat ch 91 1/2, para 3-501(a) (Smith-Hurd Supp 1990) (mental health counseling)
23. See, e.g., Jehovah's Witnesses v King County Hospital, 278 FSupp 488 (WD Wash 1967), affd, 390 US 598 (1968)
24. Wilson v Lehman, 379 SW2d 478, 479 (Ky 1964)
25. Rennie v Klein, 462 FSupp 1131 (DNJ 1978), modified, 653 F2d 836 (3d Cir 1981), vacated, 458 US 1119 (1982), on remand, 720 F2d 266 (3d Cir 1983)
26. Black HC: Black's Law Dictionary, 6th Edition. St Paul, NM, West, 1990, p 779
27. Rozovsky FA: Consent to Treatment: A Practical Guide. Boston, MA, Little, Brown, 1984, pp 87–122
28. Devinsky P, Bear DM: Varieties of aggressive behavior in patients with temporal lobe epilepsy. Am J Psychiatry 141:651–655, 1984
29. Snider WD, Simpson DM, Nielsen S, et al: Neurological complications of acquired immune deficiency syndrome: analysis of 50 patients. Ann Neurol 14: 403–418, 1983
30. Carlson RJ: Frontal lobe lesions masquerading as psychiatric disturbances. Canadian Psychiatric Association Journal 22:315–318, 1977

31a. Appelbaum PS, Lidz CW, Meisel A: Informed Consent: Legal Theory and Clinical Practice. New York, Oxford University Press, 1987, p 84

31b. Benesch K: Legal issues in determining competence to make treatment decisions, in Legal Implications of Hospital Policies and Practices. Edited by Miller RD. San Francisco, CA, Jossey-Bass, 1989, pp 97–105

32. Folstein MF, Folstein SW, McHugh PR: "Mini-Mental State": a practical method of grading the cognitive state of patients for the clinician. J Psychiatr Res 12:189–198, 1975
33. Frasier v Department of Health and Human Resources, 500 So2d 858, 864 (La Ct App 1986)
34. Aponte v United States, 582 FSupp 555, 566-69 (D PR 1984)
35. In re Quinlin, 70 NJ 10, 355 A2d 647, cert denied, 429 US 922 (1976); in re Conroy, 98 NJ 321, 486 A2d 1209 (1985)
36. Cruzan v Director, Missouri Depart of Health, 110 S Ct 2841 (1990)
37. Weir RF, Gostin L: Decisions to abate life-sustaining treatment for nonautonomous patients: ethical standards and legal liability for physicians after Cruzan. JAMA 264:1846–1853, 1990
38. Union Pacific Ry Co v Botsford, 141 US 250, 251 (1891); Schloendorff v Society of New York Hosp, 211 NY 125, 105 NE 92 (1914)
39. In re Conroy, 98 NJ 321, 486 A2d 1209, 1222-23 (1985)
40. Tune v Walter Reed Army Medical Hosp, 602 FSupp 1452 (DDC 1985); Bartling v Superior Court, 163 Cal App 3d 186, 209 Cal Rptr 220 (1984); Bouvia v Superior Court, 179 Cal App 3d 1127, 225 Cal Rptr 297 (1986); in re Farrell, 108 NJ 335, 529 A2d 404 (1987); in re Peter, 108 NJ 365, 529 A2d 419 (1987); in re Jobes, 108 NJ 365, 529 A2d 434 (1987)

41a. Marsh FH, Staver A: Physician authority for unilateral DNR orders. J Leg Med 12:115–165, 1991

41b. Schwartz HR: Do not resuscitate orders: the impact of guidelines on clinical practice, in Geriatric Psychiatry and the Law. Edited by Rosner R, Schwartz HR. New York, Plenum Press, 1987, pp 91–100

42. Council on Ethical and Judicial Affairs, American Medical Association: Guidelines for the appropriate use of do-not-resuscitate orders. JAMA 265:1868–1871, 1991
43. Solnick PB: Proxy consent for incompetent nonterminally ill adult patients. J Leg Med 6:1–49, 1985
44. Simon RI: Clinical Psychiatry and the Law. Washington, DC, American Psychiatric Press, 1987, pp 500–504
45. LaPuma J, Orentlicher D, Moss RJ: Advance directives on admission: clinical implications and analysis of the Patient Self-Determination Act of 1990. JAMA 266:402–405, 1991
46. Cruzan v Director, Missouri Dept of Health, 110 S Ct 2841, 2857 n 2 (1990)
47. Cruzan v Director, Missouri Dept of Health, 110 S Ct 2841, 2858 n 3 (1990)
48. Mishkin B: Decisions in Hospice. Arlington, VA, National Hospice Organization, 1985
49. T. G. Gutheil, October 1985, personal communication
50. Brakel SJ, Parry J, Weiner BA: The Mentally Disabled and the Law, 3rd Edition. Chicago, IL, American Bar Foundation, 1985, p 370
51. Regan M: Protective services for the elderly: commitment, guardianship, and alternatives. William and Mary Law Review 13:569–573, 1972
52. Sale B, Powell DM, Van Duizend R: Disabled Persons and the Law: State Legislative Issues, 1982, p 461
53. Sale B, Powell DM, Van Duizend R: Disabled Persons and the Law: State Legislative Issues, 1982, p 462
54. Sale B, Powell DM, Van Duizend R: Disabled Persons and the Law: State Legislative Issues, 1982, pp 461–462
55. Overman W, Stoudemire A: Guidelines for legal and financial counseling of Alzheimer's Disease patients and their families. Am J Psychiatry 145:1495–1500, 1988
56. Mishkin B: Determining the capacity for making health care decisions. Adv Psychosom Med 19:151–166, 1989
57. Uniform Guardianship and Protective Proceeding Act (UGPPA). Section 1-101(7); see also Uniform Probate Code (UPC) Section 5-101
58. Simon RI: Clinical Psychiatry and the Law. Washington, DC, American Psychiatric Press, 1987, p 451; citing, Addington v Texas, 441 US 418 (1979)
59. Perr IN: The clinical considerations of medication refusal. Legal Aspects of Psychiatric Practice 1:5–8, 1984
60. Gutheil TG, Appelbaum PS: Substituted judgment and the physician's ethical dilemma: with special reference to the problem of the psychiatric patient. J Clin Psychiatry 41:303–305, 1980
61. President's Commission for the Study of Ethical Problems in Medicine and Biomedical and Behavioral Research: Making Health Care Decisions, Vol 1: (A Report on the Ethical and Legal Implications of Informed Consent in the Patient-Practitioner Relationship). Washington, DC, Superintendent of Documents, October 1982
62. Klein J, Onek J, Macbeth J: Seminar on Law in the Practice of Psychiatry. Washington, DC, Onek, Klein & Farr, 1983, p 28
63. Zito JM, Lentz SL, Routt WW, et al: The treatment review panel: a solution to treatment refusal? Bull Am Acad Psychiatry Law 12:349–358, 1984
64. Hassenfeld IN, Grumet B: A study of the right to refuse treatment. Bull Am Acad Psychiatry Law 12: 65–74, 1984
65. Lewis DO, Pincus JH, Feldman M, et al: Psychiatric, neurological, and psychoeducational characteristics of 15 death row inmates in the United States. Am J Psychiatry 143:838–845, 1986
66. Bethea v United States, 365 A2d 64, (DC 1976) cert denied, 433 US 911 (1977)
67. Melton GB, Petrilla J, Poythress NG, et al: Psychological Evaluations for the Courts. New York, Guilford, 1987, p 128
68. Dusky v United States, 362 US 402 (1960)
69. M'Naughten's Case, 10 Cl F 200, 8 Eng Rep 718 (HL 1943); United States v Brawner, 471 F2d 969 (DC Cir 1972)
70. Note, Mental Aberration and Post Conviction Sanctions, 15 Suffolk University Law Review: 1219 (1981); State v Hehman, 110 Ariz 459, 520 P2d 507 (1974); Commonwealth v Robinson, 494 Pa 372, 431 A2d 901 (1981)
71. Ford v Wainwright, 477 US 399 (1986); Note, The eighth amendment and the execution of the presently incompetent. Stanford Law Review 32:765, 1980
72. Neely v United States, 150 F2d 977 (DC Cir), cert denied 326 US 768 (1945)
73. American Psychiatric Association: Diagnostic and Statistical Manual of Mental Disorders, 3rd Edition, Revised. Washington, DC, American Psychiatric Association, 1987
74. Reich J, Wels J: Psychiatric diagnosis and competency to stand trial. Compr Psychiatry 26:421–432, 1985
75. Wilson v United States, 391 F2d 460, 463 (DC Cir 1968)
76. McGarry AL: Competency to Stand Trial and Mental Illness (a monograph sponsored by the Center for Studies of Crime and Delinquency, National Institute of Mental Health, DHEW Publ No (HSM) 73–910). Washington, DC, U.S. Government Printing Office, 1973 p 73
77. Taylor MA, Sierles FS, Abrams R: The neuropsychiatric evaluation, in The American Psychiatric Press Textbook of Neuropsychiatry. Edited by Hales RE, Yudofsky SC. Washington DC, American Psychiatric Press, 1987, pp 3–16
78. United States v David, 511 F2d 355 (DC Cir 1975)
79. Blackstone W: Commentaries, Vol 4. pp 24–25 (1769); Coke E: Third Institute, 6th Edition. 1680
80. McDonald v United States, 312 F2d 847, 851 (DC 1962)
81. Bethea v United States, 365 A2d 64 (DC 1976) cert denied, 433 US 911 (1977); United States v Shorter, 343 A2d 569 (DC 1975)
82. The Comprehensive Crime Control Act of 1984, Publ. No. 98-473, Stat. 1840
83. 18 USC. Section 20(a)

84. Moyer KE: The Psychobiology of Aggression. New York, Harper & Row, 1976
85. Dalton K: Once A Month: Premenstrual Syndrome. Pomona, CA, Hunter House, 1979
86. Monroe RR: Brain Dysfunction in Aggressive Criminals, Lexington, MA, Lexington Books, 1978
87a. Elliot FA: Neurological findings in adult minimal brain dysfunction and the dsycontrol syndrome. J Nerv Ment Dis 170:680–687, 1982
87b. Melton GB, Petrila J, Poythress NG, et al: Psychological Evaluation for the Courts. New York, Guilford, 1987, p 128
88. Black HC: Black's Law Dictionary, 6th Edition, St Paul, MN, West, 1990, p 134
89. Fain v Commonwealth, 78 Ky 183 (1879); HM Advocate v Fraser, 4 Couper 70 (1878)
90. Low P, Jeffries J, Bonnie R: Criminal Law: Cases and Materials. Mieola, NY, Foundation Press, 1982, pp 152–154
91. Devinsky P, Bear DM: Varieties of aggressive behavior in temporal lobe epilepsy. Am J Psychiatry 141: 651,653, 1984
92. Elliot FA: Neurological aspects of antisocial behavior, in The Psychopath. Edited by Reid WH. New York, Brunner/Mazel, 1978
93. Blumer D: Psychiatric Aspects of Epilepsy. Washington, DC, American Psychiatric Press, 1984
94. People v White, 117 Cal App 3d 270, 172 Cal Rptr 612 (1981)
95. Blinder M: My examination of Dan White. Am J Forensic Psychiatry 11:12–22, 1981–1982
96. Kaplan HI, Saddock BJ: Comprehensive Textbook of Psychiatry, 5th Edition, Vol 2. Baltimore, MD, Williams & Wilkins, 1989, pp 1219–1220
97. Wilson JD, Braunwald E, Isselbacher KJ: Harrison's Principles of Internal Medicine, 12th Edition, Vol 2. New York, McGraw-Hill, 1991, p 1759
98. See e.g., Annotation [malpractice in connection with electroshock treatment] 94 ALR 3rd 317 (1979); Annotation [physician's liability to third person for prescribing drug to known drug addict] 42 ALR 4th 586 (1985)
99. American Psychiatric Association: The Practice of Electroconvulsive Therapy: Recommendations for Treatment, Training and Privileging: A Task Force Report of the American Psychiatric Association. Washington, DC, American Psychiatric Association, 1990
100. American Psychiatric Association: Tardive dyskinesia: summary of the task force report of the American Psychiatric Association. Am J Psychiatry 137:1163–1165, 1980
101. Stone v Proctor, 259 NC 633, 131 SE2d 297 (1963)
102. Joint Commission on Accreditation of Healthcare Organizations: Consolidated Standards Manual for Child, Adolescent, and Adult Psychiatric, Alcoholism and Drug Abuse Facilities and Facilities Serving the Mentally Retarded/Developmentally Disabled (1989). Chicago, IL, Joint Commission on Accreditation of Healthcare Organizations, 1988
103. Simon RI: Clinical Psychiatry and The Law. Washington, DC, American Psychiatric Press, 1987, p 34
104. Witherell v Weimer, 148 Ill App 3d 32, 499 NE2d 46 (1986) Revised on other grounds, 118 Ill2d 515 NE2d 68 (1987); Gowan v United States, 601 FSupp 1297 (D Or 1985)
105. Doerr v Hurley Medical Center, No 82-674-39 NM (Mich Aug (1984); Callan v Norland, 114 Ill App 3d 196, 448 NE2d 651 (1983)
106. American Psychiatric Association: Clinical perspectives. Managing Aggression in Elderly Patients 3:9–10, July 1990
107. Yudofsky SC, Silver JM, Schneider SE: Pharmacologic treatment of aggression. Psychiatric Annals 17: 397–407, 1987
108. Yudofsky SC, Silver JM, Schneider SE: Pharmacologic treatment of aggression. Psychiatric Annals 17: 397–407, 1987
109. Taylor MA, Sierles FS, Abrams R: The neuropsychiatric evaluation, in Textbook of Neuropsychiatry. Edited by Hales RE, Yudofsky SC. Washington, DC, American Psychiatric Press, 1987, pp 3–16
110. Rosse RB, Owen CM, Morihisa JM: Brain Imaging and Laboratory Testing in Neuropsychiatry, in Textbook of Neuropsychiatry. Edited by Hales RE, Yudofsky SC. Washington, DC, American Psychiatric Press, 1987, pp 17–39
111. Rosse RB, Owen CM, Morihisa JM: Brain Imaging and Laboratory Testing in Neuropsychiatry, in Textbook of Neuropsychiatry. Edited by Hales RE, Yudofsky SC. Washington, DC, American Psychiatric Press, 1987, pp 17–39
112. Psychiatry claims closed. Psychiatric News, April 3, 1987, p 11
113. Hogan DB: The Regulation of Psychotherapists, Vol III. Cambridge, MA, Ballinger, 1979, p 382
114. Blanchard v Levine, No D 014550 Fulton Cty Super Ct (Ga 1985); Shaughnessy v Spray, No A7905-02395 Multnomah Cty Cir Ct (Or, Feb 16, 1983)
115. See, e.g., Chaires v St John's Episcopal Hosp, No 20808/75 NY Cty Sup Ct (NY Feb 21, 1984); Clifford v United States, No 82-5002 USDC (SD 1985); Kilgore v County of Santa Clara, No 397-525 (Santa Clara Cty Super Ct Cal 1982)
116. Moran v Botsford General Hospital, No 81-225-533 Wayne Cty Cir Ct (Mich Oct 1, 1984); Wright v State, No 83-5035 Orleans Parish Civ Dist Ct (La April 1986); Karasik v Bird, 98 AD2d 359, 470 NYS2d 605 (1984)
117. Jeste DV: Madness, movements, and malpractice: what a mess! Paper presented at the annual meeting of the American Academy of Psychiatry and the Law, San Diego, CA, October 1990
118. Gardos G, Cole JO: Overview: public health issues in tardive dyskinesia. Am J Psychiatry 137:776–781, 1980
119. Klawans HL, Barr A: Prevalence of spontaneous lingual-facial–buccal dyskinesia in the elderly. Neurology 32:558–559, 1982; Kane JM, Weinhold P, Kinon B, et al: Prevalence of abnormal involuntary movements ("spontaneous dyskinesia") in the normal elderly. Psychopharmacology 77:105–108, 1982
120. Hyde v University of Michigan Bd of Regents, 426 Mich 223, 393 NW2d 847 (1986)

121. Hyde v University of Michigan Bd of Regents, 426 Mich 223, 393 NW2d 847 (1986)
122. Dovido v Vasquez, No 84-674 CA(L)(H) 15th Jud Dist Cir Ct, Palm Beach Cty (Fla Apr 4, 1986)
123. Clites v State, 322 NW2d 917 (Iowa Ct App 1982)
124. Radank v Heyl, No F4-2316 Wisc Comp Bd (1986); Frasier v Department of Health and Human Resources, 500 So2d 858 (La Ct App 1986); Rivera v NYC Health and Hospitals, No 27536/82 New York Sup Ct (NY 1988)
125. Yudofsky SC, Silver JM, Schneider SE: Pharmacologic treatment of aggression. Psychiatric Annals 17: 397–407, 1987
126. O'Connell RA: A review of the use of electroconvulsive therapy. Hosp Community Psychiatry 33:469–473, 1982
127. Weiner RD: The psychiatric use of electrically induced seizures. Am J Psychiatry 136:1507–1517, 1979
128. Perr IN: Liability and electroshock therapy. J Forensic Sci 25:508–513, 1980; Krouner LW: Shock therapy and psychiatric malpractice: the legal accommodation to a controversial treatment. J Forensic Sci 20: 404–415, 1975
129. Smith JT: Medical Malpractice: Psychiatric Care. Colo Springs, CO, Shepards-McGraw Hill, 1986, p 68; Holton v Pfingst, 534 SW2d 786, 789 (Ky 1976)
130. Howe v Citizens Memorial Hosp, 426 SW2d 882 (Tex Civ App 1968), revised 436 SW2d 115 (Tex 1968)
131. Perlin ML: Mental Disability Law: Civil and Criminal, Vol 3. Charlottesville, VA, Michie, 1989, pp 47–48
132. Tardiff K, Sweillam A: Assault, suicide and mental illness. Arch Gen Psychiatry 73:164–169, 1980
133. Tardiff K, Sweillam A: Assaultive behavior among chronic inpatients. Am J Psychiatry 139:212–215, 1982; Reid HW, Bollinger MF, Edwards G: Assaults in hospitals. Bull Am Acad Psychiatry Law 13:13–14, 1985
134. Tarasoff v Regents of the University of California, 17 Cal 3d 425, 131 Cal Rptr 14, 551 P2d 334 (1976)
135. Simon RI: Concise Guide to Clinical Psychiatry and the Law. Washington, DC, American Psychiatric Press, 1988, pp 99–121
136. Simon RI: Clinical Psychiatry and the Law. Washington, DC, American Psychiatric Press, 1987, pp 236–247
137. Zeldow PB, Taub HA: Evaluating psychiatric discharge and aftercare in a VA medical center. Hosp Community Psychiatry 32:57–58, 1981
138. Simon RI: Clinical Psychiatry and the Law. Washington, DC, American Psychiatric Press, 1987, pp 119–120
139. Simon RI: Concise Guide to Clinical Psychiatry and the Law. Washington, DC, American Psychiatric Press, 1988, pp 117
140. Johnson ID: Reports to the National Practitioner Data Bank. JAMA 265:407–411, 1991
141. Walzer RS: Impaired physicians: an overview and update of legal issues. J Leg Med 11:131–198, 1990
142. Frankowski RF, Anngers JF, Whitman S: Epidemiological and descriptive studies, part I: the descriptive epidemiology of head trauma in the United States, in Central Nervous System Trauma Status Report—1985. Edited by Becker DP, Poulishock JT. Washington, DC, National Institute of Neurological and Communicative Disorders and Stroke, 1985, pp 23–43
143. Clifton GL: Head injury incidence and organization of pre-hospital care, in Head Injury: Principles of Modern Management. Edited by Appel SH. Princeton, NJ, Geigy Pharmaceuticals, 1982, pp 3–5
144. Strasburger LH: "Crudely, without any finesse:" the defendant hears his psychiatric evaluation. Bull Am Acad Psychiatry Law 15:229–233, 1987
145 American Psychiatric Association: Principles of Medical Ethics With Annotions Especially Applicable to Psychiatry. Washington, DC, American Psychiatric Association, 1989, p 6
146. American Academy of Psychiatry and the Law Ethical Guidelines for the Practice of Forensic Psychiatry. Adopted May 1987, revised October 1989, Section IV.
147. Simon RI: The psychiatrist as a fiduciary: avoiding the double agent role. Psychiatric Annals 17:622–626, 1987

❑ APPENDIX 33–1

LIVING WILL DECLARATION

INSTRUCTIONS: Consult this column for guidance.	To My Family, Doctors, and All Those Concerned with My Care I, ______________________, being of sound mind, make this statement as a directive to be followed if I become unable to participate in decisions regarding my medical care.
This declaration sets forth your directions regarding medical treatment.	If I should be in an incurable or irreversible mental or physical condition with no reasonable expectation of recovery, I direct my attending physician to withhold or withdraw treatment that merely prolongs my dying. I further direct that treatment be limited to measures to keep me comfortable and to relieve pain.
You have the right to refuse treatment you do not want, and you may request the care you do want.	These directions express my legal right to refuse treatment. Therefore I expect my family, doctors, and everyone concerned with my care to regard themselves as legally and morally bound to act in accord with my wishes, and in so doing to be free of any legal liability for having followed my directions.
You may list specific treatments you do *not* want. For example: Cardiac resuscitation Mechanical respiration Artificial feeding/fluids by tube Otherwise, your general statement, top right, will stand for your wishes.	I especially do not want: ______________________ ______________________ ______________________ ______________________ ______________________ ______________________ ______________________
You may want to add instructions for care you *do* want—for example, pain medication; or that you prefer to die at home if possible.	Other instructions/comments: ______________________ ______________________ ______________________ ______________________
	Proxy Designation Clause: Should I become unable to communicate my instructions as stated above, I designate the following person to act in my behalf: Name ______________________ Address ______________________
If you want, you can name someone to see that your wishes are carried out, but you do not have to do this.	If the person I have named above is unable to act on my behalf, I authorize the following person to do so: Name ______________________ Address ______________________ This Living Will Declaration expresses my personal treatment preferences. The fact that I may have also executed a document in the form recommended by state law should not be construed to limit or contradict this Living Will Declaration, which is an expression of my common-law and constitutional rights.
Sign and date here in the presence of two adult witnesses, who should also sign.	Address: ______________ Address: ______________ ______________ ______________ Signed: ______________ Date: ______________ Witness: ______________ Witness: ______________ Keep the signed original with your personal papers at home. Give signed copies to your doctors, family, and to your proxy. Review your Declaration from time to time; initial and date it to show it still expresses your intent.

Note. This document is meant to be used in states that do not have natural death statutes. Each of the 39 jurisdictions with a statute has its own form for this purpose.

Source. Reprinted with permission from the Society for the Right to Die, 250 West 57th Street, New York, NY 10107.

APPENDIX 33–1 (Continued)

DURABLE POWER OF ATTORNEY FOR HEALTH CARE

Information About This Document

This is an important legal document. Before signing this document it is vital for you to know and understand these facts:

- This document gives the person you name as your agent the power to make health care decisions for you if you cannot make decisions for yourself.
- Even after you have signed this document, you have the right to make health care decisions for yourself so long as your are able to do so. In addition, even after you have signed the document, no treatment may be given to you or stopped over your objection.
- You may state in this document any types of treatment that you do not desire and those that you want to make sure you receive.
- You have the right to revoke (take away) the authority of your agent by notifying your agent or your health care provider orally or in writing of this desire.
- If there is anything in this document that you do not understand, you should ask for an explanation.

You will be given a copy of this document after you have signed it, and a copy will be sent to each person you name as your agent or alternate agent.

Durable Power of Attorney for Health Care

I, ______________________________ hereby appoint:

______________________________	______________________________
Name	Home Address
______________________________	______________________________
Home Telephone Number	
______________________________	______________________________
Work Telephone Number	

as my agent to make health care decisions for me if and when I am unable to make my own health care decisions. This gives my agent the power to consent to giving, withholding, or stopping any health care, treatment, service, or diagnostic procedure. My agent also has the authority to talk with health care personnel, get information, and sign forms necessary to carry out those decisions.

If the person named as my agent is not available or is unable to act as my agent, then I appoint the following person(s) to serve in the order listed below:

______________________________	______________________________
Name	Home Address
______________________________	______________________________
Home Telephone Number	
______________________________	______________________________
Work Telephone Number	

By this document I intend to create a power of attorney for health care which shall take effect upon my incapacity to make my own health care decisions and shall continue during that incapacity.
My agent shall make health care decisions as I direct below or as I make known to him or her in some other way.

(a) STATEMENT OF DESIRES CONCERNING LIFE-PROLONGING CARE, TREATMENT, SERVICES, AND PROCEDURES:

____

____

____

____

____

____

DURABLE POWER OF ATTORNEY FOR HEALTH CARE

(b) SPECIAL PROVISIONS AND LIMITATIONS:

____

____

____

____

____

____

BY SIGNING HERE I INDICATE THAT I UNDERSTAND THE PURPOSE AND EFFECT OF THIS DOCUMENT.

I sign my name to this form on ______________________________
(date)

at: ______________________________

______________________________(address).

____
(You sign here)

WITNESSES

I declare that the person who signed or acknowledged this document is personally known to me, that he/she signed or acknowledged this durable power or attorney in my presence, and that he/she appears to be of sound mind and under no duress, fraud, or undue influence. I am not the person appointed as agent by this document, nor am I the patient's health care provider or an employee of the patient's health care provider.

First Witness

Signature: ______________________________

Home Address: ______________________________

Print Name: ______________________________

Date: ______________________________

Second Witness

Signature: ______________________________

Home Address: ______________________________

Print Name: ______________________________

Date: ______________________________

(AT LEAST ONE OF THE ABOVE WITNESSES MUST ALSO SIGN THE FOLLOWING DECLARATION.)

I further declare that I am not related to the patient by blood, marriage, or adoption, and, to the best of my knowledge, I am not entitled to any part of his/her estate under a will now existing or by operation of law.

Signature: ______________________________

Signature: ______________________________

Source. Reprinted with permission from the National Hospice Organization, Arlington, Virginia.

❑ APPENDIX 33–2

HEALTH CARE PROXY

About the Health Care Proxy

This is an important legal form. Before signing this form, you should understand the following facts:

1. This form gives the person you choose as your agent the authority to make all health care decisions for you, except to the extent you say otherwise in this form. "Health care" means any treatment, service, or procedure to diagnose or treat your physical or mental condition.
2. Unless you say otherwise, your agent will be allowed to make all health care decisions for you, including decisions to remove or provide life-sustaining treatment.
3. Unless your agent knows your wishes about artificial nutrition and hydration (nourishment and water provided by a feeding tube), he or she will not be allowed to refuse or consent to those measures for you.
4. Your agent will start making decisions for you when doctors decide that you are not able to make health care decisions for yourself.

You may write on this form any information about treatment that you do not desire and/or those treatments that you want to make sure you receive. Your agent must follow your instructions (oral and written) when making decisions for you.

If you want to give your agent written instructions, do so right on the form. For example, you could say:

> *If I become terminally ill, I* ***do/don't*** *want to receive the following treatments: . . . .*
>
> *If I am in a coma or unconscious, with no hope of recovery, then I* ***do/don't*** *want . . . .*
>
> *If I have brain damage or a brain disease that makes me unable to recognize people or speak and there is no hope that my condition will improve, I* ***do/don't*** *want . . . .*
>
> *I have discussed with my agent my wishes about____and I want my agent to make all decisions about these measures.*

Examples of medical treatments about which you may wish to give your agent special instructions are listed below. This is **not** a complete list of the treatments about which you may leave instructions.

- artificial respiration
- artificial nutrition and hydration (nourishment and water provided by feeding tube)
- cardiopulmonary resuscitation (CPR)
- antipsychotic medication
- electric shock therapy
- antibiotics
- psychosurgery
- dialysis
- transplantation
- blood transfusions
- abortion
- sterilization

Talk about choosing an agent with your family and/or close friends. You should discuss this form with a doctor or another health care professional, such as a nurse or social worker, before you sign it to make sure that you understand the types of decisions that may be made for you. You may also wish to give your doctor a signed copy. **You do not need a lawyer to fill out this form.**

You can choose any adult (over 18), including a family member or close friend, to be your agent. If you select a doctor as your agent, he or she may have to choose between acting as your agent or as your attending doctor; a physician cannot do both at the same time. Also, if you are a patient or resident of a hospital, nursing home, or mental hygiene facility, there are special restrictions about naming someone who works for that facility as your agent. You should ask staff at the facility to explain those restrictions.

You should tell the person you choose that he or she will be your health care agent. You should discuss your health care wishes and this form with your agent. Be sure to give him or her a signed copy. Your agent cannot be sued for health care decisions made in good faith.

Even after you have signed this form, you have the right to make health care decisions for yourself as long as you are able to do so, and treatment cannot be given to you or stopped if you object. You can cancel the control given to your agent by telling him or her or your health care provider orally or in writing.

Filling Out the Proxy Form

Item (1) Write your name and the name, home address, and telephone number of the person you are selecting as your agent.

Item (2) If you have special instructions for your agent, you should write them here. Also, if you wish to limit your agent's authority in any way, you should say so here. If you do not state any limitations, your agent will be allowed to make all health care decisions that you could have made, including the decision to consent to or refuse life-sustaining treatment.

Item (3) You may write the name, home address, and telephone number of an alternate agent.

Item (4) This form will remain valid indefinitely unless you set an expiration date or condition for its expiration. This section is optional and should be filled in only if you want the health care proxy to expire.

Item (5) You must date and sign the proxy. If you are unable to sign yourself, you may direct someone else to sign in your presence. Be sure to include your address.

Two witnesses at least 18 years of age must sign your proxy. The person who is appointed agent or alternate agent cannot sign as a witness.

Source. Reprinted from Appointing Your Health Care Proxy: New York State's Proxy Law. New York State Department of Health, 1991.

HEALTH CARE PROXY

(1) I,____

hereby appoint____
(name, home address, and telephone number)

as my health care agent to make any and all health care decisions for me, except to the extent that I state otherwise. This proxy shall take effect when and if I become unable to make my own health care decisions.

(2) Optional instructions: I direct my agent to make health care decisions in accord with my wishes and limitations as stated below, or as he or she otherwise knows. (Attach additional pages if necessary.)

____

____

____

(Unless your agent knows your wishes about artificial nutrition and hydration [feeding tubes], your agent will not be allowed to make decisions about artificial nutrition and hydration. See instructions for samples of language you could use.)

(3) Name of substitute or fill-in agent if the person I appoint above is unable, unwilling, or unavailable to act as my health care agent.

____
(name, home address, and telephone number)

(4) Unless I revoke it, this proxy shall remain in effect indefinitely, or until the date or conditions stated below. This proxy shall expire (specific date or conditions, if desired):

____

(5) Signature____

Address____

Date____

Statement by Witnesses (must be 18 or older)

I declare that the person who signed this document is personally known to me and appears to be of sound mind and acting of his or her own free will. He or she signed (or asked another to sign for him or her) this document in my presence.

Witness 1____

Address____

Witness 2____

Address____

INDEX